Professional Nurse:

1993

Nursing Drug Reference

Guy's Hospital

Professional Nurse:
1993
Nursing Drug
Reference

Edited by Anne Joshua, BPharm, DipClinPharm, MRPharmS
and Theo King, RGN
With a team of Pharmacists and Nurses from
Guy's Hospital

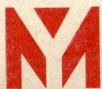

Published by
Mosby–Year Book Europe Ltd
Brook House
2–16 Torrington Place
London WC1E 7LT

ISBN 0 7234 1896 9

For full details of all Mosby–Year Book Europe Ltd titles please write to
Mosby–Year Book Europe Ltd, Brook House, 2–16 Torrington Place, London
WC1E 7LT, England.

A CIP record for this book is available from the British Library.

This book is based on an original work by Linda Skidmore-Roth, RN, MSN,
NP published in the USA on an annual basis by Mosby–Year Book as *Mosby's
Nursing Drug Reference.*

Printed by BPCC Hazell Books Ltd, Aylesbury, England

A note to the reader:

This book is intended to help nurses and midwives understand drug
protocols and the management of patients under given drug regimens.
This book should not be used as a prime source for prescribing and
dispensing drugs. Guy's Hospital, the Editors, Contributors and the
Publisher have undertaken reasonable endeavours to check dosage and
nursing content for accuracy. Because the science of clinical pharmacology is continually advancing, our knowledge base continues to
expand. Therefore, we recommend that the reader should always
check the manufacturer's product information for changes in dosage
or administration before administering any medication. This is particularly important with new or rarely used drugs.

Contents

The contributors

The Editors and Publisher would like to thank the following for their contributions to the *1993 Nursing Drug Reference*

Caroline Alexander, BSc, RGN
Helen Archibald, RGN, RM,
   ENB 997
Stephanie Barnes, MSc,
   MRPharmS
Peter Barr, BPharm, MRPharmS
Paul Blake, BPharm,
   MRPharmS
Catherine Bouchard, BPharm,
   MPhil, MRPharmS
Lisa Burnapp, RGN, ENB 136,
   ENB 998
Laura Byers, RGN
Claire Chaplin, RGN, DN
Mary Crawshaw, RGN, RM,
   ENB 124, ENB 998, DPSN
Steve Cook, BPharm, BSc,
   MPhil, MRPharmS
Louise Farrow, RGN, ENB 237,
   ENB 998
Susanna Gilmour-White,
   BPharm, MRPharmS
Joy Godden, RGN
Gillian Gooby, RGN, CHSM
Marian Howell, RGN, ENB 100
Maria Joyce, RGN, RM,
   ENB 997, DMS
Purmjit Kaur, RGN, OND
Margaret Kelly, RGN
Martin Knowles, BPharm, MSc,
   MRPharmS
Daphne Leedham, RGN, OHND
Catherine Lewis, RGN
Catrin Lord, BPharm,
   MRPharmS
Douglas MacClean, BSc, Dip
   Clin Pharm, MRPharmS
Beverley McGrath, RGN
Gillian Meade, RGN, ENB 225

Wendy Menon, RGN, ENB 338,
   ENB 998
Jacqueline Paterson, RGN,
   ENB 338
Judith Pickering, RGN, RN
   (Ohio)
Avril Platt, BPharm, MRPharmS
Julie Quinn, RGN
Rashne Ruston, RGN, ENB 100
Sheila Sawtell, RGN
Jonathan Simms, BPharm,
   MRPharmS
Richard Spooner, RGN
Rebecca Stroud, RGN, ENB 100
Paul Turnstall, BPharm,
   MRPharmS
Peter Wilson, RGN, RMN
Caroline Yarnell, RGN, ENB
   100, City & Guilds 730

With special thanks to:
Mandy Beaumont, RGN
Maxwell Summerhayes,
   BPharm, PhD, MRPharmS

The Publisher is also grateful to
the following who helped in the
early stages of the development
of the book:
Eileen Barber, Christine Brooker,
Steve Chaplin, Dinah Gould, Ann
Harris, Genitha Lloyd, Pat Mills,
Richenda Milton-Thompson,
Graham North, Marion Richardson
and Verena Tschudin.

Foreword

There are a number of excellent reference books on drugs in use in the UK, but all have been produced primarily with the clinician and pharmacist in mind, and there has been a lack of information tailored to the needs of nurses and midwives.

With the development of the professional role of the nurse, and with the coming of nurse prescribing, this gap has become more apparent. We therefore welcome the opportunity to contribute to the preparation and publication of a UK version of *Mosby's Nursing Drug Reference*, which has been in use in the USA for some years.

The unique feature of this book is the inclusion of 'Nursing Considerations' in each monograph, giving practical information of value to nurses and midwives when administering drugs and observing their actions, and in the contact with patients, their families or carers.

Roger W. Horne, *Director of Pharmacy*
Wilma MacPherson, *Director of Nursing*
Guy's Hospital
November 1992

Editors' preface

In 1983 the Lewisham and North Southwark District Formulary Committee for Guy's and Lewisham Hospitals issued its first *District Formulary*, following the introduction two years earlier of a new type of *British National Formulary (BNF)* by the Joint Formulary Committee of the British Medical Association and the Royal Pharmaceutical Society of Great Britain (formerly the Pharmaceutical Society of Great Britain).

Both publications were intended as pocket book references for those health professionals concerned with the prescribing, dispensing and administration of medicines. The Guy's and Lewisham Trust also produces a separate prescribing guide for paediatric medicines.

The *Professional Nurse: 1993 Nursing Drug Reference* from Guy's Hospital has been designed to provide advice and drug information for the nurse and midwife consistent with the nursing process and as such is a unique development not addressed by these previous publications. The intention is to produce a new edition every year so that the most up-to-date information on new and existing drugs is available to nurses and midwives.

Anne Joshua, BPharm, DipClinPharm, MRPharmS
Theo King, RGN

Introduction

This book has been produced to provide a quick reference to essential drug information. It is intended for use in the clinical situation by the practicing nurse, midwife or student. The guiding principle is to give the reader easy access to drug information and highlight the nursing considerations relating to medication which assist in the nursing process.

Now more than ever, nurses and midwives need to be aware of, and have access to, up-to-date drug information. This reference will be an annual publication which will help satisfy this need. Used in conjunction with their skills in evaluating the patient's (for patient read patient(s)/client(s) where this is more appropriate) response to the medication, and in communicating with the patients and their carers, this book will equip nurses and midwives to plan and improve care.

The Department of Health's intention is to implement nurse prescribing in the UK by the end of 1993. The specially trained nurse should be able to prescribe from a nurse's formulary according to certain criteria. As a result nurses should be aware of, and have easy access to, up-to-date information on the dosage, use and administration of these drugs. The restrictions on prescribing do not apply to the supply and administration of certain medicinal products by a certified midwife in the course of her professional practice. These products are specifically related to their use for procedures in childbirth. *See* Appendix 1.

The *Nursing Drug Reference* has been prepared by a team of nurses, midwives and pharmacists from various clinical specialties within the hospital and community care settings. The information is based on their clinical and pharmacological knowledge, confirmed by reference to the *British National Formulary*, Manufacturer's Product Data Sheets and *Martindale*, 29th edition and other background reading which is listed in the bibliography. Each drug is presented in the form of a monograph and arranged in alphabetical order by generic name. The proprietary or trade name(s) for each drug are listed below the generic name.

The drugs are those primarily used in adult medicine, but where appropriate, doses for children have been included. All the drugs are available in the UK. Currently some preparations available in the other European countries are not routinely available in the UK, and vice versa. The centralised control and licensing of drugs for Europe is still a few years away, but will eventually affect the choice of drugs available to be prescribed and how they will be monitored in the future.

Some drugs and preparations may be prescribed for use in circumstances outside the product licence. In these cases the principal responsibility rests with the prescriber but in practice there is a duty of care on both the pharmacist and the nurse or midwife. The uses stated in each monograph in this book are those for which the drug is licensed in the UK. In addition some proprietary drugs or preparations are not available on NHS prescription. These have been designated with the symbol, NHS However, it may be possible for certain individuals to obtain these black-listed preparations on NHS prescription in special circumstances. Where newer drugs have been included, a symbol ▼ has been included beside the drug's generic name to designate that it requires the prescriber to report all suspected reactions to the Committee on Safety of Medicines.

The information contained in each monograph should not be used in isolation. Multiple drug therapies and disease states will affect the patient's drug handling capacity and response to treatment. Each patient should be evaluated according to his or her own individual needs. A team approach with prescriber, pharmacist, patient and nurse should ensure that the patient receives the optimum therapy for his or her condition.

We recommend that readers should always check manufacturer's product information for any changes in dosage or administration before administering any medication. The local treatment protocol and the local pharmacy are useful additional sources of information which should be consulted.

How to use this book

Each monograph starts with the generic name of the drug. The prefix 'co' indicates that the medication is a compound preparation. Following the generic name, the most commonly used proprietory or trade name(s) are included. These are the brand names of specific drugs. The statement 'combination product' or 'many combination products' will be included where there are one or more combination products of the drug available.

The following information is then provided for each drug, wherever possible, for the safe and effective use of each drug:

Functional and chemical classification
Here all known broad functional and chemical classifications are given. The functional classes are used to enable the reader to recognise similarities between drugs or other drugs in the same functional class but which are different chemically.

Legal class

The symbols showing the legal class are used to indicate any restrictions which apply to the prescribing, dispensing and storage of such medicines:

GSL   General Sales List Medicine
P   Pharmacy Medicine
POM   Prescription Only Medicine
CD   Controlled Drug subject to the prescription requirements of the Misuse of Drugs Act 1971.

Controlled drugs are listed under five schedules of the Misuse of Drugs Regulations (1985). There are mandatory requirements which cover ordering, storage and recording of these drugs by the nurse or midwife. Of these, the most important are Schedule 2 drugs, CD(Sch2)POM, e.g. diamorphine injection. For further details see:

Pearce, M. E. (1984)*Medicines and Poisons Guide*, 4th edn, Sect. 1.9: The Pharmaceutical Press.
Medicines, Ethics and Practice, (1992), No. 9, October: Royal Pharmaceutical Society of Great Britain.

Action
The pharmacological action of the drug and its mechanism are described briefly.

Uses
This section sets out the purpose for which the drug has been granted a UK product licence.

Dosages and routes
The dosage and routes are given for adults and children according to the UK product licence. However, some of the doses shown may differ from those in current medical practice. Where differences do occur it is suggested that the reader seeks specialist advice including the Manufacturer's Product Data Sheet.

All available forms are included: tablets, capsules, modified-release formulations, lozenges, aerosols, sprays, injectables (IV, IM, SC), solutions, creams, ointments, lotions, gels, shampoos, elixirs, suspensions and suppositories.

Side effects/adverse reactions
These are grouped by body system without emphasis being given to the frequency or severity of the reaction.

The symbol ▼ at the top of the drug monograph designates that it is a newer drug which requires prescribers to report all suspected reactions to the Committee on Safety of Medicines (CSM), i.e., to report any adverse or unexpected event, however minor, which could conceivably be attributed to the drug.

Contraindications
Contraindications are instances in which the specified drug, absolutely, should NOT be used.

Precautions
This section warns of potential clinical problems associated with the drug. These may vary according to the brand of drug to be used, and the manufacturer's recommendations.

Pharmacokinetics
Metabolism, absorption, distribution and elimination are provided for all dosage forms where known. Each patient handles a particular drug according to his or her own individual parameters. Disease states will affect the pharmacokinetics of a drug.

Interactions/incompatibilities

Interactions are those clinical effects which occur as a result of more than one medication being given during a course of treatment. Interactions will still occur whether medication is given concurrently or sequentially. Incompatibilities include those pharmaceutical interactions which occur in infusion solutions, syringes, tubing or injection vials on dilution of the drug when more than one drug is given at the same time. This section also includes drug, food and smoking interactions.

Clinical assessment

This section covers procedures which are likely to be initiated by the clinician. However, in high dependency units, such as intensive or coronary care, some of the tests and procedures may be undertaken by nurses.

Laboratory test interferences

Data on laboratory test interferences are dependent on the type of test used in the laboratory, the body fluid being analysed and the drug salt/ester. Tests can vary between laboratories.

Treatment of overdose

Brief information is given about antidotes and other treatments for drug overdose wherever appropriate. Appendix 3 gives the details of national poisons information services.

NURSING CONSIDERATIONS

Five headings appear under Nursing Considerations: these are Assess, Administer, Perform/provide, Evaluate, and Teach patient/family. Nursing considerations are consistently grouped under these headings to help the nurse or midwife to plan care.

It is assumed that good basic nursing care is provided by nurses to all patients. There has been minimal reiteration of general nursing points and reminders have only been given where it has been felt that it would be helpful to the reader. Readers are advised to study the entire monograph on the drug and not just the nursing section. Details of dosage are given in the pharmacological section and are not repeated in the nursing section.

Assess

This identifies the minimum baseline assessment which should be made before administration of the drug under consideration.

Administer

Points of particular importance are noted here relating to care during the administration of the drug.

Perform/provide

This section identifies action to be taken associated with the administration of the drug. Storage of drugs and medicines should be in accordance with the Medicines Act 1968; only special storage requirements have been included in the monograph. It is essential that nurses and midwives understand the storage required for controlled drugs. They are referred to the Misuse of drugs Act 1971 and the Misuse of Drugs Regulations 1985. Certain preparations should be stored under specific environmental conditions, e.g. refrigerated storage.

Evaluate

This section highlights the reassessment of the patient's condition after, and sometimes during, the administration of the medication in question. It also acts as a prompt to the nurse when writing care notes on the patient.

Teach patient/family

This section contains a variety of information that a patient or his/her family or carer need to know about the continued use of the drug. This includes the general effects on the patient as well as any side effects. This information is of increasing importance as trained staff relinquish their responsibility and self-care or care by relatives becomes more important. An assumption is made that all nurses and midwives will remind patients and their families of the need for safe storage of medicines as well as their proper use.

Appendices

Various appendices are included for further reference including:

1: Exemptions from the Controls on Retail Sale: Midwives
2: Guide to therapeutic drug monitoring
3: District and regional drug information services
4: Immunisation against infectious diseases
5: Weights, measures and units
6: Weight conversion table
7: Height/weight - adults (desirable)
8: Height/weight - children (desirable)
9: Blood normal values
10: Urine normal values

Indexes

Two indexes have been included. The first lists in alphabetical order all the generic drugs and the proprietory brand names included in this book. The second index groups the generic drugs into their functional classes. This means that drugs which have similar properties can be compared together.

Every attempt has been made to be consistent in terms of style. Some drugs within the same therapeutic group may differ in the presentation of the information.

Thanks are due to all the nurses, midwives and pharmacists who contributed to this book at all stages prior to publication. Their enthusiasm and determination made this first edition possible.

We would welcome comments from readers of this book, via the publishers, so that we may continue to provide current and useful information in future editions.

A note to the reader:

This book is intended to help nurses and midwives understand drug protocols and the management of patients under given drug regimens. This book should not be used as a prime source for prescribing and dispensing drugs. Guy's Hospital, the Editors, Contributors and the Publisher have undertaken reasonable endeavours to check dosage and nursing content for accuracy. Because the science of clinical pharmacology is continually advancing, our knowledge base continues to expand. Therefore, we recommend that the reader should always check the manufacturer's product information for changes in dosage or administration before administering any medication. This is particularly important with new or rarely used drugs.

Abbreviations used

ACE	angiotensin converting enzyme
ACTH	adrenocorticotrophic hormone
ADH	antidiuretic hormone
AIDS	auto-immune deficiency syndrome
APTT	activated partial thromboplastin time
ATP	adenosine triphosphate
BCG	Bacillus Calmette-Guerin vaccine
BMR	basal metabolism rate
BP	blood pressure
CCF	congestive cardiac failure
CD	controlled drug
CNS	central nervous system
CO_2	carbon dioxide
CSF	cerebrospinal fluid
CSM	Committee on Safety of Medicines
CTG	cardiotocograph
CV	cardiovascular
CVA	cerebrovascular accident
CVP	central venous pressure
D&C	dilatation and curettage
DNA	deoxyribonucleic acid
DOA	dead on arrival
DOB	date of birth
DTP	Diptheria, Tetanus, Pertussis vaccine
ECT	electroconvulsive therapy
ECG	electrocardiogram
EDTA	ethylenediaminetetraacetic acid
EEG	electroencephalogram
EENT	eye, ear, nose and throat
ELECT	electrolytes
ENDO	endocrine
ESR	erthrocyte sedimentation rate
exam	examination
FSH	follicle-stimulating hormone
GABA	gamma-aminobutyric acid
GFR	glomerular filtration rate
GI	gastrointestinal
G6PD	glucose-6 phosphate dehydrogenase
GSL	general sales list medicine
GU	genitourinary
Gyn	gynaecology
HAEM	haematology
Hb	haemoglobin
HCG	human chorionic gonadotropin
H_2O	water
HDL	high density lipoprotein
HDU	high density unit
HIV	Human Immunodeficiency Virus
HPA	hypothalamic-pituitary-adrenal

HRT	hormone replacement therapy
ICU	intensive care unit
ID	identification/intradermally
IgG	immunoglobulin G
IM	intramuscular
INTEG	integument
IPV	inactivated polio vaccine
IUD	intrauterine contraceptive device
IV	intravenous
IVP	intravenous pyelogram
K	potassium
LDL	low density lipoprotein
LH	luteinizing hormone
LMP	last menstrual period
MAOIs	monoamine oxidase inhibitors
META	metabolic
MI	myocardial infarction
MICs	minimum inhibitor concentrations
MISC	miscellaneous
MS	motor sensory
Na	sodium
neg	negative
NHS	not available on NHS prescription
NIDDM	non-insulin-dependent diabetes mellitus
NSAIDs	non-steroidal anti-inflammatory drugs
O_2	oxygen
OPV	oral polio vaccine
P	pharmacy medicine
PABA	para-aminobenzoic acid
PAS	para-aminosalicylic acid
PCV	packed cell volume
pH	hydrogen ion concentration
POM	prescription only medicine
postop	postoperatively
preop	preoperatively
prep	preparation
PVC	polyvinyl chloride
RBC(s)	red blood count or cell(s)
REC	rectal
REM	rapid eye movement
RESP	respiratory
Rh factor	Rhesus factor
RNA	ribonucleic acid
SC	subcutaneous
SGOT	serum glutamic oxalo-acetic transaminase
SROM	spontaneous rupture of membranes
SYST	systemic
STD	sexually transmitted disease
TB	tuberculosis
TPN	total parenteral nutrition
TSH	thyroid-stimulating hormone

TT	thrombin time
UV	ultraviolet
VLDL	very low density lipoprotein
VMA	vanillylmandelic acid
WBC	white blood count or cell(s)

°C	degrees celsius (centigrade)
hr / hrly	hour/hourly
IU	International Units
mEq	milliequivalent
min	minute
temp	temperature
°	degree
%	percent
=	equal
▼	'new drug': report all reactions to CSM

See also Appendix 5: Weights, measures and units.

Individual drugs

acebutolol

Sectral
Func. class.: Antihypertensive, anti-anginal, anti-arrhythmic
Chem. class.: Cardioselective β-blocker
Legal class.: POM

Action: Has anti-arrhythmic and intrinsic sympathomimetic activity. Blocks effects of excessive catecholamine stimulation resulting from stress. Competitively blocks stimulation of cardiac β-adrenergic receptors, decreases heart rate, which decreases O_2 consumption in myocardium; inhibits β-2 receptors in bronchial system at high doses. Lowers blood pressure in hypertensive subjects

Uses: Hypertension, tachyarrhythmias, prophylaxis of angina pectoris

Dosage and routes:
Hypertension
• *Adult:* By mouth 400 mg once daily or in 2 divided doses, may be increased to desired response, maximum 800 mg daily
Arrhythmias
• *Adult:* By mouth 400−1200 mg daily as required in 2−3 divided doses. Dosage reduction necessary in moderate to severe renal impairment
Angina
• *Adult:* Initially 400 mg daily, adjust as required, maximum 1200 mg daily, withdraw by gradual dose reduction

Available forms include: Capsules 100 mg, 200 mg; tablets 400 mg; all acebutolol as the hydrochloride

Side effects/adverse reactions:
CV: Profound hypotension, bradycardia, congestive heart failure, cold extremities, postural hypotension, 2nd or 3rd degree heart block

CNS: Insomnia, fatigue, dizziness, mental changes, memory loss, hallucinations, depression, lethargy, drowsiness, nightmares, catatonia
GI: Nausea, diarrhoea, vomiting
RESP: Bronchospasm, dyspnoea, wheezing

Contraindications: Hypersensitivity to acebutolol or β-blockers, cardiogenic shock, atrioventricular block, bradycardia, uncontrolled heart failure, reversible obstructive airways disease (unless compelling clinical reasons)

Precautions: Pregnancy, lactation, renal impairment, chronic obstructive pulmonary disease, BP 100/60 or below

Pharmacokinetics:
By mouth: Peak 2−4 hr; drug and metabolites are excreted in urine, protein binding 5%−15%, combined plasma half-life of drug and metabolite is 7−10 hr

Interactions/incompatibilities:
• Verapamil: should not be used with nor within several days of acebutolol, risk of asystole, severe hypotension and heart failure
• Effect reduced by: non-steroidal anti-inflammatory agent
• Increased side effects: cardiac glycosides, antidiabetics, clonidine, anaesthetics, sympathomimetics
• Reduces effect of: xanthine bronchodilators

Clinical assessment:
• Anaesthetist must be informed that patient is on acebutolol
• Baseline measurements in renal and liver function tests before therapy begins
• Reduce dosage in renal dysfunction
• Maximal anti-arrhythmic effect may not be achieved until 3 hr after oral dose

Lab. test interferences: Some

patients develop anti-nuclear factor titres

Treatment of overdose: 1 mg atropine sulphate IV without delay. If insufficient follow by slow IV injection of isoprenaline (5 mcg per min). Monitor constantly until response occurs. If no response, IV glucagon 10−20 mg may produce dramatic improvement. Cardiac pacing if bradycardia becomes severe. Consider use of vasopressors, diazepam, phenytoin, lignocaine, digoxin and bronchodilators. Acebutolol can be removed from blood by haemodialysis

NURSING CONSIDERATIONS
Assess:
• Baseline weight, pulse and BP
Administer:
• Before meals or at night. Tablet may be crushed or swallowed whole
• If single daily dose take at breakfast
Perform/provide:
• Weight daily (monitor fluid balance if significant increase)
• 4 hrly BP and pulse − report significant changes in rhythm and rate
Evaluate:
• Observe for signs of dehydration
• Observe for ankle oedema daily
• Evaluate therapeutic response: decreased BP after 1−2 weeks
Teach patient/family:
• Not to take unprescribed cold remedies (may contain α-adrenergic stimulants)
• How to take pulse, and advise when to inform clinician if rate is low
• To report dizziness, confusion, fever, breathlessness, swollen ankles
• To avoid driving or operating machines if dizzy
• To avoid alcohol, smoking and excess salt in diet

acetazolamide/ acetazolamide sodium

Diamox
Func. class.: Diuretic; carbonic anhydrase inhibitor
Chem. class.: Sulphonamide derivative
Legal class.: POM

Action: Inhibits carbonic anhydrase activity in proximal renal tubules to decrease reabsorption of water, sodium, potassium and bicarbonate; decreases carbonic anhydrase in CNS, increasing seizure threshold; decreases aqueous humour in eye, which lowers intraocular pressure
Uses: Open-angle glaucoma, pre-operative management of closed-angle glaucoma, epilepsy (petit mal, grand mal, mixed), oedema associated with pre-menstrual tension or drug induced oedema, obesity, and congestive heart failure in each case where fluid retention a problem. Also Ménière's, hydrocephalus in the infant
Dosage and routes:
• By mouth, IV or IM (IM preferably avoided because of alkaline pH)
Glaucoma
• *Adult:* 250−1000 mg daily. Divided doses if greater than 250 mg daily
• *Modified release* (adult only): 500 mg night and morning
• *Child:* 125−750 mg daily in divided doses
• *Elderly:* See precautions
Abnormal retention of fluid (adult only): 125−375 mg single morning dose. Acetazolamide is often given alternating with rest days
Epilepsy
• *Adult:* 250−1000 mg daily in divided doses

• *Child:* 125–750 mg daily in divided doses

Change over from other medication should be gradual

Available forms include: Tablets (scored) 250 mg; capsules modified release 500 mg (sustet); injection IM/IV 500 mg (as sodium salt)

Side effects/adverse reactions:

GU: Hypokalaemia, polydipsia and polyuria

CNS: Drowsiness, paraesthesia of extremities and face, depression, headache, dizziness, stimulation, fatigue, irritability, ataxia

GI: Anorexia, GI upsets, thirst

EENT: Myopia, loss of hearing

INTEG: Flushing

RESP: Hyperpnoea

Contraindications: Hypersensitivity to sulphonamides, idiopathic renal hyperchloraemic acidosis, adrenal gland failure, precoma associated with hepatic cirrhosis, renal insufficiency, electrolyte imbalances (hyponatraemia, hypokalaemia), Addison's disease, long-term use in chronic congestive angle-closure glaucoma, marked kidney and liver disease

Precautions: Pregnancy, chronic obstructive pulmonary disease, emphysema, lactation, elderly, urinary tract obstruction, liver dysfunction, precarious electrolyte balance. Increased dose does not increase diuresis. Discontinue drug if loss of hearing

Pharmacokinetics:

By mouth: Onset ½–1 hr, peak 2–4 hr, duration 6–12 hr

By mouth – sustained release: Onset 2 hr, peak 8–12 hr, duration 18–24 hr

IV: Onset 2 min, peak 15 min, duration 4–5 hr

65% absorbed if fasting (oral), 75% absorbed if given with food; half-life 2½–5½ hr; excreted unchanged by kidneys (80% within 24 hr)

Interactions/incompatibilities:

• Potentiates effects of: folic acid antagonists, hypoglycaemics, oral anticoagulants

• Increased side effects: cardiac glycosides, hypotensives, aspirin, phenytoin

• Increased elimination of lithium

• If hypokalaemia occurs: amiodarone, disopyramide, cardiac glycosides, flecainide, quinidine toxicity is increased, action of lignocaine, mexiletine, tocainide is antagonised, increased risk of ventricular arrhythmias with pimozide and sotalol

• Increased risk of hypokalaemia with other diuretics, corticosteroids, corticotrophin and carbenoxolone

Clinical assessment:

• Take blood for measurement of potassium, sodium, chloride, urea, blood glucose levels and creatinine.

• Prescribe morning dosage to avoid sleep disturbance as this drug is a diuretic

• Evaluate therapeutic response: intraocular pressure should decrease as excess aqueous humour is drained

• Give potassium supplement if potassium is less than 3 mmol/litre

• Monitor fluid and electrolyte state

• Periodic blood cell counts recommended

• May need dose adjustments of cardiac glycosides or hypotensive agents administered with acetazolamide

Lab. test interferences: Possibly interferes with theophylline assay

Treatment of overdose: No specific antidote. Supportive measures with correction of electrolyte and fluid balance. Force fluids

NURSING CONSIDERATIONS
Assess:

• Baseline BP lying and standing; weight
• Electrolytes: potassium, sodium, chloride; also blood glucose levels, serum creatinine, blood pH
Administer:
• Orally or intravenously if possible; IM injections are painful
• In the morning to avoid disrupting sleep, especially if given as a diuretic
• Potassium supplement if potassium levels fall below 3.0 mmol/litre
• With food if nausea occurs; absorption may be reduced
Evaluate:
• Weigh daily and maintain fluid balance chart to determine urinary output; effectiveness of drug may be reduced if used daily
• BP lying and standing: postural hypotension may occur
• Therapeutic response indicated by: reduction in oedema and CVP daily if medication is given for congestive cardiac failure; or decrease in intraocular pressure if used to treat glaucoma
• Signs of metabolic acidosis indicated by drowsiness and restlessness
• Signs of hypokalaemia: postural hypotension, malaise, fatigue, tachycardia, leg cramps and weakness
• Confusion, especially in the elderly
Teach patient/family:
• To increase fluid intake to 2−3 litres daily unless contraindicated
• To rise slowly when standing to avoid postural hypotension
• To inform the clinician of sore throat, bleeding, bruising, paresthesiae, tremors, pain or rashes
• To avoid driving or operating machinery if drowsiness occurs
• To report skin rash or loss of hearing (stop medication)

acetylcholine chloride (ophthalmic)

Miochol
Func. class.: Miotic, cholinergic
Chem. class.: Quaternary ammonium compound
Legal class.: POM

Action: Intense, immediate miosis (pupil constriction) by causing contraction of sphincter muscle of iris
Uses: Anterior segment surgery; cataract removal, peripheral iridectomy, penetrating keratoplasty
Dosage and routes:
• *Adult and child:* Instil 0.5−2 ml of a 1% sol in anterior chamber of eye (instillation by physician)
Available forms include: Solution 1% (with Mannitol 3%)
Side effects/adverse reactions:
CV: Hypotension, bradycardia
EENT: Blurred vision, lens opacities, lacrimation
Contraindications: Hypersensitivity, when miosis is undesirable
Precautions: Acute cardiac failure, bronchial asthma
Pharmacokinetics:
Instil: Miosis occurs immediately, duration 10 min
NURSING CONSIDERATIONS
Administer:
• Mix solution with powder and shake vial well to dissolve
• Clean stopper with alcohol before administration
• Use reconstituted solution immediately; unused portion must be discarded
Evaluate:
• Pulse and blood pressure
• Patient safety: in view of artificial pupil constriction ensure patient is accompanied if mobile
Teach patient/family:
• To report visual disturbances such as blurring or loss of sight,

difficulty breathing, sweating or flushing

---

acetylcysteine

Fabrol

Func. class.: Mucolytic

Chem. class.: Amino acid L-cysteine derivative

Legal class.: POM, ~~NHS~~ except for abdominal complications associated with cystic fibrosis

---

Action: Decreases viscosity of secretions by breaking disulphide links of mucoproteins

Uses: Reduction of sputum viscosity in bronchitis and other respiratory conditions associated with the production of viscous mucus; abdominal complications associated with cystic fibrosis

Dosage and routes:

Respiratory conditions

• *Adult:* By mouth, 200 mg 3 times daily, initially 5−10 days extended up to 6 months if necessary

• *Child up to 2 yr:* By mouth, 200 mg daily; 2−6 yr, 200 mg twice daily

Maintenance in cystic fibrosis

• *Child up to 2 yr:* By mouth, 100−200 mg 3 times daily; 2−6 yr, 200 mg 3 times daily

• *Adult:* By mouth, 200 or 400 mg 3 times daily

Acute treatment of abdominal complications associated with cystic fibrosis

• By mouth, 800 mg 3 times daily. In severe cases up to 18 g daily have been used

Available forms include: Granules 200 mg

Side effects/adverse reactions:

No major side effects when given orally

Precautions: Pregnancy, diabetes: each sachet of Fabrol contains equivalent of 2.7 g sucrose

Interactions: Amoxycillin, doxycillin and erythromycin can be administered concurrently. Other antibiotics or drugs should be given 1−2 hr apart

Clinical assessment:

• Take account of sucrose content in diabetes

Treatment of overdose: No specific antidote. General supportive measures and symptomatic treatment

NURSING CONSIDERATIONS

Assess:

• Baseline vital signs and blood sugar levels in diabetics

• Respiratory status; rate, rhythm; note any shortness of breath, wheeze

• Amount of sputum produced and viscosity

Administer:

• Pre-meal, within ½−1 hr for better absorption and to decrease nausea. Reconstitute with water

Perform/provide:

• Suction to remove excess bronchial secretions

• Mouthwashes to maintain good oral hygiene

Evaluate:

• Record vital signs; palpitations may occur

• Blood sugar level assessment − contains 2.7 g sucrose. (Caution in diabetics)

• Respiratory status; absence of purulent secretions, nature of sputum, coughing rate. If wheeze occurs withhold medicine and inform clinician

Teach patient/family:

• To avoid driving or operating machinery until effects of drug have stabilised

• To avoid alcohol and other CNS depressants as they enhance sedative properties of the drug

• That unpleasant odour will decrease after repeated use

• To avoid smoking, smoky atmospheres, perfume, dust, environmental pollutants, aerosols

---

acetylcysteine

Parvolex
Func. class.: Antidote
Chem. class.: Amino acid
L-cysteine derivative
Legal class.: POM

Action: Increases hepatic-reduced glutathione, which is necessary to inactivate toxic metabolites in paracetamol overdose or by acting as an alternative substrate for the toxic paracetamol metabolite
Uses: Paracetamol toxicity
Dosage and routes:
• *Adult and child:* By IV infusion, in glucose 5%, initially 150 mg/kg in 200 ml over 15 min, followed by 50 mg/kg in 500 ml over 4 hr, then 100 mg/kg in 1000 ml over 16 hr
Available forms include: Injection 200 mg/ml, 10 ml ampoule
Side effects/adverse reactions:
INTEG: Rash
MISC: Anaphylaxis 15−60 min after infusion commenced
Contraindications: Hypersensitivity
Precautions: Asthma, history of bronchospasm, pregnancy
Pharmacokinetics: Contact Poisons Centre for information about paracetamol overdose
Incompatibilities:
• Do not use with iron, copper, rubber, nickel
Clinical assessment:
• Obtain arterial blood gas estimations for increased CO_2 retention in asthmatic patients
• Liver function tests must be performed and dose must be received within 15 hr of overdose
• Monitor plasma potassium concentration
Treatment of overdose: There is a theoretical risk of hepatic encephalopathy. There is no specific treatment, and general supportive measures should be carried out
NURSING CONSIDERATIONS:
Assess:
• Baseline vital signs
Administer:
• By IV infusion in glucose 5%
Evaluate:
• Vital signs at regular intervals as anaphylaxis can occur up to 60 min after start of infusion
• Skin — observe for rash

---

acipimox

Olbetam
Func. class.: Hypolipidaemic agent
Chem. class.: Nicotinic acid group
Legal class.: POM

Action: Lowers both cholesterol and triglyceride concentrations by inhibiting synthesis; increases high-density lipoproteins, inhibits release of fatty acids from adipose tissue
Uses: Hyperlipidaemias of types IIa, IIb and IV in patients who have not responded adequately to diet and other measures
Dosage and routes:
• *Adult:* 500−750 mg by mouth daily, in divided doses, maximum 1200 mg daily (with meals). Reduce dose in renal impairment
Available forms include: Capsules 250 mg
Side effects/adverse reactions:
CNS: Flushing
INTEG: Itching, rashes, erythema, sensation of heat
CV: Skin vasodilation
Contraindications: Peptic ulcer, hypersensitivity, pregnancy, lactation
Precautions: Modification of diet is preferred before treatment of

hyperlipidaemia. Reduce dose in renal impairment
Pharmacokinetics: Rapidly and completely absorbed orally. Peak plasma concentration within 2 hr; not bound to plasma protein; half-life 2 hr, excreted unchanged in the urine
Clinical assessment:
• Monitor plasma triglyceride and cholesterol levels
• Assess renal function
Treatment of overdose: If toxic effects observed, administer supportive and symptomatic treatment
NURSING CONSIDERATIONS
Assess:
• BP and weight
Administer:
• With or soon after food
Perform/provide:
• Measures to reduce effects of itching and vasodilation, e.g. cotton clothes
• Observe for side effects
Teach patient/family:
• To understand the importance of concurrent cholesterol lowering diet and maintenance of ideal weight
• To understand the importance of not smoking, avoiding alcohol, and of positive stress management
• That they may feel malaise, GI upsets, flushing and warmth

---

acrivastine

Semprex
Func. class.: Antihistamine
Chem. class.: Derivative of triprolidine
Legal class.: POM

Action: Competitive histamine H_1 antagonist, providing symptomatic relief of allergy
Uses: Allergic rhinitis including hayfever, urticaria

Dosage and routes:
• *Adults and children over 12 yr:* By mouth 8 mg 3 times daily
Available forms include: Capsules 8 mg
Side effects/adverse reactions:
Lacks significant anticholinergic effects. Low penetration of CNS
CNS: Drowsiness, headache
GU: Urinary retention
Contraindications: Renal impairment, hypersensitivity to acrivastine or triprolidine, elderly
Precautions: Pregnancy, lactation, driving or operating machinery. Alcohol, other CNS depressants may produce reduced mental alertness
Pharmacokinetics: Peak plasma concentration 1.5 hr; onset of effect 1 hr, maximum 2 hr, duration 8 hr; half-life 1.5 hr; excreted in urine
Interactions/incompatibilities:
Effects potentiated by alcohol, other CNS depressants, tricyclic antidepressants, antimuscarinics
Treatment of overdose: No experience of overdosage. Appropriate supportive therapy, including gastric lavage, should be initiated if indicated
NURSING CONSIDERATIONS
Administer:
• Orally, 3 times a day
Perform/provide:
• Observe for side effects — drowsiness, headaches or urinary retention
• Observe for signs of hypersensitivity
Evaluate:
• Mental alertness/drowsiness
• Urinary output (may cause urinary retention)
• Alleviation of allergic symptoms
Teach patient/family:
• Warn patient drowsiness rare but can occur — may affect driving or operating machinery. Alcohol may enhance this effect

• To avoid alcohol with medication
• To avoid driving or operating machinery

---

acyclovir (topical)

Zovirax
Func. class.: Antiviral
Chem. class.: Synthetic purine analogue
Legal class.: POM

Action: Interferes with viral DNA replication
Uses: Treatment of herpes simplex virus infections of the skin including initial and recurrent genital herpes and herpes labialis. DO NOT USE IN THE EYES
Dosage and routes: Apply topically to lesions every 4 hr (5 times daily) for 5 days
Available forms include: Cream 5% in an aqueous cream base 2 g or 10 g tube
Side effects/adverse reactions:
INTEG: Transient burning or stinging on application. Erythema or mild drying of the skin
Contraindications: Hypersensitivity to acyclovir or propylene glycol
Precautions: Avoid contact with eyes and mucous membranes, pregnancy, lactation
Pharmacokinetics: Absorption of acyclovir is usually slight following topical application
Interactions: None reported for topical application
Incompatibilities: Should not be diluted
Treatment of overdose: No untoward effects expected if entire contents of 10 g tube were ingested orally; acyclovir is dialysable
NURSING CONSIDERATIONS
Assess:
• Fluid balance

Administer:
• Apply after cleansing the local area with soap and water. Dry thoroughly
• Repeat 4 hrly
• Avoid contact with mucous membranes and eyes
• Apply sufficient medication to completely cover lesions
Perform/Provide:
• Fluids, boiled sweets, mouthwashes for dry mouth
• Store preparation below 25°C
Evaluate:
• Observe patient for signs of allergic reaction e.g. burning, stinging, swelling, redness
• Observe for therapeutic response as indicated by decrease in size and number of lesions
Teach patient/family:
• To wear gloves when applying topical medication
• To wash hands before and after each application
• To avoid use of other topical creams, lotions and ointments unless ordered by clinician

---

acyclovir (ophthalmic)

Zovirax Ophthalmic Ointment
Func. class.: Antiviral
Chem. class.: Synthetic purine analogue
Legal class.: POM

Action: Interferes with viral DNA replication
Uses: Treatment of herpes simplex keratitis
Dosage and routes: Adults, children and elderly 1 cm ribbon of ointment inside lower conjunctival sac 5 times a day (approximately 4 hrly intervals) omitting nighttime application. Continue for at least 3 days after healing is complete

Available forms include: Eye ointment 3% 4.5 g tube

Side effects/adverse reactions:
EENT: Transient mild stinging, superficial punctate keratopathy, local irritation and inflammation (blepharitis, conjunctivitis)

Contraindications: Hypersensitivity to acyclovir

Precautions: For ophthalmic use only, pregnancy, lactation

Pharmacokinetics: Rapidly absorbed into aqueous humour. Clinically insignificant levels found in urine

Interactions: None known for application to eye

Lab. test interferences: None reported

Treatment of overdose: No untoward effects expected if the entire contents of the tube containing 135 mg acyclovir were ingested orally

NURSING CONSIDERATIONS
Administer:
• After washing hands. Cleanse crust or discharge from eyes before application
• Ensure separate application for each eye and wash hands between applications to avoid cross infection
Evaluate:
• Therapeutic response; absence of redness; inflammation
• Allergy, itching, lacrimation, redness and swelling
Teach patient/family:
• To wear gloves and handle carefully
• To use exactly as prescribed
• Not to use make up
• That drug container should not touch eye
• To report adverse reaction
• That drug may cause blurred vision when ointment applied
• To avoid using flannels and towels which may cause reinfection

• Not to use other people's flannels and towels
• To wash hands carefully after application

---

acyclovir (oral)

Zovirax
Func. class.: Antiviral
Chem. class.: Synthetic purine analogue
Legal class.: POM

Action: Interferes with viral DNA replication

Uses: Herpes simplex and varicella-zoster

Dosage and routes
Herpes simplex
• *Adult:* By mouth 200 mg 5 times daily, usually for 5 days. (Use 400 mg for immunocompromised)
• *Child under 2 yr:* Half adult dose, over 2 yr adult dose
Prevention of recurrence
• *Adult:* By mouth 200 mg 4 times daily or 400 mg twice daily possibly reduced to 200 mg 2 or 3 times daily and interrupted every 6−12 months
Prophylaxis for immunocompromised
• *Adult:* By mouth 200−400 mg 4 times daily
Varicella-zoster
• *Adult:* By mouth 800 mg 5 times daily for 7 days

Available forms include: Tablets 200 mg, 400 mg, 800 mg; suspension 200 mg in 5 ml

Side effects/adverse reactions:
GI: Nausea, vomiting, diarrhoea, abdominal pains
INTEG: Rashes

Contraindications: Hypersensitivity to acyclovir

Precautions: Pregnancy, lactation, elderly, renal impairment. Maintain adequate hydration

Pharmacokinetics: Only partially absorbed from the gut. Bioavailability is very low when given orally. In normal adults terminal plasma half-life is 2.9 hr. Excreted mainly unchanged by the kidney. In children, renal impairment and the elderly, the excretion pattern differs

Interactions: Probenecid reduces acyclovir excretion (increased plasma concentrations and risk of toxicity)

Clinical assessment: Check for renal impairment; dosage adjustment may be necessary for patients with herpes zoster

Treatment of overdose: Unlikely that serious toxic effects would occur if a dose of up to 5 g were taken on a single occasion. No data on higher doses—closely observe patient. Acyclovir is dialysable

NURSING CONSIDERATIONS

Assess:
• Fluid balance
• Ask patient about any allergies before treatment and record on care plan/nursing notes
• Adequate hydration in elderly patients receiving high doses for herpes zoster

Perform/provide:
• Urinic testing, particularly for protein before and during medication

Evaluate:
• Maintain fluid balance chart. Report haematuria, oliguria, fatigue, weakness, which may indicate nephrotoxicity. Test urine for protein during treatment
• Pay particular attention to patients with known renal disease and inform clinician immediately if side effects occur
• Evaluate therapeutic response indicated by absence of painful, itching lesions
• Observe bowel pattern before and during treatment. Report severe abdominal pain with bleeding to clinician: drug should then be discontinued
• Observe skin for rashes, urticaria, itching

Teach patient/family:
• That for maximal effectiveness drug should be taken at the first sign of infection e.g. pain, irritation
• That patient has herpes; they could become infected
• Acyclovir does not cure infection, just controls symptoms
• To report sore throat, fever, fatigue could indicate secondary infection
• That drug must be taken at regular intervals throughout the day to maintain therapeutic blood levels for about 10 days
• To report side effects e.g. bruising, bleeding, fatigue, malaise to clinician; may indicate blood dyscrasias

---

acyclovir sodium

Zovirax IV for Intravenous Infusion
Func. class.: Antiviral
Chem. class.: Synthetic purine analogue
Legal class.: POM

Action: Interferes with viral DNA replication
Uses: Herpes simplex and Varicella-zoster
Dosage and routes:
Slow intravenous infusion:
• *Adult:* 5 mg/kg over 1 hr, repeated every 8 hr; doubled in zoster in the immunocompromised, and in simplex encephalitis
• *Child 3 months−12 yr:* 250 mg/m^2 doubled in the immunocompromised and in simplex encephalitis
Dosage should be adjusted accord-

ing to creatinine clearance in renal impairment

Available forms include: Powder acyclovir sodium 250 mg and 500 mg. Reconstitute with water for injections or sodium chloride 0.9% to a concentration of 25 mg/ml

Side effects/adverse reactions:

CNS: Confusion, hallucinations, agitation, tremors, somnolence, psychosis, convulsions, coma, fever

HAEM: Decrease in haematological indices

GI: Nausea, vomiting, increase in liver related enzymes

GU: Renal impairment, increase in blood urea and creatinine levels

INTEG: Rashes

Contraindications: Hypersensitivity to acyclovir

Precautions: Abnormal renal function, dehydration, not to be given orally, pregnancy, lactation

Pharmacokinetics: In normal adults terminal plasma half-life is 2.9 hr. Most of the drug is excreted unchanged by the kidney. In children, renal impairment and the elderly, the excretion pattern differs

Interactions/incompatibilities:

• Zidovudine: extreme lethargy with IV acyclovir

• Probenecid reduces excretion (risk of toxic plasma concentrations)

Clinical assessment:

• Maintain adequate hydration

• Monitor renal function during treatment

Treatment of overdose: Single doses of up to 80 mg per kg have been accidentally administered with no adverse consequences. Acyclovir is dialysable

NURSING CONSIDERATIONS

Assess:

• Hydration and fluid balance

• Renal and hepatic function

• Check for hypersensitivity, abnormal renal function, pregnancy, lactation

Administer:

• Reconstitute 250 mg drug powder with 10 ml sterile water for injections; shake; use within 12 hr; infuse over at least 1 hr to prevent nephrotoxicity

• By slow intravenous infusion over 1 hr following reconstitution and dilution

Perform/provide:

• Maintain fluid balance chart. Report haematuria, oliguria, fatigue, weakness, which may indicate nephrotoxicity. Test urine for protein during treatment

• Pay particular attention to patients with known renal disease and inform clinician immediately if side effects occur

• Store at room temperature for no more than 12 hr after reconstitution

• Ensure adequate fluid intake (2 litres/24 hr) to prevent renal damage

Evaluate:

• IV site as phelebitis is likely to occur when given peripherally

• By assessment of clinical symptoms

• Hepatic and renal function

Teach patient/family:

• That for maximal effectiveness drug should be taken at the first sign of infection e.g. pain, irritation

• That patient has herpes; they could become infected

• Acyclovir does not cure infection, just controls symptoms

• To report sore throat, fever, fatigue, which could indicate secondary infection

• That drug must be taken at regular intervals throughout the day to maintain therapeutic blood levels for about 10 days

• To report side effects e.g. bruising, bleeding, fatigue, malaise to clinician; may indicate blood dyscrasias

---

adrenaline

Min-I-Jet Adrenaline
Func. class.: Adrenergic agonist
Chem. class.: Sympathomimetic amine
Legal class.: POM

Action: Activates α- and β-adrenergic receptors producing increased contractility and heart rate, peripheral vasoconstriction or vasodilation
Uses: 1 in 1000: emergency treatment of acute anaphylaxis
1 in 10,000: cardiac arrest
Dosage and routes:
Cardiac arrest
• Adrenaline 1 in 10,000 (1 mg per 10 ml) — 10 ml by central intravenous injection
Acute anaphylaxis
• IM route, volume of 1 in 1000 (1 mg/ml) injection:
• *Adult:* 0.5−1 ml
• *Child:* Under 1 yr 0.05 ml, 1 yr 0.1 ml, 2 yr 0.2 ml, 3−4 yr 0.3 ml, 5 yr 0.4 ml, 6−12 yr 0.5 ml. May need to use half recommended dose in underweight children
Available forms include:
• Injection 1 in 1000 (adrenaline 1 mg/ml as acid tartrate), 0.5 ml, 1 ml
• Injection 1 in 10,000 (adrenaline 100 mcg/ml as acid tartrate) 10 ml
• Min-I-Jet 1 in 1000 (adrenaline 1 mg/ml as hydrochloride) 0.5 ml, 1 ml
• Min-I-Jet 1 in 10,000 (adrenaline 100 mcg/ml as hydrochloride) 3 ml, 10 ml
Side effects/adverse reactions:
CNS: Anxiety, tremor, headache
CV: Tachycardia, cold extremities, arrhythmias

EENT: Dry mouth
In overdose: Cerebral haemorrhage, pulmonary oedema
Precautions: Hyperthyroidism, diabetes mellitus, ischaemic heart disease, hypertension, elderly
Interactions: Risk of hypertension and/or arrhythmias: MAOIs (concomitant administration and up to 3 weeks after MAOIs), tricyclic antidepressants, cyclopropane, halothane, β-blockers, doxapram, dopexamine
Treatment of overdose: Supportive measures — prompt injection of rapidly-acting α-adrenergic blocking agent (e.g. phentolamine) followed by a β-blocker (e.g. propranolol). Rapidly acting vasodilators (e.g. glyceryl trinitrate) have been used

NURSING CONSIDERATIONS
Administer:
• Into central vein by pumped, continuous infusion in mcg/kg/min
• Correct hypovolaemia prior to and during administration
Perform/provide:
• CVP monitoring is advisable
• Continuous ECG monitoring during administration
• BP and pulse every 5 min; arterial pressure monitoring advised if adrenaline given by infusion
• Detailed patient observation; preferably in HDU or ICU environment
• Ensure infusion reservoir is replaced before emptied to avoid hypotension
• Do not use discoloured solutions
• Emergency equipment
Evaluate:
• Fluid balance
• Drug should be titrated against response until prescribed blood pressure is achieved
• Paraesthesias and coldness of extremities, peripheral blood flow may decrease

• Monitor peripheral and central temperatures
• Injection site: extravasation — inform medical staff immediately; find alternative access — if necessary stop infusion and observe blood pressure
• Therapeutic response — increased BP with stabilisation

Teach patient/family:
• Reason for drug administration and careful monitoring

---

adrenaline (inhaler)

Medihaler-epi
Func. class.: Adrenergic agonist
Chem. class.: Sympathomimetic amine
Legal class.: POM

Action: Activates α- and β-adrenergic receptors producing vasoconstriction, bronchodilatation, relief of mucosal congestion and causes cardiac stimulation. By inhalation: relaxes bronchial smooth muscle, constricts bronchial mucosal vessels, relieves congestion and oedema

Uses: Adjunct to anaphylaxis treatment only

Dosage and routes:
• *Adult:* minimum dose of 20 puffs inhaled
• *Child:* 10−15 puffs under supervision

Available forms include: Aerosol inhalation adrenaline acid tartrate 280 mcg/metered inhalation

Side effects/adverse reactions:
GI: Gastric pain

Precautions: Use with caution if cardiac disease, hypertension, hyperthyroidism. Tolerance develops after prolonged use. Pregnancy

Pharmacokinetics: By inhalation: onset 1 min

Interactions: Risk of hypertension and/or arrhythmias: MAOIs (concomitant administration and up to 3 weeks after MAOIs), tricyclic antidepressants, cyclopropane, halothane, β-blockers, doxapram, dopexamine

Clinical assessment:
• Check inhaler technique
• Monitor for tolerance after repeated use of inhaler

Treatment of overdose: Acute poisoning: immediate IV injections of quick-acting sympatholytics (e.g. phentolamine or piperoxan)

NURSING CONSIDERATIONS

Perform/provide:
• Monitor respiratory pattern
• Provide reassurance and comfortable patient environment to maximise respiratory function

Evaluate:
• Heart and respiratory rate, general appearance
• Response to administration by reduction in bronchospasm (and acuteness of asthma attack)

Teach patient/family:
• Correct inhalation technique

---

adrenaline HCl/ adrenaline borate complex

Epifrin, Eppy, Simplene
Func. class.: Mydriatic
Chem. class.: Sympathomimetic amine
Legal class.: P or POM

Action: Reduces production of aqueous humour and increases outflow

Uses: Primary open angle glaucoma

Dosage and routes:
• *Adult*: One or two drops in affected eye(s) once or twice daily. Less frequently if necessary

Available forms include: Eye drops 0.5%, 1%. Product specific salts

Side effects/adverse reactions:
CNS: Headache, browache
EENT: Severe smarting and redness of the eye; blurred vision, photophobia, eye pain. After prolonged use — pigmentary deposits
Contraindications: Closed angle glaucoma, patients with narrow angle prone to angle block with mydriatics, hypersensitivity to any component of preparation, soft contact lenses (some products only)
Precautions: Hypertension, heart disease, pregnancy, lactation, evaluate anterior chamber angle before initiating therapy, aneurysms, arrhythmia or tachycardia, hyperthyroidism, cerebral arteriosclerosis, diabetes mellitus. Discontinue if visual acuity deteriorates in aphakic patients. Soft contact lenses. Do not drive or operate machinery if have blurred vision
Pharmacokinetics:
INSTIL: Onset 1 hr, peak 4–8 hr, duration 12–24 hr
Interactions: Risk of hypertension and arrhythmias, MAOIs (concomitant administration and up to 3 weeks after MAOIs), tricyclic antidepressants (or within several days of their discontinuation) cyclopropane, halothane, β-blockers, doxapram, dopexamine
Incompatibilities: Soft contact lenses (some products)
Clinical assessment:
• Assess visual acuity in aphakic patients
• Tonometer readings during long-term treatment
• Evaluate anterior chamber angle prior to treatment
Treatment of overdose: Treatment of severe toxic reaction — immediate IV α-adrenoreceptor blocking agent (5–10 mg phentolamine) followed by β-adreno-

receptor blocking agent (2.5–5 mg propranolol)
NURSING CONSIDERATIONS
Assess:
• BP, pulse, respirations
• Visual acuity
Evaluate:
• Allergic reaction: itching, oedema of eyelids, eye discharge; drug should be discontinued
Teach patient/family:
• Report change in vision, blurring or loss of sight, trouble breathing, sweating, flushing
• Method of instillation: pressure on lacrimal sac for 1 min, do not touch dropper to eye
• That long-term therapy may be required if using for glaucoma
• Some smarting and redness of the eye may occur. Report to clinician if this occurs

albumin, human serum 4.5%/5%/20%/25%

Albuminar-5, -20, -25; Human Albumin solution 4.5%, 20% (Immuno); Albutein 5%, 20%, 25%; Buminate 5%, 20%; Zenalb 4.5%, 20%; Albumin solution 20% (SNBTS)
Func. class.: Blood derivative
Chem. class.: human plasma protein
Legal class.: POM

Action: Exerts osmotic pressure on tissue fluids, which expands volume of circulating blood
Uses: Isotonic solutions (4%–5% protein): acute or subacute loss of plasma volume (e.g. burns, pancreatitis, trauma, complications of surgery) plasma exchange
Concentrated solutions (15%–25% protein): severe hypoalbuminaemia associated with low

plasma volume and generalised oedema where salt and water restriction with plasma volume expansion are required, adjunct in treatment of hyperbilirubinaemia by exchange transfusion in newborn, priming heart-lung machines

Dosage and routes:

For intravenous use. Seek clinician's advice. For dosage and rate of administration

Available forms include: Varying size vials from 50 ml to 1 litre for isotonic; 5 ml to 100 ml for concentrated

Side effects/adverse reactions:

GI: Nausea, vomiting, increased salivation

CNS: Fever, chills

CV: Hypotension, tachycardia

Contraindications: Hypersensitivity, cardiac failure, severe anaemia, premature infants, dialysis patients, defects in clotting mechanism

Precautions: Lack of albumin deficiency, pregnancy, history of cardiac or circulatory (including hypertensive) disease, risk of further haemorrhage or shock due to rise in BP, correct any dehydration if necessary, watch for circulatory overload, seek clinician's advice for use in renal and hepatic disease

Pharmacokinetics: In hyponutrition states metabolized as protein energy source

Interactions/incompatibilities:

Protein hydrolysates, amino acid mixtures, solutions containing alcohol

Clinical assessment:

• Check for hypersensitivity, defects in clotting, cardiac failure or disease, severe anaemia, circulatory disease (including hypertension)

Lab. test interferences: Blood samples taken during or shortly after infusion show lower lab. test results (e.g. haematocrit). No interference with rhesus factor determination, thrombocyte function, blood coagulation

Treatment of overdose: Interrupt infusion immediately and watch patient's haemodynamic parameters carefully: Give any specific treatment necessary. Administration of large quantities of albumin should be supplemented with red cell concentrates or replaced by whole blood

NURSING CONSIDERATIONS

Assess:

• Haemodynamic stability and correction of hypovolaemia

Administer:

• Intravenous infusion — rate/volume according to clinician's advice, patient response and blood picture

• Within 4−8 hr of opening

Perform/provide:

• Appropriate storage facilities

• Observation of CVP/pulmonary wedge pressure, BP, heart rate, respirations, and temp, as often as patient's condition dictates

• Accurate fluid balance — NB: watch for possible deterioration in urinary output

Evaluate:

• Monitor BP

• Monitor any dehydration, watch for circulatory overload

• Therapeutic response: increased CVP and BP, decreased oedema, increased serum albumin (within normal limits)

• Allergic response, rash, itching, chills, flushing, urticaria, nausea, vomiting, hypotension, requires discontinuation of infusion, use of new lot if therapy reinstituted

• Overdose: circulatory overload, haemodilution. Increased CVP and BP recordings, distended neck veins, cyanosis, abnormal respiratory pattern, frothy sputum and blood

Teach patient/family:
• If appropriate, explain reason for treatment and possible adverse reactions so that these may be identified early and treated

---

alcuronium chloride

Alloferin
Func. class.: Non-depolarising muscle relaxant
Chem. class.: Derivative of toxiferine, a curare alkaloid
Legal class.: POM

Action: Causes relaxation by competing with acetylcholine as the neurotransmitter
Uses: Medium duration muscle relaxation during surgery and anaesthesia
Dosage and routes:
• *Adult:* Intravenous injection 200−250 mcg/kg (higher dose used for longer procedures) when non-potentiating anaesthetic agents used, then incremental doses of one-sixth to one-quarter of initial dose as required
• *Child over 28 days:* 125−200 mcg/kg
Available forms include: Injection IV 5 mg/ml (2 ml amp)
Side effects/adverse reactions:
CV: Tachycardia, decreased BP
Contraindications: Myasthenia gravis, hypersensitivity, pregnancy, porphyria, myasthenic (Eaton-Lambert) syndrome
Precautions: Reduce dose in renal impairment, pregnancy, hepatic disease, poliomyelitis, Duchenne muscular dystrophy, neurofibromatosis, amyotrophic lateral sclerosis, hypothermia, carcinomatosis. Anaesthetist must be present to control patient's ventilation, disturbed serum protein levels, acidosis, correct electrolyte or acid-base disturbances before administration, and correct any lack of effect
Pharmacokinetics: Laryngeal relaxation achieved within 90−120 seconds, muscle relaxation persists for 20−40 min. Half-life 3.3 hours; excreted unchanged in urine
Interactions/incompatibilities:
• Effects increased by: antibiotics of the polymixin and aminoglycoside groups, lincomycin, azlocillin, mezlocillin, nifedipine, verapamil, lithium, parenteral magnesium, clindamycin, volatile anaesthetics, quinidine, β-blockers, phenytoin, penicillamine, narcotic analgesics, ganglion-blocking agents, diazepam, high concentrations of magnesium ions
• Effects decreased by: neostigmine, pyridostigmine, demecarium and ecothiopate eye drops, high concentrations of calcium, potassium and sodium ions; do not mix with thiopentone
• Adverse effects produced by: IV dantrolene and IV verapamil (hypotension, myocardial depression, hyperkalaemia)
Treatment of overdose:
Continue artificial ventilation; reverse neuromuscular blockade with IV injection of prostigmine 1−5 mg (child 50−70 mcg/kg) plus atropine 400−1250 mcg (child 20−30 mcg/kg); observe patient until neuromuscular function is restored. Do not leave unattended until adequate spontaneous respiration is present
NURSING CONSIDERATIONS
Assess:
• Baseline pulse, blood pressure and vital signs
• Check history of sensitivity or myasthenia gravis, porphyria, pregnancy
• Test for urea and electrolytes, blood gases and pH if appropriate
• Ensure acid-base/electrolyte dis-

turbances are corrected before administration

• Airway and respirations constantly; temperature

Administer:

• Make up with water for injection, if require dilute solution, immediately before administration; do not mix with thiopentone

Perform/provide:

• In theatre or intensive care unit

• Perform IV administration in the presence of an experienced anaesthetist

• Provide equipment for intubation/resuscitation

Evaluate:

• Therapeutic response

• Observe for muscle spasms, rashes

Teach patient/family:

• The effects of the drug and communication strategies where drug is used to facilitate ventilation in intensive care

---

alfentanil

Rapifen, Rapifen Concentrate, Rapifen Intensive Care

Func. class.: Opioid analgesic
Chem. class.: Opioid, synthetic
Legal class.: CD (Sch 2), POM

Action: Inhibits ascending pain pathways in limbic system, thalamus, midbrain, hypothalamus

Uses: Analgesia especially during short operative procedure and outpatient surgery; enhancement of anaesthesia; analgesic and respiratory depressant in assisted respiration

Dosage and routes:

Spontaneous respiration

• *Adult:* IV injection, initially up to 500 mcg over 30 seconds, supplement with increments of 250 mcg

• *Child:* Not recommended

Assisted ventilation

• *Adult and child:* IV injection, initially 30−50 mcg/kg, supplement with increments of 15 mcg/kg. Discontinue dosage at least 10 min before end of surgery

IV infusion, initially 50−100 mcg/kg over 10 min or as a bolus then maintenance 0.5−1.0 mcg/kg/min. Discontinue infusion at least 30 min before end of surgery. (Supplement with IV bolus if necessary)

Available forms include: Injection 500 mcg per ml (2 ml, 10 ml amps) 5 mg per ml (as hydrochloride) (1 ml amps with sodium chloride and water for injection)

Side effects/adverse reactions:

CNS: Dizziness

GI: Nausea, vomiting

CV: Bradycardia, hypotension

RESP: Respiratory depression

MS: Rigidity

Contraindications: Obstructive airways disease or respiratory depression if not ventilating. Intolerance to alfentanil. Concurrent administration of monoamine oxidase inhibitors or within 2 weeks of their discontinuation. Administration in labour or before clamping of the cord during Caesarean section due to the possibility of respiratory depression in the new-born infant

Precautions: Reduce dose in elderly, hypothyroidism and chronic liver disease. Respiratory depression may persist or recur during postoperative period. Adequate spontaneous breathing must be established before leaving recovery room. Hypovolaemic patients, concomitant β-blocker or sedative medication. Reduced dose and extended interval may be required with concomitant use of erythromycin or cimetidine. Following cessation of Rapifen Intensive Care patient should be closely observed for at least 6 hr. Respiratory depression occurs following doses in excess of 1 mg. Seek clinician's advice on taking measures to avoid muscle rigidity

Pharmacokinetics: Half-life 1–2 hr. Peak analgesic and respiratory depressant effects occur within 90 seconds. Analgesia lasts up to 10 min

Interactions/incompatibilities:
• Cimetidine and erythromycin can inhibit alfentanil clearance leading to increased plasma levels
• Increased effects: hypnotics, CNS depressants

Treatment of overdose: Anticholinergics (e.g. atropine or glycopyrrolate)

Oxygen administration (assisted or controlled ventilation may be required)

IV neuromuscular blocking agent Maintain body temperature and adequate fluid intake. Observe patient for 24 hr

Specific narcotic antagonist (e.g. naloxone) should be available to treat respiratory depression. All the effects of alfentanil may be antagonised if necessary by a specific narcotic antagonist such as naloxone

NURSING CONSIDERATIONS
Assess:
• Respiratory function if unventilated. If ventilated, maintenance of adequate analgesia/anaesthesia
• CNS function: dizziness, drowsiness, hallucinations, euphoria, level of consciousness and pupil reactions
• Fluid balance: decreasing urine output may indicate urinary retention

Administer:
• By prescribed bolus injection with maintenance infusion as prescribed, with assisted ventilation
Perform/provide:

• Dilute before use and for infusion
• Resuscitation equipment and narcotic antagonist (e.g. naloxone) in case of respiratory depression
Evaluate:
• Response to treatment: maintenance of anaesthesia
• Allergic reactions: rash, urticaria
• Respiratory function: respiratory depression, rate and depth. Notify clinician if rate falls below 12 respirations per minute

---

allopurinol

Aloral, Aluline, Caplenal, Rimapurinol, Xanthomax, Cosuric, Hamarin, Zyloric, also others with no proprietary name
Func. class.: Antigout
Chem. class.: Enzyme inhibitor
Legal class.: POM

Action: Decreases uric acid levels by inhibiting xanthine oxidase
Uses: Gout prophylaxis, hyperuricaemia, management of some renal stones
Dosage and routes:
• *Adult:* By mouth initially 100–300 mg/day then 200–600 mg/day depending on severity
• *Child:* 10–20 mg/kg/day
• For dose in elderly, renal impairment and dialysis—seek clinician's advice
Available forms include: Tablets 100, 300 mg
Side effects/adverse reactions:
SYST: Generalised hypersensitivity reactions, withdraw drug. Initial exacerbation of acute gouty attacks
GI: Nausea, vomiting
INTEG: Fever, rashes (sometimes with fever) withdraw drug
Contraindications: Hypersensitivity, acute gout
Precautions: Pregnancy, lactation,

renal disease, hepatic disease. Maintain adequate fluid intake (2 litres per day)

Asymptomatic hyperuricaemia. Withdraw immediately and permanently at first sign of intolerance

Neoplastic conditions — allopurinol should be commenced before cytotoxics

Administer prophylactic colchicine or NSAID (not aspirin or salicylates) until at least 1 month after hyperuricaemia corrected. Do not start therapy during or immediately after a gout attack

Pharmacokinetics:
By mouth: Peak 2−4 hr; excreted in faeces, urine, half-life 1−3 hr, terminal half-life 18−30 hr

Interactions/incompatibilities:
• Increased effects of: 6-mercaptopurine, azathioprine, cyclophosphamide, chlorpropamide, coumarin anticoagulants
• Effectiveness decreased by: salicylates, and uricosuric agents
• Renal calculi with: vitamin C

Lab. test interferences: Liver function tests

Clinical assessment:
• Monitor uric acid levels twice weekly. Levels should be 6 mg/dl
• Perform full blood count, blood urea and creatinine and serum aspartate aminotransferase levels before treatment commences, then monthly
• Check for any hypersensitivity, pregnancy, lactation, renal and hepatic disease
• For initial treatment prophylactic colchicine or NSAID (not aspirin or salicylate) should be prescribed
• Commence treatment a few days before anti-neoplastic therapy

Treatment of overdose: Adequate hydration to facilitate excretion. Dialysis if considered necessary. If taken with mercaptopurine or azathioprine inform clinician

NURSING CONSIDERATIONS
Assess:
• Fluid balance; increase fluid intake to at least 2 litres per 24 hr to prevent formation of renal calculi on clinical advice
• Diet: discourage offal, sardines, salmon, pulses, gravies (high purine foods)

Administer:
• With meals to prevent gastrointestinal symptoms

Perform/provide:
• Sieve urine to detect renal calculi if calculi suspected

Evaluate:
• Therapeutic effectiveness e.g. decreased joint pain.

Teach patient/family:
• To report skin rashes, stomatitis, malaise, fever; aching; drug may have to be discontinued
• To avoid driving or handling machinery if drowsiness occurs
• To avoid alcohol, caffeine as they increase uric acid levels
• To avoid vitamin C preparations as renal calculi may develop

allyloestrenol

Gestanin
Func. class.: Progestogen
Chem. class.: Synthetic progestogen
Legal class.: POM

Action: Suppresses uterine motility, maintains pregnancy. Orally active progestogen

Uses: Threatened or habitual abortion, threatened premature labour

Dosage and routes: By mouth
Threatened abortion
• 5 mg 3 times daily for 5−7 days, extended if necessary, followed by gradual reduction in dose unless symptoms return

Habitual abortion
• 5−10 mg daily as soon as pregnancy is diagnosed and continued for at least 1 month after critical period ends
Threatened premature labour
• Dosage determined individually; high doses (up to 40 mg daily) have been used
Available forms include: Tablets 5 mg
Side effects/adverse reactions:
GI: Nausea and vomiting
Contraindications: Abnormal liver function. Porphyria
Interactions: Cyclosporin plasma concentration increased due to inhibition of metabolism
Clinical assessment:
• Liver function tests: bilirubin, alkaline phosphatase during long-term treatment
NURSING CONSIDERATIONS
Assess:
• BP at start of therapy, fluid balance, weight
Administer:
• With food or milk
Perform/provide:
• Blood/urine glucose monitoring in diabetes mellitus
Observe:
• Oedema and weight gain, clay coloured stools/dark urine etc
Evaluate:
• Vaginal bleeding
Teach patient/family:
• To inform clinician about: weight gain, per vaginum loss, jaundice, light coloured stools, nausea and vomiting, headaches and breast lumps
• To perform breast examination
• If diabetic, to monitor glucose carefully
• To avoid over exposure to sunlight

alprazolam

Xanax
Func. class.: Anxiolytic
Chem. class.: Benzodiazepine
Legal class.: CD (Sch 4) POM

Action: Depresses subcortical levels of CNS, including limbic system, reticular formation
Uses: Short-term treatment of moderate or severe anxiety and anxiety associated with depression
Dosage and routes: By mouth
• *Adult:* 250−500 mcg 3 times daily increasing if necessary to a total of 3 mg daily
• *Elderly or in the presence of debilitating disease:* 250 mcg 2 to 3 times daily to be gradually increased if needed and tolerated
• Review treatment regularly— reassess dosage at intervals of no more than 4 weeks. Treatment should be tapered off gradually
Available forms include: Tablets scored 250 mcg, 500 mcg
Side effects/adverse reactions:
CNS: Drowsiness, sedation, unsteadiness and ataxia, impaired alertness, confusion, amnesia, dependence
EENT: Blurred vision
Contraindications: Hypersensitivity to benzodiazepines, acute pulmonary insufficiency
Precautions: Elderly, debilitated, hepatic disease, renal disease, chronic respiratory disease, lactation, pregnancy, psychosis, depression, labour, alcoholism, other CNS depressants, not for use under 18 years of age, personality disorders, loss or bereavement
Pharmacokinetics:
By mouth: Onset 30 min, peak 1−2 hr, duration 4−6 hr, therapeutic response 2−3 days, metabolised by liver, excreted by kidneys, breast milk, half-life

12−15 hr; can get accumulation

Interactions/incompatibilities:

• Increased effects: alcohol, anaesthetics, opioid analgesics, antidepressants, clonazepam, antihistamines, antipsychotics, CNS depressants

Treatment of overdose: Induce vomiting and/or gastric lavage, vital sign, supportive care

NURSING CONSIDERATIONS

Assess:

• Dosage to be assessed regularly
• Baseline BP (lying, standing), pulse

Administer:

• With food or milk for GI symptoms
• Crushed if patient is unable to swallow medication whole

Perform/provide:

• Mouthwashes, frequent sips of water for dry mouth
• Assistance with ambulation during beginning therapy; drowsiness/dizziness occurs
• Safety measures, including side-rails
• Check to see oral medication has been swallowed

Evaluate:

• Therapeutic response: decreased anxiety, restlessness, sleeplessness
• Mental status: mood, alertness, affect, sleeping pattern, drowsiness, dizziness
• Physical dependency, withdrawal symptoms: headache, nausea, vomiting, muscle pain, weakness after long-term use
• Fluid balance, may indicate renal dysfunction
• Suicidal tendencies

Teach patient/family:

• That drug may be taken with food
• That drug is not to be used for everyday stress or longer than 4 months, unless directed by clinician
• To avoid non-prescribed preparations unless approved by clinician
• To avoid driving, activities that require alertness, since drowsiness may occur
• To avoid alcohol or other psychotropic medications, unless prescribed by clinician
• Not to discontinue medication abruptly after long-term use
• That drowsiness might worsen at beginning of treatment
• To see general practitioner/clinician each time a new supply is required (repeat prescriptions are not recommended)

---

alteplase INN

Actilyse

Func. class.: Fibrinolytic
Chem. class.: Tissue-type plasminogen activator (rtPA)
Legal class.: POM

Action: Accelerates conversion of plasminogen to plasmin; binds to fibrin, converts plasminogen in thrombus to plasmin, which leads to local fibrinolysis of clot. Alteplase is relatively inactive until it binds to fibrin

Uses: Fibrinolytic therapy of acute thrombotic coronary artery occlusion

Dosage and routes:

• *Adult:* IV 100 mg over 3 hr as 10 mg over 1−2 min, 50 mg over 1 hr, 40 mg over 2 hr. Patients under 67 kg receive 1.5 mg/kg in same proportions (10%, 50% and 40% of the total dose respectively). Treatment should be initiated within 6 hr of acute myocardial infarction

Available forms include: Powder for reconstitution 50 mg (29 million IU) per vial and 20 mg (11.6 million IU per vial)

Side effects/adverse reactions:
SYST: GI and GU bleeding, bleeding at site of injection, intracerebral haemorrhage, retroperitoneal bleeding, surface bleeding, nausea, vomiting
CV: Accelerated idioventricular rhythm associated with repofusion of the coronary artery
Contraindications: History of cerebrovascular disease or uncontrolled hypertension, known bleeding diathesis. Within 10 days of major surgery, severe internal bleeding episodes, or trauma or puncture of major non-compressible blood vessels. Acute pancreatitis, bacterial endocarditis, severe liver disease including hepatic failure, cirrhosis, portal hypertension (oesophageal varices) and active hepatitis, prolonged or traumatic resuscitation, active peptic ulcer
Precautions: Pregnancy, pay special attention to potential bleeding sites. Avoid IM injections, venepuncture and arterial puncture if possible, children, diabetes mellitus, diabetic retinopathy, severe renal impairment, avoid non-essential manipulation of patient. Anti-arrhythmic therapy should be available
Pharmacokinetics: Cleared by liver, 80% cleared within 10 min of administration
Interactions/incompatibilities:
• Increased risk of bleeding with prior or concomitant administration of anticoagulant
Treatment of overdose: Terminate infusion. If serious bleeding occurs fresh frozen plasma or fresh whole blood should be infused. Administer synthetic antifibrinolytic agents if necessary
NURSING CONSIDERATIONS
Assess:
• ECG, baseline temperature and neurological assessment
• Electrolytes — particular potassium (precipitates ectopics etc)
• Contraindications in patient
Administer:
• Reconstitute with diluting agent provided, then add sterile physiological saline and dilute up to 1:5 if required
• Heparin after thrombolytic treatment has been discontinued, thrombin time or activated partial thromboplastin time less than 2 times baseline (about 3−4 hr)
• Within 6 hr of coronary occlusion for best results
• As prescribed by clinician
Perform/provide:
• Continuous ECG monitoring for arrhythmias/reperfusion dysrhythmias
• Emergency resuscitation equipment if anaphylaxis or cardiac arrest occurs
• Close observation of all IV puncture sites; urine; stools for evidence of haemorrhage — inform medical staff immediately
• Analgesics for the control of central chest pain (diamorphine/GTN)
• Issue card to patient stating time and nature of fibrinolytic administration. 1 hr post-administration
Evaluate:
• Vital signs: ½−1 hrly pulse respiration and BP
• Bleeding/haemorrhage during and immediately post-infusion: haematuria, haematemesis, bleeding from mucous membranes, epistaxis, ecchymosis
• ECG
Teach patient/family:
• To report any signs of bleeding, chest pain or malaise to nursing staff immediately
• Information concerning immediate and longer term counselling as to myocardial infarction, throughout hospital stay

aluminum acetate (otic, topical)

Func. class.: Astringent
Chem. class.: Aluminum salt
Legal class.: P

Action: Precipitate protein, form superficial protective layer
Uses: Suppurating an exudative eczema or wounds, treats inflammation in otitis externa
Dosage and routes:
• *Topical lotion 0.65%:* Use undiluted as a wet dressing
• *Ear drops 13% and 8%:* Instil into meatus or apply on gauze wick kept saturated with ear drops
Available forms include: Topical lotion 0.65%; ear drops 13%, 8%
Side effects/adverse reactions:
INTEG: Irritation, increasing inflammation
Contraindications: Tight, occlusive dressing
Interactions/incompatibilities:
• Inhibits action of topical collagenase ointment
• Soap decreases action
NURSING CONSIDERATIONS
Administer:
• Apply as moist dressings to the affected area. Avoid tight packing
Evaluate:
• Observe area to receive topical application carefully for irritation, rashes, dryness and breaks in the skin
Teach patient/family:
• To discontinue use if irritation occurs
• To avoid using near eyes
• To retain ear drops by lying with affected ear uppermost for 10 min after instillation

aluminium hydroxide

Alu-Cap, ~~NHS~~ Aludrox
Func. class.: Antacid, phosphate-binder
Chem. class.: Aluminum salt
Legal class.: GSL or P

Action: Neutralises gastric acidity, adsorbs phosphates in GI tract
Uses: Antacid, hyperphosphataemia in chronic renal failure
Dosage and routes: By mouth
Antacid
• *Adult:* Suspension 5−10 ml 4 times a day between meals and at night
• *Child 6−12 yr:* up to 5 ml 3 times daily
• *Adult:* Tablets 500−1000 mg chewed 4 times daily and at night
Alu-Cap
• *Adult:* 1 capsule 4 times daily and at night. Not suitable as antacid for children
Hyperphosphataemia in renal failure
• Mixture 20−100 ml as required
Alu-Cap
• *Children and adult:* 2−10 g/day as required with meals
Available forms include: Capsules 475 mg; tablets 500 mg; mixture 4%
Side effects/adverse reactions:
GI: Constipation
Contraindications: Hypersensitivity to this drug or aluminium products; hypophosphataemia
Precautions: Renal impairment can cause aluminium accumulation. Watch for phosphate depletion. Porphyria
Pharmacokinetics:
By mouth: Onset 20−40 min, excreted in faeces and some in urine
Interactions/incompatibilities:
• Increased excretion: aspirin
• Reduced absorption: ciproflox-

acin, isoniazid, norfloxacin, oflox-
acin, tetracyclines, rifampicin,
phenytoin, diflunisal, pivampicillin, itraconazole, ketoconazole,
fosinopril, chloroquine, hydroxychloroquine, penicillamine
• Absorption of biphosphonates
reduced
Clinical assessment:
• Monitor phosphate levels as
phosphate is bound in gastrointestinal system by drug
Treatment of overdose: Gastric
lavage, mild aperient if required
NURSING CONSIDERATIONS
Administer:
• In cases of hyperphosphataemia,
administer with or immediately
before food, dose according to
blood levels
• For antacid relief (optimum up
to 2 hr), administer 1 hr after meals
Perform/provide:
• Give stool softeners as pre-
scribed if constipated
• Test urine for pH
Evaluate:
• Therapeutic response: relief of
pain/dyspepsia (antacid), relief of
pruritis (hyperphosphataemia)
• Observe for pain, symptoms of
dyspepsia
• Symptoms of hyperphospha-
taemia: e.g. persistent pruritis
• Signs of constipation
Teach patient/family:
• To drink at least 2 litres/day
unless contraindicated
• To avoid foods rich in phos-
phates e.g. dairy products, eggs,
fruits
• Inform prescribing clinician
regarding current medication
• High fibre diet unless
contraindicated
• Appropriate administration
technique
• To observe for side effects or
signs of possible sub-therapeutic
dosage

amantadine HCl

Symmetrel, Mantadine
Func. class.: Anti-viral, anti-
parkinsonian agent
Chem. class.: Tricyclic amine
Legal class.: POM

Action: Inhibits viral replication.
Prevents uncoating of viral nucleic
acid and penetration of virus into
host; potentiates dopaminergic
activity in CNS
Uses: Prophylaxis or treatment of
influenza type A, herpes zoster,
Parkinson's disease
Dosage and routes:
Herpes zoster
• *Adult:* 100 mg twice daily for 14
days. Repeat course if necessary
for post-herpetic neuralgia
Influenza type A
• *Adult:* 100 mg twice daily for 5–
7 days. Prophylaxis 100 mg twice
daily for as long as required
(usually 7–10 days)
• *Child 10–15 yr:* 100 mg daily
Parkinson's disease
• *Adult:* By mouth 100 mg daily
or twice daily, second dose not
later than 4 pm, maximum 400 mg
daily
Available forms include: Capsules
100 mg; syrup 50 mg/5 ml
Side effects/adverse reactions:
CNS: Dizziness, anxiety, hallucinations, convulsions, inability to
concentrate, insomnia
CV: Peripheral oedema
INTEG: Skin discolouration
EENT: Blurred vision
GI: Nausea, vomiting, consti-
pation, dry mouth
Contraindications: Hypersensi-
tivity, epilepsy, gastric ulceration
or history of ulceration, severe
renal disease
Precautions: Confusion, halluci-
natory states, recurrent eczema.
Renal impairment, liver disease,

psychosis, congestive heart failure. Pregnancy, lactation, elderly. Avoid abrupt withdrawal

Pharmacokinetics:

By mouth: Peak plasma levels 4 hr, half-life 24 hr, not metabolised, excreted in urine (90%) unchanged, excreted in breast milk

Interactions/incompatibilities:

• Increased antimuscarinic side effects with: antimuscarinics

• Reduced antiparkinsonian action with: methyldopa, meticosine, antipsychotics, metoclopramide, reserpine, tetrabenazine

Treatment of overdose: No specific antidote. Supportive measures aimed at symptoms of excessive central stimulation

NURSING CONSIDERATIONS

Assess:

• Allergies before commencing treatments and reaction to each administration of the drug. Note allergies in patient records and care plan and notify all staff responsible for drug administration

• Weight and fluid balance

Administer:

• Preferably before exposure to influenza and for 10 days after contact

• At least 4 hr before retiring to avoid insomnia

• After meals for better absorption and to avoid gastric upset

Evaluate:

• Therapeutic response: apyrexia, failure to develop malaise, cough, dyspnoea in infection: tremors, shuffling gait in Parkinson's disease

• For aggravation of side effects of anti-parkinsonian drugs

• Fluid balance, report urinary frequency and hesitancy

• Weight daily

• Bowel pattern before and during treatment

• Rashes, photosensitivity, after administration of drug

• Rate and depth of respirations, wheezing, tightness in chest, limb oedema

Teach patient/family:

• To alter position slowly to avoid postural hypotension

• All aspects of drug therapy: need to report breathlessness, weight gain, dizziness, lack of concentration, dysuria, behavioural changes

• To avoid situations where alertness is essential if there are CNS effects or blurred vision

• To take the drug exactly as prescribed, since parkinsonian crisis may occur if it is discontinued abruptly

---

amikacin sulphate

Amikin
Func. class.: Antibiotic
Chem. class.: Aminoglycoside
Legal class.: POM

Action: Interferes with protein synthesis in bacterial cell by binding to ribosomal subunit, which causes misreading of genetic code; inaccurate peptide sequence forms in protein chain, causing bacterial death

Uses: Serious gram-negative infection due to gentamicin-resistant organisms, e.g. some strains of *P. aeruginosa*, *E. coli*, *Enterobacter*, *Acinetobacter*, *Providencia*, *Citrobacter*, *Serratia*, *Proteus*

Dosage and routes:

• *Adult and child:* IM, slow IV injection, IV infusion 15 mg/kg/day in 2 doses

• *Neonate and premature infant:* initial loading dose 10 mg/kg then 15 mg/kg/day in 2 doses

• Severe urinary tract infection

(not due to *Pseudomonas* spp)
Adult: 7.5 mg/kg/day in 2 doses
• Life-threatening infection or pseudomonal infection: *Adult:* up to 1.5 g/day (500 mg 8 hrly) maximum 15 g total dose
• Reduce dose and/or decrease frequency in renal impairment. Other routes of administration: seek clinician's advice
Available forms include: Injection 50, 250 mg/ml
Side effects/adverse reactions:
GU: Oliguria, nephrotoxicity, azotaemia, renal irritation
CNS: Headache, numbness, paraesthesia, fever
EENT: Ototoxicity, deafness, tinnitus, vertigo
GI: Nausea, vomiting
INTEG: Rash
Contraindications: Mild to moderate infections, myasthenia gravis, hypersensitivity to aminoglycosides, pregnancy, renal or ear damage by previous drug therapy
Precautions: Renal impairment, lactation, hearing deficits, elderly, poor hydration. Renal irritation, prior administration of nephrotoxic and/or ototoxic agents
Pharmacokinetics:
IM: Onset rapid, peak 1 hr
IV: Onset immediate, peak 30 min
Plasma half-life 2−3 hr; not metabolised, excreted unchanged in urine
Interactions/incompatibilities:
• Increased risk of nephrotoxicity: cephalosporins, colistin, polymyxin, capreomycin, vancomycin, amphotericin, cyclosporin, cisplatin, diuretics
• Enhanced effects of: nondepolarising muscle relaxants
• Severe hypocalcaemia: bisphosphonates
• Do not mix in solution or syringe with other drugs
Clinical assessment:
• Monitor plasma concentrations

of drug 1 hr after IV or IM injection when levels should peak and just before next dose when levels should trough. Plasma levels should be 2−4 times greater than bacteriostatic level. 1 hr (peak) concentration should not exceed 30 mg/litre, pre-dose (trough) concentration should be less than 10 mg/litre
• Prescribe to be given at regular intervals to maintain plasma concentrations
• Assess for signs of renal impairment by creatinine clearance tests, blood urea and creatinine levels; lower dosage should be given for renal impairment
Treatment of overdose: Haemodialysis or peritoneal dialysis, monitor serum levels of drug
NURSING CONSIDERATIONS
Assess:
• Weight before treatment commences: dose is usually calculated on ideal body weight, but may be calculated on actual body weight
• Fluid balance
Administer:
• Administer IM injection into large muscle mass, rotate injection sites
• Ensure drug is given at regular intervals as prescribed to maintain blood levels
• Bicarbonate, to keep urine alkaline if drug prescribed for urinary tract infection, as drug is most effective in an alkaline environment. Bladder wash out may be used
Perform/provide:
• Monitor vital signs during infusion, observe for hypotension, change in pulse
• Obtain specimen for culture and sensitivity testing before treatment commences to identify causative organism
• Encourage patient to drink 2−3 litres fluid daily to prevent renal damage

• Flush line with normal saline after infusion

Evaluate:

• Urinalysis daily for proteinuria casts. Report sudden change in urinary output

• Observe IV site for signs of thrombophlebitis e.g. pain, redness, swelling. Inform clinician if thrombophlebitis occurs

• Therapeutic effectiveness

• Record temperature, observe wounds for signs of infection

• For signs of deafness e.g. tinnitus, vertigo. Audiometric testing may be necessary

• Observe for dehydration: concentrated urine, decrease in skin elasticity, dry mucous membranes

• Secondary infection, pyrexia, malaise, redness, pain, swelling, perineal itching, stomatitis, change in cough or sputum, diarrhoea

• Vestibular dysfunction: nausea, vomiting, dizziness, headache and report: drug may have to be discontinued if severe

Teach patient/family:

• To report headache, dizziness, symptoms of secondary infection, renal impairment

• To report hearing loss, tinnitus, feeling of 'fullness' in head

---

amiloride HCl

Midamor, Berkamil, Amilospare, many combination products

Func. class.: Potassium-sparing diuretic

Chem. class.: Pyrazine

Legal class.: POM

Action: Acts primarily on distal tubule, secondarily by inhibiting reabsorption of sodium. Reduces excretion of potassium

Uses: Oedema, potassium conservation with thiazide and loop diuretics in hypertension, congestive heart failure, hepatic cirrhosis with ascites

Dosage and routes:

Adult: By mouth initially 10 mg daily or 5 mg twice daily, maximum 20 mg daily. Cirrhosis with ascites, initially 5 mg daily. Contraindicated in children. Monitor dose carefully in elderly

Available forms include: Tablets 5 mg, sugar-free oral solution 5 mg in 5 ml

Side effects/adverse reactions:

ELECT: Hyponatraemia, hyperkalaemia

CNS: Confusion

GI: Nausea, dry mouth, anorexia, abdominal pain, flatulence

INTEG: Rash

CV: Orthostatic hypotension

Contraindications: Anuria, hyperkalaemia, diabetic nephropathy, hypersensitivity, acute renal failure, severe renal disease, pregnancy, lactation, potassium supplements, potassium-conserving agents, use in children

Precautions: Ascites, hepatic disease, renal impairment, acidosis, diabetes mellitus, elderly, cardiac oedema, potassium-rich diet

Pharmacokinetics:

By mouth: Onset 2 hr, peak 6−10 hr, duration 24 hr; excreted in urine, faeces, excreted in breast milk, half-life 6−9 hr

Interactions/incompatibilities:

• Reduced renal clearance of lithium

• Increased risk of hyponatraemia with chlorpropamide in combination with thiazide diuretic

• Increased risk of hypokalaemia in combination with angiotensin−converting enzyme inhibitor

Clinical assessment:

• Monitor electrolytes; blood potassium, sodium and chloride.

• Order medication to be given in the morning to avoid diuretic effect at night

• Assess therapeutic response e.g. oedema of feet, legs, sacral area daily if drug is given for congestive cardiac failure

Lab. test interferences:
Interfere: Glucose tolerance test. Discontinue at least 3 days before test

Treatment of overdose: Discontinue therapy. No antidote. Induce emesis or gastric lavage. Symptomatic and supportive treatment for dehydration, electrolyte imbalance, hyperkalaemia

NURSING CONSIDERATIONS
Assess:
• Fluid balance, weight, BP
Administer:
• In early morning to avoid nocturia
• With food if nausea occurs; absorption may be decreased slightly
Perform/provide:
• Weigh daily; maintain fluid balance chart
• BP (standing and lying) 6-hrly
Evaluate:
• Drowsiness and restlessness (signs of metabolic acidosis) and confusion, especially in the elderly
• Relief of dyspnoea and oedema
• Rashes, pyrexia daily
Teach patient/family:
• To increase fluid intake 2–3 litre daily unless contraindicated
• To rise slowly from lying or sitting position
• About adverse reactions
• To take medication as prescribed
• To avoid potassium-rich foods, e.g. oranges, bananas
• To inform prescribing clinician about current medication

amino acid solution

Aminoplasmal, Aminoplex, Branched Chain Aminoacids, FreAmine III, Hepanutrin, Nephramine, Perifusin, Primene, Synthamin, Vamin
Func. class.: Nutrition, intravenous
Chem. class.: Amino acids
Legal class.: POM

Action: Required for anabolism to maintain structure, decrease catabolism, promote healing
Uses: Supplemental or total parenteral nutrition (TPN) when adequate feeding via alimentary tract is not possible
Dosage and routes:
• Intravenous infusion
• Seek advice from clinician, dietician and pharmacist; folic acid, vitamin, electrolyte and mineral supplements may be necessary
Available forms include: Vary in composition of amino acids, often contain energy source and/or electrolytes
Side effects/adverse reactions:
GI: Nausea, cholestasis, abnormal liver function tests, portal tract fibrosis
GU: Hypercalciuria
ENDO: Hyperglycaemia, osteomalacia
INTEG: Phlebitis at injection site
Contraindications: Hypersensitivity, severe electrolyte imbalances, anuria, severe liver disease, errors of amino acid metabolism, acidosis, advanced renal disease (no dialysis available), severe uraemia, hyperhydration, disturbed protein metabolism, cardiac insufficiency
Precautions: Renal disease, pregnancy, children, diabetes mellitus, congestive cardiac failure, liver disease, electrolyte retention,

cardiac disease, drug therapy requiring electrolyte monitoring, energy supply necessary

Interactions/incompatibilities:
Seek specialist advice

Clinical assessment:
• Before therapy commences ensure adequate circulating volume, liver and renal function, absence of acidosis or hypoxaemia and check vitamin B_{12} status
• Monitor plasma electrolytes, circulating volume, blood glucose, acid-base, fluid balance and nutritional status throughout treatment
• Monitor ECG for potassium replacement needs
• Monitor blood urea nitrogen in addition in renal impairment
• Monitor plasma phenylalanine in infants

Treatment of overdose: Reduce rate of infusion or stop

NURSING CONSIDERATIONS

Assess:
• Fluid balance

Administer:
• Via dedicated, tunnelled central venous feeding line for long-term use i.e. Hickman line. Central venous access preferable to avoid phlebitis and extravasation
• TPN in combination with dextrose to promote (protein synthesis) anabolism
• Immediately after the freshly prepared solution has been received from pharmacy, using strict aseptic technique

Perform/provide:
• Urinalysis for glucose 6 hrly
• Blood glucose estimations are more accurate
• Monitor drip rate/infusion rate carefully. The infusion must never be speeded up; pulmonary oedema and hyperglycaemia will result
• Store all solutions according to manufacturer's instructions; slight variations may be necessary according to exact nature of solution

• Change dressing over intravenous site as necessary. Using strict aseptic technique

Evaluate:
• Infusion site for extravasation: inflammation, local oedema, necrosis, pain, hardening or tenderness; the site will need to be changed immediately
• Monitor respiratory function 4 hrly, observing respiratory rate and depth
• Monitor temperature 4 hrly. If infection is suspected the infusion must be discontinued and swabs from the tubing and container sent to the bacteriology laboratory for culture
• Hyperammonaemia: nausea, vomiting, malaise, tremors, anorexia, convulsions
• Therapeutic response: weight gain, resolution of jaundice if patient has hepatic dysfunction, increased serum albumin levels
• Urinary creatinine clearance and nitrogen excretion with 24 hr urine collection twice a week

Teach patient/family:
• Why intravenous nutrition is necessary
• If chills, sweating are experienced they should be reported at once
• If the patient is to be discharged with intravenous nutrition in the community *all* aspects of nutrition must be taught, preferably by a specialist nurse or dietitian

----

aminoglutethimide

Orimeten
Func. class.: Antineoplastic, adrenal steroid inhibitor
Chem. class.: Enzyme inhibitor, glutethimide analogue
Legal class.: POM

Action: Inhibits conversion of

androgens to oestrogens in the peripheral tissues

Uses: Advanced breast cancer in postmenopausal or oophorectomised women, advanced prostate cancer (palliative). Cushing's syndrome due to malignant disease

Dosage and routes:

• *Adult:* By mouth, breast or prostate cancer: initially 250 mg daily increasing at weekly intervals to maximum 250 mg 4 times daily (lower doses may be adequate), in conjunction with a glucocorticoid. Cushing's syndrome due to malignant disease: 250 mg daily increasing gradually to 1 g daily in divided doses

Available forms include: Tablets 250 mg scored

Side effects/adverse reactions:

HAEM: Thombocytopenia, leucopenia, agranulocytosis, pancytopenia

GI: Nausea, vomiting, diarrhoea

INTEG: Rash

RESP: Allergic alveolitis

METAB: Altered thyroid function

CNS: Dizziness, somnolence, lethargy, unsteadiness, fever

Contraindications: Hypersensitivity, pregnancy, lactation, children, porphyria

Pharmacokinetics: Half-life (long term therapy), 7 hr, peak plasma concentration 1−2 hr, metabolised in liver, excreted in urine

Interactions/incompatibilities:

• Aminoglutethimide accelerates metabolism of certain drugs: nicoumalone, warfarin, digitoxin, dexamethasone, theophylline, oral antidiabetics

Clinical assessment:

• Full blood count, platelet count every 2−3 weeks initially

• Prescribe hydrocortisone to replace drug-induced adrenal steroid production

• Response to stress may be impaired

Treatment of overdose: Remove tablets from GI tract. Supportive treatment to maintain fluid and electrolyte balance, IV steroids if needed. Symptoms may recur

NURSING CONSIDERATIONS

Assess:

• Fluid balance if GI symptoms occur

• BP and temperature

Perform/provide:

• Medication by oral route if possible: avoid IM, IV and subcutaneous injections to prevent infection

• Antacid before drug and at bedtime as ordered

• Antiemetic as prescribed before drug to prevent vomiting

• Skin care

• Nutritious diet with iron and vitamin supplements

Evaluate:

• Temperature 4 hrly; may indicate beginning of infection, but only in first few days as early toxicity then settles

• Food preferences

• For side effects; including early toxicity (dizziness, somnolence, lethargy), tumour flare (spinal cord compression, increased bone pain), nausea, vomiting

Teach patient/family:

• That drowsiness, drug fever and morbilliform eruption often settle spontaneously

• To report side effects to nurse or clinician

• That masculinisation can occur but is reversible after discontinuing treatment

aminophylline (theophylline ethylenediamine)

Phyllocontin Continus, Pecram, Amnivent
Func. class.: Bronchodilator
Chem. class.: Xanthine
Legal class.: Injection POM; Tablets P

Action: Relaxes smooth muscle of respiratory system, may have anti-inflammatory action in respiratory system

Uses: Reversible airways obstruction, status asthmaticus. In adults, cardiac asthma and left ventricular or congestive cardiac failure

Dosages and routes:
• *Adult:* By mouth
100−300 mg 3 to 4 times daily − modified-release preparations usually 1 tablet twice daily; slow IV infusion 500 mcg/kg/hr; IV injection 250−500 mg (5 mg/kg) over 20 min
• *Child:* Slow IV injection 5 mg/kg over 20 min. Maintenance IV infusion 6 months−9 yr 1 mg/kg/hr, 10−16 yr 800 mcg/kg/hr
Narrow margin between therapeutic and toxic dose
Available forms include: Tablets 100 mg, modified release 100, 225, 350 mg, Injection IV 25, mg/ml; 10 ml amp. Some modified release are hydrate salt

Side effects/adverse reactions:
CNS: Insomnia, convulsions, headache, stimulation
CV: Palpitations, tachycardia, arrhythmias
GI: Nausea, vomiting, diarrhoea, dyspepsia
Contraindications: Hypersensitivity to xanthines and ethylenediamine. Porphyria. Do not give with ephedrine in children

Precautions: Elderly, congestive heart failure, hepatic disease, cardiac disease, hypokalaemia, smoking, alcohol, viral infections, epilepsy, lactation, fever, keep to same brand of tablet, pregnancy
Pharmacokinetics:
IV: Peak 30 min. Bioavailability of different oral preparations varies greatly
Interactions/incompatibilities:
• Do not mix in syringe with other drugs
• Increased plasma theophylline levels: thiabendazole, ciprofloxacin, enoxacin, erythromycin, norfloxacin, isoniazid, viloxazine, diltiazem, verapamil, disulfiram, interferons, combined oral contraceptives, cimetidine, possibly influenza vaccine
• Reduced plasma theophylline levels: rifampicin, carbamazepine, barbiturates, phenytoin, primidone, aminoglutethimide, sulphinpyrazone, alcohol, smoking
• Increased risk of side effects: β-blockers, lithium, respiratory stimulants, fenoterol, pirbuterol, reproterol, rimiterol, ritodrine, salbutamol, salmeterol, terbutaline, tulobuterol, allopurinol, isoprenaline, halothane, lomustine, glucagon, other xanthines, ephedrine, steroids, diuretics, hypoxia
Clinical assessment:
• Monitor theophylline blood levels (therapeutic level is 10−20 mg/litre); toxicity may occur with small increase above 20 mg/litre
• Monitor serum potassium levels in severe asthma − potentially serious hypokalaemia may result from concomitant treatment with β₂-adrenoceptor stimulants, theophylline and derivatives, corticosteroids, and diuretics, and by hypoxia
• Check whether theophylline was

given recently and if modified release preparation. Measure theophylline plasma concentrations before instituting aminophylline therapy if patient has been taking oral theophylline preparations

• Once patient is stabilised on one modified-release product, do not change to another preparation without retitration and clinical assessment

Treatment of overdose: *Oral*: empty stomach. Monitor ECG, maintain fluid balance. Administer oral activated charcoal. In severe poisoning use charcoal-column haemoperfusion. Symptomatic treatment. NB: modified-release preparations will release aminophylline for several hours. If hypokalaemia, give potassium chloride by mouth or slow IV infusion. Monitor plasma potassium. Control convulsions by IV diazepam or if necessary thiopentone sodium

NURSING CONSIDERATIONS
Administer:
• Do not mix in syringe with other drugs
• Oral preparations after meals to decrease gastrointestinal symptoms; absorption may be affected
• Modified-release tablets should be swallowed whole and not chewed

Evaluate:
• Cardiac rhythm and rate during IV infusion
• Fluid balance: if diuresis occurs, dehydration may result in elderly or children
• Response to treatment; decreased dyspnoea, respiratory rate, depth
• Allergic reactions e.g. rash, urticaria and inform clinician, who may discontinue drug

Teach patient/family:

• To avoid medicines that have not been prescribed; those containing ephedrine will increase CNS stimulation
• To avoid driving and operating machinery; dizziness may occur
• To be aware of possible side effects and to know when to contact clinician
• If gastrointestinal upset occurs to take dose with about 200 ml of water, and avoid food since absorption may be decreased

---

amiodarone HCl

Cordarone X
Func. class.: Anti-arrhythmic (Class III)
Chem. class.: Iodinated benzofuran derivative
Legal class.: POM

Action: Delays repolarisation by prolonging action potential and refractory period

Uses: Wolff-Parkinson-White syndrome. Atrial flutter and fibrillation, supraventicular and ventricular tachycardias and recurrent ventricular fibrillation when other drugs ineffective or contraindicated

Dosage and routes:
• *Adult:* By mouth initially 200 mg 3 times daily for 1 week then twice daily for 1 week then 200 mg daily for maintenance
• Initiate under hospital or specialist supervision
• IV infusion via central venous catheter up to 5 mg/kg over 20−120 min under ECG, maximum 1.2 g in 24 hr

Available forms include: Tablets scored 100, 200 mg; Injection 50 mg/ml, 3 ml amp for dilution

Side effects/adverse reactions:
CNS: Headache, benign raised

intracranial pressure, nightmares, vertigo, sleeplessness, peripheral neuropathy, myopathy
GI: Hepatotoxicity
CV: Bradycardia, sinus arrest, anaphylaxis on rapid injection
INTEG: Rash, photosensitivity
EENT: Microdeposits in cornea
ENDO: Hyperthyroidism or hypothyroidism
RESP: Pulmonary fibrosis, dyspnoea, pulmonary alveolitis
Contraindications: Evidence or history of thyroid dysfunction, sinus bradycardia, atrio-ventricular block (unless pacemaker fitted) sino-atrial heartblock, IV contraindicated in severe respiratory failure, circulatory collapse or severe arterial hypotension, congestive heart failure, iodine sensitivity, lactation, pregnancy, porphyria
Precautions: Sinus node dysfunction, severe conduction disturbances, heart failure, elderly, renal impairment
Too high dose may produce severe bradycardia and conduction disturbances
Pharmacokinetics:
By mouth: Onset 1−3 weeks, peak 2−10 hr; half-life 53 days; much interpatient variation; metabolised by liver, strongly protein-bound
IV: onset 1−30 min, duration 1−3 hr
Interactions/incompatibilities:
• Increased effect of: disopyramide, flecainide, procainamide, quinidine and other anti-arrhythmics, nicoumalone, warfarin, phenytoin
• Increased risk of side effects: B-blockers, diltiazem, verapamil, digoxin, cimetidine, general anaesthesia
• Toxicity increased if hypokalaemia with acetazolamide, loop diuretics, thiazides

Clinical assessment:
• Obtain blood for potassium, sodium and chloride estimations.
• Perform liver function tests; aspartate aminotransferase, alanine aminotransferase, bilirubin and alkaline phosphatase
• Monitor for hypovolaemia
• Reduce dose slowly with ECG monitoring
• During long-term therapy— monitor eyes, thyroid function, liver function
• Inform anaesthetist about amiodarone therapy, when appropriate
Lab. test interferences: Some thyroid function tests
Treatment of overdose: Gastric lavage and general supportive measures. Monitor patient and give β-adrenoceptor stimulants or glucagon if bradycardia. Prolonged surveillance
NURSING CONSIDERATIONS
Administer:
• Infusion should be diluted as directed in 5% glucose solution. Amiodarone infusion may reduce drop size and, if appropriate, make adjustments to rate of infusion. At the discretion of the clinician, slow IV injection can be administered in extreme clinical emergency
Perform/provide:
• Patient will require continuous cardiac monitoring during IV therapy to determine drug effectiveness, check for premature ventricular contraction, other dysrhythmias
Evaluate:
• For rebound hypertension after 1−2 hr
• Changes in BP, bradycardia
• Hypothyroidism e.g. lethargy, dizziness, constipation, enlarged thyroid, oedema of extremities, cool, dry skin
• Hyperthyroidism: restlessness,

tachycardia, eyelid puffiness, weight loss, frequency of urine, menstrual irregularities, dyspnoea, warm, moist skin
• For dyspnoea, fatigue, cough, fever, chest pain may indicate pneumonitis
Teach patient/family:
• All aspects of drug therapy, side effects and when to report to clinician
• To report side effects immediately
• To protect the skin against ultra violet and visible light by using total sunblock
• That skin discolouration is reversible
• That dark glasses may be needed for photophobia and that drivers may be dazzled by headlights at night (micro-deposits in eyes)
• That metallic taste may be noted

amitriptyline HCl

Tryptizol, Lentizol, Domical, Elavil
Func. class.: Antidepressant, tricyclic
Chem. class.: Tertiary amine
Legal class.: POM

Action: Blocks reuptake of nor-adrenaline, serotonin into nerve endings, increasing action of nor-adrenaline, serotonin on nerve cells. Mode of action in depression not known
Uses: Depression, nocturnal enuresis in children
Dosage and routes:
Depression:
• *Adult:* By mouth initially 50–75 mg daily increasing as required to maximum 200 mg daily, IM/IV 10–20 mg 4 times daily
• *Adolescent/geriatric:* By mouth initially 25–50 mg daily

• Not recommended for treatment of *depression* in children under 16 yr
Nocturnal enuresis:
• *Child:* 7–10 yr: 10–20 mg at night, 11–16 yr: 25–50 mg at night. Maximum duration 3 months
Available forms include: Tablets 10, 25, 50 mg, capsules modified release 25, 50, 75 mg, mixture 10 mg (as embonate)/5 ml; injection 10 mg/ml (10 ml vial)
Side effects/adverse reactions:
HAEM: Agranulocytosis, thrombocytopenia, eosinophilia, leucopenia, purpura
CNS: Convulsions, confusion, sedation, tremors, hypomania, behavioural disturbances (especially children)
GI: Dry mouth, nausea, black tongue, paralytic ileus, increased appetite, jaundice, constipation, weight gain (occasionally loss)
GU: Difficulty with micturition, interference with sexual function
INTEG: Rash, sweating
CV: Orthostatic hypotension, tachycardia, arrhythmias, syncope
EENT: Blurred vision
METAB: Blood sugar changes
Contraindications: Hypersensitivity to tricyclic antidepressants, lactation, arrhythmias, coronary artery insufficiency, recovery phase of myocardial infarction, heart block, severe liver disease, children less than 6 yr, co-administration with MAOIs, mania, porphyria
Precautions: Suicidal patients, convulsive disorders, prostatic hypertrophy, schizophrenia, elderly, diabetes mellitus, psychoses, severe depression, manic depression, anaesthesia, increased intraocular pressure, narrow-angle glaucoma, urinary retention, hepatic disease, hyperthyroidism, thyroid medication or

anticholinergic agents, electro-shock therapy, elective surgery, pregnancy, cardiovascular disorders. Avoid abrupt cessation

Pharmacokinetics:

By mouth/IM: Onset 45 min, peak 2−12 hr, therapeutic response 2−4 weeks; metabolised by liver, excreted in urine/faeces, excreted in breast milk, half-life 10−50 hr

Interactions/incompatibilities:

• Enhanced effect: Alcohol, anaesthetics, MAOIs (stop for at least 2 weeks before starting tricyclics), fluoxetine, antiepileptics, antihistamines

• Increased side effects: Antimuscarinics, phenothiazines, anxiolytics, hypnotics, diltiazem, verapamil, disulfiram, diuretics, oral contraceptives, adrenaline noradrenaline, ephedrine, isoprenaline, phenylephrine, phenyl-propanolamine, methylphenidate

• Reduced effect of: sublingual nitrates

• Amitriptyline increases response to alcohol, barbiturates and other CNS depressants

• Reduced antidepressant effect: barbiturates

Clinical assessment:

• Perform full blood count, differential white blood count, cardiac enzymes if patient is receiving treatment long-term

• Liver function tests; aspartate aminotransferase, alanine aminotransferase, bilirubin, creatinine

• Perform ECG for flattening of T wave, bundle branch block, atrioventricular block, dysrhythmias in cardiac patients

Treatment of overdose:

Symptomatic and supportive treatment. Emesis, gastric lavage, activated charcoal. ECG, close cardiac monitoring for at least 5 days. Maintain open airway, fluid intake. Regulate body temperature. IV physostigmine salicylate if clinic-ally indicated (not for routine use). Administer anticonvulsant (non-barbiturate). Dialysis of no value. Manage circulatory shock and metabolic acidosis

NURSING CONSIDERATIONS

Assess:

• Baseline BP (lying, standing) and pulse

• Weight

Administer:

• At bedtime if over-sedation occurs during day; entire dose may be taken at bedtime; elderly may not be able to tolerate dosage once daily

• Increase fluid and fibre in diet if constipated. Urinary retention may occur, especially in children

• Give with food or milk for GI symptoms

Perform/provide:

• Mouth care and frequent sips of water for dry mouth

• Help when patient takes exercise at beginning of therapy since drowsiness/dizziness occurs

• Checking to ensure that oral medication is swallowed

Evaluate:

• BP (lying, standing), pulse 4 hrly; if systolic BP falls 20 mmHg withhold drug and inform clinician; take vital signs in all patients with cardiovascular disease

• Weight weekly; appetite may increase with drug

• Extrapyramidal symptoms in elderly e.g. rigidity, dystonia, akathisia

• Mental status: mood, clarity of thought/mental alertness, affect, increase in psychiatric symptoms e.g. depression, panic

• Withdrawal symptoms: headache, nausea, vomiting, muscle pain, weakness; do not usually occur unless drug is discontinued abruptly

• Alcohol consumption: if alcohol

is consumed inform clinician and withhold dose until morning

Teach patient/family:
• Therapeutic effects may take 2−3 weeks
• Caution when driving or operating machinery because of drowsiness, dizziness, blurred vision
• To avoid alcohol, other CNS depressants
• Not to discontinue medication suddenly after long term use; may cause nausea, headache, vomiting
• To avoid strong sunshine
• Careful supervision for risk of suicide

---

amlodipine besylate

Istin

Func. class.: Antihypertensive, anti-anginal
Chem. class.: Dihydropyridine
Legal class.: POM

Action: Calcium slow channel blocker; relaxes vascular smooth muscle; reduces total ischaemic burden

Uses: Hypertension, prophylaxis of angina

Dosage and routes:
• *Adult and elderly:* Hypertension and angina
By mouth: Initially 5 mg daily up to a maximum of 10 mg daily
• *Children:* Not recommended in patients less than 18 yr
Available forms include: Tablets 5, 10 mg

Side effects/adverse reactions:
GI: Nausea
CNS: Headache, fatigue, dizziness
INTEG: Flushing
CV: Oedema

Contraindications: Hypersensitivity to dihydropyridines such as nifedipine, nicardipine, and isradipine. Pregnancy, lactation, or women of childbearing potential unless effective contraception is used

Precautions: Hepatic insufficiency

Pharmacokinetics:
By mouth: Half-life 35−50 hr, peak 6−12 hr. Excreted mainly as inactive metabolites in urine. Highly plasma protein bound

Treatment of overdose: Gastric lavage. Treat symptomatically for excessive peripheral vasodilation, systemic hypotension. Monitor cardiac and respiratory function, elevate extremities, monitor circulating fluid volume and urine output. If no contraindication, vasoconstrictor may be useful. Not dialysable

NURSING CONSIDERATIONS

Assess:
• Baseline BP
Administer:
• With or without food
Evaluate:
• Therapeutic response: decreased anginal pain
• If used as antihypertensive, record BP regularly. Note: full effect may not be seen for 10−14 days
Teach patient/family:
• To report immediately if pregnancy is suspected
• To report headaches, dizziness, parasthesia
• To avoid hazardous activities until stabilised on drug or dizziness no longer a problem

---

amoxycillin

Amoxil, Almodan
Func. class.: Broad spectrum antibiotic
Chem. class.: Aminohydroxy penicillin
Legal class.: POM

Action: Interferes with cell wall replication of susceptible organisms; the cell wall, rendered osmotically unstable, swells, and bursts from osmotic pressure. Bactericidal

Uses: Include: urinary-tract infections, otitis media, chronic bronchitis, invasive salmonellosis, gonorrhoea, typhoid fever, dental prophylaxis, septicaemia

Dosage and routes:
• *Adult:* By mouth, 250 mg every 8 hr, doubled in severe infections
• *Child up to 10 yr:* 125 mg every 8 hr, doubled in severe infections
Severe or recurrent purulent respiratory infection
• *Adult:* 3 g every 12 hr
• *Child 2−5 yr:* 750 mg every 12 hr, 5−10 yr 1.5 g every 12 hr
Short-course oral therapy
• Dental abscess 3 g repeated after 8 hr
• Urinary tract infection 3 g repeated after 10−12 hr
• Gonorrhoea single dose of 3 g with probenecid 1 g
• Otitis media: *Child 3−10 yr:* 750 mg twice daily for 2 days
Parenteral administration
• *Adult:* IM. 500 mg every 8 hr *Child:* 50−100 mg/kg daily in divided doses
• IV injection or infusion
• *Adult:* 500 mg every 8 hr increased to 1 g every 6 hr *Child:* 50−100 mg/kg daily in divided doses

Available forms include: Capsules 250, 500 mg; powder for oral suspension, 125, 250 mg/5 ml; injection 250, 500 mg, 1 g vial for reconstitution. Dispersible sugar-free tablets 500 mg. Powder for sugar-free syrup 125, 250 mg/5 ml. Powder for paediatric suspension 125 mg/1.25 ml. Sugar-free sachets 750 mg, 3 g. Injection is sodium salt, oral preparations as trihydrate

Side effects/adverse reactions:
GI: Nausea, diarrhoea, indigestion

INTEG: Rashes (discontinue treatment)
MISC: Angioedema, anaphylaxis
Contraindications: Hypersensitivity to penicillins
Precautions: Hypersensitivity to cephalosporins. History of allergy, glandular fever, lactation, renal impairment, chronic lymphatic leukaemia, HIV-infection

Interactions/incompatibilities:
• Do not mix with blood products, protein hydrolysates, IV lipid emulsions, or aminoglycosides in same syringe
• Enhances effect of: warfarin, phenindione, probenecid
• Risk of reduced contraceptive effect: combined oral contraceptives

Pharmacokinetics:
By mouth: Peak 1−2 hr, duration 6−8 hr; half-life 1−1⅓ hr, metabolised in liver, excreted in urine, enters breast milk

Clinical assessment:
• Injection contains sodium which may restrict use if salt restricted or problems with fluid balance
Treatment of overdose: Maintain adequate fluid intake and urinary output−crystalluria possible. Removed by haemodialysis

NURSING CONSIDERATIONS
Assess:
• Obtain specimen for bacteriology laboratory for culture and sensitivity testing before treatment commences and after course is completed
• Ask patient about allergies before treatment commences and record on drug chart
Perform/provide:
• Adequate fluid intake (2 litres daily) if diarrhoea occurs
Evaluate:
• Therapeutic response
• Temperature 4 hrly; observe condition of discharging wounds

• Bowel pattern before and during treatment
• Skin rashes (often related to penicillin allergy)
• Respiratory rate, character, wheezing, tightness in chest
• Observe patient with known renal impairment carefully; toxicity may develop rapidly
Teach patient/family:
• To take oral amoxycillin with a full glass of water
• All aspects of drug therapy: the entire course must be completed unless advised otherwise by clinician
• That medication must be taken regularly to maintain blood levels
• To wear Medic Alert Identity if allergic to penicillins
• To report any diarrhoea to nurse or clinician

---

amphotericin (oral)

Fungilin
Func. class.: Antifungal
Chem. class.: Amphoteric polyene macrolide
Legal class.: POM

Action: Increases cell membrane permeability in susceptible organisms by binding sterols; decreases potassium, sodium and nutrients in cell
Uses: Intestinal candidosis, oral and perioral fungal infections, suppression of intestinal reservoir of *C. albicans*
Dosage and routes:
Intestinal candidosis
• *Adult:* By mouth, 100–200 mg every 6 hr
Oral and perioral infections
• *Adult:* Lozenges, dissolve one lozenge slowly in mouth 4 times daily. If infection is severe increase to 8 daily. May require 10–15 days
• *Adult, infant, child*: Suspension, place 1 ml in mouth after food and retain near lesions 4 times daily for 14 days
For further child doses seek advice from clinician/pharmacist
Available forms include: Tablets 100 mg; suspension 100 mg/ml; lozenges 10 mg
Side effects/adverse reactions: Few reported side effects when given orally, gastrointestinal upsets after long courses at high dose
Contraindications: No known contraindications
Precautions: No special precautions apply
Pharmacokinetics: Negligible absorption from GI tract
Interactions/incompatibilities:
• Decreased effect of: miconazole
Treatment of overdose: No systemic toxicity from oral overdose
NURSING CONSIDERATIONS
Evaluate:
• Therapeutic response
• Decreasing urinary output, concentrated urine and inform clinician immediately
Teach patient/family:
• That drug may need to be taken for 2 weeks to 3 months to clear infection

---

amphotericin intravenous

Fungizone, AmBisome ▼
Func. class.: Antifungal
Chem. class.: Amphoteric polyene macrolide
Legal class.: POM

Action: Increases cell membrane permeability in susceptible organisms by binding sterols; decreases potassium, sodium and nutrients in cell
Uses: Progressive, potentially fatal systemic fungal infections
Dosage and routes:
• By slow intravenous infusion

over at least 6 hr, 250 mcg/kg daily, gradually increased if tolerated to 1 mg/kg daily; maximum (severe infection) 1.5 mg/kg daily or on alternate days. *Note* Prolonged treatment usually necessary; if interrupted for longer than 7 days recommence at 250 mcg/kg daily and increase gradually

• Liposomal amphotericin by IV infusion, where toxicity precludes use of conventional amphotericin, initially 1 mg/kg daily as a single dose increased gradually if necessary to 3 mg/kg daily as a single dose

Available forms include:

Fungizone: Powder for reconstitution 50 mg as sodium deoxycholate complex

AmBisome: Powder for reconstitution 50 mg encapsulated in liposomes

Side effects/adverse reactions:

EENT: Tinnitus, deafness, diplopia, blurred vision, transient vertigo

INTEG: Flushing, phlebitis, skin rash

CNS: Headache, fever, chills, peripheral neuropathy, convulsions, malaise

CV: Cardiovascular toxicity

GU: Hypokalaemia, permanent renal impairment, anuria, oliguria, abnormal renal function

GI: Nausea, vomiting, anorexia, diarrhoea, cramps, abnormal liver function (discontinue), dyspepsia, weight loss, gastroenteritis, acute liver failure

MS: Arthralgia, myalgia, generalised pain, weakness

HAEM: Normochromic, normocytic anaemia, thrombophlebitis, blood disorders, coagulation problems

SYST: Anaphylaxis

Contraindications: Hypersensitivity

Precautions: Renal disease, close supervision necessary, pregnancy, abnormal liver function, other drug therapy, frequent change of injection site

Pharmacokinetics:

IV: Peak 1–2 hr, initial half-life 24 hr, excreted very slowly in urine, highly bound to plasma proteins

Interactions/incompatibilities:

• Increased nephrotoxicity: other nephrotoxic drugs e.g. aminoglycosides, cisplatin, vancomycin, cyclosporin, polymyxin B, cephalothin, cytotoxic drugs

• Increased hypokalaemia following amphotericin therapy potentiates toxicity and/or actions of: cardiac glycosides, skeletal muscle relaxants

• Amphotericin-induced potassium loss increased by corticosteroids

• Do not give other drugs in same infusion or same cannula

• Antagonism: miconazole

• Do not mix in sodium solutions or diluent with preservatives

• Dextrose of pH below 4.2

Clinical assessment:

• Perform full blood count, potassium, sodium, calcium and magnesium levels weekly

• Drug is nephrotoxic: monitor blood urea nitrogen, serum creatinine for renal toxicity

• Commence treatment only after culture and sensitivity tests are positive for the infection suspected; drug should be used only for life-threatening conditions

• Symptomatic treatment for adverse reactions

• Perform liver function tests; discontinue therapy if increasing bromsulphalein, alkaline phosphatase and bilirubin levels indicate hepatotoxicity

NURSING CONSIDERATIONS

Assess:

• Baseline vital signs, fluid balance and weight

Administer:
• Administer after diluting with 10 ml sterile water, then dilute with 500 ml of 0.5% glucose solution to concentration of 0.1 mg/ml
• Aseptic technique for handling — no preservative
• Do not reconstitute with sodium chloride solutions. Use only recommended diluent
• Do not use initial concentrate or infusion solution if there is any evidence of precipitation
• Check IV site 8 hrly for signs of inflammation

Perform/protect:
• Protect from light during infusion
• Store away from moisture and light; diluted solution is stable for 24 hr

Evaluate:
• Vital signs every 15−30 min during first infusion
• Fluid balance chart; be alert for decreasing urinary output, concentrated urine and inform clinician immediately
• Weight weekly. Inform clinician if weight increases by more than 1 kg in a week or if there is evidence of oedema
• Patient's condition; temperature, malaise, rash
• Allergic reaction and report to clinician, who may discontinue drug or order antihistamines (mild reaction) or adrenaline (severe reaction), pethidine for rigors
• Anorexia, drowsiness, weakness, decreased reflexes, increased urinary output, thirst, paraesthesiae (signs of hypokalaemia)
• Hearing impairment and vestibular dysfunction e.g. tinnitus, vertigo, hearing loss (rare)

Teach patient/family:
• That drug may need to be taken for 2 weeks to 3 months to clear infection
• To recognise side effects and report them to clinician immediately

---

ampicillin/ampicillin sodium/ampicillin trihydrate

Amfipen,   Penbritin,   Vidopen, Rimacillin
Func. class.: Broad spectrum antibiotic
Chem. class.: Aminopenicillin
Legal class.: POM

Action: Interferes with cell wall replication of susceptible organisms; the cell wall, rendered osmotically unstable, swells, bursts from osmotic pressure. Bactericidal

Uses: Include the following infections: ear, nose, throat, urinary tract, gastrointestinal, gynaecological, bronchitis, pneumonia, peritonitis, gonorrhoea, septicaemia, endocarditis, enteric fever, meningitis

Dosage and routes:
Systemic infections
• *Adult:* By mouth 250 mg−1 g 6 hrly 30 min before food, IM/IV 500 mg 4−6 hrly
• *Child:* under 10 yr: half adult dose
Meningitis
• *Adult:* IV 2 g 6-hrly
• *Child:* IV 150 mg/kg/day in divided doses
Gonorrhoea
• *Adult:* By mouth 2 g given with 1 g probenecid as a single dose
Also used intraperitoneal, intrapleural, intra-articular, extraperitoneal in conjunction with systemic therapy

Available forms include: Powder for preparing injection IV, IM 250, 500 mg; capsules 250, 500 mg; powder for oral syrup or suspension 125, 250 mg/5 ml; paediatric suspension 125 mg/1.25 ml. Contain ampicillin base, sodium or trihydrate salt depending on preparation

Side effects/adverse reactions:

GI: Nausea, diarrhoea

INTEG: Rashes (discontinue treatment)

Contraindications: Hypersensitivity to penicillins

Precautions: Lactation; hypersensitivity to cephalosporins; history of allergy, renal impairment, erythematous rashes common in glandular fever, chronic lymphatic leukaemia, HIV-infection

Pharmacokinetic:

By mouth: Peak 1−2 hr

IV: Peak 5 min

IM: Peak 1 hr

Half-life 50−110 min; metabolised in liver, excreted in urine, bile, faeces, breast milk, food can interfere with absorption

Interactions/incompatibilities:

• Enhances effect of: phenindione, warfarin, oral contraceptives

• Allopurinol increases risk of skin reactions

• Increased penicillin concentrations when used with: aspirin, probenicid

• Do not mix with blood products, proteinaceous fluids or lipid emulsions

• Do not mix with aminoglycosides in syringe, IV fluid or giving set

Clinical Assessment:

• Test for renal impairment if problem suspected

Treatment of overdose: Problems unlikely. Treat symptomatically

NURSING CONSIDERATIONS

Assess:

• Obtain specimen for bacteriology laboratory for culture and sensitivity testing before treatment commences and after course is completed. Consider resistance

• Any known allergies and record on care plan/nursing notes

Administer:

• Before food (action decreased by the presence of food in the gut)

• With full glass of water

Perform/provide:

• Adequate fluid intake (2 litres daily) if diarrhoea occurs

Evaluate:

• Observe patients with known renal impairment carefully; toxicity may develop rapidly

• Temperature 4 hrly

• Therapeutic response

• Bowel pattern before and during treatment

• Skin rashes (drug may be discontinued)

Teach patient/family:

• To take oral ampicillin on empty stomach with a full glass of water

• All aspects of drug therapy: the entire course must be completed unless advised otherwise by clinician

• To report any side effects

• Drug must be taken regularly to maintain blood levels

• To wear Medic Alert Identity if allergic to penicillins

• To report any diarrhoea to nurse or clinician

---

amsacrine

Amsidine

Func. class.: Antineoplastic agent

Chem. class.: Acridine derivative

Legal class.: POM

Action: Inhibits DNA synthesis and may modify cell membrane function; active throughout entire cell cycle

Uses: Second-line treatment in refractory acute myeloid leukaemia

Dosage and routes:

• Seek clinician's advice. Reduce

dose in impaired liver or renal function

Available forms include: Injection 50 mg/ml plus diluent to prepare concentrated solution of 5 mg/ml (as lactate) (must be diluted in 500 ml dextrose 5% before administration)

Side effects/adverse reactions:

HAEM: Leucopenia, pancytopenia, haemorrhage, infections, myelosuppression

GI: Nausea, vomiting, stomatitis, oesophagitis

CNS: Seizures

SYST: Abnormal liver function tests, jaundice

GU: Haematuria, anuria

CARDIAC: Ventricular tachycardia, congestive heart failure, cardiac arrest

INTEG: Local tissue irritation, necrosis, phlebitis, alopecia

Contraindications: Pre-existing bone marrow suppression induced by chemotherapy or radiotherapy, children under 12 yr

Precautions: Pregnancy, wear polythene gloves while handling (irritant to skin), use glass syringes, renal or hepatic impairment

Pharmacokinetics:
Half-life 7 hr; metabolised in liver and excreted as metabolites in bile

Interactions/incompatibilities:
• Incompatible with sodium chloride solutions and plastic (use glass ' syringes) protect from sunlight
• Increased risk of cardiotoxicity: diuretics, aminoglycosides and other nephrotoxic drugs, previous anthracycline therapy

Clinical assessment:
• Monitor CNS, cardiac, liver, kidney, bone marrow functions
• Ensure that potassium serum is normal.
• Perform frequent full blood counts
• Perform ECG

• Monitor urea, electrolytes, creatinine clearance
• Evaluate effects on condition

Treatment of overdose: Supportive treatments; monitor blood picture closely. If necessary administer appropriate blood products

NURSING CONSIDERATIONS

Assess:
• Temperature 4 hrly for infection, vital signs 4 hrly for arrhythmias. Fluid balance — report less than 30−60 ml urine/hr

Administer:
• In accordance with local policies for cytotoxics
• After reconstitution using manufacturer's instructions: wear polyethene gloves, use glass equipment and dilute in 500 ml 5% dextrose
• To be handled by trained staff (non-pregnant) in a designated area, wearing gloves and eye protection
• Handle with great care: causes irritation of skin and tissues leading to necrosis
• Accidents: staff should be aware of first aid measures e.g. wash skin with soap and water
• Correct disposal of equipment/ excess solution as per manufacturer's instructions
• Slow IV injection (60−90 min) using correct gauge needle

Evaluate:
• IV site for leakage, pain and phlebitis
• For infection/inflammation; neutropenia (temperature, pulse, respiration 4 hrly)
• Fluid balance, BP and daily weight
• Mouth 8 hrly for infection
• Bleeding/bruising 8 hrly for thrombocytopenia
• Fits
• Jaundice, itchy, dark urine, light stools
• Haematuria and anuria

- Oedema, pain and dysphagia
- Effects of alopecia

Perform/provide:
- Analgesia, antiemetics, antibiotics, sedatives, antiuric acid drugs and transfusions as prescribed
- Storage out of sunlight, stable for 8 hr at room temperature
- Asepsis/isolation as appropriate
- Mouth care—fizzy mouth wash, gentle teeth cleaning and oral toilet; observe for mucositis
- Warm compresses for injection (IV) site
- Support/counselling—changes in body image

Teach patient/family:
- Need for isolation and high standard of hygiene
- Effects of drug
- That hair may be lost during treatment and wig or hairpiece may make patient feel better (available free on NHS); tell patient that new hair may be different in colour, texture
- Importance of mouth examination and reporting any effects e.g. bleeding, mouth ulcers
- Avoid food/drink that may irritate mouth

amylobarbitone/ sodium

Amytal, Sodium Amytal, combination product
Func. class.: Sedative/hypnotic (intermediate acting)
Chem. class.: Barbiturate
Legal class.: CD (Sch 3) POM

Action: Depresses activity in brain cells primarily in reticular activating system in brainstem, also selectively depresses neurons in posterior hypothalamus, limbic structures; able to decrease seizure activity by inhibition of epileptic activity in CNS

Uses: Severe intractable insomnia in patients already taking barbiturates; parenteral, status epilepticus

Dosage and routes:
- *Adult:* By mouth
Amylobarbitone 100−200 mg at bedtime,
Amylobarbitone sodium 60−200 mg at bedtime
Status epilepticus
- By IM injection (maximum 5 ml at any one site) 0.25−1 g (maximum 500 mg)
- By IV infusion (maximum 50 mg/min) 0.25−1 g (maximum 1 g)

Available forms include: Amylobarbitone tablets 50 mg, Amylobarbitone sodium capsules 60, 200 mg, injection 500 mg

Sides effects/adverse reactions:
CNS: Lethargy, drowsiness, hangover, dizziness, paradoxical excitement, confusion, pain, sedation, memory defects, vertigo, headache, ataxia
GI: Nausea, vomiting
INTEG: Hypersensitivity skin reactions, skin eruptions
CV: Circulatory collapse
RESP: Depression, apnoea

Contraindications: Hypersensitivity to barbiturates, respiratory disease, uncontrolled pain, pregnancy lactation, liver impairment, porphyria, children, young adults, drug/alcohol abusers, elderly, debilitated

Precautions: Labour, depression, suicidal tendencies, hepatic disease, renal disease, shock, respiratory depression. Withdraw gradually after long use, addiction potential, cumulative effect, borderline hypoadrenal function

Pharmacokinetics:
By mouth: Onset 30−60 min, duration 6−8 hr
Metabolised by liver, excreted mainly in urine, some in faeces

and breast milk highly protein bound, half-life 20−25 hr

Interactions/incompatibilities:
• Increased CNS depression: alcohol, monoamine oxidase inhibitors, sedatives, narcotics, CNS depressants, antiepileptics, tranquillisers
• Increased metabolism of: tricyclic antidepressants, clonazepam, disopyramide, quinidine
• Decreased effect of: oral anticoagulants, corticosteroids, griseofulvin, phenytoin, digitoxin, cyclosporin, theophylline, thyroxine, oral contraceptives, rifampicin, gestrinone, tibolone, chloramphenicol doxycycline, metronidazole, chlorpromazine, isradipine, nicardipine, nifedipine
• Antagonism of anticonvulsant effect: antidepressants, antipsychotics
• Enhanced effects, reductions in plasma concentrations possible − antiepileptics or enhanced toxicity

Clinical assessment:
• Measure amylobarbitone plasma levels if on repeated IV/IM doses

Treatment of overdose: Symptomatic and supportive. Gastric lavage, monitor vital signs. IV fluids. Maintain BP, body temperature, adequate respiratory exchange. Haemodialysis.

NURSING CONSIDERATIONS
Assess:
• Vital signs every 30 minutes for 2 hours after intravenous injection
• Barbiturate or other dependency

Administer:
• If intramuscular injection is inavoidable inject deeply into a large muscle to prevent tissue necrosis and abscesses
• Only after all other measures for insomnia have proven ineffective
• After mixing with sterile water for injection. The drug must be used within 30 minutes of preparation

• Administer intravenously at 50 mg/min. The drug should be given only by someone who has received full training in the use of intravenous additives and only with emergency equipment available
• 30 minutes to an hour before bedtime if used to treat insomnia
• Give on an empty stomach to enhance absorption for oral doses

Perform/provide:
• Supervision to mobile patients once the drug is given
• Necessary safety precautions e.g. cotsides. Ensure that the patient has a nightlight and knows how to summon the nurse quickly
• With resuscitative equipment available

Evaluate:
• Therapeutic response; ability to sleep throughout the night without early morning wakening
• Mental status: mood, whether oriented in time and place, memory (long and short term)
• Habituation to dependency on drug: increasingly frequent requests for medication, shaking, anxiety
• Barbiturate toxicity hypotension, bronchospasm, cold clammy skin, cyanosis of the lips, insomnia, nausea, vomiting, hallucinations, delirium, weakness. Mild symptoms may occur/persist 10−12 hours after receiving the drug .
• Respiratory: respiratory depression, rate, depth and rhythm. Withhold drug if respirations are less than 1 per minute or if pupils are dilated
• Blood dyscrasias: pyrexia, sore throat, bruising, rashes, jaundice, epistaxis

Teach patient/family:
All points for treatment of insomnia:
• Hangover is to be expected

• Use of the drug is permitted only for short term treatment of insomnia that it will probably become ineffective after 2 weeks
• Drug dependency may result if used for extended periods (45−90 days depending on dose)
• To avoid driving, handling machinery etc
• To avoid alcohol or other CNS depressants: severe depression of the CNS may otherwise occur
• Not to stop taking the drug abruptly after long term use; dose should be reduced gradually over a period of 1−2 weeks
• To inform G.P. that a barbiturate has been prescribed
• That insomnia may recur after short-term use, but further doses are not indicated, as this will improve within 1−3 nights
• Benefits may not be noted until 2 nights after commencing drug
• Other additional measures to combat insomnia (reading, exercise, warm bath, hot milk, drinks, television, deep breathing exercises)
• Self hypnosis as a form of meditation
• That drug must be kept well out of children's reach

ancrod

Arvin

Func. class.: Anticoagulant
Chem. class.: Enzymatic principle, derived from the venom of the Malayan pit viper
Legal class.: POM ('named-patient' basis)

Action: Reduces plasma fibrinogen by cleavage of fibrin; reduces blood viscosity but has no effect on established thrombi

Uses: Deep-vein thrombosis, prevention of postoperative thrombosis ('named-patient' basis only)

Dosage and routes:
• *Adult: IV infusion:* 2−3 units/kg in 50−500 ml sodium chloride 0.9% over 4−12 hr (usually 6−8 hr) then by infusion or slow IV injection, 2 units/kg every 12 hr, initial infusion *must* be given slowly
• *Adult: SC injection*, for prophylaxis of deep-vein thrombosis, 280 units immediately after surgery, then 70 units daily for 4 days (fractured femur) or 8 days (hip replacement)

Available forms include: Injection, 70 units/ml 1 ml amp (available only on 'named-patient' basis)

Sides effects/adverse reactions:
• Drugs for anaphylaxis and antidote should be available. Alternatively reconstituted freeze-dried fibrinogen or 1 litre fresh frozen plasma
HAEM/CV: Haemorrhage, thrombocytopenia (stop treatment if thrombocytopenia), massive intravascular formation of unstable fibrin if drug not given slowly
INTEG: Alopecia, hypersensitivity reactions
MS: Osteoporosis if use is prolonged
SYST: Hypersensitivity reactions
Contraindications: Haemophilia and other bleeding disorders, peptic ulcer, cerebral aneurysm, severe hypertension, liver disease, recent surgery of eye or nervous system, coronary thrombosis, severe infection, disseminated intravascular coagulation, pregnancy, lactation, hypersensitivity, septicaemia
Precautions: Renal colic, cardiovascular disease, uraemia, resistance may develop, stroke

Pharmacokinetics: Duration 12–24 hours. May be necessary to give antidote — see Treatment of overdose

Interactions/incompatibilities:
• Avoid administration with dextrans, aminocaproic acid

Clinical assessment:
• Clotting function, aim for 2–3 mm clot after 2 hr standing or directly measure plasma fibrinogen concentrations
• Plasma fibrinogen, full blood count, prior to therapy. Platelet count also if treatment longer than 5 days

Treatment of overdose: Antidote (ancrod antivenom), reconstituted freeze-dried fibrinogen or fresh frozen plasma. For anaphylaxis adrenaline, antihistamines, corticosteroids

NURSING CONSIDERATIONS

Assess:
• Vital signs, fluid balance

Administer:
• After diluting in 50–500 ml sodium chloride
• Slowly (induction dose over at least 4 hr) and maintenance 10–50 ml/5 min

Perform/provide:
• Refrigerated storage at 4–8°C; do not freeze
• Emergency equipment in case of anaphylaxis

Evaluate:
• Observe for bleeding

Teach patient/family:
• To report any signs of haemorrhage immediately

---

anistreplase (APSAC)

Eminase

Func. class.: Thrombolytic enzyme
Chem. class.: Enzyme complex
Legal class.: POM

Action: An anisoylated complex of streptokinase with human plasminogen, the precursor of the natural fibrinolytic enzyme plasmin. Acylation of the plasminogen molecule retards its conversion to plasmin, but it does not affect its binding to fibrin. After IV injection deacylation produces enzymatically active plasminogen-streptokinase activator complex. This converts plasminogen to plasmin within the thrombus

Uses: Treatment of acute myocardial infarction

Dosage and routes:
• *Adult:* Slow IV injection 30 units single dose over 4 to 5 min, administered as soon as possible after the onset of symptoms and preferably within 6 hours

Available forms include: IV injection 30 units/vial, powder for reconstitution

Side effects/adverse reactions:
HAEM: Bleeding
GI: Nausea, vomiting
INTEG: Flushing, allergic reactions
CV: Bradycardia, hypotension (transient), anaphylaxis (uncommon)
CNS: Fever

Contraindications: Hypersensitivity, surgery or major trauma within previous 10 days, recent (previous 2 months) neurosurgical procedures or recent traumatic cardiopulmonary resuscitation, active peptic ulcer or internal bleeding (previous 6 months), cerebrovascular accident, bleeding diathesis, severe hypertension, intracranial neoplasms or aneurysm, menorrhagia

Precautions: Risk of bleeding increased. Risk of emboli with intramural ventricular thrombi or thrombi within abdominal aneurysms or enlarged left atrium with atrial fibrillation. Arrhythmias may develop. Patients over 70 yr. Pregnancy, lactation, external chest compression, recent or concurrent anticoagulant therapy. Keep invasive procedures to a minimum e.g. cardiac catheterization. Repeated therapy (or streptokinase therapy) from 5 days−12 months previously

Lab. test interferences: For 24−48 hr after therapy
Decreased plasma fibrinogen and plasminogen concentrations
Increased fibrin degradation products

Treatment of overdose: Transfusion with packed cells or whole blood if necessary−or cryoprecipitate or purified clotting factor concentrates. Tranexamic acid or aprotinin competitively inhibit fibrinolytic action

NURSING CONSIDERATIONS

Assess:
• All baseline vital signs, ECG

Administer:
• Mix solution with normal saline as recommended
• Infuse via peripheral line over 30 minutes
• As soon as thrombi identified; value of treatment within first 12 hr is established
• Cryoprecipatate or fresh, frozen plasma if bleeding occurs. Control local bleeding with pressure
• Loading dose at beginning of therapy may require increase loading doses
• Heparin therapy after thrombolytic therapy is discontinued, TT or APTT less than 2 times control (about 3−4 hr)

• After reconstituting, do not shake. Have available antiarrhythmic therapy for bradycardia and/or ventricular irritability
• About 10% patients have high streptococcal antibody titres requiring increased loading doses

Perform/provide:
• Bed rest during entire course of treatment
• Avoidance of any other invasive procedures: injection, rectal temperature
• Treatment of fever with paracetamol or aspirin
• Pressure for 30 seconds to minor bleeding sites; inform clinician if this does not attain haemostasis; apply pressure dressing
• Pain relief as required
• Emergency resuscitation equipment if cardiac arrest occurs
• Continuous ECG monitoring for reperfusion arrhythmias

Evaluate:
• 12 lead ECG before and after drug administration
• Vital signs, BP, pulse, respiration, neurological signs, at least 4 hrly; temperature or other indications of internal bleed, cardiac rhythm following intracoronary administration
• Electrolytes, particularly potassium and magnesium
• Allergy: fever, rash, itching, chills; mild reaction may be treated with antihistamines
• For bleeding during first hr of treatment: haematuria, haematemesis, bleeding from mucous membranes, epistaxis, ecchymosis

Teach patient/family:
• Issue advice card stating that malaise or signs of bleeding need to be reported to clinician
• Provide information concerning immediate and long-term counselling provisions for myocardial infarction problems

anti-D (Rh$_o$) immunoglobulin, human

Partobulin
Func. class.: Immunising agent
Chem. class.: IgG
Legal class.: POM

Action: Suppresses immune response of non-sensitised Rh$_o$ negative patients who are exposed to Rh$_o$ positive blood

Uses: To prevent a rhesus-negative mother from forming antibodies to fetal rhesus-positive cells which may pass into maternal circulation during childbirth, abortion or miscarriage. Transfusion of rhesus-incompatible blood. Also given in threatened miscarriage when blood loss has occurred

Dosage and routes:
Rh exposure/postabortion
• Ideally within 72 hr. Intramuscular injection
• *Adult:* 500 units following birth of rhesus-positive infant; 250 units if before 20 weeks gestation
After transfusion
Consult clinician
Available forms include: Injection IM single use vial or preloaded syringe

Side effects/adverse reactions:
Well tolerated generally without reactions

Contraindications: Intravenous administration. Rh$_o$(D) positive individuals or neonates

Precautions: Active immunisation with live virus vaccines should be postposed until 3 months after last anti-D dose. If administration is essential, seek clinician's advice. If anti-D needs to be given within 2–4 weeks of live virus vaccination, efficacy of vaccination may be impaired

Lab. test interference: Previous anti-D therapy (even months before) may affect Rh$_o$(D) antibody levels. Additional antibodies (e.g. rubella) in anti-D may give false positive tests for such antibodies

Treatment of overdose: No problems anticipated in rhesus-negative individuals

NURSING CONSIDERATIONS

Administer:
• After sending neonate's cord blood to lab after delivery for cross match and type. Infant must be rhesus-positive, with rhesus-negative mother
• IM only
• Rhesus-negative clients routinely given anti-D in termination of pregnancy and miscarriage (rhesus status of fetus is not available)
• Only equal lot numbers of drug, cross-match

Perform/provide:
• Storage in refrigerator

Evaluate:
• Allergic reaction: rash, urticaria, nausea, fever, wheezing
• Therapeutic response in threatened miscarriages

Teach patient/family:
• How the therapy works
• That after subsequent deliveries doses may be needed if the baby is rhesus-positive or fetal blood group is not known

ascorbic acid (vitamin C)

~~NHS~~ Redoxon
Func. class.: Water-soluble vitamin
Legal class.: GSL
POM (Injection)

Action: Needed for collagen synthesis, antioxidant, carbohydrate metabolism

Uses: Vitamin C deficiency, prevention and treatment of scurvy

Dosage and routes:
Scurvy
• *Adult:* By mouth, IM, IV or subcutaneous not less than 250 mg/day in divided doses
Deficiency prophylactic 25−75 mg daily
Available forms include: Tablets 25, 50, 100, 200, 500 mg; tablets effervescent 1000 mg; injection IM/IV/subcutaneous 100 mg/ml 5 ml amp
Side effects/adverse reactions:
Large doses only
GI: Nausea, vomiting, diarrhoea, anorexia, heartburn, cramps
GU: Oxalate renal stones
HAEM: Haemolytic anaemia in patients with G-6-PD
Contraindications:
None significant
Precautions: Hyperoxaluria
Pharmacokinetics:
Readily absorbed from GI tract. Metabolised in liver, metabolites and unused amounts excreted in urine (unchanged), excreted in breast milk. Removed by haemodialysis
Clinical assessment:
• Monitor blood ascorbic acid levels if severe deficiency is present, e.g., scurvy
Lab. test interferences:
• False positive, negatives in tests involving oxidation and reduction reactions
• Plasma, faeces and urine may be affected
NURSING CONSIDERATIONS
Assess:
• Fluid balance
Perform/provide:
• Diet with high content of vitamin C e.g. citrus fruit, vegetables
Evaluate:
• Continued signs of deficiency e.g. anorexia, pallor, joint pain, hyperkeratosis, petechiae
• Injection sites for inflammation
Teach patient/family:

• That foods rich in vitamin C should be included in diet
• Extra vitamin C is needed if patient smokes or takes oral contraceptives

---

aspirin

Caprin, Platet, Solprin, Nuseals Aspirin, Angettes 75, many combination products
Func. class.: Minor analgesic
Chem. class.: Salicylate
Legal class.: Aspirin BP Tablets packsize more than 25 P; tablets packsize 25 GSL

Action: Inhibition of prostaglandin synthesis; antipyretic action results from inhibition of hypothalamic heat-regulating centre, inhibits platelet aggregation
Uses: Mild to moderate pain or fever; pain and inflammation in rheumatic disease and other musculoskeletal disorders; prophylaxis of cerebrovascular disease or myocardial infarction
Dosage and routes:
Arthritis
• *Adult:* By mouth 0.3−1 g every 4 hr, maximum 8 g daily in acute conditions
Pain/fever
• By mouth 300−900 mg every 4−6 hr, maximum 4 g daily
Thromboembolic disorders, prophylaxis
• *Adult:* By mouth 75−300 mg daily
Available forms include: Tablets 75, 100, 300, 600 mg in various formulations
Side effects/adverse reactions:
HAEM: Increased bleeding time
GU: Urate kidney stones
CNS: Confusion
GI: Nausea, vomiting, GI bleeding, ulceration, diarrhoea, heartburn, anorexia

INTEG: Rash, urticaria
EENT: Tinnitus, subconjunctival haemorrhage, vertigo
RESP: Wheezing, bronchospasm
Contraindications: Hypersensitivity to salicylates, GI bleeding and ulceration, bleeding disorders, children under 12 yr except for juvenile arthritis, lactation, not for treatment of gout, mifepristone therapy
Precautions: G6PD-deficiency, hepatic disease, renal disease, allergic disease, asthma, pregnancy, dehydration, elderly, history of GI ulceration, gout, hypertension
Pharmacokinetics: Onset 15–30 min, peak 1–2 hr, by mouth duration 4–6 hr but values depend on formulation
Metabolized by liver, excreted by kidneys, excreted in breast milk, half-life 1–3½ hr
Interactions/incompatibilities:
• Decreased effects of aspirin: antacids, adsorbents, urinary alkalinisers
• Increased effects and toxicity of: anticoagulants, insulin, methotrexate, phenytoin, sodium valproate, acetazolamide
• Decreased effects of: probenecid, spironolactone, sulphinpyrazone
• Increased effect of aspirin: metoclopramide
• Avoid aspirin until 8–12 days after mifepristone
Clinical assessment:
• Monitor patients with hypertension for bleeding
• Monitor blood clotting picture
Treatment of overdose: Gastric lavage, forced alkaline diuresis, monitor electrolytes, ventricular systole. Haemodialysis in severe cases. Restore acid-base balance. Observe patient for at least 24 hr
NURSING CONSIDERATIONS
Assess:
• Pre-existing conditions, omit if known gastric ulcer or bleeding
• Prior drug history: there are many drug interactions
Administer:
• With food or milk to decrease gastric symptoms
Perform/provide:
• Repositioning to decrease pain
• Cool cloth for fever
Evaluate:
• Relief of pain (if reason for prescription)
• Hepatotoxicity: dark urine, clay-colored stools, yellowing of skin, sclera, itching, abdominal pain, fever, diarrhoea if patient is on long-term therapy
• Allergic reactions: rash, urticaria; if these occur, drug may need to be discontinued
• Renal dysfunction: decreased urine output
• Ototoxicity: tinnitus, ringing, roaring in ears; audiometric testing needed before, after long-term therapy
• Visual changes: blurring, halos, corneal, retinal damage
• Oedema in feet, ankles, legs
Teach patient/family:
• To report any symptoms of hepatotoxicity, renal toxicity, visual changes, ototoxicity, allergic reactions (long-term therapy)
• Not to exceed recommended dosage; acute poisoning may result
• To read label on other non-prescribed drugs; many contain aspirin
• That the therapeutic response may take 2 weeks (arthritis)
• To avoid alcohol ingestion; GI bleeding may occur
• To store in child-proof container and out of reach of children

atenolol

Antipressan, Tenormin, Atenix, Totamol, Vasaten
Func. class.: Antihypertensive, antianginal
Chem. class.: Selective β-blocker
Legal class.: POM

Action: Competitively blocks stimulation of β-adrenergic receptors, produces negative chronotropic, inotropic activity (decreases rate of SA node discharge, increases recovery time), slows conduction of atrioventricular node decreases heart rate, decreases O_2 consumption in myocardium. Cardioselective, without intrinsic sympathomimetic and membrane stabilising activities
Uses: Hypertension, cardiac dysrhythmias, acute phase after myocardial infarction, angina pectoris
Dosage and routes:
• *Adult:* By mouth, hypertension 50 mg daily, angina 100 mg daily in 1 or 2 doses, arrhythmias 50−100 mg daily
• Reduce dose in renal impairment
• By IV injection, arrhythmias, 2.5 mg at 1 mg/min. Repeat at 5 min intervals, maximum 10 mg
• By IV infusion, arrhythmias, 150 mcg/kg over 20 min. Repeat every 12 hr if required. Early intervention within 12 hr of infarction, 5−10 mg by slow IV injection then by mouth 50 mg after 15 min, 50 mg after 12 hr, then 100 mg daily
Available forms include: Tablets 25, 50, 100 mg, syrup 25 mg/5 ml. Injection 500 mcg/ml
Side effects/adverse reactions:
CV: Cold extremities
MS: Muscle fatigue
INTEG: Rash
EENT: Dry burning eyes

Contraindications: Hypersensitivity to β-blockers, cardiogenic shock, heart block (2nd, 3rd degree), congestive heart failure cardiac failure (uncontrolled), children
Precautions: Myasthenia gravis, pregnancy, lactation, diabetes mellitus, renal disease. Reversible obstructive airways disease, asthma, well compensated heart failure, poor cardiac reserve, anaesthesia. Avoid abrupt withdrawal. NB: verapamil treatment, clonidine.
Pharmacokinetics dynamics:
By mouth. Peak 2−4 hr; half-life 6−7 hr, excreted unchanged in urine, protein binding 3%
Interactions/incompatibilities:
• Increased effect: alcohol, anaesthetics, antihypertensives (NB: clonidine), anxiolytics and hypnotics, diuretics
• Increased side effects: mefloquine, diltiazem, nifedipine, verapamil, cardiac glycosides, antiarrhythmics, anti-diabetics
• Reduced effects: oestrogens, combined oral contraceptives, sympathomimetics, carbenoxolone, xamoterol, NSAIDS
Clinical assessment:
• Obtain baseline data of renal function before treatment commences
• Assess time lapse since infarction
• Prescribe reduced dosage for patients with known renal disease
• Evaluate therapeutic response (fall in BP) after 1−2 weeks
• Monitor respiratory function if appropriate
Lab test interferences:
Interference: Glucose/insulin tolerance tests
Treatment of overdose: IV atropine, follow if necessary with IV glucagon. Follow by IV prenalterol or dobutamine if required

NURSING CONSIDERATIONS

Assess:
- Fluid balance and weight
- Apex and radial pulses before dose is given
- Monitor peak flow rate (PEFR) in patients with reversible airways obstruction

Administer:
- Crushed or whole tablets before meals and at bedtime

Evaluate:
- Weight and fluid balance daily
- Pulse and BP at least 4 hrly
- Legs and feet for oedema daily
- Signs of dehydration e.g. loss of skin elasticity, dry mucous membranes
- Respiratory rate, rhythm, depth

Teach patient/family:
- That drug must not be discontinued suddenly, but should be reduced gradually over a period of 2 weeks
- Not to take other non-prescribed medicines without the clinician's permission
- To report bradycardia, dizziness, confusion, depression, fever
- How to take pulse and explain that this must be done at home. Ensure patient knows when to contact clinician
- To avoid alcohol, smoking, salt
- To reduce weight if necessary and take sufficient exercise
- To carry Medic Alert Card. (Alerts patient is taking drug and any known allergies)
- To avoid driving or operating machinery if dizzy

atracurium besylate

Tracrium
Func. class.: Non-depolarising muscle relaxant
Chem. class.: Biquaternary non-chlorine diester
Legal class.: POM

Action: Inhibits transmission of nerve impulses by binding with cholinergic receptor sites, antagonising action of acetylcholine

Uses: Facilitation of endotracheal intubation, skeletal muscle relaxation during mechanical ventilation, surgery, or general anaesthesia. Caesarean section

Dosage and routes:
- *Adult and child over 1 month:* IV initially 300−600 mcg/kg then 100−200 mcg/kg as required; IV infusion 300−600 mcg/kg/hr

Available forms include: Injection IV 10 mg/ml, 2.5 ml, 5 ml, 25 ml ampoules

Side effects/adverse reactions:
CV: Transient hypotension
RESP: Respiratory depression
INTEG: Flushing

Contraindications: Hypersensitivity

Precautions: Pregnancy, cardiovascular disease, lactation, electrolyte imbalances, myasthenia gravis, hypothermia, neuromuscular disease, only under anaesthetist supervision

Pharmacokinetics:
IV: Onset 2 min, duration 15−35 min; half-life 2 min, 29 min (terminal), excreted in urine, faeces (metabolites). Duration not affected by impaired renal, hepatic or circulatory function

Interactions/incompatibilities:
- Increased neuromuscular blockade: aminoglycosides, clindamycin, lincomycin, quinidine, azlocillin, mezlocillin, propranolol, nifedipine, verapamil, par-

enteral magnesium, polypeptide antibiotics, lithium, inhalation anaesthetics
• Do not mix with barbiturates or any alkaline agent in solution or syringe
• Do not administer depolarising muscle relaxant to prolong neuro-muscular block
• Hypotension, myocardial depression, hyperkalaemia with: IV dantrolene and verapamil
• Decreased neuromuscular blockade: demecarium and eco-thiopate eye drops, neostigmine, pyridostigmine
Treatment of overdose: (or delayed recovery) Administer atropine and neostigmine. Maintain artificial ventilation as required
NURSING CONSIDERATIONS
Assess:
• BP, pulse, respirations, temperature, airway, strength of hand-grip until fully recovered
• Fluid balance chart; check for urinary retention, frequency, hesitancy
• Previous anaesthetic history to ensure patient has not had myasthenia gravis
• Test for urea and electrolytes, blood gases and pH if appropriate
Administer:
• IV, slowly (onset 1−2 min)
• Only under medical supervision of an anaesthetist
• Allow 90 seconds after initial administration before endotracheal tube is inserted
Perform/provide:
• Flush cannula before and after use
• Do not mix with barbiturates
Evaluate:
• Airway status, strength of hand-grip, ability to raise head from pillow, reduced facial movement
Teach patient/family:
• About effects of drug, weakness, loss of muscle tone

atropine sulphate

Min-I-Jet, Atropine sulphate
Func. class.: Antimuscarinic, para-sympatholytic
Chem. class.: Belladonna alkaloid
Legal class.: POM or P depending on preparation

Action: Competes for acetyl-choline receptors at parasympath-etic neuroeffector sites; increases cardiac output, heart rate by blocking vagal stimulation in heart
Uses: Bradycardia, anticholine-sterase insecticide poisoning, blocking cardiac vagal reflexes, decreasing secretions before surgery, antispasmodic, with neostig-mine for reversal of competitive neuromuscular block
Dosage and routes:
• Seek advice from clinician
Available forms include: Tablets 600 mcg; injection 600 mcg/ml, 1 ml; injection 100 mcg/ml, 5 ml, 10 ml
Side effects/adverse reactions:
GU: Retention, hesitancy
GI: Dry mouth, constipation, difficulty in swallowing, thirst
CV: Bradycardia followed by tachycardia, palpitations, arrhythmias
INTEG: Dry skin, flushing
EENT: Blurred vision, photo-phobia, glaucoma, dilatation of pupils
Contraindications: Hypersensitivity to belladonna alkaloids, closed-angle glaucoma
Precautions: Pregnancy, elderly, urinary retention, prostatic enlargement, tachycardia, cardiovascular disease, paralytic ileus, ulcerative colitis, pyloric stenosis, lactation
Pharmacokinetics:
IV: Peak 2−4 min
IM: Peak 30 min

Half-life 2−3 hr, incompletely metabolised in liver, excreted in breast milk, excreted in urine unchanged and as metabolites
Interactions/incompatibilities:
• Decreased effects of: phenothiazines, ketoconazole, sublingual nitrates
• Increased side effects: other drugs with antimuscarinic effects, nefopam, disopyramide, tricyclics, MAOIs, antihistamines, phenothiazines, amantadine
• Delayed absorption: mexiletine
• Decreased GI effects: cisapride, metoclopramide, domperidone
Treatment of overdose: If overdose by mouth: aspiration, lavage or induction of emesis. Activated charcoal to reduce absorption. Supportive therapy. Neostigmine or carbachol antagonises only peripheral effects

NURSING CONSIDERATIONS
Administer:
• Intravenously usually as a bolus injection, directly into vein, can be repeated 4−6 hr later
• Intramuscularly, subcutaneously, orally as prescribed
Perform/provide:
• Frequent drinks to prevent dry mouth when taking oral medication
Evaluate:
• Cardiac rate, rhythm, character; blood pressure, respirations
• Input and output of fluids, check for urinary retention
• For bowel sounds; check for constipation
• Pulse, respiration and blood pressure especially during intravenous infusion; monitor with electrocardiograph
• Dry mouth, dry skin, urinary retention, dilation of pupils
• Therapeutic response, increase in cardiac output, decrease in secretions before surgery and parkinsonism

• Allergy to atropine sulphate — rash on face upper trunk, rapid respirations, tachycardia, hyperpyrexia
• Effect of any other drug therapy
Teach patient family:
• To report blurred vision, chest pain, palpitations
• That long term medication may be required to improve cardiac output

---

atropine sulphate (ophthalmic)

Isopto Atropine, Minims
Func. class.: Mydriatic, cycloplegic
Chem. class.: Belladonna alkaloid
Legal class.: POM

Action: Blocks response of iris sphincter muscle, muscle of accommodation of ciliary body to cholinergic stimulation, resulting in dilation of pupil, paralysis of accommodation
Uses: Iritis, uveitis, cycloplegic refraction
Dosage and routes:
• *Adult:* Refraction (1%) instil 1 drop into each eye twice daily for 1 or 2 days before examination
Uveitis (1%) instil 1 or 2 drops into the eye(s) 4 times daily or as required
• *Children:* Refraction (1%) instil 1 drop twice daily for 1−3 days before examination and 1 hr before. Eye ointment 1% preferred for children under 5 yr — apply twice daily for 3 days before examination
Uveitis (1%) instil 1 drop into the eye(s) up to 3 times daily
Available forms include: Eye ointment 1%; eye drops 1% 5, 10 ml, Minim 1%

Side effects/adverse reactions:
SYST: Constipation, vomiting, giddiness, flushing, dry skin, dry mouth, abdominal discomfort (infants: abdominal distention), bradycardia followed by tachycardia, palpitations and arrhythmias, urinary urgency, difficulty and retention
EENT: Increased intraocular pressure, stinging, sensitivity to light. Prolonged use — irritation, hyperaemia, oedema, conjunctivitis
INTEG: Contact dermatitis, rash (in children)

Contraindications: Hypersensitivity, glaucoma or tendency to glaucoma, soft contact lenses (some preparations), pregnancy, lactation, children under 3 months

Precautions: Darkly pigmented iris more resistant to dilation

Pharmacokinetics:
Instil: Peak 30−40 min (mydriasis), 60−180 min (cycloplegia), duration 6−12 days

Interactions/incompatibilities:
Effects enhanced by other drugs with antimuscarinic properties

Treatment of overdose: Supportive treatment. Infants and small children — keep body surface moist. Accidental ingestion — induce emesis/gastric lavage

NURSING CONSIDERATIONS
Evaluate:
• Observe for resolution of inflammation, pupil dilation
• Withhold dose if eye pain occurs and inform clinician

Teach patient/family:
• To report visual disturbances e.g. loss of sight, difficulty breathing, sweating, hot flushes
• That blurring is inevitable but will decrease with repeated use of drops and ointment
• How to administer eyedrops; protect eyes from bright illumination during dilation
• To avoid driving, operating machinery until able to see
• To wait 5 min before instilling other eyedrops
• Not to blink more than usual
• Not to get the preparation in a child's mouth and to wash their own hands and the child's hands following administration

auranofin

Ridaura
Func. class.: Gold salt
Chem. class.: Orally active gold complex
Legal class.: POM

Action: Anti-inflammatory action unknown, may decrease phagocytosis, lysosomal activity or decrease prostaglandin synthesis; decreases concentration of rheumatoid factor, immunoglobulins

Uses: Active progressive rheumatoid arthritis when NSAIDs ineffective alone

Dosage and routes: Seek specialist advice
• *Adult:* By mouth 3 mg twice daily, single 6 mg dose if well tolerated, may increase to 9 mg/day in 3 divided doses after 6 months, discontinue if no effect after further 3 months

Available forms include: Tablets 3 mg

Side effects/adverse reactions:
HAEM: Thrombocytopenia agranulocytosis, aplastic anaemia, leucopenia, granulocytopenia
INTEG: Rash, pruritus, alopecia
GI: Diarrhoea, abdominal cramping, stomatitis, nausea, vomiting, other GI symptoms, metallic taste

GU: Proteinuria, haematuria
EENT: Conjunctivitis
RESP: Pulmonary fibrosis
Contraindications: Hypersensitivity to gold, necrotising enterocolitis, bone marrow aplasia, children, lactation, pregnancy, porphyria, pulmonary fibrosis, exfoliative dermatitis, systemic lupus erythematosus, blood dyscrasias, progressive renal disease, severe hepatic disease
Precautions: Elderly, allergic conditions, eczema, ulcerative colitis, renal impairment, rash, drugs causing blood disorders, liver dysfunction, inflammatory bowel disease, history of bone marrow depression
Pharmacokinetics:
By mouth: Absorbed by GI tract, peak 2 hr, steady state 8–12 weeks, excreted in urine, faeces
Interactions/incompatibilities:
None known
Clinical assessment:
• Perform urine tests monthly. Proteinuria may necessitate withdrawal
• Annual chest X-ray — watch for breathlessness, dry cough
• Perform monthly full blood counts (including total and differential white cell and platelet counts) drug should be discontinued if platelets less than 100,000/mm^3. Monitor gold toxicity e.g. decreased Hb, white blood count and platelets
• Perform liver function tests; renal function tests
• Monitor for GI bleeding, rash, pruritus, stomatitis, metallic taste
Treatment of overdose: Induce vomiting or gastric lavage. Supportive treatment; chelating agents may be indicated
NURSING CONSIDERATIONS
Assess:
• Fluid balance

Evaluate:
• Therapeutic response to treatment; ability to move joints with less pain
• Urine for haematuria, proteinuria
• Stools for diarrhoea
• Respiratory status; inform clinician of dyspnoea, wheezing
• Allergic reaction e.g. rash, dermatitis, pruritus. (Drug may be discontinued if side effects are pronounced.)
Teach patient/family:
• To use a mouthwash for mild stomatitis
• To avoid hot, spicy foods and those that are highly acidic
• A soft toothbrush should be used
• That drug must be taken exactly as prescribed to be effective
• That diarrhoea is common, but if blood appears in stools or urine, the clinician must be informed at once
• To report skin conditions, stomatitis, fatigue, jaundice; these may indicate blood dyscrasias
• That therapeutic effect may take 3–4 months
• To practice contraception and avoid becoming pregnant

azathioprine

Azamune, Berkaprine, Imuran, Immunoprin
Func. class.: Immunosuppressant
Chem. class.: Purine analogue
Legal class.: POM

Action: Produces immunosuppression by inhibiting purine synthesis in cells, interferes with nucleic acid synthesis
Uses: Organ transplants to prevent rejection, refractory rheumatoid arthritis and other refractory diseases, autoimmune conditions

(when steroids inadequate) e.g. chronic active hepatitis, haemolytic anaemia, systemic lupus erythematosus

Dosage and routes:
Adult and child:
Prevention of rejection
• By mouth or slow IV injection, loading dose of up to 5 mg/kg then maintenance 1.0–4.0 mg/kg daily; IV *only* if oral not practical
Other conditions
• Seek specialist advice

Available forms include: Tablets 25, 50 mg; injection IV 50 mg vial (sodium salt)

Side effects/adverse reactions:
GI: Nausea, vomiting, stomatitis, anorexia, oesophagitis, pancreatitis, hepatotoxicity, jaundice
HAEM: Leucopenia, thrombocytopenia, anaemia, pancytopenia, increased mean corpuscular volume, red cell haemoglobin content, myelosuppression
INTEG: Rash
MS: Arthralgia, muscle wasting, muscle pain
CV: Cardiac dysrhythmia, hypotension
CNS: Malaise, dizziness, rigors. Transplant patients also receiving steroids: hair loss, increased susceptibility to infection

Contraindications: Hypersensitivity to azathioprine or 6-mercaptopurine, pregnancy (seek specialist advice)

Precautions: Renal disease, hepatic disease, elderly, recent/concommitant cytostatic agents

Pharmacokinetics: Metabolised in liver, excreted in urine (active metabolite)

Interactions/incompatibilities:
• Increased action of this drug: allopurinol, oxipurinol, thiopurinol
• Increased effect of: depolarising muscle relaxants

• Decreased effect of: non-depolarising muscle relaxants

Clinical assessment:
• Blood studies: complete blood counts (including platelets) at least weekly initially
• Watch for manifestations of bone marrow depression: infections, bruising, bleeding
• Examine skin for tumours regularly in transplant recipients
• Liver function studies

Treatment of overdose: (Chronic and acute) Symptomatic. Gastric lavage. Monitor blood picture and liver function

NURSING CONSIDERATIONS

Assess:
• Temperature, pulse baseline

Administer:
• IV preparation slowly and diluted, or flushed well with normal saline after administration
• With prophylactic medication (e.g. oral nystatin for stomatitis) if required to protect against side effects

Evaluate:
• Temperature, pulse daily (for pyrexia)
• For signs of nausea, vomiting, damage to oral/oesophageal mucosae, rash, muscle-wasting, pain, arthralgia
• For signs of infection, bone marrow suppression

Teach patient/family:
• About all side effects and report immediately
• Increased potential risk of infection—avoid contact with people who have obviously infective illnesses
• Record daily temperature
• Inform prescribing clinician of any medication already taken, e.g. allopurinol

azlocillin sodium

Securopen
Func. class.: Antipseudomonal
antibiotic
Chem. class.: Ureidopenicillin
Legal class.: POM

Action: Interferes with cell wall
replication of susceptible organisms; the cell wall, rendered
osmotically unstable, swells, bursts
from osmotic pressure
Uses: Infections due to *Pseudomonas aeruginosa* especially
respiratory and urinary tract and
septicaemia
Dosage and routes:
• *Adult:* IV injection 2 g every
8 hr, IV infusion 5 g 8 hrly
• *Premature infant:* IV injection
50 mg/kg 12 hrly. *Neonate:* IV
injection 100 mg/kg 12 hrly. *Infant:*
IV injection 7 days-1 yr 100 mg/kg
8 hrly
• *Child 1–14 yr:* IV injection
75 mg/kg 8 hrly. Reduce dose in
renal impairment
Available forms include: Powder for
injection 500 mg, 1 g, 2 g.
Powder for infusion 5 g. All as
sodium salt
Side effects/adverse reactions:
HAEM: Increased bleeding time
INTEG: Local irritation, rashes,
pruritus
GI: Nausea, vomiting, diarrhoea,
pseudomembranous colitis
SYST: Anaphylaxis
Contraindications: Hypersensitivity to penicillins and cephalosporins
Precautions: Pregnancy, neonates,
renal impairment
Pharmacokinetics: Half-life 55–
70 min, metabolised in liver,
(limited extent), excreted in urine,
bile, breast milk (small amount)
Interactions/incompatibilities:
• Increased penicillin concentrations when used with:
probenicid
• Prolonged neuromuscular
blockade: vecuronium and other
non-depolarising muscle relaxants
• Anti-coagulants: need more
frequent monitoring
• Reduced contraceptive effect:
oral contraceptives
• Incompatibility in solution:
seek pharmacist's advice before
mixing
Treatment of overdose: Standard
monitoring and supportive
measures. Reduce serum levels by
dialysis
NURSING CONSIDERATIONS
Administer:
• Seek pharmacist's advice before mixing (incompatibility in
solutions)
• For doses of 2 g or less administer
as IV bolus injection. Larger doses
infuse over 20–30 min
• Dilute injection in appropriate
infusion solutions e.g. glucose 5%
sodium chloride 0.9%
Perform/provide:
• Check IV site for local irritation
• Observe for skin rashes and
pruritus
Teach patient/family:
• To observe for bruising or bleed-
ing if taking anti-coagulants

bacampicillin HCl

Ambaxin
Func. class.: Broad spectrum
antibiotic
Chem. class.: Aminopenicillin
ester
Legal class.: POM

Action: Interferes with cell wall
replication of susceptible organisms; the cell wall, rendered osmotically unstable, swells, bursts
from osmotic pressure
Uses: Respiratory tract infec-

tions, skin, urinary tract infections; effective for Gram-positive cocci, Gram-negative cocci, Gram-negative bacilli

Dosage and routes:
• *Adult:* By mouth 400−800 mg 2 or 3 times daily
• Uncomplicated gonorrhoea 1.6 g as a single dose with probenecid 1 g
• *Child:* By mouth over 5 yr 200 mg 3 times daily
Available forms include: Tablets, scored 400 mg

Side effects/adverse reactions:
Sensitivity reactions: (discontinue treatment) rashes, urticaria, fever, joint pain, angioedema, anaphylactic shock
HAEM: Anaemia, increased bleeding time, bone marrow depression, granulocytopenia
GI: Nausea, vomiting, diarrhoea, increased aspartate aminotransferase, rarely pseudomembranous colitis, increased alanine aminotransferase, abdominal pain, glossitis, colitis
GU: Oliguria, proteinuria, haematuria, vaginitis, moniliasis, glomerulonephritis
CNS: Lethargy, hallucinations, anxiety, depression, twitching, coma, convulsions
META: Hypokalaemia, alkalosis

Contraindications: Hypersensitivity to penicillins

Precautions: Pregnancy, renal impairment, history of allergy, lactation, risk of erythematous rashes particularly high in glandular fever, lymphatic leukaemia and HIV infection. Possibility of superinfection with mycotic organisms or bacterial pathogens. Renal, hepatic and haemopoietic function should be monitored during prolonged therapy

Pharmacokinetics:
Period of onset: 30−60 min, duration 5−6 hr, hydrolysed to am-picillin in gut wall and plasma, metabolised in liver, excreted in urine

Interactions/incompatibilities:
• Phenindione and warfarin: prothrombin time can be prolonged
• Small risk of reduced contraceptive effect with combined oral contraceptives
• Decreased antimicrobial effectiveness of this drug: tetracyclines, erythromycins
• Increased penicillin concentrations when used with: aspirin, probenicid

Lab. test interferences: Interferes with tests for amino acids, serum-albumin and glucose

Clinical assessment:
• Liver studies: aspartate aminotransferase, alanine aminotransferase
• Renal studies: urinalysis, protein, blood
• Culture, sensitivity before drug therapy; drug may be taken as soon as culture is taken

Treatment of overdose: Problems of overdose unlikely to be encountered

NURSING CONSIDERATIONS

Assess:
• Bowel pattern
• Fluid balance
• Allergies before initiation of treatment; reaction of each medication; highlight allergies on chart
• Check for pregnancy, history of allergy, lactation, glandular fever, lymphatic leukaemia, HIV infection, other medication
• Any patient with compromised renal system, since drug is excreted slowly in poor renal system function; toxicity may occur rapidly

Administer:
• After culture and sensitivity completed

Perform/provide:

• Adrenaline, suction, tracheostomy set, endotracheal intubation equipment on unit
• Adequate intake of fluids (2 litres) during diarrhoea episodes

Evaluate:
• For therapeutic effectiveness:
• Bowel pattern before, during treatment
• Fluid balance; report haematuria, oliguria since penicillin in high doses is nephrotoxic
• Skin eruptions after administration of penicillin to 1 week after discontinuing drug
• Respiratory status: rate, character, wheezing, tightness in chest

Teach patient/family:
• Aspects of drug therapy: culture may be taken after completed course of medication
• To report sore throat, fever, fatigue (could indicate superimposed infection)
• To wear or carry a Medic Alert ID if allergic to penicillins
• To notify nurse of diarrhoea

---

baclofen

Lioresal
Func. class.: Skeletal muscle relaxant, central acting
Chem. class.: GABA chlorophenyl derivative
Legal class.: POM

Action: Antispastic agent acting at spinal level. GABA derivative. Depresses monosynaptic and polysynaptic reflex transmission probably by activating GABA neurotransmission. Neuromuscular transmission is unaffected. Reduces painful flexor spasms and spontaneous clonus. Antinociceptive effect

Uses: Spinal cord injury, spasticity in multiple sclerosis, motor neurone disease

Dosage and routes:
• *Adult:* By mouth 5 mg 3 times daily, gradually increased to a maximum of 100 mg daily
• *Child:* By mouth, 0.75−2 mg/kg daily (over 10 yr maximum 2.5 mg/kg daily) or 2.5 mg 4 times daily increased gradually according to age to maintenance: 1−2 yr 10−20 mg daily, 2−6 yr 20−30 mg daily, 6−10 yr 30−60 mg daily

Available forms include: Tablets 10 mg; sugar-free liquid 5 mg/5 ml

Side effects/adverse reactions:
CNS: Dizziness, weakness, fatigue, drowsiness, headache, disorientation, insomnia, paraesthesiae, tremors, hallucinations, nightmares, convulsions, increased spasticity, muscular hypotonia, muscular pain, daytime sedation, mental confusion, euphoria, depressive states
MS: Myalgia, muscular weaknesses, ataxia
EENT: Nasal congestion, blurred vision, accommodation disorders
CV: Hypotension, chest pain, palpitations, cardiovascular depression
GI: Nausea, constipation, vomiting, increased aspartate aminotransferase, alkaline phosphatase, abdominal pain, dry mouth, anorexia, retching, diarrhoea, alteration in taste, deterioration in liver function tests
GU: Urinary frequency, dysuria, enuresis
INTEG: Rash, pruritus, hyperhidrosis
RESP: Respiratory depression

Contraindications: Hypersensitivity, peptic ulceration, porphyria
Precautions: Psychotic disorders, schizophrenia, confusional states, epilepsy, antihypertensive therapy, cerebrovascular accident, respiratory, hepatic or renal impairment, hypertonic bladder sphincter, diabetes mellitus, preg-

nancy, elderly, spastic states of cerebral origin.

Pharmacokinetics:
Peak ½−1½ hr. Half life 3−4 hr Serum protein binding approximately 30%. Eliminated largely in unchanged form via kidneys

Interactions/incompatibilities:
Increased effect: tricyclic antidepressants. Increased sedation: alcohol, CNS depressants. Aggravation of hyperkinetic symptoms: lithium. Increased effect of: antihypotensives. Increased toxicity: ibuprofen, levodopa with carbidopa

Clinical assessment:
• Perform EEG for patients with history of epilepsy

Lab. test interferences:
Increase: Aspartate aminotransferase, alkaline phosphatase, blood glucose, SGOT

Treatment of overdose: No specific antidote. Induce vomiting, gastric lavage; comatose patients should be intubated prior to gastric lavage. Administration of activated charcoal. If necessary, saline aperient. In respiratory depression, administration of artificial respiration, also measures in support of cardiovascular functions. Generous quantities of fluid should be given, possibly with a diuretic. If convulsions occur, diazepam should be administered cautiously IV

NURSING CONSIDERATIONS
Administer:
• With food or milk to reduce gastric symptoms

Perform/provide:
• Mouthcare, mouthwashes for dry mouth
• Help during standing/walking if dizziness or drowsiness occurs

Evaluate:
• Effectiveness of drug indicated by decreased pain and spasticity
• Urinary output; watch for urinary retention, frequency, hesitancy
• Allergic reactions e.g. rash, fever, respiratory distress
• Weakness, numbness · in extremities
• Psychological dependency e.g. increased need for medication, more frequent requests for medication, increased pain
• CNS depression; dizziness, drowsiness, psychiatric symptoms

Teach patient/family:
• Medication must not be discontinued suddenly; hallucinations, spasticity, tachycardia will occur. Drug must be discontinued slowly over 1−2 weeks
• Not to take with alcohol or other CNS depressants
• To avoid driving or operating machinery if dizzy or drowsy
• To avoid medicines that have not been prescribed, especially cough linctuses, antihistamines
• To take with food/milk
• Some benefits after 2−3 hr, but full benefits after several weeks
• To report any urinary problems
• Ask patient about fits/seizures if a known epileptic; this drug may induce seizures

---

BCG (bacillus Calmette-Guérin vaccine)

Func. class.: Vaccine
Chem. class.: Live attenuated strain derived from bovine *Mycobacterium tuberculosis*
Legal class.: POM

Action: Stimulates the development of immunity to the bacillus *Mycobacterium tuberculosis*
Uses: Active immunisation against tuberculosis
Dosage and routes: Intradermal injection 0.1 ml (infants under 3 months, 0.05 ml) by operators

skilled in the technique. Percutaneous vaccine *not* recommended

Available forms include:
• BCG vaccine
• BCG vaccine, Isoniazid-Resistant
• BCG vaccine, Percutaneous

Side effects/adverse reactions:
INTEG: Mild discomfort at injection site; prolonged ulceration or subcutaneous abscess formation due to faulty injection technique; rash, induration, pain
SYST: Mild fever and malaise, lymphadenopathy. Anaphylactic reactions are rare

Contraindications: Tuberculoprotein hypersensitivity, HIV-positive and other immunocompromised patients, existing acute illness; pregnancy, systemic treatment with corticosteroids, immunosuppressive treatment, malignant disease, pyrexia, infected dermatoses, eczema at injection site, radiotherapy and irradiation tumours of reticuloendothelial system, generalised septic skin conditions. For time lapse between stopping drug therapy and having BCG — refer to clinician

Precautions: Do not give within 3 weeks (or minimum 10 days) of other live vaccines; do not administer other vaccines in the same arm as BCG for at least 3 months

Pharmacokinetics: Seroconversion occurs within 8–14 weeks

Clinical assessment:
• Measles or rubella infection can cause tuberculin positive patients to revert temporarily and become tuberculin negative
• Perform skin test for sensitivity. Newborn infants require no skin test. When BCG is given to infants there is no need to delay primary immunisations including polio

NURSING CONSIDERATIONS
Administer:
• Nurses must be fully competent in the technique of intradermal injection
• After preparation according to manufacturer's instruction using sodium chloride or water for injection
• Do not shake. Allow to stand for 1 min. Draw up twice to ensure homogenous solution. Once prepared protect from light and use within 4 hr
• If the injection site is swabbed with alcohol, allow to dry before administration of vaccine to prevent contamination
• Use syringe fitted with a short bevel gauge 25 needle. The use of jet injectors is not recommended
• Give intradermally in the arm over the insertion of the deltoid muscle. The thigh can be used in females for cosmetic reasons but is not recommended in neonates
• Record date, name of vaccine, dose, route, site and batch number of vaccine and sodium chloride or water in patient's notes

Perform/provide:
• Incinerate excess vaccine or treat with disinfectant such as strong hypochlorite solution

Teach patient/family:
• To leave open to facilitate healing or, if discharging, cover with dry, non-occlusive dressing. Avoid abrasion e.g. by tight clothing
• To expect some mild discomfort
• To expect small swelling after 1 week, ulcer at 3 weeks which heals after 6–12 weeks. Scar is initially red and later becomes white
• To see clinician in event of pain, swelling, discharge or increasing fever
• High risk workers e.g. nurses, to contact clinician or occupational health department after 6 weeks for follow-up to confirm immunity, if indicated

beclomethasone dipropionate (inhaled)

Becotide 50, Becotide 100, Becotide 200, Becodisks, Becotide Rotacaps, Becloforte, AeroBec, AeroBec Forte
Func. class.: Synthetic corticosteroid
Chem. class.: Beclomethasone diester
Legal class.: POM

Action: Reduces inflammation by depression of migration of polymorphonuclear leucocytes, fibroblasts, reversal of increased capillary permeability and lysosomal stabilisation. At normal therapeutic doses the inhaled preparation lacks systemic side effects
Uses: Treatment and prophylaxis of asthma
Dosages and routes:
• *By inhalation of powder* Becodisks/Rotacaps: *Adult:* 200 mcg 3 to 4 times daily or 400 mcg twice daily. Maximum dose 1 mg daily
• *Child*: 100 mcg 2 to 4 times daily or 200 mcg twice daily
• *By aerosol inhalation:* Becotide, AeroBec: *Adult:* 200 mcg twice daily or 100 mcg 3 to 4 times daily (in more severe cases initially 600−800 mcg daily)
• *Child*: 50−100 mcg 2 to 4 times daily
• AeroBec Forte: Becloforte: *Adult:* 500 mcg twice daily or 250 mcg 4 times daily. Maximum 500 mcg 3 to 4 times daily. Not indicated for children
Available forms include:
Aerosol inhalation: 50 mcg per metered inhalation (Becotide 50, AeroBec, breath-actuated unit AeroBec Autohaler) 200 inhalations; 100 mcg per metered inhalation (Becotide 100) 200 inhalations; 200 mcg per metered inhalation (Becotide 200) 200 inhalations
Rotacaps containing powder for inhalation: 100, 200, 400 mcg
Becodisks containing 8 powder blisters per disk: 100, 200, 400 mcg
Becloforte, AeroBec Forte aerosol 250 mcg per metered inhalation
Becloforte VM (2 Becloforte inhaler plus volumatic spacer)
Side effects/adverse reactions:
EENT: Dry mouth, candidiasis of mouth and throat (treat with topical antifungal therapy whilst still continuing inhaler), hoarseness or throat irritation
RESP: Potential for paradoxical bronchospasm (discontinue treatment immediately and institute alternative therapy)
Contraindications: Hypersensitivity to beclomethasone, active or quiescent pulmonary tuberculosis, status asthmaticus (primary treatment), non-asthmatic bronchial disease
Precautions: Pregnancy, lactation, poor inhalation technique. After transfer from oral corticosteroid therapy may need to reinstate systemic therapy during periods of stress, infection or when airway obstruction or mucus prevent drug access to smaller airways. Use regularly. No adrenal suppression likely until doses of 1500 mcg per day. Reduced plasma cortisol levels reported at doses of 2000 mcg per day
Pharmacokinetics:
Inhalation: Onset 10 min, excreted in faeces (metabolites), half-life 3−15 hr, metabolised in lungs, liver, GI system
Incompatibilities: None significant
Clinical assessment:
• Check inhalation technique, advise to use regularly
• Candidiasis is reduced with 'spacer' apparatus and also

responds to antifungal lozenges without discontinuing treatment
• Assess adrenal function periodically
• Becloforte — advise carry steroid card. Do not stop abruptly
Treatment of overdose: Inhalation of large amounts of drug over a short time — no special emergency action needed. Continue treatment at recommended dose. Hypothalamic-pituitary-adrenal (HPA) function recovers in a day or two. Excessive use over a long time could lead to adrenal suppression, transfer to oral corticosteroid therapy and when condition is stabilised return to inhaled therapy at recommended dose. Then withdraw oral steroids gradually
NURSING CONSIDERATIONS
Administer:
• With correct technique and equipment e.g. Spacer
Perform/provide:
• Mouthcare, mouthwashes to counteract dryness and reduce risk of fungal colonisation
Evaluate:
• By recording peak flow pre- and post-administration. Assess for paradoxical bronchospasm
Teach patient/family:
• Correct technique of administration
• To wash inhaler with warm water after use and dry thoroughly
• If mouth and/or throat problems occur after use advise to rinse mouth thoroughly with water immediately after inhalation
• To carry identity as a steroid user
• To report if the drug no longer seems effective, as the dose may need readjusting
• All aspects of drug taking and side effects, including Cushingoid symptoms
• To recognise symptoms of adrenal insufficiency e.g. nausea,

anorexia, fatigue, dizziness, dyspnoea, weakness, joint pain, depression
• To seek advice if not well, particularly nausea, anorexia, joint pain

beclomethasone dipropionate (nasal)

Beconase Nasal Spray, Beconase Aqueous Nasal Spray
Func. class.: Synthetic corticosteroid
Chem. class.: Beclomethasone diester
Legal class.: POM

Action: Anti-inflammatory properties in nasal passages
Uses: Treatment and prophylaxis of seasonal or perennial rhinitis
Dosage and routes:
• *Adult and child over 6 yr:* Apply 100 mcg (2 puffs) into each nostril twice daily or 50 mcg (1 puff) 3 to 4 times daily. Maximum 8 puffs daily
Available forms include: Aerosol 50 mcg per inhalation, aqueous spray 50 mcg per spray
Side effects/adverse reactions:
EENT: Dryness, nasal irritation, burning, sneezing
Contraindications: Hypersensitivity to any components, children under 6 yr
Precautions: Pregnancy, lactation, infections of nasal passages and paranasal sinuses, systemic steroid therapy, prolonged use in children
Pharmacokinetics:
INSTIL: Readily absorbed; peak, concentration, other data have not been determined
Treatment of overdose: Inhalation of large amounts over a short time — no special emergency action needed. Continue treatment at the recommended dose. Hypothalamic-

pituitary-adrenal (HPA) function recovers in a day or two

NURSING CONSIDERATIONS
Administer:
• After cleaning top of aerosol with warm water and drying thoroughly
• After cleaning/blowing nose
Perform/provide:
• Storage in a cool place, do not puncture or incinerate
Evaluate:
• Condition of nasal passages during long term treatment for changes in mucous membrane
Teach patient/family:
• To clear nasal passages before administration, use decongestant if needed, shake inhaler, invert, tilt head backwards, insert nozzle into nostril away from septum, hold other nostril closed, depress activator, inhale through nose and exhale through mouth
• When Beconase *Aerosol* administered as 2 puffs, the 1st puff should be directed at the upper and the 2nd puff at the lower part of the nasal cavity
• If sneezing occurs nasal passages should be cleared and dose repeated
• To continue treatment if mild nasal bleeding occurs; it is usually transient
• How to use and to read manufacturer's instructions

bendrofluazide

Aprinox, Berkozide Neo-NaClex, Centyl, combination product
Func. class.: Diuretic
Chem. class.: Thiazide
Legal class.: POM

Action: Acts on distal tubule by increasing excretion of water, sodium, chloride, potassium
Uses: Oedema, hypertension

Dosage and routes:
• *Adult:* By mouth: oedema, initially 5−10 mg in the morning, daily or on alternate days, maintenance 2.5−10 mg 1−3 times weekly; hypertension: 2.5 mg in the morning
Available forms include: Tablets 2.5, 5 mg
Side effects/adverse reactions:
GU: Polyuria, uraemia, glycosuria, impotence, thirst
CNS: Dizziness, weakness
GI: Nausea, vomiting, anorexia, hepatic encephalopathy, constipation, diarrhoea, cramps, pancreatitis, GI irritation
INTEG: Rash, purpura, photosensitivity
META: Hyperglycaemia, hyperuraemia, increased plasma cholesterol
HAEM: Neutropenia, thrombocytopenia
CV: Orthostatic hypotension
ELECT: Hypokalaemia, hypochloraemic alkalosis, hypercalcaemia, hyponatraemia, hypomagnesaemia, hyperuricaemia, gout
Contraindications: Hypersensitivity to thiazides or sulphonamides, anuria, lactation, lithium, pregnancy, hypercalcaemia, Addison's disease, porphyria, severe hepatic/renal failure, diabetic ketoacidosis
Precautions: Hypokalaemia, renal/hepatic impairment, elderly, gout, lupus erythematosus, diabetes mellitus, prostatic hypertrophy
Pharmacokinetics:
Period of onset: Onset 2 hr, peak 4 hr, duration 6−12 hr
Excreted some in urine 3−6 hr, excreted in breast milk
Interactions/incompatibilities:
• Increased effect/toxicity: lithium, non-depolarising skeletal muscle relaxants, NSAIDs, chlorpropamide

• Decreased effects of: anti-diabetics
• Decreased absorption of thiazides: cholestyramine, colestipol (give at least 2 hr apart)
• Increased action of: halothane
• Enhanced hypotensive effects: barbiturates, alcohol, MAOIs, narcotics, antihypertensives
• If hypokalaemia: Increased side effects/toxicity: amiodarone, disopyramide, flecainide, quinidine, pimozide, sotalol, cardiac glycosides, allopurinol. Decreased effect: lignocaine, mexiletine, tocainide
• Antagonise diuretic effect: NSAIDs, corticosteroids, oestrogens, combined oral contraceptives, carbenoxolone
• Increased risk of hypokalaemia: indapamide, corticosteroids, other diuretics, carbenoxolone ACTH, acetazolamide, NSAIDs
• Increased risk of postural hypotension: tricyclics
• Risk of hypercalcaemia: calcium salts

Clinical assessment:
• Electrolytes: potassium, sodium, calcium, magnesium, chloride; include blood urea nitrogen, blood sugar, serum creatinine, blood pH, and uric acid
• Potassium replacement if necessary
• Monitor renal function throughout therapy
• Monitor insulin requirement of diabetic patients
• Monitor blood lipids
• Test for glycosuria

Lab. test interferences:
• Estimation of serum protein-bound iodine
• Tests of parathyroid function

Treatment of overdose: Lavage if recently taken orally, activated charcoal. Monitor electrolyte and fluid balance, BP, renal function. Avoid cathartics. Symptomatic and supportive treatment. No specific antidote

NURSING CONSIDERATIONS
Assess:
• Baseline BP, weight, fluid balance

Administer:
• In the morning to avoid interference with sleep if using drug as a diuretic
• With food if nausea occurs; absorption may be decreased slightly

Evaluate:
• Weight, fluid balance daily to determine fluid loss; effect of drug may be decreased if used daily
• Rate depth, rhythm of respiration, effect of exertion
• BP lying, standing; postural hypotension may occur
• Glucose in urine if patient is diabetic
• Improvement in oedema of feet, legs, sacral area daily if medication is being used in congestive cardiac failure
• Improvement in CVP and BP recordings
• Signs of metabolic acidosis: drowsiness, restlessness
• Signs of hypokalaemia: postural hypotension, malaise, fatigue, tachycardia, leg cramps, weakness
• Rashes, pyrexia daily
• Confusion especially in elderly; observe carefully

Teach patient/family:
• To increase fluid intake to 2−3 litres daily unless contraindicated; to rise slowly from lying or sitting position
• To notify clinician of muscle weakness, cramps, nausea, dizziness, joint pain (gout)
• Drug may be taken with food or milk
• That blood sugar may be increased in diabetics
• To take early in day to avoid nocturia

benorylate

Benoral
Func. class.: Non-narcotic analgesic
Chem. class.: Aspirin and paracetamol ester
Legal class.: P

Action: Blocks pain impulses in CNS by inhibition of prostaglandin synthesis; antipyretic action results from inhibition of hypothalamic heat-regulating centre to produce vasodilation to allow heat dissipation

Uses: Mild to moderate pain and inflammation in rheumatic disease and other musculoskeletal disorders, including arthritis; fever

Dosage and routes:
• *Adult:* By mouth *Rheumatic diseases* 4−8 g divided into 2−3 doses with food as needed
• *Mild to moderate pain and pyrexia:* 2 g twice daily with food
Available forms include: Tablets 750 mg, granules 2 g/sachet, suspension 2 g/5 ml. 2 g benorylate is equivalent to 1.15 g aspirin and 0.97 g paracetamol

Side effects/adverse reactions:
HAEM: Rare blood dyscrasias, increased prothrombin time
CNS: Stimulation, drowsiness, dizziness, confusion, convulsion, headache, flushing, hallucinations, coma (in large doses)
GI: Nausea, vomiting, GI bleeding, diarrhoea, heartburn, anorexia, hepatitis
INTEG: Rash, urticaria, bruising
EENT: Tinnitus, hearing loss
RESP: Wheezing
ENDO: Hypoglycaemia

Contraindications: Hypersensitivity to salicylates and paracetamol, GI bleeding, bleeding disorders, children under 12 yr (except for Still's disease) association with Reye's syndrome, lactation, acute renal disease

Precautions: Anaemia, hepatic disease, renal disease, Hodgkin's disease, pregnancy, elderly, dehydration, peptic ulcer

Pharmacokinetics: Benorylate metabolised to salicylate and paracetamol by esterases after absorption. Metabolised by liver, excreted by kidneys, excreted in breast milk

Interactions/incompatibilities:
• Decreased effects of this drug: antacids, steroids, urinary alkalinisers
• Increased effects of salicylate: carbonic anhydrase inhibitors
• Increased blood loss: alcohol, heparin
• Increased effects of: anticoagulants, insulin, methotrexate
• Decreased effects of: probenecid, frusemide
• Decreased blood sugar levels: salicylates

Clinical assessment:
• Liver function tests: enzymes, aspartate aminotransferase, alanine aminotransferase, bilirubin, creatinine if problem anticipated
• Renal function studies: blood urea, urine creatinine if patient has renal impairment, problem anticipated
• Prior drug history; there are many drug interactions

Lab. test interferences:
Increase: Coagulation studies, liver function studies

Treatment of overdose: Measure serum levels of salicylate and paracetamol; lavage, activated charcoal, monitor electrolytes, vital signs, forced alkaline diuresis, correction of acid-base balance. May have to use IV acetylcysteine or oral methionine to correct paracetamol overdose if given within 10−12 hr of drug ingestion
NURSING CONSIDERATIONS

Assess:
• Fluid balance, weight
Administer:
• With food or milk to decrease gastric symptoms; give with or after meals
Perform/provide:
• Repositioning to decrease pain
• Cooling for fever
Evaluate:
• Fluid balance; decreasing output may indicate renal failure (long-term therapy)
• Hepatotoxicity: dark urine, clay-coloured stools, yellowing of skin, sclera, itching, abdominal pain, fever, diarrhoea if patient is on long-term therapy
• Oedema in feet, ankles, legs
Teach patient/family:
• To take with food or milk
• To report any symptoms of hepatotoxicity, renal toxicity, visual changes, ototoxicity, allergic reactions (long-term therapy)
• Not to exceed recommended dosage; acute poisoning may result
• To read label on other non-prescribed drugs; many contain aspirin or paracetamol
• That therapeutic response takes 2 weeks (arthritis)
• To avoid alcohol; GI bleeding may occur
• Report indigestion or black tarry stools

---

benzathine penicillin

Penidural
Func. class.: Antibiotic, broad-spectrum
Chem. class.: Penicillin
Legal class.: POM

Action: Interferes with cell wall replication of susceptible organisms; osmotically unstable cell wall swells, bursts from osmotic pressure

Uses: A depot form of benzyl-penicillin used in mild to moderate bacterial infections due to susceptible organisms
Dosage and routes:
• *Adult:* By mouth 458 mg 3 or 4 times a day
• *Children over 5 yr:* By mouth 229 mg 3 or 4 times a day
• *Children less than 5 yr:* By mouth about 77–154 mg 3 or 4 times a day
Available forms include: Oral suspension 229 mg/5 ml; oral drops, 115 mg/ml
Side effects/adverse reactions:
HAEM: Haemolytic anaemia, increased bleeding time, granulocytopenia
GI: Nausea, diarrhoea, sore mouth, heartburn
INTEG: Rash, urticaria, angio-edema (signs of hypersensitivity)
SYST: Anaphylaxis, joint pains, fever (hypersensitivity)
Contraindications: Hypersensitivity to penicillins
Precautions: History of allergy, renal impairment
Pharmacokinetics: Half-life 30–60 min, excreted in urine, faeces, breast milk
Interactions/incompatibilities:
• Possibly decreased antimicrobial effect of penicillin: tetracyclines, erythromycins, chloramphenicol
• Increased antimicrobial effectiveness of penicillins: aminoglycosides
• Increased penicillin concentrations: aspirin, probenecid
Lab. test interferences:
False positive: Urine glucose, urine protein
Treatment of overdose: Supportive care
NURSING CONSIDERATIONS
Assess:
• Bowel pattern
• Fluid balance
• Patch test to assess allergy,

usually done when penicillin is only
drug of choice, or patient gives
history of allergy
• Any patient with compromised
renal system since drug is excreted
slowly in poor renal system function; toxicity may occur rapidly
Administer:
• On an empty stomach for best
absorption
• Drug after culture and sensitivity
has been completed
Perform/provide:
• Resuscitation equipment
• Adequate fluid intake (2 litres
daily) during diarrhoea episodes
Evaluate:
• Fluid balance; report haematuria, oliguria since penicillin in
high doses is nephrotoxic
• Therapeutic response: absence
of fever, purulent drainage, redness inflammation
• Bowel pattern during treatment
• Skin eruptions after administration of penicillin to 1 week after
discontinuing drug
• Respiratory status: rate,
character, wheezing, tightness in
chest
• Allergies before initiation of
treatment, reaction of each medication; highlight allergies on
nursing care plan
Teach patient/family:
• To take complete course
• To take oral penicillin on empty
stomach with full glass of water
• Culture may be taken after completed course of medication
• To report sore throat, fever,
fatigue; could indicate superimposed infection
• To wear or carry ID if allergic to
penicillins
• To notify nurse of diarrhoea

benzhexol

Artane, Broflex
Func. class.: Antimuscarinic
Chem. class.: Synthetic tertiary
amine
Legal class.: POM

Action: Decreases cholinergic
function in CNS, correcting the
imbalance in cholinergic and
dopaminergic function and
reducing extrapyramidal effects
Uses: Parkinsonian symptoms,
drug-induced extrapyramidal
symptoms (except tardive dyskinesia)
Dosage and routes:
• *Adult:* By mouth 1 mg daily increased by 1−2 mg every 3−5 days
until symptoms controlled, to a
total of 5−15 mg daily in 3−4
divided doses
Available forms include: Tablets 2,
5 mg; elixir 5 mg/5 ml
Side effects/adverse reactions:
CNS: Confusion, anxiety, restlessness, irritability, delusions, hallucinations, dizziness
EENT: Blurred vision, photophobia, dilated pupils, difficulty
swallowing
CV: Palpitations, tachycardia
GI: Dryness of mouth, constipation, nausea, vomiting, abdominal distress, paralytic ileus
GU: Urinary retention
Contraindications: Hypersensitivity, tardive dyskinesia
Precautions: Hypertension, cardiac
disorders, liver or kidney disorders, elderly, arteriosclerosis,
prostatic hypertrophy, narrow-
angle glaucoma, myasthenia gravis,
GI/GU obstruction, risk of abuse
Pharmacokinetics:
By mouth: Onset 1 hr, peak
2−3 hr, duration 6−12 hr, excreted
in urine
Interactions/incompatibilities:

• Increased anticholinergic effects: antihistamines, tricyclic antidepressants, MAOIs, phenothiazines, amantadine, nefopam, disopyramide

NURSING CONSIDERATIONS

Assess:
• Fluid balance
• Bowel patterns
• Age of patient — over 65 yr slightly more sensitive and require smaller amounts of drugs

Administer:
• Orally following the dosage regimen for suitable gradual introduction
• At bedtime if a single daily dose is given
• After food to prevent nausea, or before food to reduce dry mouth

Perform/provide:
• Frequent drinks to prevent a dry mouth

Evaluate:
• Therapeutic response: decreased rigidity of muscle spasm, tremors slow movement, excessive salivation. Relieving depression and mental inertia
• Input and output of fluids, observe for retention
• Minor side effects — dryness of mouth, constipation, urinary retention, blurring of vision
• Optimal response with minimal side effects

Teach patient/family:
• Not to discontinue medication without medical advice. Dose changes by gradual increments and tapered off slowly
• Not to take any other drugs without medical advice

benzoyl peroxide

Acetoxyl, Acnegel, Benoxyl, Benzagel, Nericur, Panoxyl
Func. class.: Antiseptic, keratolytic
Legal class.: P

Action: Antibacterial activity especially against predominant bacteria causing acne. Also keratolytic and sebostatic

Uses: Acne vulgaris

Dosage and routes:
• *Adult:* Topical. Apply to affected area once or twice daily. Start with lower strengths. Children under 12 yr — seek clinician's or pharmacist's advice

Available forms include: Topical cleansers, lotions, creams, gels 2.5%, 5%, 10%

Side effects/adverse reactions:
INTEG: Local skin irritation, reddening, scaling, increased peeling in first few weeks (discontinue temporarily)

Contraindications: Hypersensitivity to benzoic acid derivatives

Precautions: Avoid contact with eyes, mouth and mucous membranes; may bleach fabrics. Care on sensitive areas (e.g. neck)

Pharmacokinetics:
Topical: 50% absorbed through skin, metabolised to benzoic acid, excreted in urine

Interactions/incompatibilities:
None known

NURSING CONSIDERATIONS

Perform/provide:
• Gloves to apply, then wash hands immediately to avoid irritation

Evaluate:
• Effectiveness, indicated by decreased acne
• Other factors which help or aggravate condition
• Allergic reaction e.g. rash, irri-

tation, dermatitis; use should be discontinued

Teach patient/family:
• To avoid application to unaffected skin, nose, eyes, mucous membranes
• To discontinue if rash develops
• May cause transitory warmth or stinging over area treated
• May stain hair or clothing. Avoid contact
• Cosmetics may be used over treated area
• That some dryness and peeling is to be expected

---

benztropine mesylate

Cogentin
Func. class.: Antimuscarinic
Chem. class.: Tertiary amine
Legal class.: POM

Action: Antagonises central cholinergic activity, which decreases involuntary movements

Uses: Parkinsonism, drug-induced extrapyramidal symptoms (not tardive dyskinesia)

Dosage and routes:
Parkinsonism
• *Adult:* By mouth 0.5−1 mg daily usually at bedtime, gradually increased to maximum 6 mg daily as necessary. Usual maintenance dose 1−4 mg daily in single or divided doses

Extrapyramidal symptoms
• *Adult:* IM/IV injection 1−2 mg; repeated if symptoms reappear

Available forms include: Tablets 2 mg (scored); injection IM, IV 1 mg/ml (2 ml)

Side effects/adverse reactions:
CNS: Confusion, anxiety, numbness of fingers, disorientation memory impairment, listlessness, hallucinations, exacerbation of pre-existing psychotic symptoms, sedation, depression, dizziness

EENT: Blurred vision, dilated pupils
INTEG: Allergic rash, anhidrosis
CV: Tachycardia
GI: Dryness of mouth, constipation, nausea, vomiting
GU: Hesitancy, retention, dysuria

Contraindications: Hypersensitivity, child under 3 yr

Precautions: Pregnancy, elderly, lactation, tachycardia, prostatic hypertrophy, narrow-angle glaucoma, myasthenia gravis, GI obstruction, abnormalities of sweating, children. May impair ability/alertness for driving etc. Cumulative action. Mental disorders, cardiovascular disease, urinary retention, hepatic/renal impairment. Do not withdraw abruptly, liable to abuse

Pharmacokinetics:
IM/IV: Onset 15 min, duration 6−10 hr
By mouth: Onset 1 hr, duration 6−10 hr

Interactions/incompatibilities:
• Antagonism of GI effect: cisapride, domperidone, metoclopramide
• Increased antimuscarinic side effects: other drugs with antimuscarinic effects, nefopam, disopyramide tricyclics, MAOIs, antihistamines, phenothiazines, amantadine
• Reduced absorption: ketoconazole
• Decreased plasma levels: phenothiazines
• Reduced effect: sublingual nitrates

Treatment of overdose: Induce emesis or gastric lavage if recent ingestion. Physostigmine salicylate to reverse anticholinergic symptoms. Symptomatic and supportive treatment. Possible use of short-acting barbiturate for CNS excitement (NB: subsequent depression, also avoid convulsant stimulants), artificial respiration, local miotic, ice bags, vasopressor, fluids, darkened room

NURSING CONSIDERATIONS

Administer:

• At bedtime to avoid drowsiness during day

• With or after meals to prevent gastric upset; may be given with fluids other than water

• Parenteral dose slowly. Patient should stay in bed for at least 1 hr afterwards

Perform/provide:

• Mouthcare and mouthwashes to relieve dry mouth

Evaluate:

• Response to drug; parkinsonism, extrapyramidal symptoms e.g. shuffling gait, muscle rigidity, involuntary movements should decrease

• Dose may need to be increased or changed in the event of tolerance or long term treatment

• Urinary output; retention may occur

• Fluid intake, fibre in diet and encourage exercise if constipation occurs

• GI problems—especially paralytic ileus

• Worsening of mental symptoms during early treatment e.g. CNS depression, change in mood or affect

Teach patient/family:

• Drug must not be discontinued suddenly, but gradually over 1 week

• To avoid driving or operating machinery as drowsiness may occur

• To avoid medicines that have not been prescribed, especially those for coughs and colds and antihistamines

• Not to be taken with alcohol

benzylpenicillin (Penicillin G)

Crystapen, combination products
Func. class.: Antibiotic, broad-spectrum
Chem. class.: Penicillin
Legal class.: POM

Action: Interferes with cell wall replication of susceptible organisms; osmotically unstable cell wall swells, bursts from osmotic pressure

Uses: Bacterial infections due to susceptible organisms, including tonsillitis, otitis media, erysipelas, streptococcal endocarditis, meningococcal and pneumococcal meningitis, prophylaxis in limb amputation, diphtheria, gas gangrene, gonococcal infections, syphilis, tetanus

Dosage and routes:

Mild-moderate infections

• *Adult:* IM or slow IV injection 0.6−1.2 g daily in 2−4 divided doses, increased up to 2.4 g daily if necessary

• *Child:* 1 month−12 yr 10−20 mg/kg daily in 4 divided doses

• *Neonate:* 30 mg/kg daily in 2−4 divided doses

Bacterial endocarditis

• Slow IV injection or infusion up to 7.2 g daily in 4−6 divided doses

Meningitis

• *Child 1 month−12 yr:* Slow IV injection or infusion 20−40 mg/kg daily in 4−6 divided doses

• *Neonate:* 60−90 mg/kg daily in 3−4 divided doses

Available forms include: Injection IV/IM 600 mg

Side effects/adverse reactions:

HAEM: Haemolytic anaemia, increased bleeding time, granulocytopenia

GI: Nausea, diarrhoea, sore mouth, heartburn

INTEG: Rash, urticaria, angio-edema (signs of hypersensitivity)

CNS: Convulsions, encepha-lopathy, and paralysis (high/intrathecal dosage)

META: Hypokalaemia, hyper-natraemia

SYST: Anaphylaxis, joint pains, fever (hypersensitivity)

Contraindications: Hypersensitivity to penicillins

Precautions: History of allergy, renal impairment

Pharmacokinetics:

IM: Peak 12−24 hr, half-life 0.5 hr. Metabolised in liver, excreted in faeces, breast milk

Interactions/incompatibilities:

• Possibly decreased antimicrobial effectiveness of penicillin: tetra-cyclines, erythromycins, chlor-amphenicol

• Increased antimicrobial effec-tiveness of penicillin: amino-glycosides

• Increased penicillin concen-trations when used with: aspirin, probenecid

Lab. test interferences:

False positive: Urine glucose, urine protein

Treatment of overdose: Supportive care; blood levels reduced by haemodialysis

NURSING CONSIDERATIONS

Assess:

• Patch test to assess allergy, when penicillin is only drug of choice or history of allergy to penicillins

• Bowel pattern

• Fluid balance

Administer:

• Drug after culture and sensitivity has been completed

Perform/provide:

• Emergency resuscitation kit in case of anaphylaxis

• Adequate fluid intake (2 litres daily) during diarrhoea episodes

• Aseptic technique during IV/IM injection

• Observe IV injection site for inflammation

Evaluate:

• Therapeutic effectiveness: ab-sence of fever, draining wounds

• Fluid balance, report haema-turia, oliguria since penicillin in high doses is nephrotoxic

• Any patient with compromised renal system since drug is excreted slowly in poor renal system func-tion; toxicity may occur rapidly

• Bowel pattern before and during treatment

• Skin eruptions after adminis-tration of penicillin to 1 week after discontinuing drug

• Respiratory status: rate, charac-ter, wheezing, tightness in chest

• Allergies before initiation of treatment, reaction of each medi-cation; highlight allergies on nursing care plan

Teach patient/family:

• Aspects of drug therapy, includ-ing need to complete course of medication to ensure organism death; culture may be taken after completed course

• To report sore throat, fever, fa-tigue; could indicate superimposed infection

• To wear or carry Medic Alert ID if allergic to penicillins

• To notify nurse of diarrhoea

• To report any rash

---

betahistine hydrochloride

Serc

Func. class.: Vasodilator
Chem. class.: Histamine analogue
Legal class.: POM

Action: Reduces endolymphatic pressure

Uses: Vertigo, tinnitus, hearing loss associated with Meniere's disease

Dosage and routes:

• *Adult:* By mouth initially 16 mg 3 times daily, maintenance 24−48 mg daily in divided doses

Available forms include: Tablets, 8, 16 mg

Side effects/adverse reactions:
GI: Nausea

Contraindications:
Phaeochromocytoma

Precautions: Asthma, pregnancy

Pharmacokinetics: Peak 3−5 hr. Excreted in urine (metabolites)

Interactions/incompatibilities:
Antihistamines − antagonism (theoretical)

Treatment of overdose: Symptomatic management; gastric lavage may be indicated

NURSING CONSIDERATIONS

Administer:
• With food or after food

Perform/provide:
• Storage in original package

Evaluate:
• Benefits of therapy
• Side effects

Teach patient/family:
• About side effects; headache, nausea and rash and need to inform clinician
• Not to remove from pack until just before taking dose (tablets are hygroscopic)

---

betamethasone/ betamethasone sodium phosphate

Betnelan, Betnesol

Func. class.: Synthetic corticosteroid

Chem. class.: Glucocorticoid, long-acting

Legal class.: POM

Action: Decreases inflammation by suppression of migration of polymorphonuclear leucocytes, fibroblasts, reversal of increased capillary permeability and lysosomal stabilisation

Uses: Suppression of inflammatory, auto-immune, and allergic disease, adrenal hyperplasia, cerebral oedema, severe shock, immunosuppression

Dosage and routes:
• *Adult:* By mouth 0.5−5 mg/daily in divided doses; IM or IV infusion 4−20 mg (as sodium phosphate) up to 4 times in 24 hr
• *Child:* less than 1 yr: Slow IV injection 1 mg; 1−5 yr: 2 mg; 6−12 yr: 4 mg

Available forms include: Tablets 500 mcg (as base or sodium phosphate); Injection 4 mg/ml (as sodium phosphate)

Side effects/adverse reactions:
INTEG: Acne, poor wound healing, flushing, bruising, skin thinning

CNS: Depression, mental disturbances, headache, raised intracranial pressure, mood changes

CV: Thromboembolic disorders

MS: Fractures, osteoporosis, weakness, muscle wasting

GI: Gastrointestinal disturbances, peptic ulcer, increased appetite, pancreatitis

EENT: Oral fungal infections, increased intraocular pressure, cataract

ENDO: Hyperglycaemia, adrenal suppression, growth retardation (children)

MISC: Increased susceptibility to infection, moon face (Cushingoid symptoms)

Contraindications: Hypersensitivity, systemic infection (untreated), live virus vaccine immunisation

Precautions: Psychosis, hypertension, congestive heart failure, surgery or intercurrent illness, elderly, peptic ulcer, pregnancy, diabetes mellitus, glaucoma, osteoporosis, seizure disorders, myasthenia gravis; withdrawal should be gradual

Pharmacokinetics:

Period of onset: Onset 1−2 hr, peak 1 hr, duration 3 days

IM/IV: Onset 10 min, peak 4−8 hr, duration 1−1½ days

Metabolised in liver, excreted in urine as steroids

Interactions/incompatibilities:

• Decreased action of betamethasone: cholestyramine, colestipol, barbiturates, rifampicin, ephedrine, phenytoin, theophylline

• Possibly decreased effects of: anticonvulsants, antidiabetics, antihypertensives, diuretics, non-steroidal anti-inflammatory agents

• Increased effects of anticoagulants

Clinical assessment:

• Assess blood potassium levels and blood sugar levels while on long term treatment

• Prescribe lowest effective dose

• Prescribe in a single dose to be given in the morning to prevent adrenal suppression

NURSING CONSIDERATIONS

Assess:

• Baseline BP, weight and fluid balance

Administer:

• Injections after shaking solution

• IM injections deeply into large muscle, rotate sites, use 19G needle

• Orally with food or milk to decrease GI symptoms

Evaluate:

• Weight daily. Inform clinician if weekly gain greater than 2 kg

• BP 4 hrly and pulse. Inform clinician of chest pain

• Fluid balance chart. Be alert for decreasing urinary output and oedema

• Response to treatment; decreased respiratory embarrassment, decreased inflammation

• Temperature; drug may mask signs of infection even after course has been completed

• Signs of potassium depletion e.g. paraesthesiae, fatigue, nausea, vomiting, depression, polyuria, dysrhythmias, weakness

• Cardiac symptoms e.g. oedema, hypotension

• Aggression, behavioural change, change in mood or affect

Teach patient/family:

• To carry identity as a steroid user

• Clinician must be informed if response to drug decreases; dose may need adjustment

• Drug must not be discontinued suddenly or adrenal crisis may result

• Medicines should be avoided unless prescribed, particularly aspirin, cough or cold mixtures containing alcohol

• All aspects of treatment and recognition of Cushingoid symptoms

• To recognise symptoms of adrenal insufficiency e.g. nausea, anorexia, fatigue, dizziness, dyspnoea, weakness, joint pain

---

betamethasone dipropionate

Diprosone

Func. class.: Topical corticosteroid

Chem. class.: Synthetic fluorinated agent

Legal class.: POM

Action: Possesses antipruritic, anti-inflammatory actions

Uses: Psoriasis, eczema, severe dermatitis and inflammatory skin disorders

Dosage and routes:

• *Adult and child:* Apply thinly to affected area once or twice daily

Available forms include: Ointment

0.05%; cream 0.05%; lotion 0.05%

Side effects/adverse reactions:
INTEG: Acne, hypertrichosis, perioral dermatitis, hypopigmentation, atrophy, striae, secondary infection

Contraindications: Hypersensitivity to corticosteroids, long-term therapy, rosacea, acne, perioral dermatitis, tuberculosis, viral skin infection, untreated fungal or bacterial skin infection

Precautions: Pregnancy, large areas of broken skin

NURSING CONSIDERATIONS
Administer:
• Only to affected areas; do not get in eyes
• Leave uncovered or use light dressing; do not cover with occlusive dressing
• Only to dermatoses; do not use on weeping, denuded, or infected area
• Apply thinly

Perform/provide:
• Cleansing before application of drug
• Treatment for a few days after area has cleared

Evaluate:
• Therapeutic response: absence of severe itching, patches on skin, flaking
• Temperature; if fever develops, drug should be discontinued

Teach patient/family:
• To avoid sunlight on affected area; burns may occur
• That ointment is not curative; rebound exacerbation may occur when discontinued

betamethasone valerate

Betnovate, Betnovate-RD
Func. class.: Topical corticosteroid
Chem. class.: Synthetic fluorinated agent (potent)
Legal class.: POM

Action: Possesses antipruritic, anti-inflammatory actions

Uses: Psoriasis, eczema, contact dermatitis, pruritus and other severe inflammatory skin disorders unresponsive to less potent corticosteroids

Dosage and routes:
• *Adult and child:* Apply thinly to affected area two or three times daily—for child see precautions
Available forms include: Ointment 0.025%, 0.1%; cream 0.025%, 0.1%; lotion 0.1%; scalp application 0.1%

Side effects/adverse reactions:
SYST: Prolonged use, large amounts, extensive area: hypercorticism, Hypothalamic-pituitary-adrenal (HPA) axis suppression
INTEG: Acne, hypertrichosis, perioral dermatitis, spread of untreated infection, thinning, dilatation of superficial blood vessels, striae, depigmentation, vellus hair

Contraindications: Dermatoses in children under 1 yr. Hypersensitivity to corticosteroids or other constituents, scalp/skin infections, rosacea, acne, perioral dermatitis, peri-anal and genital pruritus, ulcerative conditions

Precautions: Pregnancy, lactation, psoriasis, secondary infection, children, avoid long-term continuous therapy especially on face. Avoid eyes

Interactions/incompatibilities: None known

NURSING CONSIDERATIONS
Administer:

• To affected areas wearing gloves. Do not get in eyes
• Cover treated area with occlusive dressing (only if prescribed), change 12 hrly. Occlusive dressings will increase absorption and systemic side effects
• Apply only to affected area, avoid raw, weeping or infected areas

Perform/provide:
• Cleansing before application
• Continued treatment for a few days after inflammation has resolved

Evaluate:
• Temperature daily; if fever develops clinician should be informed and treatment should discontinue
• Monitor quantity of preparation used — more than 100 g per week of 0.1% likely to cause adrenal suppression
• In childhood or on face — limit use to 5 days, do not use occlusive dressings
• Monitor adrenal function if prolonged use
• Response to treatment; itching and flaking should subside

Teach patient/family:
• Must avoid exposing treated area to strong sunshine; sunburn may occur
• To use sparingly
• To avoid eyes
• That ointment is not curative; rebound exacerbation may occur when discontinued

---

betaxolol hydrochloride

Kerlone
Func. class.: Antihypertensive
Chem. class.: Cardioselective β-blocker
Legal class.: POM

Action: Preferentially blocks cardiac β-adrenergic receptors, reducing response to sympathetic stimulation

Uses: Hypertension

Dosage and routes:
By mouth, 20 mg daily increased to 40 mg daily if required; 10 mg daily in elderly patients
Available forms include: Tablets, 20 mg

Side effects/adverse reactions:
RESP: Bronchospasm
CV: Bradycardia, heart failure, peripheral vasoconstriction, exacerbation of Raynaud's disease or intermittent claudication, paraesthesiae, hypotension, atrioventricular block, cardiac insufficiency
EENT: Dry eyes
GI: Disturbances
SYST: Fatigue

Contraindications: Uncontrolled heart failure, second or third degree heart block, cardiogenic shock, bradycardia (less than 50/min); history of asthma or obstructive airways disease

Precautions: Pregnancy, breast feeding; avoid abrupt withdrawal in angina; reduced dose in renal impairment; history of cardiovascular disease; diabetes mellitus; inform anaesthetist before general anaesthesia

Pharmacokinetics: Peak plasma concentration within 4–6 hr. Half-life 16–20 hr, excreted in urine as unchanged drug and metabolites

Interactions/incompatibilities:
Toxicity enhanced by myocardial depressants or drugs which depress atrioventricular conduction such as verapamil and related calcium channel blockers

Treatment of overdose: Atropine for bradycardia; supportive care

NURSING CONSIDERATIONS

Assess:
• Baseline BP (lying and standing) and pulse, respirations

• For history of chronic obstructive airways disease/asthma

Administer:

• Orally with full glass of water

Perform/provide:

• BP (lying and standing), pulse for bradycardia

Evaluate:

• Therapeutic response: reduction in blood pressure to required level

• Side effects e.g. headache, weight gain, bradycardia

Teach patient/family:

• Not to stop drug unless advised by clinician

• To change position slowly to avoid dizziness

• About possible sleep disturbances/nightmares, GI upsets and cold extremities

betaxolol HCl (ophthalmic)

Betoptic

Func. class.: Antihypertensive, ocular

Chem. class.: Cardioselective β-blocker

Legal class.: POM

Action: Reduces intra-ocular pressure, probably by reducing the rate of production of aqueous humour

Uses: Chronic simple glaucoma, ocular hypertension

Dosage and routes:

• *Adult:* Instil one drop into affected eye(s) twice daily

Available forms include: Eyedrops 0.5% (base)

Side effects/adverse reactions:

EENT: Eye irritation, transitory dry eyes, tearing, allergic blepharo-conjunctivitis

Contraindications: Sinus bradycardia greater than first-degree block, history of cardiogenic shock, overt cardiac failure, hypersensitivity, children

Precautions: Concurrent systemic beta-blocker or adrenergic psychotropic therapy, diabetes, thyrotoxicosis, general anaesthesia, soft contact lenses, pregnancy, lactation, asthma, history of obstructive air-ways disease, systemic absorption may occur

Pharmacokinetics: Systemic absorption may occur; extensively metabolised and excreted in urine; half-life 17 hr

Interactions/incompatibilities: If significant systemic absorption occurs:-

• Greatly enhances hypertensive effects of adrenaline, noradrenaline, amphetamines, phenylephrine, phenylpropanolamine and other sympathomimetic amines

• Increases toxicity of: calcium antagonists, anti-arrhythmic drugs, rauwolfia alkaloids, mefloquine, cardiac glycosides, sotalol

• Increased risk of vasoconstriction with ergotamine

• Mydriasis when given with adrenaline

• Increased hypotensive effect: alcohol, anaesthetics, antihypertensives, anxiolytics, hypnotics, diuretics

• Increased effect of: anti-diabetics

• Increased risk of withdrawal hypertension of clonidine

• Reduced effect of xamoterol and reduced β-blockade

Clinical assessment:

• Check history of cardiac conditions, asthma and chronic obstructive airways disease

Treatment of overdose: Flush from eye(s) with warm tap water

NURSING CONSIDERATIONS

Administer:

• Using correct technique to instil drops

Perform/provide:

- Care for dryness of eyes
- Safe environment if visually handicapped

Evaluate:
- Pulse 4 hrly, respirations
- Intra-ocular pressure every 4 weeks at different times of day
- Side effects especially those affecting the eye

Teach patient/family:
- Correct method of instilling eye drops and care of equipment
- To report: eye irritation, visual changes, breathing problems, sweating, flushing, rashes
- Blurred vision will decrease with continued use. Withdraw slowly
- To discard after 4 weeks of opening eye-drops

---

bezafibrate

Bezalip, Bezalip-Mono
Func. class.: Hypolipidaemic agent
Chem. class.: Clofibrate analogue
Legal class.: POM

Action: Decreases serum triglycerides, reduces LDL-cholesterol, raises HDL-cholesterol
Uses: Severe hyperlipidaemia or hypertriglyceridaemia resistant to modification of diet

Dosage and routes:
- By mouth, 200 mg 3 times daily; may be reduced to twice daily in hypertriglyceridaemia; modified-release tablets, 400 mg daily in evening

Available forms include: Tablets, 200 mg; modified-release tablets 400 mg

Side effects/adverse reactions:
GI: Nausea, abdominal discomfort
GU: Impotence (rare)
INTEG: Pruritus, urticaria
SYST: Hypersensitivity
MS: Myositis

Contraindications: Severe renal or hepatic impairment, primary biliary cirrhosis, hypoalbuminaemia, gallbladder disease, nephrotic syndrome, pregnancy, lactation, hypersensitivity
Precautions: Anticoagulant therapy, moderate renal impairment
Pharmacokinetics: Peak plasma concentrations 2 hr, progressive hypolipidaemic response over several weeks. Half-life 2 hr, excreted in urine

Interactions/incompatibilities:
- May increase effects of: anticoagulant, antidiabetic agents

NURSING CONSIDERATIONS
Administer:
- In the evening with food, swallowed whole and not chewed if modified release

Perform/provide:
- Smaller meals if 'fullness' a problem

Evaluate:
- Side-effects including pruritus

Teach patient/family:
- To continue with other measures — maintain ideal weight, low fat diet, no smoking, stress management and reduce alcohol intake. Encourage compliance
- To avoid pregnancy

---

bisacodyl

~~NHS~~ Dulcolax
Func. class.: Laxative, stimulant
Chem. class.: Diphenylmethane
Legal class.: P

Action: Acts directly on intestine by increasing motor activity
Uses: Short-term treatment of constipation, bowel or rectal preparation for surgery, examination

Dosage and routes:
Constipation
- *Adult:* By mouth, 5–10 mg at night, increased if necessary to 15–20 mg; rectal 10 mg in the morning

• *Child:* By mouth, 5 mg at night; rectal 5 mg in the morning
Bowel preparation
• *Adult:* By mouth 10 mg at night for 2 days before procedure, plus 10 mg by rectum 1 hr before procedure if necessary
Available forms include: Enteric coated tablets 5 mg; suppository 5, 10 mg
Side effects/adverse reactions:
GI: Cramps, diarrhoea, rectal burning (suppositories)
META: Hypokalaemia, electrolyte and fluid imbalances (prolonged or excessive use)
Contraindications: Hypersensitivity, intestinal obstruction
Precautions: Children, inflammatory bowel disease, rectal fissures, ulcerated haemorrhoids
Pharmacokinetics:
Tablets taken after food act in 10−12 hr
Suppositories produce a motion within 20−60 min of insertion
Partially absorbed, metabolised by liver, excreted in urine, bile, faeces, breast milk
NURSING CONSIDERATIONS
Assess:
• Normal bowel function/pattern
Administer:
• Alone to enhance absorption; should not be taken within an hour of other drugs, antacids, cimetidine or milk
Evaluate:
• Response; bowel action should result
Perform/provide:
• Inform clinician if cramping, rectal bleeding, nausea or vomiting occur; drug should be discontinued
Teach patient/family:
• Tablets should be swallowed whole; they should not be chewed
• Bowel movements do not always occur daily
• Laxatives should not be used long term; bowel tone will be lost

• Tablets should not be taken if there is abdominal pain, nausea, vomiting
• To tell clinician if constipation is not relieved or if symptoms of electrolyte imbalance occur: muscle cramps, pain, weakness, dizziness
• Of dietary changes to avoid constipation

bisoprolol fumarate

Emcor, Monocor
Func. class.: Antihypertensive and anti-anginal agent
Chem. class.: Cardioselective β-blocker
Legal class.: POM

Action: Preferentially blocks β-adrenoceptors in the heart, reducing response to sympathetic stimulation. Some action on peripheral vasculature
Uses: Hypertension, angina
Dosage and routes:
• By mouth 10 mg daily (5 mg daily adequate in some patients); maximum dose, 20 mg daily
Available forms include: Tablets, 5, 10 mg
Side effects/adverse reactions:
RESP: Bronchospasm
CNS: Headache, dizziness, paraesthesia, sleep disturbances
CV: Bradycardia, exacerbation of Raynaud's disease or intermittent claudication, hypotension, atrioventricular block, cardiac insufficiency
EENT: Dry eyes
INTEG: Rashes, sweating
GI: Disturbances
SYST: Lassitude
Contraindications: Untreated heart failure, second or third degree heart block, cardiogenic shock, severe bradycardia (less

than 50/min), severe hypotension, severe asthma

Precautions: Pregnancy, breast feeding, prolonged PR conduction interval, poor cardiac reserve, peripheral circulatory disease, diabetes mellitus, obstructive airways disease; avoid abrupt withdrawal in angina; reduce dose in renal or hepatic impairment; inform anaesthetist before general anaesthesia

Pharmacokinetics: Half-life 10–12 hr, metabolised in liver and excreted in urine as inactive metabolites and unchanged drug

Interactions/incompatibilities:

• Increased effects of bisoprolol: anaesthetics, other antihypertensives, diuretics, cimetidine

• Possibly increased toxicity: anti-arrhythmics, calcium channel blockers, cardiac glycosides, sympathomimetics (hypertension), ergotamine

• Increased effects of: antidiabetic agents

• Decreased effects of bisoprolol: NSAIDs, corticosteroids, oestrogens, oral contraceptives, rifampicin

Treatment of overdose: Supportive symptomatic care

NURSING CONSIDERATIONS

Assess:
• Baseline BP (lying and standing) and pulse
• Respirations

Administer:
• With a full glass of water

Perform/provide:
• BP (lying and standing), pulse (for bradycardia) 4-hrly

Evaluate:
• Weight gain, GI upsets and other side effects
• Therapeutic response: reduction in BP to required level
• Reduction in chest pain

Teach patient/family:

• Do not stop unless advised by clinician
• Sleep disturbances and nightmares may occur
• To report any side effects e.g. cold extremities

bleomycin sulphate

Func. class.: Antineoplastic
Chem. class.: Glycopeptide antibiotic
Legal class.: POM

Action: Inhibits synthesis of DNA, RNA, protein; replication is decreased by binding to DNA, which causes strand splitting; drug is phase specific in the G_2 and M phases

Uses: Squamous cell carcinoma, Hodgkin's disease and other lymphomas, malignant effusion of serous cavities, testicular teratoma, malignant melanoma

Dosage and routes: Dosage varies with indication and concomitant therapy and should be individualised for each patient. Usual dose ranges:

• *Adult:* IM/IV 15–60 units weekly, total dose usually no greater than 500 units; IV infusion 15 units daily for 10 days or 30 units daily for 5 days; intracavity, for malignant effusions, 60 units/100 ml sodium chloride 0.9%

• *Elderly:* IM/IV 15–30 units weekly, total dose usually no greater than 100–300 units

Available forms include: Injection 15 units

Side effects/adverse reactions:
SYST: Anaphylaxis, fever
GI: Nausea, anorexia, stomatitis
INTEG: Rash, hyperkeratosis, nail changes, alopecia, hyperpigmentation
RESP: Fibrosis (potentially fatal), pneumonitis, wheezing

CV: Hypotension, thrombophlebitis

Contraindications: Hypersensitivity, pregnancy, lactation, reduced lung function, pulmonary infection

Precautions: Renal impairment, respiratory disease, lymphoma (increased risk of anaphylaxis)

Pharmacokinetics: Half-life 2 hr when creatinine clearance is 35 ml/min; for lower clearance, half-life is increased. Metabolised in tissues (except lung, skin), 50% excreted in urine (unchanged)

Interactions/incompatibilities:
• Increased toxicity: other antineoplastics or radiation therapy
• Risk of respiratory failure if general anaesthetic given with high inspired oxygen concentrations; particularly if cummulative dose of bleomycin is more than 100 units

Clinical assessment:
• Obtain chest X-ray before treatment commences and weekly throughout treatment and for one month after

NURSING CONSIDERATIONS
Assess:
• Baseline temperature
Administer:
• Antiemetic 30–60 min before drug as prescribed to prevent vomiting
• Analgesia for stomatitis as ordered
• As a freshly prepared solution; discard that is unused
Perform/provide:
• Encouragement for deep breathing exercises taught by physiotherapist
• Mouthwashes 3–4 times daily and gentle mouth care; a soft tooth brust and unwaxed dental floss should be used
• Support in bed to facilitate breathing
Evaluate:
• Dyspnoea, unproductive cough, chest pain, tachypnoea, fatigue, tachycardia, pallor, lethargy
• Food preferances
• Effects of alopecia on body image; discuss feelings about body changes
• Oral mucosa 8 hrly for dryness, sores, ulceration, white patches, bleeding, dysphagia
• Injection site for local irritation, pain, burning, discolouration
• Severe allergic reaction e.g. rash, pruritus, urticaria, purpuric skin lesions, itching, hot flushes can occur 3–5 hr post administration

Teach patient/family:
• Any side effects must be reported to clinician or nurse
• Any respiratory changes or coughing must be reported
• That hair may be lost during treatment but a wig or hair piece may be worn (available free on NHS). New hair may be different in colour or texture
• That mouth should be examined once a day; bleeding, white spots, ulcers should be reported
• That short-term pain can be experienced

---

botulism antitoxin

Func. class.: Trivalent antitoxin
Chem. class.: Antitoxin globulins
Legal class.: POM

Action: Neutralises toxins A, B and E produced by the bacterium *Clostridium botulinum* types A, B, and E

Uses: Post-exposure prophylaxis and treatment of botulism

Dosage and routes:
• *Prophylaxis:* IM injection 20 ml as soon as possible after exposure
• *Treatment:* Slow IV infusion, 20 ml diluted to 100 ml with 0.9% sodium chloride, then 10 ml 2–

4 hr later if necessary; further doses at intervals of 12–24 hr

Available forms include: Available from designated holding centres

Side effects/adverse reactions:

SYST: Hypersensitivity

Precautions: Asthma, allergic rhinitis, other allergic conditions; ineffective in infantile botulism

Clinical assessment: Previous history of antitoxin administration or allergic conditions should be checked before administration; prior sensitivity test should be carried out (using diluted antitoxin if history of allergy)

NURSING CONSIDERATIONS

Administer:

• IM or slow IV infusion as directed by clinician

Teach patient/family:

• That there may be mild discomfort at the injection site

---

bretylium tosylate

Bretylate, Min-I-Jet Bretylium Tosylate

Func. class.: Anti-arrhythmic (class II/III)

Chem. class.: Quaternary ammonium compound

Legal class.: POM

Action: Inhibits release of noradrenaline in postganglionic nerve endings; prolongs duration of cardiac action potential

Uses: Ventricular arrhythmias resistant to other treatment

Dosage and routes:

• *Adult:* IM 5 mg/kg repeated after 6–8 hr if required then 5–10 mg/kg every 6–8 hr; slow IV injection 5–10 mg/kg over 8–10 min, repeated after 1–2 hr if required to maximum dose 30 mg/kg; maintenance 1–2 mg/min by IV infusion or IM dose as above

Available forms include: Injection (IV, IM, IV infusion) 50 mg/ml

Side effects/adverse reactions:

GI: Nausea, vomiting

CV: Hypotension, transient hypertension, tachycardia, ectopic beats, bradycardia

MS: Tissue necrosis at injection site (restrict volume at any site to 5 ml)

Contraindications: Hypersensitivity, digitalis toxicity, phaeochromocytoma

Precautions: Renal disease, pulmonary hypertension, severe aortic stenosis

Pharmacokinetics:

IV: Onset 5 min

IM: Onset ½–2 hr, peak 6–9 hr, duration 24 hr

Half-life 4–17 hr, excreted unchanged by kidneys (70%–80% in 24 hr), not metabolised

Interactions/incompatibilities:

• Increased effects of bretylium: other antiarrhythmics

• Increased effects of: sympathomimetics

• Toxicity: digitalis

Clinical assessment:

• Patient requires cardiac monitoring

Treatment of overdose: Supportive symptomatic care; extreme caution if catecholamines considered necessary for hypotension (effects may be enhanced, use only under expert supervision)

NURSING CONSIDERATIONS

Assess:

• Baseline vital signs and ECG

Administer:

• By slow injection 8–10 min or infusion as prescribed

• To patient on strict bed rest, under close supervision

Perform/provide:

• Resuscitation equipment in case of further cardiac arrhythmias

• In cardiac arrest, must continue resuscitation for further 20 min to ensure action

- Continuous ECG monitoring in high dependency area

Evaluate:
- For rebound hypertension after 1 hr
- Frequency of ventricular arrhythmia
- Response to treatment and continuation of arrhythmias
- BP and vital signs — correct hypovolaemia, hypotension or hypertension
- Electrolyte balance: as exacerbation of arrhythmias
- For side effects

---

bromocriptine mesylate

Parlodel
Func. class.: Dopamine agonist
Chem. class.: Ergot alkaloid derivative
Legal class.: POM

Action: Inhibits prolactin release by activating postsynaptic dopamine receptors; activation of dopamine receptors could be reason for improvement in Parkinson's disease

Uses: Female infertility, Parkinson's disease, suppression of postpartum lactation, galactorrhoea or hypogonadism caused by hyperprolactinaemia, cyclic mastalgia and menstrual disorders, acromegaly, prolactinoma

Dosage and routes:
Parkinson's disease
- By mouth initially 1−1.25 mg at night for 1 week, then 2−2.5 mg at night for 1 week, increasing by 2.5 mg weekly increments as required to an optimum dosage range 10−40 mg daily in divided doses
Suppression of lactation
- By mouth: 2.5 mg daily for 2−3 days then 2.5 mg twice daily for 14 days

Galactorrhoea, infertility, hypogonadism
- By mouth: 1−1.25 mg at night increased by 1−2.5 mg at 2−3 day intervals to 7.5 mg daily in divided doses, maximum 30 mg daily
Cyclic benign breast disease, menstrual disorder
- By mouth: 1−1.25 mg at night, increased gradually to 2.5 mg twice daily
Acromegaly, prolactinoma
- By mouth: 1−1.25 mg at night increased gradually to 5 mg or more 6-hrly, maximum 30 mg daily
Available forms include: Capsules 5, 10 mg; tablets 1, 2.5 mg

Side effects/adverse reactions:
EENT: Blurred vision, diplopia, dry mouth, nasal congestion
CNS: Headache, dizziness, drowsiness, excitation, confusion, psychotic reactions, hallucinations, dyskinesias
GU: Incontinence
GI: Nausea, vomiting, constipation, dry mouth, GI haemorrhage, retroperitoneal fibrosis
RESP: Pleural effusions
CV: Orthostatic hypotension, cold-induced digital vasospasm, arrhythmias

Contraindications: Hypersensitivity to ergot, porphyria, toxaemia of pregnancy, post-partum hypertension

Precautions: Pregnancy, lactation, hepatic disease, cardiovascular disease, history of psychosis

Pharmacokinetics:
Period of onset: Peak 1−3 hr, duration 4−8 hr, 90%−96% protein bound, half-life 3−8 hr, metabolised by liver (inactive metabolites), excreted in urine, faeces

Interactions/incompatibilities:
- Decreased action of bromocriptine: phenothiazines, haloperidol, droperidol, domperidone, metoclopramide, oral contraceptives
- Possibly increased action of

bromocriptine: erythromycin
• Increased toxicity: Alcohol
Clinical assessment:
• Monitor for pituitary enlargement, especially during pregnancy
• Gynaecological assessment including cervical/endometrial cytology every 6 months in postmenopausal and every 12 months in premenopausal women if on long-term therapy
• Assess acromegalic patients for peptic ulceration before therapy
• Observe patients on long-term high dose therapy for signs of retroperitoneal fibrosis or pleural effusion
NURSING CONSIDERATIONS
Assess:
• BP before, during and after treatment
Administer:
• Orally following the dosage regimen for suitable gradual introduction
• With food to prevent nausea and vomiting. Not suitable under 15 yr
Evaluate:
• Therapeutic responses: Parkinson's disease: decreased dyskinesia, slow movement, excessive salivation; female infertility: pregnancy; suppression of lactation; menstrual disorders
• Optimal response with minimum side effects
Teach patient/family:
• To stand-up slowly to prevent postural hypotension
• To use other forms of contraception if oral contraceptives have been used or if female of childbearing age
• That gynaecological assessment is necessary including cervical and endometrial cytology; 6-monthly for post-menopausal, annually for regular menstruation
• That therapeutic response may not be immediate, up to 2 months galactorrhoea, amenorrhoea

• That alcohol should not be taken
• Not to drive or operate machinery if dizziness occurs

---

budesonide

Pulmicort, Rhinocort
Func. class.: Corticosteroid
Chem. class.: Non-halogenated synthetic corticosteroid
Legal class.: POM

Action: Reduces inflammation in bronchial or nasal mucosae, leading to reduction in oedema and mucus secretion. At normal therapeutic doses the inhaled preparation lacks systemic side effects
Uses: Chronic airways obstruction, especially in asthma not controlled by bronchodilators and/or antiallergic agents; allergic and vasomotor rhinitis
Dosage and routes:
Asthma
• *Adults:* Inhalation (metered dose) 200 mcg twice daily, increased if necessary to maximum 1600 mcg daily; nebuliser inhalation 1−2 mg twice daily, reduced to 0.5−1 mg twice daily for maintenance
• *Children:* Inhalation (metered dose) 50−400 mcg twice daily; nebuliser inhalation 0.5−1 mg twice daily, reduced to 0.25−0.5 mg twice daily for maintenance
Rhinitis
• Nasal spray 100 mcg into each nostril twice daily or 200 mcg per nostril once daily, reduced to half these doses once symptoms controlled
Available forms include: Metered dose inhaler 50, 200, and 400 mcg/inhalation; nasal spray 50 and 100 mcg/dose
Side effects/adverse reactions:
EENT: Candidiasis of mouth

or throat, coughing, irritation, hoarseness, sneezing and slight haemorrhage after intranasal administration
META: Slight adrenal suppression (high dose)
Contraindications: Hypersensitivity
Precautions: Respiratory tract infection (especially tuberculosis), pregnancy, lactation, steroid dependence
Pharmacokinetics: Therapeutic effect usually within 10 days

NURSING CONSIDERATIONS
Assess:
• Peak flow, respiration, wheezing before administration and 4 hrly after administration
• BP
• Weight
Administer:
• After cleaning/blowing nose (nasal route)
• With correct technique and equipment
Perform/provide:
• Mouth care, provide fluids and mouth washes for dry mouth
• Inspect mouth and throat for candidiasis, oedema, inflammation
Evaluate:
• Breathing: less wheezing and dyspnoea
Teach patient/family:
• Always to carry a steroid card for high dose.
• That improvement takes 3−7 days
• Not to stop unless advised by clinician and to maintain regular use
• To see clinician if condition worsens
• Proper administration techniques
• About side effects which include adrenal suppression
• That drug is not effective during an asthma attack

bumetanide

Burinex, combination products
Func. class.: Loop diuretic
Chem. class.: Sulphonamide derivative
Legal class.: POM

Action: Acts on ascending loop of Henle by increasing excretion of chloride, sodium
Uses: Oedema, oliguria such as that associated with renal failure
Dosage and routes:
• *Adult:* By mouth 1 mg in the morning repeated if required after 6−8 hr, refractory cases may need up to 5 mg or more daily; IV injection 1−2 mg repeated if necessary after 20 min; IV infusion 2−5 mg in 500 ml fluid over 30−60 min; IM 1 mg initially adjusted according to response
• *Elderly:* 0.5 mg daily may be sufficient
Available forms include: Tablets 1, 5 mg; injection 0.5 mg/ml; oral liquid 1 mg/5 ml
Side effects/adverse reactions:
GU: Gynaecomastia
META: Hypokalaemia, hypochloraemic alkalosis, hyponatraemia, hyperuricaemia, hypocalcaemia
CNS: Headache, fatigue, dizziness
GI: Nausea, diarrhoea, vomiting, cramps, upset stomach, abdominal pain, acute pancreatitis, altered liver enzyme values
EENT: Loss of hearing, tinnitus
INTEG: Rash, pruritus, Stevens-Johnson syndrome
MS: Cramps, arthralgia, myalgia
ENDO: Hyperglycaemia
HAEM: Thrombocytopaenia, granulocytopenia
CV: Hypotension, circulatory collapse
Contraindications: Hypersensitivity to sulphonamides, anuria or

oliguria developing during treatment, hepatic coma

Precautions: Severe electrolyte depletion, severe renal disease, pregnancy, lactation, elderly, diabetes mellitus, gout, low-salt diets

Pharmacokinetics:

Period of onset: Onset ½−1 hr, duration 4 hr
IM: Onset 40 min, duration 4 hr
IV: Onset 5 min, duration 2−3 hr
Excreted by kidneys, liver

Interactions/incompatibilities:

• Increased toxicity: lithium, antiarrhythmics, aminoglycosides, carbenoxolone, cardiac glycosides, cephalosporins, corticosteroids, other diuretics, NSAIDs, tricyclic antidepressants, vancomycin
• Increased effects of: antihypertensives
• Decreased effects of: antidiabetics
• Decreased diuretic effect: corticosteroids, oestrogens, oral contraceptives, NSAIDs

Clinical assessment:

• Regular checks of serum electrolytes and electrolyte replacement where indicated

Treatment of overdose: Supportive symptomatic care

NURSING CONSIDERATIONS

Assess:

• Baseline BP, weight, fluid balance

Administer:

• In the morning to avoid nocturia
• With food if nausea occurs: absorption may decrease slightly

Evaluate:

• Response to drug; oedema in feet, legs, sacral area if drug is used for congestive cardiac failure
• Daily weight
• Fluid balance chart; effectiveness of drug may decrease if used every day
• Rate, depth, rhythm of respiration and effect of exertion

• BP lying and standing; postural hypotension may occur
• Urine for glucose if patient is diabetic
• Improvement in CVP and BP recordings
• For signs of myalgia, rashes, purpura, gynaecomastia joint pains (early gout)
• For signs of metabolic acidosis e.g. drowsiness, restlessness
• For signs of hypokalaemia e.g. postural hypotension, fatigue, tachycardia, leg cramps, weakness
• Elderly people are particularly likely to become confused: observe carefully

Teach patient/family:

• That fluid intake should be increased to 2−3 litres daily unless contraindicated.
• To rise slowly from sitting or lying position
• To inform prescribing clinician if taking any other medication
• Possible adverse reactions e.g. muscle cramps, weakness, nausea, dizziness
• That gastric symptoms may be counteracted by taking tablets with food or milk
• To take tablets early in day to prevent nocturia
• Blood sugar may rise in diabetes

---

bupivacaine HCl

Marcain
Func. class.: Local anaesthetic
Chem. class.: Amide
Legal class.: POM

Action: Competes with calcium for sites in nerve membrane that control sodium transport across cell membrane; decreases rise of depolarisation phase of action potential
Uses: Epidural anaesthesia, peripheral nerve block

Dosage and routes:
• As a 0.25–0.75% solution. Dose depends on route and nature of anaesthesia
Available forms include: Injection 0.25%, 0.5%, 0.75%; injection with adrenaline 0.25%, 0.5%; with glucose (80 mg/ml) 5 mg/4 ml
• Test dose in epidural anaesthesia
Side effects/adverse reactions:
CNS: Lightheadedness, dizziness, convulsions, loss of consciousness, drowsiness
CV: Myocardial depression, cardiac arrest, arrhythmias, bradycardia, hypotension
GI: Nausea, vomiting
EENT: Numbness of tongue (warning sign of systemic toxicity)
INTEG: Rash, urticaria, allergic reactions
RESP: Respiratory arrest, anaphylaxis
Contraindications: Hypersensitivity, IV regional anaesthesia, hypovolaemia, complete heart block; epidural use contraindicated in CNS disease, coagulation disorders, shock, pyogenic skin infection; solutions with adrenaline contraindicated for appendages and in thyrotoxicosis, severe heart disease
Precautions: Elderly, debilitated, pregnancy, cardiovascular disease, epilepsy, respiratory impairment, hepatic disease
Pharmacokinetics:
Onset 4–17 min, duration 4–8 hr, excreted in urine (metabolites), metabolised by liver
Treatment of overdose: Supportive, symptomatic care; prolonged resuscitation may be needed in cardiac arrest
NURSING CONSIDERATIONS
Assess:
• If used as epidural infusion assess patient position; extent of anaesthesia and unilateral/bilateral effect depending on level of epidural cannula
• Baseline BP
Perform/provide:
• Nursing supervision to detect and provide assistance for daily living activities
• Hospital policy will indicate who may/may not refill epidurals/epidural infusions
• Emergency equipment
• Discard any solution not used
Evaluate:
• BP, pulse, respiration throughout treatment, possibility of hypotension, tachycardia, respiratory depression and neurological disturbance
• Degree of anaesthesia throughout procedure
• For allergic reaction e.g. rash, urticaria, itching

---

buprenorphine HCl

Temgesic
Func. class.: Opioid analgesic
Chem. class.: Thebaine derivative
Legal class.: POM (Sch 3) CD

Action: Inhibits ascending pain pathways in limbic system, thalamus, midbrain, hypothalamus
Uses: Moderate to severe pain
Dosage and routes:
• *Adult:* Sublingual 200–400 mcg every 6–8 hr as necessary; IM/slow IV injection 300–600 mcg every 6–8 hr
• *Child:* Sublingual, 16–25 kg bodyweight: 100 mcg, 25–37.5 kg, 100–200 mcg, 37.5–50 kg, 200–300 mcg; IM/slow IV injection 3–6 mcg/kg every 6–8 hr, maximum 9 mcg/kg
Available forms include: Sublingual tablets 200, 400 mcg; injection 300 mcg/ml
Side effects/adverse reactions:
CNS: Drowsiness, dizziness, con-

fusion, lightheadedness, headache, euphoria, depression, dependence, hallucinations
GI: Nausea, vomiting, cramps
RESP: Respiratory depression
INTEG: Sweating
Contraindications: Hypersensitivity
Precautions: History of drug abuse, opioid dependence (may provoke withdrawal due to partial antagonist action), respiratory depression, hepatic impairment, pregnancy, labour
Pharmacokinetics:
IM: Onset 10−30 min, peak ½ hr, duration 3−4 hr
IV: Onset 1 min, peak 5 min
Metabolised in liver, excreted in faeces, urine; half-life 2½−3½ hr
Interactions:
• Increased effect/toxicity: alcohol, other opioids, sedatives/hypnotics, antipsychotic agents, MAOIs, other CNS depressants
• Decreased effects of: cisapride, domperidone, metoclopramide
Treatment of overdose: Supportive symptomatic care; naloxone (other opioid antagonists) may not be completely effective in reversing symptoms
NURSING CONSIDERATIONS:
Assess:
• Respiratory function as potential respiratory depressant
• Pain control and appropriateness of analgesic
• Need for anti-emetic
Administer:
• Sublingually or by IM/IV route as prescribed
• As prescribed, when or before pain recurs
Perform/provide:
• Safe environment (potent analgesic). Patient to refrain from mobilising until drug has taken effect in case of dizziness
Evaluate:
• Effectiveness of pain control
• For CNS and respiratory depression: support and inform clinician
Teach patient/family:
• That tablets should not be swallowed or chewed
• Not to exceed recommended frequency of administration
• To report dizziness, drowsiness, etc., to medical staff

---

buserelin

Suprefact
Func. class.: Hormone agonist
Chem. class.: Gonadotrophin-releasing hormone analogue
Legal class.: POM

Action: Causes initial stimulation of LH release by the pituitary gland followed by a decrease in LH secretion and reduced production of testosterone
Uses: Metastatic prostate cancer
Dosage and routes:
• Subcutaneous injection, 500 mcg 8-hrly for 7 days; then by nasal spray, 100 mcg into each nostril 6 times daily
Available forms include: Injection 1 mg (as acetate)/ml; spray 100 mcg (as acetate)/metered spray
Side effects/adverse reactions:
CV: Hot flushes, thrombosis, pulmonary embolism
CNS: Headache, loss of libido, transient increase in pain, mental depression
EENT: Transient nasal irritation and nosebleed (nasal spray)
GU: Impotence, gynaecomastia
SYST: Disease flare, anaphylaxis
INTEG: Urticaria, erythema (hypersensitivity)
Contraindications: Surgical removal of testes, tumours unresponsive to hormone manipulation, hypersensitivity
Precautions: Concomitant anti-

androgen such as cyproterone acetate may be commenced 3 days before buserelin and continued for at least 3 weeks to prevent disease flare

Clinical assessment:

• Monitor testosterone levels for response to therapy

• Evaluate for possible spinal cord compression or ureteric obstruction if disease flare occurs

NURSING CONSIDERATIONS

Assess:

• Testerone level before and during initial treatment

Administer:

• Subcutaneously for 7 days. Then intranasal spray, one spray dose into each nostril before and after each meal (6 times a day) as maintenance therapy

• If required to prevent disease flare, prophylactic use of anti-androgen drugs is used 3 days before buserelin treatment and continued for at least 3 weeks after

Perform/provide:

• Adequate pain relief

Evaluate:

• Therapeutic response: decreased pain often after an initial increase in pain which is transient

• If no improvement, but decreased testerone — shows tumours not sensitive to hormone therapy. Alternative therapy required

• Increased pain may include cord compression

• Side effects: hot flushes, nose bleeds, loss of potency, depressed libido, growth of male breasts

Teach patient/family:

• How to spray into each nostril

• To discard container after 7 days use

• That regular administration is necessary for any benefits

• That body changes will occur, including enlarged breasts, loss of libido, hot flushes

• That nose bleeds do not effect absorption and are usually transient

• To see clinician immediately if urinary difficulties or pain increases or altered sensations occurs; sign of cord compression

---

busulphan

Myleran

Func. class.: Antineoplastic alkylating agent

Chem. class.: Methane sulphonate derivative

Legal class.: POM

Action: Alkylates DNA, preventing cell replication; mode of action not completely established

Uses: Chronic myeloid leukaemia

Dosage and routes:

• *Adult:* By mouth induction of remission: 60 mcg/kg daily to maximum 4 mg/day, discontinue when WBC $20,000-25,000/mm^3$ or platelets less than $100,000/mm^3$; maintenance $0.5-2$ mg daily

Available forms include: Tablets 500 mcg

Side effects/adverse reactions:

HAEM: Thrombocytopaenia, leucopenia, pancytopenia, haemorrhage, delayed or irreversible bone marrow depression

GI: Nausea, vomiting, diarrhoea, hepatotoxicity

GU: Sterility, amenorrhoea, gynaecomastia

INTEG: Hyperpigmentation, rash, erythema

RESP: Fibrosis, pneumonitis (may be progressive and fatal)

EENT: Cataracts

CNS: Convulsions (high doses)

META: Pseudo-Addisonian syndrome

Precautions: Radiotherapy or concomitant chemotherapy, non-malignant disorders (probable carcinogen, mutagen), pregnancy (teratogen)

Pharmacokinetics: Well absorbed orally, excreted in urine, excreted in breast milk

Interactions/incompatibilities:
• Increased toxicity: other antineoplastics or radiation, oxygen (may exacerbate pulmonary effects)

Clinical assessment:
• Blood tests: total and differential blood count at least weekly
• Periodic monitoring of pulmonary function

Treatment of overdose: Supportive; monitor blood counts, give infusion products, filgrastim as appropriate

NURSING CONSIDERATIONS

Assess:
• Weight before treatment
• Fluid balance
• Full blood count before and weekly during treatment. Special attention to platelets and WBC
• Signs of infection, fever, cough, cold

Administer:
• Orally, tailor dosage and length of course to patient for induction and remission
• Antibiotic prophylaxis for suspected infection
• Antiemetics, antacids as required

Perform/provide:
• Protective isolation and medical asepsis if low WBC
• Dietary advice

Teach patient/family:
• Need for protective isolation
• To report any bleeding of skin, bowels and excessive bruising immediately
• That in females and gynaecomastia in males amenorrhoea may occur, but is reversible after treatment has been discontinued
• That regular blood tests are essential
• That changes in breathing, coughing must be reported

calcitriol (1,25-Dihydroxy-cholecalciferol)

Rocaltrol

Func. class.: Parathyroid agent (calcium regulator)
Chem. class.: Vitamin D
Legal class.: POM

Action: Increases intestinal absorption of calcium and phosphate, regulates bone mineralisation, increases renal tubular absorption of phosphate

Uses: Correction of calcium and phosphate abnormalities in renal osteodystrophy

Dosage and routes:
• *Adult:* initially 1−2 mcg/day increased by increments of 0.25−0.5 mcg to 2−3 mcg/day as required

Available forms include: Capsules 0.25, 0.5 mcg

Side effects/adverse reactions:
CVS: Cardiac arrhythmias
CNS: Headache, apathy, somnolence, overt psychosis (rarely)
HAEM: Hypercalcaemia
GI: Nausea, vomiting, anorexia, paralytic ileus, abdominal pain
GU: Polyuria, hypercalciuria, nocturia; dehydration; thirst

Contraindications: Hypercalcaemia, metastatic calcification

Precautions: Pregnancy (use not established, potential benefit versus possible hazard), lactation (not known if enters human milk)

Pharmacokinetics:
Period of onset: Peak 4 hr, duration 15−20 days, half-life 12−22 days

Interactions/incompatibilities:
• Phosphate binding agents; dosage may need to be modified

Clinical assessment:
• Blood urea nitrogen, urinary calcium, aspartate aminotransferase, alanine aminotransferase,

cholesterol, creatinine, uric acid, chloride, magnesium, electrolytes, urine pH, phosphate. Serum calcium should be kept at 2.12−2.65 mmol/litre, vitamin D 3−30 ng/ml, phosphate 0.8−1.5 mmol/litre

• For increased blood level since toxic reactions may occur rapidly

Treatment of overdose: Gastric lavage up to 8 hr after ingestion; discontinue drug in hypercalcaemia; general supportive measures; rehydration and induced diuresis in severe hypercalcaemia

NURSING CONSIDERATIONS:

Assess:
• Fluid balance
• Calcium sufficiency
• Weight, rate and respirations

Administer:
• By mouth, may be adjusted depending on serum calcium level

Perform/provide:
• Restriction of sodium, potassium if required
• Restriction of fluids if required for chronic renal failure

Evaluate:
• For dry mouth, polyuria, bone pain, muscle weakness, headache, fatigue, tinnitus, change in loss of consciousness, irregular pulse, dysrhythmias, increased respirations, anorexia, nausea, vomiting, cramps, abdominal pain, constipation, tetany, fitting; may indicate hypercalcaemia
• Renal status: decreased urinary output (oliguria, anuria), oedema in extremities, weight gain, periorbital oedema, dyspnoea
• Changes in weight
• Nutritional status

Teach patient/family:
• The symptoms of hyper- and hypocalcaemia
• About foods rich in calcium
• To avoid products with sodium
• To avoid products with potassium in chronic renal failure

• To avoid non-prescribed medicines containing calcium, potassium, or sodium in chronic renal failure
• All aspects of drug: action, side effects, dose, when to notify clinician
• To avoid all preparations containing vitamin D
• To inform prescribing clinician of current medication
• To seek advice if pregnant

calcium chloride/calcium gluconate/calcium lactate

Func. class.: Electrolyte replacements — calcium supplement
Legal class.: Injection POM, oral P/GSL

Action: Cation needed for maintenance of nervous, muscular and skeletal enzyme reactions, normal cardiac contractility, coagulation of blood; affects secretory activity of endocrine, exocrine glands

Uses: Prevention and treatment of hypocalcaemia, hypermagnesaemia, hypoparathyroidism, neonatal tetany, cardiac toxicity caused by hyperkalaemia

Dosage and routes:

Osteoporosis
• 20 mmol calcium daily

Hypocalcaemic tetany
• IV initially 2.25 mmol then infusion IV 9 mmol daily

Cardiac arrest
• IV 10 ml 10% calcium chloride injection

Available forms include: Many, check with local pharmacy

Side effects/adverse reactions:
CVS: Bradycardia, arrhythmias
GI: Nausea, vomiting, anorexia, constipation
GU: Polyuria, thirst
CNS: Headache, coma, lethargy, muscle weakness

HAEM: Hypercalcaemia
MISC: Irritation after IV injection
Contraindications: Hypercalcaemia, digitalis toxicity, ventricular fibrillation, renal calculi
Precautions: Pregnancy, lactation, children, renal disease, respiratory disease, cor pulmonale, digitalised patient, respiratory failure
Interactions/incompatibilities:
• Large IV doses of calcium may precipitate arrhythmias; risk of hypercalcaemia with thiazides
• Antibacterials: reduced absorption of tetracyclines
• Biphosphonates; reduced absorption

NURSING CONSIDERATIONS
Assess:
• Continuous vital signs
Administer:
• Slowly through a large vein cannula. There is a risk of tissue necrosis if given via a peripheral vein.
• Calcium chloride should not be given through the same IV line as bicarbonate salts due to precipitation
• May be given IM in emergencies only when IV route unavailable
• Oral calcium to be given after meals or with milk
• Continuous ECG and blood pressure monitoring while administering
Perform/provide:
• Seizure precautions: padded side rails, decreased stimuli, (noise, light); place airway suction equipment, padded mouth gag if calcium levels are low
Evaluate:
• Cardiac status: rate, rhythm, CVP
• Therapeutic response: decreased twitching, paraesthesias, muscle spasms, absence of tremors, convulsions, dysrhythmias, dyspnoea, laryngospasm, negative Chvostek's sign, Trousseau's sign

• Baseline ECG for decreased QT and T wave inversion: hypercalcaemia, drug should be reduced or discontinued
• Total bound calcium levels during treatment (2.10−2.60 mmol/litre is normal level, providing albumin levels are normal)
Teach patient/family:
• To remain recumbent ½ hr after IV dose
• To add calcium-rich foods to diet: dairy products, shellfish, dark green leafy vegetables; and decrease oxalate-rich and zinc-rich foods: nuts, legumes, chocolate, spinach, rhubarb

capreomycin

Capastat
Func. class.: Antitubercular
Chem. class.: S. carpreolus polypeptide antibiotic
Legal class.: POM

Action: Inhibits RNA synthesis, decreases tubercle bacilli replication
Uses: Pulmonary tuberculosis resistant to first-line drugs, as adjunctive
Dosage and routes:
• *Adult:* IM 1 g daily (not more than 20 mg/kg) for 60−120 days then 1 g 2−3 times weekly
Available forms include: Powder for injection 1 g (1,000,000 units)
Side effects/adverse reactions:
INTEG: Pain, irritation, sterile abscess at injection site, rash, urticaria
CNS: Headache, vertigo, fever, neuromuscular blockade with large doses
EENT: Tinnitus, deafness, ototoxicity
GU: Proteinuria, decreased cre-

atinine clearance, increased blood urea nitrogen, tubular necrosis, hypokalaemia, alkalosis, haematuria, albuminuria, nephrotoxicity
HAEM: Eosinophilia, leucocytosis, leucopaenia, thrombocytopenia (rarely)
Contraindications: Hypersensitivity, pregnancy
Precautions: Renal disease, hearing impairment, allergy history, hepatic disease, lactation
Pharmacokinetics:
IM: Peak 1−2 hr, half-life 4−6 hr; excreted in urine unchanged
Interactions/incompatibilities:
• Increased toxicity: aminoglycosides, polymyxin, colistin, vancomycin
• Cytotoxics: increased risk of nephrotoxicity and ototoxicity with cisplatin
Clinical assessment:
• Liver studies weekly: aspartate aminotransferase, alanine aminotransferase, bilirubin, potassium
• Renal status: before therapy, weekly blood urea nitrogen, creatinine output, urinalysis
• Blood levels of drug
• Audiometry and assessment of vestibular functions before and during treatment
Treatment of overdose: Symptomatic and supportive therapy is required. Activated charcoal rather than lavage or emesis. Rehydration and haemodialysis are effective
NURSING CONSIDERATIONS
Administer:
• Give IM in large muscle mass, rotating sites. Observe for pain or induration at injection site
• Reconstituted solutions may be stored for 14 days in a refrigerator or 48 hr at room temp
• With other antituberculars
• After sputum culture every month is completed (to detect resistance)

• Reduced dosage in renal impairment
Evaluate:
• Therapeutic response: decreased dyspnoea, fatigue
• Ototoxicity: tinnitus, vertigo, change in hearing; audiometric testing should be done before, during, after treatment
• Hepatic status: decreased appetite, jaundice, dark urine, fatigue
Teach patient/family:
• That compliance with dosage schedule, length is necessary
• Side effects: hearing loss, change in urine or urinary habits

captopril

Capoten, Acepril
Func. class.: Antihypertensive
Chem. class.: Angiotensin converting enzyme inhibitor
Legal class.: POM

Action: Selectively suppresses renin-angiotensin-aldosterone system; inhibits angiotensin converting enzyme, prevents conversion of angiotensin I to angiotensin II, reducing vasoconstriction
Uses: Mild to moderate hypertension, first-line treatment alone or with thiazide; severe resistant hypertension, where standard therapy is ineffective; adjunctive treatment of congestive heart failure with diuretics and digitalis where appropriate
Dosage and routes:
Hypertension
• *Adult:* Initial dose alone, 12.5 mg twice daily; with thiazide, in elderly or in renal impairment, initially 6.25 mg twice daily (1st dose at night); maintenance 25−50 mg twice daily, maximum 50 mg twice daily (rarely 3 times daily in severe hypertension)
Congestive heart failure
• *Adult:* By mouth with thiazide,

initially 6.25−12.5 mg 3 times daily under supervision in hospital, maintenance 25 mg 3 times daily (maximum 50 mg 3 times daily)

Available forms include: Tablets 12.5, 25, 50 mg

Side effects/adverse reactions:

CV: Tachycardia, hypotension

GU: Dysuria, nocturia, proteinuria, nephrotic syndrome, acute reversible renal failure, polyuria, oliguria, urinary frequency

HAEM: Neutropenia, anaemia, thrombocytopenia, hyperkalaemia

INTEG: Rash, pruritus, photosensitivity

RESP: Bronchospasm, cough

CNS: Paraesthesia of hands

MISC: Angioedema of face, lips, mucous membranes, tongue and extremeties

Contraindications: Hypersensitivity, pregnancy, lactation, heart block, aortic stenosis, outflow obstruction, potassium-sparing diuretics, renovascular disease, porphyria

Precautions: Dialysis patients, hypovolaemia, leukaemia, blood dyscrasias, congestive cardiac failure, renal disease, diuretics with first dose may cause hypotension, hypotension with low sodium diet, dialysis or dehydration

Pharmacokinetics:

Period of Onset: Peak 1 hr; duration 2−6 hr; half-life 6−7 hr, metabolised by liver, metabolites, excreted in urine; crosses placenta, excreted in breast milk

Interactions/incompatibilities:

• Increased hypotension: diuretics, other antihypertensives, ganglionic blockers, adrenergic blockers

• Increased toxicity: potassium-sparing diuretics, lithium, NSAIDs, cyclosporin

• Do not use with vasodilators, hydralazine, prazosin

• Allopurinol, procainamide: Stevens-Johnson syndrome reported

• Azathioprine, cyclophosphamide: blood dyscrasias in patients with renal failure

• Probenecid: reduced renal clearance

Clinical assessment:

• Blood studies: neutrophils, decreased platelets

• Renal studies: protein, blood urea nitrogen, creatinine, watch for increased levels that may indicate nephrotic syndrome

• Baselines in renal, liver function tests before therapy begins

• Potassium levels, although hyperkalaemia rarely occurs

Lab. test interferences

False positive: Urine acetone

Treatment of overdose: Monitor BP and if hypotension give volume expansion. Removed by dialysis

NURSING CONSIDERATIONS

Assess:

• BP, apex/radial baselines

Administer:

• With patient in supine position if hypotensive

• IV infusion of sodium chloride 0.9% (as prescribed) to expand fluid volume if severe hypotension occurs

Perform/provide:

• Supine or Trendelenburg position for severe hypotension

Evaluate:

• BP ¼ hrly for 1½ hr, starting 1 hr after 1st dose. Continue if BP drops

• Apex/radial baselines before and after first dose. Report any significant change

• Daily urinalysis for protein (first morning specimen) 24 hr urine collection if positive.

• Assess ankle oedema daily

• Therapeutic response: decrease in BP in hypertensives, decreased signs of cardiac failure

• *Observe for:* Allergic reaction

(rash, fever, pruritus, urticaria); drug should be stopped if anti-histamines fail to help. Renal symptoms (polyuria, oliguria, frequency)

Teach patient/family:
• Not to discontinue drug abruptly
• Not to use non-prescribed (cough, cold, or allergy) products unless directed by clinician
• Prescribed doses should be continued even if the patient feels better. Rise to sitting/standing position slowly to reduce effect of postural hypotension
• Inform clinician if mouth ulcers, sore throat, fever, palpitations, chest pain, or ankle oedema occur
• May experience dizziness or fainting during first days of therapy

---

carbamazepine

Tegretol
Func. class.: Anticonvulsant
Chem. class.: Iminostilbene derivative
Legal class.: POM

Action: Inhibits nerve impulses by limiting influx of sodium ions across cell membrane in motor cortex
Uses: Tonic-clonic, complex-partial, mixed seizures; trigeminal neuralgia; prophylaxis of manic depressive psychosis in patient unresponsive to lithium therapy
Dosage and routes:
Seizures
• *Adult and child over 15 yr:* Initially 100–200 mg once or twice daily gradually increased to 800–1,200 mg daily, maximum 1,600 mg daily
• *Child under 15 yr:* By mouth 10–15 yr 600–1,000 mg daily 5–10 yr 400–600 mg daily 1–5 yr 200–400 mg daily under 1 yr 100–200 mg daily

Manic depressive illness
• Initially 400 mg daily in divided doses increased until symptoms controlled; usual range 400–600 mg daily maximum 1.6 g daily
Trigeminal neuralgia
• *Adult:* By mouth 100 mg twice daily, may increase 100 mg every 12 hr until pain subsides, not to exceed 1.6 g/day; maintenance (not prophylaxis) 200 mg 3 to 4 times daily
Available forms include: Tablets 100, 200, 400 mg; 'chewtabs' 100, 200 mg; liquid 100 mg/5 ml
Side effects/adverse reactions:
HAEM: Thrombocytopenia, agranulocytosis, leucocytosis, neutropenia, aplastic anaemia, eosinophilia, leucopenia, thrombo-embolism
CNS: Drowsiness, dizziness, confusion, fatigue, headache, somnolence, ataxia, states of confusion and agitation (in the elderly)
GI: Nausea, constipation, diarrhoea, anorexia, vomiting, increased liver enzymes, hepatitis
INTEG: Rash, Stevens-Johnson syndrome, urticaria
EENT: Tinnitus, dry mouth, blurred vision, diplopia, nystagmus, conjunctivitis
GU: Proteinuria, hyponatraemia
MISC: Lymph node enlargement, fever
Contraindications: Hypersensitivity to carbamazepine, atrioventricular conduction abnormality
Precautions: Hepatic disease, renal disease, cardiac disease, pregnancy, lactation, elderly, blood counts and liver function tests prior to initial therapy
Pharmacokinetics:
Period of onset: Onset slow, peak 4–8 hr, metabolised by liver, excreted in urine, faeces, excreted in breast milk, half-life 14–16 hr
Interactions/incompatibilities:

- Toxicity: erythromycin, cimetidine, isoniazid, dextropropoxyphene, lithium, verapamil
- Decreased effects of: oral anticoagulants, phenytoin, primidone, oral contraceptives, cyclosporin, theophylline
- Do not administer with or within 2 weeks of MAOI therapy

Clinical assessment:
- Renal studies: urinalysis, blood urea nitrogen, urine creatinine
- Blood studies: RBC, haematocrit, Hb, reticulocyte counts weekly for 4 weeks then monthly; if myelosuppression occurs, drug should be discontinued
- Hepatic studies: aspartate aminotransferase, alanine aminotransferase, bilirubin, creatinine
- Drug levels during initial treatment; should remain at 4−14 mg/litre (caution in the range of 8−14 mg/litre)

Lab. test interferences:
Decrease: Thyroid function tests

Treatment of overdose: Lavage, activated charcoal as appropriate

NURSING CONSIDERATIONS

Administer:
- If chewable tablets, tell patient to chew tablet, not swallow it whole

Perform/provide:
- Hard sweets, frequent rinsing of mouth to relieve dryness of mouth
- Assistance with ambulation during early part of treatment if dizziness occurs

Evaluate:
- Therapeutic response: decreased seizure activity, record in care plan evaluation
- Side effects: usually disappear spontaneously 7−14 days after initiating therapy
- Mental status: mood, alertness, affect, behavioural changes; if mental status changes notify medical staff

- Eye problems: need for ophthalmic examinations before, during, after treatment (slit lamp, fundoscopy, tonometry)
- Allergic reaction: purpura, red raised rash, if these occur, medication should be discontinued
- Blood dyscrasias: fever, sore throat, bruising, rash, jaundice
- Toxicity: bone marrow depression, nausea, vomiting, ataxia, diplopia, cardiovascular collapse, Stevens-Johnson syndrome

Teach patient/family:
- To carry ID card or Medic-Alert bracelet
- To avoid driving, other activities that require alertness, early in treatment
- To avoid alcohol ingestion; convulsions may result
- Not to discontinue medication quickly after long-term use
- Urine may turn pink to brown depending on dose
- All aspects of drug: action, use, side effects, adverse reactions, when to notify clinician

---

carbenicillin

Pyopen
Func. class.: Antibiotic, antipseudomonal
Chem. class.: Penicillin
Legal class.: POM

Action: Inhibits bacterial cell wall synthesis producing non-viable cell; bactericidal.

Uses: Infections due to *Pseudomonas aeruginosa* and *Proteus* spp

Dosage and routes:
Pseudomonas aeruginosa
- *Adult:* By slow IV infusion or rapid IV infusion 5 g 4−6 hrly; by IM injection 2 g 6-hrly
- *Child:* By slow IV infusion or rapid IV infusion 200−400 mg/kg

daily in divided doses; by IM injection 100 mg/kg daily in divided doses

Proteus spp

• *Adult:* By slow IV injection or rapid IV infusion 5 g 6-hrly; by IM injection 1–2 g 6-hrly

• *Child:* By slow IV injection or rapid IV infusion 250 mg/kg in divided doses or IM injection 50–100 mg/kg in divided doses

Available forms include: Vials 1 g, 5 g

Side effects/adverse reactions:

GI: Nausea, vomiting, diarrhoea

INTEG: Skin rashes, haemorrhage (rarely)

Contraindications: Penicillin hypersensitivity

Precautions: Pregnancy and lactation

Pharmacokinetics: Peak plasma concentration 15 min after IV injection; half-life 1–1.5 hr, excreted unchanged in the urine

Incompatibilities:

• Intravenous lipid emulsions

• Intravenous aminoglycosides

Clinical assessment:

• Dosage may need to be reduced when renal function impaired

• Monitor electrolytes; high sodium content in 5 g vial

Treatment of overdose: Removed by haemodialysis

NURSING CONSIDERATIONS

Assess:

• Baseline observations

Administer:

• After samples have been sent for culture and sensitivity

• By IV infusion, slow or rapid depending on severity of condition

• Immediately after reconstitution

NB. Must not be mixed with aminoglycosides

Evaluate:

• Therapeutic response

• For side effects

• Signs of anaphylaxis

carbimazole

Neo-mercazole

Func. class.: Antithyroid agent

Chem. class.: Imidazoline

Legal class.: POM

Action: Inhibits production of thyroid hormones after metabolism to methimazole

Uses: Hyperthyroidism, preparation for thyroidectomy and radio-iodine treatment

Dosage and routes:

• *Adult:* By mouth initially 20–60 mg daily in 2–3 doses until euthyroid. Maintenance, 5–15 mg daily or, in combination with 50–150 mcg/day thyroxine, 20–60 mg daily. Maintenance therapy should be continued for up to 18 months

• *Child:* 15 mg daily according to response

Available forms include: Tablets, 5, 20 mg

Side effects/adverse reactions:

HAEM: Agranulocytosis, neutropenia

CNS: Headache

GI: Nausea, gastric distress

INTEG: Rashes, pruritus, alopecia

MS: Arthralgia

SYST: Jaundice

Contraindications: Hypersensitivity, lactation

Precautions: Pregnancy

Pharmacokinetics: Converted to active metabolite, producing peak plasma concentration after 0.5–1 hr. Clinical improvement seen after 1–3 weeks. Half-life 3 hr, excreted in urine

Clinical assessment:

• Perform ECG

• Prescribe antihistamines for rashes

• Stop prior to thyroid surgery and prescribe iodine

• Evaluate level of thyroid function, be alert to hypothyroid states occurring
• Evaluate possibility of bone marrow suppression
• Full blood count and platelets (if sore throat reported)
• Measure thyroid function — T3, T4, TSH

Lab. test interferences:
Increase: aspartate aminotransferase, alanine aminotransferase

NURSING CONSIDERATIONS
Assess:
• Baseline ECG, pulse and BP
Administer:
• Once daily (same time) with food
• Discontinue prior to use of ^{131}I (3 or 4 weeks before)
Perform/provide:
• Measures to minimise pruritus e.g. cotton clothes
Evaluate:
• Pulse (sleeping), temperature 4 hrly, BP, daily weight, mouth and throat
• For hypothyroidism, oedema, weight gain in excess (weight daily for first week)
• Other side effects e.g. sore throat, nausea, headaches, rashes, pruritus, arthralgia (rarely), alopecia, agranulocytosis, jaundice
Teach patient/family:
• Report sore throat, mouth lesions, fever, rashes
• That breast feeding is contraindicated unless neonatal development is monitored closely
• To check pulse and increases in weight

---

carboplatin

Paraplatin
Func. class.: Antineoplastic agent
Chem. class.: Cisplatin analogue
Legal class.: POM

Action: Platinum forms cross-links between strands DNA. Not cell specific

Uses: Advanced ovarian carcinoma of epithelial origin, small cell carcinoma of lung, other sensitive tumours

Dosage and routes:
• *Adult:* IV infusion 400 mg/m^2 as single dose; reduce by 20–25% if risk factors (e.g. prior myelosuppression) present
Available forms include: Injection, powder for reconstitution/solution 50, 150, 450 mg

Side effects/adverse reactions:
EENT: High tone hearing loss, tinnitus
CNS: Peripheral neuropathy
META: Hypomagnesaemia, hypocalcaemia, hypokalaemia, abnormal liver function tests
GI: Nausea and vomiting, altered taste
GU: Nephrotoxity
HAEM: Thrombocytopenia, leucopenia, anaemia
SYST: Fever, chills

Contraindications: Severe renal impairment (creatinine clearance less than 20 ml/min), severe myelosuppression, hypersensitivity to platinum compounds or mannitol, pregnancy, lactation

Precautions: Reduce dose in renal impairment

Pharmacokinetics: Free platinum excreted in urine predominantly within 24 hr; half-life 24 hr, depressed blood count 14–21 days post-treatment

Interactions/incompatabilities:
Toxicity enhanced by other nephrotoxic and myelosuppressive agents

Clinical assessment:
• Neurological assessment, hearing test. Check sensitivity to platinum and mannitol. Only used by experienced clinicians. Do not repeat under 4 weeks. Do not give if myelosuppression severe. Anti-

emetics, anti-bacterial drugs, anti-uric acid drugs, Transfusion as required
• Evaluate blood results, tumour regression, extent of side effects
• *Renal function*: urea, creatinine clearance, uric acid. Full blood count at nadir and prior to treatment. Liver function tests: aspartate aminotransferase, alanine aminotransferase, bilirubin, alkaline phosphatase — monthly. Electrolytes — especially magnesium, calcium before each treatment

Treatment of overdose:
Monitor blood count, supportive therapy as required

NURSING CONSIDERATIONS
Assess:
• Temperature, pulse, respiration and BP, respirations and cough, fluid balance, test urine
• Weight

Administer:
• Following procedures in local cytotoxic policy
• Reconstitute immediately before use with water for injection, sodium chloride 0.9% or dextrose 5%
• Give IV over 15−60 min

Perform/provide:
• Reconstituted drug stable for 8 hr at room temperature, 24 hr refrigerated
• Avoid subcutaneous and IM injections where possible
• Other drugs as prescribed e.g. antiemetics, pre-medication, antimicrobials
• Antiemetics before and during treatment as nausea is severe with initial therapy
• Protection from infection: asepsis/isolation as required
• Fluids (2−3 litres), toast, dry biscuits as vomiting subsides. Ascertain food preferences and provide diet low in purines
• Mouth care: fizzy mouth washes, teeth cleaning and oral toilet
• Help with mobilisation if neurological side effects exist

Evaluate:
• For infection (temperature, pulse, respiration)
• Mouth 8 hrly (infection)
• Other signs of infection/inflammation
• Bruising or bleeding
• Tetany: corpopedal spasm
• Report urine output less than 30−60 ml hrly
• Extent of side effects and effectiveness of measures to minimise them

Teach patient/family:
• Reasons for protective isolation and high standard of hygiene
• Importance of reporting side effects
• Mouth examination for infection, ulcers etc
• Signs of cytopenia

---

carmustine (BCNU)

BiCNU
Func. class.: Antineoplastic alkylating agent
Chem. class.: Nitrosourea
Legal class.: POM

Action: Alkylates DNA, RNA; is able to inhibit enzymes that allow synthesis of amino acids in proteins
Uses: Brain tumours such as glioblastoma, brainstem glioma, medulloblastoma, astrocytoma, ependymoma and metastatic brain tumours, multiple myeloma, Hodgkin's disease, other lymphomas

Dosage and routes:
• *Adult:* IV 200 mg/m^2 every 6 weeks, adjusted according to WBC, other drugs
Available forms include: Injection

powder for reconstitution 100 mg
IV

Side effects/adverse reactions:

HAEM: Delayed myelosuppression, thrombocytopenia, leucopenia, anaemia

GI: Nausea, vomiting, hepatic toxicity

GU: Decrease in kidney size, azotaemia, renal failure

RESP: Pulmonary infiltrate, fibrosis

INTEG: Burning, intense flushing, suffusion of the conjunctiva

Contraindications: Hypersensitivity, leucopenia, thrombocytopenia, pregnancy, lactation

Pharmacokinetics: Degraded within 15 min, crosses blood-brain barrier, 70% excreted in urine as metabolites within 96 hr, 10% excreted as CO_2, fate of 20% is unknown

Interactions/incompatibilities:

• Increased toxicity: other antineoplastics, or radiation

Clinical assessment:

• Pulmonary function tests, chest X-ray films before, during therapy; chest film should be obtained regularly during treatment

• Renal function studies: blood urea nitrogen, serum uric acid, urine creatinine clearance before, during therapy

Treatment of overdose:

Monitor blood count, supportive therapy as required—transfusion products, filgrastim

NURSING CONSIDERATIONS

Assess:

• Full blood count, differential, platelet count weekly; withhold drug if WBC is less than 4000 or platelet count is less than 75,000; notify clinician of results

Administer:

• After ensuring clinician is aware of blood results

• Antiemetic 30—60 min before giving drug to prevent vomiting

• Antibiotics for prophylaxis of infection if indicated

Perform/provide:

• Storage in refrigerator

• Avoid contact with skin. Wash off thoroughly if contact occurs

• Strict medical asepsis, protective isolation if WBC levels are low

• Administer as an infusion. Painful as a bolus injection

• Increase fluid intake to 2—3 litres daily to prevent urate deposits, calculi formation

• Rinsing of mouth 3 or 4 times daily with water, prescribed mouthwashes; brushing of teeth 2 or 3 times daily with soft brush or cotton tipped applicators for stomatitis; use unwaxed dental floss

• Warm compresses at injection site for inflammation if indicated

Evaluate:

• Monitor temperature 4 hrly (in neutrophic patients only, may indicate beginning infection)

• Bleeding: haematuria due to thrombocytopenia, bruising or petechiae, mucosa or orifices 8 hrly

• Dyspnoea, rales, unproductive cough, chest pain, tachypnoea

• Food preferences; list likes, dislikes

• Inflammation of mucosa, breaks in skin

• Severity of nausea/vomiting (often severe)

Teach patient/family:

• Of protective isolation precautions if indicated due to neutropenia

• To report any complaints or side effects to nurse or clinician

• To report any changes in breathing or coughing

• Good mouth care and to report any bleeding, white spots, or ulceration in mouth to clinician; tell patient to examine mouth daily

carteolol HCl (ophthalmic)

Teoptic
Func. class.: Anti-hypertensive, Ocular
Chem. class.: Non-selective β-blocker
Legal class.: POM

Action: Non-selective β-adrenergic blocking agent
Uses: Ocular hypertension, chronic open-angle glaucoma, some secondary glaucomas
Dosage and routes:
• *Adult:* One drop of the 1% solution instilled into the affected eye(s) twice daily. If inadequate use 2% solution
• *Children:* Not recommended
Available forms include: Eye-drops 1%, 2%
Side effects/adverse reactions:
SYST: May cause systemic effects if absorbed
EENT: Ocular irritation, burning, pain, dryness, blurred vision, hyperaemia, diffuse superficial keratitis
Contraindications: Asthma or history of obstructive airways disease, uncompensated cardiac failure, pregnancy
Precautions: Sinus bradycardia, 2nd or 3rd degree atrioventricular block, cardiogenic shock, right ventricular insufficiency due to pulmonary hypertension or congestive heart failure, diabetes mellitus
NURSING CONSIDERATIONS
Assess:
• Ability of patient to instil drops
Administer:
• Into lacrymal sac
Perform/provide:
• Storage in refrigerator
Evaluate:
• Therapeutic response
• For allergic reactions-occular irritation, pain, burning
Teach patient/family:
• Instillation method
• That drop must not be used by anyone else
• To discard drops after 28 days
• To store in refrigerator

cefotaxime sodium

Claforan
Func. class.: Antibiotic, broad-spectrum
Chem. class.: Cephalosporin (3rd generation)
Legal class.: POM

Action: Inhibits bacterial cell wall synthesis, rendering cell wall osmotically unstable
Uses: Septicaemia, infections of respiratory tract, urinary tract, soft tissue, bone and joint, gonococcal infections, meningitis, surgical prophylaxis, obstetric and gynaecological infections
Dosage and routes:
• *Adult:* IM/IV 1 g 8 hrly, life threatening infection 2 g 8 hrly, maximum 12 g daily
Gonorrhoea
• 1 g as a single dose
Urinary tract
• 1 g every 12 hr
• *Neonate:* 50 mg/kg daily in 2−4 doses, severe infections 150−200 mg/kg daily
• *Child:* 100−150 mg/kg daily in 2−4 doses, severe infections up to 200 mg/kg daily
• *Intravenous infusion:* 1−2 g over 20−60 min
Available forms include: Powder for injection IM/IV, 500 mg, 1 g, 2 g
Side effects/adverse reactions:
CNS: Fever
GI: Diarrhoea, rises in liver transaminase and alkaline phosphatase

GU: Candidiasis
HAEM: Eosinophilia, leucopenia, neutropenia, haemolytic anaemia, granulocytopenia, agranulocytosis
INTEG: Rash, injection site pain, phlebitis

Contraindications: Hypersensitivity to cephalosporins

Precautions: Hypersensitivity to penicillins, severe renal dysfunction, pregnancy, lactation

Pharmacokinetics:
IV: Onset 5 min
IM: Onset 30 min
Half-life 1 hr, 35%−65% is bound to plasma proteins, 40%−65% is eliminated unchanged in urine in 24 hr, 25% eliminated as metabolites excreted in breast milk (small amounts)

Interactions/incompatibilities:
• Increased toxicity: aminoglycosides, frusemide, probenecid, vancomycin

Clinical assessment:
• Nephrotoxicity: increased blood urea nitrogen, creatinine
• Blood studies: aspartate aminotransferase, alanine aminotransferase, full blood count, haematocrit, bilirubin, lactic dehydrogenase, alkaline phosphatase, Coombs' test monthly if patient is on long-term therapy
• Electrolytes: potassium, sodium, chloride monthly if the patient is on long-term therapy

Lab. test interferences: False positive to glucose with reducing methods

Treatment of overdose: Serum levels decreased by peritoneal dialysis or haemodialysis

NURSING CONSIDERATIONS
Assess:
• Fluid balance
• Bowel pattern
Administer:
• After culture and sensitivity completed
Evaluate:

• Therapeutic response
• Bowel pattern daily; if severe diarrhoea occurs, drug should be discontinued; may indicate pseudomembranous colitis
• IV site for extravasation or phlebitis, change site 72 hrly
• Urine output; if decreasing, notify clinician; may indicate nephrotoxicity
• Allergic reactions: rash, urticaria, pruritus, chills, fever, joint pain, angioneurotic òedema; may occur few days after therapy begins
• Bleeding: ecchymosis, bleeding gums, haematuria, blood in faeces daily
• Overgrowth of infection: perineal itching, fever, malaise, redness, pain, swelling, drainage, rash, diarrhoea, change in cough, sputum

Teach patient/family:
• To use live yogurt to maintain intestinal flora, decrease diarrhoea
• To report sore throat, bruising, bleeding, joint pain; may indicate blood dyscrasias (rare)
• To be aware of side effects
• Diabetics may get false values when testing urine

---

cefoxitin

Mefoxin
Func. class.: Antibiotic, broad spectrum
Chem. class.: Cephamycin
Legal class.: POM

Action: Inhibits bacterial cell wall synthesis rendering cell wall osmotically unstable
Uses: Susceptible bacterial infections causing: peritonitis, intra-abdominal and intrapelvic infections, gonorrhoea and septicaemia; infections of: female genital tract, urinary tract, respiratory tract, bones, joints, skin and

soft tissues. Gram-negative and Gram-positive susceptible pathogens both aerobic and anaerobic

Dosage and routes:
• IM, slow IV, or IV infusion, 1−2 g every 6−8 hr, maximum 12 g daily
• *Child:* Up to 1 week, 20−40 mg/kg every 12 hr; 1−4 weeks, 20−40 mg/kg every 8 hr; over 1 month, 20−40 mg/kg every 6−8 hr

Available forms include: Powder for injections; 1, 2 g vial

Side effects/adverse reactions:
CNS: Fever
GI: Nausea and vomiting, pseudomembranous colitis, transient increased aspartate aminotransferase, alanine aminotransferase, alkaline phosphatase and jaundice
GU: Increased creatinine and blood urea, acute renal failure
HAEM: Eosinophilia, leucopenia, granulocytopenia; neutropenia, thrombocytopenia, and bone marrow depression
CV: Hypotension
INTEG: Thrombophlebitis, pain, induration, tenderness, rash, exfoliative dermatitis, urticaria, pruritus, anaphylaxis

Contraindications: Hypersensitivity to cephalosporins
Precautions: Hypersensitivity to penicillins, pregnancy, lactation, renal disease (dosage reduction necessary) GI disease

Pharmacokinetics:
IV: Peak 3 min
IM: Peak 15−60 min
Half-life 1−2 hr, 33%−55% bound by plasma proteins, 90%−100% eliminated unchanged in urine; crosses blood-brain barrier, eliminated in milk, not metabolised

Interactions:
Probenecid: reduced excretion of cefoxitin

Lab. test interferences:
• False positive reaction to glucose in the urine
• False high creatinine with Jaffe technique
• False high corticosteroid level with Porter Silber method
• Positive Coombs' test

Treatment of overdose: Not absorbed from GI tract so reaction on accidental ingestion is unlikely. After injection no known antidote is available, give supportive treatment

NURSING CONSIDERATIONS
Assess:
• Bowel pattern
• Fluid balance
Administer:
• After samples taken for culture and sensitivity
• IV route by slow bolus injection
Evaluate:
• Fluid balance daily
• Bowel pattern daily; if severe diarrhoea occurs, drug may be discontinued, (risk of pseudomembranous colitis)
• IV site for extravasation or phlebitis; change site every 72 hr
• Urine output; if decreasing, notify clinician as may indicate nephrotoxicity
• For allergic reactions; rash, urticaria, pruritus, chills, fever, joint pain, angioneurotic oedema; may occur a few days after therapy begins
• For bleeding; ecchymosis, bleeding gums, haematuria, stool Hb daily
• False positive Coombs' test (diabetics)
• For overgrowth of infection; perineal itching, fever, malaise, pain redness, swelling, drainage, rash, diarrhoea, change in cough, sputum
• Therapeutic response:
Teach patient/family:
• To report sore throat, bruising, bleeding, joint pain; may indicate blood dyscrasias (rare)

ceftazidime

Fortum

Func. class.: Antibiotic, broad-spectrum
Chem. class.: Cephalosporin (3rd generation)
Legal class.: POM

Action: Bactericidal through inhibition of bacterial cell wall synthesis. Resistant to majority of beta-lactamases

Uses: Active against a wide range of organisms including:

Gram-negative: *Haemophilus influenzae, Escherichia coli, Proteus mirabilis, Proteus vulgaris, Proteus rettgeri, Klebsiella pneumoniae, Klebsiella* spp, *Citrobacter* spp, *Enterobacter* spp, *Salmonella* spp, *Shigella* spp, *Actinobacter* spp, *Neisseria gonorrhoeae, Neisseria meningitidis, Serratia* spp, *Pseudomonas aeruginosa, Pseudomonas* spp (other), *Morganella morganii, Providencia* spp, *Yersinia enterocolitica, Pasteurella multocida*

Gram positive: *Streptococcus pneumoniae, Streptococcus pyogenes, Streptococcus* spp, *Staphylococcus aureus, Staphylococcus epidermitis, Micrococcus* spp

Anaerobic strains: *Streptococcus* spp, *Peptostreptococcus* spp, *Propionibacterium* spp, *Fusobacterium* spp, *Bacteroides* spp, *Clostridium perfringens*

Upper, lower, serious respiratory tract, urinary tract, skin, gonococcal, intra-abdominal infections, septicemia, meningitis

Dosage and routes:

• *Adult:* IM, IV or infusion 1 g 8 hrly or 2 g every 12 hr, severe infections 2 g every 8–12 hr, less severe infections e.g. urinary tract infections 500 mg–1 g 12 hrly. Elderly usual maximum 3 g daily
• *Child:* IV up to 2 months 25–60 mg/kg daily in 2 divided doses, over 2 months 30–100 mg/kg daily in 2–3 divided doses. Meningitis, immunocompromised or fibrocystic children up to 150 mg/kg daily in 3 divided doses

Cystic fibrosis: Pseudomonal lung infection
• *Adult:* Normal renal function 100–150 mg/kg daily in 3 divided doses
• *Child:* Up to 150 mg/kg daily in 3 divided doses

Available forms include: Injection vials of 250 mg, 500 mg, 1 g and 2 g

Side effects/adverse reactions:

CNS: Headache, dizziness, weakness, paraesthesia, hyperactivity, confusion

GI: Nausea, vomiting, diarrhoea, pain, bad taste, colitis (possibly pseudomembranous colitis) transient hepatitis and cholestatic jaundice

GU: Vaginitis, candidiasis, reversible interstitial nephritis

HAEM: Leucopenia, thrombocytopenia, neutropenia, lymphocytosis, agranulocytosis, eosinophilia, transient elevation of blood urea, blood urea nitrogen and/or serum creatinine

INTEG: Maculopapular or urticarial rash

MISC: Allergic reactions: fever, pruritus, etc, rarely angioedema, anaphylaxis

Contraindications: Hypersensitivity to cephalosporins, porphyria

Precautions: Penicillin allergy, renal impairment (reduce dosage – seek specialist advice), pregnancy, breastfeeding, concurrent treatment with nephrotoxic drugs, overgrowth of non-susceptible organisms, possible antagonism with concurrent treatment with chloramphenicol

Pharmacokinetics:

IV/IM: Peak 1 hr, half-life ½–1 hr, 90% bound by plasma

proteins, 80% eliminated unchanged in urine, excreted in breast milk

Interactions/incompatibilities:
• Possible increased toxicity with aminoglycosides
• Do not mix with vancomycin, aminoglycosides in same giving set

Lab. test interferences:
• *False positive:* Coombs' test (about 5% patients) leading to interference with blood cross matching
• *Slight interference:* with Benedict's, Fehling's and Clinitest

Treatment of overdose: Supportive measures. Dialysis reduces serum levels

NURSING CONSIDERATIONS

Assess:
• Fluid balance
• Bowel pattern

Administer:
• After specimens have been obtained for bacteriological culture and sensitivity

Evaluate:
• Response to treatment indicated by apyrexia and resolution of all signs and symptoms of infection
• Bowel pattern daily. If severe diarrhoea occurs the drug must be discontinued as this may be indicative of pseudomembranous colitis
• Intravenous site for extravasation, infection and phlebitis
• Urinary output. Inform clinician of oliguria as this may indicate nephrotoxicity
• Allergic reactions: rash, urticaria, pruritus, chills and fever which may develop within a few days of commencement of treatment
• Bleeding: ecchymosis, bleeding gums, haematuria, melaena
• Secondary infection indicated by perineal irritation, pyrexia, malaise, inflammation, discharge, rash, diarrhoea, productive cough

Teach patient/family:
• To inform clinician/nurse of sore throat, bruising, bleeding and joint pain which may indicate blood dyscrasias

cefuroxime sodium/ cefuroxime axetil

Zinacef, Zinnat
Func. class.: Antibiotic, broad-spectrum
Chem. class.: Cephalosporin (2nd generation)
Legal class.: POM

Action: Bactericidal through inhibition of bacterial cell wall synthesis, resistant to majority of beta-lactamases

Uses: Active against a wide range of organisms including:
Gram negative: *Haemophilus influenzae, Escherichia coli, Neisseria* spp, *Proteus mirabilis, Klebsiella* spp, *Proteus rettgeri, Enterobacter* spp, *Salmonella typhi, Salmonella typhimurium, Salmonella* spp, *Shigella* spp, *Bordetella pertussis*
Gram positive: *Staphylococcus aureus, Staphylococcus epidermitis, Streptococcus pyogenes, Streptococcus mitis, Clostridium* spp
Respiratory tract, urinary tract, skin, bone, joint, soft tissue, gynaecological and obstetric, ear, nose and throat, gonococcal infections, septicaemia, meningitis, surgical prophylaxis

Dosage and routes:
• *Adult:* By mouth with or after food 250 mg twice daily. Bronchitis, pneumonia 500 mg twice daily IM, IM 750 mg every 6−8 hr, severe infections 1.5 g every

6−8 hr. Single doses over 750 mg IV only

Gonorrhoea:

• Uncomplicated, by mouth 1 g as a single dose. IM 1.5 g as a single dose (divided between 2 sites)

• *Child:* By mouth over 5 years 125 mg twice daily. *Otitis media*, if necessary, 250 mg twice daily. IM, IV 30−100 mg/kg daily in 3−4 divided doses (2−3 divided doses in neonates)

Meningitis

• *Adult:* 3 g IV every 8 hr

• *Child:* 200−240 mg/kg daily in 3−4 divided doses reduced to 100 mg/kg daily after 3 days or on clinical improvement

• *Neonate:* 100 mg/kg daily reduced to 50 mg/kg daily

Surgical prophylaxis

• 1.5 g IV at induction, then supplemented depending on surgery — seek specialist advice

Available forms include:

Injection: IM, IV 250, 750 mg, 1.5 g cefuroxime as cefuroxime sodium

Tablets: 125, 250 mg cefuroxime as cefuroxime axetil

Side effects/adverse reactions:

CNS: Headache, dizziness, confusion, agitation

GI: Nausea, vomiting, diarrhoea, pseudomembranous colitis, transient hepatitis, cholestatic jaundice

GU: Candidiasis, reversible interstitial nephritis

HAEM: Eosinophilia, leucopenia, neutropenia, thrombocytopenia

INTEG: Maculopapular and urticarial rash

MISC: Allergic reactions, fever, anaphylaxis, pruritus, erythema multiforme, toxic epidermal necrolysis

Contraindications: Hypersensitivity to cephalosporins, porphyria (seek specialist advice)

Precautions: Penicillin sensitivity, renal impairment (reduce dosage), pregnancy, breast-feeding, concurrent treatment with potent diuretics, aminoglycosides and other nephrotoxic drugs, overgrowth of non-susceptible organisms

Pharmacokinetics:

IV: Peak 3 min

IM: Peak 30−45 min

Half-life 1−2 hr, 33%−50% bound to plasma proteins, 90%−100% eliminated unchanged in urine, crosses blood-brain barrier, excreted in breast milk, not metabolised

Interactions/incompatibilities:

• Possible increased toxicity with aminoglycosides

• Do not mix with aminoglycosides in same giving set

Lab. test interferences:

• *False positive:* Coombs' test leading to interference with blood cross matching

• *Slight interference:* with Benedict's, Fehling's, and Clinitest

Treatment of overdose: Supportive measures. Dialysis reduces serum levels

NURSING CONSIDERATIONS

Assess:

• Bowel pattern

• Fluid balance

Administer:

• With food

• After specimens have been obtained for culture and sensitivity

Evaluate:

• Therapeutic response

• Bowel pattern daily; if severe diarrhoea occurs, drug should be discontinued; may indicate pseudomembranous colitis

• IV site for extravasation, phlebitis; change site 72 hrly

• Urine output: if decreasing, notify clinician may indicate nephrotoxicity

• Allergic reactions: rash, urticaria, pruritus, chills, fever, joint pain, angioneurotic oedema; may occur few days after therapy begins
• Bleeding: ecchymosis, haematuria, stools daily
• Overgrowth of infection: perineal itching, fever, malaise, redness, pain, swelling, drainage, rash, diarrhoea, change in cough, sputum

Teach patient/family:
• Be aware of side effects
• To use yoghurt to maintain intestinal flora, decrease diarrhoea
• To take all medication prescribed for length of time ordered
• To report sore throat, bruising, bleeding, joint pain; may indicate blood dyscrasias (rare)

---

cephalexin monohydrate

Ceporex, Keflex
Func. class.: Antibiotic, broad-spectrum
Chem. class.: Cephalosporin (1st generation)
Legal class.: POM

Action: Inhibits bacterial cell wall synthesis, rendering cell wall osmotically unstable
Uses: Active against a wide range of organisms including:
Gram negative: *Haemophilus influenzae, Escherichia coli, Proteus mirabilis, Klebsiella* spp, *Moraxella catarrhalis*
Gram positive: *Streptococcus pneumoniae, Streptococcus* spp, *Staphylococcus* spp
Respiratory tract, urinary tract, skin, bone, joint, soft tissue, gynaecological and obstetric, dental, ear, nose and throat and gonococcal infections
Dosage and routes:
• *Adult:* By mouth 250 mg 6 hrly or 500 mg every 8−12 hr increasing to 1−1.5 g every 6−8 hr for severe infections
• *Child:* By mouth under 1 yr 125 mg every 12 hr, 1−5 yr 125 mg every 8 hr, 6−12 yr 250 mg every 8 hr, or 25 mg/kg daily in divided doses, doubled for severe infections
Available forms include: Capsules 250, 500 mg, tablets 250, 500 mg, 1 g, syrup 125, 250, 500 mg/5 ml, suspension 125, 500 mg/5 ml, drops 125 mg/1.25 ml

Side effects/adverse reactions:
CNS: Headache, dizziness, agitation, confusion, hallucinations
GI: Nausea, vomiting, diarrhoea, pain, dyspepsia, pseudomembranous colitis, transient hepatitis and cholestatic jaundice
GU: Vaginitis, candidiasis, reversible interstitial nephritis
HAEM: Thrombocytopenia, eosinophilia, neutropenia
INTEG: Maculopapular or urticarial rash
MISC: Allergic reactions: fever, pruritus, angioedema, anaphylaxis, erythema multiforme, toxic epidermal necrolysis
Contraindications: Hypersensitivity to cephalosporins, porphyria
Precautions: Penicillin sensitivity, renal impairment (reduce dosage), overgrowth of non-susceptible organisms, pregnancy, breast-feeding, concurrent treatment with nephrotoxic drugs
Pharmacokinetics:
Period of onset: Peak 1 hr, duration 6−8 hr, half-life 30−72 min, 5%−15% bound to plasma proteins, 90%−100% eliminated unchanged in urine, excreted in breast milk
Interactions/incompatibilities:
• Possible increased toxicity with aminoglycosides, probenecid
Lab. test interferences:
False positive: Coombs' test leading to interference with blood

cross matching, Benedict's test, Fehling's test and Clinitest

Treatment of overdose: Supportive measures, dialysis reduces serum levels

NURSING CONSIDERATIONS

Assess:
- Bowel pattern
- Fluid balance

Administer:
- With food if needed, for GI symptoms
- After specimens have been obtained culture and sensitivity

Evaluate:
- Therapeutic response
- Bowel pattern daily, if severe diarrhoea occurs, drug should be discontinued; may indicate pseudomembranous colitis
- IV site for extravasation, phlebitis; change site 72 hrly
- Urine output: if decreasing, notify clinician; may indicate nephrotoxicity
- Allergic reactions: rash, urticaria, pruritus, chills, fever, joint pain, angioneurotic oedema, may occur few days after therapy begins
- Bleeding: ecchymosis, bleeding gums, haematuria, melaena
- Overgrowth of infection: perineal itching, fever, malaise, redness, pain, swelling, drainage, rash, diarrhoea, change in cough, sputum

Teach patient/family:
- To use yoghurt or buttermilk to maintain intestinal flora, decrease diarrhoea
- To take all medication prescribed for length of time ordered
- To report sore throat, bruising, bleeding, joint pain; may indicate blood dyscrasias (rare)
- To be aware of side effects
- Diabetics may get false values when testing urine

cephazolin sodium

Kefzol
Func. class.: Antibiotic, broad-spectrum
Chem. class.: Cephalosporin (1st generation)
Legal class.: POM

Action: Inhibits bacterial cell wall synthesis rendering cell wall osmotically unstable

Uses: Active against a wide range of organisms including:
Gram negative: *Escherichia coli, Klebsiella* spp, *Proteus mirabilis, Haemophilus influenzae, Enterobacter aerogenes*
Gram positive: *Streptococcus pneumoniae, Staphylococcus aureus, Staphylococcus epidermidis*
Upper, lower respiratory tract, genito-urinary tract, skin and soft tissue, bone and joint, biliary tract infections, septicaemia, endocarditis and surgical prophylaxis

Dosage and routes:
- *Adult:* IM, IV 0.5−1 g every 6−12 hr
- *Child:* 25−50 mg/kg daily in divided doses, increasing to 100 mg/kg daily in severe infections
Available forms include: Injection IM, IV 500 mg, 1 g cephazolin as sodium salt

Side effects/adverse reactions:
CNS: Headache, dizziness, paraesthesia
GI: Nausea, vomiting, diarrhoea, anorexia, oral candidiasis, symptoms of pseudomembranous colitis, transient hepatitis, cholestatic jaundice
GU: Candidiasis, vaginitis, pruritus
HAEM: Leucopenia, thrombocytopenia, neutropenia, eosinophilia
INTEG: Rash
MISC: Allergic reactions, fever, anaphylaxis

Contraindications: Hypersensitivity to cephalosporins, porphyria, safety in prematures and infants under 1 month not established

Precautions: Penicillin allergy, renal impairment (reduce dosage), pregnancy, breast feeding, concurrent treatment with potent diuretics, aminoglycosides and other nephrotoxic drugs, overgrowth of non-susceptible organisms

Pharmacokinetics:
IM: Peak ½−2 hr, half-life 1−2 hr
IV: Peak 10 min, half-life 30 min, eliminated unchanged in urine

Interactions/incompatibilities:
• Possible increased toxicity with aminoglycosides, probenecid, potent diuretics
• Do not mix with other antibiotics, including aminoglycosides in same giving set

Lab. test interferences:
False positive: Coombs' test (leading to interference with blood cross matching), Benedict's, Fehling's and Clinitest

Treatment of overdose: Supportive measures. Dialysis reduces serum levels

NURSING CONSIDERATIONS
Assess:
• Bowel pattern
• Fluid balance
Administer:
• After culture and sensitivity completed
Evaluate:
• Therapeutic response: decreased fever, malaise, chills
• Bowel pattern daily; if severe diarrhoea occurs drug should be discontinued; may indicate pseudomembranous colitis
• IV site for extravasation or phlebitis, change site 72 hrly
• Urine output: if decreasing, notify clinician (may indicate nephrotoxicity)

• Allergic reactions: rash, urticaria, pruritus, chills, fever, joint pain, angioedema; may occur few days after therapy begins
• Bleeding: ecchymosis, bleeding gums, haematuria, melaena
• Overgrowth of infection: perineal itching, fever, malaise, redness, pain, swelling, drainage, rash, diarrhoea, change in cough, sputum

Teach patient/family:
• To use yoghurt or buttermilk to maintain intestinal flora, decrease diarrhoea
• To report sore throat, bruising, bleeding, joint pain; may indicate blood dyscrasias (rare)
• To be aware of other side effects
• Diabetics may get false values when testing urine

---

cephradine

Velosef
Func. class.: Antibiotic, broad-spectrum
Chem. class.: Cephalosporin (1st generation)
Legal class.: POM

Action: Inhibits bacterial cell wall synthesis, rendering cell wall osmotically unstable
Uses: Active against a wide range of organisms including:
Gram negative: *Haemophilus influenzae, Escherichia coli, Proteus mirabilis, Klebsiella* spp, *Shigella* spp, *Salmonella* spp, *Neisseria* spp
Gram positive: *Staphylococcus aureus, Streptococcus pneumoniae, Streptococcus pyogenes, Streptococcus faecalis*
Respiratory tract, urinary tract, skin and soft tissue, gastrointestinal tract infections, surgical prophylaxis, septicaemia, endocarditis, bone and joint infections

Dosage and routes:
• *Adult:* By mouth 250−500 mg every 6 hr or 0.5−1 g every 12 hr
• *Child:* By mouth 25−50 mg/kg daily in divided doses
• *Adult:* IM, IV or by IV infusion 0.5−1 g every 6 hr, severe infections increase to 8 g daily
• *Child:* IM IV or by IV infusion 50−100 mg/kg daily in 4 divided doses
Available forms include: Injection 500 mg, 1 g; capsules 250, 500 mg; syrup 250 mg/5 ml
Side effects/adverse reactions:
CNS: Headache, dizziness, confusion, nervousness
GI: Nausea, vomiting, diarrhoea, dyspepsia, pseudomembranous colitis, abdominal pain, transient hepatitis, cholestatic jaundice
GU: Vaginitis, candidiasis, reversible interstitial nephritis
HAEM: Leucopenia, eosinophilia, thrombocytopenia
INTEG: Skin rashes
MISC: Allergic reactions: fever, pruritus, anaphylaxis, erythema multiform, toxic epidermal necrolysis
Contraindications: Hypersensitivity to cephalosporins, porphyria
Precautions: Penicillin sensitivity, renal impairment (reduce dosage) overgrowth of non-susceptible organisms, pregnancy, breast-feeding, concurrent treatment with nephrotoxic drugs
Pharmacokinetics:
Period of onset: By mouth: Peak 1 hr
IV: Peak 5 min
IM: Peak 1 hr
Half-life 36−54 min, 20% bound to plasma proteins, 60%−90% eliminated unchanged in urine, excreted in breast milk
Interactions/incompatibilities:
• Possible increased toxicity with aminoglycosides, probenecid
Lab. test interferences:

False positive: Coomb's test leading to interference with blood cross matching, Benedict's test, Fehling's test and Clinitest
Treatment of overdose: Supportive measures. Dialysis reduces serum levels
NURSING CONSIDERATIONS
Assess:
• Bowel patterns
• Fluid balance
Administer:
• With food if needed, for GI symptoms
• After specimens have been obtained culture and sensitivity
Evaluate:
• Therapeutic response
• Bowel pattern daily; if severe diarrhoea occurs, drug should be discontinued; may indicate pseudomembranous colitis
• IV site for extravasation, phlebitis; change site 72 hrly
• Urine output: if decreasing, notify clinician; may indicate nephrotoxicity
• Allergic reactions: rash, urticaria, pruritus, chills, fever, joint pain, angioneurotic oedema; may occur few days after therapy begins
• Bleeding: ecchymosis, bleeding gums, haematuria, stool haem daily
• Overgrowth of infection: perineal itching, fever, malaise, redness, pain, swelling, drainage, rash, diarrhoea, change in cough, sputum
Teach patient/family:
• Management of diet
• Not to discontinue medication except on medical instruction
• To report sore throat, bruising, bleeding, joint pain; may indicate blood dyscrasias (rare)
• To be aware of other side effects
• Diabetics may get false values when testing urine

cetirizine

Zirtek
Func. class.: Antihistamine
Chem. class.: Active metabolite of
hydroxyzine
Legal class.: POM

Action: Potent antihistamine; a
selective H_1-antagonist for
symptomatic relief of allergy
Uses: Allergic rhinitis, urticaria
Dosage and routes: By mouth
10 mg daily or 5 mg twice daily
Available forms include: Tablets,
10 mg
Side effects/adverse reactions:
EENT: Dry mouth
CNS: Drowsiness, headache,
dizziness, agitation
GI: Discomfort
Contraindications: Not recom-
mended in children under 12,
lactation, pregnancy
Precautions: Do not exceed the
recommended dose if driving or
operating machinery, halve dose
in renal impairment
Pharmacokinetics: Peak plasma
concentration at 0.5−1 hr; half-
life 9 hr
Interactions/incompatabilities:
• Drowsiness potentiated by
alcohol
Treatment of overdose: Gastric
lavage with the usual supportive
measures
NURSING CONSIDERATIONS
Evaluate:
• Nasal secretions/rash, level of
side effects
Perform/provide:
• Fluids, boiled sweets, fruit for
dry mouth
• Safe environment if drowsiness
occurs
Teach patient/family:
• May cause drowsiness, if this
occurs not to drive or operate
machinery
• To avoid alcohol.

chenodeoxycholic acid

Chendol, Chenofalk
Func. class.: Dissolution of gall-
stones
Chem. class.: Natural human bile
acid
Legal class.: POM

Action: Reduces biliary cholesterol
secretion and saturation of cholesterol in bile allowing solubilisation
of gallstones
Uses: Dissolution of radiolucent
gallstones
Dosage and routes:
• By mouth 10−15 mg/kg daily in
divided doses or single dose at bedtime. Treatment is from 3 months
to 2 yr depending on gallstone size
and continued for 3 months after
dissolution
Available forms include: Tablets
250 mg; capsules 125, 250 mg
Side effects/adverse reactions:
GI: Diarrhoea, transient rises in
liver transaminases
INTEG: Pruritus
Contraindications: Radio-opaque
gallstones, non-functioning gall
bladder, chronic liver disease, inflammatory bowel disease, biliary
colic, biliary obstruction, gastric
or duodenal ulcer, liver cirrhosis,
pregnancy, children
Precautions: Consider other
methods of contraception by
women than oral contraceptives as
they may increase the lithogen-
icity of bile
Pharmacokinetics: Metabolised by
liver, excreted in faeces (metab-
olite/unchanged drug)
Interactions/incompatibilities:
• Concurrent administration of
cholestyramine, colestipol, aluminium antacids, charcoal may
bind chenodeoxycholic acid and
interfere with absorption
NURSING CONSIDERATIONS
Assess:

• Baseline vital signs and fluid balance

Administer:
• With meals for better absorption
• Antidiarrhoeals if necessary

Perform/provide:
• Increased fluids, fibre, encouragement to exercise, to decrease constipation

Evaluate:
• Therapeutic response; absence of epigastric pain, gallstones on diagnostic testing
• Assess cardiac status; check for dysrhythmias, increased rate, palpitations
• Fluid balance; check for urinary retention or hesitancy
• For GI complaints; nausea, vomiting, anorexia, diarrhoea; (if diarrhoea is severe, drug may need to be decreased)

Teach patient/family:
• That stone dissolution may take 3 months−2 yr; therapy is discontinued after 18 months if gallstones still intact
• To notify clinician if pregnancy is likely

---

chloral betaine

Welldorm (tablets)
Func. class.: Hypnotic
Chem. class.: Chloral hydrate derivative
Legal class.: POM

Action: CNS depressant
Uses: Short-term treatment of insomnia
Dosage and routes: By mouth
• *Adult:* 0.7−1.4 g (equivalent to 414−828 mg of chloral hydrate) at night; maximum 5 tablets (3.5 g, equivalent to 2 g chloral hydrate) daily
Available forms include: Tablets 707 mg (equivalent to chloral hydrate 414 mg)

Side effects/adverse reactions:
CNS: Drowsiness the following day; headache, excitement, delirium, dependence
GI: Gastric irritation, flatulence
GU: Renal damage on prolonged use, ketonuria
INTEG: Rashes
Contraindications: Gastritis, severe cardiac disease, marked hepatic or renal impairment, porphyria
Precautions: History of drug abuse or personality disorder; respiratory disease; pregnancy, lactation; reduce dose in elderly or debilitated patients; avoid prolonged use and abrupt withdrawal
Pharmacokinetics: Converted to chloral hydrate and ultimately to trichlorethanol (half-life 7−11 hr). Onset of action within 30 minutes

Interactions/incompatibilities:
• Effects enhanced by: other CNS depressants, including alcohol
• May increase the effects of: coumarin anticoagulants
Treatment of overdose: Gastric lavage, haemoperfusion; supportive treatment

NURSING CONSIDERATIONS
Administer:
• With water 20 min prior to bedtime
• Avoid contact with skin/mucous membranes

Perform/provide:
• Safe environment: cot sides, help with mobilisation

Evaluate:
• Rashes
• Observe for any abnormal bleeding
• Signs of dependence
• Sleep pattern improvement

Teach patient/family:
• They may be drowsy next day; if affected not to drive or operate machinery
• Report side effects — rash, headache

- That nightmares may occur
- To take with full glass of water
- That tolerance may occur
- About encouraging normal sleep patterns: exercise in day, milk drink, warm bath, relaxation techniques, books/TV etc.
- Not to discontinue medication abruptly

---

chloral hydrate

Noctec, Welldorm (elixir)
Func. class.: Hypnotic
Chem. class.: Chloral derivative
Legal class.: POM

Action: Metabolite trichlorethanol believed to have central depressant effect which induces sleep

Uses: Short-term treatment of insomnia

Dosage and routes:
- *Adult:* 0.5−1 g, 15−30 min before bedtime with plenty of water. Maximum 2 g
- *Child:* 30−50 mg/kg, maximum 1 g per day

Available forms include: Capsules 500 mg; tablets chloral betaine 707 mg (equivalent to 414 mg chloral hydrate), syrup 143 mg/5 ml

Side effects/adverse reactions:
HAEM: Eosinophilia, leucopenia
CNS: Excitement, headache, delirium, lightheadedness, ataxia, paranoia
INTEG: Allergic skin reactions
CV: Hypotension, dysrhythmias
RESP: Depression (in children)
GI: Gastric irritation, abdominal distension, flatulence

Contraindications: Marked hepatic or renal impairment, severe cardiac disease, gastritis, hypersensitivity to chloral hydrate or triclofos, pregnancy, lactation, porphyria

Precautions: Causes drowsiness, possibility of habituation

Pharmacokinetics:
Period of onset: Onset 30 min−1 hr, duration 4−8 hr. Metabolised by liver, excreted by kidneys (inactive metabolite) and faeces, excreted in breast milk; half-life 8−11 hr; metabolite is highly protein bound

Interactions/incompatibilities:
- Increased action of anticoagulants, increased action of both drugs with alcohol, benzodiazepines, other hypnotics and anxiolytics
- When chloral hydrate is followed by IV frusemide variable blood pressure including hypertension, sweating, hot flushes may result

Clinical assessment:
- Monitor prothrombin time if patients on anticoagulants. Watch for habituation if on long-term treatment and delirium on sudden withdrawal

Lab. test interferences: Possible false positive results in some tests for glucose, measurement of urinary 17-hydroxycorticosteroids, possible raised results in blood urea determinations

Treatment of overdose: Gastric lavage or induction of vomiting to empty the stomach. Supportive measures must be used; in severe poisoning haemoperfusion or dialysis may be beneficial

NURSING CONSIDERATIONS
Administer:
- After trying conservative measures for insomnia
- ½−1 hr before bedtime for insomnia
- On empty stomach with full glass of water or juice for best absorption and decrease corrosion (do not chew); after meals to decrease GI symptoms if using for sedation

Perform/provide:

• Checking to see oral medication swallowed
• Assistance with ambulation after receiving dose
• Safety measure: siderails, night-light, callbell within easy reach
Evaluate:
• Therapeutic response: ability to sleep at night, decreased amount of early morning awakening if taking drug for insomnia
• Mental status: mood, alertness, affect, memory (long, short)
• Physical dependency: more frequent requests for medication, shakes, anxiety
• Respiratory dysfunction: respiratory depression, character, rate, rhythm; hold drug if respirations are less than 12/min or if pupils are dilated (rare)
• Blood dyscrasias: fever, sore throat, bruising, rash, jaundice, epistaxis (rare)
• Previous history of substance abuse, cardiac disease, or gastritis
Teach patient/family:
• To avoid driving or other activities requiring alertness
• To avoid alcohol ingestion or CNS depressants; serious CNS depression may result
• Not to discontinue medication quickly after long-term use; drug should be tapered over 1–2 weeks
• That effects may take 2 nights for benefits to be noticed
• Alternate measures to improve sleep (reading, exercise several hours before bedtime, warm bath, warm milk, TV, self-hypnosis, deep breathing)

chlorambucil

Leukeran
Func. class.: Antineoplastic alkylating agent
Chem. class.: Nitrogen mustard
Legal class.: POM

Action: Interferes with cell replication by alkylating DNA, RNA; inhibits enzymes that allow synthesis of proteins
Uses: Chronic lymphocytic leukaemia, Hodgkin's disease, certain forms of non-Hodgkin's lymphoma, Waldenstrom's macroglobulinaemia, advanced ovarian adenocarcinoma, breast cancer

Dosage and routes:
• *Adult and child:* As single agent by mouth usually 100–200 mcg/kg daily for 4–8 weeks
Available forms include: Tablets 2, 5 mg

Side effects/adverse reactions:
CNS: Seizures, peripheral neuropathy
HAEM: Bone marrow suppression, jaundice
GI: Nausea, vomiting, diarrhoea, oral ulceration
MISC: Hypersensitivity
RESP: Fibrosis, pneumonia
GU: Sterile cystitis
Contraindications: Teratogenic, avoid in first trimester if possible. Use balanced against benefit. Avoid breast feeding
Precautions: Used only by experienced physicians, monitor blood counts, patients given other cytotoxic agents or recent radiotherapy, impaired renal function
Pharmacokinetics: Well absorbed orally, metabolised in liver, excreted in urine; half-life 2 hr
Interactions/incompatibilities:
• Increased toxicity: other antineoplastics or radiation

• Reduce dosage if patients receiving phenylbutazone

Clinical assessment:
• Ensure full blood count, differential, platelet count weekly; notify clinician of results
• Pulmonary functions test, chest X-ray films before, during therapy; chest film should be obtained at intervals during treatment
• Renal function studies: blood urea nitrogen, serum uric acid, urine creatinine clearance before, during therapy
• Liver function tests before, during therapy (bilirubin, aspartate aminotransferase, alanine aminotransferase, lactic dehydrogenase) as needed or monthly

Treatment of overdose: Monitor blood picture, institute general supportive measures; blood transfusion, filgrastim if necessary

NURSING CONSIDERATIONS
Administer:
• Following local cytotoxic policy
• Other medications by oral route; if possible avoid IM, subcutaneous, IV routes to prevent infections
• Other medication e.g. antacid, antiemetic, allopurinol, antibiotics, as ordered
• Antiemetics before and during treatment
• With food

Perform/provide:
• Strict medical asepsis, protective isolation if WBC levels are low
• Special skin care
• Increase fluid intake to 2–3 litres daily to prevent urate deposits, calculi formation
• Diet low in purines: offal (kidney, liver), dried beans, peas, to maintain alkaline urine

Evaluate:
• Fluid balance; report fall in urine output of 30 ml/hr
• Monitor temperature and BP 4 hrly in bone marrow depression
• Unexpected bleeding: e.g. haematuria, bruising or petechiae
• Yellowing of skin, sclera, dark urine, clay-coloured stools, itchy skin, abdominal pain, fever, diarrhoea
• Signs and symptoms of infection, particularly in the chest
• Effects of alopecia on body image; discuss feelings about body changes (rare)

Teach patient/family:
• Protective isolation precautions
• To report any complaints or side effects to nurse or clinician
• To report any changes in breathing or coughing
• That hair may be lost during treatment; a wig or hairpiece may make patient feel better (obtainable free on NHS); new hair may be different in colour, texture (rare)
• That impotence or amenorrhoea can occur but is generally reversible after discontinuing treatment

---

chloramphenicol/ chloramphenicol palmitate/ chloramphenicol sodium succinate

Chloromycetin, Kemicetine
Func. class.: Antibacterial/antirickettsial
Chem. class.: Dichloroacetic acid derivative
Legal class.: POM

Action: Interferes with protein synthesis in intact bacterial cells to exert a mainly bacteriostatic effect
Uses: Active against a wide range of organisms including:
Gram-negative, particularly *Salmonella typhi, Haemophilus influenzae, Neisseria meningitidis*
Gram-positive, *Streptococcus pneumoniae, Rickettsia* spp, *Myco-*

plasma spp, *Vibro* spp., *Chlamydia* spp of the Psittacosis—Lymphogranuloma group

Dosage and routes:
• *Adults and children over 2 weeks:* By mouth, IV or infusion 50 mg/kg daily in 4 divided doses
• For severe infections—septicaemia, meningitis—may be doubled. Reduce high doses as soon as clinically indicated
• *Infants under 2 weeks:* 25 mg/kg daily in 4 divided doses

Available forms include: Injection IV 300 mg, 1.0, 1.2 g; capsules 250 mg; oral suspension 125 mg/5 ml

Side effects/adverse reactions:
HAEM: Aplastic anaemia, bone marrow depression, hypoplastic anaemia, thrombocytopenia, agranulocytosis, leucopenia
EENT: Optic neuritis, blindness
GI: Nausea, vomiting, diarrhoea, dry mouth, glossitis, stomatitis, enterocolitis, pruritus ani
INTEG: Erythema multiforme
CU: Haemoglobinuria (nocturnal)
MISC: Grey's syndrome in newborn: abdominal distension with or without vomiting, pallid cyanosis, vasomotor collapse, irregular respiration

Contraindications: Hypersensitivity, toxic reaction to drug, pregnancy, breast feeding, porphyria, trivial infections, administration IV during labour

Precautions: Reduce dose in impaired hepatic or renal function, overgrowth of non-susceptible organisms, carry out blood studies

Pharmacokinetics:
Period of onset: IV: Peak 1—2 hr, duration 8 hr, half-life 1½—4 hr, conjugated in liver, excreted in urine (up to 15% as free drug), breast milk, faeces

Interactions/incompatibilities:
• Enhanced effects of: coumarin anticoagulants (nicoumalone, warfarin), some hypoglycaemic agents (e.g. tobutamide), phenytoin
• Reduced action of chloramphenicol: rifampicin, phenobarbitone
• Half-life prolonged by: paracetamol
• Avoid myelossuppressive drugs, increased risks of blood disorders

Treatment of overdose: Empty stomach if oral dosage (excess of 12 capsules or 120 ml suspension), then supportive measures as necessary. After IV dosage, supportive measures as necessary

NURSING CONSIDERATIONS
Assess:
• Allergies before treatment, reaction of each medication; note allergies on chart, in bright red letters; alert all people giving medication
• Bowel patterns
• Fluid balance

Administer:
• After specimens have been obtained for culture and sensitivity
• IV slowly over at least 1 min
• Reconstituted solution should be used once only
• Oral form on empty stomach with full glass of water

Perform/provide:
• Storage: reconstituted solution at room temperature for up to 30 days
• Ensure emergency equipment available should anaphylaxis occur
• Adequate intake of fluids (2 litres daily) during diarrhoea episodes
• Record/be aware of fluid balance in view of possible renal impairment
• Care of IV site: look for phlebitis extravasation, etc

Evaluate:
• Therapeutic response: decreased temperature, negative culture and sensitivity

• Bowel pattern before, during treatment
• Skin eruptions, itching
• Respiratory status: rate, character, wheezing, tightness in chest
• Signs of bone marrow suppression. Ensure blood studies reviewed at regular intervals
• Neonates for beginning of Grey's syndrome: cyanosis, abdominal distention, irregular respiration, failure to feed; drug should be discontinued immediately

Teach patient/family:
• Aspects of drug therapy: need to complete entire course of medication to ensure organism death; culture may be taken after complete course of medication
• To report sore throat, fever, fatigue, unusual bleeding, bruising; could indicate bone marrow depression (may occur weeks or months after termination of drug)
• That drug must be taken in equal intervals around clock to maintain blood levels
• To wear or carry identification if allergic to this drug
• To notify nurse of diarrhoea
• To be aware of all side effects

chloramphenicol (ophthalmic)

Chloromycetin,   Snophenicol, Minims chloramphenicol
Func. class.: Anti-infective
Chem. class.: Dichloroacetic acid derivative
Legal class.: POM

Action: Bacteriostatic action by interference with protein synthesis in intact bacterial cells. Antibacterial action effective against virtually all bacterial pathogens causing eye disease
Uses: Infection of eye
Dosage and routes:

Adult and child: Instil 2 drops every 2 hr then reduce frequency as infection controlled; continue for 48 hr after healing. Apply ointment at night if drops are being used or 3−4 times daily if ointment used alone
Available forms include: Eye drops 0.5%, eye ointment 1%
Side effects/adverse reactions:
EENT: Transient stinging, burning sensations, overgrowth of non-susceptible organisms
HAEM: Aplastic anaemia (rare)
Contraindications and precautions: Hypersensitivity

NURSING CONSIDERATIONS
Administer:
• After washing hands, cleanse crusts or discharge from eye before application
• Apply pressure to lacrimal sac for 1 min to prevent systemic absorption
• Apply ointment topically inside lower eye lid (to conjunctival sac)
Perform/provide:
• Storage at room temperature, protect from light
Evaluate:
• Therapeutic response: absence of redness, inflammation, tearing
• Allergy: itching, lacrimation, redness, swelling
Teach patient/family:
• To use drug exactly as prescribed
• That drug container tip should not be touched to eye
• To use separate applicator for each eye
• Wash hands between applications to reduce risk of cross-infection
• Not to use eye makeup, towels, washcloths, eye medication of others; reinfection may occur
• That drug may cause blurred vision when ointment is applied
• To report itching, increased redness, burning, stinging, swelling; drug should be discontinued

chloramphenicol (ear drops)

Func. class.: Broad-spectrum antibiotic
Chem. class.: Dichloroacetic acid derivative
Legal class.: POM

Action: Interferes with protein synthesis in intact bacterial cells
Uses: Bacterial infection in external ear (otitis externa)

Dosage and routes:
• *Adult and child:* Instil into ear 2−3 drops 2−3 times daily
Available forms include: Ear drops 5%, 10% in propylene glycol

Side effects/adverse reactions:
EENT: Itching, irritation in ear
INTEG: Rash, urticaria, contact dermatitis, burning
Contraindications: Hypersensitivity, perforated eardrum
Precautions: Avoid prolonged use, high incidence of sensitivity reactions to propylene glycol

NURSING CONSIDERATIONS
Administer:
• After removing impacted cerumen by irrigation with 0.5% bicarbonate of soda or 0.9% sodium chloride
• After cleaning stopper with alcohol
• After warming solution to body temperature

Evaluate:
• Therapeutic response: decreased ear pain
• For redness, swelling, pain in ear, which indicates superimposed infection

Teach patient/family:
• Method of instillation, using aseptic technique, including not touching dropper to ear
• That dizziness may occur after instillation

• To avoid prolonged use
• About side effects

chlordiazepoxide HCl

NHS Librium
Func. class.: Anti-anxiety
Chem. class.: Benzodiazepine
Legal class.: CD Benz POM

Action: Action via GABA receptors depressing subcortical levels of CNS, including limbic system, reticular formation
Uses: Short term management of anxiety, adjunct in acute alcohol withdrawal

Dosage and routes:
Anxiety
• *Adult:* By mouth 30 mg daily in divided doses, up to 60−100 mg daily in divided doses if necessary
Alcohol withdrawal
• *Adult:* By mouth 25−100 mg repeated 2−4 hrly if required
• *Children:* Not to be used
• *Elderly:* Half adult dose
Available forms include: Capsules 5, 10 mg; tablets 5, 10, 25 mg

Side effects/adverse reactions:
CNS: Drowsiness, sedation, unsteadiness, ataxia, confusion, headache, vertigo
GI: Upsets—diarrhoea, constipation, salivation changes
INTEG: Rashes
EENT: Visual disturbances
HAEM: Blood disorders and jaundice reported
GU: Urinary retention
MISC: Changes in libido
Contraindications: Respiratory depression, acute pulmonary insufficiency, hypersensitivity to benzodiazepines, phobic or obsessional states, chronic psychoses
Precautions: Chronic pulmonary

insufficiency, psychosis, marked personality disorder, muscle weakness, drug abuse, pregnancy, lactation. Reduce dose in elderly, debilitated, hepatic and renal impairment. Avoid prolonged use and sudden withdrawal. Alteration of performance at skilled tasks e.g. driving

Pharmacokinetics:
Period of onset: Onset 30 min, peak ½ hr, duration 4−6 hr, metabolised by liver, excreted by kidneys, in breast milk, half-life 5−30 hr

Interactions/incompatibilities:
• Increased effects of this drug: CNS acting drugs: neuroleptics, tranquillisers, antidepressants, hypnotics, analgesics, anaesthetics, alcohol, disulfiram, ulcer healing drugs e.g. cimetidine

Treatment of overdose: Gastric lavage if soon after ingestion. In hospital IV flumazenil as antidote in emergency situations. Take supportive measures. Do not use barbiturates if excitation occurs

NURSING CONSIDERATIONS

Assess:
• Baseline BP and fluid balance

Administer:
• With food or milk for GI symptoms
• Crush tablets if patient is unable to swallow medication whole
• Boiled sweets, frequent sips of water for dry mouth

Perform/provide:
• Check to see oral medication has been swallowed
• Assistance with ambulation during initial therapy, since drowsiness/dizziness occurs
• Safety measure, including siderails

Evaluate:
• Therapeutic response: decreased anxiety, restlessness, sleeplessness

• BP (lying, standing), pulse; if systolic BP drops 20 mmHg, withhold drug, notify clinician
• Fluid balance, may indicate renal dysfunction
• Mental status: mood, alertness, affect, sleeping pattern, drowsiness, dizziness
• Physical dependency, withdrawal symptoms: headache, nausea, vomiting, muscle pain, weakness after long-term use
• Suicidal tendencies

Teach patient/family:
• That drug may be taken with food
• Not to be used for everyday stress or used longer than 4 months, unless directed by clinician
• Avoid non-prescribed preparations unless approved by clinician
• To avoid driving, activities that require alertness; drowsiness may occur
• To avoid alcohol ingestion or other psychotropic medications, unless prescribed by clinician
• Not to discontinue medication abruptly after long-term use
• To rise slowly or fainting may occur
• That drowsiness might worsen at beginning of treatment

chlorhexidine gluconate

Bacticlens, Chlorasept, Hibidil, Hibiscrub, Hibisol, Hibitane 5% concentrate, Hibitane gluconate 20% Phiso-med, Rotarsept, Unisept
Func. class.: Disinfectant
Chem. class.: Polychlorinated phenol derivative
Legal class: GSL, P

Action: Antimicrobial agent effective against a wide range of

vegetative Gram-positive and Gram-negative bacteria
Uses: Surgical scrub, skin cleanser, bladder irrigation, wound cleanser, disinfection of surfaces, instruments, obstetrics
Dosage and route:
• *Adult and child:* seek specialist advice
Available forms include: Soap, solution, spray, cream, bladder irrigation
Side effects/adverse reactions:
INTEG: Irritation, sensitivity, dryness, dermatitis
MISC: Rare generalised allergic reactions
Contraindications: Hypersensitivity to chlorhexidine, use on brain, meninges, middle ear, eye or other sensitive tissues
Precautions: Bladder irrigations of concentrated solutions may cause haematuria
Interactions/incompatibilities:
Soaps and other anionic materials
Treatment of overdose: Ingestion: gastric lavage using milk, gelatin or mild soap. Supportive measures as necessary
NURSING CONSIDERATIONS
Administer:
• Topically to body areas only. Avoid contact with face, lips, eyes and mouth, all mucous membranes
• Only to adults; repeated use may lead to systemic absorption
Evaluate:
• Area of body involved; irritation, rash, breaks, redness, dryness, itching
Teach patient/family:
• To report itching, irritation, dizziness, headache, confusion; discontinue use immediately

chlormethiazole edisylate

Heminevrin
Func. class.: Hypnotic
Chem. class.: Non-benzodiazepine
Legal class.: POM

Action: Hypnotic, sedative and anticonvulsant properties via effects on catecholaminergic and GABAergic systems
Uses: Alcohol withdrawal, severe insomnia, restlessness and agitation in the elderly
IV Infusions: Pre-eclamptic toxaemia, eclampsia, status epilepticus, acute alcohol withdrawal, sedation during regional anaesthesia
Dosage and routes:
Severe insomnia
• By mouth, 1–2 capsules at bedtime, 5–10 ml syrup
Restlessness/agitation in elderly
• By mouth, 1 capsule or 5 ml syrup 3 times a day
Alcohol withdrawal
• *Adult:* By mouth, initially 2–4 capsules, repeated if necessary in several hours; day 1, 9–12 capsules in 3 or 4 divided doses; day 2, 6–8 capsules in 3 or 4 divided doses; day 3, 4–6 capsules in 3 or 4 divided doses; then gradually reduced. Total treatment not to exceed 9 days. 5 ml of syrup can be substituted for each capsule. IV infusion, dose controlled by patient's response — seek specialist advice. Not recommended for use in children
Available forms include: Capsules, 192 mg base; syrup, 250 mg/5 ml, (therapeutically equivalent to 1 capsule); intravenous infusion 0.8% (8 mg/ml)
Side effects/adverse reactions:
RESP: Respiratory depression
HAEM: Thrombophlebitis

EENT: Sneezing, conjunctival irritation
CNS: Headache, confusion, paradoxical excitement, dependence
GI: Gastrointestinal disturbances
CV: Cardiovascular depression
SYSTEM: Hypersensitivity

Contraindications: Sensitivity to chlormethiazole, acute pulmonary insufficiency, alcoholics who continue to drink, lactation, pregnancy especially in first and last trimesters

Precautions: Cardiac or respiratory disease, chronic respiratory insufficiency, reduce dose in elderly, debilitated and in patients with hepatic or renal impairment, history of drug abuse, personality disorder, avoid prolonged use or abrupt withdrawal. Causes drowsiness; patients so affected should not drive or operate machinery

Pharmacokinetics: Peak plasma concentration within 15−45 min; extensively metabolised in liver

Interactions/incompatibilities:
• Increased effects: CNS depressants e.g. tranquillisers, alcohol, anaesthetics, etc
• Increase in blood/plasma levels given with: cimetidine
• Sinus bradycardia: propranolol
• Adverse neonatal reactions: maternal administration of chlormethiazole and diazoxide

Clinical assessment:
• Monitor constantly when continuously infused. Danger in high doses as patient may pass into deep unconsciousness with risk of mechanical airway obstruction

Treatment of overdose: Symptomatic basis, similar principles as barbiturate overdosage. Secure airway, give oxygen, take supportive measures

NURSING CONSIDERATIONS

Assess:
• Establish baseline of BP, pulse and respiration rates

Administer:
• Orally—ensuring patient compliance with treatment
• IV over 5−10 mins
• Use glass equipment for small children, in adults use Teflon IV cannula and change giving set every 24 hr

Perform/provide:
• Safe environment: cot sides, help with mobilisation
• Facilities for intubation and resuscitation
• Eye care; if irritation occurs check that no alcohol is consumed
• Constant monitoring of vital signs when given IV

Evaluate:
• Therapeutic effect
• Vital signs and conscious level (check by reducing IV rate during prolonged treatment) and continuous heart monitoring
• For acute confusion states resulting from hypoxia
• Side effects
• Thrombophlebitis at administration site

Teach patient/family:
• Not to take any alcohol
• That drug may cause drowsiness which persists into the next day. If this occurs not to drive or operate machinery
• That side effects include GI upsets, sneezing, headache
• About encouraging normal sleep patterns: exercise in day, milk drink, warm bath, relaxation techniques, TV/books
• Ensure patient is aware of importance of regime

chloroquine phosphate, chloroquine sulphate

Avloclor, Nivaquine

Func. class.: Antimalarial
Chem. class.: Synthetic 4-amino-quinoline derivative
Legal class.: POM but if for the prophylaxis of malaria P

Action: Inhibits parasite replications. Mechanism is unclear but there is interference with parasitic synthesis of nucleoproteins and influence on haemoglobin digestion

Uses: Treatment, prophylaxis and suppression of malaria caused by *Plasmodium vivax*, *Plasmodium ovale* and *Plasmodium falciparum* (some strains), rheumatoid arthritis, discoid and systemic lupus erythematosus, light sensitive skin eruptions, amoebic hepatitis and abscess

Dosage and routes:
Malaria prophylaxis
• *Adult:* By mouth 300 mg (base) weekly on same day; begin 2 weeks before journey and continue for 4 weeks after return
• *Child less than 5 weeks:* 12.5% adult dose; 6 weeks–11 months, 25% adult dose; 1–5 yr, 50% adult dose; 6–12 yr, 75% adult dose
Malaria (benign) treatment
• *Adult:* By mouth 600 mg (base) then 300 mg after 6–8 hr, and 300 mg on subsequent 2 days
• *Child:* By mouth 10 mg/kg then 5 mg/kg after 6–8 hr, and 5 mg/kg on subsequent 2 days
• *Adult and child:* Slow IV infusion in sodium chloride 0.9% injection 10 mg/kg base over 8 hr followed by three 8-hr infusions of 5 mg/kg base; seek specialist advice for further information
Amoebic hepatitis

• *Adult:* By mouth 600 mg (base) daily for 2 days then 150 mg twice daily for 2–3 weeks
Rheumatoid arthritis
• *Adult:* By mouth 150 mg (base) at bedtime
Systemic lupus erythematosus
• *Adult:* By mouth 150 mg (base) until maximum improvement then smaller maintenance dosage
• *Child:* 3 mg/kg (base) per day
Light sensitive skin eruptions
• *Adult:* By mouth 150–300 mg (base) daily
• *Child:* By mouth 3 mg/kg (base) daily
Available forms include: Tablets (phosphate) 250 mg; tablets (sulphate) 200 mg; both equivalent to chloroquine base 150 mg. Syrup (sulphate) 68 mg/5 ml; equivalent to base 50 mg/5 ml. Injection (sulphate) 54.5 mg/1 ml; equivalent to base 40 mg/1 ml

Side effects/adverse reactions:
CV: ECG changes, hypotension, cardiac arrhythmias
INTEG: Pruritus, depigmentation, skin eruptions, alopecia, bleaching of hair pigment
CNS: Headache, psychosis, anxiety, personality changes
EENT: Blurred vision, irreversible retinal damage, difficulty in accommodation, corneal opacities, retinal degeneration
GI: Disturbances including nausea, vomiting, diarrhoea
HAEM: Thrombocytopenia, agranulocytosis, aplastic anaemia, neutropenia

Contraindications: No absolute contraindications

Precautions: Porphyria, hepatic and renal impairment, alcoholism, pregnancy (when malaria treatment outweighs the risks), irreversible retinal damage, psoriasis, neurological disorders especially epilepsy, G6PD deficiency, children, hypersensitivity, avoid concurrent therapy with hepatotoxic drugs

Pharmacokinetics:
Period of onset: Peak 1−2 hr, half-life 3−5 days, metabolised in the liver, excreted in urine, faeces, breast milk

Interactions/incompatibilities:
• Reduced absorption: antacids
• Increased plasma concentration: cimetidine
• Chloroquine possibly increases plasma concentration of digoxin
• Antagonism of effects of: neo-stigmine and pyridostigmine

Clinical assessment:
• Ensure blood counts taken and examination for ocular disturbances if patient on extended treatment

Treatment of overdose: Induce vomiting, gastric lavage urgently. Institute resuscitation measures: protect airway and if necessary provide artificial ventilation. Reduce absorption of remaining chloroquine using activated charcoal. Seek specialist advice for further information

NURSING CONSIDERATIONS
Administer:
• Before or after meals at same time each day to maintain drug level

Perform/provide:
• Storage in tight, light-resistant containers at room temperature; injection should be kept in cool environment

Evaluate:
• Allergic reactions: pruritus, rash, urticaria
• Blood dyscrasias: malaise, fever, bruising, bleeding (rare)
• For ototoxicity (tinnitus, vertigo, change in hearing)
• For toxicity: blurring vision, difficulty focusing, headache, dizziness, knee, ankle reflexes; drug should be discontinued immediately

Teach patient/family:
• To use sunglasses in bright sunlight to decrease photophobia
• To report hearing, visual problems, fever, fatigue, bruising, bleeding, which may indicate blood dyscrasias
• Warn against driving or operating machinery on first taking drug as visual disturbances can occur
• About side-effects that should be reported immediately
• The importance of continuing drug therapy for 4 weeks, after return, for malaria prophylaxis
• To seek immediate replacement if medication is misplaced
• To be aware of malarial risk in area of travel (also quinine resistence)

---

chlorothiazide

Saluric
Func. class.: Diuretic
Chem. class.: Thiazide; sulphonamide derivative
Legal class.: POM

Action: Increases excretion of water by inhibiting sodium reabsorption at beginning of distal tubule

Uses: Oedema, hypertension

Dosage and routes:
Oedema
• Initially 0.5−1 g once or twice a day, maintenance 0.5−1 g daily or on alternate days, or less frequently
Hypertension
• 0.5−1 g daily in single or divided doses

Available forms include: Tablets 500 mg

Side effects/adverse reactions:
GU: Impotence, glycosuria
CNS: Paraesthesia, headache, dizziness, vertigo, weakness
GI: Nausea, vomiting, anorexia,

constipation, diarrhoea, cramps, pancreatitis, gastric irritation, jaundice, salivary gland inflammation
EENT: Yellow vision, blurred vision
INTEG: Rash, urticaria, purpura, photosensitivity
HAEM: Aplastic anaemia, haemolytic anaemia, leucopenia, agranulocytosis, thrombocytopenia
CV: Hypotension, orthostatic hypotension
MISC: Hypokalaemia, hypochloraemia, hyponatraemia, hyperglycaemia, hyperuricaemia, renal dysfunction, interstitial nephritis, renal failure, muscle spasm, anaphylactic reactions
RESP: Respiratory distress: pneumonitis, pulmonary oedema
Contraindications: Hypersensitivity to thiazides or sulphonamides, anuria, severe renal or hepatic impairment, Addison's disease, hypercalcaemia, breast feeding, porphyria
Precautions: Fluid and electrolyte imbalance, hypokalaemia, diabetes, gout, pregnancy, renal and hepatic impairment, lupus erythematosus, allergy, bronchial asthma
Pharmacokinetics:
Period of onset: Onset 2 hr, peak 4 hr, duration 6−12 hr; excreted in breast milk
Interactions/incompatibilities:
• Increased toxicity: lithium, non-depolarising skeletal muscle relaxants, digitalis, NSAIDs, amiodarone, disopyramide, flecainide, quinidine, corticosteroids, corticotrophin
• Decreased effects of: antidiabetics
• Decreased absorption of chlorothiazide: cholestyramine, colestipol
• Decreased hypotensive response: indomethacin

• Enhanced hypotensive response: angiotensin-converting enzyme inhibitors
• Hypercalcaemia: calcium salts
• Potentiate orthostatic hypotension: alcohol, barbiturates, narcotics
• Additive effect: other hypertensives
• Decreased arterial responsiveness to pressor amines e.g. adrenaline
Clinical assessment:
• Monitor for signs of electrolyte depletion: hypokalaemia, hypochloraemia, hyponatraemia, dehydration
Lab. test interferences: Parathyroid function tests: possibility of interference as thiazides may affect calcium metabolism
Treatment of overdose: Symptomatic and supportive therapy. Recent ingestion: emesis or gastric lavage. Treat dehydration, electrolyte imbalance, hepatic coma and hypotension. Oxygen or artificial respiration if impaired respiration
NURSING CONSIDERATIONS
Assess:
• Baseline BP, weight, fluid balance
Administer:
• In morning to avoid interference with sleep if using drug as a diuretic
• Potassium replacement as prescribed if potassium is less than 3.0 mmol/l
• With food if nausea occurs; absorption may be decreased slightly
Evaluate:
• Weight, fluid balance daily to determine fluid loss; effect of drug may be decreased if used daily
• BP lying, standing; postural hypotension may occur
• Glucose in urine if patient is diabetic
• Improvement in oedema of feet, legs, sacral area daily if medication

is being used in congestive cardiac failure

• Improvement in CVP 8 hrly
• Signs of metabolic acidosis: drowsiness, restlessness
• Signs of hypokalaemia: irregular pulse, postural hypotension, malaise, fatigue, tachycardia, leg cramps, weakness
• Rashes, raised temperature
• Confusion, especially in elderly; take safety precautions if needed

Teach patient/family:

• To increase fluid intake 2−3 litres daily unless contraindicated
• To rise slowly from lying or sitting position
• To report muscle weakness, cramps, nausea, dizziness
• Drug may be taken with food or milk
• That blood sugar may be increased in diabetics
• To take early in day to avoid nocturia

---

chlorpheniramine maleate

Alunex, Piriton
Func. class.: Antihistamine
Chem. class.: Alkylamine derivative
Legal class.: Oral dosage forms P; injection POM

Action: Acts on blood vessels, GI system, respiratory system, by competing with histamine for H_1-receptor site; decreases allergic response by blocking histamine

Uses: By oral route for symptomatic relief from allergic conditions responsive to antihistamines such as hay fever, rhinitis, urticaria. By injection for emergency treatment of anaphylactic reactions

Dosage and routes:

• *Adult:* By mouth 4 mg four to six hrly (maximum daily: 24 mg), SC/IM 10−20 mg, maximum 40 mg/24 hr; IV 10−20 mg with 5−10 ml blood over 1 min
• *Child 6−12 yr:* By mouth 2 mg four to six hrly (maximum daily 12 mg), 2−5 yr: 1 mg four to six hrly (maximum daily 6 mg), 1−2 yr: 1 mg twice daily

Available forms include: Tablets 4 mg; syrup 2 mg/5 ml; injection IM, SC, IV 10 mg/ml

Side effects/adverse reactions:

CNS: Various degrees of sedation; dizziness, poor coordination, inability to concentrate, excitation, headaches
CV: Hypotension, palpitations, tachycardia, arrhythmias
RESP: Increased thick secretions, chest tightness
HAEM: Haemolytic and other blood dyscrasias
INTEG: Urticaria, photosensitivity, exfoliative dermatitis
GI: Dry mouth, nausea, vomiting, diarrhoea, anorexia, constipation
EENT: Blurred vision
GU: Urinary retention

Contraindications: Hypersensitivity to H_1-receptor antagonists, patients treated with monoamine oxidase inhibitors within 14 days, premature infants, neonates

Precautions: Pregnancy, breast feeding, narrow angle glaucoma, urinary retention, prostatic hypertrophy, hepatic or cardiovascular disorders

Pharmacokinetics:

Period of onset: Onset 20−60 min, duration 8−12 hr; detoxified in liver, excreted by kidneys, (metabolites/free drug), half-life 20−24 hr

Interactions/incompatibilities:

• Increased CNS depression: alcohol, tricyclic antidepressants, anxiolytics, hypnotics
• Antagonism: betahistine — theoretical

• Enhancement of antimuscarinic effects: MAOIs. Avoid within 2 weeks of MAOI treatment.
• Additive antimuscarinic action: atropine, tricyclic antidepressants
• Causes drowsiness; patients so affected should not drive or operate machinery
Clinical assessment:
• Monitor response and watch for side effects
Lab. test interferences: May suppress positive skin test results and hence stopped several days before the test
Treatment of overdose: Administer ipecacuanha syrup or perform gastric lavage, then activated charcoal or cathartics to minimise absorption, take supportive measures
NURSING CONSIDERATIONS
Administer:
• IV; slowly over 1 min
• With meals if GI symptoms occur; absorption may slightly decrease
Perform/provide:
• Frequent sips of water, rinsing of mouth for dryness
Evaluate:
• Therapeutic response: absence of running or congested nose or rashes
• Fluid balance; be alert for urinary retention, frequency, dysuria; drug should be discontinued if these occur
• Blood dyscrasias: thrombocytopenia, agranulocytosis (rare)
• Respiratory status: rate, rhythm, increase in bronchial secretions, wheezing, chest tightness
• Cardiac status: palpitations, increased pulse, hypotension, CNS stimulation
Teach patient/family:
• All aspects of drug use; to notify clinician if confusion, sedation, hypotension occurs
• To avoid driving or other hazardous activity if drowsiness occurs

• To avoid concurrent use of alcohol or other CNS depressants

chlorpromazine HCI

Largactil
Func. class.: Neuroleptic
Chem. class.: Phenothiazine-derivative
Legal class.: POM

Action: Depresses cerebral cortex, hypothalamus, limbic system, which control activity aggression; blocks neurotransmission produced by dopamine at synapse; exhibits antagonism of α-adrenergic, cholinergic effects
Uses: Schizophrenia and other psychoses, mania and hypomania, short term adjunctive management of violent or dangerously impulsive behaviour, severe anxiety, psychomotor agitation, excitement, intractable hiccup, nausea and vomiting, induction of hypothermia
Dosage and routes:
Psychoses
• *Adult:* By mouth initially 25 mg 3 times daily or 75 mg at night increasing as required to 75–300 mg daily, maximum 1 g daily; IM 25–50 mg 6–8 hrly; rectal 100 mg 6–8 hrly
• *Child:* IM, by mouth 1–5 yr, 500 mcg/kg 4–6 hrly, maximum 40 mg daily; 6–12 yr, 33%–50% adult dose, maximum 75 mg daily
Nausea and vomiting of terminal illness
• *Adult:* By mouth 10–25 mg 4–6 hrly as needed; IM 25 mg initially then 25–50 mg 3–4 hrly; rectal 100 mg every 6–8 hr as needed
• *Child:* By mouth 1–5 yr, 0.5 mg/kg 4–6 hrly, maximum 40 mg daily, IM 0.5 mg/kg 6–8 hrly; 6–12 yr by mouth 0.5 mg/

kg 4−6 hrly, maximum 75 mg daily, IM 0.5 mg/kg 6−8 hrly

Intractable hiccups

• *Adult:* By mouth 25−50 mg 3 or 4 times a day; IM 25−50 mg (used only if oral dose does not work); and if this fails IV infusion 25−50 mg in 500−1000 ml sodium chloride injection infused slowly

Available forms include: Tablets 10, 25, 50, 100 mg; syrup 25 mg/5 ml, 100 mg/5 ml; suppositories 100 mg; injection IM, IV 25 mg/ml

Side effects/adverse reactions:

RESP: Nasal stuffiness, respiratory depression

CNS: Extrapyramidal symptoms: pseudoparkinsonism, acute dystonias or dyskinesias, akathisia, tardive dyskinasia, agitation, drowsiness, apathy

HAEM: Leucopenia, agranulocytosis, anaemia

INTEG: Contact skin sensitisation, rash, photosensitivity

CV: Arrhythmias, ECG changes, tachycardia

GI: Dry mouth, constipation

ENDO: Galactorrhoea, gynaecomastia, amenorrhoea, impotence, weight gain

EENT: Blurred vision

MISC: Impaired liver function, hypothermia

Contraindications: Pregnancy unless clinician considers essential, bone-marrow depression, closed-angle glaucoma, coma caused by CNS depressants

Precautions: Pregnancy, breast feeding, cardiovascular and cerebrovascular disease, elderly, respiratory disease, hepatic or renal dysfunction, epilepsy, Parkinson's disease, hypothyroidism, phaeochromocytoma, myasthenia gravis, prostate hypertrophy, leucopenia, acute infections, history of jaundice. Monitor for eye defects and abnormal skin pigmentation on prolonged use. Avoid abrupt withdrawal. May cause drowsiness, do not drive or operate machinery

Pharmacokinetics:

Period of onset: By mouth: onset erratic, peak 2−4 hr. Duration: may be detected for up to 6 months after last dose

IM: Onset 15−30 min, peak 15−20 min. Duration: may be detected for up to 6 months after last dose

IV: Onset 5 min, peak 10 min. Duration: may be detected for up to 6 months after last dose

REC: Onset erratic, peak 3 hr

Metabolised by liver, excreted in urine (metabolites), enters breast milk; 95% bound to plasma proteins; elimination half-life 10−20 hr

Interactions/incompatibilities:

• Oversedation: other CNS depressants, alcohol, barbiturates, other sedatives

• Enhanced hypotensive effect: antihypertensive drugs, anaesthetics

• Decreased absorption with: antacids

• Increased anticholinergic effects: other anticholinergics

• Decreased effects of: levadopa, amphetamine, clonidine, guanethidine, adrenaline, antiparkinsonian agents

• Reduced antipsychotic effect: anticholinergics

• Reduced response to hypoglycaemic agents

• Possible transient metabolic encephalopathy with simultaneous administration of desferrioxamine

• Increased toxicity with lithium

Lab. test interferences:

False positive: Pregnancy tests, thyroid function tests, Coombs' test

Interferes with: Adrenal medullary tests

Interferes with estimation for: 5-

hydroxyindole-acetic acid, blood urea, urinary ketones and steroids, porphobilinogen and vitamin B_{12}

Treatment of overdose: Gastric lavage up to 6 hr after ingestion. Induction of vomiting unlikely to be any use. Give activated charcoal and supportive measures. Seek specialist advice

NURSING CONSIDERATIONS

Assess:
• Baseline BP (lying and standing)
• For hoarding or giving of medication to other patients

Administer:
• Being aware that drug can cause contact sensitisation
• Drug in liquid form if hoarding is suspected (ensure drug is swallowed)
• Stagger IM injection sites if more than 4 ml is used

Perform/provide:
• Decreased noise input by dimming lights, avoiding loud noises
• Supervised ambulation until stabilised on medication; do not involve in strenuous exercise because fainting is possible; patient should not stand still for long periods of time
• Increased fluids to prevent constipation
• Sips of water, frequent rinsing for dry mouth

Evaluate:
• Therapeutic response: decrease in emotional excitement, hallucinations, delusions, paranoia, reorganisation of patterns of thought, speech
• Effect, orientation, loss of consciousness, reflexes, gait, co-ordination, sleep pattern disturbances
• BP standing and lying; report drops of 30 mmHg; pulse and respirations 4 hrly during initial treatment
• Dizziness, faintness, palpi-

tations, tachycardia on rising
• Extrapyramidal symptoms including akathisia (inability to sit still, no pattern to movements), tardive dyskinesia (bizarre movements of the jaw, mouth, tongue, extremities), pseudoparkinsonism (rigidity, tremors, pill rolling, shuffling gait)
• Skin turgor daily
• Constipation, urinary retention daily; if these occur, increase bulk, water in diet

Teach patient/family:
• That orthostatic hypotension occurs often, and to rise from sitting or lying position gradually
• To remain lying down after IM injection for at least 30 min
• To avoid saunas, hot showers, or hot baths since hypotension may occur
• To avoid abrupt withdrawal of this drug
• To avoid non-prescribed preparations (cough, hayfever, cold) unless approved by clinician since serious drug interactions may occur; avoid use with alcohol or CNS depressants; increased drowsiness may occur
• To use a sunscreen during sun exposure to prevent photosensitivity
• Regarding compliance with drug regimen
• About necessity for meticulous oral hygiene since oral candidiasis may occur
• To report sore throat, malaise, fever, bleeding, mouth sores

chlorpropamide

Diabinese, Glymese
Func. class.: Oral hypoglycaemic
Chem. class.: Sulphonylurea (1st generation)
Legal class.: POM

Action: Causes functioning β-cells in pancreas to synthesise and release insulin, leading to drop in blood glucose levels; not effective if patient lacks functioning β-cells; effects outside the pancreas may also play a role in action

Uses: Stable, mild to moderately severe maturity onset diabetes (diabetes mellitus, type II diabetes), diabetes insipidus

Dosage and routes:
Diabetes mellitus
• By mouth 250 mg daily initially, with breakfast, adjusted according to response. Recommended maximum daily dose is 500 mg. Elderly patients 100−125 mg daily initially but alternative drug used if possible

Diabetes insipidus
• *Adult:* up to 350 mg daily
• *Child:* up to 200 mg daily

Available forms include: Tablets 100, 250 mg

Side effects/adverse reactions:
CNS: Headache, weakness, dizziness
GI: Cholestatic jaundice, nausea, vomiting, diarrhoea
HAEM: Leucopenia, thrombocytopenia, agranulocytosis, aplastic anaemia, pancytopenia, haemolytic anaemia
INTEG: Sensitivity reactions leading to transient rashes, dermatitis, photosensitivity
ENDO: Hypoglycaemia

Contraindications: Hypersensitivity to sulphonylureas, breast feeding, hepatic disease, renal insufficiency, insulin dependant (juvenile) diabetes mellitus, diabetic ketoacidosis, pregnancy, surgery, severe infection or trauma, serious impairment of hepatic, renal or thyroid function

Precautions: Severe hypoglycaemic reactions, lactation

Pharmacokinetics:
Period of onset: Completely absorbed by GI route, onset 1 hr, peak 3−6 hr, duration 24 hr, half-life 36 hr, metabolised in liver, excreted in urine (metabolites and unchanged drug), breast milk, 90%−95% is plasma protein bound

Interactions/incompatibilities:
• Increased effects of chlorpropamide by drugs that are highly protein bound: NSAIDs, salicylates, sulphonamides, chloramphenicol, probenecid, coumarins, also MAOIs, β-blockers
• Alcohol intolerance with chlorpropamide may produce a disulfiram−alcohol interaction
• Decreased effectiveness and hyperglycaemia may be caused by calcium channel blockers, corticosteroids, oral contraceptives, thiazide and other diuretics, isoniazid, oestrogens, thyroid preparations, phenytoin, nicotinic acid and symphathomimetics
• Cyclophosphamide may alter diabetic control in some patients

Treatment of overdose: Acute poisoning, empty the stomach by aspiration and lavage; no loss of consciousness treat with oral glucose; severe reaction with coma use 50% glucose intravenously followed by 10% glucose as a continuous infusion; blood glucose level to be maintained above 5.6 mmol/l. In case hypoglycaemia recurs monitor patient over several days

NURSING CONSIDERATIONS

Assess:

• Blood glucose prior to administration

Administer:

• Drug 30 min before breakfast and ensure dietary allowance is consumed to prevent hypoglycaemia

Evaluate:

• Therapeutic response: decrease in polyuria, polydipsia, polyphagia, clear alertness, absence of dizziness, stable gait

• Hypoglycaemic/hyperglycaemic reaction that can occur soon after meals

Teach patient/family:

• That all food included in diet plan must be eaten in order to prevent hypoglycaemia

• To take drug in morning to prevent hypoglycaemic reactions at night

• That this drug must be continued on daily basis; explain consequence of discontinuing drug abruptly

• Symptoms of hypo- and hyperglycaemia, what to do about each

• To test urine glucose levels with reagent strip approximately 2 hr after each meal as appropriate

• To use capillary blood glucose test while on this drug as appropriate

• To check for symptoms of cholestatic jaundice: dark urine, pruritus, yellow sclera; if these occur, clinician should be notified

• That diabetes is life-long illness, drug will not cure disease

• To carry Medic-Alert ID and/or Diabetic card for emergency purposes

• To seek clinician's advice about taking other medicines

chlortetracycline HCl

Aureomycin

Func. class.: Broad spectrum antibiotic

Chem. class.: Tetracycline

Legal class.: POM

Action: Interferes with bacterial cell synthesis

Uses: Respiratory tract infection; sexually-transmitted disease, acne; infection due to *Chlamydia*, *Brucella*, *Mycoplasma*, *Rickettsia* spp

Dosage and routes:

• *Adult:* By mouth 250−500 mg 6 hrly; topical apply 3 times a day; eye apply 2-hrly

Available forms include: Capsules 250 mg; eye ointment 1%; ointment, cream 3%

Side effects/adverse reactions:

Side effects following topical application are mild and transient.

GU: Nephrotoxicity

CNS: Headache, benign intracranial hypotension

GI: Nausea, vomiting, diarrhoea, anorexia, hepatotoxicity, enterocolitis

HAEM: Eosinophilia, neutropenia, thrombocytopenia, haemolytic anaemia

INTEG: Rash, urticaria, photosensitivity; stinging, burning at site of topical application

Contraindications: Hypersensitivity to tetracyclines

Precautions: Over growth of resistant organisms may occur with long-term use

Interactions/incompatibilities:

• Decreased absorption of tetracycline: antacids, dairy products, iron, quinalpril, calcium salts, sucralfate, bismuth, zinc

• Increased effect of: oral anticoagulants

- Decreased effect: penicillins
- Nephrotoxicity enhanced by: methoxyflurane
- Reduced effect of: oral contraceptives

Treatment of overdose:
After oral ingestion: Gastric lavage, administer milk or antacid, supportive treatment

NURSING CONSIDERATIONS
Administer:
- Enough medication to completely cover lesions (topical)
- After cleansing with soap and water and drying well before each topical application
- Orally 1 hr before or 2 hr after ferrous or milk products; 3 hr after antacid

Evaluate:
- Allergic reaction: burning, stinging, swelling, redness (topical)
- Therapeutic response: decrease in size, number of lesions (topical)
- Negative blood cultures following oral therapy

Teach patient/family:
For topical application:
- To use gloves when applying a cream ointment
- To avoid use of non-prescribed creams, ointments, lotions unless directed by clinician
- To wash hands before, after each application
- To avoid touching or squeezing lesions to prevent spread of infection

For oral medication:
- To avoid milk products administered at same time as tetracycline
- Avoid sun exposure since burns may occur; sunscreen does not decrease photosensitivity
- That all prescribed medication must be taken to prevent superimposed infection

---

chlorthalidone

Hygroton
Func. class.: Diuretic
Chem. class.: Thiazide-related; sulphonamide derivative
Legal class.: POM

Action: Acts on distal tubule by increasing excretion of water, sodium, chloride, potassium
Uses: Oedema, hypertension, diabetes insipidus
Dosage and routes:
Oedema
- By mouth: Initially 50 mg daily or 100−200 mg alternate days, reduced for maintenance
Hypertension
- By mouth: 25−50 mg daily
Diabetes insipidus
- By mouth: Initially 100 mg twice a day reduced to 50 mg daily for maintenance, where possible
Available forms include: Tablets 50 mg
Side effects/adverse reactions:
GU: Uraemia, glycosuria
CNS: Drowsiness, paraesthesia, dizziness
GI: Nausea, vomiting, anorexia, constipation, diarrhoea, cramps, pancreatitis, hepatitis
EENT: Blurred vision
INTEG: Rash, urticaria
META: Hyperglycaemia, hyperuraemia, increased creatinine
HAEM: Aplastic anaemia, haemolytic anaemia, leucopenia, agranulocytosis, thrombocytopenia
CV: Irregular pulse, orthostatic hypotension
ELECT: Hypokalaemia, hypercalcaemia, hyponatraemia, hypochloraemia, hypomagnesaemia
Contraindications: Hypersensitivity to thiazides or sulphonamides, severe renal or hepatic

disease, hypercalcaemia, Addison's disease, symptomatic hyperuricaemia

Precautions: Hypokalaemia, renal disease, pregnancy, hepatic disease, gout, lupus erythematosus, diabetes mellitus, coronary or cerebral arteriosclerosis, lactation, hyperlipidaemia

Pharmacokinetics:
Period of onset: Onset 2 hr, peak 6 hr, duration 24−72 hr; excreted unchanged by kidneys, enters breast milk, half-life 35−55 hr

Interactions/incompatibilities:
• Increased toxicity: lithium, digitalis, carbenoxolone, corticosteroids, corticotrophin, NSAIDs
• Increased effects of: antihypertensive drugs (e.g. guanethidine, methyldopa, β-blockers, vasodilators, calcium antagonists and angiotensin-converting enzyme inhibitors), non-depolarizing skeletal muscle relaxants
• Decreased effects of: antidiabetics, disopyramide
• Decreased absorption of thiazides: cholestyramine, colestipol
• Decreased hypotensive response: NSAIDs

Clinical assessment:
• Electrolytes: potassium, sodium, chloride; include blood urea nitrogen, blood sugar, full blood count, serum creatinine, blood lipids (in hyperlipidaemic patients)

Treatment of overdose: Lavage, emesis or activated charcoal, monitor electrolytes and blood pressure, and give supportive treatment

NURSING CONSIDERATIONS
Assess:
• Baseline BP standing, lying; respirations, weight, fluid balance
Administer:
• Orally. In morning to avoid interference with sleep if using as a diuretic

• Potassium replacement may be required in severe cases of oedema, hepatic cirrhosis and in long-term therapy
• With food if nausea occurs; absorption may be decreased slightly
Evaluate:
• Weight during initial treatment: fluid balance to determine fluid loss.
• Initial effect of drug, increase or decreasing−then reduce where possible to a maintenance dose
• Rate, depth, rhythm of respiration, effect of exertion
• Effect of any other drugs taken e.g. digoxin may need to be reduced in congestive cardiac failure
• BP lying, standing; postural hypotension may occur
• Regular urinalysis
• Improvement in oedema of feet, legs, sacral area daily if medication is being used in congestive heart failure
• Improvement in CVP 8 hrly
• Signs of metabolic acidosis: infrequent and mild; usually resolve spontaneously or following temporary reduction of dosage
• Signs of hypokalaemia: postural hypotension, malaise, fatigue, tachycardia, leg cramps, weakness
• Rashes
• Confusion, especially in elderly; electrolyte balance (precarious)
Teach patient/family:
• To increase fluid intake to 2−3 litres daily unless contraindicated.
• To rise slowly from lying or sitting position
• To notify clinician of muscle weakness, cramps, nausea, dizziness, gout, increase in oedema
• Drug may be taken with food or milk if nausea occurs
• To take in morning for oedema
• To test urine

134

cholera vaccine

cholera vaccine

Func. class.: Vaccine
Chem. class.: Killed suspension of
Vibrio cholerae
Legal class.: POM

Action: Stimulates antibodies to causative organism of cholera
Uses: Provides some protection against the bacterium *Vibrio cholerae*
Dosage and routes:
• Two doses, minimum 1 week, preferably 4 weeks apart; deep subcutaneous or IM injection
• *Adult:* First dose, 0.5 ml; 2nd dose, 1.0 ml
• *Child 1–5 yr:* First dose, 0.1 ml; 2nd dose, 0.3 ml
• *Child 5–10 yr:* First dose, 0.3 ml; 2nd dose, 0.5 ml
Available forms include: Multidose injection 10 ml, single dose 1.5 ml
Side effects/adverse reactions:
CNS: Headache
INTEG: Mild discomfort at injection site
NERV: Neuritis, polyneuritis
SYST: Mild fever and malaise
Contraindications: Existing acute illness, hypersensitivity, infants less than 1 yr
Precautions: Pregnancy
Pharmacokinetics: Immunity persists for 6 months
Clinical assessment:
• Immune status
NURSING CONSIDERATIONS
Assess:
• Active or suspected infection
• History of allergies or known hypersensitivity to any component
Administer:
• Deep subcutaneous or IM route. To reduce reactions use the intradermal route after repeated doses
• At least 1 week between doses and preferably 4 weeks
• Shake well prior to use

• Discard unused vaccine at the end of session
Perform/provide:
• Store at 2–8°C, protect from light. Record details (lot numbers) of vaccine and patient
• Ensure correct documentation completed
• Facilities for dealing with anaphylaxis
Evaluate:
• Reaction to vaccination
• Level of patient understanding for further precautions against cholera
Teach patient/family:
• That general food/water hygiene is still required
• That full immunity is not immediate, unless it is a booster dose
• Remind that documents needed in some countries
• Recommend further dose in 6 months if living in endemic area
• Warn about general malaise, raised temperature and mild discomfort at site

cholestyramine

Questran, Questran A
Func. class.: Hypolipidaemic
Chem. class.: Bile acid sequestrant
Legal class.: POM

Action: Adsorbs, combines with bile acids to form insoluble complex that is excreted through faeces; loss of bile acids lowers cholesterol levels
Uses: Primary hyperlipidemia; pruritus associated with biliary obstruction; diarrhoea caused by ileal resection, radiation, vagotomy, Crohn's disease, vagal neuropathy
Dosage and routes:
• *Adult:* By mouth. Hyperlipidaemia, diarrhoea 12–24 g daily,

maximum 36 g daily. Pruritus 4−8 g daily

• *Child 6−12 yrs:* Initial dose based on following calculation (child's weight in kg × adult dose) ÷ 70. Subsequent dosage adjustment may be necessary where clinically indicated

Available forms include: Powder 4 g

Side effects/adverse reactions:

GI: Constipation, abdominal pain, nausea, faecal impaction, aggravation of haemorrhoids, flatulence, vomiting, diarrhoea

INTEG: Rash, irritation of perianal area

HAEM: Decreased vitamin A, D, K leading to increased bleeding tendency, hyperchloremic acidosis

Contraindications: Hypersensitivity, complete biliary obstruction

Precautions: Pregnancy, lactation, children under 6 yr

Pharmacokinetics:

Period of onset: Maximum effect in 2 weeks; excreted in faeces

Interactions/incompatibilities:

• Decrease absorption of phenylbutazone, warfarin, thiazides, digitalis, penicillins, tetracyclines, phenobarbitone, folic acid, corticosteroids, iron, thyroxine, clindamycin, trimethoprim, chenodeoxycholic acid, anticoagulants, paracetamol, vitamins A, D, K

• Decreased activity of oral vancomycin

Clinical assessment:

• Cardiac glycoside level, if both drugs are being administered

• Clotting time if anticoagulants are being co-administered

• Serum cholesterol, triglyceride levels, electrolytes if on extended therapy

NURSING CONSIDERATIONS

Assess:

• For signs of vitamin A, D, K deficiency

Administer:

• Drug before meals, at bedtime; give all other medications 1 hr before cholestyramine or 4−6 hr after cholestyramine to avoid poor absorption

• Drug sprinkled on food or stirred into beverage; let stand for 2 min

• May result in excess foaming if mixed with carbonated drinks (use large glass)

Evaluate:

• Bowel pattern daily; increase bulk, water in diet if constipation develops

• Therapeutic response: decreased triglyceride, cholesterol level (hyperlipidaemia); diarrhoea, pruritus (excess bile)

Teach patient/family:

• Symptoms of hypothrombinaemia: bleeding mucous membranes, dark tarry stools, petechiae; report immediately

• Stress patient compliance since toxicity may result if doses are missed

• That risk factors should be decreased: high fat diet, smoking, alcohol consumption, absence of exercise

• That non-prescribed preparations should be avoided unless directed by clinician

choline magnesium trisalicylate

Trilisate

Func. class.: Anti-inflammatory analgesic

Chem. class.: Salicylate

Legal class.: P

Action: Prevents inflammation and pain impulse production by peripheral and CNS inhibition of prostaglandin synthesis; antipyretic action results from inhibition of hypothalamic heat-regulating centre

Uses: Rheumatoid arthritis, osteoarthritis

Dosage and routes:

• *Adult:* By mouth 0.5−1.5 g twice a day

Available forms include: Tablets 500 mg

Side effects/adverse reactions:

HAEM: Thrombocytopenia, agranulocytosis, leucopenia, neutropenia, haemolytic anaemia, increased bleeding time

CNS: Stimulation, drowsiness, dizziness, confusion, convulsions, headache, flushing, hallucinations, coma

GI: Nausea, vomiting, GI bleeding, diarrhoea, heartburn, anorexia, hepatitis

INTEG: Rash, urticaria, bruising

EENT: Tinnitus, hearing loss

CV: Rapid pulse, pulmonary oedema

RESP: Wheezing, hyperpnoea

ENDO: Hypoglycaemia, hyponatraemia, hypokalaemia

Contraindications: Hypersensitivity to salicylates, GI bleeding, haemophilia, active peptic ulcer, children less than 12 yr

Precautions: Anaemia, hepatic disease, renal disease, Hodgkin's disease, pregnancy, lactation, gastritis

Pharmacokinetics:

Period of onset: Onset 15−30 min, peak 1−2 hr, duration 4−6 hr, metabolised by liver, excreted by kidneys, excreted in breast milk, half-life 1−3½ hr

Interactions/incompatibilities:

• Decreased effects of this drug: antacids, steroids, urinary alkalinisers

• Increased effects of this drug: metoclopramide

• Increased blood loss: alcohol, heparin

• Increased effects of: anti-coagulants, insulin, methotrexate, phenytoin, sulphonylurea hypoglycaemics

• Decreased effects of: probenecid, spironolactone, sulfinpyrazone

• Toxic effects: Digoxin, acetazolamide

Clinical assessment:

• Liver function studies: aspartate aminotransferase, alanine aminotransferase, bilirubin, if patient is on long-term therapy

• Renal function studies: blood urea nitrogen, serum creatinine if patient is on long-term therapy

• Blood studies: Full blood count, Hb, prothrombin-time if patient is on long-term therapy

Lab. test interferences:

Increase: Coagulation studies, liver function studies, serum uric acid, amylase, CO_2, urinary protein

Decrease: Serum potassium, protein bound iodine, cholesterol

Treatment of overdose: Lavage with sodium bicarbonate solution 5%, monitor electrolytes and vital signs

NURSING CONSIDERATIONS

Assess:

• Baseline weight and fluid balance

Administer:

• Crushed or whole; chewable tablets may be chewed

• 30 min before or 2 hr after meals

Perform/provide:

• Repositioning to decrease pain

• Cool cloth for fever

Evaluate:

• Fluid balance; decreasing output may indicate renal failure (long-term therapy)

• Hepatotoxicity: dark urine, clay-coloured stools, yellowing of skin, sclera, itching, abdominal pain, fever, diarrhoea if patient is on long-term therapy

• Allergic reactions: rash, urti-

caria; if these occur, drug may need to be discontinued
• Renal dysfunction: decreased urine output
• Ototoxicity: tinnitus, ringing, roaring in ears
• Visual changes: blurring, halos, corneal, retinal damage
• Oedema in feet, ankles, legs
• Prior drug history; there are many drug interactions
• Weight changes

Teach patient/family:
• To report any symptoms of hepatotoxicity, renal toxicity, visual changes, ototoxicity, allergic reactions (long-term therapy)
• Not to exceed recommended dosage; acute poisoning may result
• To read label on other non-prescription drugs; many contain aspirin and should not be taken
• That therapeutic response takes 2 weeks (arthritis)
• To avoid alcohol ingestion; GI bleeding may occur
• To record weight daily

---

choline theophyllinate

Choledyl, Sabidal SR
Func. class.: Spasmolytic
Chem. class.: Choline salt of theophylline
Legal class.: P

Action: Relaxes smooth muscle of respiratory system by blocking phosphodiesterase, which increases cyclic-AMP; 64% theophylline

Uses: Relief and prevention of bronchospasm in asthma, chronic bronchitis and emphysema

Dosage and routes:
• *Adult and child over 12 yr:* tablets, 100−400 mg 6 hrly; modified-release tablets 424 mg, one morning and two evening

• *Child 3−6 yr:* 62.5−125 mg 8 hrly
• *Child 6−12 yr:* tablets, 300−400 mg daily in divided doses. Adjust doses to desired response, therapeutic level

Available forms include: Elixir 62.5 mg/5 ml; tablets 100, 200 mg, modified-release tablets 424 mg

Side effects/adverse reactions:
CNS: Anxiety, restlessness, insomnia, dizziness, convulsions, headache, lightheadedness
CV: Palpitations, sinus tachycardia, hypotension
GI: Nausea, vomiting, anorexia, diarrhoea, bitter taste, dyspepsia
RESP: Increased rate
INTEG: Flushing, urticaria

Contraindications: Hypersensitivity to xanthines, tachydysrhythmias

Precautions: Elderly, congestive cardiac failure, cor pulmonale, hepatic disease, active peptic ulcer disease, hyperthyroidism, hypertension, children, cardiac disease

Pharmacokinetics:
Rapid absorbtion, metabolised in liver, excreted in urine, breast milk

Interactions/incompatibilities:
• Decreased action of this drug: phenytoin, rifampicin, aminoglutethimide, carbamazepine smoking, alcohol
• Increased action of this drug: cimetidine, erythromycin, allopurinol, propranolol, oral contraceptives, influenza vaccine, β-adrenergic agonists
• Cardiotoxicity: ephedrine and other sympathomimetics

Clinical assessment:
• Assess therapeutic blood levels; toxicity may occur with small increase above therapeutic level peak serum levels not greater than 20 mcg/ml, optimum is 10−20 mcg/ml

Treatment of overdose: Induced emesis or gastric lavage, activated charcoal, saline laxative and in severe cases (usually serum theophylline of 40 mg/litre or more) charcoal haemoperfusion. For fall in blood pressure nurse in head down position. Monitor and correct electrolyte imbalances

NURSING CONSIDERATIONS
Administer:
• After meals to decrease GI symptoms
Evaluate:
• Therapeutic response: absence of dyspnoea, wheezing
• Fluid balance: if diuresis occurs, dehydration may result in elderly or children
• Respiratory rate, rhythm, depth; notify clinician of abnormalities
• Allergic reactions: rash, urticaria; if these occur, inform clinician and withhold further doses
Teach patient/family:
• To check non-prescribed medications, current prescription medications for ephedrine, which will increase stimulation
• To avoid hazardous activities; dizziness may occur
• On all aspects of drug therapy: dosage, routes, side effects, when to notify the clinician
• If GI upset occurs, to take drug with 200 ml water; avoid food; absorption may be decreased

---

chorionic gonadotrophin, human

Gonadotrophon LH, Profasi
Func. class.: Human chorionic gonadotrophin
Chem. class.: Polypeptide hormone
Legal class.: POM

Action: Stimulates production of gonadal steroids, stimulates ovulation from developed follicles
Uses: Infertility, anovulation, hypogonadism, non-obstructive cryptorchidism

Dosage and routes:
Infertility/anovulation
• *Adult:* IM 10,000 U 1 day after last dose of menotrophin
Hypogonadism
• *Adult:* IM 500–2000 U 2 or 3 times a week for minimum 4 months, when menotrophin may be added if required
Cryptorchidism
• *Child (boy 4–9 yr):* IM 500–1000 U alternate days for several weeks
Available forms include: Powder for injection 500, 1000, 2000, 5000 U
Side effects/adverse reactions:
CNS: Headache, depression, fatigue, anxiety, irritability
GU: Gynaecomastia, early puberty, oedema, ectopic pregnancy, multiple pregnancy
INTEG: Pain at injection site
Contraindications: Hypersensitivity, pituitary hypertrophy/tumour, early puberty, prostatic cancer
Precautions: Where fluid retention may be dangerous: asthma, migraine, convulsive disorders, cardiac disease, renal disease
Pharmacokinetics:
IM: Peak 6 hr, half-life 11–24 hr, excreted by kidneys
Interactions/incompatibilities: None known
Treatment of overdose: Conservative support required for ovarian hyperstimulation
NURSING CONSIDERATIONS
Assess:
• Baseline BP, weight, fluid balance
Administer:
• Only after clomiphene citrate has been tried on anovulatory client
• After reconstitution with solvent enclosed in package
Evaluate:

• Weight weekly; notify clinician if weekly weight gain is more than 2 kg
• BP
• Be alert for decreasing urinary output, increasing oedema
• Oedema, hypertension
Teach patient/family:
• All aspects of drug usage
• That some lower abdominal pain may occur 36 hr after administration
• Advise best time to have intercourse — about 36 hr after injection
• To report persistant or severe abdominal pain, abdominal distension or breathlessness immediately
• To report symptoms of ectopic pregnancy: dizziness, pain on one side or shoulder, pallor, weak thready pulse, haemorrhage (shock may proceed rapidly)
• To report facial, axillary, pubic hair, change in voice, penile enlargement, acne in male, abdominal pain, distention, vaginal bleeding in women. (Changes only for long-term use)

---

cimetidine

Tagamet
Func. class.: Antihistamine — H$_2$ receptor
Chem. class.: Imidazole derivative
Legal class.: POM

Action: Antagonises histamine at H$_2$ receptor site in parietal cells, which inhibits gastric acid secretion
Uses: Treatment and prophylaxis of benign gastric and duodenal ulcer; Zolinger-Ellison syndrome; reflux oesophagitis
Dosage and routes:
Gastric/duodenal ulcer
• *Adult:* By mouth, 400 mg twice a day or 800 mg at night for 4−6 weeks, maximum 2.4 g daily.

Parenteral 200 mg IM or 200−400 mg IV 4−6 hrly
• *Child:* 20−30 mg/kg daily in divided doses
Prophylaxis
• *Adult:* 400−800 mg daily
Reflux oesophagitis
• *Adult:* 400 mg 4 times a day for 4−8 weeks
Zollinger-Ellison syndrome
• *Adult:* 400 mg 4 times a day increased as required, normal maximum 2.4 g daily
Available forms include: Tablets 200, 400, 800 mg; liquid 200 mg/5 ml; injection 200 mg; infusion 400 mg in 100 ml 0.9% sodium chloride; chewable tablets 200 mg; suspension 200 mg/5 ml; soluble tablets 400 mg
Side effects/adverse reactions:
CNS: Headache, depression, dizziness, anxiety, weakness, psychosis, tremors, convulsions, confusion
GI: Diarrhoea, abdominal cramps, paralytic ileus, jaundice, altered bowel habit
GU: Gynaecomastia, galactorrhoea, impotence, interstitial nephritis
CV: Bradycardia, tachycardia
HAEM: Agranulocytosis, thrombocytopenia, neutropenia, aplastic anaemia, increase in bleeding time
INTEG: Urticaria, rash, alopecia, sweating, flushing, exfoliative dermatitis
Precautions: Pregnancy, lactation, hepatic disease, renal disease
Pharmacokinetics:
Period of onset: Peak 1−1½ hr after oral administration, half-life 1½ hr; metabolised by liver, excreted in urine (unchanged), enters breast milk
Interactions/incompatibilities:
• Increased toxicity: fluorouracil, flecainide, disopyramide, pethidine, metronidazole, quinine, metformin, metoprolol, pro-

pranolol, phenytoin, quinidine, theophylline, tricyclic antidepressants, lignocaine, anticoagulants, carbamazepine
• Decreased action of this drug: rifampicin

Clinical assessment:
• Blood urea nitrogen, creatinine; plasma phenytoin levels in patients on both drugs

Treatment of overdose: Gastric lavage or forced emesis

NURSING CONSIDERATIONS

Assess:
• Fluid balance ratio
• Temperature, pulse, respiration and BP

Administer:
• With meals for prolonged drug effect
• IV slowly (over 30 min); arrhythmias may occur

Teach patient/family:
• About side effects
• That gynaecomastia, impotence may occur, but is reversible after treatment is ended
• Avoid driving or other hazardous activities until patient is stabilised on this medication
• Give dietary advice
• To avoid non-prescribed preparations: aspirin, cough, cold preparations
• Inform clinician if pregnancy is suspected

---

ciprofloxacin

Ciproxin
Func. class.: Broad spectrum antibiotic
Chem. class.: Fluoroquinolone
Legal class.: POM

Action: Inhibits the enzyme DNA gyrase, preventing bacterial synthesis of functional DNA
Uses: Infection due to Gram-negative or Gram-positive bacteria, including those resistant to other antibiotics. Anaerobic bacteria, *Ureaplasma* and some *Mycobacteria* are normally less susceptible

Dosage and routes:
Uncomplicated urinary tract infections
• *Adult:* By mouth 250 mg 12 hrly; IV 100 mg 12 hrly
Complicated/severe urinary tract infections
• *Adult:* By mouth 500 mg 12 hrly; IV 200 mg 12 hrly
Respiratory, bone, skin, joint infections
• *Adult:* By mouth 250−750 mg 12 hrly; IV 200 mg 12 hrly
Available forms include: Tablets 250, 500 mg (as hydrochloride); injection 100, 200 mg (as lactate)

Side effects/adverse reactions:
CNS: Headache, dizziness, fatigue, insomnia, depression, restlessness, confusion, convulsions
GI: Nausea, abdominal pain, flatulence, heartburn, vomiting, diarrhoea, oral candidiasis, dysphagia, increased alanine aminotransferase, aspartate aminotransferase
INTEG: Rash, pruritus, urticaria, photosensitivity, flushing, fever, chills
MS: Blurred vision, tinnitus

Contraindications: Hypersensitivity to quinolones
Precautions: Pregnancy, lactation, children, severe renal disease, history of convulsive disorder

Pharmacokinetics:
Period of onset: Peak 1 hr, half-life 3−4 hr; excreted in urine as active drug, metabolites

Interactions/incompatibilities:
• Decreased absorption: magnesium antacids, aluminium hydroxide, iron salts
• Increased serum levels of ciprofloxacin: probenecid
• Increased theophylline levels when used with ciprofloxacin

• Prolonged bleeding time when administered with anticoagulants

Clinical assessment:

• Serum theophylline levels in patients receiving both drugs

Treatment of overdose: Gastric lavage

NURSING CONSIDERATIONS

Assess:

• Fluid balance and urinary pH. pH of less than 5.5 is ideal

Administer:

• After a clean midstream specimen of urine has been obtained for bacterial culture and sensitivity tests

• Advise patient to limit intake of highly alkaline foods, drugs, and dairy products, peanuts, vegetables, antacids and sodium bicarbonate

Evaluate:

• Response to treatment indicated by decreased dysuria, frequency, urgency and negative bacteriological test results, which suggest that infection has resolved

• Allergic reactions: fever, rash, urticaria, pruritus

• CNS symptoms: headache, dizziness, fatigue, insomnia, depression

Teach patient/family:

• Avoid antacids containing magnesium or aluminium until at least 4 hr after taking the drug

• To avoid sunlight or use suncare preparations as photosensitivity occurs

• Fluid intake must be increased to 3 litres daily to avoid crystallisation and renal calculi

• If dizziness occurs ambulant patients require careful supervision

• The full course of treatment must be completed

• The clinician must be informed if adverse reactions occur

• Medication must be taken with food or milk to reduce gastric irritation

• Effects of alcohol can be enhanced

---

cisapride

Prepulsid

Func. class.: Gastrointestinal prokinetic agent

Chem. class.: Methoxybenzamide

Legal class.: POM

Action: Cisapride probably acts by enhancing the release of acetylcholine at the level of the myenteric plexus in the gut wall

Uses: Treatment of symptoms (e.g. heartburn, regurgitation) and mucosal lesions associated with gastro-oesophageal reflux. Relief of symptoms (e.g. nausea, early satiety, anorexia, bloating, epigastric pain) of impaired gastric motility secondary to disturbed and delayed gastric emptying associated with diabetes, systemic sclerosis and autonomic neuropathy

Dosage and routes:

Gastro-oesophageal reflux

• *Adult:* By mouth 10 mg 3 or 4 times a day for 12 weeks

Impaired gastric motility

• *Adult:* By mouth 10 mg 3 or 4 times a day for at least 6 weeks

• *Children (below 12 yr):* Not recommended

Available forms include: Tablets 10 mg (as monohydrate)

Side effects/adverse reactions:

CNS: Headache, lightheadedness, convulsions

GI: Abdominal cramps, borborygmi, diarrhoea

Contraindications: Pregnancy; gastrointestinal haemorrhage, mechanical obstruction, perforation.

Precautions: Elderly, renal or

hepatic impairment, lactation. Accelerates gastric emptying so gastric absorption of concomitant drugs can be diminished, while intestinal absorption is increased. Plasma levels of drugs needing careful titration e.g. anti-convulsants

Pharmacokinetics: Rapidly absorbed, peak 1−2 hr, elimination half-life 10 hr, metabolised by liver, excreted in urine, faeces. Cisapride is extensively bound to plasma proteins

Treatment of overdose: Gastric lavage, close observation and general supportive measures

NURSING CONSIDERATIONS

Assess:
• Bowel pattern before treatment

Administer:
• 15 to 30 min before a meal. When an additional dose is required to control night-time symptoms, the tablet should be taken at bedtime

Evaluate:
• Reduction of symptoms.
• Bowel pattern during treatment

Teach patient/family:
• Not to take non-prescribed medicines
• To inform clinician if pregnancy occurs

---

cisplatin

Platosin

Func. class.: Antineoplastic alkylating agent
Chem. class.: Platinum complex
Legal class.: POM

Action: Alkylates DNA, RNA; inhibits enzymes that allow synthesis of proteins

Uses: Advanced bladder cancer, lung cancer, stomach cancer, adjunctive in metastatic testicular cancer, adjunctive in metastatic ovarian cancer

Dosage and routes:
• Single-agent: IV infusion 50−120 mg/m^2 every 3−4 weeks, or 15−20 mg/m^2 daily for 5 days every 3−4 weeks

Available forms include: Injection IV, 1.0 mg/ml; 10, 25, 50, 100 mg vials. Powder for preparing IV solution; 10, 50 mg vials

Side effects/adverse reactions:
EENT: Tinnitus, hearing loss, vestibular toxicity
HAEM: Thrombocytopenia, leucopenia, pancytopenia
CV: Cardiac abnormalities
GI: Nausea, vomiting, diarrhoea, weight loss
GU: Renal tubular damage, renal insufficiency, impotence, sterility, amenorrhoea, gynaecomastia, hyperuraemia
INTEG: Alopecia, dermatitis, peripheral neuropathy
CNS: Convulsions
RESP: Fibrosis
META: Hypomagnesaemia, hypocalcaemia, hypokalaemia, hypophosphataemia

Contraindications: Hypersensitivity, dehydration, renal impairment, hearing disorders, depressed bone marrow function, pregnancy, lactation

Precautions: Live vaccines, radiation therapy within 1 month, chemotherapy within 1 month, thrombocytopenia

Pharmacokinetics: Mainly excreted in urine; half-life of unbound, active drug 1 hr

Interactions/incompatibilities:
• Increased toxicity: aminoglycosides

Clinical assessment:
• Full blood count, differential, platelet count weekly; withhold drug if WBC is less than 2000, or platelet count is less than 75,000; notify clinician of results
• Renal function studies: blood urea nitrogen, serum uric acid,

urine creatinine clearance before, during therapy

Treatment of overdose:
Monitor blood count, renal function, electrolytes. Correct electrolyte imbalances; transfusion products, filgrastim as needed

NURSING CONSIDERATIONS
Assess:
• Baseline vital signs

Administer:
• Following local cytotoxic policy
• Avoiding use of aluminium equipment as cisplatin is degraded on contact

Perform/provide:
• Strict medical asepsis, protective isolation if WBC levels are low
• Strict fluid balance with forced diuresis for patients on high doses
• Antiemetics before and during treatment
• Sedation during treatment (usually haloperidol and lorazepam)
• Storage protected from light, at room temperature, for 20 hr once reconstituted
• Special skin care
• Increase fluid intake to 2−3 litre/daily to prevent urate deposits, calculi formation
• Diet low in purines: offal (kidney, liver), dried beans, peas to maintain alkaline urine

Evaluate:
• Weight
• Temperature and blood pressure 4 hrly when neutropenic. Changes may indicate start of infection
• Fluid balance; report fall in urine output of 30 ml/hr
• Bruising, bleeding due to thrombocytopenia, cytopenia
• Nausea and vomiting
• Diarrhoea
• Fluid overload
• Signs of infection
• Dyspnoea, râles, unproductive cough, chest pain, tachypnoea
• Urinalysis changes indicate nephrotoxicity
• Effects of alopecia on body image, discuss feelings about body changes
• Yellowing of skin, sclera, dark urine, clay-coloured stools, itchy skin, abdominal pain, fever, diarrhoea
• Joint or stomach pain, oedema in feet and legs, shaking
• Inflammation of mucosa, breaks in skin

Teach patient/family:
• Protective isolation precautions
• To report any complaints or side effects to clinician
• That impotence or amenorrhoea can occur, reversible after discontinuing treatment
• To report any changes in breathing or coughing
• That hair may be lost during treatment; a wig or hairpiece may make patient feel better (available free on NHS); new hair may be different in colour, texture
• The possibility of tinnitus and peripheral neuropathy
• Good mouth care
• That a bland diet may reduce the metallic taste

---

clemastine fumarate

Tavegil
Func. class.: Antihistamine H_1-receptor antagonist
Chem. class.: Ethanolamine derivative
Legal class.: P

Action: Acts on blood vessels, GI tract, respiratory system by competing with histamine for H_1-receptor site; decreases allergic response by blocking histamine
Uses: Allergy symptoms, rhinitis, angioneurotic oedema, urticaria

Dosage and routes:
• *Adult and child over 12 yr:* By mouth 1 mg twice a day
• *Child 1 to 3 yr:* 250−500 mcg twice a day; 3 to 6 yr 500 mcg twice a day; 6 to 12 yr: 500−1000 mcg twice a day
Available forms include: Tablets 1 mg; elixir 500 mcg/5 ml

Side effects/adverse reactions:
CNS: Dizziness, drowsiness, poor coordination, fatigue, anxiety, euphoria, confusion, paraesthesia, neuritis
CV: Hypotension, palpitations, tachycardia
RESP: Increased thick secretions, wheezing, chest tightness
GI: Dry mouth, nausea, vomiting, anorexia, constipation, diarrhoea
INTEG: Rash, urticaria, photosensitivity
GU: Retention
EENT: Blurred vision, dilated pupils, tinnitus, nasal stuffiness, dry nose, throat, mouth

Contraindications: Hypersensitivity to H_1-receptor antagonists, pregnancy, lactation, hepatic disease

Precautions: Increased intraocular pressure, renal disease, bronchial asthma, stenosed peptic ulcers, prostatic hypertrophy, bladder neck obstruction, acute asthma attack, lower respiratory tract disease

Pharmacokinetics:
Period of onset: Peak 5−7 hr, duration 10−12 hr or more; metabolised in liver, excreted by kidneys

Interactions/incompatibilities:
• Increased CNS depression: barbiturates, narcotics, hypnotics, tricyclic antidepressants, alcohol, betahistine, anticholinergics, antiparkinsonian drugs, e.g. benzhexol
• Increased effect of this drug: MAOIs

Treatment of overdose: Administer ipecacuanha syrup or lavage, diazepam for convulsions, vasopressors

NURSING CONSIDERATIONS

Administer:
• With meals if GI symptoms occur; absorption may slightly decrease

Perform/provide:
• Boiled sweets, gum, frequent rinsing of mouth for dryness

Evaluate:
• Therapeutic response: absence of running or congested nose or rashes
• Fluid balance; be alert for urinary retention, frequency, dysuria; drug should be discontinued if these occur
• Blood dyscrasias: thrombocytopaenia, agranulocytosis (rare)
• Respiratory status: rate, rhythm, increase in bronchial secretions, wheezing, chest tightness
• Cardiac status: palpitations, increased pulse, hypotension

Teach patient/family:
• All aspects of drug use; to notify clinician if confusion, sedation, hypotension occur
• To avoid driving or other hazardous activity if drowsiness occurs
• To avoid concurrent use of alcohol or other CNS depressants
• To change position slowly, as drug may cause dizziness, hypotension (elderly)

clindamycin HCl/ clindamycin palmitate HCl/clindamycin phosphate

Dalacin C, Dalacin T
Func. class.: Antibacterial
Chem. class.: Lincomycin derivative
Legal class.: POM

Action: Binds to 50S subunit of

bacterial ribosomes, suppresses protein synthesis

Uses: Infections caused by staphylococci, streptococci, pneumococci, *Rickettsia* spp, *Fusobacterium* spp, *Actinomyces*, spp, *Peptostreptococcus*, spp, *Bacteroides* spp, topically in acne vulgaris

Dosage and routes:
• *Adults:* By mouth 150−450 mg 6-hrly; IM IV 0.6−2.7 g daily in 2−4 doses; topically as a thin film twice a day
• *Child:* By mouth 3−6 mg/kg, 6 hrly, IM/IV 15−40 mg/kg daily (minimum 300 mg daily) in 3−4 doses

Available forms include: Injection 150 mg/ml; capsules 75, 150 mg; oral suspension 75 mg/5ml; topical lotion and solution 0.1%

Side effects/adverse reactions:
HAEM: Leucopenia, eosinophilia, agranulocytosis, thrombocytopenia
GI: Nausea, vomiting, abdominal pain, diarrhoea, pseudomembranous colitis. Increased aspartate aminotransferase, alanine aminotransferase, bilirubin, alkaline phosphatase, jaundice
GU: Vaginitis
INTEG: Rash, urticaria, pruritus, erythema, pain, abscess at injection site, skin irritation, contact dermatitis, Gram-negative folliculitis and stinging of the eyes after topical administration

Contraindications: Hypersensitivity to this drug or lincomycin, diarrhoeal states

Precautions: Renal disease, liver disease, GI disease, pregnancy, lactation

Pharmacokinetics:
Period of onset: Oral: peak 45 min
IM: Peak 3 hr. Half-life 2½ hr, metabolised in liver, excreted in urine, bile, faeces as active/inactive metabolites, crosses placenta, excreted in breast milk

Interactions/incompatibilities:
• Increased neuromuscular blockade: non-depolarising muscle relaxants
• Decreased action of: pyridostigmine, neostigmine

Clinical assessment:
• Any patient with compromised renal system; drug is excreted slowly in poor renal system function; toxicity may occur rapidly
• Liver studies: aspartate aminotransferase, alanine aminotransferase. Drug excreted more slowly in hepatic impairment and may be hepatotoxic
• Blood studies: During long-term therapy WBC, RBC, platelets; drug should be discontinued if bone marrow depression occurs

Treatment of overdose: No specific treatment. Not removable from circulation by dialysis

NURSING CONSIDERATIONS
Assess:
• Bowel patterns
• Fluid balance
• Allergies before treatment, reaction of each medication; note allergies on chart in bright red letters; notify all people giving drugs
• Culture and sensitivity before drug therapy; drug may be used as soon as culture is taken
• BP, pulse in patient receiving drug parenterally

Administer:
• IV by infusion only; do not administer bolus dose
• IM deep injection; rotate sites
• Orally with at least 250 ml water

Perform/provide:
• Storage at room temperature (capsules) and up to 2 weeks (reconstituted solution)
• Adrenaline, suction, endotracheal intubation, equipment on unit/ward
• Adequate intake of fluids (2 litres) during diarrhoea episodes

Evaluate:
• Therapeutic response: decreased temperature, negative culture and sensitivity
• Bowel pattern during treatment
• Skin eruptions, itching, dermatitis after administration
• Respiratory status: rate, character, wheezing, tightness in chest

Teach patient/family:
• To take oral drug with full glass of water; may be taken with food if GI symptoms occur
• Aspects of drug therapy: need to complete entire course of medication to ensure organism death
• To report sore throat, fever, fatigue; could indicate superimposed infection
• That drug must be taken in equal intervals around clock to maintain blood levels
• To wear or carry ID if allergic to this drug
• To notify nurse of diarrhoea

---

clobetasol propionate

Dermovate
Func. class.: Topical corticosteroid
Chem. class.: Synthetic fluorinated agent, group I potency (very potent)
Legal class.: POM

Action: Antipruritic and anti-inflammatory properties
Uses: Psoriasis, eczema, contact dermatitis, lichen planus, discoid lupus erythematosus; usually reserved for short-term treatment of severe dermatoses that have not responded to less potent formulation

Dosage and routes:
• *Adult and child:* Apply sparingly to affected area twice daily for up to 4 weeks, reducing frequency
Available forms include: Ointment

0.05%; cream 0.05%; scalp application 0.05%

Side effects/adverse reactions:
INTEG: Burning, irritation, acne, folliculitis, hypertrichosis, perioral dermatitis, hypopigmentation, atrophy, striae, miliaria, allergic contact dermatitis, secondary infection
META: Adrenocortical suppression

Contraindications: Hypersensitivity, skin infection, rosacea, acne, perioral dermatitis
Precautions: Pregnancy, lactation, viral infections, bacterial infections

NURSING CONSIDERATIONS
Administer:
• Only to affected areas; do not get in eyes
• Leaving uncovered or lightly covered; occlusive dressing is not recommended
• Only to dermatoses; do not use on weeping, denuded, or infected area

Perform/provide:
• Cleansing to remove bacteria and cream before application of drug
• Treatment for a few days after area has cleared

Evaluate:
• Therapeutic response: absence of severe itching, patches on skin flaking
• Temperature, if fever develops, drug should be discontinued

Teach patient/family:
• To avoid sunlight on affected area; photosensitivity may occur
• To limit treatment to 14 days using less than 50 g a week
• To report any side-effects

clofibrate

Atromid-S
Func. class.: Hypolipidaemic
Chem. class.: Aryloxyisobutyric acid derivative
Legal class.: POM

Action: Reduces blood levels of very low density lipoproteins, low density lipoproteins and triglycerides by reducing synthesis or increasing clearance. Increases high density lipoprotein-cholesterol

Uses: Type III hyperlipidaemia, severe hypertriglyceridaemia in types IIb, IV and V

Dosage and routes:
• *Adult:* By mouth 1.5−2 g daily in divided doses

Available forms include: Capsules 500 mg

Side effects/adverse reactions:
GI: Nausea, vomiting, dyspepsia, increased liver enzymes, flatulence, hepatomegaly, gastritis, increased cholelithiasis

INTEG: Rash, urticaria, pruritus, dry hair and skin, alopecia

HAEM: Leucopenia, anaemia, eosinophilia

CNS: Fatigue, weakness, headache

GU: Decreased libido, impotence, dysuria, proteinuria, oliguria

MS: Myalgias, arthralgias, myositis

CV: Angina, dysrhythmias, thrombophlebitis, pulmonary emboli

Contraindications: Severe hepatic disease, severe renal disease, primary biliary cirrhosis, pregnancy, lactation, gall bladder disease, gall stones

Precautions: Peptic ulcer, nephrotic syndrome

Pharmacokinetics:
Period of onset: Peak 2−6 hr, plasma protein binding greater than 90%; half-life 6−25 hr, excreted in urine, metabolised in liver

Interactions/incompatibilities:
• Increased effects of: sulphonylureas, anticoagulants, phenytoin

Clinical assessment:
• Renal and hepatic function in patients on long-term therapy

Lab. test interferences:
Increase: Serum protein-bound iodine
Decrease: Urinary VMA

Treatment of overdose: Symptomatic

NURSING CONSIDERATIONS
Evaluate:
• A wide range of adverse reactions; including nausea, vomiting, rashes, fatigue, weakness, angina, headaches

Teach patient/family:
• To take tablets regularly, toxicity may occur from missed doses
• To report bleeding mucous membranes or dark tarry stools immediately (signs of hypothrombinaemia)
• To report GU symptoms i.e. decreased libido, impotence, dysuria, proteinuria, oliguria
• That birth control should be practiced whilst taking the drug
• To reduce other risk factors i.e. high fat diet, smoking, lack of exercise

clomiphene citrate

Clomid, Serophene
Func. class.: Ovulation stimulant
Chem. class.: Non-steroidal triethylamine derivative
Legal class.: POM

Action: Increases LH, FSH, which increase maturation of ovarian follicle, ovulation, development of corpus luteum

Uses: Anovulatory infertility

Dosage and routes:
• *Adult:* By mouth 50 mg daily for 5 days from 5th day of cycle; if no ovulation occurs double dose for next cycle; maximum 6 cycles
Available forms include: Tablets 50 mg
Side effects/adverse reactions:
EENT: Blurred vision, diplopia, photophobia, scotomata
HAEM: Haemolytic anaemia
CNS: Headache, depression, restlessness, anxiety, nervousness, fatigue, insomnia
GI: Nausea, vomiting, constipation, increased appetite, abdominal pain
INTEG: Rash, dermatitis, urticaria, alopecia, hot flushes
GU: Polyuria, frequency, birth defects, spontaneous abortions, multiple ovulation, breast pain, oliguria, ovarian hyperstimulation
Contraindications: Hypersensitivity, pregnancy, hepatic disease, undiagnosed vaginal bleeding, endometrial cancer, ovarian cyst
Precautions: Depression
Pharmacokinetics: Readily absorbed; metabolised in liver, excreted in faeces, stored in fat, half-life 5−7 days
Interactions/incompatibilities: None known
NURSING CONSIDERATIONS
Administer:
• At same time each day to maintain drug level
Teach patient/family:
• That multiple births are slightly more common after drug is taken
• To notify clinician if low abdominal pain occurs, may indicate ovarian cyst, cyst rupture (miscarriage rate is slightly higher)
• Visual symptoms (blurring, spots) may occur rarely and should be reported to clinician; drug will be stopped
• Mucus awareness (temperature taking is rarely accurate)

• Suggest intercourse alternate days when mucus appears ovulatory
• If pregnancy is suspected, clinician must be notified immediately

---

clomipramine hydrochloride

Anafranil, Anafranil SR
Func. class.: Antidepressant
Chem. class.: Tricyclic antidepressant
Legal class.: POM

Action: Inhibits neuronal reuptake of neurotransmitters noradrenaline and serotonin within CNS; precise mechanism of antidepressive action uncertain
Uses: Depressive illness, adjunctive treatment of obsessional/phobic states, cataplexy associated with narcolepsy
Dosage and routes:
• By mouth, initially 10 mg daily, increased gradually as necessary to 30−150 mg in divided doses or as single dose at bedtime, higher doses may be required; elderly patients 10 mg daily, up to 30−75 mg maximum
• IM injection: up to 150 mg daily
• IV infusion: initially 25−50 mg to test tolerance, increased by 25 mg daily until optimum therapeutic dose is reached
Available forms include: Capsules, 10, 25, 75 mg; syrup, 25 mg/5 ml; injection, 25 mg/2 ml; tablets modified-release 75 mg
Side effects/adverse reactions:
HAEM: Agranulocytosis, leucopenia, eosinophilia, purpura, thrombocytopenia, jaundice
CNS: Sedation, blurred vision, tremor, confusion, hypomania, behavioural disturbances, convulsions

META: Blood sugar level changes in diabetics or weight changes
GI: Nausea, dry mouth, black tongue, paralytic ileus
GU: Difficulty with micturition, changes in sexual function
INTEG: Sweating, rashes
CV: Arrhythmias, postural hypotension, tachycardia, syncope

Contraindications: Recent myocardial infarction, heart block, cardiac failure, any cardiac arrhythmia, severe liver impairment, concurrent use of MAOIs, narrow angle glaucoma, urinary retention, mania, porphyria

Precautions: Diabetes, cardiac disease, epilepsy, pregnancy, hepatic impairment, thyroid disease, psychoses; avoid abrupt cessation of therapy; caution in anaesthesia, elderly, bladder neck obstruction, lactation

Pharmacokinetics: Onset of effect over 2−4 weeks. Half-life 17−28 hr. Converted in liver to active metabolite; excreted in urine

Interactions/incompatibilities:
• Increased toxicity: MAOIs within 3 weeks of stopping therapy, anaesthetic agents
• Decreased effects of guanethidine, bethanidine, debrisoquine, clonidine, methyldopa
• Potentiation of adrenaline, ephedrine, isoprenaline, noradrenaline, phenylephrine, phenylpropanolamine
• Sedation potentiated by alcohol, other CNS depressants
• Plasma levels decreased by barbiturates, and increased by methylphenidate, neuroleptics
• Effects enhanced by thyroid hormones

Clinical assessment:
• Check that MAOIs have not been taken in last 3 weeks
• Caution prescribing with anaesthesia
• Full blood count, white cell differential monthly for first 4 months, thereafter if problems suspected

Treatment of overdose: Gastric lavage, activated charcoal; nurse in intensity therapy unit monitoring ECG. Supportive treatment

NURSING CONSIDERATIONS
Assess:
• Baseline BP; all vital signs in patient with cardiovascular disease
• Weight

Administer:
• IV use dilute in 0.9% sodium chloride or 5% dextrose and mix well. Initially 25−50 mg in 200−500 ml in 2 hr IV
• Orally at bedtime if drowsiness occurs, check dose taken. Divide dose in the elderly. Not with alcohol

Perform/provide:
• Counselling for sexual problems
• Fluids and fibre for constipation
• Mouth care as required for dryness
• Measures to minimise effects of sweating e.g. change linen
• Checks that retention has not occurred
• Safe environment; get patient up slowly; help with mobilisation

Evaluate:
• BP (lying and standing) 4 hrly plus other vital signs in cardiovascular disease
• Weight weekly (may lose/gain)
• Other side effects
• Mood, sleeping pattern
• Suicidal tendencies

Teach patient/family:
• To swallow whole, not to be chewed
• Patient must not drive or operate machinery if drug causes drowsiness
• To avoid alcohol
• That medication takes 2−3 weeks to work; not to stop taking drug suddenly
• The importance of reporting side

effects such as sore throat, mouth lesions and fever
• About problems with sexual functions

---

clonazepam

Rivotril
Func. class.: Anticonvulsant
Chem. class.: Benzodiazapine derivative
Legal class.: CD Benz POM

Action: Prevents generalisation of convulsive activity and raises seizure threshold
Uses: All clinical forms of epilepsy including; absence, atypical absence, akinetic, myoclonic seizures, status epilepticus
Dosage and routes:
• *Adult:* By mouth initially 1 mg at night, 0.5 mg in the elderly, gradually increased over 2−4 weeks to 4−8 mg daily
• *Child under 1 yr:* Initially 250 mcg daily by mouth increased to 0.5−1 mg; 1−5 yr, 250 mcg daily by mouth increased to 1−3 mg; 5−12 yr, 0.5 mg daily by mouth increased to 3−6 mg
Status epilepticus
• *Adult:* Slow IV injection 1 mg over 30 seconds
• *Child:* 500 mcg over 30 seconds. Clonazepam can also be infused in sodium chloride or dextrose solutions
Available forms include: Tablets 0.5, 2 mg; injection 1 mg/ml
Side effects/adverse reactions:
HAEM: Thrombocytopenia, leucocytosis, eosinophilia
CNS: Drowsiness, dizziness, confusion, behavioural changes, tremors, insomnia, headache, suicidal tendencies
GI: Nausea, constipation, polyphagia, anorexia, abnormal liver function tests, diarrhoea

INTEG: Rash, alopecia, hirsutism
EENT: Increased salivation, nystagmus, diplopia, abnormal eye movements, sore gums
RESP: Respiratory depression, dyspnoea, congestion
CV: Palpitations, bradycardia
Contraindications: Hypersensitivity to benzodiazepines, acute pulmonary insufficiency; respiratory depression
Precautions: Open-angle glaucoma, chronic respiratory disease, lactation, pregnancy, porphyria
Pharmacokinetics:
Period of onset: Peak 1−2 hr, metabolised by liver, excreted in urine, half-life 18−50 hr
Interactions/incompatibilities:
• Increased CNS depression: alcohol, barbiturates, narcotics, antidepressants, other anticonvulsants
• Decreased effect of this drug: carbamazepine phenytoin, phenobarbitone
Clinical assessment
• Renal studies: blood urea nitrogen, urine creatinine
• Blood studies: RBC, haematocrit, Hb, WBC, platelet
• Hepatic studies: alanine aminotransferase, aspartate aminotransferase, bilirubin
Treatment of overdose: Lavage. Supportive treatment. Antagonism with flumazenil in non-epileptic patients
NURSING CONSIDERATIONS
Administer:
• IV; slowly (1 mg over 30 secs); infused in sodium chloride or dextrose
• With food, milk to decrease GI symptoms
Perform/provide:
• Assistance with ambulation during early part of treatment; dizziness occurs
Evaluate:

• Therapeutic response: decreased seizure activity, document on patient's chart
• Mental status: mood, alertness, affect, behavioural changes; if mental status changes, notify clinician
• Allergic reaction: red raised rash; if this occurs, drug should be discontinued
• Blood dyscrasias: may cause fever, sore throat, bruising, rash, jaundice
• Toxicity: bone marrow depression, nausea, vomiting, ataxia, diplopia, cardiovascular collapse

Teach patient/family:
• To avoid driving, other activities that require alertness
• To avoid alcohol ingestion or CNS depressants, increased sedation may occur
• Not to discontinue medication quickly after long-term use; taper off over several weeks
• All aspects of the drug: action, use, side effects, adverse reactions, when to notify clinician

---

clonidine HCl

Catapres, Dixarit, Catapres Perlongets
Func. class.: Antihypertensive
Chem. class.: Central α-adrenergic agonist
Legal class.: POM

Action: Inhibits sympathetic vasomotor centre in CNS, which reduces impulses in sympathetic nervous system; blood pressure decreases, pulse rate, cardiac output decreases

Uses: Hypertension, migraine prophylaxis, menopausal flushing

Dosage and routes:
Hypertension
• *Adult:* By mouth 50−100 mcg 3 times a day increased every 2−3 days, usual maximum 1.2 mg daily or 1−3 modified-release tablets of 250 mcg daily in divided doses; slow IV injection 150−300 mcg, maximum 750 mcg in 24 hr for hypertensive crisis

Migraine prophylaxis, menopausal flushing
• 50 mcg twice daily increased after 2 weeks to 75 mcg twice a day if required

Available forms include: Tablets 25 mcg, 100 mcg; modified-release tablets 250 mcg; IV injection 150 mcg

Side effects/adverse reactions:
CV: Hypotension, orthostatic palpitations, rebound hypertension after sudden withdrawal
CNS: Drowsiness, sedation, headache, fatigue, nightmares, insomnia, mental changes, anxiety, depression, hallucinations, delirium
GI: Nausea, vomiting, malaise, constipation, dry mouth
INTEG: Rash, alopecia, facial pallor, pruritus, oedema, chilblains
EENT: Taste change, parotid pain
ENDO: Hyperglycaemia
MS: Muscle/joint pain, leg cramps
GU: Impotence, dysuria, nocturia, gynaecomastia

Contraindications: Hypersensitivity
Precautions: Myocardial infarction (recent), chronic renal failure, Raynaud's disease, thyroid disease, depression, pregnancy, lactation

Pharmacokinetics:
Period of onset: Peak 3−5 hr; half-life 6−20 hr, metabolised by liver, 70% excreted in urine (50% unchanged, 20% inactive metabolites), crosses blood-brain barrier, excreted in breast milk

Interactions/incompatibilities:
• Increased CNS depression: narcotics, sedatives, alcohol, anaesthetics

• Decreased hypotensive effects: tricyclic antidepressants, MAOIs, α-adrenergic blockers
• Increased hypotensive effects: diuretics
• Increased bradycardia: β-blockers, cardiac glycosides

Clinical assessment:
• Increased risk of withdrawal hypertension: β-blockers, tricyclic antidepressants
• Baselines in renal, liver function tests before therapy begins

Treatment of overdose: Gastric lavage, supportive treatment, administer an α-adrenergic blocking drug e.g. phentolamine for severe overdose

NURSING CONSIDERATIONS
Administer:
• 1 hr before meals
• IV infusion of 0.9% sodium chloride (as prescribed) to expand fluid volume if severe hypotension occurs (according to local policy)
Evaluate:
• Therapeutic response: decrease in BP
• Signs of chronic cardiac failure
• Renal symptoms: polyuria, oliguria, frequency
Teach patient/family:
• To take dose 1 hr before meals
• Not to discontinue drug abruptly; rebound rise in BP may follow causing raised BP, anxiety, headache, insomnia, tachycardia, tremors, nausea, sweating
• That drug may cause dizziness, fainting, lightheadedness during first few days of therapy
• Stress patient compliance with dosage schedule even if feeling better
• Not to use non-prescription (cough, cold, or allergy) products unless directed by clinician
• Not to stop drug unless directed by clinician
• Patient to avoid sunlight or wear sunscreen if in sunlight, photosensitivity may occur
• Notify clinician of: mouth sores, sore throat, fever, swelling of hands or feet, irregular heartbeat, chest pain, signs of angioneurotic oedema
• Excessive perspiration, dehydration, vomiting; diarrhoea may lead to fall in BP — consult clinician if these occur
• May cause skin rash or impaired perspiration

---

clotrimazole (topical)

Canesten
Func. class.: Local antifungal
Chem. class.: Imidazole derivative
Legal class.: P

Action: Interferes with fungal DNA replication; binds sterols in fungal cell membrane, which increases permeability, leaking of cell nutrients
Uses: Tinea pedis, tinea cruris, tinea corporis, tinea versicolor, *Candida albicans* infection of the vagina, vulva. Dermatophyte infections of the skin
Dosage and routes:
• *Adult and child:* Topical: apply to affected area twice a day for at least 2 weeks for candidal infections and 1 month for dermatophyte infections; Intravaginal: 1 tablet at night for 1 (500 mg), 3 (200 mg) or 6 (100 mg) nights, or 1 application of cream (10%) at night for 1 night or 1 application of cream (2%) for 6 nights
Available forms include: Cream, powder, solution, spray 1%; vaginal tablets 100, 200, 500 mg, vaginal cream 2%, 10%
Side effects/adverse reactions:
INTEG: Rash, urticaria, stinging, burning

Contraindications: Hypersensitivity
Precautions: Pregnancy, lactation
NURSING CONSIDERATIONS
Administer:
• After cleansing with soap, water before each application, dry well
• Enough medication to cover lesions completely
• 1 filled applicator or 1 tablet deep-intravaginally each night; 500 mg as a single dose
Evaluate:
• Allergic reaction: burning, stinging, swelling, redness
• Therapeutic response: decrease in size, number of lesions, in itching or white patches around vulva
Teach patient/family:
• To wash hands before, after each application
• To apply with glove to prevent further infection
• To avoid use of non-prescription creams, ointments, lotions unless directed by clinician
• Cream should be applied daily to the partner's penis to prevent re-infection in vaginal, vulval infections

---

clozapine

Clozaril
Func. class.: Antipsychotic agent
Chem. class.: Dibenzodiazepine
Legal class.: POM

Action: Rapid acting sedative antipsychotic. Weak dopamine antagonist properties, potent α-adrenergic blocker, anticholinergic, antihistaminic
Uses: In patients who are non-responsive to, or intolerant of, conventional neuroleptics
Dosage and routes:
• *Adult:* The dose must be adjusted individually. By mouth 25–50 mg on the first day. The dose may then be increased in daily increments of 25–50 mg to a maximum of 300 mg daily. Judicious increments (not exceeding 100 mg) are permissible up to 900 mg daily. In most patients, efficacy can be expected with 200–450 mg daily in divided doses. After achieving maximum therapeutic benefit many patients can be maintained on a lower dose. Careful downward titration to 150–300 mg daily in divided doses is recommended. Up to 200 mg can be given as a single evening dose
• *Elderly:* By mouth initial dose 25 mg, increasing in increments of 25 mg daily
Available forms include: Tablets 25, 100 mg
Side effects/adverse reactions:
INTEG: Skin reactions
GI: Hypersalivation, gastrointestinal disturbances, dry mouth, cholestasis, increases in hepatic enzymes
CV: Tachycardia, ECG changes, arrhythmias, postural hypotension
CNS: Drowsiness, fatigue, transient autonomic reactions, EEG changes and lowering of the seizure threshold, rarely delirium, extrapyramidal symptoms, neuroleptic malignant syndrome, disturbances in temperature regulation
HAEM: Neutropenia, unexplained leucocytosis
Contraindications: History of drug-induced neutropenia/agranulocytosis; myeloproliferative disorders; alcoholic and toxic psychoses; drug intoxication; comatose conditions and other forms of severe CNS depression; severe hepatic or renal disease; pregnancy; lactation; children; co-administration drugs causing agranulocytosis
Precautions: Prostatic enlargement, narrow-angle glaucoma, paralytic ileus, renal disease

Pharmacokinetics: 90−95% absorption of oral doses 50−60% first pass metabolism. Peak plasma levels 2.1 hr post-dose. Hepatic metabolism. Half life 6−26 hr

Interactions/incompatibilities:
• Enhanced toxicity to blood: co-trimoxazole, chloramphenicol, sulphonamides, pyrazolone analgesics, phenylbutazone, penicillamine, carbamazepine, cytotoxic agents
• Enhanced risk of neuroleptic malignant syndrome: lithium
• Enhanced toxicity of: warfarin
• Enhanced CNS effects of: narcotics, benzodiazepines, alcohol, antihistamines MAOIs
• Enhanced activity of: anticholinergic, hypotensive drugs

Clinical assessment:
• If the white blood cell count falls below 3000/mm^3 and/or the absolute neutrophil count drops below 1500/mm^3 the drug must be withdrawn and the patient closely monitored
• In the event of an infection, or routine WBC count between 3000 and 3500/mm^3 and/or a neutrophil count between 1500 and 2000/mm^3 the patient should be re-evaluated immediately
• Should either count decline further, clozapine must be withdrawn at once. Otherwise, treatment may continue provided that leucocytes and granulocytes are checked at least twice weekly until it is certain that they are stable
• If the WBC count falls below 1000/mm^3 after drug withdrawal and/or neutrophils decrease below 500/mm^3 the patient should be referred immediately for specialised care
• In patients with a history of seizures, or with cardiovascular, renal or liver disease, the initial dose should be low and any increase should be slow

• Regular monitoring of liver function tests in patients with liver disease
• Warfarin levels in patients receiving both drugs

Treatment of overdose: Gastric lavage, activated charcoal, supportive measures. Close medical supervision for at least 4 days; possible delayed reactions

NURSING CONSIDERATIONS

Assess:
• Patients must be registered with the Clorazil Patient Monitoring Service
• Initiation of treatment must be in hospital inpatients, who must have a normal white blood cell and differential blood count
• Only patients with normal findings may receive the drug

Perform/provide:
• Blood count should be repeated every week for the first 18 weeks, and then at 2 weeks intervals for the duration of the therapy

Teach patient/family:
• If treatment is to be stopped, a gradual dose reduction over 1 to 2 weeks is recommended. Abrupt discontinuation carries the risk of rebound psychosis
• That they must ensure regular blood test undertaken whilst on this medication this may restrict holidays
• To contact the clinician immediately if any kind of infection begins to develop

cocaine HCl (ophthalmic)

Cocaine Eye-drops, Combination product
Func. class.: Local anaesthetic
Chem. class.: Ester
Legal class.: CD POM

Action: Prevents generation and transmission of pain impulses along neurones; produces local vasoconstriction

Uses: Local anaesthetic

Dosage and routes: Topical solutions of 4−10% (greater than 4% not recommended due to systemic effects)

Available forms include: Eye-drops, 4%

Side effects/adverse reactions:

SYST: Absorption after topical application, hypersensitivity

CNS: Dependence, stimulation, excitement, tremor, convulsions

CV: Bradycardia, tachycardia, hypotension, hypertension, ventricular fibrillation

EENT: Blurred vision, corneal damage, ulceration

Contraindications: Hypersensitivity to ester local anaesthetics

Precautions: Cardiovascular disease, thyrotoxicosis, hypertension, porphyria

Pharmacokinetics: Rapid onset of anaesthesia, duration at least 30 min

Interactions/incompatibilities:

• Toxicity increased by: sympathomimetics (adrenaline), MAOIs

Clinical assessment:

• Evaluate effects on eye such as keratitis

NURSING CONSIDERATIONS

Perform/provide:

• Proper storage and administration according to CD regulations (abuse/misuse)

• Storage in a cool place

Evaluate:

• Therapeutic effect

• Side effects

Teach patient/family:

• Effects of drug

• Not to attempt to drive until effects of drug have worn off

co-careldopa (levodopa/carbidopa)

Sinemet, Sinemet LS, Sinemet-Plus, Sinemet CR

Func. class.: Antiparkinson agent

Legal class.: POM

Action: Decarboxylation of levodopa to dopamine, which increases dopamine levels in brain. Carbidopa prevents peripheral breakdown of levodopa

Uses: Parkinsonism

Dosage and routes:

• *Adult:* By mouth initially, 100−125 mg (expressed as levodopa) 3−4 times daily adjusted according to response; usual maintenance 0.75−1.5 g daily in divided doses after food

Available forms include: Tablets (mg carbidopa/mg levodopa) 10/100, 12.5/50, 25/100; modified-release 50/200

Side effects/adverse reactions:

HAEM: Haemolytic anaemia, transient leucopenia/thrombocytopenia

CNS: Choreiform involuntary movements, fatigue, headache, anxiety, twitching, numbness, weakness, confusion, agitation, insomnia, nightmares, psychosis, hallucinations, hypomania, depression, dizziness, peripheral neuropathy

GI: Nausea, vomiting, anorexia, abdominal distress, bitter taste, transient rises in liver enzymes, GI bleeding

INTEG: Sweating, alopecia, flushing

CV: Orthostatic hypotension, tachycardia, hypertension, palpitation, arrhythmias

MISC: Reddish colouration of urine and other body fluids

Contraindications: Concurrent use of MAOIs (except selegiline), hypersensitivity, narrow-angle glaucoma, previous history of or active malignant melanoma, psychosis, drug-induced parkinsonism

Precautions: Renal disease, cardiovascular disease, hepatic disease, peptic ulcer, diabetes, pregnancy

Pharmacokinetics (of levodopa component):

By mouth: Peak 1−3 hr, metabolised in gut, liver, kidney, excreted in urine (metabolites), plasma half-life 45−65 min. Dose required 20−40% of that given without carbidopa

Interactions/incompatibilities:

• Hypertensive crisis: MAOIs (except selegiline) or within 21 days of stopping

• Dysrhythmias: cyclopropane, halogenated hydrocarbon anaesthetics

• Increased effects of: guanethidine, methyldopa, other antihypertensives

• Decreased effect of: antipsychotics

• Effects of co-careldopa reduced by: benzodiazepines, metoclopramide, domperidone, iron

Clinical assessment:

• Adjust dosage depending on patient response

• Hepatic, haematological, renal, cardiovascular, psychiatric surveillance during prolonged therapy

• Domperidone for nausea

Lab. test interferences:

False positive: Urine ketones (dipstick)

False negative: Urine glucose (glucose oxidase method)

Treatment of overdose: Gastric lavage, ECG monitoring, supportive treatment

NURSING CONSIDERATIONS

Administer:

• Drug to be given until patient is starved (before surgery)

• Follow exact prescribing times to ensure maximum therapeutic effect

• With meals; limit protein taken with drug

Perform/provide:

• Assistance with ambulation during beginning therapy

• Testing for diabetes mellitus, acromegaly if on long-term therapy

Evaluate:

• Mental status: affect, mood, behavioural changes, depression, assess suicidal tendencies

• Therapeutic response: decrease in involuntary movements; diminution of early morning stiffness

Teach patient/family:

• To change positions slowly to prevent orthostatic hypotension

• To report side effects: twitching, eye spasms; indicate overdose

• To use drug exactly as prescribed; if drug is discontinued abruptly, parkinsonian crisis may occur

• That urine, sweat may darken

codeine phosphate

Func. class.: Narcotic analgesic

Chem. class.: Opioid, phenanthrene derivative

Legal class.: P or POM (tablets, syrup), CD POM (injection)

Action: Inhibits ascending pain pathways in CNS, increases pain threshold, alters pain perception

Uses: Moderate to severe pain, non-productive cough, diarrhoea

Dosage and routes:

Pain

• *Adult:* By mouth 30−60 mg 4-hrly, maximum 240 mg daily; IM 30−60 mg every 4 hr when necessary

• *Child (1−12 yr):* By mouth 3 mg/kg daily in divided doses 4-hrly

Cough
- *Adult:* By mouth 15−30 mg 3 or 4 times a day
- *Child (1−5 yr):* By mouth 3 mg 3 or 4 times a day

Available forms include: Injection IM, 60 mg/ml; tablets 15, 30, 60 mg, syrup 15 mg/5 ml, 3 mg/5 ml

Side effects/adverse reactions:
CNS: Drowsiness, sedation, dizziness, agitation, dependency, lethargy, restlessness
GI: Nausea, vomiting, anorexia, constipation
RESP: Respiratory depression, respiratory paralysis
CV: Bradycardia, palpitations, orthostatic hypotension, tachycardia
GU: Urinary retention
INTEG: Flushing, rash, urticaria

Contraindications: Hypersensitivity to opioids, respiratory depression, increased intracranial pressure, seizure disorders, severe respiratory disorders

Precautions: Elderly, cardiac dysrhythmias

Pharmacokinetics: Onset 15−30 min, peak 1−2 hr, duration 4−6 hr; metabolised by liver, excreted by kidneys, excreted in breast milk, half-life 2½−4 hr

Interactions/incompatibilities:
- CNS depression may be increased with other CNS depressants: alcohol, narcotics, sedative/hypnotics, antipsychotics, skeletal muscle relaxants

NURSING CONSIDERATIONS

Administer:
- With antiemetic if nausea, vomiting occur
- With milk or food for less severe GI symptoms

Perform/provide:
- Assistance with walking
- Safety measures: call bell, cot sides

Evaluate:
- Level of pain
- Need for analgesia
- Cough: type, duration, ability to expectorate
- CNS changes, dizziness, drowsiness, hallucinations, restlessness, agitation, mood changes, level of consciousness
- Fluid balance; check for decreasing output; may indicate urinary retention
- Skin rashes, itching, facial flushing
- Respiratory changes: respiratory depression, check rate and depth
- Physical dependence

Teach patient/family:
- To report any symptoms of CNS changes
- To observe for itching, rashes, facial flushing
- That physical dependency may result when used for extended periods of time
- To change position slowly as hypotension may occur
- To avoid hazardous activities such as driving or operating machinery if drowsiness or dizziness occurs
- To avoid alcohol unless directed by clinician
- To take a high fibre diet as constipation may occur

colchicine

Func. class.: Antigout agent
Chem. class.: Colchicum autumnale alkaloid
Legal class.: POM

Action: Inhibits microtubule formation in leucocytes, which decreases phagocytosis in joints
Uses: Acute gout, short-term prophylaxis of gout when commencing allopurinol therapy
Dosage and routes:
Prophylaxis

• *Adult:* By mouth 500 mcg twice or three times a day

Treatment

• *Adult:* By mouth initially 1 mg then 500 mcg every 2−3 hr, max total dose 10 mg; do not repeat within 3 days

Available forms include: Tablets 500 mcg

Side effects/adverse reactions:

HAEM: Agranulocytosis, thrombocytopenia, aplastic anaemia, pancytopaenia

CNS: Headache, drowsiness, neuritis, dizziness

GI: Nausea, vomiting, anorexia, malaise, metallic taste, cramps, peptic ulcer, diarrhoea, abdominal pain

GU: Renal damage

EENT: Retinopathy, cataracts

INTEG: Stomatitis, fever, chills, dermatitis, pruritus, purpura, erythema, alopecia

Contraindications: Hypersensitivity

Precautions: Severe cardiac, GI or renal disease, blood dyscrasias, pregnancy, lactation

Pharmacokinetics:

Period of onset: Peak ½−2 hr, half-life 20 min, deacetylated in liver, excreted in faeces (metabolites/active drug)

Clinical assessment:

• Full blood count, platelets, reticulocytes before, 3 monthly during therapy

NURSING CONSIDERATIONS

Administer:

• On empty stomach only, to facilitate absorption

Evaluate:

• Therapeutic response: decreased stone formation on x-ray, decreased pain in kidney region, absence of haematuria; decreased pain in joints

• Toxicity: diarrhoea, vomiting abdominal pain, rashes, blood dyscrasias

• Fluid balance; observe for decrease in urinary output

Teach patient/family:

• To avoid alcohol, non-prescription preparations that contain alcohol; skin rashes may occur

• To report any pain, redness, or hard area often in lower limb joints; any signs of toxicity

• Stress patient compliance with medical regimen; bone marrow depression may occur

colistin sulphate

Colomycin

Func. class.: Antibacterial

Chem. class.: Polymixin

Legal class.: POM

Action: Interacts with phospholipids, penetrates cell wall; changes occur immediately in bacterial cytoplasmic membrane causing leakage of essential intracellular metabolites

Uses: Infections caused by *Pseudomonas* spp, *Enterobacter* spp, *E. coli*, *Klebsiella* spp, *Shigella* spp, *Haemophilus* spp, *Salmonella* spp, *Serratia* spp, *Bordetella* spp, *Vibrio cholerae*, bowel sterilisation in neutropenic patients

Dosage and routes:

• *Adult:* IM/IV injection/infusion/nebulised 2 million units 8-hrly. By mouth (for bowel sterilisation) 1.5−3 million units every 8 hr

• *Child:* By mouth 15−30 kg, 0.75−1.5 million units 8-hrly; under 15 kg body-weight, 0.25−0.5 million units 8-hrly

Available forms include: Tablets 1.5 million units; oral powder for suspension 250,000 units/5 ml; powder for IM, IV injection 500,000 units/vial, 1 million units/vial; powder for topical administration 1 g

Side effects/adverse reactions:
INTEG: Pruritus, urticaria, rash, pain at injection site
RESP: Arrest, dyspnoea
GU: Nephrotoxicity
CNS: Paresthaesia, dizziness, ataxia, slurred speech, psychosis, coma, drug fever, confusion
EENT: Blurred vision
Contraindications: Hypersensitivity
Precautions: Elderly, pregnancy, renal failure
Pharmacokinetics:
Poorly absorbed by mouth
IM: Peak 2 hr, duration less than 12 hr
IV: Peak 2 hr, duration less than 12 hr Half-life 1½–8 hr IM, IV; excreted in urine (active drug, metabolites)
Interactions/incompatibilities:
• Increased neurotoxicity, nephrotoxicity: cephalothin, aminoglycosides, amphotericin B, polymyxin, vancomycin
• Increased neuromuscular blockade: tubocurarine, decamethonium, suxamethonium, gallamine
Clinical assessment:
• Liver studies: aspartate aminotransferase, alanine aminotransferase
• Renal studies: urinalysis, protein, blood, blood urea nitrogen, creatinine
• Drug level in impaired hepatic, renal systems (10–15 mcg/ml)
Treatment of overdose: Renal insufficiency, muscle weakness and apnoea may result. Supportive treatment. Increase drug elimination by mannitol diuresis, prolonged haemodialysis or peritoneal dialysis
NURSING CONSIDERATIONS
Assess:
• Fluid balance
• Bowel pattern
• Allergies before treatment, reaction of each medication; note allergies on chart, in bright red letters; advise all people giving medication
• Any patient with compromised renal system; drug is excreted slowly in poor renal system function; toxicity may occur rapidly
• Culture and sensitivity before drug therapy; drug may be used as soon as culture is taken
Administer:
• IV by infusion only; do not administer bolus dose
• IM deep injection; rotate sites
• Orally with at least 200 ml water
• Nebuliser: 2 million units 8 hrly nebulised for 10–20 min. Mix with 2–4 ml sterile water or sodium chloride 0.9% (nebulise with compressor to generate a flow of at least 8 litres/min)
• If nebulised: isolate patient and use an aerosol concentration device (e.g. Mizer System 22) to prevent general contamination of ward environment and protect other patients/staff from exposure
Perform/provide:
• Colistin oral solution; can be stored in refrigerator for up to 2 weeks, protect from light
• Ensure that emergency equipment is available on unit; respiratory arrest has occurred following IM dose
• Adequate intake of fluids (2 litres) during diarrhoea episodes
Evaluate:
• Therapeutic response: decreased temperature, negative culture and sensitivity
• BP, pulse in patient receiving drug parenterally
• Bowel pattern during treatment
• Skin eruptions, itching, dermatitis
• Respiratory status: rate, character, wheezing, tightness in chest
Teach patient/family:
• To take oral drug with full glass

of water, may be taken with food if GI symptoms occur
• Aspects of drug therapy: need to complete entire course of medication to ensure organism death; culture may be taken after completed course of medication
• To report sore throat, fever, fatigue; could indicate superimposed infection
• That drug must be taken in equal intervals around clock to maintain blood levels
• To notify nurse of diarrhoea

---

co-phenotrope, diphenoxylate HCl with atropine sulphate (diphenoxylate HCl 2.5 mg with atropine sulphate 25 mcg)

Lomotil, Diarphen
Func. class.: Antidiarrhoeal
Chem. class.: Diphenoxylate — phenylpipeoridine derivative, opiate agonist. Atropine — antimuscarinic alkaloid
Legal class.: POM

Action: Inhibits gastric motility by acting on mucosal receptors responsible for peristalsis
Uses: Adjunct to rehydration in acute diarrhoea; control of stool formation after colostomy/ileostomy; relief of symptoms in chronic mild ulcerative colitis
Dosage and routes: By mouth
• *Adult:* 4 tablets or 20 ml followed by 2 tablets or 10 ml every 6 hr
• *Children under 4:* not recommended
• *4–8 yr:* 1 tablet or 5 ml 3 times a day
• *9–12 yr:* 1 tablet or 5 ml 4 times a day
• *13–16 yr:* 2 tablets or 10 ml 3 times a day

Available forms include: Tablets 2.5/0.025 mg; liquid 2.5/0.025 mg in 5 ml
Side effects/adverse reactions:
CNS: Malaise, lethargy, sedation, somnolence, confusion, dizziness, depression, restlessness, euphoria, hallucinations, headache, flushing, hyperthermia
ALLERGIC: Anaphylaxis, angiooedema, urticaria, pruritus
GI: Paralytic ileus, toxic megacolon, nausea, vomiting, anorexia, abdominal discomfort
EENT: Blurred vision, dry mouth
INTEG: Dry skin and mucous membranes
CVS: Tachycardia
GU: Urinary retention
Contraindications: Hypersensitivity, severe liver disease, pseudomembranous enterocolitis, intestinal obstruction, glaucoma, children less than 4 yr, electrolyte imbalances
Precautions: Ulcerative colitis, lactation, Down's syndrome, renal disease
Pharmacokinetics:
Period of onset: Onset 45–60 min, peak 2 hr, duration 3–4 hr, half-life 2½ hr; metabolised in liver to active, inactive metabolites; excreted in urine, faeces, breast milk
Interactions/incompatibilities:
• Do not use with or within 14 days of MAOIs; hypertensive crisis may occur
• Increased action of: alcohol, narcotics, barbiturates, other CNS depressants
Clinical assessment:
• Electrolyte balance (potassium, sodium, chloride and appropriate fluid intake)
Treatment of overdose: Danger of narcosis (respiratory depression) or atropine poisoning (i.e. hyperthermia, tachycardia, lethargy, coma). Treat respiratory depression with naloxone and con-

sider gastric lavage and activated charcoal. Observe for at least 48 hr

NURSING CONSIDERATIONS
Assess:
- Bowel pattern
- Fluid balance

Administer:
- For 48 hr only

Evaluate:
- Therapeutic response: return to normal bowel habit
- Bowel pattern before; for rebound constipation after termination of medication
- Response after 48 hr; if no response, drug should be discontinued
- Hydration status — if unable to produce adequate urinary output, IV fluids may be necessary
- Dehydration in children
- Abdominal distention, toxic megacolon, which may occur in ulcerative colitis

Teach patient/family:
- Avoid non-prescribed products unless directed by clinician; may contain alcohol
- Inform of side effects and advise to contact clinician if any occur
- Not to exceed recommended dose

cortisone acetate

Cortistab, Cortisyl
Func. class.: Glucocorticoid, short-acting
Chem. class.: Corticosteroid, synthetic
Legal class.: POM

Action: Decreases inflammation by suppression of migration of polymorphonuclear leucocytes, fibroblasts, reversal of increased capillary permeability and lysosomal stabilisation
Uses: Adrenal insufficiency

Dosage and routes:
- *Adult:* 12.5−50 mg daily in divided doses
- *Child:* 5−25 mg daily in divided doses
Available forms include: Tablets 5, 25 mg
Side effects/adverse reactions:
INTEG: Acne, poor wound healing, ecchymosis, bruising, petechiae
CNS: Depression, flushing, sweating, headache, mood changes, euphoria, insomnia
CV: Thrombophlebitis, embolism, tachycardia, congestive cardiac failure, hypertension
HAEM: Thrombocytopenia
MS: Fractures, osteoporosis, weakness, proximal myopathy, growth retardation in children
GI: Diarrhoea, nausea, abdominal distention, GI haemorrhage, increased appetite, pancreatitis
EENT: Fungal infections, increased intraocular pressure, blurred vision
META: Hyperglycaemia, hypokalaemia
Contraindications: Systemic fungal infection, hypersensitivity
Precautions: Psychosis, idiopathic thrombocytopenia, pregnancy, diabetes mellitus, glaucoma, osteoporosis, epilepsy, peptic ulceration, congestive cardiac failure, myasthenia gravis, hypertension
Pharmacokinetics:
Period of onset: Peak 2 hr, duration 1½ days
Interactions/incompatibilities:
- Decreased action of this drug: cholestyramine, barbiturates, rifampicin, phenytoin
- Decreased effects of: anticoagulants, anticonvulsants, anti diabetics, toxoids, vaccines
- Increased side effects: alcohol, salicylates, indomethacin, amphotericin B

Clinical assessment:
• Plasma cortisol levels during long-term therapy
• Potassium, blood glucose; hypokalaemia and hyperglycaemia

NURSING CONSIDERATIONS

Assess:
• BP, pulse, fluid balance, weight

Administer:
• Titrated dose, use lowest effective dose
• In one dose in morning to prevent adrenal suppression
• With food or milk to decrease GI symptoms

Perform/provide:
• Assistance with ambulation in patient with bone tissue disease to prevent fractures

Evaluate:
• Therapeutic response: ease of respirations, decreased inflammation
• Glycosuria while on long-term therapy
• Weight daily, notify clinician of weekly gain greater than 2 kg
• BP 4 hrly, pulse, notify clinician if chest pain occurs
• Fluid balances; be alert for decreasing urinary output and increasing oedema
• Infection: increased temperature; drug masks symptoms of infection
• Potassium depletion: paraesthesias, fatigue, nausea, vomiting, depression, polyuria, dysrhythmias, weakness
• Oedema, hypotension, cardiac symptoms
• Mental status: affect, mood, behavioural changes, aggression

Teach patient/family:
• That a steroid medication card should be carried at all times
• To notify clinician if therapeutic response decreases; dosage adjustment may be needed
• Not to discontinue this medication abruptly or adrenal crisis can result
• To avoid non-prescription products: salicylates, alcohol in cough products, cold preparations unless directed by clinician
• Teach patient all aspects of drug usage, including Cushingoid symptoms
• Symptoms of adrenal insufficiency: nausea, anorexia, fatigue, dizziness, dyspnoea, weakness, joint pain

co-trimoxazole (sulphamethoxazole and trimethoprim)

Bactrim, Septrin, Comixco, Fectrim, Laratrim, Comox
Func. class.: Anti-infective
Chem. class.: Combined sulphonamide and synthetic pyrimidine derivative
Legal class.: POM

Action: Sulphamethoxazole interferes with bacterial biosynthesis of proteins by competitive antagonism of PABA when adequate levels are maintained; trimethoprim blocks synthesis of tetrahydrofolic acid; this combination blocks 2 consecutive steps in bacterial synthesis of essential nucleic acids, protein
Uses: Urinary tract infections, otitis media, chronic prostatitis, shigellosis, *Pneumocystis carinii* pneumonitis, chronic bronchitis
Dosage and routes:
• *Adult:* By mouth 960 mg 12-hrly, maximum 1.44 g 12-hrly, 480 mg 12 hrly if treated for more than 14 days; IV infusion 960 mg twice a day, maximum 1.44 g 12 hrly, 960 mg 8 hrly
• *Child:* By mouth 6 weeks–6 months, 120 mg twice a day,

6 months−6 yr, 240 mg twice a day, 6−12 yr, 480 mg twice a day
Gonorrhoea
• By mouth 1.92 g 12-hrly for 2 days, or 2 doses of 2.4 g 8 hr apart
Pneumocystis carinii pneumonitis
• *Adult and child:* 120 mg/kg daily in divided doses
Available forms include: Tablets 20 mg trimethoprim 100 mg sulphamethoxazole (120 mg); 80 mg trimethoprim/400 mg sulphamethoxazole (480 mg), 160 mg trimethoprim/800 mg sulphamethoxazole (960 mg); suspension 240 mg/5 ml, 480 mg/5 ml; IV injection 96 mg/ml, IM 320 mg/ml
Side effects/adverse reactions:
SYST: Anaphylaxis
GI: Nausea, vomiting, abdominal pain, stomatitis, hepatitis, glossitis, pancreatitis, diarrhoea, enterocolitis
CNS: Headache, confusion, insomnia, hallucinations, depression, vertigo, fatigue, anxiety, convulsions, drug fever, chills
HAEM: Leucopenia, neutropenia, thrombocytopenia, agranulocytosis, haemolytic anaemia, megaloblastic anaemia (due to trimethoprim)
INTEG: Rash, dermatitis, urticaria, Stevens-Johnson syndrome, erythema multiforme, photosensitivity, pain, inflammation at injection site
GU: Renal failure, toxic nephrosis, increased blood urea nitrogen, creatinine, crystalluria
CV: Allergic myocarditis
Contraindications: Hypersensitivity to trimethoprim or sulphonamides, pregnancy at term, megaloblastic anaemia, liver damage, blood disorders, renal insufficiency, infants up to 6 weeks, premature infants
Precautions: Pregnancy, lactation, renal disease, elderly, G-6-PD deficiency, impaired hepatic func-

tion, possible folate deficiency, severe allergy, bronchial asthma
Pharmacokinetics:
Period of onset: Rapidly absorbed, peak 1−4 hr; half-life 8−13 hr, excreted in urine (metabolites and unchanged), breast milk, highly bound to plasma proteins
Interactions/incompatibilities:
• Increased effect of: sulphonylurea hypoglycaemic agents, phenytoin, methotrexate, thiopentone
• Increased anticoagulant effects: oral anticoagulants
• Decreased renal excretion of: methotrexate
• Decreased hepatic clearance of: phenytoin
• Increased nephrotoxic effect: cyclosporin
• Increased anti-folate effect: pyrimethamine
Clinical assessment:
• Kidney function studies: blood urea nitrogen, creatinine, urinalysis if on long-term or high dose therapy
Treatment of overdose:
• Gastric lavage within 1 hr. Calcium folinate, general supportive measures
NURSING CONSIDERATIONS
Assess:
• Fluid balance
Administer:
• After specimens taken for culture and sensitivity
• With resuscitative equipment available; severe allergic reactions may occur
• With full glass of water to maintain adequate hydration; increase fluids to 2 litres daily to decrease crystallisation in kidneys
• Medication after culture and sensitivity; repeat culture and sensitivity after full course of medication completed (allow 5 days after end of course before re-culture)

Evaluate:
• Therapeutic response: absence of pain, fever, culture and sensitivity negative
• Blood dyscrasias: skin rash, fever, sore throat, bruising, bleeding, fatigue, joint pain
• Allergic reaction: rash, dermatitis, exfoliation, urticaria, pruritus, dyspnoea
• Note colour, character, pH of urine if drug administered for urinary tract infections; if urine is highly acidic, alkalinisation may be needed

Teach patient/family:
• To take each oral dose with full glass of water to prevent crystalluria
• To complete full course of treatment to prevent superimposed infection
• To avoid non-prescription medications (aspirin, vitamin C) unless directed by clinician
• To notify clinician if skin rash, sore throat, fever, mouth sores, unusual bruising, bleeding occur
• To seek advice if there is any possibility of pregnancy

---

crisantaspase

Erwinase
Func. class.: Antineoplastic
Chem. class.: Asparaginase enzyme
Legal class.: POM

Action: Indirectly inhibits protein synthesis in tumour cells; breaks down L-asparagine which tumour cells are unable to synthesise
Uses: Acute lymphoblastic leukaemia in combination with other antineoplastics
Dosage and routes:
In combination
• *Adult:* IM, subcutaneous, IV 200 IU/kg (variable doses used)
Available forms include: Injection 10,000 IU
Side effects/adverse reactions:
HAEM: Thrombocytopenia, leucopenia, anaemia
GI: Nausea, vomiting, anorexia, cramps, stomatitis, hepatotoxicity, pancreatitis
GU: Urinary retention, renal failure, glycosuria, polyuria, azotaemia
INTEG: Rash, urticaria, chills, fever
ENDO: Hyperglycaemia
RESP: Anaphylaxis
CNS: Neuritis, dizziness, headache, coma, depression, fatigue, confusion, hallucinations
Contraindications: Hypersensitivity, pregnancy, pancreatitis
Precautions: Renal disease, hepatic disease, lactation
Pharmacokinetics: Half-life 4−9 hr, terminal 1.4−1.8 hr
Clinical assessment:
• Perform full blood count and platelet count weekly
• Perform tests for blood urea, uric acid, electrolytes and creatinine clearance before and during treatment
• Perform liver function tests before and during treatment
• Obtain blood for Hb and haematocrit as these may be reduced
• Prescribe antiemetics
• Prescribe allopurinol to maintain uric acid levels
• Prescribe antibiotics as prophylaxis against infection
NURSING CONSIDERATIONS
Assess:
• Baseline observations including BP and weight
• Urinalysis for hyperglycaemia if pancreatitis suspected
Administer:
• Following local cytotoxic policy
Perform/provide:

- Strict hygienic precautions; protective isolation may be necessary if white blood cell count becomes low
- Encouragement for deep breathing exercises as taught by physiotherapist
- Increased fluid intake to 2–3 litres daily to prevent formation of renal calculi (urate deposits)
- Diet low in purines e.g. offal, pulses to maintain alkaline urine
- Nutritious diet with iron and vitamin supplements. Advice of dietician may be sought
- Mouthcare. Encourage frequent mouthwashes and the use of a soft toothbrush to avoid stomatitis. Unwaxed dental floss should be used
- Care of skin
- Support in bed to facilitate breathing

Evaluate:
- Fluid balance; report decrease in urinary output to below 30 ml/hr to clinician
- Temperature and BP 4 hrly if neutropenic
- 8 hrly for signs of bleeding e.g. haematuria, occult blood in stools, melaena, bruising, petechiae, perianal lesions
- Signs of chest infection e.g. dyspnoea, increased respiratory rate, fatigue, lethargy
- Food preferences
- Joint and abdominal pain, shaking, oedema in feet and legs
- Jaundice e.g. skin discolouration, yellow sclera, dark urine, clay-coloured stools, itchy skin, fever, diarrhoea
- Oral mucosa 8 hrly for dryness, sores or ulceration, infection, pain, bleeding, dysphagia
- Inflammation at injection site
- Symptoms of severe allergic reaction e.g. rash, pruritus, urticaria, purpuric skin lesions, itching, hot flushes

- Diarrhoea, signs of acidosis and dehydration
- General malaise
- Observe for anaphylaxis

Teach patient/family:
- Need for protective isolation
- To report side effects to nurse or clinician
- To report any changes in respiration, breathing
- To avoid foods containing citric acid, and those that are very spicy
- Good mouthcare
- Possibility of side effects

---

cyclizine HCl, cyclizine lactate

Valoid

Func. class.: Antiemetic, antihistamine

Chem. class.: H_1-receptor antagonist, piperazine derivative

Legal class.: Tablets P; Injection POM

Action: Acts centrally by blocking chemoreceptor trigger zone, which is turn acts on vomiting centre

Uses: Nausea, vomiting, including drug-induced, radiation-induced, post-operative; vertigo, motion sickness, labyrinthine disorders

Dosage and routes:
- *Adult:* By mouth IM/IV 50 mg 3 times a day
- *Child 6–12 yr:* By mouth 25 mg 3 times a day
- Not licensed for subcutaneous route

Available forms include: Tablets 50 mg as hydrochloride: injection 50 mg/ml as lactate

Side effects/adverse reactions:

CNS: Drowsiness, dizziness, restlessness, insomnia

EENT: Dry mouth, blurred vision

MISC: tachycardia, urinary retention, constipation

Contraindications: Hypersensitivity to cyclizine
Precautions: Children, narrow-angle glaucoma, urinary retention, lactation, prostatic hypertrophy, elderly, pregnancy, shock
Pharmacokinetics:
Duration 4−6 hr, other pharmacokinetics not known
Interactions/incompatibilities:
• May increase effect of: alcohol, tranquilisers, narcotics, anticholinergic agents
• Decreased effects of: betahistine
Treatment of overdose: Gastric lavage and general supportive measures
NURSING CONSIDERATIONS
Assess:
• Temperature, pulse, respiration, BP; check patients with cardiac disease regularly
Administer:
• Intramuscularly, intravenously, orally; subcutaneously in infusion pumps especially in terminal symptom control (not a licensed indication)
Perform/provide:
• If in subcutaneous pump observe at least 4 hrly for skin irritation
Evaluate:
• Signs of toxicity of other drugs or masking of symptoms of disease: brain tumour, intestinal obstruction
• Observe for drowsiness, dizziness
• May be irritant to skin especially if used as subcutaneous route
Teach patient/family:
• To avoid hazardous activities or activities requiring alertness including driving as drug can cause drowsiness; dizziness may occur; that assistance with ambulation may be needed
• That a false negative result may occur with skin testing; skin testing procedures should not be scheduled for 4 days after discontinuing use

• Avoid alcohol, other CNS depressants

---

cyclopenthiazide

Navidrex
Func. class.: Diuretic
Chem. class.: Thiazide
Legal class.: POM

Action: Inhibits reabsorption of sodium chloride and water at the distal tubule; reduces peripheral vascular resistance
Uses: Oedema, hypertension, congestive heart failure
Dosage and routes:
Oedema, congestive heart failure
• *By mouth* initially 0.5−1 mg in morning, maintenance 500 mcg on alternate days
Hypertension
• 250−500 mcg in morning. Maximum dose, 1.5 mg daily
Available forms include: Tablets, 500 mcg
Side effects/adverse reactions:
HAEM: Thrombocytopenia, hypokalaemia
EENT: Photosensitivity
META: Hyperuricaemia, hyperglycaemia
GU: Impotence, glycosuria
INTEG: Rashes
Contraindications: Hypercalcaemia, renal failure, Addison's disease, porphyria, concurrent lithium therapy
Precautions: Pregnancy, diabetes, gout, renal or hepatic impairment, hyperlipidaemia
Pharmacokinetics: Diuresis induced within 1−2 hr, duration 12 hr
Interactions/incompatibilities:
• Increased cardiac glycoside toxicity due to hypokalaemia
• Antagonism of insulin and oral antidiabetic agents

• Antagonism of effects by NSAIDs

• Increased hypokalaemia with ACTH, corticosteroids

Clinical assessment:

• Frequent checks on potassium levels

• Review of hypoglycaemic requirement in known diabetics

Treatment of overdose: Induction of vomiting and gastric lavage, check BP and electrolytes, IV fluids and electrolyte replacement

NURSING CONSIDERATIONS

Administer:

• In the morning with food

Perform/provide:

• Potassium rich diet, high fibre to avoid constipation

• Help with getting up, patient should rise slowly

• Monitor diabetics carefully

• Counselling for sexual problems

Evaluate:

• Fluid balance, pulse 4 hrly; risk of potassium depletion

• Weight daily, BP (lying/standing) daily; possibility of postural hypotension

• Test urine for glucose

• Irregular heart rate

• Muscle fatigue/spasm

• Oedema/dry skin

• Bruising

• Rashes

• Effects on urinary output/oedema

• Insulin requirements in known diabetics

Teach patient/family:

• About possibility of impotence (reversible)

• To use a sunscreen

• To rise slowly

• To report side effects including painful joints

• Dietary advice on potassium, salt, fibre intake

• To seek advice about drug interactions

cyclopentolate HCl (ophthalmic)

Mydrilate, Minims Cyclopentolate Hydrochloride

Func. class.: Mydriatic, cycloplegic, anticholinergic

Legal class.: POM

Action: Dilates the pupil and paralyses the ciliary muscle

Uses: Diagnostic purposes for fundoscopy and cycloplegic refraction, dilating the pupil in inflammatory conditions of the iris and uveal tract

Dosage and routes:

Refraction

• *Adults:* Instil one drop of a 0.5% solution and repeat after 15 min if necessary

• *Child: 6−16 yr* Instil one drop of a 1% solution 40 min before examining the eye; under 6 yr, instil one or two drops as above

Uveitis

• *Adult:* Instil one or two drops of a 0.5% solution up to 4 times a day

• *Child:* At the discretion of the prescriber

Deeply pigmented eyes may require a 1% solution

Available forms include: 0.5%, 1% solution in multi-use bottles; 0.5%, 1% Minims

Side effects/adverse reactions:

CV: Tachycardia, flushing (infants: abdominal distention, irregular pulse, respiratory depression)

EENT: Blurred vision, temporary burning sensation on instillation, eye dryness, photophobia, conjunctivitis, increased intraocular pressure

CNS: (In children), psychotic reaction, behavior disturbances, ataxia, restlessness, hallucinations, somnolence, disorientation, grand mal seizures; confusion, fever

GI: Abdominal distention, vomiting, dry mouth
Contraindications: Hypersensitivity, infants less than 3 months, local or systemic glaucoma, conjunctivitis, paralytic ileus, soft contact lenses (Minims may be used)
Precautions: Prostatic enlargement, coronary insufficiency, cardiac failure
Pharmacokinetics:
INSTIL: Peak 30−60 min (mydriasis), 25−74 min (cyclopegia), duration ¼−1 day
Interactions/incompatibilities:
• Enhanced effects with: other anti-muscarinic agents
Treatment of overdose: Supportive measures, induce vomiting and gastric lavage if accidentally ingested

NURSING CONSIDERATIONS
Evaluate:
• Therapeutic response
• Side effects particularly in very young and elderly
Perform/provide:
• Storage in a cool place
• Clear explanation of effect of drug
Teach patient/family:
• To report change in vision, blurring, or loss of sight, trouble breathing, sweating, flushing
• Method of instillation: pressure on lacrimal sac for 1 min, do not touch dropper to eye
• That blurred vision will decrease with repeated use of drug
• That drug may sting when instilled
• Wear dark sunglasses for photophobia
• Not to do hazardous tasks until able to see clearly (up to 4 hr)

cyclophosphamide

Endoxana
Func. class.: Cytotoxic alkylating agent
Chem. class.: Nitrogen mustard
Legal class.: POM

Action: Alkylates DNA, RNA; inhibits enzymes that allow synthesis of proteins; is also responsible for cross linking DNA strands
Uses: Leukaemias, lymphomas and a wide range of solid tumours. May be used alone or in combination with other cytotoxic agents
Dosage and routes:
• *Adult:* Variable, depending on patient's condition, regimen and tumour; conventional dose IV or by mouth 100−300 mg daily, or 500 mg−1 g weekly IV, high dose IV 20−40 mg/kg every 10−20 days
Available forms include: Powder for injection IV 100, 200, 500 mg, 1 g; tablets 50 mg
Side effects/adverse reactions:
CV: Cardiotoxicity (high doses)
HAEM: Thrombocytopenia, leucopenia, pancytopenia
GI: Nausea, vomiting, diarrhoea, weight loss, colitis, hepatotoxicity
GU: Haemorrhagic cystitis, haematuria, neoplasms, amenorrhoea, azoospermia, impotence, sterility, ovarian fibrosis
INTEG: Alopecia, dermatitis
RESP: Fibrosis, pneumonitis
CNS: Headache, dizziness
Contraindications: Hypersensitivity, haemorrhagic cystisis, porphyria, acute infections, bone marrow aplasia
Precautions: Radiation therapy, pregnancy, bone marrow depression, renal failure, liver failure
Pharmacokinetics: Metabolised by liver to active compound, excreted in urine; half-life 4−6½

hr; 50% bound to plasma proteins

Interactions/incompatibilities:
- Increased hypoglycaemic effects of sulphonylurea compounds
- Potentiation of suxamethonium effects
- Increased bone marrow depression: allopurinol

Clinical assessment:
- Full blood count, differential, platelet count weekly
- Pulmonary function tests, chest X-ray films before, during therapy
- Renal function studies: blood urea nitrogen, serum uric acid, urine creatinine clearance before, during therapy
- Liver function test before during therapy
- Prescribe mesna (with high dose therapy), anti-emetics

Treatment of overdose: Early gastric lavage if drug in tablet form. Supportive measures e.g. broad-spectrum antibiotics, blood transfusions, IV mesna (if recognised early), maintenance of fluid balance

NURSING CONSIDERATIONS

Assess:
- Urinalysis for blood
- Weight, fluid balance

Administer:
- In accordance with local cytotoxic policy
- Intravenously or orally as prescribed
- Other medications by oral route; if possible avoid IM, subcutaneous, IV routes to prevent infections
- Antacid before oral administration, give drug on an empty stomach if possible
- Prescribed antiemetics before and during administration of cyclophosphamide
- IV infusion over 2–3 min using 21-, 23-, 25-gauge needle
- Topical or systemic analgesics for pain
- Local or systemic drugs for infection as prescribed

Perform/provide:
- Protective isolation if/when neutropenic
- Deep breathing exercises with patient 3 or 4 times a day
- Increase fluid intake to 3 litres daily to prevent urate deposits, calculi formation
- Mouth care; brushing of teeth with soft brush or cotton-tipped applicators for stomatitis; use unwaxed dental floss
- Warm compresses at injection site for inflammation
- Urinalysis for blood

Evaluate:
- Fluid balance (report fall in urine output of 30 ml/hr)
- Monitor temperature and BP 4 hrly when neutropenic; hourly if temperature is above 38°C
- Bleeding in any site or tissue
- Signs and symptoms of cytopenia and haemorrhagic cystitis
- Dyspnoea, rales, unproductive cough, chest pain, tachypnoea
- Food preferences; list likes, dislikes
- Effects of alopecia on body image, discuss feelings about body changes
- Yellowing of skin, sclera, dark urine, clay-coloured stools, itchy skin, abdominal pain, fever, diarrhoea
- Oedema in feet, joint pain, stomach pain, shaking
- Inflammation of mucosa, breaks in skin
- Buccal cavity 8 hrly for dryness, sores or ulceration, white patches, oral pain, bleeding, dysphagia
- Symptoms indicating severe allergic reaction: rash, pruritus, urticaria, purpuric skin lesions, itching, flushing
- Tachypnoea, ECG changes, dyspnoea, oedema, fatigue

Teach patient/family:

- Protective isolation precautions
- To report any complaints or side effects to nurse or clinician
- That impotence or amenorrhoea can occur, but is reversible after discontinuing treatment
- To report any changes in breathing or coughing
- That hair may be lost during treatment; a wig or hairpiece may make patient feel better (available free on NHS); new hair may be different in colour, texture
- Dietary advice
- To report any bleeding, white spots or ulcerations in mouth to clinician; tell patient to examine mouth 6 hrly

---

cycloserine

Func. class.: Antibiotic, antitubercular
Chem. class.: D-alanine analogue
*Legal class.:*POM

Action: Inhibits cell wall synthesis, decreases tubercle bacilli replication
Uses: In combination with other drugs, tuberculosis resistant to first-line drugs
Dosage and routes:
- *Adult:* By mouth 250 mg 12-hrly, maximum 1 g daily
- *Children:* Start at 10 mg/kg daily and adjust according to blood levels and clinical response
Available forms include: Capsules 250 mg
Side effects/adverse reactions:
INTEG: Dermatitis, photosensitivity
CV: Congestive cardiac failure, dysrhythmias
CNS: Headache, anxiety, drowsiness, tremors, convulsions, lethargy, depression, confusion, psychosis, aggression

META: Changes in liver function tests
HAEM: Megaloblastic anaemia
Contraindications: Hypersensitivity, severe renal disease, alcoholism (chronic), depression, severe anxiety or neurosis, epilepsy
Precautions: Pregnancy, children
Pharmacokinetics:
Period of onset: Peak 3–4 hr; excreted unchanged in urine, excreted in breast milk
Interactions/incompatibilities:
- May increase toxicity: ethionamide, isoniazid, alcohol
- Increased plasma level of: phenytoin
Clinical assessment:
- Liver studies every week: aspartate aminotransferase, alanine aminotransferase, bilirubin
- Renal status: before therapy and every month: blood urea nitrogen, creatinine, urinary output, specific gravity, urinalysis
- Blood levels of drug; keep below 30 mcg/ml or toxicity may occur
Lab. test interferences:
Increase: Aspartate aminotransferase, alanine aminotransferase
Treatment of overdose: Administer vitamin B_6, anticonvulsants, O_2, assisted respiration, activated charcoal to reduce absorption, haemodialysis in life-threatening acute toxicity
NURSING CONSIDERATIONS
Administer:
- After culture and sensitivity is completed every month to detect resistance
Evaluate:
- Mental status often: affect, mood, behavioural changes, psychosis may occur
- Hepatic status: decreased appetite, jaundice, dark urine, fatigue
Teach patient/family:
- Avoid alcohol while taking drug

- That compliance with dosage schedule, length is necessary
- To report neurotoxicity: confusion, headache, drowsiness, tremors, paraesthesia, mental changes
- To avoid hazardous activities if drowsiness or dizziness occurs

---

cyclosporin

Sandimmun
Func. class.: Immunosuppressant
Chem. class.: Fungus-derived peptide
Legal class.: POM

Action: Produces immunosuppression by blocking resting lymphocytes and inhibiting lymphokine production and release

Uses: Organ transplants (including allogeneic bone marrow transplants) to prevent rejection, prophylaxis and treatment of graft-versus-host disease

Dosage and routes:
Organ transplants
- *Adult and child:* By mouth 14–17.5 mg/kg several hours before surgery then daily for 1–2 weeks, reduce daily dosage by 2 mg/kg at monthly intervals to 6–8 mg/kg a day then adjust according to blood levels

Bone marrow transplant, graft-versus-host disease
- IV initially 3–5 mg/kg on the day before surgery and continuing until oral therapy starts within 2 weeks; by mouth 12.5 mg/kg daily for 3–6 months then gradually decrease to zero

Available forms include: Oral solution 100 mg/ml; injection (concentrate for IV infusion) 50 mg/ml (1 ml, 5 ml ampoules), capsules 25, 50, 100 mg

Side effects/adverse reactions:
GI: Nausea, vomiting, diarrhoea, anorexia, oral candidiasis, gum hyperplasia, hepatotoxicity
INTEG: Rash, acne, hirsutism
ELECT: Hyperkalaemia
CNS: Tremors, headache
GU: Albuminuria, haematuria, proteinuria, renal impairment

Contraindications: Hypersensitivity

Precautions: Severe renal disease, severe hepatic disease

Pharmacokinetics: Peak 4 hr, highly protein bound, half-life (biphasic) 1.2 hr, 25 hr; metabolised in liver, excreted in faeces, excreted in breast milk

Interactions/incompatibilities:
- Increased action of this drug: diltiazem, erythromycin, nicardipine, progestogens, verapamil, ketoconazole, itraconazole, danazol
- Decreased action of this drug: phenytoin, rifampicin, phenobarbitone, carbamazepine, primidone, octreotide
- Increased nephrotoxicity: amphotericin B, aminoglycosides
- Increased hyperkalaemia: enalapril, captopril, potassium supplements, potassium-sparing diuretics
- Increased myopathy: simvastatin, pravastatin

Clinical assessment:
- Renal function, urea and electrolytes, creatinine at least monthly during treatment, 3 months after treatment
- Liver function studies: alkaline phosphatase, aspartate aminotransferase, alanine aminotransferase, bilirubin
- Drug blood levels during treatment

NURSING CONSIDERATIONS

Administer:
- As part of immunosuppressive regime

• With milk or meals to avoid GI upset and for palatability
• At prescribed time for accurate monitoring of serum levels and taking account of these values
• With oral nystatin for potential *Candida* infections (at least 6 weeks of therapy)

Perform/provide:
• Store and administer liquid preparation in glass containers

Evaluate:
• Toxicity: reduced urinary output and/or dark urine, jaundice, pruritus, pale stools
• Hypersensitivity; severe tremor of hands, nausea, vomiting, diarrhoea

Teach patient/family:
• To report any signs of infection immediately (fever, sore throat general malaise)
• Importance of minimising exposure to infection
• Importance of continuity and accurate administration of medication
• Not to breast feed
• To use contraceptive measures during treatment, and for 12 weeks after ending therapy
• To avoid direct sunlight; use sunscreen and protective measures

---

cyproheptadine HCl

Periactin

Func. class.: Antihistamine
Chem. class.: H_1-receptor antagonist, piperidine derivative
Legal class.: P

Action: Acts on blood vessels, GI, respiratory system by competing with histamine for H_1-receptor site; decreases allergic response by blocking histamine

Uses: Allergy symptoms, rhinitis, pruritus, stimulation of appetite, migraine

Dosage and routes:
Allergy and pruritus
• *Adult:* By mouth 4 mg, 3 or 4 times a day, maximum 32 mg daily
• *Child 7–14 yr:* By mouth 4 mg 2 or 3 times a day, not to exceed 16 mg daily
• *Child 2–6 yr:* By mouth 2 mg 2 or 3 times a day, not to exceed 12 mg daily

Appetite stimulation
• *Adult:* By mouth 4 mg 3 times a day or 12 mg in the evening
• *Child 7–14 yr:* Not more than 12 mg daily
• *Child 2–6 yr:* Not more than 8 mg daily

Migraine
• By mouth, 4 mg repeated after 30 min if required; maintenance 4 mg every 4–6 hr

Available forms include: Tablets 4 mg; syrup 2 mg/5 ml

Side effects/adverse reactions:
CNS: Dizziness, drowsiness, poor coordination, fatigue, anxiety, euphoria, confusion, paraesthesia, neuritis, increased appetite
CV: Hypotension, palpitations, tachycardia
RESP: Increased thick secretions, wheezing, chest tightness
GI: Dry mouth, nausea, vomiting, anorexia, constipation, diarrhoea
INTEG: Rash, urticaria, photosensitivity
GU: Retention, dysuria, frequency
EENT: Blurred vision, dilated pupils, tinnitus, nasal stuffiness, dry nose, throat, mouth

Contraindications: Hypersensitivity to H_1-receptor antagonists, acute asthma attack, lower respiratory tract disease, stenosing peptic ulcer, glaucoma, neonate, premature infant, lactation, symptomatic prostatic hypertrophy, bladder neck obstruction, GI obstruction, elderly or debilitated patients, urinary retention, MAOIs

Precautions; Increased intraocular pressure, renal disease, cardiac disease, hypertension, bronchial asthma, seizure disorder, hyperthyroidism, pregnancy

Pharmacokinetics:
By mouth: duration 4−6 hr, metabolised in liver, excreted by kidneys, excreted in breast milk

Interactions/incompatibilities:
• Increased CNS depression: barbiturates, narcotics, hypnotics, tricyclic antidepressants, alcohol
• Increased effect of this drug: MAOIs

Clinical assessment:
• Full blood count during long term therapy

Lab. test interferences: Reduces hypoglycaemia-induced growth hormone secretion

Treatment of overdose: Induce emesis or gastric lavage, plus supportive therapy

NURSING CONSIDERATIONS
Administer:
• With meals if GI symptoms occur; absorption may slightly decrease

Perform/provide:
• Frequent drinks and mouth washes for dryness

Evaluate:
• Therapeutic response: absence of running or congested nose or rashes
• Fluid balance: observe for urinary retention, frequency, dysuria; drug should be discontinued if these occur
• Respiratory status: rate, rhythm, increase in bronchial secretions, wheezing, chest tightness
• Cardiac status: palpitations, increased pulse, hypotension

Teach patient/family:
• All aspects of drug use; notify the clinician if confusion, sedation, hypotension occurs
• Driving or operation of machinery may be impaired
• To avoid concurrent use of alcohol or other CNS depressants

---

cyproterone acetate

Androcur, Cyprostat
Func. class.: Anti-androgen with progestogenic activity
Chem. class.: Steroid
Legal class.: POM

Action: Antagonises the effects of androgens by blocking androgen receptors; reduces gonadotrophin secretion by negative feedback

Uses: Control of severe hypersexuality or sexual deviation in men; palliative treatment of prostatic carcinoma

Dosage and routes:
• Hypersexuality: 50 mg twice daily, prostatic carcinoma: 200−300 mg daily in 2−3 doses

Available forms include: Tablets, 50 mg

Side effects/adverse reactions:
META: Weight gain, changes in hair pattern, gynaecomastia, galactorrhoea, benign breast nodules
GU: Inhibition of spermatogenesis, abnormal sperm, reduced menstrual flow, intermenstrual bleeding
GI: Liver abnormalities, hepatic tumours, nausea, vomiting
MS: Osteoporosis, may arrest bone maturation in young men
SYST: Severe fatigue, lassitude
CNS: Headache, changed libido, depression
INTEG: Chloasma, patchy body hair growth, lightening of hair colour

Contraindications: Patients under 18 yr; liver disease, malignant or wasting disease (excluding prostatic cancer), severe depression, history of thromboembolic disorders, ineffective in chronic alcoholism, pregnancy, lactation, sickle cell anaemia, abnormal vaginal bleeding of unknown cause.

Precautions: Diabetes mellitus, adrenocortical insufficiency, hypertension, abnormal liver function

Pharmacokinetics: Peak plasma concentration within 3−10 hr, excreted as metabolites in faeces and urine

Interactions/incompatibilities:
• Effects diminished by: alcoholism
• Risk of chloasma increased by: UV light and strong sunlight

Clinical assessment:
• Full blood count, Hb (hypochronic anaemia)
• Liver function tests, adrenal function, blood glucose (especially diabetics)
• Check history of alcohol abuse, hepatic tumours and thrombo-embolic conditions
• Obtain fully informed consent

Treatment of overdose: Gastric lavage, symptomatic treatment

NURSING CONSIDERATIONS
Assess:
• Baseline weight
Administer:
• With or after food
Evaluate:
• Weight—weekly; fluctuations may occur
Teach patient/family:
• That reversible male infertility may occur
• To avoid alcohol
• That ability to drive or operate machinery may be impaired; causes drowsiness at first
• That hair pattern may change,

skin becomes dry and gynaecomastia may occur
• Tiredness may be a problem

---

cytarabine (ARA-C, cytosine arabinoside)

Alexan, Cytosar
Func. class.: Cytotoxic antimetabolite
Chem. class.: Pyrimidine nucleoside
Legal class.: POM

Action: Competes with physiological substrate, inhibits DNA synthesis; interferes with cell replication at S phase, directly before mitosis

Uses: Acute myeloid leukaemia, acute lymphoblastic leukaemia, chronic myeloid leukaemia, and in combination for non-Hodgkin's lymphomas

Dosage and routes:
Different doses apply for induction and maintenance of remission. Seek specialist advice for details. Cytarabine may be given by IV injection, infusion or subcutaneous injection. Doses and routes depend on tumour type and concurrent drug treatment

Available forms include: Injection IV 100, 500 mg; 20, 100 mg/ml

Side effects/adverse reactions:
HAEM: Thrombophlebitis, bleeding, thrombocytopenia, leucopenia, myelosuppression, anaemia
GI: Nausea, vomiting, anorexia, diarrhoea, stomatitis, hepatotoxicity, abdominal pain, haematemesis, GI haemorrhage
EENT: Sore throat, conjunctivitis
GU: Urinary retention, renal failure, hyperuricaemia
INTEG: Rash, fever, freckling, cellulitis
RESP: Pneumonia, dyspnoea

CV: Chest pain, cardiopathy
CNS: Neuritis, dizziness, headache, personality changes, coma
CYTARABINE SYNDROME: Fever, myalgia, bone pain, chest pain, rash, conjunctivitis, malaise (6−12 hr after administration)
Contraindications: Hypersensitivity, pregnancy, lactation
Precautions: Renal disease, hepatic disease, bone marrow depression
Pharmacokinetics:
IV: Distribution half-life 10 min, elimination half-life 1−3 hr
Interactions/incompatibilities:
• Increased toxicity: radiation or other antineoplastics
• Decreased effects of: oral digoxin
Clinical assessment:
• Full blood count (RBC, PCV, Hb), differential, platelet count weekly
• Renal function studies: blood urea nitrogen, serum uric acid, urine creatinine clearance, electrolytes before and during therapy
• Liver function tests before and during therapy: bilirubin, alanine aminotransferase, aspartate aminotransferase, alkaline phosphatase, as needed or monthly
• Blood uric acid levels during therapy

NURSING CONSIDERATIONS
Administer:
• Follow local cytotoxic policy
• Direct IV infusion using appropriate gauge needle
• Continuous IV infusion over 5−10 days
• Subcutaneously (reconstituted with small amount of diluent)
• All other medication as prescribed including antiemetics, antibiotics and analgesics; antiemetics before and during treatment
Perform/provide:
• Good aseptic technique when administering and/or connecting to IV line
• Subcutaneous injection: charge site for each injection
• Increase fluid intake to 2−3 litres a day to prevent urate deposits and calculi formation, unless contraindicated
• Mouthcare, brushing of teeth with soft brush or cotton-tipped applicators for stomatitis; use unwaxed dental floss
• Observe subcutaneous injection sites for skin irritation
• Warm compresses at injection site for inflammation, pain
Evaluate:
• Fluid balance; report fall in urine output to below 30−50 ml/hr
• Temperature, pulse, respiration and BP if neutropenic 4 hrly; fever may indicate infection
• Fever, flu-like symptoms, myalgia, bone pain, chest pain, rash, conjunctivitis, malaise
• Bleeding in any site or tissue
• Dyspnoea, unproductive cough, chest pain, tachypnoea, fatigue, increased pulse, pallor, lethargy, personality changes, with high doses
• Oedema in feet, joint pain, abdominal pain, shaking
• Inflammation of mucosa, breaks in skin
• Yellowing of skin, sclera, dark urine, clay-coloured stools, itchy skin, abdominal pain, diarrhoea
• Signs of stomatitis
• GI symptoms: frequency of stools, cramping
• Acidosis, signs of dehydration: rapid respirations, poor skin turgor, decreased urine output, dry skin, restlessness, weakness
Teach patient/family:
• Protective isolation precautions
• To report signs of stomatitis, bleeding from any source, or feelings of malaise

- Dietary advice
- Major side effects of drug

dacarbazine

DTIC-Dome
Func. class.: Antineoplastic, alkylating agent
Chem. class.: Cytotoxic triazine
Legal class.: POM

Action: Alkylates DNA, RNA; inhibits enzymes that allow synthesis of proteins; also responsible for cross-linking DNA strands

Uses: Hodgkin's disease, sarcomas, neuroblastoma, malignant melanoma. Also used in combination with other cytotoxic agents; carcinoma—colon, ovary, breast, lung, testicular teratoma, solid tumors in children

Dosage and routes:
• *Adult:* IV 2−4.5 mg/kg for 10 days repeated after 4 weeks, or 250 mg/m² for 5 days repeated after 3 weeks, or total dose at once
Available forms include: Injection IV 100, 200 mg

Side effects/adverse reactions:
HAEM: Thrombocytopenia, leucopenia, anaemia
GI: Nausea, anorexia, vomiting, diarrhoea, hepatotoxicity
CNS: Facial paraesthesia, flushing, fever, malaise, anaphylaxis
INTEG: Alopecia, dermatitis, pain at injection site, photosensitivity reactions

Contraindications: Lactation hypersensitivity, pregnancy
Precautions: Radiation therapy
Pharmacokinetics: Metabolised by liver, excreted in urine; half-life 35 min, terminal 5 hr, 5% protein bound

Clinical assessment:
• Full blood count, differential, platelet count weekly; withhold drug if WBC is less than 4.0 × 10⁹/litre or platelet count is less than 75 × 10⁹/litre
• Liver function tests before, during therapy (bilirubin, aspartate aminotransferase, alanine aminotransferase, lactic dehydrogenase) as needed or monthly

NURSING CONSIDERATIONS
Assess:
• Temperature, pulse, respiration
Administer:
• Other medications by oral route if possible; avoid IM, subcutaneous, IV routes to prevent infections and bruises but only if thrombocytopenic. IV route used if central line *in situ*
• Anti-emetic 30−60 min before giving drug to prevent vomiting
• Antibiotics for prophylaxis of infection only when indicated
• Slow IV infusion using appropriate gauge needle. NB: handle with *great* care—very irritant to tissues and skin
• Observe for extravasation (vesicant drug)
Perform/provide:
• Strict medical asepsis, protective isolation if WBC levels are low
• Special skin care
• Increase fluid intake to 2−3 litres daily to prevent urate deposits, calculi formation
• Warm compresses at injection site for inflammation
Evaluate:
• Bleeding: haematuria, bruising or petechiae, mucosa or orifices 8 hrly
• Food preferences; list likes, dislikes
• Effects of alopecia on body image, discuss feelings about changes in body image
• Yellowing of skin, sclera, dark urine, clay-coloured stools, itchy skin, abdominal pain, fever, diarrhoea

• Inflammation of mucosa, breaks in skin

Teach patient/family:
• Of protective isolation precautions
• To report any complaints or side effects to nurse or clinician

---

dactinomycin (actinomycin D)

Cosmegen Lyovac
Func. class.: Antineoplastic
Chem. class.: Cytotoxic antibiotic
Legal class.: POM

Action: Inhibits DNA, RNA, protein synthesis; derived from *Streptomyces parrullus*; replication is decreased by binding to DNA, which causes strand splitting; cell cycle nonspecific

Uses: Sarcomas, melanomas, trophoblastic tumours in women, testicular cancer, Wilms' tumour, rhabdomyosarcoma, experimental indication include Ewing's sarcoma, oestrogenic sarcoma

Dosage and routes:
• *Adult:* IV 500 mcg daily for 5 days, repeat after 3 weeks if required
• *Child:* IV 15 mcg/kg daily for 5 days, or a total dose of 2500 mcg/m² given IV over 1 week
• Dose for adults and children not to exceed 15 mcg/kg or 400–600 mcg/m² daily for 5 days; stop drug until bone marrow recovery, then repeat cycle (not within 3 weeks)

Available forms include: Injection IV 500 mcg containing 20 mg mannitol

Side effects/adverse reactions:
HAEM· Thrombocytopenia, leucopenia, myelosuppression, aplastic anaemia
GI: Nausea, vomiting, anorexia, stomatitis, hepatotoxicity, abdominal pain, diarrhoea, gastrointestinal ulceration
INTEG: Rash, alopecia, pain at injection site, folliculitis, acne
EENT: Cheilitis, ulcerative stomatitis, dysphagia, oesophagitis
CNS: Malaise, fatigue, lethargy, fever
MS: Myalgia
META: Hypocalcaemia

Contraindications: Hypersensitivity, chickenpox, herpes infections, children under 12 months

Precautions: Renal disease, hepatic disease, pregnancy, lactation, bone marrow depression

Pharmacokinetics: Half-life 36 hr
IV: onset 2–5 min, concentrates in kidneys, liver, spleen; does not cross blood-brain barrier, excreted in bile and urine

Interactions/incompatibilities:
• Increased toxicity: other antineoplastics or radiation

Clinical assessment:
• Full blood count, differential, platelet count weekly; withhold drug if WBC is less than 4.0×10^9/litre or platelet count is 75×10^9/litre; notify clinician of these results
• Renal function studies: urea, serum uric acid, creatinine clearance, electrolytes before, during therapy
• Liver function tests before, during therapy: bilirubin, aspartate aminotransferase, alanine aminotransferase, alkaline phosphatase, as needed or monthly

NURSING CONSIDERATIONS

Assess:
• Baseline vital signs and fluid balance

Administer:
• Other medications by oral route if possible; avoid IM, subcutaneous, IV routes to prevent infections and bruises

• Anti-emetic 30−60 min before giving drug to prevent vomiting
• Slow IV infusion using appropriate gauge needle
• Topical or systemic analgesics for pain
• Local or systemic drugs for infection
• Transfusion for anaemia
• Antispasmodic for GI symptoms
• In accordance with local cytotoxic policy
NB: Care with handling, very irritant to tissues
Perform/provide:
• Strict medical asepsis, protective isolation if WBC levels are low
• Nutritious diet (as tolerated by the patient)
• Scrupulous care of the mouth
• Warm compresses at injection site for inflammation; check for extravasation
Evaluate:
• Fluid balance; report fall in urine output to less than 30−50 ml/hr
• Temperature, pulse, respiration 4 hrly; fever may indicate infection
• Bleeding: haematuria, bruising, petechiae, mucosa or orifices 8-hrly
• Food preferences; nutritional status
• Effects of alopecia on body image; discuss feelings about in body image changes
• Oedema in feet; joint, abdominal pain; shaking
• Inflammation of mucosa, breaks in skin
• Yellowing of skin, sclera, dark urine, clay-coloured stools, itchy skin, abdominal pain, fever, diarrhoea
• Buccal cavity for dryness, sores, ulceration, white patches, oral pain, bleeding, dysphagia; 8-hrly
• Local irritation, pain, burning at injection site
• Symptoms indicating severe allergic reaction: rash, pruritus, urticaria, purpuric skin lesions, itching, flushing
• GI symptoms: frequency of stools, cramping
• Acidosis, signs of dehydration: rapid respirations, poor skin turgor, decreased urine output, dry skin, restlessness, weakness
Teach patient/family:
• Why protective isolation precautions are necessary
• To report any complaints, side effects to nurse or clinician
• That hair may be lost during treatment and wig or hairpiece may make patient feel better (available free on NHS); tell patient that new hair may be different in colour, texture
• To avoid foods which irritate mucosa
• To report any bleeding, white spots, ulcerations in mouth to clinician; tell patient to examine mouth daily

---

danazol
Danol
Func. class.: Androgen
Chem. class.: α-Ethinyl testosterone derivative
Legal class.: POM

Action: Decreases FSH, LH, which are controlled by pituitary; this leads to amenorrhoea/anovulation, atrophy of endometrial tissue. Inhibition of enzymes of steroidgenesis
Uses: Endometriosis, benign breast disorders, menorrhagia, gynaecomastia, mastalgia
Dosage and routes:
Endometriosis
• *Adult:* By mouth initial dose 400 mg in 2−4 doses, adjusted as required, for 6 months
Benign breast disorders

- *Adult:* By mouth initially 300 mg daily, adjusted according to response, for 3−6 months

Gynaecomastia
- *Adolescents:* 200 mg daily for 6 months, increased to 400 mg according to response
- *Adults:* 400 mg, daily in divided doses for 6 months

Mastalgia
- 200−300 mg daily according to symptoms for 3−6 months

Menorrhagia
- 200 mg daily for 3 months

Available forms include: Capsules 100, 200 mg

Sides effects/adverse reactions:
HAEM: Erythrocytosis, polycythaemia, eosinophillia, leucopenia
INTEG: Rash, acneiform lesions, oily hair, skin, flushing, sweating, acne vulgaris, alopecia, hirsutism
CNS: Dizziness, headache, fatigue, tremors, paraesthesias, flushing, sweating, anxiety, lability, insomnia
MS: Cramps, spasms
CV: Increased BP, tachycardia, hypertension
GU: Haematuria, amenorrhoea, vaginitis, decreased libido, decreased breast size, clitoral hypertrophy, testicular atrophy
GI: Nausea, vomiting, constipation, weight gain, cholestatic jaundice
EENT: Carpal tunnel syndrome, conjunctival oedema, nasal congestion, voice changes, visual disturbances
ENDO: Abnormal glucose tolerance test
Contraindications: Hypersensitivity, pregnancy, lactation, genital bleeding (abnormal), porphyria, androgen dependant tumour, thromboembolic disease
Precautions: Migraine headaches, seizure disorders, diabetes mellitus, renal disease, cardiac disease, hepatic disease

Pharmacokinetics: Half life 4.5 hr, metabolised in liver, metabolites excreted in urine

Interactions/incompatibilities:
- Increased effects of: oral antidiabetics, cyclosporin, alphacalcidol, carbamazepine
- Increased prothrombin time: anticoagulants potentiated
- Reduced effect of: antihypotensives due to promotion of fluid retention
- Decreased effects of: insulin

Clinical assessment:
- Potassium, blood sugar, urine glucose while on long-term therapy
- Haematological monitoring
- Liver function studies: aspartate aminotransferase, alanine aminotransferase, alkaline phosphatase

Lab. test interferences:
Increase: LDL-cholesterol; uptake of tri-iodothyronine
Decrease: HDL-cholesterol, thyroid binding globulin

NURSING CONSIDERATIONS
Assess:
- Baseline weight and fluid balance
Administer:
- With food or milk to decrease GI symptoms
Perform/provide:
- Help with physiotherapy exercise for patients who are immobile
Evaluate:
- Therapeutic response: decreased pain in endometriosis, decreased size, pain in benign breast disorders
- Weight daily; notify clinician if weekly weight gain more than 2.5 kg
- Fluid balance; observe for urine retention, increasing oedema
- Oedema, hypertension, cardiac symptoms, jaundice
- Mental status: affect, mood, behavioural changes, aggression, sleep disorders, depression

• Signs of virilisation: deepening of voice, decreased libido, facial hair (may not be reversible)
Teach patient/family:
• Notify clinician if therapeutic response decreases
• Not to discontinue medication abruptly but to taper over several weeks
• All aspects of drug usage
• Women to report menstrual irregularities, that amenorrhoea usually occurs but menstruation resumes 2−3 months after termination of therapy
• Routine breast self-examination, report any increase in nodule size
• Drug should induce anovulation; reversible within 60−90 days after drug is discontinued

---

dantrolene sodium

Dantrium, Dantrium Intravenous
Func. class.: Skeletal muscle relaxant, direct acting
Legal class.: POM

Action: Interferes with the release of calcium in muscle therefore preventing contraction
Uses: Spasticity in multiple sclerosis, stroke, spinal cord injury, cerebral palsy. Intravenously for malignant hyperthermia
Dosage and routes:
Spasticity
• *Adult:* By mouth initially 25 mg daily increasing weekly over 7 weeks, to maximum of 100 mg 4 times a day
• *Child:* Not recommended
Malignant hyperthermia
• *Adult and child:* IV 1 mg/kg, may repeat to total dose of 10 mg/kg; if relapse occurs, repeat administration at last effective dose
Available forms include: Capsules 25, 100 mg; powder for injection IV 20 mg/vial

Side effects/adverse reactions:
CNS: Dizziness, fatigue, drowsiness, malaise, headache, seizures, insomnia
EENT: Visual disturbance
MS: Muscle weakness
GI: Nausea, constipation, vomiting, transient diarrhoea, increased aspartate aminotransferase, alkaline phosphatase, hepatotoxicity, hepatitis
GU: Urinary frequency, incontinence, urinary retention, haematuria, crystalluria
INTEG: Acneiform rash
Contraindications: Hypersensitivity; children; where spasticity is useful; hepatic dysfunction, acute skeletal muscle spasm
Precautions: Impaired cardiac, renal disease, hepatic disease, obstructive lung disease, pregnancy
Pharmacokinetics:
Period of onset: Peak 5 hr, highly protein bound, half-life 8 hr, metabolised in liver, excreted in urine (metabolites)
Interactions/incompatibilities:
• Increased CNS depression: alcohol, tricyclic antidepressants, narcotics, barbiturates, sedatives, hypnotics
• Increased risk of liver damage: oestrogens
• Hyperkalaemia: verapamil with IV dantrolene
Clinical assessment:
• EEG in epileptic patients; poor seizure control has occurred in patients taking this drug
• Hepatic function by frequent determination of aspartate aminotransferase, alanine aminotransferase, bilirubin, alkaline phosphate
Treatment of overdose: Induce emesis in conscious patient, gastric lavage, dialysis
NURSING CONSIDERATIONS
Assess:
• Fluid balance

• Liver function before, after 6 weeks and periodically
• Attainable therapeutic goals
Administer:
• Intravenously (usually in hospital) for malignant hyperthernia; inject directly into vein rapidly
• Orally with meals. To increase dosages at recommended rate until optimum response with minimum side effects
Perform/provide:
• Help with mobility
Evaluate:
• Therapeutic response: attained physical goal, decreased pain, spasticity
• Fluid balance, retention, frequency, hesitancy
• For increased epileptic seizure activity
• Any adverse effects: drowsiness, dizziness, malaise, headache, nausea, diarrhoea usually transient
• Incontinence more common in elderly
• Signs of jaundice, report immediately
• Psychological dependency: increased need for medication, frequent requests for medication, increased pain
Teach patient/family:
• Not to discontinue medication without medical advice. Drug should be tapered off slowly
• To take other medication only if directed by clinician
• That alcohol should not be taken
• To avoid driving or use of machinery until therapy is established
• To notify clinician if there is any yellowing in skin, clay coloured stools, dark urine

dapsone

Func. class.: Antibiotic, leprostatic
Chem. class.: Sulphone
Legal class.: POM

Action: Competitive inhibition of bacterial replication of folic acid from PABA
Uses: Leprosy, dermatitis herpetiformis
Dosage and routes:
Leprosy
• *Adult:* By mouth 1−2 mg/kg daily with rifampicin and/or clofazimine for 6 months to 2 yr
Dermatitis herpetiformis
• 50−400 mg daily
Available forms include: Tablets 50, 100 mg; combination product with pyrimethamine, *Maloprim*, for malaria prophylaxis
Side effects/adverse reactions:
INTEG: Allergic dermatitis, Stevens-Johnson syndrome, exfoliative dermatitis
CV: Tachycardia
CNS: Headache, anxiety, insomnia, tremors, lethargy, depression, confusion, psychosis, aggression
EENT: Blurred vision, optic neuritis, photophobia
HAEM: Haemolytic anaemia, agranulocytosis, methaemoglobinaemia
GI: Anoxeria, nausea, vomiting, hepatitis
Contraindications: Hypersensitivity to sulphones, severe anaemia, porphyria
Precautions: Cardiac or pulmonary disease, hepatic disease, glucose-6-phosphate dehydrogenase deficiency, pregnancy, breast-feeding
Pharmacokinetics: Complete absorption, half-life 20−30 hr; metabolite highly protein bound
Interactions/incompatibilities:
• Increased action of dapsone: probenecid, folic acid antagonists

• Decreased action of dapsone: rifampicin

Clinical assessment:

• Liver function weekly; aspartate aminotransferase, alanine aminotransferase, bilirubin
• Renal function, urea, creatinine
• Blood levels of drug
• Full blood count

Treatment of overdose: Gastric lavage, aspiration. Administration of activated charcoal. Treat methaemoglobinaemia with methylene blue 1−2 mg/kg IV

NURSING CONSIDERATIONS

Assess:

• Baseline temperature
• Fluid balance, specific gravity, urinalysis

Administer:

• With meals to decrease GI symptoms
• Anti-emetic if vomiting occurs
• After culture and sensitivity is completed; repeat monthly to detect resistance

Perform/provide:

• Infants to be kept with mothers infected with leprosy, breastfeeding during drug therapy is encouraged. NB: Small risk of haemolytic anaemia in infants

Evaluate:

• Temperature, if less than 38°C, drug should be reduced
• Mental status often: affect, mood, behavioural changes; psychosis may occur
• Hepatic status: decreased appetite, jaundice, dark urine, fatigue
• Urinalysis, specific gravity monthly

Teach patient/family:

• That therapeutic effects may occur after 3−6 months of drug therapy
• That compliance with dosage schedule, length is necessary
• That scheduled appointments must be kept or relapse may occur

dehydrocholic acid

Func. class.: Biliary stimulant
Chem. class.: Unconjugated oxidised acid
Legal class: P

Action: Facilitates drainage from gallbladder by increasing volume, water content, flow of low-viscosity diluted bile

Uses: Post biliary tract surgery, to flush common duct and drainage tube and wash away small calculi obstructing bile flow

Dosage and routes:

• *Adult:* By mouth 250−750 mg 3 times a day
Cholecystography
• 500−750 mg 4 hrly for 12 hr before and after procedure
Available forms include: Tablets 250 mg

Contraindications: Complete biliary obstruction, chronic liver disease, occlusive hepatitis

Precautions: Asthma, prostatic hypertrophy, hepatitis, child under 12 years, elderly, pregnancy

Pharmacokinetics:

Period of onset: Concentrated in liver, excreted in bile

NURSING CONSIDERATIONS

Administer:

• With fluids

Teach patient/family:

• About effect of drug and use before and after cholecystography

demeclocycline HCl

Ledermycin, combination products
Func. class.: Antibiotic, broad-spectrum
Chem. class.: Tetracycline
Legal class.: POM

Action: Inhibits protein synthesis, phosphorylation in microorganisms by binding to 30S ribosomal subunits, reversibly binding to 50S ribosomal subunits

Uses: Gram-positive/Gram-negative bacteria, protozoa, rickettsia, mycoplasma, infections; inappropriate ADH syndrome, acne

Dosage and routes:
• *Adult:* By mouth 150 mg 6 hrly or 300 mg 12 hrly, atypical pneumonia 900 mg daily in 3 divided doses, 6 days total

Inappropriate ADH syndrome
• *Adult:* 900−1200 mg daily in divided doses then 600−900 mg daily as maintenance

Available forms include: Tablets 300 mg; capsules 150 mg

Side effects/adverse reactions:
HAEM: Eosinophilia, neutropenia, thrombocytopenia, leucocytosis, haemolytic anaemia
EENT: Dysphagia, glossitis, decreased calcification of deciduous teeth, oral candidiasis
GI: Nausea, vomiting, diarrhoea, anorexia, enterocolitis, hepatotoxicity, flatulence, abdominal cramps, epigastric burning, stomatitis, pseudomembranous colitis
CV: Pericarditis
GU: Increased blood urea nitrogen, polyuria, polydipsia, renal failure, nephrotoxicity
INTEG: Rash, urticaria, photosensitivity, increased pigmentation, exfoliative dermatitis, pruritus, angioedema, exacerbation of systemic lupus erythematosus

Contraindications: Hypersensitivity to tetracyclines, children under 12 yr, pregnancy, renal failure, systemic lupus erythematosus

Precautions: Renal disease, hepatic disease, lactation

Pharmacokinetics:
Period of onset: Peak 3−6 hr, half-life 10−17 hr, excreted in urine and faeces, excreted in breast milk, 36%−91% bound to serum protein

Interactions/incompatibilities:
• Decreased effect of this drug: antacids, sodium bicarbonate, dairy products, oral iron, calcium, zinc, magnesium, aluminium
• Increased effect: anticoagulants
• Decreased effect: penicillins, oral contraceptives

Clinical assessment:
• Blood studies, full blood count, urea, creatinine, prothrombin time, aspartate aminotransferase, alanine aminotransferase

Treatment of overdose: No antidote. Gastric lavage, administration of milk, antacids

NURSING CONSIDERATIONS

Assess:
• Fluid balance

Administer:
• On empty stomach 1 hr before, or 2 hr after meals with a glass of water
• After culture and sensitivity obtained
• 2 hr before or after laxative or iron (ferrous) products; 3 hr after antacid

Evaluate:
• Therapeutic response: decreased temperature, absence of lesions, negative culture and sensitivity
• Allergic reactions: rash, itching, pruritus, angioedema
• Nausea, vomiting, diarrhoea; administer anti-emetic, antacids as ordered
(NB: antacids reduce absorption of tetracyclines)
• Overgrowth of infection: increased temperature, malaise, redness, pain, swelling, drainage, perineal itching, diarrhoea, changes in cough, sputum

Teach patient/family:
• To avoid sun exposure since burns may occur; sunscreen does not seem to decrease photosensitivity

• That diabetics should avoid use of Clinistix Diastix for urine glucose testing
• All prescribed medication must be taken to prevent superimposed infection
• To avoid milk products

---

desferrioxamine mesylate

Desferal
Func. class.: Chelating agent
Chem. class.: Siderochrome
Legal class.: POM

Action: Binds iron ions (ferric ions), and aluminium ions to form water-soluble complex that is removed by kidneys
Uses: Acute iron intoxication, chronic iron overload, aluminium overload, corneal rust stains and occular siderosis
Dosage and routes:
Acute
• *Adult and child:* By mouth 50−100 ml 10% solution after lavage, then IM 1−2 g every 3−12 hrly, to maximum 6 g in 24 hr, or IV 15 mg/kg/hr to maximum 80 mg/kg in 24 hr
Chronic
• *Adult and child:* IM 500 mg−1 g daily initially, usual daily dose 20−40 mg/kg. Subcutaneous infusion 20−40 mg/kg over 8−24 hr 3−7 times a week. All dosage regimens and routes dependant on individual needs
Aluminium overload
• Individual doses determined by patient's needs
Haemodialysis/haemofiltration
• 1 g IV over 1 hr during last hr of third dialysis
CAPD
• 1 g once or twice week−IV, subcutaneous, IM, intraperitoneal
Corneal rust stains and occular siderosis

• 10% eye drop prepared from injection, applied 4−6 times daily
Available forms include: Powder for injection IV, IM, subcutaneous 500 mg/vial
Side effects/adverse reactions:
INTEG: Urticaria, erythema, pruritus, pain at injection site, fever
CNS: Dizziness, convulsions
MS: Leg cramps
HAEM: Thrombocytopenia
CV: Hypotension, tachycardia
GI: Diarrhoea, abdominal cramps
EENT: Blurred vision, night or colour blindness, visual field defects, hearing disturbance
GU: Dysuria, pyelonephritis
SYST: Anaphylaxis, infection
Contraindications: Hypersensitivity, renal impairment (dialysis may be necessary)
Precautions: Pregnancy, lactation
Pharmacokinetics: Excreted by kidneys as complex, unchanged drug
Interactions/incompatibilities:
• Prolonged unconsciousness with prochlorperazine
• Vitamin C: enhanced excretion of iron
Clinical assessment:
• Renal function tests: urea, creatinine, creatinine clearance
• Monitor serum iron levels
Treatment of overdose:
Supportive measures, reduce dose, remove excess by dialysis
NURSING CONSIDERATIONS
Assess:
• Vital signs. Observe for hypotension
• Fluid balance
• Weight
• Monitor disturbance in vision, hearing
Administer:
• Injection diluted according to each route of administration. Follow dosage regimen appropri-

ate to each patient; duration depends on condition
• When adrenaline and resuscitation equipment available for acute therapy in case of anaphylaxis
Perform/provide:
• Drugs and equipment for resuscitation
Evaluate:
• Allergic reactions: rash, urticaria; if these occur, drug should be discontinued
• Side effects
• For hypotension
Teach patient/family:
• That blood tests and treatment may continue for several months with chronic iron overload
• How to manage subcutaneous infusion for long term therapy

---

desipramine HCl

Pertofran
Func. class.: Antidepressant, tricyclic
Chem. class.: Dibenzazepine, secondary amine
Legal class.: POM

Action: Blocks reuptake of noradrenaline, serotonin into nerve endings, increasing action of noradrenaline, serotonin in nerve cells
Uses: Depression
Dosage and routes:
• *Adult:* By mouth initially 75 mg in divided doses for 3 days, increasing to 150–200 mg daily in divided doses or single dose at night
• *Elderly:* By mouth 25 mg daily, increase as necessary
Available forms include: Tablets 25 mg
Side effects/adverse reactions:
HAEM: Agranulocytosis, thrombocytopenia, eosinophilia, leucopenia

CNS: Dizziness, drowsiness, confusion, headache, anxiety, tremors, agitation, weakness, insomnia, nightmares, increased psychiatric symptoms
GI: Constipation, dry mouth, nausea, vomiting, increased appetite, cramps, epigastric distress, jaundice, hepatitis, stomatitis
GU: Retention, disturbance in sexual function
INTEG: Rash, urticaria, sweating, pruritus, photosensitivity
CV: Orthostatic hypotension, ECG changes, tachycardia, hypertension, palpitations
EENT: Blurred vision, tinnitus, mydriasis, ophthalmoplegia
Contraindications: Recovery phase of myocardial infarction, heart block or other cardiac arrhythmias, narrow-angle glaucoma, severe liver disease, mania, child less than 12 yr, urinary retention
Precautions: Suicidal patients, severe depression, convulsive disorders, prostatic hypertrophy, elderly, pregnancy, lactation, avoid abrupt cessation of therapy
Pharmacokinetics:
Period of onset: Steady state 2–11 days; metabolised by liver, excreted by kidneys, half-life 7–62 hr
Interactions/incompatibilities:
• Increased effect of this drug: neuroleptics, methylphenidate
• Decreased effects of this drug: barbiturates
• Decreased effects of: guanethidine, clonidine, indirect acting sympathomimetics (ephedrine)
• Increased effects of: direct acting sympathomimetics (adrenaline), alcohol, benzodiazepines, CNS depressants
• Hyperpyretic crisis, convulsions, hypertensive episode: MAOIs
• Anaesthetics: increased effects of arrhythmia and hypotension

Clinical assessment:
• Blood studies; full blood count WBC and differential cardiac enzymes (if receiving long term therapy)
• Hepatic studies; aspartate aminotransferase, alanine aminotransferase, bilirubin, creatinine
• ECG for flattening of T-wave, bundle branch block, atrioventricular block, dysrhythmias in cardiac patients

Treatment of overdose: ECG monitoring, induce emesis, lavage, activated charcoal, administer IV diazepam for convulsions

NURSING CONSIDERATIONS
Assess:
• Baseline pulse, weight

Administer:
• Increased fluids, fibre in diet if constipation, urinary retention occur
• With food or milk for GI symptoms
• Dosage at bedtime if oversedation occurs during day; may take entire dose at bedtime; elderly may not tolerate once daily dosing
• Frequent sips of water for dry mouth

Perform/provide:
• Assistance with ambulation during beginning therapy since drowsiness/dizziness may occur

Evaluate:
• BP (lying, standing), pulse; take vital signs 4 hrly in patients with cardiovascular disease
• Weight weekly, appetite may increase with drug
• Blurred vision
• Mental status: mood, alertness, affect, suicidal tendencies, an increase in psychiatric symptoms: depression, panic
• Urinary retention, constipation
• Withdrawal symptoms: headache, nausea, vomiting, muscle pain, weakness; do not usually occur unless drug was discontinued abruptly
• Alcohol consumption; increases sedative effect

Teach patient/family:
• That therapeutic effects may take 2−3 weeks
• Use caution in driving or other activities requiring alertness because of drowsiness, dizziness, blurred vision
• To avoid alcohol ingestion, other CNS depressants
• Do not discontinue medication quickly after long-term use, may cause nausea, headache, malaise
• Wear sunscreen or large hat since photosensitivity occurs

---

desmopressin acetate

DDAVP, Desmospray
Func. class.: Pituitary hormone
Chem. class.: Synthetic antidiuretic hormone analogue peptide
Legal class.: POM

Action: Promotes reabsorption of water by action on renal tubular epithelium, contracts smooth muscles, causing vasoconstriction with a pressor
Uses: Haemophilia, von Willebrand's disease prior to surgery, pituitary diabetes insipidus, nocturnal enuresis
Dosage and routes:
Diabetes insipidus
• *Adult:* Intranasally 10−40 mcg daily as a single dose or in divided doses; IM/IV 1−4 mcg daily
• *Child:* Intranasally 5−30 mcg daily; IM/IV 0.4 mcg daily
Haemophilia/von Willebrand's disease
• 0.3−0.4 mcg/kg IV infusion ½−1½ hr before surgery
Primary nocturnal enuresis
• *Adult and child over 7 yr:*

Intranasally 20–40 mcg at night
Available forms include: Intranasal spray 10 mcg/metered dose and drops 100 mcg/ml; injection IV, IM 4 mcg/ml

Side effects/adverse reactions:

EENT: Nasal irritation, congestion, rhinitis (all after intranasal use)

GI: Nausea, cramps

CV: Increased BP

SYST: Water retention, hyponatraemia, hypersensitivity reactions

INTEG: Pallor

Contraindications: Hypersensitivity, nephrogenic diabetes insipidus

Precautions: Pregnancy, asthma, hypertension, renal impairment, cystic fibrosis, cardiovascular disease

Pharmacokinetics:

NASAL: Onset 1 hr, peak 1–5 hr, duration 8–20 hr, half-life 0.4–4 hr, excreted in breast milk

Interactions/incompatibilities:

• Decreased response to desmopressin: alcohol

• Increased response to desmopressin: carbamazepine, chlorpropamide, fludrocortisone

Clinical assessment:

• Withdraw for at least 1 week for reassessment after 3 months treatment of enuresis

• Monitor fluid balance when starting therapy; body weight, serum electrolytes at regular intervals during

NURSING CONSIDERATIONS

Assess:

• Baseline BP and pulse when to be given IV

Evaluate:

• Therapeutic response: absence of severe thirst, decreased urine output, osmolality

• Pulse, BP when giving drug IV

• Weight daily, check for oedema in extremities

• Intranasal use: nausea, congestion, cramps, headache, usually decreased with decreased dose

Teach patient/family:

• Technique for nasal instillation: to insert tube into nasal cavity to instil drug

• Avoid non-prescribed products: response; do not use with alcohol

• All aspects of drug: action, side effects, dose, when to notify clinician

---

dexamethasone/ dexamethasone phosphate/ dexamethasone sodium phosphate

Decadron, Decadron Shock-Pak

Func. class.: Corticosteroid

Chem. class.: Glucocorticoid, long-acting

Legal class.: POM

Action: Decreases inflammation by suppression of migration of polymorphonuclear leucocytes, fibroblasts, reversal of increase capillary permeability and lysosomal stabilisation; anti-emetic

Uses: Inflammation, allergies, neoplasms, cerebral oedema, shock, arthritis, chemotherapy-induced nausea and vomiting

Dosage and routes:

Inflammation

• *Adult:* By mouth 0.5–9 mg daily preferably as a single morning dose; IM or IV 0.5–20 mg

• *Child:* IM or IV 200–500 mcg/kg daily

Shock

• *Adult:* IV 2–6 mg/kg repeated after 2–6 hr if required

Cerebral oedema

• *Adult:* IV 10 mg initially, then 4 mg IM 6 hrly for 2–10 days, reduce dose gradually

Acute life threatening cerebral oedema, use high dose IV schedule. Seek specialist advice

Intra-articular/intrabursally/into tendon sheaths
• *Adult:* 0.4−4 mg every 3 days − 3 weeks depending on response and condition being treated

Anti-emesis with chemotherapy
• *Adult:* IV 5−20 mg 30 min prior to chemotherapy then 2−4 mg 2 or 3 times a day by mouth as required

Notes: Many other treatment schedules in use
Courses longer than 5 days should be tailed-off, not stopped abruptly
Available forms include: Tablets 0.5, 2 mg; injection IV (as sodium phosphate) 5 mg/ml, (as phosphate) 4 mg/ml, (as dexamethasone) 20 mg/ml

Side effects/adverse reactions:
INTEG: Acne, poor wound healing, ecchymosis, petechiae, striae, skin atrophy, hirsutism, increased sweating, allergic skin reactions, tingling in perineum after rapid IV injection
CNS: Depression, flushing, headache, mood changes, convulsions, vertigo, psychosis
CV: Hypertension, circulatory collapse, thrombophlebitis, embolism
MS: Fractures, osteoporosis, weakness, growth retardation (children), myopathy
GI: Nausea, abdominal distention, GI haemorrhage, increased appetite, pancreatitis, gastric/duodenal ulcer, dyspepsia
EENT: Increased intraocular pressure, blurred vision, cataracts
ENDO: Cushingoid state, adrenocortical suppression, decreased glucose tolerance
GU: Menstrual irregularities, fluid retention, sodium retention, hypokalaemia
Contraindications: Hypersensitivity

Precautions; Psychosis, amoebiasis, fungal and certain viral infections, live viral vaccines, gastro-intestinal ulceration, pregnancy, diabetes mellitus, glaucoma, osteoporosis, seizure disorders, ulcerative colitis, chronic cardiac failure, myasthenia gravis, Cushing's syndrome, renal impairment, hypertension, migraine, latent tuberculosis, incomplete growth, lactation, cerebral malaria

Pharmacokinetics: Well absorbed by mouth, metabolised in liver and kidneys, excreted in urine, plasma half-life 190 min
Dexamethasone 4 mg/ml = dexamethasone phosphate 4.8 mg/ml = dexamethasone sodium phosphate 5 mg/ml

Interactions/incompatibilities:
• Decreased action of dexamethasone: barbiturates, rifampicin, ephedrine, phenytoin, aminoglutethimide
• Decreased effects of: antidiabetics, antihypertensives, isoniazid, vaccines
• Increased side effects of: salicylates, indomethacin, amphotericin B, digitalis preparations, diuretics, live viral vaccines
• Increased action of dexamethasone: oestrogens

Clinical assessment:
• Electrolytes especially potassium in patients on potassium-lowering drugs or cardiac glycosides
• Review requirements for hypoglycaemic agents/oral anti-coagulants in co-treated patients

Treatment of overdose:
Symptomatic treatment

NURSING CONSIDERATIONS
Assess:
• Baseline vital signs
Administer:
• Titrated dose, use lowest effective dose

- IM injection deeply in large mass
- Rotate sites, avoid deltoid, use 19G needle
- In one morning dose to prevent adrenal suppression
- Avoid subcutaneous administration, damage may be done to tissue
- If treatment lasts more than 5 days reduce dose slowly when stopping

Perform/provide:
- Assistance with ambulation in patient with bone tissue disease to prevent fractures

Evaluate:
- Weight daily, notify clinician of weekly gain more than 2 kg
- BP and pulse, 4 hrly
- Fluid balance; be alert for decreasing urinary output and increasing oedema
- Therapeutic response: ease of respirations, decreased inflammation
- Infection: increased temperature, WBC even after withdrawal of medication; drug masks symptoms of infection
- Potassium depletion: parasthesia, fatigue, nausea, vomiting, depression, polyuria, dysrhythmias, weakness
- Oedema hypotension, cardiac symptoms
- Blood/urine glucose especially in diabetic patients
- Mental status: affect, mood behavioural changes, aggression

Teach patient/family:
- That steroid user card must be carried
- Notify clinician if therapeutic response decreases; dosage adjustment may be needed
- Not to discontinue this medication abruptly or adrenal crisis can result
- Avoid non-prescribed products: salicylates, alcohol in cough products, cold preparations unless directed by clinician
- All aspects of drug usage, including Cushingoid symptoms
- Symptoms of adrenal insufficiency: nausea, anorexia, fatigue, dizziness, dyspnoea, weakness, joint pain
- To report any chest pain
- Inform any clinician, dentist or therapist of drug regimen

---

dexamethasone (ophthalmic)

Maxidex, combination products
Func. class.: Anti-inflammatory, ophthalmic
Chem. class.: Glucocorticoid, long acting
Legal class.: POM

Action: Anti-inflammatory, resulting in decreased pain, photophobia

Uses: Inflammation of eye, lids, conjunctiva, cornea, uveitis, iridocyclitis, allergic conditions, burns, foreign bodies. May be combined with antibiotics

Dosage and routes:
- *Adult and child:* Instil 1−2 drops into conjunctival sac ½−4 hrly depending on condition

Available forms include: Ophthalmic suspension 0.1%, several combination products

Side effects/adverse reactions:
EENT: Increased intraocular pressure, poor corneal wound healing, increased possibility of corneal infection, decreased acuity, visual field defects, cataracts
MISC: Systemic glucocorticoid action may be seen with intensive use

Contraindications: Hypersensitivity, acute superficial herpes simplex, fungal/viral diseases of the eye or conjunctiva, ocular tuberculosis, infections of the eye, undiagnosed red eye

Precautions: Corneal abrasions, glaucoma

Clinical assessment:

• Check intraocular pressure and lens clarity regularly during long-term therapy

NURSING CONSIDERATIONS

Administer:

• Only to dermatoses; do not use on weeping, denuded or infected areas

• Only to affected areas

• After thoroughly cleansing area to be treated

• Apply wearing gloves; wash hands well before and after application

Perform/provide:

• Treatment for a few days after area has cleared

Evaluate:

• Therapeutic response: improved vision, decrease inflammation

• Temperature; if pyrexia develops, treatment should be discontinued

• Allergic reactions: redness, itching, swelling, lacrimation

• Therapeutic response: absence of swelling, redness, exudate

• Development of side effects such as increased intraocular pressure

Teach patient/family:

• Not to use other non-prescribed products unless approved by clinician

• Instillation method: pressure on lacrimal sac for 1 min

• Not to share eye medications with others

• Discard eyedrops 28 days after opening

dexamphetamine sulphate

Dexedrine

Func. class.: Cerebral stimulant
Chem. class.: Amphetamine
Legal class.: CD (Sch 2) POM

Action: Increases release of noradrenaline, dopamine from neurones

Uses: Narcolepsy; attention deficit disorder with hyperactivity in children under the supervision of a clinician specialising in child psychiatry

Dosage and routes:

• *Adult:* By mouth 10 mg daily in divided doses, increased by 10 mg daily at weekly intervals to maximum 60 mg daily if needed

• *Elderly:* By mouth starting dose 5 mg daily increased by 5 mg daily at weekly intervals if needed

• *Child 3−5 yr:* By mouth 2.5 mg daily, increased by 2.5 mg daily at weekly intervals to maximum 20 mg daily in divided doses if needed

• *Child over 6 yr:* By mouth 5−10 mg daily in divided doses, increased by 5 mg daily at weekly intervals to maximum 40 mg daily if needed

Available forms include: Tablets 5 mg

Side effects/adverse reactions:

CNS: Hyperactivity, insomnia, restlessness, talkativeness, dizziness, headache, chills, stimulation, dysphoria, irritability, aggressiveness, dependence, psychosis, tremor

GI: Nausea, vomiting, anorexia, dry mouth, diarrhoea, constipation, weight loss, cramps

GU: Impotence, change in libido

CV: Palpitations, tachycardia, hypertension, cardiomyopathy

INTEG: Urticaria, sweating

ENDO: Growth retardation in children

Contraindications: Hypersensitivity to sympathomimetic amines, hyperthyroidism, moderate to severe hypertension, glaucoma, parkinsonism, drug abuse, cardiovascular disease, anxiety, porphyria, pregnancy, breast feeding, within 14 days of MAOI therapy

Precautions: Gilles de la Tourette's disorder, anorexia, unstable personality, mild hypertension

Pharmacokinetics:
Period of onset: Onset 30 min, peak 1−3 hr, duration 4−20 hr, metabolised by liver, excreted by kidneys, breast milk, elimination half-life 12−13 h

Interactions/incompatibilities:
• Hypertensive crisis: MAOIs or within 14 days of MAOIs inhibitors
• Increased effect of dexamphetamine: acetazolamide, antacids, sodium bicarbonate
• Decreased effects of dexamphetamine: ascorbic acid, ammonium chloride
• Decreased effects of: guanethidine, other antihypertensives

Treatment of overdose: Gastric lavage, no specific antidote, supportive treatment including diazepam for convulsions. Elimination increased by forced acid diuresis

NURSING CONSIDERATIONS
Assess:
• Weight and height in children and monitor growth rates
• Diet, check for food allergies especially 'E' numbers in children
• Pulse, blood pressure and respiration, before treatment

Administer:
• Orally following the dosage regimen for suitable gradual introduction
• Optimum response at smallest dose
• Do not give late in the day to avoid interference with sleep

Perform/provide:
• Frequent drinks to prevent a dry mouth

Evaluate:
• Therapeutic response: increased mental attention, decreased drowsiness
• Over stimulation; hyperactivity insomnia, restlessness, talkativeness, palpitation, tachycardia
• Drug dependency may occur as tolerance develops. Larger dose for some effect. Treatment should be stopped gradually
• Growth rate, height in children (maybe decreased)

Teach patient/family:
• To follow suitable diet, avoiding foods that may increase irritability, combined with rest and exercise
• That alcohol should be avoided
• Not to discontinue medication without medical advise. Drug should be tapered off slowly
• To take other medication only if directed by clinician. The effect of dexamphetamine is increased and decreased by several drugs
• To avoid driving or use of machinery until therapy established

dextran

Gentran, Lomodex, Rheomacrodex, Macrodex, Dextraven
Func. class.: Plasma volume expander
Chem. class.: Low molecular weight polysaccharide
Legal class.: POM

Action: Similar to human albumin, expands plasma volume
Uses: Expand plasma volume, prophylaxis of embolism, thrombosis, emergency blood substitute in haemorrhage

Dosage and routes:
- *Adult:* IV infusion initially 500–1000 ml, up to 2500–3000 ml over several days according to patient's needs. Seek specialist advice for treatment regimens

Available forms include: 10% dextran 40 in 0.9% sodium chloride or 5% dextrose; 6% dextran 70 in 0.9% sodium chloride or 5% dextrose; 6% dextran 110 in 0.9% sodium chloride or 5% dextrose

Side effects/adverse reactions:
HAEM: Decreased haematocrit, increased bleeding/coagulation times
INTEG: Rash, urticaria, pruritus, angioneurotic oedema
RESP: Wheezing, dyspnoea, bronchospasm, pulmonary oedema
GU: Renal failure
GI: Nausea, vomiting
SYST: Anaphylaxis, other allergic reactions

Contraindications: Hypersensitivity, renal failure, severe congestive cardiac failure, extreme dehydration

Precautions: Bleeding disorders, pregnancy

Pharmacokinetics:
IV: Expands blood volume 1–2 times the amount infused, excreted in urine and faeces, low molecular weight dextrans largely excreted unchanged. Dextran 110 metabolised in tissues, half-life depends on product

Interactions/incompatibilities:
- May precipitate weak acid drugs, avoid adding drugs to dextrans if possible

Clinical assessment:
- Blood grouping and crossmatching, biochemical tests prior to administration of dextran to avoid interference

Lab. test interferences:
False increase: Blood glucose (using acid reagents), urinary protein

Interferes: Blood typing/crossmatching, some bilirubin assays, total protein using Biuret reagent

Treatment of overdose: Stop or slow infusion, supportive treatment

NURSING CONSIDERATIONS

Assess:
- Baseline vital signs including ECG and CVP (if possible)
- Fluid balance

Administer:
- After crossmatching, if blood is to be given also

Perform/provide:
- Discard part-used units

Evaluate:
- Vital signs every 5 min for 30 min
- CVP during infusion
- Urine output hrly; watch for increase in urinary output which is common; if output does not increase, infusion should be decreased or discontinued
- Allergy: rash, urticaria, pruritus, wheezing, dyspnoea, bronchospasm, drug should be discontinued immediately
- Circulatory overload: increased pulse, respiration, dyspnoea, wheezing, chest tightness, chest pain
- Dehydration after infusion: decreased output, increased temperature, poor skin turgor, increased specific gravity, dry skin

dextromoramide

Palfium
Func. class.: Narcotic analgesic
Chem. class.: Pyrrolidine derivative
Legal class.: CD (Sch 2) POM

Action: Potent narcotic analgesic acting at CNS opiate receptors
Uses: Severe acute pain, short

duration of action makes it unsuitable for chronic pain control

Dosage and routes:
• By mouth, 5 mg increasing to 20 mg when required
• Subcutaneous/IM injection, 5 mg increasing to 15 mg when required
• Rectal suppositories, 10 mg, when required

Available forms include: Tablets, 5, 10 mg; injection 5, 10 mg/ml (as tartrate); suppositories, 10 mg (as tartrate)

Side effects/adverse reactions:
RESP: Respiratory depression, cough suppression
CNS: Drowsiness, alteration of pupillary responses, hallucinations, vertigo, mood changes
GI: Nausea, reduced motility, constipation
GU: Urinary retention
INTEG: Pain and tissue damage at injection site, sweating, rashes
SYST: Tolerance, dependence
CV: Hypotension, palpitation

Contraindications: Childbirth, respiratory depression, within 21 days of taking MAOIs, head injury, raised intracranial pressure

Precautions: History of drug abuse, dosage may need to be reduced for elderly or debilitated patients, hypothyroidism, pregnancy, lactation, hypotension, decreased respiratory reserve, asthma, renal impairment, liver damage

Pharmacokinetics: Onset of analgesia within 20−30 min, duration 2−3 hr

Interactions/incompatibilities:
• Risk of hypertensive crisis with: MAOIs or within 21 days of stopping them
• Increased effect of: hypnotics, other CNS depressants

Clinical assessment:
• Co-prescribe laxatives, antiemetic if needed

• Switch to longer acting agent if prolonged analgesia needed

Treatment of overdose: Gastric lavage if recently ingested; specific antagonist: naloxone; supportive treatment

NURSING CONSIDERATIONS

Assess:
• Baseline vital signs
• Pain levels
• Respirations, BP, pulse, pupils and conscious level 4 hrly

Administer:
• With an antiemetic if needed

Perform/provide:
• Proper storage and administration of drug according to CD regulations (abuse/misuse)
• Help with physiotherapy as required
• Fluids and fibre for constipation
• Safe environment: assist with mobilisation, cot sides
• Local treatment to site of injection

Evaluate:
• Side effects
• Response (short duration only, 2−3 hr)

Teach patient/family:
• Not to use machinery or mobilise without assistance
• To take no alcohol.
• Warn about dependence.
• May cause dizzy turns and sweating if ambulant. To rest supine after first few doses
• To store securely

---

dextrose (*D*-glucose)

Func. class.: Caloric
Chem. class.: Monosaccharide
Legal class.: POM (injection) GSL (powder)

Action: Essential component of carbohydrate metabolism
Uses: Increases intake of calories, maintains fluid balance in patients

unable to maintain adequate intake orally

Dosage and routes:
• *Adult and child:* By mouth, IV depends on individual requirements

Available forms include: Injection 5%, 10%, 20%, 25%, 50% IV; powder

Side effects/adverse reactions:
NB: Seen mainly in diabetic patients or with hypertonic (greater than 5%) solutions; 5% dextrose infusion/oral dextrose are without adverse effects

CNS: Confusion, loss of consciousness, dizziness

CV: Hypertension, congestive cardiac failure, pulmonary oedema

GU: Glycosuria, osmotic diuresis with hypertonic solutions

META: Hyperglycaemia, rebound hypoglycaemia, hyperosmolar syndrome, hyperosmolar hyperglycaemic nonketotic syndrome, electrolyte disturbances

INTEG: Chills, flushing, warm feeling, extravasation necrosis with hypertonic solutions

Contraindications: Hyperglycaemia. Hypertonic solutions: delirium tremens with dehydration, haemorrhage (cranial/spinal), anuria

Clinical assessment:
• Electrolytes (potassium, sodium, calcium, chloride, magnesium), blood glucose, ammonia, phosphate for acute therapy

NURSING CONSIDERATIONS

Assess:
• Respiratory function 4-hrly
• Temperature 4 hrly for increased fever, indicating infection; if infection suspected, infusion is discontinued, tubing, infusion bag/container cultured
• Urine glucose 6 hrly using Clinistix, Keto-Diastix, which are not affected by infusion substances
• Nutritional status: consult dietician

Administer:
• Solutions stronger than 5% by central venous line; use peripheral route for stronger solutions only under direction of clinician

Perform/provide:
• Care of central line using aseptic technique
• Infusion of these solutions should not be rapid or very prolonged

Evaluate:
• Injection site for extravasation: redness along vein, oedema at site, necrosis, pain, hard tender, area; site should be changed immediately
• Therapeutic response: increased weight

Teach patient/family:
• Reason for dextrose infusion

---

diamorphine hydrochloride

Func. class.: Narcotic analgesic
Chem. class.: Diacetyl derivative of morphine
Legal class.: CD (Sch 2) POM

Action: Potent narcotic analgesic acting at CNS opiate receptors. Inhibits ascending pain pathways in CNS, increases pain threshold, alters pain perception

Uses: Severe pain, particularly in terminal illness; acute pulmonary oedema; myocardial infarction

Dosage and routes:
Acute pain
• *Adult:* Subcutaneous/IM injection, 5 mg (maximum 10 mg for large patients) repeated 4 hrly if necessary; by slow IV injection quarter to half of corresponding IM dose

Chronic pain
• *Adult:* By mouth, subcutaneous, IM; 5–10 mg 4 hrly, may be in-

creased according to need; IM dose should be approximately half oral dose for treating same level of pain

Pulmonary oedema
• *Adult:* Slow IV injection (1 mg/min) 2.5−5 mg

Myocardial infarction:
• *Adult:* Slow IV injection (1 mg/min), 5 mg followed by 2.5−5 mg if necessary; reduce dose by half in elderly or frail patients

Available forms include: Tablets, 10 mg; injection, powder for reconstitution, 5, 10, 30, 100, 500 mg ampoules; extemporaneously prepared oral liquids

Side effects/adverse reactions:
RESP: Respiratory depression, cough suppression
EENT: Miosis
META: Hypothermia
CNS: Drowsiness, alteration of pupillary responses, hallucinations, vertigo, mood changes
GI: Nausea, reduced motility, constipation, vomiting, anorexia, cramps, dry mouth
GU: Urinary retention
INTEG: Pain and tissue at injection site, sweating, urticaria, pruritis, flushing
SYST: Tolerance, dependence
CV: Hypotension, palpitations, bradycardia

Contraindications: Respiratory depression, within 21 days of taking MAOIs, head injury, raised intracranial pressure, paralytic ileus, hypersensitivity

Precautions: History of drug abuse, pregnancy, childbirth, lactation, hypotension, hypothyroidism, decreased respiratory reserve, asthma, renal impairment, liver damage; dosage may need to be reduced for elderly or debilitated patients

Pharmacokinetics: Ultimately converted by hepatic metabolism to morphine, excreted in urine, duration of action about 4 hr

Interactions/incompatibilities:
• Risk of hypotensive crisis given within 21 days of: monoamine-oxidase inhibitors
• Potentiation of: Hypnotics, other CNS depressants, alcohol
• Absorption of mexiletine may be delayed by opiates and cisapride action antagonised

Clinical assessment:
• Must be given 4 hrly in chronic pain
• IV route no more than 1 mg/min
• Prescribe anti-emetic as required
• Prescribe prophylactic laxative

Treatment of overdose: Gastric lavage; specific antagonist: naloxone 0.4−2 mg IV at 2 to 3 min intervals up to 10 mg, supportive treatment

NURSING CONSIDERATIONS

Assess:
• Baseline pulse, respirations, BP
• Fluid balance
• When pain is beginning to return; determine dosage interval by patient response

Administer:
• Before pain becomes too severe
• With an anti-emetic if nausea and vomiting

Perform/provide:
• Safe environment: help with mobilisation
• Fluids and fibre (constipation)

Evaluate:
• Side effects
• Changes in BP and respiratory rate
• Need for additional analgesia, physical dependence
• Therapeutic response: decrease in pain

Teach patient/family:
• Effects of drug
• No alcohol
• May cause dizziness
• That dependency may result if dose taken is more than that required to relieve pain
• Withdrawal symptoms may

occur if high dosage reduced too quickly: nausea, vomiting, cramps, fever, faintness, anorexia
• Need for secure storage
• Not to mobilise without assistance

---

diazepam

Tensium, Rimapam, Atensine, Diazemuls, Stesolid, Valium
Func. class.: Anxiolytic, anticonvulsant, muscle relaxant
Chem. class.: Benzodiazepine
Legal class.: CD (Sch 4) POM (oral preparations only prescribable generically on NHS)

Action: Depresses subcortical levels of CNS, including limbic system, reticular formation
Uses: Anxiety, insomnia, acute alcohol withdrawal, adjunct in seizure disorders, induction and IV sedation, muscle spasm
Dosage and routes:
Anxiety/convulsive disorders
• *Adult:* By mouth 2−10 mg 3 times daily; 5−15 mg at night for insomnia associated with anxiety
• *Child:* By mouth 1−5 mg at bedtime for night terrors/somnambulism
Muscle spasms
• *Adult:* By mouth 2−15 mg daily in divided doses
Cerebral spasticity
• *Adult:* By mouth 2−60 mg daily in divided doses
• *Child:* By mouth 2−40 mg daily in divided doses
Tetanus
• *Adult/child:* IV (slow) 100−300 mcg/kg 1−4 hrly followed by IV infusion (or some dose via nasogastric tube) 3−10 mg/kg over 24 hr according to response
Status epilepticus
• *Adult:* IM, IV (slow) 10−20 mg, repeat after 0.5−1 hr if needed.

Then slow IV infusion to maximum 3 mg/kg in 24 hr. Rectally 10 mg, repeat after 5 min if needed
• *Child:* IM/IV (slow) 200−300 mcg/kg. Rectally, over 3 yr 10 mg, 1−3 yr 5 mg; repeat after 5 min if needed
• *Elderly:* Halve normal adult doses
Surgical sedation/premedication
• *Adult:* IV (slow) 100−200 mcg/kg; rectally 10 mg
• *Child:* IV (slow) as adult, rectally, over 3 yr 10 mg, 1−3 yr 5 mg
• *Elderly:* Halve normal adult doses
Available forms include: Tablets 2, 5, 10 mg; IM/IV injection 5 mg/ml; suppositories 10 mg; syrup 2 mg/5 ml; rectal tubes 5, 10 mg
Side effects/adverse reactions:
CNS: Dizziness, drowsiness, confusion, headache, anxiety, tremors, stimulation, fatigue, depression, insomnia, hallucinations, ataxia, dependence, amnesia, vertigo, changed libido
GI: Constipation, dry mouth, nausea, anorexia, diarrhoea
INTEG: Rash, dermatitis, itching, pain and thrombophlebitis after injection
CV: Orthostatic hypotension, hypotension
EENT: Blurred vision
RESP: Respiratory depression, apnoea
HAEM: Blood dyscrasias
Contraindications: Hypersensitivity to benzodiazepines, psychosis, acute pulmonary insufficiency, phobic or obsessional states, respiratory depression
Precautions: Elderly, debilitated, hepatic disease, renal disease, respiratory disease, muscle weakness, history of drug abuse, pregnancy, lactation
Pharmacokinetics:

By mouth: Onset 30 min, peak 1−2 hr

IM: Onset 15−30 min, absorption erratic

IV: Onset 1−5 min

Metabolised by liver, excreted by kidneys, breast milk, half-life 20−50 hr, active metabolite, half-life 30−200 hr

Interactions/incompatibilities:

• Increased effects of diazepam with: CNS depressants, alcohol, cimetidine, disulfiram

• Incompatible with all drugs in solution or syringe

Clinical assessment:

• Dependence potential, use for shortest possible period

Treatment of overdose: Gastric lavage, specific antidote: flumazenil, supportive care, vital signs

NURSING CONSIDERATIONS

Assess:

• Baseline vital signs

• BP, pulse, respiration if IV administration

Administer:

• IV slowly into large vein to decrease risk of extravasation

• Orally with food or milk for GI symptoms

• Crushed if patient is unable to swallow medication whole

• IM route, erratic absorption

• Rectally if unable to take oral medication

Perform/provide:

• Frequent sips of water for dry mouth

• Help with walking during beginning therapy, since drowsiness/dizziness occurs

• Safety measures, including cot sides

• Check to see oral medication has been swallowed

Evaluate:

• Therapeutic response: decreased anxiety, restlessness, insomnia, muscular spasm, spasticity

• Mental status: mood, sensorium, affect, sleeping pattern, drowsiness, dizziness

• Physical dependency, withdrawal symptoms: headache, nausea, vomiting, muscle pain, weakness after long-term use

• Suicidal tendencies in depressed patients

Teach patient/family:

• Not to be used for everyday stress or used longer than 4 months, unless directed by clinician

• Avoid non-prescribed preparations unless approved by clinician

• Avoid driving, activities that require alertness; drowsiness may occur

• Avoid alcohol ingestion or other psychotropic medications, unless prescribed by clinician

• Do not discontinue medication abruptly after long-term use

• Rise slowly or fainting may occur

• Drowsiness might worsen at beginning of treatment

• To seek psychiatric help if depressed

---

diazoxide

Eudemine

Func. class.: Antihypertensive

Chem. class.: Benzothiadiazine

Legal class.: POM

Action: Vasodilation of arteriolar smooth muscle by direct relaxation producing a reduction in blood pressure with concomitant increases in heart rate, cardiac output

Uses: Hypertensive crisis when urgent decrease of diastolic pressure required

Dosage and routes:

• *Adult:* IV bolus 150−300 mg repeated up to 4 times in 24 hr

• *Child:* IV bolus 5 mg/kg

Available forms include: Injection IV 300 mg/20 ml

Side effects/adverse reactions:

CV: Hypotension, T wave changes, angina pectoris, palpitations, supraventricular tachycardia, oedema, rebound hypertension, bradycardia

CNS: Extrapyramidal symptoms, cerebral infarction

GI: Nausea, vomiting, dry mouth

INTEG: Rash, burning at injection site

HAEM: Thrombocytopenia, leucopenia, haemolytic anaemia

ENDO: Hyperglycaemia, ketoacidotic coma

META: Sodium, water retention

Contraindications: Hypersensitivity to thiazides

Precautions: Pregnancy, labour, aortic coarctation or arteriovenous shunt, dissecting aortic aneurysm, lactation, impaired cerebral or cardiac circulation, children, impaired renal function, low plasma proteins

Pharmacokinetics:

IV: Onset 1–2 min, peak 5 min, duration 3–12 hr

Half-life 20–36 hr, metabolised in liver excreted slowly in urine, crosses blood-brain barrier, placenta

Interactions/incompatibilities:

• Do not mix with any drug in syringe or solution

• Increased effects of: warfarin, other coumarins, antihypertensives, diuretics

• Increased hyperglycaemia/hyperuricaemia when given with: thiazides, diuretics

• Decreased pharmacological effects of: hypoglycaemic agents

Clinical assessment:

• Electrolytes (potassium, sodium, chloride), glucose, carbon dioxide, full blood count

• Treat hypoglycaemia with tolbutamide, exceptionally insulin

• Control sodium, water retention with diuretic

Treatment of overdose: Supportive treatment including insulin for hypoglycaemia, IV fluids for hypotension

NURSING CONSIDERATIONS

Assess:

• Baseline BP and weight

Administer:

• IV injection must be administered rapidly and not exceed 30 seconds

• Patient in recumbent position, keep in that position for 1 hr after administration

Evaluate:

• Therapeutic response: decreased BP, primarily diastolic pressure

• BP every 5 min for 2 hr, then hrly for 2 hr, then 4 hrly

• Pulse, jugular venous distention 4 hrly

• Fluid balance

• Oedema in feet, legs daily

• Skin turgor, dryness of mucous membranes for hydration status

• Rales, dyspnoea, orthopnoea

• IV site for extravasation

• Signs of congestive cardiac failure, dyspnoea, oedema wet rales

• Postural hypotension, take BP sitting, standing 4 hrly

---

diclofenac sodium

Voltarol, Rhumalgan, Valenac, Volraman, Diclozip

Func. class.: Non-steroidal anti-inflammatory agent

Chem. class.: Phenylacetic acid derivative

Legal class.: POM

Action: Inhibits prostaglandin synthesis; possesses analgesic, anti-inflammatory, antipyretic properties

Uses: Acute, chronic rheumatoid arthritis, renal colic, osteoarthrosis, ankylosing spondylitis, gout, acute musculoskeletal disorders; post-operative pain, juvenile chronic arthritis

Dosage and routes:

• *Adult:* By mouth 25−50 mg 8−12 hrly; modified-release, 100 mg daily; rectal, 100 mg daily, usually at night; IM 75 mg once or twice a day for 2 days maximum. Total daily dose should not exceed 150 mg

• *Child over 1 yr:* 1−3 mg/kg daily in divided doses

Available forms include: Tablets enteric coated 25, 50 mg; modified-release, 100 mg; dispersible 50 mg (as base); suppositories 12.5, 100 mg; injection IM 75 mg/3 ml

Side effects/adverse reactions:

GI: Nausea, anorexia, vomiting, diarrhoea, jaundice, hepatitis, constipation, flatulence, cramps, dry mouth, peptic ulcer, GI bleeding, dyspepsia, colitis, pancreatitis, stomatitis

CNS: Dizziness, drowsiness, fatigue, tremors, confusion, insomnia, anxiety, depression, paraesthesia, muscle weakness, headache, psychosis

CV: Peripheral oedema, palpitations, hypertension, fluid retention, chest pain

INTEG: Purpura, rash, pruritus, sweating, erythema, petechiae, photosensitivity, alopecia; suppositories only: ano-rectal irritation. Pain at injection site

GU: Nephrotoxicity: haematuria, oliguria, azotaemia, nephrotic syndrome, papillary necrosis

HAEM: Blood dyscrasias, epistaxis, bruising

EENT: Tinnitus, hearing loss, blurred vision, taste disturbances

RESP: Dyspnoea, haemoptysis, pharyngitis, bronchospasm, laryngeal oedema, rhinitis

Contraindications: Hypersensitivity to aspirin or other NSAIDs, active or suspected peptic ulcer or gastrointestinal bleeding; asthma. Do not use suppositories in inflammatory conditions of anus, rectum, sigmoid colon. Porphyria

Precautions: Pregnancy, bleeding disorders, history of GI disorders, cardiac, hepatic or renal disorders, recovery from major surgery, elderly

Pharmacokinetics:

By mouth: Peak 1−4 hr, elimination half-life 1−2 hr, 90% bound to plasma proteins, metabolised in liver excreted in urine

Interactions/incompatibilities:

• Increased anticoagulant effect: oral anticoagulants (low risk)

• Increased toxicity of: cyclosporin

• Increased plasma levels of diclofenac: probenecid

• Increased plasma levels of: methotrexate, lithium, cardiac glycosides

• Reduced effects of: antihypertensives

• Altered requirements for: oral antidiabetics

Clinical assessment:

• Renal, hepatic function at intervals during long-term therapy

• Changes in clotting parameters if diclofenac started/stopped during treatment with oral anticoagulants

Treatment of overdose: Gastric lavage, activated charcoal, symptomatic and supportive treatment

NURSING CONSIDERATIONS

Administer

• With food and/or milk

Evaluate:

• Effectiveness of drug regarding movement of joints and stiffness

• Bruising, fatigue, bleeding and impaired healing, indigestion or black tarry stool (indicates possible blood dyscrasia)

Teach patient/family:

• To be effective drug must be taken until the course is complete

- To inform clinician/nurse of bleeding bruising, fatigue and malaise — blood dyscrasias could occur
- To avoid aspirin and alcohol
- To take with food, milk or antacids to avoid gastric irritation
- To be careful/avoid driving as drowsiness and dizziness may occur
- To report any unresolved indigestion
- How to administer suppositories

dienoestrol

Ortho Dienoestrol
Func. class.: Oestrogen
Chem. class.: Non-steroidal synthetic oestrogen
Legal class.: POM

Action: Applied topically, reverses post-menopausal and other atrophic changes to vagina and vulva

Uses: Atrophic vaginitis, kraurosis vulvae

Dosage and routes:
- *Adult:* Vaginal cream 0.01% 1–2 applicatorfuls daily for 1–2 weeks, then gradually reduce to half dose for 1–2 weeks then to 1 application 1–3 times weekly
Available forms include: Vaginal cream 0.01%

Side effects/adverse reactions:
CNS: Dizziness, headache, migraines, depression
CV: Hypertension, thrombophlebitis, oedema, thromboembolism, stroke, pulmonary embolism, myocardial infarction. Risks of CV effects small in post-menopausal women
GI: Nausea, vomiting, diarrhoea, pancreatitis, cramps, increased appetite, cholestatic jaundice
EENT: Contact lens intolerance, increased myopia, astigmatism
GU: Amenorrhoea, cervical erosion, breakthrough bleeding, dysmenorrhoea, vaginal candidiasis, endometrial hypertrophy/carcinoma, irritation at administration site, change in cervical secretions, increase in size of fibromyomata
INTEG: Rash, urticaria, acne, oily skin, seborrhoea, purpura, melasma
META: Folic acid deficiency, weight gain, hypercalcaemia, hyperglycaemia
ENDO: Breast tenderness, enlargement, secretion

Contraindications: Breast cancer, thromboembolic disorders, oestrogen-dependent cancer, genital bleeding (abnormal, undiagnosed), pregnancy, severe liver disease, porphyria, uterine fibromyomata

Precautions: Hypertension, asthma, gall-bladder disease, congestive cardiac failure, diabetes mellitus, bone disease predisposing to hypercalcaemia, depression, migraine headache, convulsive disorders, hepatic disease, family history of cancer of the breast or reproductive tract, contact lenses

Pharmacokinetics:
Topical: Significant absorption, degraded in liver, excreted in urine, excreted in breast milk

Interactions/incompatibilities:
- Decreased action of: oral anticoagulants, oral hypoglycaemics, antihypertensives
- Increased toxicity of: tricyclic antidepressants, cyclosporin, (raised blood levels)
- Increased action of: corticosteroids

Clinical assessment:
- Liver function studies
- Regular measurement of blood pressure

NURSING CONSIDERATIONS

Assess:
• Baseline weight and fluid balance
Administer:
• At bedtime for better absorption
• Titrated dose, use lowest effective dose, to prevent adverse reactions
• Dosage reduction should continue at 3–6 month intervals
Evaluate:
• Weight daily; notify clinician of weekly weight gain more than 2 kg
• BP 4 hrly
• Fluid balance, be alert for decreasing urinary output and increasing oedema
• Oedema, hypertension, cardiac symptoms, jaundice
• Mental status; affect, mood, behavioural changes, aggression
• Hypercalcaemia
Teach patient/family:
• How to fill applicator and insert cream
• Report breast lumps, vaginal bleeding, oedema, jaundice, dark urine, clay coloured stools, dyspnoea, headache, blurred vision, abdominal pain, numbness or stiffness in legs, chest pain

---

diflunisal

Dolobid
Func. class.: Non-steroid antiinflammatory drug
Chem. class.: Salicylate
Legal class.: POM

Action: Inhibits prostaglandin synthesis; possesses analgesic, antiinflammatory, antipyretic actions
Uses: Mild to moderate pain including osteoarthritis and rheumatoid arthritis
Dosage and routes:
Pain/fever
• *Adult:* By mouth 500–1500 mg daily in 2–3 divided doses

Available forms include: Tablets 250, 500 mg
Side effects/adverse reactions:
HAEM: Thrombocytopenia, granulocytosis, haemolytic anaemia, increased prothrombin time
GU: Renal impairment, dysuria
CNS: Stimulation, drowsiness, dizziness, confusion, convulsions, headache, flushing, hallucinations, coma, insomnia, anxiety, paraesthesia
GI: Nausea, vomiting, GI bleeding, diarrhoea, heartburn, anorexia, hepatitis, ulceration, liver damage, stomatitis
INTEG: Rash, urticaria, exfoliative dermatitis
EENT: Tinnitus, hearing loss, blurred vision
CV: Rapid pulse, oedema
RESP: Wheezing, bronchospasm
Contraindications: Hypersensitivity to salicylates or NSAIDs, GI bleeding, children, pregnancy, lactation, asthma, peptic ulcer
Precautions: Bleeding disorders, hepatic disease, renal disease, Hodgkin's disease, history of GI ulceration
Pharmacokinetics:
Period of onset: Onset 30–60 min, peak 2–3 hr, metabolised by liver, excreted by kidneys, 99% protein bound, excreted in breast milk, plasma half-life 7–11 hr (dose dependent)
Interactions/incompatibilities:
• Decreased effects of diflunisal: aluminium antacids
• Increased effects of: anticoagulants
• Decreased effects of: antihypertensives, diuretics
• Increased toxicity of: methotrexate, cyclosporin, lithium, indomethacin
Clinical assessment:
• Liver function studies if toxicity suspected
• Renal function studies: blood

urea creatinine if impairment suspected
• Changes in clotting parameters in patients already receiving oral anticoagulants, or if diflunisal withdrawn from such patients
Treatment of overdose: Gastric lavage, activated charcoal, monitor electrolytes, vital signs, supportive treatment

NURSING CONSIDERATIONS
Assess:
• Baseline fluid balance
• Prior drug history; there are many drug interactions
Administer:
• As whole tablets: not to be crushed or chewed
• With food or milk to decrease gastric symptoms
Perform/provide:
• Repositioning to decrease pain
• Cool cloth for fever
Evaluate:
• Fluid balance; decreasing output may indicate renal failure (long-term therapy)
• Hepatotoxicity: dark urine, clay-coloured stools, yellowing of skin, sclera, itching, abdominal pain, fever, diarrhoea if patient is on long-term therapy
• Allergic reactions: rash, urticaria; if these occur, drug may need to be discontinued
• Ototoxicity: tinnitus, ringing, roaring in ears; audiometric testing is needed before, after long-term therapy
• Visual changes: blurring, halos, corneal, retinal damage
• Oedema in feet, ankles, legs
Teach patient/family:
• To report any symptoms of hepatotoxicity, renal toxicity, visual changes ototoxicity, allergic reactions (long-term therapy)
• Not to exceed recommended dosage; acute poisoning may result
• To read label on other non-prescribed drugs; many contain aspirin
• That therapeutic response takes 2 weeks (arthritis)
• To avoid alcohol ingestion; GI bleeding may occur

digitoxin

Func. class.: Antidysrhythmic, cardiac glycoside
Chem. class.: Digitalis preparation
Legal class.: POM

Action: Acts by influx of calcium ions from extracellular to intracellular cytoplasm, increasing force of contraction and cardiac output
Uses: Congestive heart failure, atrial fibrillation, atrial flutter, atrial tachycardia
Dosage and routes:
• *Adult:* By mouth 50−200 mcg daily
• *Loading dose (if required):* By mouth 600 mcg, followed by 400 mcg after 4−6 hr, then 200 mcg every 6 hr up to a maximum of 1.6 mg, or 200 mcg twice daily for 4 days
• *Child:* Seek specialist advice
Available forms include: Tablets 100 mcg
Side effects/adverse reactions:
CNS: Headache, drowsiness, apathy, confusion, disorientation, fatigue, depression, hallucinations
CV: Dysrhythmias, bradycardia, atrioventricular block
GI: Nausea, vomiting, anorexia, abdominal pain, diarrhoea, intestinal ischaemia/necrosis
EENT: Blurred vision, yellow-green halos, photophobia, diplopia
MS: Muscular weakness
ENDO: Gynaecomastia
INTEG: Skin rashes
Contraindications: Hypersensi-

tivity to digitalis, supraventricular arrhythmias caused by Wolff-Parkinson-white syndrome

Precautions: Renal disease, hepatic disease, acute myocardial infarction, atrioventricular block, severe respiratory disease, hypothyroidism, elderly (reduce dose), electrolyte disturbances (especially hypokalaemia), cardioversion

Pharmacokinetics:

By mouth: Onset about 120 min, peak effect about 12 hr, duration variable, half-life 5−7 days, metabolised in liver, excreted in urine

Interactions/incompatibilities:

• Drugs increasing hypokalaemia and risk of digitoxin toxicity: diuretics, amphotericin B, corticosteroids, lithium, carbenoxolone

• Blood levels of digitoxin increased: spironolactone, verapamil, diltiazem, possibly other calcium antagonists

• Decreased blood levels of digitoxin: aminoglutethimide, barbiturates, anti-epileptics, rifampicin, cholestyramine, colestipol

• Increased risk of cardiac toxicity: β-blockers, suxamethonium, verapamil

• *Caution advised for those drugs interacting with digoxin*

Clinical assessment:

• Electrolytes (prior to treatment; if toxicity suspected; if patient at risk of renal/electrolyte abnormalities): potassium, sodium, chloride, calcium; renal function studies: urea, creatinine

• Monitor drug levels (therapeutic level 10−30 mcg/litre) once treatment stabilised; if toxicity suspected

Treatment of overdose: Gastric lavage if ingestion recent, activated charcoal, correct any hypokalaemia, treat arrhythmias with non-cardiac glycoside drugs, consider administration of specific antibody fragments, monitor ECG continuously

NURSING CONSIDERATIONS

Assess

• BP, respiration, pulse

• Pulse is taken prior to each dose of digitoxin. If radial or apex pulse is less than 60 withhold drug and retake pulse after 1 hr; if pulse less than 60 notify clinician

• Weigh before and regularly during treatment

• Fluid balance; check for oedema and retention

Administer:

• Orally using the lowest effective dose

• Potassium supplements if prescribed for potassium levels less than 3.0 mmol/litre

Evaluate:

• Cardiac status: apical pulse, character, rate, rhythm

• Therapeutic response: decreased weight, oedema, pulse, respiration and increased urine output

Teach patient/family:

• Visual changes, headache

• To report symptoms of toxicity, oedema

• To only take other medication on clinicians advice

• To take own pulse and contact clinician if it falls below 60

• Not to take antacid at the same time

• Not to stop drug abruptly; teach all aspects of drug

---

digoxin

Lanoxin, Lanoxin-PG

Func. class.: Antidysrhythmic, cardiac glycoside

Chem. class.: Digitalis preparation

Legal class.: POM

Action: Acts by influx of calcium ions from extracellular to intracellular cytoplasm; increases cardiac contractility and cardiac output

Uses: Congestive heart failure, atrial fibrillation, atrial flutter, atrial tachycardia

Dosage and routes:
• *Adult:* By mouth 62.5−500 mcg daily (higher dose divided)
• *Loading dose (if required):* By mouth 1−1.5 mg in divided doses over 24 hr, or 250−500 mcg (higher dose divided) for 1 week; IV infusion, 0.5−1.0 mg infused over at least 2 hr
• *Child:* Seek specialist advice
• Avoid IM route; causes painful local reactions

Available forms include: Elixir 50 mcg/ml; tablets 62.5, 125, 250 mcg; injection 100, 250 mcg/ml

Side effects/adverse reactions:
CNS: Headache, drowsiness, apathy, confusion, disorientation, fatigue, depression, hallucinations
CV: Dysrhythmias, bradycardia, atrioventricular block
GI: Nausea, vomiting, anorexia, abdominal pain, diarrhoea, intestinal ischaemia/necrosis
EENT: Blurred vision, yellow-green halos, photophobia, diplopia
MS: Muscular weakness
ENDO: Gynaecomastia
INTEG: Skin rashes

Contraindications: Hypersensitivity to digitalis, supraventricular arrhythmias caused by Wolff-Parkinson-white syndrome

Precautions: Renal disease, acute myocardial infarction, atrioventricular block, hypothyroidism, elderly (reduce dose), electrolyte disturbances (especially hypokalaemia), cardioversion

Pharmacokinetics:
IV: Onset 5−30 min, peak 1−5 hr, duration variable, half-life 1.5 days excreted in urine, therapeutic range in plasma 1.5−3 mcg/litre

Interactions/incompatibilities:
• Drugs increasing risk of hypokalaemia and digoxin toxicity: diuretics, amphotericin B, corticosteroids, lithium, carbenoxolone
• Increased blood levels of digoxin: spironolactone, quinidine, verapamil, nifedipine, diltiazem, amiodarone, quinine, prazosin, erythromycin, tetracyclines, quinine, nicardipine
• Decreased blood levels of digoxin: anticholinergics, neomycin, sulphasalazine, certain cytotoxics, cholestyramine, colestipol
• Increased risk of cardiotoxicity: β-blockers, verapamil, suxamethonium, IV calcium

Clinical assessment:
• Electrolytes (prior to treatment; if toxicity suspected; if patient at risk of renal/electrolyte abnormality): potassium, sodium, chloride, calcium; renal function studies, urea, creatinine
• Drug levels (therapeutic levels 1.5−3.0 mcg/litre) once therapy stabilised; if toxicity suspected

Treatment of overdose: Gastric lavage if ingestion recent, correct any hypokalaemia, treat arrhythmias with non-cardiac glycoside drugs, consider administration of digoxin-specific antibody fragments, monitor ECG continuously

NURSING CONSIDERATIONS

Assess:
• BP, respiration, pulse
• Apex and radical pulse for 1 min before each dose: if below 60, take again in 1 hr; if greater than 60, call clinician and withhold drug
• Fluid balance, weight; check for oedema and retention

Administer:
• Orally using the lowest effective dose
• Potassium supplements if prescribed for potassium levels less

than 3.0 mmol/litre
Evaluate:
• Cardiac status: pulse, character, rate, rhythm at least once a day
• Therapeutic response: decreased weight, oedema, pulse, respiration and increased urine output
• For weight gain
• Apex beat and pulse: inform clinician of discrepancy
Teach patient/family:
• Not to stop drug abruptly; teach all aspects of drug
• Visual changes, headache
• To report symptoms of toxicity, oedema
• To only take other medication on clinician's advice
• To take own pulse and contact clinician if it falls below 60
• Not to take antacid at the same time

---

digoxin-specific antibody fragments (Fab)

Digibind
Func. class.: Antidote to digoxin toxicity
Chem. class.: Fragments of sheep antibody to digoxin
Legal class.: POM

Action: Fragments bind to free digoxin; reverses digoxin toxicity by enhancing excretion and removal from site of action
Uses: Life-threatening digoxin or digitoxin toxicity, overdose with other digitalis derivatives
Dosage and routes:
• *Adult:* IV dosage used to counteract digoxin or digitoxin overdose is calculated in 2 ways depending on the time lapsed following ingestion
1. *An acutely ingested dose*
dose of digoxin or digitoxin (mg)

$\times$ 0.8 $\times$ 60 = dose of Fab required (mg)
2. *A dose ingested longer than 6 hr ago*
Digoxin
plasma (serum) concentration (ng/ml) $\times$ 0.0056 $\times$ body weight (kg) $\times$ 60 = dose of Fab required (mg)
Digitoxin
plasma (serum) concentration (ng/ml) $\times$ 0.00056 $\times$ bodyweight (kg) $\times$ 60 = dose of Fab required (mg)
Available forms include: Injection 40 mg/vial
Side effects/adverse reactions:
CV: Return of symptoms controlled by cardiac glycoside
INTEG: Hypersensitivity, allergic reactions
SYST: Anaphylactic or other allergic reactions possible
Contraindications: None known
Precautions: Renal disease, pregnancy, allergy to sheep products; concurrent digoxin or digitoxin therapy
Pharmacokinetics:
IV: Peaks after completion of infusion, onset 30 min (variable); half-life biphasic 14−20 hr; prolonged in renal disease; excreted by kidneys
Lab. test interferences:
Interfere: Digoxin immunoassay
NURSING CONSIDERATIONS
Administer:
• By a bolus injection if cardiac arrest is imminent, otherwise by slow intravenous injection over 20 min using a 0.22 micron millipore filter
• Storage of the injection at 2−8°C
• Reconstituted solution should not be stored for more than 24 hr, even in refrigerator
Perform/provide:
• Nursing in ICU preferable
• Continuous monitoring of cardiac status

Evaluate:
• Response to treatment: correction of digoxin toxicity. Digoxin levels must be checked
• Watch for unmasking of symptoms controlled by cardiac glycosides

---

dihydrocodeine tartrate

DHC Continus, combination products, ~~NHS~~ DF 118
Func. class.: Narcotic analgesic
Chem. class.: Opioid related to codeine
Legal class.: POM, CD (oral formulation Sch 5; Injection Sch 2.)

Action: Narcotic analgesic acting at opiate receptors in the CNS. Inhibits ascending pain pathways in CNS, increases pain threshold, alters pain perception
Uses: Moderate to severe pain
Dosage and routes:
• *Modified-release:* 120−240 mg daily in 2 divided doses
• *Deep subcutaneous/IM injection*: up to 50 mg every 4−6 hr
• *Adult:* By mouth, 30 mg every 4−6 hr, after food, when required
• *Child over 4 yr:* By mouth 0.5−1 mg/kg every 4−6 hr
Available forms include: Tablets, 30 mg; modified-release tablets, 60, 90, 120 mg; elixir, 10 mg/5 ml; injection 50 mg/ml
Side effects/adverse reactions:
RESP: Respiratory depression, cough suppression, exacerbation/precipitation of asthma
CNS: Drowsiness, alteration of pupillary responses, hallucinations, mood changes
GI: Nausea, reduced motility, constipation, gastric irritation, vomiting, anorexia, cramps, dry mouth
EENT: Miosis

CV: Hypotension, palpatations, bradycardia
META: Hypothermia
GU: Urinary retention
INTEG: Pain at injection site, rashes
SYST: Tolerance, dependence
Contraindications: Respiratory depression, head injury, raised intracranial pressure
Precautions: History of drug abuse, asthma, pregnancy, childbirth, lactation, hypotension, hypothyroidism, renal impairment, liver damage; dosage may need to be reduced for elderly or debilitated patients
Pharmacokinetics: Well absorbed orally, metabolised in liver, excreted in urine. Elimination half-life 3.4−5.5 hr. Excreted in breast milk
Interactions/incompatibilities:
• Risk of hypertensive crisis with: MAOIs or within 21 days of stopping them
• Increased effects of: hypnotics, other CNS depressants, alcohol
Clinical assessment:
• Co-prescribe laxatives, anti-emetic if needed
• Evaluate degree of pain control
Treatment of overdose: Gastric lavage; specific antagonist: naloxone 0.4−2 mg IV at 2 to 3 min intervals up to 10 mg; supportive treatment
NURSING CONSIDERATIONS
Assess:
• Pain; to determine dosage interval appropriate for patient
• BP, pulse, respirations, pupils and conscious level
• Fluid balance
Administer:
• With an anti-emetic if nausea, vomiting
• With or after food (oral)
Perform/provide:
• Storage and administration, according to CD regulations;

diluted elixir should be protected from light; has a 14 day "life"
• Fibre/fluids (constipation)
• Safe environment: cot sides, help with mobilisation
• Local treatment for injection site
• Assistance with ambulation
Evaluate:
• Need for additional analgesia, physical dependence
• Side effects
• Therapeutic response: decrease in pain
Teach patient/family:
• That dizziness/drowsiness may occur, if affected don't drive or operate machinery
• To take with food and not to have alcohol.
• About side effects, tolerance and dependence

---

diltiazem HCl

Tildiem, Britiazem, Adizem, Tildiem Retard, Adizen-SR, Angiozem
Func. class.: Calcium channel blocker
Chem. class.: Benzothiazepine
Legal class.: POM

Action: Inhibits calcium ion influx across cell membrane during cardiac depolarisation; produces relaxation of coronary vascular smooth muscle, dilates coronary arteries
Uses: Prophylaxis and treatment of angina, hypotension
Dosage and routes:
Angina
• *Adult:* By mouth, 60 mg 3 times daily or modified-release 120 mg twice daily, increasing dose gradually to maximum 480 mg daily in divided doses
Hypertension
• *Adult:* By mouth modified-release 120 mg twice daily, increasing gradually if required to 360 mg daily
Available forms include: Tablets 60 mg; modified-release, 90, 120 mg
Side effects/adverse reactions:
CV: Bradycardia, hypotension, heart block
GI: Nausea, vomiting, gastric upset, deranged liver function studies
INTEG: Rash, pruritus, flushing, photosensitivity
CNS: Headache, fatigue, drowsiness, dizziness, anxiety, depression
Contraindications: Sick sinus syndrome, 2nd or 3rd degree heart block, hypotension, severe bradycardia, pregnancy, left ventricular failure, porphyria
Precautions: Congestive cardiac failure, mild hypotension, hepatic impairment, lactation, renal disease, mild bradycardia
Pharmacokinetics:
By mouth: Rapidly and completely absorbed, approximately 50% first-pass metabolism, half-life 3½−9 hr; metabolised by liver, excreted in urine (96% as metabolites)
Interactions/incompatibilities:
• Increased blood levels of: β-blockers, digitalis glycosides, cyclosporin, carbamazepine
• Increased cardiac toxicity given with: amiodarone, β-blockers
• Increased effects of: theophylline, antihypertensives
Treatment of overdose: Gastric lavage, observation in coronary care unit, supportive treatment
NURSING CONSIDERATIONS
Assess:
• Baseline vital signs, ECG
Administer:
• Before meals, bed time
Evaluate:
• Therapeutic response: decreased

anginal pain, reduction in BP to required level
• Cardiac status: BP, pulse, respiration, ECG
Teach patient/family:
• How to take pulse before taking drug; record or graph should be kept
• To avoid hazardous activities until stabilised on drug and dizziness is no longer a problem
• To limit caffeine consumption
• To avoid non-prescribed drugs unless directed by a clinician
• Importance of compliance to all areas of medical regimen: diet, exercise, stress reduction, drug therapy

---

dimercaprol (BAL)

Func. class.: Chelating agent
Chem. class.: Dithiol compound
Legal class.: POM

Action: Binds ions from arsenic, gold, mercury, lead, copper to form water-soluble complex removed by kidneys
Uses: Heavy metal poisoning
Dosage and routes:
• *Adult:* IM 2.5–3 mg/kg 4-hrly, for 2 days, 2–4 times on the 3rd day then once or twice a day
Available forms include: Injection IM 50 mg/ml
Side effects/adverse reactions:
CNS: Headache, paraesthesia, convulsions, coma
INTEG: Urticaria, erythema, pruritus, pain at injection site, sweating, fever (especially in children), burning sensation of lips, mouth, throat, eyes
EENT: Lacrimation, conjunctivitis, rhinorrhoea
MS: Myalgia, muscle spasm

CV: Hypertension, tachycardia
GI: Nausea, vomiting, salivation, abdominal pain
Contraindications: Hypersensitivity, hepatic insufficiency, poisoning by iron or cadmium, severe renal disease, hepatic impairment due to arsenic
Precautions: Hypertension, pregnancy, lactation
Pharmacokinetics: Metabolised by plasma enzymes, excreted by kidneys and bile as complex of heavy metal and unchanged drug. Peak plasma levels 1 hr after IM injection
Interactions/incompatibilities:
• Increased toxicity: iron, selenium, uranium, cadmium
• Urinary alkalinisers may reduce nephrotoxicity by stabilising dimercaprol-metal complexes
Clinical assessment:
• Kidney function studies: blood urea nitrogen, creatinine, creatinine clearance
• Urine: pH albumin, casts and blood
• Metal levels daily
NURSING CONSIDERATIONS
Assess:
• Baseline BP, fluid balance
Administer:
• IM in deep muscle mass; rotate injection sites
• Only when adrenaline 1:1000 is on unit for anaphylaxis
• In conjunction with the general treatment for each particular metal poison
Perform/Provide:
• If ampoule appears cloudy in cold weather, warm slightly before use
• Drugs and equipment for resuscitation
• Acetazolamide or sodium citrate to decrease pH of urine, which decreases renal damage
Evaluate:

• BP, increasing BP or tachycardia
• Monitor fluid balance, report decreases in output, weight changes
• Urine: pH, albumin, blood
• Therapeutic effect: decreased levels of metal in blood
• Increased renal impairment; renal failure will reduce effectiveness of drug
• Side effects; usually reversible, rarely necessary to stop treatment
• Severity of poisoning; determines duration of therapy
Teach patient/family:
• That breath may smell

---

dimethicone

Infacol, Windcheaters, many combination products
Func. class.: Antiflatulent
Legal class.: GSL/P (depending on product)

Action: Disperses, prevents gas pockets in GI system
Uses: Flatulence, gripes, colic or wind pains
Dosage and routes:
• *Adult and child over 12 yr:* Up to 2 g daily in divided doses after meals and at bedtime
• *Infants:* 20−40 mg before feeds
Available forms include: Capsules 100 mg; liquid 40 mg/ml
Side effects/adverse reactions:
GI: Belching, rectal flatus
Contraindications: Hypersensitivity
Pharmacokinetics: By mouth, not absorbed

NURSING CONSIDERATIONS:
Administer:
• Before each feed for infants
Evaluate:
• Therapeutic response: absence of flatulence, colic

dinoprost trometamol

Prostin F$_2$ alpha
Func. class.: Oxytocic
Chem. class.: Prostaglandin F$_2$ alpha
Legal class.: POM

Action: Stimulates uterine contractions causing abortion
Uses: Abortion during 2nd trimester
Dosage and routes:
Therapeutic abortion
• Intra-amniotic injection 40 mg, slowly
Available forms include: Intra-amniotic injection 5 mg/ml
Side effects/adverse reactions:
CNS: Headache, dizziness, fainting, convulsions, EEG changes
CV: Hypotension, cardiovascular collapse
GI: Nausea, vomiting, diarrhoea, cramps, epigastric pain
INTEG: Flushing, hot flushes, shivering, irritation at injection site
GU: Uterine rupture
RESP: Wheezing, bronchospasm
Contraindications: Hypersensitivity, uterine fibrosis, cervical stenosis, pelvic surgery, pelvic inflammatory disease (PID), hypotonic arterie inertia, placenta praevia, severe toxaemia, history of Caesarean section, fetal malpresentation, history of difficult delivery, major cephalopelvic mismatch
Precautions: Hepatic disease, renal disease, cardiac disease, asthma, anaemia, convulsive disorders, hypotension, glaucoma, multiple pregnancy, multiparity
Treatment of overdose: Symptomatic, supportive
NURSING CONSIDERATIONS
Assess:
• Baseline vital signs

Administer:
• With emergency resuscitation equipment available on unit
Evaluate:
• BP, pulse; watch for change that may indicate haemorrhage
• For length, duration of contraction; notify clinician of contractions lasting over 1 min or absence of contractions, blood loss and products passed per vaginum
Teach patient/family:
• To report increased blood loss, abdominal cramps, increased temperature, foul-smelling lochia or any side effects

---

dinoprostone

Prepidil, Prostin E_2
Func. class.: Oxytocic
Chem. class.: Prostaglandin E_2
Legal class.: POM

Action: Stimulates uterine contractions and causes vasodilation
Uses: Induction of labour, fetal death *in utero*, termination of pregnancy, missed abortion and hydatidiform mole
Dosage and routes:
Cervical softening and dilation
• Cervical gel — 500 mcg as a single dose
Induction of labour
• *Tablets* — by mouth 500 mcg followed by 0.5−1 mg (maximum 1.5 mg) at hrly intervals
• *By IV infusion* 1 mg/1 ml, dilute and infuse at 0.25 mcg/minute for 30 min and then maintain or increase
• *Vaginal gel* — 1 or 2 mg followed after 6 hr by 1−2 mg if required. Maximum 3 or 4 mg depending on induction features
• *Vaginal tablets* — posterior fornix 3 mg followed after 6−8 hr by 3 mg if labour not established, maximum 6 mg

Termination of pregnancy, missed abortion, hydatidiform mole
• By IV infusion 10 mg/1 ml — dilute and infuse at 2.5 mcg/min for 30 min and then maintain or increase to 5 mcg/min. Maintain rate for at least 4 hr before increasing further
Termination of pregnancy —
• *Extra-amniotic:* 10 mg/1 ml. Dilute to produce 100 mcg/ml and instil 1 ml then depending on response instil 1 or 2 ml at 2-hrly intervals
Note: Vaginal tablets and gel are not bioequivalent
Available forms include: Cervical gel 200 mcg/1 ml; tablets 500 mcg; intravenous solution 1 mg/ml, 10 mg/ml; extra-amniotic solution 10 mg/ml; vaginal gel 400 mcg/1 ml; vaginal tablets 3 mg
Side effects/adverse reactions:
CNS: Headache, dizziness, flushing
GI: Nausea, vomiting, diarrhoea
GU: Vaginitis, vaginal pain, vulvitis, vaginismus, shivering, uterine hypertonus
MS: Leg cramps, joint swelling, weakness, severe uterus contractions
HAEM: Raised blood cell
All dose related and more common after intravenous therapy; local tissue reaction and erythema after intravenous administration
Contraindications: No absolute contraindications, but not recommended where oxytoxic drugs generally contraindication, ruptured membranes, hypersensitivity to prostaglandins, unexplained vaginal bleeding, non-vertex presentations, pelvic infection/vaginal infections/PID
Precautions: Glaucoma, asthma, hypotonus, fetal distress
Pharmacokinetics:
Metabolised in spleen, kidney, lungs, excreted in urine

Treatment of overdose:
Supportive measures, appropriate obstetric measures as indicated

NURSING CONSIDERATIONS

Assess:
• Cervical ripening (i.e. Bishop's score)
• Fetal well-being (CTG tracing)
• Presentation
• Gestation

Administer:
• With bladder empty
• Do not give if BP high (risk of cord prolapse)
• Inserted into posterior fornix of vagina
• Useful to dip pessary in water before inserting (starts dissolving process)
• Do not use hibitane cream

Perform/provide:
• Call bell (patient to remain supine for 30 min)
• CTG tracing 20 min after insertion
• Refrigerated storage for gel

Evaluate:
• Cervical assessment according to treatment regimen as necessary (e.g. 4–8 hr)
• CTG (fetal well-being)

Teach patient/family:
• Stay supine for ½ hr
• Report spontaneous rupture of membranes or rapid fetal movements
• Painful contractions, backache may ensue

---

dipipanone hydrochloride BP

Diconal
Func. class.: Narcotic analgesic (with anti-emetic)
Chem. class.: Opioid related to methadone
Legal class.: CD (Sch 2) POM

Action: Narcotic analgesic acting at opiate receptors in CNS. Inhibits ascending pain pathways in CNS, increases pain threshold, alters pain perception

Uses: Moderate to severe pain in patients not responding to pethidine or morphine

Dosage and routes:
• *Adults:* By mouth 1 tablet 6-hrly, gradually increased to 3 tablets 6-hrly if required
Caution in elderly due to increased confusion
Available forms include: Tablets, dipipanone hydrochloride 10 mg, cyclizine hydrochloride 30 mg

Side effects/adverse reactions:
RESP: Respiratory depression, cough suppression
CV: Hypotension, bradycardia, palpatations
CNS: Drowsiness, alteration of pupillary responses, blurred vision, hallucinations, vertigo
GI: Nausea, reduced motility, constipation, dry mouth, vomiting, cramps, dry mouth
GU: Difficulty in micturition
SYST: Tolerance, dependence

Contraindications: Respiratory depression, obstructive airways disease, concurrent use of MAOIs, head injury, raised intracranial pressure

Precautions: Severe liver or kidney disease. Possibility of addiction, impaired respiration. Use of other CNS depressants, pregnancy, lactation

Pharmacokinetics: Onset of effect within 1 hr, duration 6 hr

Interactions/incompatibilities:
• Risk of hypotensive crisis given within 21 days of: Monoamine-oxidase inhibitors

Clinical assessment
• Prescribe anti-emetic as required (preparation contains cyclizine)
• Prescribe prophylactic laxative if constipated

Treatment of overdose: Respiratory depression—use naloxone 0.4−2 mg IV at 2 to 3 min intervals up to 10 mg, gastric lavage, oxygen and respiratory support if necessary

NURSING CONSIDERATIONS
Assess:
• Base line vital signs: blood pressure, pulse, respiration, pupils, consciousness level
• Fluid balance
• When pain is beginning to return; determine dosage interval by patient response
Perform/provide:
• Fluids/fibre (constipation)
• Assistance with ambulation
Evaluate:
• For changes in vital signs
• Pain, side effects (blurred vision, drowsiness)
• Therapeutic response: decrease in pain
Teach patient/family:
• That it may cause drowsiness, if affected not to drive/operate machinery. Take no alcohol
• About side effects, tolerance and dependence
• To report side effects
• Withdrawal symptoms may occur if high, long term dosage reduced too quickly: nausea, vomiting, cramps, fever, faintness, anorexia

---

dipivefrin HCl (ophthalmic)

Propine
Func. class.: Anti-hypertensive, ocular
Chem. class.: Diesterified adrenaline
Legal class.: POM

Action: Converted to adrenaline which decreases aqueous humour production and increases outflow
Uses: Chronic open angle glaucoma or occular hypertensive patient with anterior chamber open angle
Dosage and routes:
• *Adult:* Instil 1 drop 12 hrly
Available forms include: Eye drops 0.1%
Side effects/adverse reactions:
CV: Hypertension, tachycardia, arrhythmias
EENT: Burning, stinging, mydriasis, photophobia, corneal deposits, conjunctivitis
Contraindications: Closed angle glaucoma, soft contact lenses (contains benzalkonium chloride)
Precautions: Aphakia, narrow angles
Pharmacokinetics:
Instil: Onset 30 min, duration 1 hr

NURSING CONSIDERATIONS
Perform/provide:
• Storage of drug at room temperature
Teach patient/family:
• To report stinging, burning, itching, lacrimation, puffiness
• Method of instillation, including pressure on lacrimal sac for 1 min and not to touch dropper to eye
• To discard 28 days after opening
• Not to wear soft (hydrophilic) contact lenses

---

dipyridamole

Persantin
Func. class.: Coronary vasodilator, antiplatelet
Chem. class.: Pyrimidine derivative
Legal class.: POM

Action: Decreases platelet aggregation, adhesion and survival when given orally. Intravenous use causes coronary vasodilatation
Uses: Prophylaxis of thromboembolism associated with prosthetic heart valves (tablets)

Injection—myocardial imaging
Dosage and routes:
• *Tablets* 300−600 mg daily in 3 or 4 divided doses
• *Injection* 0.56 mg/kg over 4 min
Available forms include:
Tablets 25, 100 mg; injection 10 mg/2 ml
Side effects/adverse reactions:
CV: Postural hypotension, increased anginal attacks, myocardial ischaemia
CNS: Headache, dizziness, weakness, fainting, syncope
GI: Nausea, vomiting, anorexia, diarrhoea, dyspepsia
INTEG: Rash, flushing
Contraindications: Hypersensitivity, rapidly worsening angina, aortic stenosis, recent myocardial infarction. For injection only
Precautions: Pregnancy, unstable angina, aortic coagulation disorders, stenosis
Pharmacokinetics:
Period of onset: Onset 30 sec, peak 2−2½ min. Therapeutic response may take several months, metabolised in liver, excreted in bile, undergoes enterohepatic recirculation
Interactions/incompatibilities:
• Enhance effects of: anticoagulants
• Decreased effects: antacids
Treatment of overdose: Administer aminophylline for coronary vasolidatation
NURSING CONSIDERATIONS
Assess:
• Baseline vital signs, ECG
Administer:
• On an empty stomach: 1 hr before meals or 2 hr after
Evaluate:
• BP, pulse during treatment until stable; take BP lying, standing; ECG monitor may be necessary; orthostatic hypotension is common
• Therapeutic response: decreased chest pain (angina)
• Cardiac status: chest pain, what aggravates or ameliorates condition
Teach patient/family:
• That medication is not cure, may need to be taken continuously; therapeutic response may not be evident for 2−3 months
• That it is necessary to stop smoking to prevent excessive vasoconstriction
• To avoid hazardous activities until stabilised on medication; dizziness may occur

---

disopyramide

Dirythmin SA, Rythmodan, Rythmodan Retard
Func. class.: Anti-arrhythmic (Class I)
Chem. class.: Synthetic butyramide
Legal class.: POM

Action: Decreases myocardial contractility. Shortens sinus node recovery time, increases atrial/ventricular refractory time, suppresses ectopic focal activity, reduces duration of action potential between normal, infracted myocardium
Uses: Atrial or ventricular ectopic beats. Paroxysmal atrial or ventricular tachycardia. Arrhythmias post—myocardial infarction. Wolff-Parkinson-White syndrome. Maintains sinus rhythm after electro-cardioversion. Control of glycoside induced arrhythmias
Dosage and routes:
• *Adult:* By mouth 300−800 mg daily in divided doses; modified-release 250−375 mg daily maximum 900 mg daily
• By IV injection: 2 mg/kg, maximum 150 mg over not less than 5 min. Patients should respond within 10−15 min. Transfer to oral

200 mg every 8 hr for 24 hr—then 500—750 mg daily. Maintenance IV dose 0.4 mg/kg/hr up to a maximum of 800 mg. Dose adjustments needed in heart failure and impaired renal function

Available forms include: Capsules 100, 150 mg; modified-release 150, 250 mg (as phosphate); injection 50 mg/ml (as phosphate)

Side effects/adverse reactions:

GU: Retention, hesitancy

CNS: Headache, dizziness, psychosis

GI: Dry mouth, constipation, nausea, flatulence, cholestatic jaundice

CV: Hypotension, bradycardia, angina, premature ventricular contraction, tachycardia, increases QRS, QT segments, cardiac arrest, oedema, weight gain, atrioventricular block

META: Hypoglycaemia

MS: Weakness, pain in extremities

EENT: Blurred vision, dry nose, throat, eyes, narrow-angle glaucoma

HAEM: Thrombocytopenia, agranulocytosis, anaemia (rare)

Contraindications: Hypersensitivity, 2nd/3rd degree block, cardiogenic shock, congestive cardiac failure (uncompensated), series node disease without pacemaker

Precautions: Widening of QRS or prolonging of QT internal. Atrial flutter/tachycardia with block, significant heart failure, hypocalcaemia will reduce patient response. Digitalis intoxication, bundle branch block. Hypoglycaemia

Pharmacokinetics:

IV: Onset 30 min-3½ hr, peak 1—2 hr, duration 1½—8½ hr

IM: Onset 30 min, peak 60—90 min, duration 6—8 hr

Half-life 4—10 hr, metabolised in liver, excreted in faeces, urine, breast milk

Interactions/incompatibilities:

• Amiodarone—increased risk of ventricular arrhythmias

• Anti-arrhythmics—myocardial depression

• Disopyramide—plasma level increased by erythromycin, plasma level decreased by rifampicin, phenobarbitone, phenytoin

• Antimuscarinics—increased antimuscarinics side effects

• Diuretics—hypokalaemia will increase disopyramide toxicity

Clinical assessment:

• Blood levels during treatment

• Electrolytes (sodium, chloride potassium)

• Liver, kidney function studies: aspartate amino transferase alonine aminotransferase bilirubin, urea, creatinine during treatment

• ECG, check for increased QT, widening QRS; drug should be discontinued

Treatment of overdose: O_2, artificial ventilation, ECG, administer dopamine or isoprenaline for circulatory depression; administer diazepam or thiopentone for convulsions. Possibility of haemodialysis or haemoperfusion in poor renal function

NURSING CONSIDERATIONS

Assess:

• Baseline weight, pulse rate

• Consider fluid balance in heart failure

• Diabetics for signs of hypoglycaemia—regular BM stix

Administer:

• Frequent sips of water for dry mouth

• Reduced dosage slowly with ECG monitoring

Evaluate:

• BP regularly for hypotension, hypertension

• Increase in QRS, QT; report to

clinician
• For rebound hypertension after 1−2 hr
• For constipation; consider increasing fibre content of diet; possible need of laxatives
• Heart rate; respiration; rate, rhythm, character
• Assess for urinary hesitancy, frequency or retension daily
• Check for oedema daily; daily weight

Teach patient/family:
• Take drug exactly as prescribed
• Avoid alcohol or severe hypotension may occur; to avoid non-prescribed drugs or serious drug interactions may occur
• Change position slowly during early therapy to prevent fainting
• Avoid hazardous activities if dizziness or blurred vision occurs
• Stress patient compliance with drug regimen; explain to patient that this drug does not cure condition

---

distigmine bromide

Ubretid
Func. class.: Anticholinesterase
Chem. class.: Quaternary ammonium compound
Legal class.: POM

Action: Long acting inhibition of the enzymic degradation of the neurotransmitter acetylcholine and enhances neuromuscular transmission in voluntary and involuntary transmission

Uses: Post operative urinary retention. Post operative ileus and intestinal atony. Emptying of neurogenic bladder. Myasthenia gravis

Dosage and routes:
Myasthenia gravis
• *Adult:* By mouth initially 5 mg daily 30 min before breakfast, increase at intervals of 3−4 days as necessary to maximum 20 mg daily
• *Child:* Maximum 10 mg by mouth daily, according to age
Urinary retention, ileus or intestinal atony post surgery, neurogenic bladder
• 5 mg by mouth 30 min before breakfast, daily or on alternate days; IM injection, 500 mcg 12 hr after surgery, repeat every 24 hr if necessary

Available forms include: Tablets 5 mg; injection 500 mcg/ml

Side effects/adverse reactions:
GI: Nausea, increased salivation, vomiting, diarrhoea, abdominal cramps, intestinal colic
CNS: Blurred vision
INTEG: Sweating
CV: Bradycardia
SYST: Cholinergic crisis caused by accumulation of acetylcholine

Contraindications: Intestinal or urinary obstruction, recent anastomosis, severe post-operative shock, spastic or mechanical ileus, severe circulatory insufficiency, pregnancy

Precautions: Elderly patients, epilepsy, parkinsonism, asthma, cardiovascular disease, peptic ulcer, vagotonia, lactation

Pharmacokinetics: Cholinesterase maximally inhibited 9 hr after single IM dose, duration 24 hr; normal function within 48 hr

Interactions/incompatibilities:
• Absorption impaired by food
• Adverse effects enhanced by other anticholinergic agents

Clinical assessment:
• Check recent history of cardiac disease (myocardial infarction), check mechanical obstruction not cause of retention, check ileus not due to mechanical obstruction. Recent bowel anastomosis

Treatment of overdose: Atropine

for 24 hr, up to 2 mg IM, symptomatic treatment

NURSING CONSIDERATIONS

Assess:
- BP, pulse, respiration
- Fluid balance
- Extent of underlying pathology to enable accurate evaluation

Administer:
- 30 min before breakfast; absorption impaired by food

Perform/provide:
- Close supervision in early stages if used for myasthenia gravis ('crisis')
- Toilet facilities in case of disturbance in bowel habit
- Wash/change linen for sweating
- Atropine always available
- Safe environment: Cot side, Help with mobilisation directed by individual patient assessment

Evaluate:
- Side effects e.g. BP or slowed pulse, colic, problems passing urine, abdominal distention; salivation
- Improvement in urinary function, bowel movement, micturition, etc.
- Bowel sounds
- Therapeutic effect as elicited by formal assessment

Teach patient/family:
- About blurred vision. That effects last for up to 24 hr, returning to normal within 48 hr
- To take as prescribed
- Change position slowly. To report increased salivation
- About sweating, breathing (potential) problems. To carry ID card or bracelet if they have myasthenia gravis
- To seek medical advice if adverse reactions occur

---

disulfiram

Antabuse 200
Func. class.: Alcohol deterrent
Chem. class.: Aldehyde dehydrogenase inhibitor
Legal class.: POM

Action: Blocks oxidation of alcohol at acetaldehyde stage

Uses: Chronic alcoholism with appropriate supportive treatment

Dosage and routes:
- *Adult:* By mouth after a 24 hr alcohol-free period:
Day 1: no more than 4 tablets as one dose
Day 2: 3 tablets
Day 3: 2 tablets
Day 4 and 5: 1 tablet
Subsequent dose as 1 or ½ tablet daily

Available forms include: Tablets 200 mg

Side effects/adverse reactions:
CNS: Headache, drowsiness, restlessness, dizziness, fatigue, tremors, psychosis, libido reduction
GI: Nausea, vomiting, anorexia, hepatotoxicity, halitosis
INTEG: Rash, dermatitis, urticaria, peripheral neuritis
GU: Severe thirst

Contraindications: Hypersensitivity, alcohol intoxication, psychoses, hypertension, cardiac failure, coronary artery disease, CVA

Precautions: Hypothyroidism, hepatic disease, diabetes mellitus, seizure disorders, respiratory disease, diabetes mellitus, renal failure

Pharmacokinetics:
By mouth: Onset 12 hr, oxidized by liver, excreted unchanged in faeces

Interactions/incompatibilities:

• Increased effects of: tricyclic antidepressants, theophylline, oral anticoagulants, phenytoin, diazepam, chlordiazepoxide, narcotics, amphetamines
• Disulfiram reaction: alcohol, chlorpromazine, amitriptyline — both may increase intensity of alcohol reactions
• Psychosis: metronidazole, paraldehyde, isoniazid
Clinical assessment:
• Liver function studies every 2 weeks during therapy: aspartate aminotransferase, alanine aminotransferase
• Full blood count sequential multiple analysis every 3–6 months to detect any abnormality including increased cholesterol
Treatment of overdose: Low toxicity — symptomatic with gastric lavage or observation
NURSING CONSIDERATIONS
Administer:
• Once per day in the morning or bedtime if drowsiness occurs
• Only after patient has not had alcohol for more than 12 hr
Evaluate:
• Mental status: affect, mood, drug history, ability to follow treatment, abstain from alcohol
Teach patient/family:
• Effect of this drug if alcohol is taken, check patient understanding and record in nursing documentation
• That shaving lotions, creams, cough preparations, skin products must be checked for alcohol content; even in small amount, alcohol can produce a reaction
• That tolerance will not develop if treatment is prolonged
• That reaction may occur for 2 weeks after last dose
• Carry medication record card listing disulfiram therapy
• Avoid driving or hazardous tasks

if drowsiness occurs
• That disulfiram reaction occurs 10 min after drinking alcohol; characterised by violent flushing, dyspnoea, headache, palpitations, tachycardia, nausea and vomiting

---

dithranol

Alphodith, Anthianol, Dithrocream, Ditholam, Psoradoute, Psorion, Exolam, combination products
Func. class.: Anti-psoriatic/anti-eczema
Legal class.: POM/P depending on strength

Action: Inhibits epidermal cell replication by decreasing mitosis by halting nucleic protein synthesis
Uses: Subacute and chronic psoriasis
Dosage and routes:
• *Adult and child:* Topical, apply to affected area for 30–60 min. Start with low concentrations and build up
Available forms include: Topical cream 0.1%, 0.2%, 0.25%, 0.4%, 0.5%, 1%; topical ointment 0.1%, 0.25%, 0.4%, 0.5%, 1%, 2%
Side effects/adverse reactions:
INTEG: Rash on normal skin, discolouration of nails, hair, skin, clothing, burning sensation and irritation
Contraindications: Hypersensitivity, acute psoriasis
Precautions: Excessive soreness — reduce frequency. Avoid eyes and mucous membranes
Pharmacokinetics:
Topical: Absorption poor, absorbed amount excreted in urine
Interactions/incompatibilities: None known

NURSING CONSIDERATIONS
Assess:
• Urinalysis weekly for albumin and casts
Administer:
• Wear gloves to protect hands and wash hands carefully after application
• Avoid contamination of healthy surrounding skin by protection with barrier cream e.g. zinc oxide, petroleum jelly
• Cover with dressing to avoid staining of clothes
• Apply to the scalp after the application of olive oil or liquid paraffin. Remove scales with comb
• Apply at bedtime to ensure contact time of 10−12 hr
• Continue treatment for 2−4 weeks, as required
Evaluate:
• Therapeutic response: decreased itching, redness, dryness and scaling
• Observe the skin involved carefully, noting any agents that appear to aggravate the condition
Teach patient/family:
• To avoid application to surrounding healthy skin, mucous membranes and eyes
• Skin, nails and hair may assume a brown-yellow tinge if cream is applied to them
• To discontinue use if rash, urticaria or folliculitis develop

---

dobutamine HCl

Dobutrex
Func. class.: Adrenergic direct-acting β-agonist
Chem. class.: Catecholamine
Legal class.: POM

Action: Causes increased contractility and heart rate by acting on β-1 receptors in heart

Uses: Low output cardiac failure due to myocardial infarction, open heart surgery, sepsis, shock, possible alternative to exercise in stress testing
Dosage and routes:
• *Adult:* IV infusion 2.5−10 mcg/kg/min, may increase to 40 mcg/kg/min if needed. Should be given diluted and adjust according to patient response
Available forms include: Injection IV solution 12.5 mg (as hydrochloride)/ml
Side effects/adverse reactions:
CV: Palpitations, tachycardia, hypertension, angina
GI: Nausea, vomiting
Contraindications: Hypersensitivity
Precautions: Pregnancy, lactation, ventricular filling or outflow obstruction. Hypotension due to cardiogenic shock
Pharmacokinetics:
IV: Onset 1−5 min, peak 10 min, half-life 2 min, metabolised in liver (inactive metabolites), excreted in urine
Interactions/incompatibilities:
• Incompatible with alkaline solutions: sodium, bicarbonate
Treatment of overdose: Withdraw dobutamine until condition stabilises

NURSING CONSIDERATIONS
Assess:
• Heart rate, rhythm, BP, ECG, cardiac output
• Fluid balance
• Hrly urine measurement — patient may need urinary catheter. Inform clinician if output less than 30 ml/hr
• Continuous cardiac monitoring during administration
• BP and pulse after parenteral route half hrly initially. Assess dependency on stability of patient's condition and therapeutic response
Administer:

• Patients usually managed on a cardiac or intensive care unit
• May be given peripherally but ideally through a central line with pressure monitoring (or such a central line or Swan Ganz catheter) in situ
• Must be diluted as prescribed and given via intravenous pump (usually to 50 mls and given via a syringe pump)

Perform/provide:
• Storage of reconstituted solution, if refrigerated, for no longer than 48 hr

Evaluate:
• Therapeutic response: increased BP with stabilisation, increase in urinary output and effect on heart rate—or inform medical staff of lack of response

Teach patient/family:
• Reason for drug administration
• Explanation of equipment and monitors to allay fear

---

docusate sodium

Dioctyl, Norgalax Micro-enema, Fletchers' Enemette, combination products
Func. class.: Laxative
Chem. class.: Anionic surfactant
Legal class.: P

Action: Increases water penetration to soften stools for easier passage
Uses: Prevent and treat chronic constipation

Dosage and routes:
• *Adult:* By mouth up to 500 mg a day in divided doses; enema 5 ml as needed
• *Child over 3 yr:* Enema as adult
• *Child over 12 yr:* By mouth 12.5–25 mg 3 times a day
• *Infant over 6 months:* 12.5 mg 3 times a day. Give with a full glass of water

Available forms include: Tablets 100 mg; oral solution 50, 12.5 mg/ml; enema 90 mg/5 ml
Side effects/adverse reactions:
GI: Nausea, anorexia, cramps atonic colon, hypocalcaemia
Contraindications: Obstruction, nausea/vomiting, infants under 6 months
Precautions: Breast feeding
Pharmacokinetics: Onset 1–2 days
Interactions/incompatibilities:
• Mineral oil; Anthraquinones, increased absorption
Clinical assessment:
• Urine/blood electrolytes
Treatment of overdose: Fluids to replace excessive loss

NURSING CONSIDERATIONS
Assess:
• Cause of constipation; identify whether fluids, fibre or exercise is missing from lifestyle
• Fluid balance to identify fluid loss
Administer:
• Alone for better absorption; do not take within 1 hr of other drugs or within 1 hr of antacids, milk, or cimetidine
• In morning or evening (oral dose)
Evaluate:
• Therapeutic response: decrease in constipation—if diarrhoea, discontinue and seek advice
• Cramping, rectal bleeding, nausea, vomiting; if these symptoms occur, drug should be discontinued
Teach patient/family:
• Health education: to other possible means of avoiding constipation
• Swallow tablets whole; do not chew
• That normal bowel movements do not always occur daily
• Do not use in presence of abdominal pain, nausea, vomiting
• Notify clinician if constipation unrelieved or if symptoms of

electrolyte imbalance occur: muscle cramps, pain, weakness, dizziness

---

domperidone

Motilium
Func. class.: Antiemetic
Chem. class.: Substituted imidazoline
Legal class.: POM

Action: Dopamine antagonist which blocks chemoreceptor trigger zone and acts upon upper GI tract
Uses: Acute treatment of nausea and vomiting of any aetiology in adults; nausea and vomiting associated with L-dopa and bromocriptine. *Children:* Only for nausea and vomiting due to cancer chemotherapy or radiation
Dosage and routes:
• *Adults:* By mouth 10−20 mg, by rectum 1−2 suppository every 4−8 hr
• *Children:* 0.2−0.4 mg/kg 4−8 hrly orally, by rectum 1−4 suppositories a day depending on weight
Available forms include: Tablets, 10 mg; sugar-free suspension, 5 mg/5 ml; suppositories, 30 mg
Side effects/adverse reactions:
META: Raised prolactin levels, possible galactorrhoea, gynaecomastia
Precautions: Pregnancy/lactation
Pharmacokinetics: Excreted in faeces and urine as metabolites
Interactions/incompatibilities:
Effects reduced by anticholinergic agents, opioid analgesics
• Antagonises hyperprolactinaemic action of bromocriptine
• Possible enhanced GI absorption of concurrent oral drugs
Administer:

• Limit to short-term treatment only
• Orally as tablets or suspension but as suppository if frequent vomiting
• Underlying medical cause of nausea/vomiting
Lab. test interferences: *Increase:* prolactin
NURSING CONSIDERATIONS
Assess:
• Fluid balance (renal disease)
• Degree of nausea and vomiting
• Weight of children
Perform/provide:
• Cool storage for suppositories
• Mouth washes as required
• Adequate fluids by mouth or IV
Evaluate:
• Side effects related to concurrent drug therapy
• Therapeutic response: decrease in nausea/vomiting
Teach patient/family:
• About side effects of increased prolactin e.g. galactorrhoea
• That therapy is for short-term use only. Maximum usually 12 weeks

---

dopamine HCl

Intropin
Func. class.: Dopaminergic
Chem. class.: Catecholamine
Legal class.: POM

Action: At low doses causes renal and mesenteric vascular dilatation, improving renal blood flow, glomerular filtration rate and urine output. At higher doses, exerts positive inotropic effect and increases blood pressure and urine output. At very high doses, increases blood pressure by peripheral vasoconstriction
Uses: Correction of poor per-

fusion, low cardiac output, renal failure and shock due to myocardial infarction, trauma, endotoxin septicaemia, open heart surgery, heart failure

Dosage and routes:

• *Adult:* IV infusion 2−5 mcg/kg/min titrated upwards in increments of 5−10 mcg/kg/min up to 20−50 mcg/kg/min

Side effects/adverse reactions:

CNS: Headache

CV: Palpitations, tachycardia, hypertension, hypotension, ectopic beats, angina, dyspnoea resp

GI: Nausea, vomiting

Contraindications: Hypovolaemia, ventricular fibrillation, tachydysrhythmias, phaeochromocytoma

Precautions: Hypersensitivity to sulphites, extravasation-use large vein, occlusive vascular disease

Pharmacokinetics:

IV: Onset 5 min, duration up to 10 min, metabolised in liver, excreted in urine (metabolites)

Interactions/incompatibilities:

• Do not use within 2 wks of monoamine oxidase inhibitors, or hypertensive crisis may result; starting dose 1/10 of normal dose

• Dysrhythmias: general anaesthetics

• Incompatible with alkaline solutions: sodium bicarbonate

Clinical assessment:

• Therapeutic level, cardiovascular and renal parameters

• ECG during administration continuously

• CVP during infusion if possible to measure cardiac output

Treatment of overdose:

Dose reduction or discontinue; if fails consider phentolamine mesylate

NURSING CONSIDERATIONS

Assess:

• To exclude hypovolaemia: administer prescribed plasma expanders

• BP, pulse and respiration prior to administration: CVP is also valuable

• Baseline electrolytes, renal function and fluid balance

Administer:

• By infusion pump having calculated prescribed dose in mcg/kg/min

• Via central line access or large peripheral versus access as last resort

• No other medications through same line to avoid bolus doses

Perform/provide:

• Continuous cardiac monitoring: report elevations in heart rate and blood pressure, dose may require adjustment titrated against effect

• Hrly vital sign recording and fluid balance

• Resuscitation equipment available

Evaluate:

• Therapeutic response: increased urine output for example

• IV site: observe for extravasation at least hrly

• Peripheral circulation as may cause vasoconstriction

---

dothiepin hydrochloride

Prothiaden

Func. class.: Antidepressant

Chem. class.: Tricyclic antidepressant

Legal class.: POM

Action: Blocks reuptake of noradrenaline and serotonin into nerve endings, increasing action of noradrenalin, serotonin in nerve cells

Uses: Depressive illness, particularly where sedation and an anxiolytic action is required

Dosage and routes:
• *Adult:* By mouth, initially 75 mg daily in divided doses or as single dose at bedtime, increased as necessary to maximum 225 mg; elderly patients 50—75 mg maximum

Available forms include: Capsules 25 mg; Tablets 75 mg

Side effects/adverse reactions:
HAEM: Agranulocytosis, depression of bone marrow, jaundice
CNS: Sedation, blurred vision, tremor, confusion, hypomania, behavioural disturbances, convulsions
GI: Nausea, dry mouth, paralytic ileus
GU: Difficulty with micturition, changes in sexual function
INTEG: Sweating, rashes
CV: Arrhythmias, postural hypotension, tachycardia

Contraindications: Recent myocardial infarction, heart block; mania; liver disease

Precautions: Diabetes, cardiac disease, epilepsy, pregnancy, hepatic impairment, psychoses, urinary retention, elderly, narrow angle glaucoma, prostatic hypertrophy; avoid abrupt cessation of therapy; caution in anaesthesia

Pharmacokinetics:
Converted in liver to active metabolite; half-life 19—33 hr, excreted in urine. Onset of antidepressant effect 2—4 weeks, anxiolytic effect apparent within several days

Interactions/incompatibilities:
• Increased effect: alcohol, antihistamines, anxiolytics, disulfiram
• Risk of hypertension: anaesthetics, anti-hypotensives, sympathomimetics, diuretics
• Reduced effect: antiepileptics
• Risk of hypertension: MAOIs, other antidepressants

Clinical assessment:
• ECG and cardiac status
• Check no urinary retention or glaucoma
• Full blood count, WBC and differential every 4 weeks. Blood glucose

Treatment of overdose: Gastric lavage, activated charcoal, ECG, intubate, treatment for convulsions or arrhythmias

NURSING CONSIDERATIONS

Assess:
• Blood pressure (lying/standing), pulse, temperature
• Weight, fluid balance

Administer:
• At bedtime with food or as a divided dose. Ensure dose taken
• Not with alcohol
• Withdraw therapy gradually

Perform/provide:
• Fluids/fibre for constipation
• Fluids, sips of water for dry mouth
• Safe environment: Cot sides
• Help with mobilisation

Evaluate:
• Sleeping patterns
• Retention of urine
• Mood, level of confusion, mental state

Teach patient/family:
• That drug may cause drowsiness, if affected don't drive or operate machinery
• No alcohol. Warn that response may take 2—4 weeks, encourage them to persist and not stop abruptly
• About side effects: dry mouth, sore throat, weight gain, blurred vision, retention, sweating, rapid pulse, sexual problems; these should be reported
• That they must report these to clinician
• To get up slowly to avoid fainting

doxapram HCl

Dopram
Func. class.: Respiratory stimulant
Chem. class.: Analeptic agent
Legal class.: POM

Action: Respiratory stimulation through action on peripheral chemoreceptors

Uses: Acute respiratory failure, postanaesthesia respiratory stimulation

Dosage and routes:
Acute respiratory failure
• *Adult:* IV infusion 1.5 mg/min to 4.0 mg/min
Following anaesthesia
• *Adult:* IV injection, 1.0–1.5 mg/kg over 30 secs or more, repeated at 1 hrly intervals if necessary IV infusion, 2–3 mg/min according to response

Available forms include: Injection IV 20 mg/ml 5 ml ampoule; infusion 2 mg/ml, 500 ml infusion in 5% glucose

Side effects/adverse reactions:
CNS: Headache, restlessness, dizziness, confusion, paraesthesia, flushing, sweating, rigidity (clonus/generalised), depression
GI: Nausea, vomiting, anorexia, diarrhoea, hiccups
GU: Retention, incontinence
CV: Chest pain, hypotension, change in heart rate, lowered T waves, tachycardia
INTEG: Pruritus, irritation at injection site
EENT: Pupil dilation, sneezing
RESP: Laryngospasm, bronchospasm, rebound hypoventilation, dyspnoea
Contraindications: Hypersensitivity, seizure disorders, severe hypertension, severe bronchial asthma, severe dyspnoea, severe cardiac disorders, pneumothorax, pulmonary embolism, severe respiratory disease, thyrotoxicosis

Precautions: Bronchial asthma, hyperthyroidism, phaeochromocytoma, severe tachycardia, dysrhythmias, cerebral oedema, increased cerebrospinal fluid

Pharmacokinetics:
IV: Onset 20–40 sec, peak 1–2 hr, duration 5–10 hr; metabolised by liver, excreted by kidneys (metabolites)

Interactions/incompatibilities:
• Synergistic pressor effect: monoamine oxidase inhibitors, sympathomimetics
• Cardiac dysrhythmias: halothane, cyclopropane, enflurane
• Do not mix in alkaline solution including aminophylline, frusemide
• Increased skeletal muscle activity and agitation with aminophylline

Clinical assessment:
• Heart rate, blood gases before administration, every 30 mins
• Arterial oxygen tension, arterial carbon dioxide tension, oxygen saturation during treatment

Treatment of overdose:
Lavage, activated charcoal, monitor electrolytes, vital signs

NURSING CONSIDERATIONS

Assess:
• B/P, pulse and other vital signs
Administer:
• IV at prescribed infusion rate, adjust for desired respiratory response
• Only after adequate airway is established
• With oxygen, resuscitation equipment available
• Using infusion pump IV
Perform/provide:
• Discontinue infusion if side effects occur
• Frequent arterial blood gas studies and pH measurements
Evaluate:
• Therapeutic effect

• For hypertension, dysrhythmias, tachycardia, dyspnoea, skeletal muscle hyperactivity; may indicate overdosage; discontinue if these occur
• For signs of respiratory stimulation: increased respiratory rate
• Extravasation, change IV site 48 hrly
• If unsuccessful further respiratory support should be considered i.e. ventilation

---

doxazosin mesylate

Cardura
Func. class.: Antihypertensive, alpha-blocker
Chem. class.: Quinazoline
Legal class.: POM

Action: Selective competitive antagonist at post-synaptic alpha$_1$-receptor, causing vasodilatation
Uses: Hypertension, if necessary in conjunction with thiazide or beta-blocker
Dosage and routes:
• *Adult:* By mouth, 1 mg daily, if necessary increased after 1−2 weeks to 2 mg daily and thereafter to 4 mg daily; max dose 16 mg daily
Available forms include: Tablets, 1 mg, 2 mg, 4 mg
Side effects/adverse reactions:
CNS: Dizziness, vertigo, headache, fatigue, asthenia
CV: Postural hypotension, oedema
Contraindications: Hypersensitivity, lactation
Precautions: Pregnancy
Pharmacokinetics:
Peak plasma concentration within 2 hr; metabolised in liver and excreted in faeces as metabolites; half-life 22 hr. Maximum hypotensive effect 2−6 hr after administration. Highly protein bound

Clinical assessment:
• Introduce slowly
• Thiazides and β-blockers may be required as additional treatment
Treatment of overdose: Supine position, IV-volume expanders, vasopressors with care. Not removed by dialysis

NURSING CONSIDERATIONS
Assess:
• Baseline blood pressure (lying/standing), pulse, fluid balance, weight
Administer:
• First dose at bedtime
Perform/provide:
• Safe environment: get up slowly, help with mobilisation
Evaluate:
• Side effects: postural hypotension particularly at start of therapy
• Therapeutic response: reduction in BP to required level
Teach patient/family:
• Take first dose in bed
• Get up slowly to avoid postural hypotension
• Not to drive or operate machinery after first dose

---

doxepin HCl

Sinequan
Func. class.: Antidepressant, tricyclic
Chem. class.: Dibenzoxepin, tertiary amine
Legal class.: POM

Action: Blocks reuptake of noradrenaline, serotonin into nerve endings, increasing action of noradrenaline serotonin in nerve cells
Uses: Endogenous depression, especially where sedation is required
Dosage and routes:
• *Adult:* By mouth, initially 75 mg (elderly 10−50 mg) daily in 3

divided doses, increased gradually to maximum 300 mg daily in divided doses; up to 100 mg may be given as a single dose at bedtime
Available forms include: Capsules 10, 25, 50, 75 mg

Side effects/adverse reactions:
HAEM: Agranulocytosis, thrombocytopenia, eosinophilia, leucopenia
CNS: Dizziness, drowsiness, confusion, headache, anxiety, tremors, agitation, weakness, insomnia, nightmares, increased psychiatric symptoms
GI: Diarrhoea, dry mouth, nausea, vomiting, paralytic ileus, increased appetite, cramps, epigastric distress, jaundice, hepatitis, stomatitis
GU: Retention, acute renal failure
INTEG: Rash, urticaria, sweating, pruritus, photosensitivity
CV: Orthostatic hypotension, ECG changes, tachycardia, hypertension, palpitations
EENT: Blurred vision, tinnitus, mydriasis, ophthalmoplegia, glossitis

Contraindications: Hypersensitivity to tricyclic antidepressants, urinary retention, narrow-angle glaucoma, prostatic hypertrophy, severe hepatic disease, mania

Precautions: Suicidal patients, elderly, recent myocardial infarction, epilepsy, pregnancy, lactation

Pharmacokinetics:
Period of onset: Steady state 2−8 days; metabolised by liver, excreted by kidneys, excreted in breast milk, half-life 8−24 hr

Interactions/incompatibilities:
• Decreased effects of: guanethidine, debrisoquine, clonidine, indirect acting sympathomimetics (ephedrine)
• Increased effects of: direct acting sympathomimetics (adrenaline), alcohol, barbiturates, benzodiazepines, CNS depressants, thyroxine
• Hyperpyretic crisis, convulsions, hypertensive episode: monoamine oxidase inhibitors

Clinical assessment:
• Blood studies: full blood count, WBCs and differential, cardiac enzymes if patient is receiving long-term treatment
• ECG for flattening of T wave, bundle branch block, AV block, dysrhythmias in cardiac patients

Treatment of overdose
ECG monitoring, induce emesis, gastric lavage, activated charcoal, administer anticonvulsant

NURSING CONSIDERATIONS

Assess:
• Pulse and B/P, check for postural hypotension
• Weight wkly, appetite may increase with drug

Administer:
• Orally, increase dose slowly according to clinical response; dose reduction may be possible for maintenance
• With food or milk for GI symptoms
• Dosage at bedtime if oversedation occurs during day; may take entire dose at bedtime elderly may not tolerate once/day dosing
• Frequent sips of water for dry mouth

Perform/provide:
• Assistance with walking during beginning therapy since drowsiness/dizziness occurs
• Safety measures, including cot sides, primarily in elderly
• Checking to see oral medication swallowed

Evaluate:
• Therapeutic response: improved mental state
• Side effects such as dizziness, drowsiness, dry mouth, blurred vision, skin rashes
• For extrapyramidal symptoms

primarily in elderly: rigidity, dystonia, akathisia
• Mental status: mood, alertness, affect; for suicidal tendencies, an increase in psychiatric symptoms: depression, panic
• Alcohol consumption; if alcohol is consumed, withhold dose until morning

Teach patient/family:
• That therapeutic effects may take 2−3 wks
• To only take other medication if directed by clinician
• To use caution in driving or other activities requiring alertness because of drowsiness, dizziness, blurred vision
• To avoid alcohol and other CNS depressants
• Not to discontinue medication without medical supervision; gradual dosage reduction necessary
• To wear sunscreen or large hat in sunshine since photosensitivity can occur

---

doxorubicin HCl

Doxorubicin Rapid Dissolution, Doxorubicin Solution for Injection
Func. class.: Antineoplastic
Chem. class.: Antibiotic, cytotoxic
Legal class.: POM

Action: Inhibits DNA synthesis, primarily; derived from *Streptomyces peucetius;* replication is decreased by binding to DNA, which causes strand splitting; active throughout entire cell cycle
Uses: Antimitotic and cytotoxic. Produces regression in acute leukaemia, lymphomas, soft-tissue and oestrogenic sarcomas, paediatric malignancies and adult solid tumours, in particular breast and lung carcinomas. Frequently used in combination therapy

Dosage and routes: Dosage may vary according to combination therapy and disease
• *Adult:* IV infusion (inject over 2−3 mins) 60−75 mg/m^2 every 3 weeks as a single dose when used alone. Reduce to 30−40 mg/m^2 every 3 weeks if used in combination therapy. Calculated on basis of body weight: 1.2−2.4 mg/kg as a single dose every 3 weeks. Alternative regimen may give greater toxicity, 0.4−0.8 mg/kg or 20−25 mg/m^2 on each day over 3 successive days. Weekly administration leads to reduced cardiotoxicity, 20 mg/m^2 weekly. Reduce dose in elderly and impaired hepatic function
• Intra-arterial or intravesical administration is used for certain disorders. Seek specialist advice
Available forms include: Injection IV 10, 20, 50 mg

Side effects/adverse reactions:
HAEM: Thrombocytopenia, leucopenia, myelosuppression, anemia
GI: Nausea, vomiting, anorexia, mucositis, hepatotoxicity
GU: Impotence, sterility, amenorrhoea, gynaecomastia, hyperuricaemia
INTEG: Rash, necrosis at injection site, dermatitis, reversible alopecia, cellulitis, thrombophlebitis at injection site
CV: Cardiomyopathy, CCF
CNS: Fever, chills
Contraindications: Hypersensitivity, pregnancy, lactation, systemic infections sensitivity to hydroxybenzoates
Precautions: Renal, hepatic, cardiac disease, gout, bone marrow depression (severe). Accumulative dose of 450−500 mg/m^2 should only be exceeded with extreme caution due to cardiac toxicity
Pharmacokinetics: Triphasic

pattern of elimination; half-life 12 min, 3⅓ hr, 29⅔ hr, metabolised by liver, appears in breast milk, excreted in urine, bile

Interactions/incompatibilities:
• Increased toxicity: other antineoplastics or radiation
• Do not mix with other drugs in solution or syringe

Clinical assessment:
• Full blood count, differential, platelet count weekly
• Blood, urine uric acid levels
• Renal function studies: blood urea nitrogen serum uric acid, urine creatinine clearance electrolytes before, during therapy
• Liver function tests before, during therapy: bilirubin, aspartate aminotransferase, alanine aminotransferase, alkaline phosphatase as needed or monthly
• ECG; for ST-T wave changes, low QRS and T, possible dysrhythmias (sinus tachycardia, heart block)

Treatment of overdose: Supportive measures, blood transfusions, barrier nursing. Look for signs of cardiac failure

NURSING CONSIDERATIONS

Assess:
• Baseline signs, weight, fluid balance

Administer:
• In accordance with local cytotoxic policy
• Other medications by oral route if possible; avoid IM, SC, IV routes to prevent infections and bruises
• Antiemetic 30−60 min before giving drug to prevent vomiting
• Allopurinol or sodium bicarbonate to maintain uric acid levels, alkalinisation of urine
• IV infusion using appropriate, gauge needle; check for extravasation. Discord unused solution
• Topical or systemic analgesics for pain
• Antispasmodic for GI symptoms

N.B. Care with handling—very irritant to skin and oral tissues

Perform/provide:
• Strict medical asepsis and protective isolation if WBC levels are low
• Diet as tolerated
• Increased fluid intake to 2−3 L/day to prevent urate, calculi formation
• Diet low in purines: omit offal (kidney, liver), dried beans, peas to maintain alkaline urine
• Mouth care
• Warm compresses at injection site for inflammation; check for extravasation

Perform/provide:
• Storage at room temperature for 24 hr after reconstituting infusion or 48 hr refrigerated

Evaluate:
• Bleeding: haematuria, bruising or petechiae, mucosa or orifices 8 hrly
• Food preferences; list likes, dislikes
• Effects of alopecia on body image; discuss feelings about body changes
• Oedema in feet, joint, abdominal pain, shaking
• Inflammation of mucosa, breaks in skin
• Yellowing of skin, sclera, dark urine, clay-coloured stools, itchy skin, abdominal pain, fever, diarrhoea
• Buccal cavity 8 hrly for dryness, sores, ulceration, white patches, oral pain, bleeding, dysphagia
• Local irritation, pain, burning at injection site
• GI symptoms: frequency of stools, cramping
• Acidosis, signs of dehydration: rapid respirations, poor skin turgor, decreased urine output, dry skin, restlessness, weakness
• Cardiac status: B/P, pulse, character, rhythm, rate

Teach patient/family:
• Why protective isolation precautions are necessary
• To report any complaints, side effects to nurse or clinician
• That hair may be lost during treatment and wig or hairpiece may make the patient feel better (available free on NHS); tell patient that new hair may be different in colour, texture
• To avoid foods with citric acid, hot or rough texture
• To report any bleeding, white spots, ulcerations in mouth to physician; tell patient to examine mouth daily
• That urine may be red-orange for 48 hr

---

doxycycline hydrochloride

Vibramycin, Nordox, Vibramycin-D
Func. class.: Antibiotic, broad spectrum
Chem. class.: Tetracycline
Legal class.: POM

Action: Inhibits protein synthesis, prosphorylation in microorganisms by binding to 30S ribosomal subunits, reversibly binding to 50S ribosomal subunits
Uses: Effective against a wide range of Gram-positive and Gram-negative bacteria. Chlamydia trachomatis, gonorrhoea, lymphogranuloma venereum, mycoplasma, brucellosis (with rifampicin), exacerbations of chronic bronchitis, severe acne vulgaris, prostatitis and sinusitis, traveller's diarrhoea, leptospirosis
Dosage and routes:
• *Adult:* By mouth 200 mg on first day, then 100 mg daily; severe infections 200 mg daily
Acne
• 50 mg daily for 6−12 weeks
STD
• 100 mg twice daily for 7 days
Acute epididymoorchitis
• 100 mg twice daily for 10 days
Primary/secondary syphilis
• 300 mg daily in divided doses for at least 10 days
Available forms include: Tablets dispersible 100 mg; capsules 50, 100 mg
Side effects/adverse reactions:
CNS: Fever, headache, paraesthesia
HAEM: Eosinophilia, neutropenia, thrombocytopenia, leucocytosis, haemolytic anaemia
EENT: Dysphagia, glossitis, decreased calcification of deciduous teeth, abdominal pain, oral candidiasis
GI: Nausea, vomiting, diarrhoea, anorexia, enterocolitis, hepatotoxicity, flatulence, abdominal cramps, gastric burning, stomatitis, pseudomembranous colitis
CV: Pericarditis
GU: Increased blood urea nitrogen, polyuria, polydipsia, renal failure, nephrotoxicity
INTEG: Rash, urticaria, photosensitivity, increased pigmentation, exfoliative dermatitis, pruritus, angioedema
Contraindications: Hypersensitivity to tetracyclines, children less than 8 yr, pregnancy (2nd and 3rd trimester), porphyria
Precautions: Hepatic disease, lactation
Pharmacokinetics:
Period of onset: Peak 1½−4 hr, half-life 15−22 hr; excreted in bile, 25%−93% protein bound
Interactions/incompatibilities:
• Decreased effects of this drug: antacids, sodium bicarbonate,

dairy products, alkali products
- Increased effect: anticoagulants (chronic treatment)
- Decreased effects: penicillins
- Nephrotoxicity: methoxyflurane

Clinical assessment:
- Blood studies: full blood count, Pathrombin time, blood urea nitrogen, aspartate aminotransferase, alanine aminotransferase, creatinine

Treatment of overdose: Supportive measure, gastric lavage

NURSING CONSIDERATIONS
Assess:
- Baseline fluid balance

Administer:
- With food and plenty of fluids
- After culture and sensitivity obtained
- Not at the same time as antacids, calcium, iron; all decrease absorption

Perform/provide:
- Storage in tight, light-resistant container at room temperature

Evaluate:
- Therapeutic response: decreased temperature, absence of lesions, negative culture and sensitivity
- Allergic reactions: rash, itching, pruritus, angioneurotic oedema
- Nausea, vomiting, diarrhoea; administer antiemetic, antacids as ordered
- Overgrowth of infection: increased temperature, malaise, redness, pain, swelling, drainage, perineal itching, diarrhoea, changes in cough or sputum

Teach patient/family:
- Avoid sun exposure since burns may occur; sunscreen does not seem to decrease photosensitivity
- Of diabetic to avoid use of Clinistix, Diastix, for urine glucose testing
- That all prescribed medication must be taken to prevent superimposed infection
- When to take milk products in relation to dose

droperidol

Droleptan
Func. class.: Antipsychotic, neuroleptic
Chem. class.: Butyrophenone derivative
Legal class.: POM

Action: Acts on CNS at subcortical levels, produces tranquilisation, sleep
Uses: Premedication for surgery, neuroleptanalgesia, anti-emetic, emergency sedation or rapid calming the manic, agitated patient

Dosage and routes:
Neuroleptanalgesia
- *Adult:* IV 5−15 mg with narcotic analgesic at induction
- *Child:* IV 0.2−0.3 mg/kg

Premedication in anaesthesia
- *Adult:* By mouth, IM 2.5−10 mg
- *Child 2−12 yr:* IM 0.2−0.5 mg/kg; By mouth 0.3−0.6 mg/kg

Antiemetic
- *Adult:* IV, IM 5 mg post-operative
- *Child:* IV, IM 0.02−0.075 mg/kg post-operative

In cancer chemotherapy for antiemesis
- *Adults:* IM/IV 1−10 mg loading dose 30 mins before therapy then IV infusion 1−3 mg/hr or IV/IM 1−5 mg every 1−6 hr as required
- *Child:* IV/IM 0.02−0.075 mg/kg according to requirements

Emergency sedation
- *Adult:* By mouth 5−20 mg every 4−8 hr; IV 5−15 mg; IM up to 10 mg every 4−6 hr
- *Child:* By mouth, IM 0.5−1 mg daily adjusted according to response

Available forms include: Injection IM, IV 5 mg/ml, 2 ml ampoules; Tablets 10 mg; Oral liquid 1 mg/ml

Side effects/adverse reactions:

RESP: Laryngospasm, broncho-spasm

CNS: Dystonia, akathisia, flexion of arms, fine tremors, dizziness, anxiety, drowsiness, restlessness, hallucination, depression

GI: Nausea, loss of appetite, dyspepsia

ENDO: Galactorrhoea, gynaecomastia, and oligo-or amenorrhoea

CV: Tachycardia, hypotension

EENT: Upward rotation of eyes, oculogyric crisis

SYST: Chills, facial sweating, shivering

Contraindications: Hypersensitivity, pregnancy, coma, severe depression

Precautions: Elderly, cardiovascular disease (hypotension, bradydysrhythmias), epilepsy, renal disease, liver disease, Parkinson's disease, lactation

Pharmacokinetics:

IM/IV: Onset 3–10 min, peak ½ hr, duration 3–6 hr; metabolised in liver, excreted in urine as metabolites

Interactions/incompatibilities:

• Increased CNS depression: alcohol, narcotics, barbiturates, anti-psychotics, methyldopa or other CNS depressants

• Decreased effects of: amphetamines, anticonvulsants, anticoagulants, levadopa, when given with this drug

• Increased intraocular pressure: anticholinergics, antiparkinson drugs

• Increased side effects of: lithium

Clinical Assessment:

• Fluid balance and blood pressure when used in anaesthesia

• Liver and renal function

Treatment of overdose: Supportive measures combined with sedative or anti-Parkinsonian drugs, as required

NURSING CONSIDERATIONS

Assess:

• Baseline vital signs including temperature

Administer:

• Only with resuscitation equipment nearby

• IV slowly only

Perform/provide:

• Slow movement of patient to avoid orthostatic hypotension

Evaluate:

• Changes in vital signs every 10 min during IV administration, every 30 min after IM dose

• Therapeutic response: decreased anxiety, absence of vomiting during surgery

• Extrapyramidal reactions: tremor, dystonia, akathisia

• For increasing heart rate or decreasing B/P, notify clinician at once; do not place patient in Trendelenburg position or sympathetic blockade may occur causing respiratory arrest

Teach patient/family:

• Drug must not be discontinued suddenly (may cause acute withdrawal syndrome or rapid relapse)

---

dydrogesterone

Duphaston

Func. class.: Progestogen, orally active

Chem. class.: Progesterone analogue

Legal class.: POM

Action: Produces secretory endometrium in oestrogen-primed uterus but lacks androgenic or oestrogenic activity and does not inhibit ovulation

Uses: All cases of endogenous progesterone deficiency: Endometriosis, infertility, irregular menstruation, amenorrhoea, dysmenorrhoea, premenstrual syndrome, dysfunctional uterine bleeding, habitual abortion, HRT, threatened abortion

Dosage and routes:

Endometriosis
• *Adult:* By mouth 10 mg 2−3 times daily from 5th−25th day of cycle or continuously

Infertility, irregular cycles
• 10 mg twice daily from days 11−25 of cycle until conception, for at least 6 cycles

Amenorrhoea
• 10 mg twice daily from days 11−25 of cycle, with oestrogen therapy from days 1−25 of cycle

Dysmenorrhoea
• 10 mg twice daily from days 5−25 of cycle

Premenstrual syndrome
• 10 mg twice daily from days 12−26 of cycle, increased if necessary

Dysfunctional uterine bleeding
• 10 mg twice daily (with an oestrogen) for 5−7 days to arrest bleeding; 10 mg twice daily from days 11−25 of cycle (together with an oestrogen) to prevent bleeding

Habitual abortion
• 10 mg twice daily from days 11−25 of cycle until conception, then continuously until 20th week of pregnancy and then gradually reduced

Hormone replacement therapy
• With continuous oestrogen therapy, 10 mg twice daily for first 12−14 days of each calendar month; with cyclical oestrogen therapy, 10 mg twice daily for last 12−14 days of each treatment cycle

Threatened abortion
• 40 mg at once then 10 mg 8-hrly until symptoms remit; increase dose by 10 mg every 8 hr if symptoms return. Continue for 1 week after remission and gradually withdraw

Primary dysmenorrhoea
• *Child:* By mouth 10 mg twice daily at discretion of the physician

Available forms include: Tablets 10 mg

Side effects/adverse reactions:
META: Oedema, weight gain, changes in libido, breast discomfort; in treatment of habitual abortion
GU: Breakthrough bleeding may occur (increase dose)
GI: Disturbances, jaundice

Precautions: Diabetes, liver, cardiac or renal disease, hypertension, history of thromboembolism, mammary carcinoma

Pharmacokinetics: 50% of dose excreted in urine within 24 hr

Clinical assessment:
• Liver function tests, aspartate aminotransferase, alanine aminotransferase, bilirubin during long-term treatment
• Renal function − urea, creatinine

Lab. test interferences: No false positive in any diagnostic urine tests

Treatment of overdose: Gastric lavage, symptomatic treatment

NURSING CONSIDERATIONS

Assess:
• Blood pressure (at start of treatment), weight, fluid balance
• History of thrombo-embolic disorders

Administer:
• With food

Perform/provide:
• Counselling for sexual problems
• Breast examination

Evaluate:
• Oedema, weight gain
• Bleeding per vagina

- Rise in BP
- Side effects

Teach patient/family:
- Explain drug regimen in full and warn about side effects such as 'breakthrough' bleeding
- Report any of the following: weight gain, breast discomfort, pain in legs or chest, sexual problems
- About breast examination
- Diabetics should monitor glucose more often
- Need for regular follow-up and examination

before each application, dry well
- Enough medication to cover lesions completely

Perform/provide:
- Storage at room temperature in dry place

Evaluate:
- Allergic reaction: burning, stinging, swelling, redness
- Therapeutic response: decrease in size, number of lesions

Teach patient/family:
- Use medical asepsis (hand washing) before, after each application
- Avoid use of non-prescribed creams, ointments, lotions unless directed by clinician

---

econazole nitrate

Ecostatin, Gyno-Pevaryl, Pevaryl, combination product
Func. class.: Antibiotic, antifungal
Chem. class.: Imidazole derivative
Legal class.: P or POM (vaginal route)

Action: Interferences with fungal DNA replication; binds sterols in fungal cell membrane, which increases permeability, leaking of cell nutrients
Uses: *Tinea pedis*, *tinea cruris*, *tinea corporis*, *tinea versicolor*, candida infection
Dosage and routes:
- *Adult and child:* Topical apply to affected area 2 or 3 times a day depending on condition
Available forms include: Cream, 1%; pessaries 150 mg; lotion, powder, spray
Side effects/adverse reactions:
INTEG: Rash, urticaria, stinging, burning, pruritus
Contraindications: Hypersensitivity
NURSING CONSIDERATIONS
Administer:
- After cleansing with soap, water

---

edrophonium chloride

Tensilon
Func. class.: Cholinergic, anticholinesterase
Chem. class.: Quaternary ammonium compound
Legal class.: POM

Action: Inhibits destruction of acetylcholine, which increases concentration at sites where acetylcholine is released; this facilitates transmission of impulses across myoneural junction
Uses: To diagnose myasthenia gravis, antagonist of non-depolarising muscle relaxants such as tubocurarine, differentiation of myasthenic crisis from cholinergic crisis
Dosage and routes:
Tensilon test
- *Adult:* IV 1–2 mg, then 8 mg if no response; IM 10 mg
- *Child:* 0.1 mg/kg; inject 20% dose initially, if no response after 30 sec, inject remainder
Reversal of neuromuscular blockade

• *Adult and child:* IV 0.5−0.7 mg/kg with atropine over several minutes

Differentiation of myasthenic crisis from cholinergic crisis

• *Adult:* IV 2 mg 1 hr after last dose of anticholinergic agent

Available forms include: Injection IV 10 mg/ml

Side effects/adverse reactions:

INTEG: Rash, urticaria

CNS: Dizziness, headache, sweating, confusion, weakness, convulsions, uncoordination, paralysis

GI: Nausea, diarrhoea, vomiting, cramps

CV: Tachycardia

GU: Frequency, incontinence

RESP: Respiratory depression, bronchospasm, constriction

EENT: Miosis, blurred vision, lacrimation

Contraindications: Hypersensitivity, hypotension, obstruction of intestine, renal system

Precautions: Bradycardia, seizure disorders, bronchial asthma, coronary occlusion, hyperthyroidism, dysrhythmias, peptic ulcer, megacolon, poor GI motility, parkinsonism

Pharmacokinetics:

IV: Onset 30−60 sec, duration 6−24 min

IM: Onset 2−10 min, duration 12−45 min

Interactions/incompatibilities:

• Decreased action of this drug: procainamide, quinidine

• Bradycardia: digoxin

NURSING CONSIDERATIONS

Assess:

• Baseline vital signs, respiration

Administer:

• Only with atropine sulphate available for cholinergic crisis

• Only after all other cholinergics have been discontinued

• NB: only in the presence of a person skilled in intubation

Perform/provide:

• Storage at room temperature

• Resuscitation equipment available on unit

Evaluate:

• Vital signs and respiratory rate

• Therapeutic response: increased muscle strength, hand grasp, improved gait, absence of laboured breathing (if severe)

Teach patient/family:

• Wear Medicare ID specifying myasthenia gravis, and prescribed therapy

---

enalapril maleate

Innovace, combination product

Func. class.: Antihypertensive

Chem. class.: Angiotensin converting enzyme inhibitor

Legal class.: POM

Action: Selectively suppresses renin-angiotensin-aldosterone system; inhibits angiotensin-converting enzyme, prevents conversion of angiotensin I to angiotensin II

Uses: Hypertension not responsive to other hypertensive medications; adjunct to diuretics/digoxin for congestive heart failure

Dosage and routes:

Hypertension

• Adult with no concomitant diuretics, initially 5 mg daily adjusted as necessary to a maximum of 40 mg daily

• Adults with concomitant diuretic therapy and the elderly (over 65 yr), initially 2.5 mg adjusted as necessary to a maximum of 40 mg daily

Congestive heart failure

• Initially 2.5 mg daily

Available forms include: Tablets 2.5, 5, 10, 20 mg

Side effects/adverse reactions:
CV: Hypotension, chest pain, tachycardia, dysrhythmias
CNS: Insomnia, dizziness, paraesthesia, headache, fatigue, anxiety
GI: Nausea, vomiting, colitis, cramps, diarrhoea, constipation flatulence, dry mouth
INTEG: Rash, purpura, alopecia
HAEM: Agranulocytosis
EENT: Tinnitus, visual changes, sore throat, double vision, dry burning eyes, angioneurotic oedema
GU: Proteinuria, renal failure, increased frequency of polyuria or oliguria
RESP: Dyspnoea, cough, rales
Contraindications: Pregnancy
Precautions: Renal disease, hyperkalaemia, lactation
Pharmacokinetics:
Period of onset: Peak 4−6 hr; half-life 1½ hr; metabolised by liver to active metabolite, excreted in urine
Interactions/incompatibilities:
• Severe hypotension: diuretics, other antihypertensives
• Decreased effects when used with: aspirin
• Increased potassium levels: salt substitutes, potassium-sparing diuretics, potassium supplements
• May increase effects of: ergot derivatives, neuromuscular blocking agents, antihypertensives, hypoglycaemics, barbiturates, lithium, reserpine, levodopa
• Effects may be increased by: phenothiazines, diuretics, phenytoin, quinidine
Clinical assessment:
• Electrolytes: potassium, sodium chloride
• Baselines in renal liver function tests, before therapy begins
Lab. test interferences:
Interferences: Glucose/insulin tolerance tests

Treatment of overdose: Gastric lavage, IV atropine for bradycardia, IV theophylline for bronchospasm, digoxin, O_2, diuretic for cardiac failure, haemodialysis
NURSING CONSIDERATIONS
Assess:
• Baseline BP, apical/radial pulse
Administer:
• With patient in supine position if hypotension
• First dose under supervision, monitor BP for hypotension
Evaluate:
• BP, pulse 4 hrly, note rate, rhythm, quality
• Apical/radial pulse before administration; notify clinician of any significant changes
• Oedema in feet, legs daily
• Skin turgor, dryness of mucous membranes for hydration status
• Symptoms of congestive cardiac failure: oedema, dyspnoea
Teach patient/family:
• Not to discontinue drug abruptly
• Rise slowly to sitting or standing position to minimise postural hypotension
• Benefits of therapy in heart failure (such as reduction in fatigue) are often long-term rather than immediate

---

enoxacin

Comprecin
Func. class.: Antibacterial
Chem. class.: 4-quinolone
Legal class.: POM

Action: Inhibits DNA gyrase; active against Gram-negative organisms and staphylococci. It is usually active against pathogens resistant to beta-lactams and aminoglycosides

Uses: Urinary tract, genital tract, skin and soft tissue infections, shigellosis

Dosage and routes:

By mouth:

Urinary tract infections
• *Adult:* 200 mg twice daily for 3 days; severe infections 400 mg twice daily for 7−14 days

Genital tract infections
• *Adult:* 400 mg as a single dose

Chancroid
• *Adult:* 400 mg twice daily for 3 doses skin and soft tissue infections
• *Adult:* 400 mg twice a day for 7 days

Shigellosis
• *Adult:* 400 mg twice a day for 5 days

NB: In the elderly over 65 yr and in severe renal impairment (creatinine clearance less than 30 ml/min) dose should be reduced to 200 mg or 400 mg as a single dose

Side effects/adverse reactions:

GI: Nausea, vomiting, altered taste, dyspepsia, abdominal pain, dry mouth and throat, stomatitis
CNS: Fatigue, dizziness, insomnia, seizures, headache, tremor, nervousness, amblyopia, tinnitis
CV: Tachycardia, oedema
INTEG: Rash; photosensitivity

Contraindications: Hypersensitivity to quinolone antibiotics, pregnancy, breastfeeding

Precautions: Renal impairment, elderly. History for epilepsy or severe cerebral arteriosclerosis

Pharmacokinetics:

Period of onset: Peak plasma levels after 2 hr. Half-life 3−7 hr

Interactions/incompatibilities:
• Increased effect of: theophylline. Enoxacin inhibits the metabolism of theophylline. If concurrent use is necessary reduce theophylline dose by 50−75% and monitor blood levels

Clinical assessment:
• Renal and liver function tests: blood urea nitrogen, creatinine, serum aspartate aminotransferase, serum alanine transpeptidase

Treatment of overdose: Supportive measures

NURSING CONSIDERATIONS

Assess:
• Fluid balance, urinary pH

Administer:
• Once a clean-catch/midstream specimen of urine or other samples have been obtained for bacterial culture and sensitivity tests

Evaluate:
• Response to treatment indicated by decreased dysuria, frequency, urgency and negative bacteriological test results, which suggest that infection has resolved
• CNS symptoms: headache, dizziness, fatigue, insomnia, depression
• Fluid balance and urinary pH. pH of less than 5.5 is ideal if treated for urinary tract infection
• Allergic reactions: fever, rash, urticaria, pruritus

Teach patient/family:
• Avoid antacids containing magnesium or aluminium until at least 4 hr after taking the drug
• Photosensitivity occurs: patients should avoid sunlight or use suncare preparations to avoid sunburn
• Fluid intake must be increased to 3 litres daily to avoid crystallisation and renal calculi
• To limit intake of highly alkaline foods, drugs, and dairy products, peanuts, vegetables, antacids, sodium bicarbonate, and iron supplements if treated for a urinary tract infection
• If dizziness occurs ambulant patients require careful supervision

• The full course of treatment must be completed

• The clinician must be informed if adverse reactions occur

---

enoximone

Perfan

Func. class.: Inotropic agent
Legal class.: POM

Action: Phosphodiesterase inhibitor

Uses: Congestive heart failure where cardiac output reduced and filling pressure increased

Dosage and routes:

• *Adult:* Slow IV, rate not exceeding 12.5 mg/min, diluted before use

• Initially 0.5–1 mg/kg, then 500 mcg/kg every 30 min until satisfactory response or total of 3 mg/kg given. Maintenance, initial dose of up to 3 mg/kg may be repeated every 3–6 hr as required

• IV infusion: initially 90 mcg/kg/min over 10–30 min, followed by continuous or intermittent infusion of 5–20 mcg/kg/min. Total dose over 24 hr should not normally exceed 24 mg/kg

Available forms include: IV injection 5 mg/ml

Side effects/adverse reactions:

CV: Ectopic beats, less frequently ventricular tachycardia or supraventricular arrhythmias (more likely in patients with pre-existing arrhythmias), hypotension, chills, fever

CNS: Headache, insomnia, upper and lower limb pain

GU: Oliguria, urinary retention

GI: Nausea, vomiting, diarrhoea

Precautions: Heart failure associated with hypertrophic cardiomyopathy, stenotic or obstructive valvular disease or other outlet obstruction, renal impairment

NURSING CONSIDERATIONS

Assess:

• Baseline vital signs, ECG, CPV

Administer:

• Dilute before use with water for injection or sodium chloride 0.9%.

• Use immediately post dilution

• Do not use if diluted solution is not a clear yellow colour

• Avoid extravasation

• Plastic containers and syringes should be used as crystal formation occurs when glass is used

Evaluate:

• For side effects

• BP, heart rate, ECG, central venous pressure, fluid and electrolyte status, platelet count, hepatic enzymes

Perform/provide:

• Continuous monitoring (preferably in coronary care unit or intensive care unit)

---

ephedrine hydrochloride

Func. class.: Nasal decongestant
Chem. class.: Sympathomimetic
Pamine
Legal class.: P

Action: Vasoconstriction of mucosal blood vessels reduces thickness of nasal mucosa

Uses: Nasal congestion associated with colds, hayfever, sinusitis, other allergic conditions, adjunct in middle ear infections

Dosage and routes:

• *Adult and child:* Instil 1–2 drops when required

Available forms include: Solution 0.5%, 1%

Side effects/adverse reactions:

EENT: Irritation, burning, sneezing, stinging, dryness, rebound congestion

INTEG: Contact dermatitis

CNS: Anxiety, restlessness, tremors, weakness, insomnia, dizziness, fever, headache

Contraindications: Hypersensitivity to sympathomimetic amines

Precautions: Child under 3 months, elderly, diabetes, cardiovascular disease, hypertension, hyperthyroidism, prostatic hypertrophy, lactation

Interactions/incompatibilities: Minimal systemic absorption, interactions rare

• Hypertension: MAOIs, β-adrenergic blockers

• Hypotension: methyldopa, reserpine

NURSING CONSIDERATIONS

Administer:

• No more than 4 hrly

• For less than 4 consecutive days

Perform/provide:

• Environmental humidification to decrease nasal congestion, dryness

Evaluate:

• Redness, swelling, pain in nasal passages

Teach patient/family:

• Stinging may occur for a few applications; drying of mucosa may be decreased by environmental humidification

• Notify clinician if irregular pulse, insomnia, dizziness, or tremors occur

• Proper administration to avoid systemic absorption

---

ephedrine sulphate

Func. class.: Adrenergic, indirect and direct acting

Chem. class.: Sympathomimetic amine

Legal class.: P

Action: Direct bronchodilatation, relaxes bladder detrusor muscle and increases bladder sphincter tone

Uses: Nocturnal enuresis, bronchodilation

Dosage and routes:

Nocturnal enuresis

• *Child 7−8 yr:* By mouth 30 mg at night

• *9−12 yr:* 45 mg at night

• *13−15 yr:* 60 mg at night

Bronchodilator

• *Adult:* By mouth 15−60 mg 3 times a day

• *Child up to 1 yr*: By mouth 7.5 mg 3 times a day

• *1−5 yr:* 5 mg 3 times a day

• *6−12 yr:* 30 mg 3 times a day

Available forms include: Tablets 15, 30, 60 mg; syrup 4 mg/5 ml, 15 mg/5 ml

Side effects/adverse reactions:

CNS: Tremors, anxiety, insomnia, headache, dizziness, confusion, hallucinations, convulsions, CNS depression

EENT: Dry nose, irritation of nose and throat

CV: Palpitations, tachycardia, hypertension, chest pain, dysrhythmias

GI: Anorexia, nausea, vomiting

RESP: Depression

Contraindications: Hypersensitivity to sympathomimetics, narrow-angle glaucoma, elderly

Precautions: Pregnancy, cardiac disorders, hyperthyroidism, diabetes mellitus, prostatic hypertrophy

Pharmacokinetics:

By mouth: Onset 15−60 min, duration 2−4 hr

Metabolised in liver, excreted in urine (unchanged), excreted in breast milk

Interactions/incompatibilities:

• Hypertensive crisis: MAOIs or tricyclic anti-depressants

• Decreased effect of this drug: methyldopa, urinary acidifiers, rauwolfia alkaloids

• Increased effect of this drug: urinary alkalinisers

Treatment of overdose: Administer an α-blocker, then noradrenaline for severe hypotension

NURSING CONSIDERATIONS

Assess:
• Fluid balance
• Frequency of nocturnal enuresis

Perform/provide:
• Do not use discoloured solutions

Evaluate:
• For paraesthesias and coldness of extremities, peripheral blood flow may decrease
• Therapeutic response: increased BP with stabilisation
• For hypovolaemia; plasma expanders may be ordered

Teach patient/family:
• Reason for drug administration
• Avoid drinks at bedtime if nocturnal enuresis

---

ergometrine maleate

Syntometrine (combination product)
Func. class.: Oxytocic
Chem. class.: Ergot alkaloid
Legal class.: POM

Action: Stimulates uterine contractions, decreases bleeding

Uses: Treatment of haemorrhage associated with postpartum or postabortion

Dosage and routes:
• *Adult:* IM 200−500 mcg, period of onset 5−7 min; duration 45 min; IV 100−500 mcg, period of onset 1 min; by mouth 500 mcg − 1 mg, period of onset 8 min, duration 1 hr

Available forms include: Injection 500 mcg/ml; tablets 250 mcg, 500 mcg

Side effects/adverse reactions:
CNS: Headache, dizziness, fainting

CV: Hypertension, chest pain, vasoconstriction
GI: Nausea, vomiting
INTEG: Sweating
RESP: Dyspnoea
EENT: Tinnitus
GU: Cramping

Contraindications: Hypersensitivity to ergot derivatives, 1st and 2nd stages of labour, before delivery of placenta, spontaneous abortion (threatened), pelvic inflammatory disease (PID), renal, hepatic impairment

Precautions: Cardiac disease, asthma, anaemia, convulsive disorders, hypertension, glaucoma, toxaemia

Pharmacokinetics:
Metabolised in liver, excreted in urine

NURSING CONSIDERATIONS

Assess:
• Baseline BP and pulse

Administer:
• IM in deep muscle mass; rotate injection sites if additional doses are given

Evaluate:
• For side effects
• BP and pulse
• For length, duration of contraction
• Amount of blood loss per vaginum

Teach patient/family:
• To report increased blood loss, abdominal cramps, increased temperature or foul-smelling lochia when used at home

---

ergotamine tartrate

Lingraine, Medihaler-Ergotamine, combination products
Func. class.: Adrenergic agonist
Chem. class.: Ergot alkaloid
Legal class.: POM

Action: Constricts smooth muscle

in periphery, cranial blood vessels

Uses: Vascular headache attack, migraine

Dosage and routes:

• *Adult:* Sublingual 2 mg, repeat every 30 min as necessary, not to exceed 6 mg daily or 12 mg weekly; inhalation, one inhalation puff, may repeat in 5 min, not to exceed 6 puffs in 24 hr or 15 puffs in a week

Available forms include: Sublingual tablets 2 mg; inhalation 0.36 mg per dose

Side effects/adverse reactions:

CNS: Numbness in fingers, toes, headache

CV: Transient tachycardia, chest pain, bradycardia

GI: Increase or decrease in BP, nausea, vomiting

MS: Muscle pain

Contraindications: Hypersensitivity to ergot preparations, occlusion (peripheral, vascular), coronary artery disease, pregnancy, lactation, septic conditions, peptic ulcer, hypertension, children, renal, hepatic, cardiovascular disease

Pharmacokinetics:

Period of onset: Peak 30 min—3 hr; metabolised in liver, excreted as metabolites in faeces, crosses blood-brain barrier, excreted in breast milk

Interactions/incompatibilities:

• Effects of ergotamine may be potentiated by: erythromycin

• Increase vasoconstriction may occur with: concurrent use of β-blockers

NURSING CONSIDERATIONS

Assess:

• Baseline weight

• Cardiac rate and rhythm

Administer:

• At beginning of headache, dose must be titrated to patient response

• By sublingual route if possible for better, faster absorption

• With meals or after meals to avoid GI symptoms

• Only to women who are not pregnant; harm to fetus may occur

Perform/provide:

• Quiet, calm environment with decreased stimulation for noise, or bright light or excessive talking

Evaluate:

• Weight daily

• Peripheral oedema in feet, legs

• Therapeutic response: decrease in frequency, severity of headache

• For stress level, activity, recreation, coping mechanisms of patient

• Neurological status: level of consciousness blurring vision, nausea, vomiting, tingling in extremities that can precede the headache

• Ingestion of tyramine foods (pickled products, beer, wine, some cheese), food additives, preservatives, colourings, artificial sweeteners, chocolate, caffeine, which may precipitate these types of headaches

Teach patient/family:

• Not to use non-prescribed medications, serious drug interactions may occur

• Maintain dose at approved level, not to increase even if drug does not relieve headache

• Report side effects including increased vasoconstriction starting with cold extremities, then paraesthesia, weakness

• That an increase in headaches may occur when this drug is discontinued after long-term use

erythromycin (topical)

Stiemycin, Zineryt (combination product)
Func. class.: Antibacterial
Chem. class.: Macrolide antibiotic
Legal class.: POM

Action: Interferes with bacterial DNA replication to disrupt bacterial cell wall formation. Bacteriostatic
Uses: Acne vulgaris
Dosage and routes:
• *Adult and child:* Topical, apply to affected area twice daily
Available forms include: Topical solution 2%
Side effects/adverse reactions:
INTEG: Rash, urticaria, stinging, burning, pruritus, dry or oily skin
Contraindications: Hypersensitivity
Precautions: Pregnancy, lactation
NURSING CONSIDERATIONS
Administer:
• Enough medication to cover lesions completely
• After cleansing with soap, water before each application, dry well
Evaluate:
• Allergic reaction: burning, stinging, swelling, redness
• Therapeutic response: decrease in size, number of lesions
Teach patient/family:
• To apply wearing gloves to prevent further infection
• Avoid use of non-prescribed creams, ointments, lotions unless directed by clinician
• To wash hands before and after each application

erythromycin base, erythromycin ethylsuccinate, erythromycin lactobionate, erythromycin stearate, erythromycin estolate

Erythrocin, Erythroped, Erymax, Ilosone
Func. class.: Antibacterial
Chem. class.: Macrolide antibiotic
Legal class.: POM

Action: Broad spectrum bacteriostatic; interacts with phospholipids, penetrates cell wall; changes occur immediately in membrane
Uses: Wide range of infections due to Gram-positive and Gram-negative organisms in penicillin-sensitive patients or when due to *M. pneumoniae, B. pertussis, L. monocytogenes,* syphilis, Legionnaire's disease, *C. trachomatis Branhamella catarrhalis*
Dosage and routes:
Soft tissue infections
• *Adult and child over 8 yr:* By mouth 250−500 mg 6 hrly
• *Child 2−8 yr:* By mouth 250 mg 6 hrly
• *Up to 2 yr:* 125 mg 6 hrly
• *Adult and child:* IV 25 mg/kg daily in 4 divided doses. Increase to 50 mg/kg daily in severe infection. Dilute to 5 mg/ml with sodium chloride 0.9% and administer as IV infusion over 20−60 min
Syphilis
• 20 g over 10 days in divided doses
Available forms include: Base: tablets, enteric-coated 250, 500 mg; tablets, film-coated 250, 500 mg; capsules, enteric-coated 250 mg; estolate: tablets 500 mg, capsules 250 mg; suspension 125, 250 mg/5 ml; stearate:

tablets, film-coated 250, 500 mg; ethylsuccinate: tablets, film-coated, 500 mg suspension 125, 250, 500 mg/5 ml, sachets 125, 250, 500 mg

Lactobionate: injection 1 g

Side effects/adverse reactions:

INTEG: Rash, urticaria, pruritus

GI: Nausea, vomiting, diarrhoea, hepatotoxicity, abdominal pain, stomatitis, heartburn, anorexia, pruritus ani

GU: Vaginitis, moniliasis

EENT: Hearing loss, tinnitus

Contraindications: Hypersensitivity

Precautions: Pregnancy, hepatic disease

Pharmacokinetics: Peak 4 hr, duration 6 hr, half-life 1−3 hr, metabolised in liver, excreted in bile, faeces

Interactions/incompatibilities:

• Increased action of: oral anticoagulants, digoxin, theophylline, carbamazepine methylprednisolone, cyclosporin

• Decreased action of: clindamycin, penicillins

Clinical assessment:

• Liver studies: aspartate aminotransferase, alanine aminotransferase

Treatment of overdose: Withdraw drug, general supportive measures

NURSING CONSIDERATIONS

Assess:

• Bowel pattern

• Fluid balance

• Allergies before treatment; record allergies on drug chart, nursing documentation; notify all people giving drugs

• Culture and sensitivity before drug therapy is commenced; both may be repeated after treatment

Administer:

• Enteric-coated tablets may be given with food

Perform/provide:

• Adequate intake of fluids (2 litres) during diarrhoea episodes

Evaluate:

• Fluid balance report haematuria, oliguria in renal disease

• Urinalysis, protein, blood

• Bowel pattern, during treatment

• Skin eruptions, itching

• Respiratory status: rate, character, wheezing, tightness in chest; discontinue drug if these occur

Teach patient/family:

• Take oral drug with full glass of water; with food if GI symptoms occur

• Do not take with fruit juice

• Report sore throat, fever, fatigue; could indicate superimposed infection

• Notify nurse of diarrhoea

• Take at evenly spaced intervals; complete dosage regimen

---

estramustine phosphate

Estracyt

Func. class.: Antineoplastic

Chem. class.: Alkylating agent, oestrogen

Legal class.: POM

Action: Complex delivers mustine (alkylating agent) to oestrogen receptors

Uses: Prostate cancer

Dosage and routes:

• *Adult:* By mouth 0.14−1.4 g daily

Available forms include: Capsules 140 mg (as disodium salt)

Side effects/adverse reactions:

HAEM: Thrombocytopenia, leucopenia

GI: Nausea, vomiting, diarrhoea, hepatotoxicity

GU: Impotence, gynaecomastia, fluid retention

INTEG: Rash

CV: Myocardial infarction, hypertension, angina

Contraindications: Peptic ulcer, severe hepatic or cardiac disease

Precautions: Oedema, thromboembolic disorders, cardiac disorders, epilepsy, hypertension, diabetes mellitus

Pharmacokinetics:

Period of onset: Peak 1−2 hr, metabolised in liver, excreted in bile, half-life 20 hr (terminal)

Interactions/incompatibilities:
Should not be taken with milk, dairy products

Clinical assessment:
- Periodic blood count
- Liver function tests
- ECG before, during treatment

Treatment of overdose:
Blood products if necessary indicated by low blood count

NURSING CONSIDERATIONS

Assess:
- Fluid balance
- Weight before initial treatment then at regular intervals
- ECG and blood count

Administer:
- Orally with meals, adjust accordingly to response
- Suitable analgesic, antiemetic and diurectic when required
- Not to be taken with milk or dairy products

Perform/provide:
- Diet suitable to enhance each patient's good health

Evaluate:
- Therapeutic response; destruction of malignant cells, decreased malignant grown
- Input and output of fluids check for retention
- Side effects: nausea, vomiting, diarrhoea impotency, slight enlargement of breasts, fluid retention, rash, angina, myocardial infarction

Teach patient/family:
- That additional analgesia is available when required
- To report any chest pains or retention of urine immediately
- Not to take the drugs with milk or dairy products
- That nausea is often transient
- That body changes occur; impotence, and breast enlargement in men

---

ethacrynic acid

Edecrin
Func. class.: Loop diuretic
Chem. class.: Ketone derivative
Legal class.: POM

Action: Acts on loop of Henle by increasing excretion of chloride, sodium

Uses: Pulmonary oedema, oedema in congestive cardiac failure, liver disease, renal disease

Dosage and routes:
- *Adult:* By mouth 50−150 mg daily may give up to 400 mg daily; given as 2 equally divided doses
- *Child over 2 yr:* By mouth 25 mg, increased by 25 mg a day until desired effect occurs

Pulmonary oedema
- *Adult:* IV 50−100 mg given over several min or 0.5−1 mg/kg

Available forms include: Tablets 50 mg; powder for injection 50 mg

Side effects/adverse reactions:

GU: Polyuria, gynaecomastia, ejaculatory problems, renal failure, glycosuria

ELECT: Hypokalaemia, hypochloraemic alkalosis, hypomagnesaemia, hyperuricaemia, hypocalcaemia, hyponatraemia

CNS: Headache, fatigue, weakness, vertigo

GI: Nausea, diarrhoea, dry mouth, vomiting, anorexia, cramps, upset stomach, abdominal pain, acute pancreatitis, jaundice, GI bleeding

EENT: Loss of hearing, ear pain, tinnitus, blurred vision
INTEG: Rash, pruritus, purpura, Stevens-Johnson syndrome, sweating
MS: Cramps, arthritis, stiffness
ENDO: Hyperglycaemia
HAEM: Thrombocytopenia, agranulocytosis, leucopenia, neutropenia
CV: Chest pain, hypotension, circulatory collapse, ECG changes
Contraindications: Hypersensitivity to sulphonamides, anuria, hypovolaemia, children less than 2 yr, lactation, electrolyte depletion
Precautions: Dehydration, ascites, severe renal disease, pregnancy
Pharmacokinetics:
Period of onset: Onset ½ hr, peak 2 hr, duration 6−8 hr
IV: Onset 5 min, peak 15−30 min, duration 2 hr
Excreted by kidneys, half-life 30−70 min
Interactions/incompatibilities:
• Increased toxicity: lithium, non-depolarising skeletal muscle relaxants, digitalis, aminoglycosides, corticosteroids
• Increased anticoagulant activity
Clinical assessment:
• Electrolytes: potassium, sodium, chloride urea, blood sugar, serum creatinine, full blood count, pH and blood gases
Treatment of overdose: Gastric lavage if taken orally, monitor electrolytes, administer dextrose in saline

NURSING CONSIDERATIONS
Assess:
• Baseline vital signs, weight, fluid balance
Administer:
• In morning to avoid interference with sleep if using drug as a diuretic
• Potassium replacement if potassium is less than 3.0 mmol/litre
• With food, if nausea occurs, absorption may be decreased slightly
Evaluate:
• Weight, fluid balance daily to determine fluid loss; effect of drug may be decreased if used daily
• Rate, depth, rhythm of respiration, effect of exertion
• BP lying, standing; postural hypotension may occur
• Glucose in urine if patient is diabetic
• Improvement in oedema of feet, legs, sacral area daily if medication is being used in congestive cardiac failure
• Improvement in CVP 8 hrly
• Signs of metabolic acidosis: drowsiness, restlessness
• Signs of hypokalaemia: postural hypotension, malaise, fatigue, tachycardia, leg cramps, weakness
• Rashes, temperature elevation daily
• Confusion, especially in elderly, take safety precautions if needed
Teach patient/family:
• Increase fluid intake 2−3 litres daily unless contraindicated: to rise slowly from lying or sitting position
• Adverse reactions: muscle cramps, weakness, nausea, dizziness
• Take with food or milk for GI symptoms
• Take early in day to prevent nocturia

ethambutol HCl

Myambutol, combination products
Func. class.: Antitubercular
Chem. class.: Di-isopropyl-ethylene diamide derivative
Legal class.: POM

Action: Inhibits RNA synthesis,

decreases tubercle bacilli replication

Uses: Pulmonary tuberculosis as an adjunctive. Should only be used in conjunction with other antitubercular drugs

Dosage and routes:
• *Adult:* By mouth 15 mg/kg daily as a single dose
• *Child over 6 yr:* Initially 25 mg/kg daily for 60 days then 15 mg/kg daily
• In impaired renal function the dose may need to be reduced according to blood levels (2−5 mcg/1 ml)

Retreatment
• *Adult and child:* By mouth 25 mg/kg daily as single dose for 2 months with at least 1 other drug, then decrease to 15 mg/kg daily as single dose

Available forms include: Tablets 100, 400 mg; in combination with isoniazid, tablets 200, 250, 300, 365 mg

Side effects/adverse reactions:
INTEG: Dermatitis, photosensitivity
CV: Congestive cardiac failure, dysrhythmias
CNS: Headache, anxiety, drowsiness, tremors, convulsions, lethargy, depression, confusion, psychosis, aggression, numbness, paraesthesia
EENT: Blurred vision, optic neuritis, photophobia, colour blindness
HAEM: Megaloblastic anaemia, vitamin B_{12}, folic acid deficiency

Contraindications: Hypersensitivity, optic neuritis child less than 6 yr, elderly

Precautions: Pregnancy, renal disease, diabetic, retinopathy, cataracts, ocular defects

Pharmacokinetics:
Period of onset: Peak 2−4 hr, half-life 3 hr; metabolised in liver, excreted in urine (unchanged drug/inactive metabolites, faeces)

Interactions/incompatibilities:
• Increased toxicity: aminoglycosides, cisplatin, aluminium salts

Clinical assessment:
• Liver studies every week
• Renal status before therapy and every month: urea, creatinine
• Full ophthalmic examination including ophthalmoscopy, colour vision, periphery and visual acuity before and during treatment

NURSING CONSIDERATIONS

Assess:
• Urinalysis: output, specific gravity

Administer:
• After samples sent for culture and sensitivity every month to detect resistance
• With meals to decrease GI symptoms
• Anti-emetic if vomiting occurs

Perform/provide:
• Storage of drug at controlled room temperature (15−30°C); prevent access of moisture

Evaluate:
• Ocular toxicity: blurred vision, colour blindness
• Mental status often: affect, mood, behavioural changes; psychosis may occur
• Hepatic status: decreased appetite, jaundice, dark urine, fatigue

Teach patient/family:
• That compliance with dosage schedule, length is necessary
• That scheduled appointments must be kept or relapse may occur
• Report any visual changes at once

ethinyloestradiol ▼

Func. class.: Oestrogen
Chem. class.: Synthetic oestrogen
Legal class.: POM

Action: Oestrogens are needed for adequate functioning of female reproductive system; affects release of pituitary gonadotrophins, inhibits ovulation, promotes adequate calcium use in bone structures

Uses: Menopause, primary amenorrhoea, hereditary haemorrhagic telangiectasia

Dosage and routes:

Menopause
• *Adult:* By mouth 10−20 mcg daily 3 weeks on, 1 week off

Primary amenorrhoea
• *Adult:* By mouth 10 mcg on alternate days to maximum 50 mcg daily, with progestrogen for last days of the month

Haemorrhagic telangiectasia
• *Adult:* By mouth 0.5−1 mg daily

Available forms include: Tablets 10 mcg, 20 mcg, 50 mcg, 1 mg

Side effects/adverse reactions:

CNS: Dizziness, headache, migraine, depression

CV: Hypotension, thrombophlebitis, oedema, thromboembolism, stroke, pulmonary embolism, myocardial infarction

GI: Nausea, vomiting, diarrhoea, anorexia, pancreatitis, cramps, constipation, increased appetite, increased weight, cholestatic jaundice

EENT: Contact lens intolerance, increased myopia, astigmatism

GU: Amenorrhoea, cervical erosion, breakthrough bleeding, dysmenorrhoea, vaginal candidiasis, breast changes, gynaecomastia, testicular atrophy, impotence

INTEG: Rash, urticaria, acne, hirsutism, alopecia, oily skin, seborrhoea, purpura, chloasma

META: Folic acid deficiency, hypercalcaemia, hyperglycaemia

Contraindications: Breast cancer, thromboembolic disorders, oestrogen-dependent neoplasm, genital bleeding (abnormal, undiagnosed), pregnancy

Precautions: Hypertension, asthma, blood dyscrasias, gallbladder disease, congestive cardiac failure, diabetes mellitus, bone disease, depression, migraine headache, convulsive disorders, hepatic disease, renal disease, family history of cancer of breast or reproductive tract lactation

Pharmacokinetics: Metabolised in the liver, excreted in urine, excreted in breast milk

Interactions/incompatibilities:
• Decreased action of: anticoagulants, oral hypoglycaemics
• Toxicity: tricyclic antidepressants
• Decreased action of this drug: anticonvulsants, barbiturates, phenylbutazone, rifampicin
• Increased action of: corticosteroids

NURSING CONSIDERATIONS

Assess:
• Baseline BP, weight, urinalysis (in diabetics)

Administer:
• Titrated dose, use lowest effective dose
• With food or milk to decrease GI symptoms

Evaluate:
• BP 4 hrly, watch for increase caused by water and sodium retention
• Fluid balance, be alert for decreasing urinary output and increasing oedema
• Therapeutic response: absence of breast engorgement, reversal of

menopause, or decrease in tumour size in prostatic cancer
• Oedema, hypertension, cardiac symptoms, jaundice, hypercalcaemia
• Mental status: affect, mood, behavioural changes, aggression
Teach patient/family:
• To weigh weekly, report gain more than 2.5 kg

ethosuximide

Zarontin, Emeside
Func. class.: Anticonvulsant
Chem. class.: Succinimide
Legal class.: POM

Action: Inhibits spike wave formation in absence seizures (petit mal), decreases amplitude, frequency, duration, spread of discharge in minor motor seizures
Uses: Absence seizures, myoclonic seizures, atypical seizures
Dosage and routes:
• *Adult:* By mouth 250 mg twice a day initially; may increase by 250 mg every 4−7 days, not to exceed 2 g daily
• *Child under 6 yr:* By mouth 250 mg daily, adjusted as required
• *Child over 6 yr:* 500 mg daily, adjusted as required to a maximum of 2 g daily
Available forms include: Capsules 250 mg; syrup 250 mg/5 ml
Side effects/adverse reactions:
HAEM: Agranulocytosis, aplastic anaemia, thrombocytopenia, leucocytosis, eosinophilia, pancytopenia
CNS: Drowsiness, dizziness, fatigue, euphoria, lethargy, anxiety, aggressiveness, irritability, depression, insomnia
GI: Nausea, vomiting, heartburn, anorexia, diarrhoea, abdominal pain, cramps, constipation
GU: Vaginal bleeding, haematuria, renal damage
INTEG: Urticaria, pruritic erythema, hirsutism, Stevens-Johnson syndrome, systemic lupus erythematosus
EENT: Myopia, gum hypertrophy, tongue swelling, blurred vision
Contraindications: Hypersensitivity to succinimide derivatives, porphyrias
Precautions: Lactation, pregnancy, hepatic disease, renal disease
Pharmacokinetics:
Period of onset: Peak 1−7 hr, steady state 4−7 days, metabolised by liver, excreted in urine, bile, faeces, half-life 24−60 hr
Interactions/incompatibilities:
• Antagonist effect: tricyclic antidepressants (imipramine, doxepin)
• Decreased effects of: oestrogens, oral contraceptives
Clinical assessment:
• Renal studies: urinalysis, blood urea nitrogen, urine creatinine
• Blood studies: full blood count, haematocrit, Hb, reticulocyte counts every week for 4 weeks, then every month
• Hepatic studies: aspartate aminotransferase, alanine aminotransferase, bilirubin, creatinine
• Drug levels during initial treatment, therapeutic range (40−80 mcg/ml)
Lab. test interferences:
Increase: Coombs' test
Treatment of overdose: Lavage, activated charcoal, monitor electrolytes, vital signs
NURSING CONSIDERATIONS
Assess:
• Eye problems: need for ophthalmic examinations before, during, after treatment (slit lamp, ophthalmoscopy, tonometry)

Administer:
• With food, milk to decrease GI symptoms

Perform/provide:
• Frequent sips of water, mouth-washes to relieve dry mouth
• Assistance with ambulation during early part of treatment; dizziness occurs

Evaluate:
• Allergic reaction: red raised rash, exfoliative dermatitis; if these occur, drug should be discontinued
• Blood dyscrasias: fever, sore throat, bruising, rash, jaundice
• Toxicity: bone marrow depression, nausea, vomiting, ataxia, diplopia, cardiovascular collapse, Stevens-Johnson syndrome
• Therapeutic response: decreased seizure activity, document on patient's care plan
• Mental status: mood, alertness, affect, behavioural changes; if mental status changes notify clinician

Teach patient/family:
• To carry ID card or Medic-Alert bracelet stating drugs taken, condition, GP's name, phone number
• To avoid driving, other activities that require alertness
• To avoid alcohol ingestion, CNS depressants; increased sedation may occur
• Not to discontinue medication quickly after long-term use
• All aspects of drug: action, use, side effects, adverse reactions, when to notify clinician

etidronate disodium

Didronel
Func. class.: Parathyroid agent (calcium regulator)
Chem. class.: Diphosphonate
Legal class.: POM

Action: Reduces bone resorption of calcium

Uses: Paget's disease, hypercalcaemia of malignancy

Dosage and routes:
Paget's disease
• *Adult:* By mouth 5 mg/kg daily for up to 6 months. Doses above 10 mg/kg daily for up to 3 months. Doses above 20 mg/kg daily are not recommended

Hypercalcaemica of malignancy
• *IV infusion:* 7.5 mg/kg daily for 3 days, repeat course once if necessary after at least 7 days
• *By mouth:* On day after last IV dose 20 mg/kg daily for 30 days, maximum treatment period is 90 days
• Avoid food for at least 2 hr before and after oral treatment — particularly calcium containing products

Available forms include: Tablets 200 mg; injection 50 mg/ml

Side effects/adverse reactions:
GI: Nausea, diarrhoea
MS: Bone pain, hypocalcaemia, decreased mineralisation of non-affected bones
INTEG: Angioneurotic oedema/urticaria, pruritus rush

Precautions: Pregnancy, lactation, enterocolitis, children, fractures, restricted vitamin D/calcium

Pharmacokinetics: Not metabolised, excreted in urine/faeces, therapeutic response: 1—3 months

Interactions/incompatibilities:
• Antacids reduced absorption

• Aminoglycoside: severe hypo-calcaemia

Clinical assessment:

• Blood urea nitrogen, creatinine, phosphate, urine hydroxyproline uric acid, chloride, electrolytes, pH, urine calcium, magnesium, alkaline phosphatase, urinalysis, calcium, vitamin D

• Muscle spasm, laryngospasm, paraesthesia, facial twitching, nutritional status with regard calcium and phosphate, colic; may indicate hypocalcaemia

Treatment of overdose: Symptoms of hypocalcaemia; withdraw drug and correct hypocalcaemia with IV calcium gluconate

NURSING CONSIDERATIONS

Administer:

• On empty stomach with water 2 hr before meals

Evaluate:

• Fluid balance check for decreased output in renal patients

• Nutritional status, diet for sources of vitamin D (milk, some seafood), calcium (dairy products, dark green vegetables), phosphates — adequate intake is necessary

• Persistent nausea or diarrhoea

Teach patient/family:

• Avoid non-prescribed products

• All aspects of drug: action, side effects, dose, when to notify clinician

• Therapeutic response may take 1−3 months, effects persist for months after drug is discontinued

• Adequate intake of calcium, vitamin D is necessary

• Teach patient about dietary requirements

etodolac

Lodine

Func. class.: Non-steroidal anti-inflammatory drug

Chem. class.: Indoleacetic acid derivative

Legal class.: POM

Action: Inhibits prostaglandin synthesis by decreasing enzyme needed for biosynthesis; possesses analgesic and anti-inflammatory, antipyretic actions

Uses: Acute or long-term treatment of rheumatoid arthritis

Dosage and routes:

• By mouth 200 mg twice daily or 400 mg once daily; maximum dose 600 mg daily

Available forms include: Tablets 200 mg; capsules 200, 300 mg

Side effects/adverse reactions:

GI: Discomfort, bleeding, nausea, diarrhoea

CV: Angioneurotic oedema; congestive cardiac failure in elderly

CNS: Headache, dizziness, vertigo

RESP: Asthma

INTEG: Rashes

EENT: Hearing disturbances, tinnitus

META: Fluid retention

RENAL: Acute renal failure; papillary necrosis or interstitial fibrosis leading to chronic renal failure

Contraindications: Active peptic ulceration, aspirin/anti-inflammatory induced allergy or history of peptic ulcer disease or GI bleeding

Precautions: Elderly patients, asthma, renal or hepatic impairment, pregnancy

Interactions/incompatibilities:

Increased effect of: salicylates, anticoagulants, antihypertensives, cardiac glycocides, diuretics, captopril, enalpril, methotrexate

Clinical assessment:
- Hearing tests
- Check history of asthma, peptic ulcer, allergies
- H_2 receptor blockers if essential for patient with peptic ulcer
- Evaluate response and level of side effects
- Liver function tests, aspartate aminotransferase, alanine aminotransferase
- Renal function — urea, creatinine, Hb

Lab. test interference:
False positive: Bilirubin in urine
Treatment of overdose: No data available. Gastric lavage, activated charcoal and supportive treatment
NURSING CONSIDERATIONS
Administer:
- With food
- Lowest effective dose

Perform/provide:
- Help with mobility
- Safe environment (dizzy/vertigo)

Evaluate:
- Side effects such as tinnitus, bleeding
- Toxicity
- Swelling, mobility, stiffness and pain

Teach patient/family:
- To take with or after food
- Not to take other drugs unless specifically prescribed, especially aspirin or other NSAID
- No alcohol to be taken
- Report ringing in the ears, reduced urine output, abdominal pain, joint pain increase
- Report unresolved indigestion or black tarry stools

etomidate

Hypnomidate
Func. class.: Anaesthetic, general
Chem. class.: Nonbarbiturate hypnotic
Legal class.: POM

Action: Acts at level of reticular-activating system to produce anaesthesia

Uses: Induction of general anaesthesia

Dosage and routes:
• *Adult and child:* Slow IV 300 mcg/kg; IV infusion 100 mcg/kg/min until anaesthetised

Available forms include: Injection IV 2, 125 mg/ml

Side effects/adverse reactions:
GI: Nausea, vomiting (postoperatively)
CNS: Tonic movements, myoclonic movements, averting movements, pain on injection
CV: Tachycardia, hypotension, hypertension, bradycardia
ENDO: Decreases steroid production
RESP: Laryngospasm

Contraindications: Hypersensitivity, labour/delivery, reduced adrenocortical function

Precautions: Pregnancy, lactation

Pharmacokinetics:
IV: Onset 20 sec, peak 1 min, duration 3−5 min; half-life 75 min, metabolised in liver, excreted in urine

Clinical assessment:
• Plasma cortisol levels if administered over several hours (5−20 mcg/100 ml normal level of cortisol)
• Corticosteroids for severe hypotension
• Etomidate should not be used for maintenance anaesthesia

Treatment of overdose: General supportive measures

NURSING CONSIDERATIONS
Assess:
• Starvation status
• Degree of pain during adminis-tration
• Do not mix with any other drug
Administer:
• IV slowly under anaesthetic supervision
• Only with emergency trolley/ resuscitation equipment at hand
Evaluate:
• Vital signs every 10 min during IV administration
• Degree of extraneous muscle movement following injection
• Level of anaesthesia after 3−5 mins
• Cardiac and respiratory status
• Observe ECG for dysrhythmias
• IV slowly only, muscular twitch-ing is reduced with fentanyl before anaesthesia induction
• Increasing or decreasing heart rate or dysrhythmias shown on ECG
Teach/patient:
• Effect of drug; drowsiness followed by sleep

---

etoposide

Vepesid
Func. class.: Antineoplastic
Chem. class.: Semisynthetic podophyllotoxin
Legal class.: POM

Action: Inhibits mitotic activity through metaphase to mitosis; also inhibits cells from entering mitosis, depresses DNA, RNA synthesis
Uses: Leukaemias, lung, tes-ticular cancer, lymphomas, neuroblastoma
Dosage and routes:
Dosage dependent on cancer being treated and local protocols
• *Adult:* IV 60−120 mg/m^2 daily for 5 days. Do not repeat within 3 weeks. Dilute injection to 0.25 mg/ml with sodium chloride 0.9% and give over 30 min
• By mouth 120−240 mg/m^2 daily for 5 days. Do not repeat within 3 weeks
Available forms include: Injection IV 20 mg/ml; capsules 50, 100 mg
Side effects/adverse reactions:
HAEM: Thrombocytopenia, leucopenia, myelosuppression, anaemia
GI: Nausea, vomiting, anorexia, hepatotoxicity
INTEG: Rash, alopecia, phlebitis
RESP: Bronchospasm
CV: Hypotension
CNS: Headache, fever
Contraindications: Hypersensi-tivity, bone marrow depression, severe hepatic disease, severe renal disease, bacterial infection
Precautions: Renal disease, hep-atic disease, lactation, pregnancy, children, gout
Pharmacokinetics: Half-life 3 hr, terminal 15 hr, metabolised in liver, excreted in urine
Interactions/incompatibilities:
• Do not use with radiation
• Do not dilute injection with dextrose solution
Clinical assessment:
• Full blood count, differential, platelet count weekly; withhold drug if WBC is less than 4000 or platelet count is less than 100,000; notify clinician of results
• Pulmonary function tests, chest X-ray studies before, during ther-apy; chest X-ray film should be obtained every 2 weeks during treatment
• Renal function studies: blood urea nitrogen, serum uric acid, urine creatinine clearance, elec-trolytes before, during therapy
• Antibiotics, antispasmodics, analgesics as appropriate

• Liver function tests before, during therapy (bilirubin, aspartate aminotransferase, alanine aminotransferase, lactic dehydrogenase) as needed or monthly
• Transfusion for anaemia

NURSING CONSIDERATIONS

Perform/provide:

• Strict asepsis for all procedures; protective isolation if WBC levels are low
• Special care of skin
• Increase fluid intake to 2−3 litres daily to prevent urate deposits, calculi formation
• Warm compresses at injection site for inflammation, avoid extravasation
• Pain relief as required

Evaluate:

• Nausea and vomiting (worse with oral medication)
• Fluid balance, report fall in urine output of 30 ml/hr
• Bleeding: haematuria, bruising or petechiae, mucosa or orifices 8 hrly
• Dyspnoea, rales, unproductive cough, chest pain, tachypnoea, fatigue, increased pulse, pallor, lethargy
• Food preferences; list likes, dislikes
• Effects of alopecia on body image; discuss feelings about body changes
• Oedema in feet, joint pain, stomach pain, shaking
• Inflammation of mucosa, breaks in skin
• Yellowing of skin and sclera, dark urine, clay-coloured stools, itchy skin, abdominal pain, fever, diarrhoea
• Buccal cavity 8 hrly for dryness, sores or ulceration, white patches, oral pain, bleeding, dysphagia
• Local irritation, pain, burning, discolouration at injection site
• Symptoms indicating severe allergic reaction: rash, pruritus, urticaria, purpuric skin lesions, itching, flushing

Teach patient/family:

• About protective isolation precautions and rationale
• To report any complaints or side effects to nurse or clinician
• To report any changes in breathing or coughing
• That hair may be lost during treatment; a wig or hairpiece may be available on NHS; tell patient that new hair may be different in colour, texture

---

etretinate

Tigason
Func. class.: Antipsoriatic, systemic
Chem. class.: Retinoid
Legal class.: POM

Action: Reverses hyperkeratotic skin changes

Uses: Severe, extensive resistant psoriasis; palmo-plantar pustular psoriasis; severe congenital ichthyosis; keratosis follicularis

Dosage and routes:

• *Adult:* By mouth 0.75−1 mg/kg daily in divided doses, not to exceed 75 mg/day; maintenance dose 0.25−0.51 mg/kg daily

Available forms include: Capsules 10, 25 mg

Side effects/adverse reactions:

INTEG: Alopecia; peeling of palms, soles, fingertips; itching; rash; dryness; red scaling face; bruising; sunburn; pyogenic granuloma; paronychia; onycholysis; perspiration change

CNS: Fatigue, headache, dizziness, fever, pain, anxiety, amnesia, depression

EENT: Eye irritation, pain, double vision, change in lacrimation, earache, otitis externa

GI: Anorexia, abdominal pain, nausea, hepatitis, constipation,

diarrhoea, flatulence
CV: Oedema, CV obstruction, atrial fibrillation, chest pain, coagulation disorders
RESP: Dyspnoea, cough
GU: WBC in urine, proteinuria, glycosuria, increased blood urea nitrogen, creatinine, haematuria, casts, ketonuria, haemoglobinuria
ELECT: Increase or decrease potassium, calcium, phosphate, sodium, chloride
MS: Hyperostosis, bone pain, cramps, myalgia, gout, hypertonia
Contraindications: Pregnancy; hepatic or renal impairment
Precautions: Women of childbearing age; exclude possibility of pregnancy in subsequent 2 yr, children
Pharmacokinetics: 99% plasma protein binding; excreted in bile, urine; terminal half-life 120 days; accumulates in fatty tissue
Interactions/incompatibilities:
• Increased absorption of etretinate: milk or high lipid diet
Clinical assessment:
• Liver function and blood lipids (fasting value) measured at start of therapy, after first month of administration and at 3 monthly intervals thereafter
• Blood sugar levels should be checked frequently at beginning of treatment period
• Investigate any atypical musculo-skeletal symptoms; possible etretinate-induced bone changes

NURSING CONSIDERATIONS
Evaluate:
• Neurological status: headache, nausea, vomiting, visual disturbance, papilloedema
• Visual disturbance: blurring, poor nocturnal vision, decreased visual acuity. If these symptoms develop the drug must be discontinued and ophthalmic opinion sought

• Response to treatment indicated by decrease in scaling, itching and resolution of psoriasis
Teach patient/family:
• To take with food
• Not to take if pregnancy is suspected. A reliable form of contraception must be used for 2 yr after treatment is complete for women of child bearing age
• Not to take vitamin A supplements
• Wearing contact lens may be difficult/uncomfortable
• Not to donate blood either during or for at least 2 yr following discontinuation of therapy

---

famotidine

Pepcid PM
Func. class.: H_2-receptor antagonist
Chem. class.: Substituted thiazole
Legal class.: POM

Action: Competitively inhibits histamine at histamine H_2 receptor site, decreasing gastric secretion while pepsin remains at stable level
Uses: Short-term treatment of active duodenal and benign gastric ulcer, maintenance therapy for duodenal ulcer, Zollinger-Ellison syndrome, multiple endocrine adenomas
Dosage and routes:
Duodenal and gastric ulcer
• *Adult:* By mouth 40 mg at night for 4−8 weeks
Prophylaxis of duodenal ulcer relapse
• 20 mg at night
Zollinger-Ellison syndrome
• *Adult:* By mouth 20 mg 4 times a day increasing to maximum 800 mg daily as necessary
Available forms include: Tablets 20, 40 mg
Side effects/adverse reactions:

HAEM: Thrombocytopenia
CNS: Headache, dizziness, paraesthesia, seizure, depression, anxiety, somnolence, insomnia, fever
GI: Constipation, nausea, vomiting, anorexia, cramps, abnormal liver enzymes
RESP: Bronchospasm
EENT: Taste change, tinnitus, orbital oedema
INTEG: Rash
MS: Myalgia, arthralgia
GU: Decreased libido
Contraindications: Hypersensitivity
Precautions: Pregnancy, lactation, children, severe renal disease, severe hepatic function, elderly
Pharmacokinetics:
Period of onset: Peak 1–3 hr, plasma protein-binding 15%–20%; metabolised in liver (active metabolites), excreted by kidneys, half-life 2.5–3.5 hr
Clinical assessment:
• Blood counts during therapy, watch for decreasing platelets, if low, therapy may need to be discontinued and restarted after haematologic recovery

NURSING CONSIDERATIONS
Assess:
• Baseline pulse
• Fluid balance
Evaluate:
• Blood dyscrasias (thrombocytopenia): bruising, fatigue, bleeding, poor healing
Perform/provide:
• Monitor pulse frequently during administration
Teach patient/family:
• That drug must be continued for prescribed time to be effective
• To report bleeding, bruising, fatigue, malaise since blood dyscrasias do occur
• Discuss possibility of decreased libido, reversible after discontinuing therapy
• Appropriate dietary advice

---

fat emulsions

Intralipid 10%, 20%
Func. class.: Nutrition, caloric
Chem. class.: Fatty acid, long chain
Legal class.: POM

Action: Required for energy, heat production; consist of neutral triglycerides, primarily unsaturated fatty acids plus variable amounts of vitamin E
Uses: Increase calorie intake as part of balanced feeding regimen
Dosage and routes:
Adjunct to total parenteral nutrition
• *Adult:* IV infusion 500–1000 ml/24 hr 10%–20% maximum rate, 500 ml/5 hr 20%, 500 ml/3 hr 10%. Maximum 3 g fat/kg/24 hr
• *Infant:* 0.02–0.17 g fat/kg/hr; small for age/low birthweight, initially 0.5 g fat/kg/24 hr, maximum 2 g fat/kg/24 hr. Administer over 20 hr; measure blood electrolytes 4 hr later
Available forms include: Injection IV 10%, 20%
Side effects/adverse reactions:
CNS: Dizziness, headache, drowsiness, focal seizures, pyrexia
CV: Shock
GI: Nausea, vomiting, hepatomegaly, abnormal liver function tests
RESP: Dyspnoea, fat in lung tissue
HAEM: Hyperlipidaemia, hypercoagulation, thrombocytopenia, leucopenia, leucocytosis
Contraindications: Hypersensitivity, hyperlipidaemia, lipid necrosis, acute pancreatitis accompanied by hyperlipidaemia
Precautions: Severe liver disease, diabetes mellitus, thrombocytopenia, gastric ulcers, premature and term newborns
Interactions/incompatibilities:
• Do not mix with any drug, electrolytes, solutions, vitamin unless

prepared by pharmacy e.g. TPN solutions

Clinical assessment:
• Triglycerides, free fatty acid levels, platelet counts daily to prevent fat overload, thrombocytopaenia
• Liver function studies: aspartate aminotransferase, alanine aminotransferase

NURSING CONSIDERATIONS
Administer:
• Alone; do not mix with any drug, solution vitamin or electrolyte
• Carefully due to tendency of solution to coagulate and clog IV line
• Use infusion pump; do not use in-line filter; clogging will occur
Perform/provide:
• Change IV tubing at each infusion: infection may occur with old tubing
Evaluate:
• Therapeutic response: increased weight
• Nutritional status: calorie count by dietician
Teach patient/family:
• Reason for use of lipids
• How to care for parenteral feeding and IV line if on long-term therapy e.g. TPN

---

fenbufen ▼

Lederfen, Lederfen F
Func. class.: Non-steroidal anti-inflammatory drug
Chem. class.: Propionic acid derivative
Legal class.: POM

Action: Has both analgesic and anti-inflammatory effects
Uses: Pain and inflammation in rheumatic disease and other acute musculoskeletal disorders
Dosage and routes: By mouth 300 mg in morning and 600 mg at night or 450 mg twice daily

Available forms include: Tablets 300, 450 mg; effervescent tablets 450 mg; capsules 300 mg
Side effects/adverse reactions:
GI: Discomfort, bleeding, nausea, diarrhoea
CV: Angioneurotic oedema, congestive cardiac failure in elderly
CNS: Headache, dizziness, vertigo
RESP: Asthma
INTEG: Rashes
EENT: Hearing disturbances, tinnitus
META: Fluid retention
RENAL: Acute renal failure; papillary necrosis or interstitial fibrosis leading to chronic renal failure
Contraindications: Active peptic ulceration
Precautions: Elderly patients, history of peptic ulceration, allergic disorders, asthma, renal or hepatic impairment, pregnancy
Pharmacokinetics: Converted to active metabolites with half-lives of approximately 10 hr; these undergo hepatic metabolism before excretion in the urine
Interactions/incompatibilities:
• Increased risk of side effects: salicylates, anticoagulants, antihypertensives, cardiac glycosides, diuretics, captopril, enalapril, methotrexate
Clinical assessment:
• Hearing tests in impaired patients
• Check history of peptic ulcer, asthma and any allergies
• Renal function: urea, creatinine before, during treatment if problem anticipated
• Liver function tests: aspartate aminotransferase, alanine, bilirubin, alkaline phosphatase before, during treatment if problem anticipated
Treatment of overdose: Gastric lavage, symptomatic treatment
NURSING CONSIDERATIONS

Assess:
• Fluid balance (renal failure/oedema)
• Hepatic and renal studies, including fluid balance and oedema
• Respiration (asthma)
• Audio and visual ability, before and during treatment

Administer:
• Tablets and capsules orally with food or milk to decrease gastric irritation. Effervescent tablets in half a glass of water

Perform/provide:
• Help with mobility

Evaluate:
• Therapeutic response: decreased pain, stiffness, swelling in joints; increased mobility
• Signs of toxicity
• Rashes, erythema multiforme, tinnitus

Teach patient/family:
• That therapeutic response may not be immediate (2–4 weeks)
• To take other medication only if directed by clinician especially aspirin and other NSAIDs
• To report any rashes, ringing in ears, blood in stools or vomiting
• To report changes in urinary patterns

---

fenfluramine HCl

Ponderax Pacaps
Func. class.: Appetite suppressant
Chem. class.: Amphetamine derivative
Legal class.: POM

Action: Increases release of noradrenaline, dopamine in cerebral cortex to reticular activating system
Uses: Treatment of severe obesity, including severe obesity associated with maturity-onset diabetes
Dosage and routes:
• *Adult:* 60 mg capsule daily, ½ hr before a meal
Available forms include: Capsules 60 mg

Side effects/adverse reactions:
CNS: Insomnia, talkativeness, dizziness, drowsiness, headache, irritability
GI: Nausea, vomiting, anorexia, dry mouth, diarrhoea, constipation, abdominal pain
GU: Impotence, change in libido, dysuria, urinary frequency
CV: Palpitations, tachycardia, hypertension, hypotension
INTEG: Urticaria, rash, burning, sweating, chills, fever

Contraindications: Hypersensitivity to sympathomimetic amine, glaucoma, drug abuse, cardiovascular disease, alcoholism, epilepsy, depression
Precautions: Diabetes mellitus, hypertension, pregnancy, lactation, elderly

Pharmacokinetics:
Period of onset: Onset 1–2 min, duration 4–6 hr, metabolised by liver, excreted by kidneys

Interactions/incompatibilities:
• Hypertensive crisis: MAOIs or within 21 days of MAOIs
• Increased effect of this drug: acetazolamide, antacids, sodium bicarbonate, ascorbic acid, ammonium chloride, phenothiazines, haloperidol, antidepressants
• Decreased effects of this drug: barbiturates
• Decrease effects of: guanethidine, other antihypertensives

Clinical assessment:
• Full blood count; urinalysis; in diabetes, blood sugar, urine sugar, insulin changes may need to be made since eating will increase
• Height, growth rate in children (may be decreased)

Treatment of overdose: Administer fluids, haemodialysis or peritoneal dialysis; antihypertensive for increased BP; ammonium chloride for increased excretion

NURSING CONSIDERATIONS

Assess:
• Pulse, blood pressure and respirations before treatment
• Weight before, during and after treatment
• Diet
• Effect due to other drugs taken; antihypertensives check these patients more often

Administer:
• For obesity only if patient is on weight reduction programme, including dietary changes, exercise; patient will develop tolerance and weight loss won't occur without additional methods
• Orally ½ hour before a meal
• Do not give late in the day to avoid interference with sleep

Perform/provide:
• Frequent drinks to prevent a dry mouth
• Close support and supervision, especially with diet regime. (Weight reducing programme)

Evaluate:
• Therapeutic response: effective weight loss
• Side effects: insomnia, talkativeness dry mouth, diarrhoea palpitation, tachycardia
• If no weight loss occurs discontinue drug slowly
• Mental status: mood, alertness, affect, stimulation, insomnia, aggressiveness may occur
• Physical dependency: should not be used for extended time; dose should be discontinued gradually
• Withdrawal symptoms: headache, nausea, vomiting, muscle pain, weakness
• Drug tolerance will develop after long-term use
• Dosage should not be increased if tolerance develops
• Any other medication, the effect of fenfluamine may be increased

or decrease or it may decrease to effects of other drug—antihypertensives

Teach patient/family:
• To follow suitable diet and seek support if necessary
• Avoid foods that may increase irritability e.g. coffee, chocolate
• To combine diet with exercise and rest
• That alcohol should be avoided
• To avoid driving or use of machinery until therapy established
• To take other medication only if directed by clinician
• To discontinue treatment *after* six months. Drug should be tapered off slowly over several weeks

---

fenofibrate ▼

Lipantil
Func. class.: Hypolipidaemic agent
Chem. class.: Isobutyric acid derivative
Legal class.: POM

Action: Precise mechanism of action is unclear. Lowers LDL- and VLDL-cholesterol and triglycerides. Increases HDL-cholesterol
Uses: Treatment of patients with severe hyperlipidaemia (Types IIa, IIb, III, IV, V) unresponsive to diet

Dosage and routes:
• *Adult:* By mouth initially 300 mg daily in divided doses with food. Maintenance dose usually in the range 200–400 mg daily
• *Children:* 5 mg/kg body-weight daily
Available forms include: Capsules 100 mg

Side effects/adverse reactions:
GI: Gastro-intestinal disturbances, elevated liver enzymes
INTEG: Skin reactions

CNS: Headache, fatigue, vertigo
MS: Muscle cramps
GU: Sexual asthenia
Contraindications: Severe liver dysfunction, existing gall bladder disease, severe renal disorders, pregnancy, lactation, hypersensitivity
Precautions: Renal impairment. Discontinue if an adequate response is not achieved in 3 months
Pharmacokinetics: Rapidly and well absorbed; rapidly metabolised in liver to active metabolites, chiefly fenofibric acid. Drug and metabolites extensively protein bound. Plasma half-life 27 hr. Excreted in urine
Interactions/incompatibilities:
• Increased effect of oral anti-coagulants and, possibly, other protein-bound drugs
Clinical assessment:
• Lipid profile
Treatment of overdose: Gastric lavage and supportive care
NURSING CONSIDERATIONS
Assess:
• Serum lipids
Administer:
• With food
Evaluate:
• For nausea and abdominal discomfort
Teach patient/family:
• That other risk factors should be decreased: high fat diet, smoking, lack of exercise

---

fenoprofen calcium

Progesic, Fenopron
Func. class.: Non-steroidal anti-inflammatory drug
Chem. class.: Propionic acid derivative
Legal class.: POM

Action: Inhibits prostaglandin synthesis by inhibiting enzyme needed for biosynthesis; possesses analgesic, anti-inflammatory, anti-pyretic properties
Uses: Mild to moderate pain, osteoarthritis, rheumatoid arthritis, ankylosing spondylitis, pyrexia
Dosage and routes:
• *Adult:* By mouth 200−600 mg 3 or 4 times a day, not to exceed 3 g daily
Available forms include: Tablets 200, 300, 600 mg
Side effects/adverse reactions:
GI: Nausea, anorexia, vomiting, diarrhoea, jaundice, constipation, flatulence, cramps, dry mouth, peptic ulcer, bleeding, dyspepsia, jaundice, hepatitis, oral ulceration, pancreatitis, metallic taste
CNS: Dizziness, drowsiness, fatigue, tremors, confusion, insomnia, anxiety, depression
CV: Tachycardia, peripheral oedema, palpitations, dysrhythmias
INTEG: Purpura, rash, pruritus, sweating, exfoliative dermatitis, alopecia
GU: Nephrotoxicity: dysuria, haematuria, oliguria, azotaemia, cystitis, nephrotic syndrome
HAEM: Blood dyscrasias
EENT: Tinnitus, hearing loss, blurred vision
RESP: Bronchospasm in patients with history of asthma/allergy
Contraindications: Hypersensitivity, severe renal disease, active peptic ulceration
Precautions: Pregnancy, lactation, asthma, anaemia, bleeding disorders, cardiac disorders, hypersensitivity to other NSAIDs, history of peptic ulcer, gastrointestinal haemorrhage, ulcerative colitis
Pharmacokinetics:
Period of onset: Peak 2 hr, half-life 3−3½ hr, metabolised in liver, excreted in urine (metabolites), 90% protein bound, enters breast milk

Interactions/incompatibilities:
• May increase the action of: oral anticoagulants, sulphonylurea hypoglycaemics, phenytoin
• Decreased effect of: diuretics
• Enhanced toxicity of: methotrexate, lithium, cyclosporin

Clinical assessment:
• Patient at high risk of peptic ulceration or GI bleeding
• Renal and hepatic function if impairment anticipated
• Eye examinations if visual disturbances occur
• Regular hearing tests in impaired patients

Treatment of overdose: Gastric lavage, supportive treatment, correct serum electrolytes

NURSING CONSIDERATIONS

Administer:
• With or after food to decrease GI symptoms

Evaluate:
• Decreased pain and stiffness in joints. Ability to move more easily
• For tinnitus, hearing loss, blurred vision, indigestion and black tarry stools

Teach patient/family:
• Report indigestion and black tarry stools
• Take with food or milk
• Report changes in vision or hearing

---

fentanyl citrate/ droperidol combination

Thalamonol
Func. class.: General anaesthetic/ opioid analgesic
Chem. class.: Phenylpiperone derivative
Legal class.: CD(Sch 2), POM

Action: Action at subcortical levels to reduce motor activity, produces neuroleptanalgesia
Uses: Premedication, adjunct to general and regional anaesthesia, maintenance of anaesthesia

Dosage and routes:
Induction
• *Adult:* IV 6−8 ml followed by assisted ventilation
• *Child:* IM 0.4−1.5 ml
Premedication
• *Adult:* IM 12 ml 5−15 min before surgery or procedure
• *Child:* IM 0.03−0.045 ml/kg 5− 15 min before surgery or procedure
Available forms include: Injection IM, IV 0.05 mg fentanyl, 2.5 mg droperidol/ml

Side effects/adverse reactions:
RESP: Laryngospasm, bronchospasm, respiratory arrest
CNS: Dystonia, akathisia, flexion of arms, fine tremors, dizziness, anxiety, drowsiness, restlessness, hallucination, depression
CV: Tachycardia, hypotension, circulatory depression
EENT: Upward rotation of eyes, oculogyric crisis, blurred vision
INTEG: Chills, facial sweating, shivering, diaphoresis
GI: Nausea, vomiting

Contraindications: Hypersensitivity, severe depression, obstructive airways disease, treatment with MAOIs within 14 days, respiratory depression

Precautions: Elderly, increased intracranial pressure, cardiovascular disease (bradydysrhythmias), renal disease, liver disease, hypothyroidism Parkinson's disease, chronic obstructive airways disease

Pharmacokinetics:
IV: Onset 20 sec, peak 2−5 min, duration ½−2 hr
IM: Onset 7 min, duration 1−2 hr, metabolised in liver, excreted in urine metabolites (90%)

Interactions/incompatibilities:
• Increased CNS depression: alcohol, narcotics, barbiturates, antipsychotics or other CNS depressants

• Decreased effects of: amphetamines; anticonvulsants, anticoagulants
• Increased intraocular pressure: anticholinergics, antiparkinsonism drugs
• Increased side effects of: lithium
Treatment of overdose:
Administer naloxone 0.1−0.2 mg IV/IM as required to reverse effects. Respiratory support
NURSING CONSIDERATIONS
Assess:
• Baseline vital signs
Administer:
• Do not mix with barbiturates in solution
• Anticholinergics for extrapyramidal reaction
• Adult: IV followed by assisted ventilation or IM 5−15 minutes before surgery
• Child: IM route preferred
Perform/provide:
• Storage as Controlled Drug regulations and local procedures
Evaluate:
• Vital signs every 10 min during IV administration, every 30 min after IM dose
• Respiratory rate and function
• Observe for bradycardia, nausea, vomiting
• Therapeutic response: decreased anxiety, absence of vomiting, maintenance of anaesthesia
• Rigidity of skeletal muscles
• Extrapyramidal reactions: dystonia, akathisia
Teach patient/family:
• About effects of drug; drowsiness, lightheadedness
• To use deep breathing, coughing after surgery to prevent increased secretions in lungs

ferrous fumarate

Fersaday, Fersamal, many combination products
Func. class.: Haematinic
Chem. class.: Iron preparation
Legal class.: P

Action: Replaces iron stores needed for red blood cell development, energy and O_2 transport, utilisation; drug contains 33% iron
Uses: Iron deficiency anaemia
Dosage and routes:
• *Adult:* By mouth 300−600 mg of ferrous fumarate (100−200 mg of elemental iron) daily
• *Full-term infant and child:* By mouth 2.5−5 ml of Fersamal syrup (22.5−45 mg of elemental iron) twice daily
• *Premature infant:* 0.6 ml/kg daily of Fersamal syrup (5.4 mg/kg of elemental iron). Increase to 2.4 ml/kg daily (21.6 mg/kg of elemental iron)
Available forms include: Tablets 200 mg (65 mg iron), 304 mg (100 mg iron); capsules 290 mg (100 mg iron); modified-release capsules 330 mg (110 mg iron); syrup 140 mg (45 mg iron) in 5 ml
Side effects/adverse reactions:
GI: Nausea, constipation, epigastric pain, black and red tarry stools, vomiting, diarrhoea
Contraindications: Hypersensitivity, ulcerative colitis/regional enteritis, haemosiderosis/haemochromatosis, active peptic ulcer disease, haemolytic anaemia, anaemia (long-term)
Precautions: Treated or controlled peptic ulcer
Pharmacokinetics:
By mouth: Excreted in faeces, urine, skin, breast milk
Interactions/incompatibilities:
• Decreased absorption of tetra-

cycline, ciprofloxacin, quinolones, penicillamine
• Decreased absorption of iron preparations: chloramphenicol, antacids
• Increased absorption of iron preparation: ascorbic acid

Clinical assessment:
• Blood studies: haematocrit, Hb reticulocytes, bilirubin before treatment, at least monthly
• Cause of iron loss or anaemia, including salicylates, sulphonamides, antimalarials, quinidine

Lab. test interferences:
False-positive: Occult blood

Treatment of overdose: Induce vomiting; give eggs, milk until lavage can be done. Administer desferroxamime IM and orally to remove iron. Fluid replacement essential

NURSING CONSIDERATIONS
Assess:
• Nutritional status, amount of iron in diet

Administer:
• Between meals for best absorption, may give with juice; do not give with antacids or milk, delay at least 1 hr; if GI symptoms occur, give with food, absorption may be decreased
• Syrup through plastic straw to avoid discolouration of tooth enamel; dilute thoroughly
• At least 1 hr before bedtime to avoid GI pain

Evaluate:
• Therapeutic response: improvement in haematocrit, Hb, reticulocytes, decreased fatigue, weakness
• Toxicity: nausea, vomiting, diarrhoea (green then tarry stools), haematemesis, pallor, cyanosis, shock, coma
• Elimination; if constipation occurs, increase fluid intake, bulk, activity

Teach patient/family:
• That iron will change colour of stools to black or dark green
• That iron poisoning may occur if increased beyond recommended level
• Not to crush; swallow tablet whole to prevent staining of teeth
• Keep out of reach of children
• Do not substitute one iron salt for another; elemental iron content differs (e.g. 300 mg ferrous fumarate contains about 100 mg elemental iron whereas 300 mg ferrous gluconate contains only about 30 mg elemental iron)
• Avoid reclining position for 15–30 min after taking drug to avoid oesophageal corrosion
• That medication may be needed for 6 months or more
• To increase amount of iron in diet (meat, dark green leafy vegetables, dried beans, dried fruits, eggs)

---

ferrous gluconate

Fergon
Func. class.: Haematinic
Chem. class.: Iron preparation
Legal class.: P

Action: Replaces iron stores needed for red blood cell development; drug contains 11.6% iron
Uses: Iron deficiency anaemia
Dosage and routes:
Therapeutic
• *Adult:* By mouth 300–600 mg 3 times a day
• *Child 6–12 yr:* By mouth 300–900 mg daily
Prophylactic
• *Adult:* By mouth 600 mg daily
• *Child 6–12 yr:* By mouth 300–400 mg daily
Available forms include: Tablets 300 mg
Side effects/adverse reactions:
GI: Nausea, constipation, epi-

gastric pain, black and red tarry stools, vomiting, diarrhoea
INTEG: Temporarily discoloured tooth enamel, eyes
Precautions: Hypersensitivity, ulcerative colitis/regional enteritis,   haemosiderosis/haemochromatosis,   peptic   ulcer   disease, haemolytic   anaemia,   cirrhosis, anaemia (long-term)
Pharmacokinetics:
Period of onset: Excreted in faeces, urine, through skin, breast milk
Interactions/incompatibilities:
• Decreased absorption of both drugs: tetracycline, zinc salts
• Decreased absorption of iron preparations: chloramphenicol, antacids
• Decreased   absorption   of: penicillamine,   quinolone   antibiotics
• Increased   absorption   of   iron preparation: ascorbic acid
Clinical assessment:
• Blood studies: haematocrit, Hb, reticulocytes,   bilirubin   before treatment, at least monthly
• Only with vitamin E supplements to infants or haemolytic anaemia may occur
• Cause of iron loss or anaemia including   salicylates,   sulphonamides, antimalarials, quinidine
• Therapeutic response: improvement in haematocrit, Hb, reticulocytes, decreased fatigue, weakness
Lab. test interferences:
False positive: occult blood
Treatment of overdose: Induce vomiting; give eggs, milk until lavage can be done

NURSING CONSIDERATIONS

Assess:
• Cause of iron loss or deficiency
• Blood tests for haematocrit, Hb, reticulocytes, bilirubin before and monthly during treatment
• Prophylactic   or   therapeutic treatment
Administer:

• Orally about 1 hr before meals with water or juice; do not give with antacids or milk. Decreased absorption if stomach not empty
• After food if gastrointestinal symptoms occur
• At least 1 hr before bed time to diminish GI irritation
Perform/Provide:
• Store in childproof, light resistant container
• Mouth care, regular brushing teeth/dentures
Evaluate:
• Therapeutic response: improvement of haematocrit, Hb, reticulocytes, decreased fatigue, weakness
• Signs of toxicity: nausea, vomiting, diarrhoea (dark green tarry stools),   haematemesis,   pallor, cyaniosis, shock, coma
• Elimination — for   constipation, increase fluids, fibre and bulk in diet, physical activity
• Diet: increase amount of iron rich foods
Teach patient/family:
• That iron will change stools to dark green or black and often cause constipation
• That iron poisoning is dangerous, never increase recommended doses
• Keep safe from children
• To swallow whole as iron stains teeth/dentures
• Not to replace their iron tablets for others as iron contents differ
• To avoid lying down for 15–30 min after taking drug as oesophageal corrosion can occur
• To eat an iron-rich diet

ferrous sulphate

Feospan, Ferrograd, Slow-Fe
Func. class.: Haematinic
Chem. class.: Iron preparation
Legal class.: P

Action: Replaces iron stores needed for red blood cell development. Drug contains 20% iron
Uses: Iron deficiency anaemia, prophylaxis for iron deficiency in pregnancy
Dosage and routes:
Therapeutic
• *Adult:* By mouth 200−600 mg daily in divided doses
• *Child 6−12 yr:* By mouth 400 mg in divided doses
• *1−5 yr:* By mouth 240 mg in divided doses
• *Less than 1 year:* By mouth 120 mg in divided doses
Prophylactic
• *Adult:* By mouth 200 mg daily
Available forms include: Tablets 200 mg; modified release tablets 160, 325 mg; modified release capsules 150 mg
Side effects/adverse reactions:
GI: Nausea, constipation, epigastric pain, black and red tarry stools, vomiting, diarrhoea
INTEG: Temporarily discoloured tooth enamel, eyes
Precautions: Hypersensitivity, ulcerative colitis/regional enteritis, haemosiderosis/haemochromatosis, peptic ulcer disease, haemolytic anaemia, cirrhosis, anaemia (long-term)
Pharmacokinetics:
By mouth: Excreted in faeces, urine, through skin, breast milk
Interactions/incompatibilities:
• Decreased absorption of both drugs: tetracycline, zinc salts
• Decreased absorption of iron preparations: chloramphenicol, antacids
• Decreased absorption of: penicillamine
• Increased absorption of iron preparation: ascorbic acid
Clinical assessment:
• Blood studies: haematocrit, Hb, reticulocytes, bilirubin before treatment, at least monthly
• Only with vitamin E supplements to infants or haemolytic anaemia may occur
• Only after determining cause of anaemia
Lab. test interferences:
False-positive: Occult blood
Treatment of overdose: Induce vomiting, give eggs, milk until lavage can be done
NURSING CONSIDERATIONS
Assess:
• Cause of iron loss or deficiency
• Blood tests for Hb, reticulocytes, haematocrit, bilirubin before and monthly during treatment
• Prophylactic or therapeutic treatment
Administer:
• Orally about 1 hr before meals with water or juice; do not give with antacids or milk. Decreased absorption if stomach is not empty
• At least 1 hr before bed time to diminish GI irritation
• After food if gastrointestinal symptoms occur
Perform/provide:
• Store in childproof, light-resistant container
• Mouth care, regular brushing of teeth/dentures
Evaluate:
• Therapeutic response: improvement of Hb, reticulocytes, haematocrit, decreased fatigue, weakness
• Signs of toxicity: nausea, vomiting, diarrhoea (dark green tarry stools), cyanosis, pallor, haematemesis, shock, coma
• Elimination: for constipation increase fluids, fibre and bulk in diet, physical activity

- Diet: increase amount of iron rich foods

Teach patient/family:
- That iron will change stools to dark green or black and often causes constipation
- That iron poisoning is dangerous, never increase recommended doses
- Keep safe from children
- To swallow whole as iron stains teeth
- Not to replace their iron tablets for others as the iron contents differ
- To avoid lying down for 15–30 min after taking drug as oesophageal corrosion can occur
- To eat an iron rich diet

---

flavoxate HCl

Urispas
Func. class.: Spasmolytic
Chem. class.: Flavone derivative
Legal class.: POM

Action: Relaxes smooth muscles in urinary tract
Uses: Relief of nocturia, incontinence, suprapubic pain, dysuria, frequency associated with urologic conditions (symptomatic only)
Dosage and routes:
- *Adult and child under 12 yr:* By mouth 200 mg 3 times a day
Available forms include: Tablets 100 mg
Side effects/adverse reactions:
HAEM: Leucopenia, eosinophilia
CNS: Anxiety, restlessness, dizziness, convulsions, headache, drowsiness, confusion
CV: Palpitations, sinus tachycardia, hypotension
GI: Nausea, vomiting, anorexia, abdominal pain, constipation
GU: Dysuria
INTEG: Urticaria, dermatitis
EENT: Blurred vision, increased intraocular tension, dry mouth, throat
Contraindications: Hypersensitivity, achalasia GI obstruction, GI haemorrhage, GU obstruction
Precautions: Pregnancy, lactation, suspected glaucoma, children under 12 yr
Pharmacokinetics: Excreted in urine

NURSING CONSIDERATIONS
Evaluate:
- Urinary status: dysuria, frequency, nocturia, incontinence
- Allergic reactions: rash, urticaria; if these occur, drug should be discontinued
Teach patient/family:
- To avoid hazardous activities; dizziness may occur
- On all aspects of drug therapy: dosage, routes, side effects, when to notify clinician

---

flecainide acetate

Tambocor
Func. class.: Anti-arrhythmic (Class I)
Chem. class.: Lignocaine analogue
Legal class.: POM

Action: Increases electrical stimulation threshold of ventrical HIS-Purkinje system, which stabilises cardiac membrane
Uses: Ventricular tachyarrhythmias unresponsive to other therapy
Dosage and routes:
- *Adult:* By mouth 100 mg 12 hrly for 3–5 days then lowest effective dose, maximum 400 mg daily, reduce after 3–5 days. IV over 10–30 min 2 mg/kg. IV infusion initially 1.5 mg/kg/hr for 1 hr then 0.1–0.25 mg/kg/hr with blood level monitoring
Available forms include: Tablets 100 mg; injection 10 mg/ml
Side effects/adverse reactions:
CNS: Headache, dizziness, in-

voluntary movement, confusion, psychosis, restlessness, irritability, paraesthesia
EENT: Tinnitus, blurred vision, hearing loss
GI: Nausea, vomiting, anorexia
CV: Hypotension, bradycardia, angina, premature ventricular contraction, heart block, cardiovascular collapse, arrest, dysrhythmias
RESP: Dyspnoea, respiratory depression
INTEG: Rash, urticaria, oedema, swelling
Contraindications: Hypersensitivity, severe heart block, cardiogenic shock, cardiac failure
Precautions: Pregnancy, lactation, children elderly (reduce dose) renal disease, liver disease, congestive cardiac failure, respiratory depression, myasthenia gravis, cardiac pacemaker
Pharmacokinetics:
Period of onset: Peak 1 hr; half-life 7−20 hr; metabolised by liver, excreted unchanged by kidneys (10%), excreted in breast milk
Interactions/incompatibilities:
• May increase effects when used with: aminodarone cimetidine, propranolol, quinidine
• May decrease effects when used with: phenytoin
Lab. test interferences:
Increase: Creatinine phosphokinase
Treatment of overdose: O_2, artificial ventilation, ECG, administer dopamine for circulatory depression, administer diazepam or thiopentone for convulsions
NURSING CONSIDERATIONS
Assess:
• Baseline vital signs including temperature
• ECG before commencing drug
Administer:
• IV infusion diluted with 5% dextrose solution
• Cardiac monitoring in a specialist

unit or ITU for IV administration
• Close observation for potential convulsions
• 4−6 hrly BP, TPR for oral use
Perform/provide:
• ECG continuously to determine increased PR or QRS segments; if these develop, discontinue
Evaluate:
• Blood levels of drug
• Malignant hyperthermia: tachypnoea, tachycardia
• Cardiac rate, respiration: rate, rhythm, character, continuously
• Respiratory status: rate, rhythm, lung fields for rales
• CNS effects: dizziness, confusion, psychosis, paraesthesia, convulsions; drug should be discontinued
• Lung fields, bilateral rales may occur in congestive cardiac failure patient
• Increased respiration, increased pulse; drug should be discontinued
• BP continuously for fluctuations
• Temperature and pulse rate. Report changes to clinician
Teach patient/family:
• To report any nausea, shortness of breath, dizziness, palpitations, rash or hearing loss to clinician
• To avoid hazardous activities if dizziness occurs

---

fluclorolone acetonide

Topilar
Func. *class.:* Corticosteroid, topical
Chem. *class.:* Fluorinated corticosteroid
Legal class.: POM

Action: Reduces inflammation
Uses: Severe inflammatory skin disorders e.g. eczema in patients unresponsive to less potent corticosteroids
Dosage and routes:

• Apply sparingly twice daily; reduce strength and frequency as condition responds

• Undiluted: potent; Diluted: moderately potent

Available forms include: Cream, ointment 0.025% in non-aqueous base

Side effects/adverse reactions:

INTEG: Spread and worsening of untreated infection; thinning of the skin; irreversible striae atrophicae; perioral dermatitis; acne at site of application; mild depigmentation and vellus hair; increased hair growth

Contraindications:

• Untreated bacterial, fungal or viral skin infections

• Avoid if possible in infants

Clinical assessment:

• Reduce dose slowly

NURSING CONSIDERATIONS

Assess:

• Possibility of pregnancy

• Temperature

Administer:

• With appropriate anti-infective therapy for bacterial/fungal skin infections

• As a thin smear twice daily

• Use occlusion dressings if prescribed

• Avoid the eyes

Perform/provide:

• Store in cool place

Evaluate:

• Temperature 4-hrly

• Response to treatment

• Side effects

• Infection, worsening of condition

Teach patient/family:

• To apply sparingly. That nappies/plastic pants may increase absorption

• To report infection or worsening at once

• Avoid the eyes

• Not to use any other preparations

• Warn about skin changes, increased hair growth etc.

flucloxacillin

Floxapen,   Ladropen,   Stafoxil, Staphlipen

Func. class.: Penicillinase-resistant anti-staphylococcal penicillin

Chem. class.: Penicillin

Legal class.: POM

Action: Bactericidal, interferes with bacterial cell wall synthesis. Resistant to degradation by bacterial penicillinases

Uses: Treatment of infections due to Gram-positive organisms, especially β-lactamase-producing staphylococci, including skin, soft tissue and respiratory tract infections, osteomyelitis, endocarditis, meningitis and septicaemia caused by sensitive organisms

Dosage and routes:

• *Adult:* By mouth 250 mg 6 hrly, at least 30 min before food; IM, 250 mg every 6 hr; IV, 0.25−1 g every 6 hr. Doses may be doubled in severe infection

• Osteomyelitis, endocarditis: up to 8 g daily in 3 or 4 divided doses

• Surgical prophylaxis: 1−2 g IV at induction of anaesthesia followed by 500 mg by mouth, IV, IM 6-hrly for up to 72 hr

• In conjunction with systemic therapy: by nebuliser 125−250 mg 4 times a day; intrapleural 250 mg once daily; intra-articular 250−500 mg once daily

• *Child:* Under 2 yr, quarter adult dose; 2−10 yr, half adult dose

Available forms include: Capsules 250, 500 mg; oral mixture 125 mg/5 ml, 250 mg/5 ml; powder vials for preparing IV, IM, intra-articular, intrapleural injections, nebulisation solutions 250, 500 mg, 1 g

Side effects/adverse reactions:
GI: Nausea, diarrhoea, hepatitis, cholestatic jaundice, pseudo-membranous colitis
INTEG: Skin rashes
CNS: Encephalopathy (in renal impairment, excessive doses)
Contraindications: Hypersensitivity to penicillins, ocular administration, porphyria
Precautions: Pregnancy, lactation
Pharmacokinetics: Peak plasma concentration about 1 hr after oral administration, after IM injection within 30 min. Half-life 1 hr, prolonged in neonates, 50−90% excreted in urine with 6 hr
Interactions/incompatibilities:
• Do not mix with aminoglycoside antibiotics in syringe, infusion bag or giving set, or with blood products, proteinaceous solutions, lipid emulsions for IV use
Clinical assessment:
• Sensitivity of bacterial cultures
Treatment of overdose: Symptomatic
NURSING CONSIDERATIONS
Assess:
• Site of infection: take specimens for culture and sensitivity before administration
• Check previous allergic response to penicillins; identify in red on patient's notes if any known allergies
• Temperature and other vital signs
• Bowel pattern
• Fluid balance
Administer:
• By mouth: 30 min before food with full glass of water
• IV: diluted with water for injection
Perform/provide:
• Monitor for allergic response: rashes, pyrexia, airway obstruction
Evaluate:
• Therapeutic response
• Reduction of temperature

• Effectiveness of treatment
• IV site for extravasation, phlebitis
Teach patient/family:
• To take before food
• To take all medication prescribed for length of time ordered

---

fluconazole

Diflucan
Func.   class.: Orally active antifungal
Chem. class.: Triazole
Legal class.: POM

Action: Inhibits fungal enzymes necessary for the synthesis of ergosterol
Uses: Acute or recurrent vaginal candidiasis, oropharyngeal candidiasis (including in immunocompromised patients), atrophic oral candidiasis associated with dentures, systemic candidiasis, mucosal candidiasis and cryptococciosis (including cryptococcal meningitis). Prevention of relapse of cryptococcal disease in AIDS patients
Dosage and routes:
• *Adult:* By mouth or IV, vaginal candidiasis 150 mg as single dose
• Oropharyngeal candidiasis 50 mg daily for 7−14 days; maximum 14 days except in patients with severely compromised immune systems
• Atrophic oral candidiasis 50 mg daily for 14 days
• Dose for other mucosal candidal infections, 50 mg daily for 14−30 days, maximum 100 mg daily
• Candidaemia, disseminated candidiasis, other invasive candidal infections: 400 mg on day one then 200−400 mg daily according to response
• Cryptococcal meningitis and other cryptococcal infections:

400 mg on day one then 200–400 mg daily; duration in meningitis usually 6–8 weeks
• Prevention of relapse of cryptococcal meningitis in patients with AIDS: at least 100 mg daily
• Doses for all indications can be given IV/by mouth without adjustment depending on condition of patient
• *Child over 1 yr with normal renal function:* superficial candidial infection, 1–2 mg/kg daily; systemic candidial/cryptococcal infection, 3–6 mg/kg daily
Available forms include: Capsules 50, 150, 200 mg; injection 2 mg/ml, 25 ml, 100 ml vials

Side effects/adverse reactions:
GI: Nausea, abdominal discomfort, diarrhoea, flatulence, abnormalities of liver function
INTEG: Rash

Contraindications: Hypersensitivity to triazoles, lactation, pregnancy

Precautions: Renal impairment, toxicity, children

Pharmacokinetics: Rapidly and completely absorbed orally, 80% excreted unchanged in urine. Plasma half-life 30 hr

Interactions/incompatibilities:
• Potentiates effects of anticoagulants
• Increases blood levels of sulphonylurea oral hypoglycaemics and phenytoin
• Effectiveness reduced by rifampicin

Clinical assessment:
• Culture and sensitivity
• Antiemetics for nausea
• Consider stopping if liver function tests abnormal, rash develops
Treatment of overdose: Gastric lavage and supportive treatment. Removable by haemodialysis if considered necessary

NURSING CONSIDERATIONS

Assess:

• Fluid balance (renal impairment), temperature
Administer:
• With food, avoid alkalis within 2 hr
Perform/provide:
• Adequate oral hygiene if used for oral conditions
Evaluate:
• Side effects e.g. rashes, signs of liver toxicity (jaundice, pale stools)
• Therapeutic response, improvement
Teach patient/family:
• To take at regular intervals and always finish course unless told otherwise
• That long-term treatment is sometimes required
• To avoid other medicines
• Warn not to take at same time as indigestion medicines
• Inform about side effects especially jaundice, pale stools etc. See clinician if side effects occur

flucytosine

Alcobon
Func. class.: Antifungal
Chem. class.: Pyrimidine (fluorinated)
Legal class.: POM

Action: Converted to fluorouracil within fungal cell and interferes with protein synthesis
Uses: Infections with *Candida* spp (septicaemia, endocarditis, pulmonary, urinary tract infections), *Cryptococcus* spp (meningitis, pulmonary, urinary tract infections), *Torulopsis glabrata, Hansenula* spp
Dosage and routes:
• *Adult and child:* 200 mg/kg daily in 4 doses
Available forms include: Tablets

500 mg; IV infusion 10 mg/ml, 250 ml bottle

Side effects/adverse reactions:
INTEG: Rash
CNS: Headache, confusion, dizziness, sedation, hallucinations
GI: Nausea, vomiting, anorexia, diarrhoea, cramps, enterocolitis, altered liver function tests, hepatitis, bowel perforation (rare)
HAEM: Thrombocytopenia, agranulocytosis, anaemia, leucopenia, pancytopenia
GU: Increased blood urea nitrogen, creatinine
Contraindications: Hypersensitivity, pregnancy
Precautions: Renal, hepatic disease, bone marrow depression, blood dyscrasias, radiation/chemotherapy
Pharmacokinetics:
Period of onset: Peak 2½−6 hr, half-life 3−6 hr, excreted in urine (unchanged), well-distributed to CSF, aqueous humour, joints
Interactions/incompatibilities:
• Synergism: Amphotericin B
Clinical assessment:
• Blood studies: full blood count, including platelets at regular intervals
• Drug level during treatment in renal impairment; therapeutic level 25−50 mcg/ml, maximum 80 mcg/ml
• Prescribe drug only after culture and sensitivity confirms organism, drug needed to treat condition
• Few tablets at a time to decrease nausea, vomiting over 15 min
• Therapeutic response: decreased fever, malaise, rash, negative culture for infecting organism
• For renal toxicity: increasing blood urea nitrogen, serum creatinine; if serum creatinine greater than 1.7 mg/100 ml, dosage may be reduced
• For hepatotoxicity: check regularly for increasing aspartate aminotransferase, alanine aminotransferase, alkaline phosphatase
• For blood dyscrasias, fatigue, bruising, malaise, dark urine

NURSING CONSIDERATIONS
Assess:
• Baseline vital signs
• After samples taken for culture and sensitivity tests
Perform/provide:
• Symptomatic treatment as ordered for adverse reactions: aspirin, antihistamines, antiemetics, antispasmodics
Evaluate:
• Vital signs every 15−30 min during first infusion, note changes in pulse and BP
• Therapeutic response
• For side effects
Teach patient/family:
• That long-term therapy may be needed to clear infection (1−2 months depending on type of infection)
• To report symptoms of blood dyscrasias; fatigue, bruising, malaise, dark urine

---

fludrocortisone acetate

Florinef
Func. class.: Corticosteroid
Chem. class.: Mineralocorticoid
Legal class.: POM

Action: Mimics endogenous adrenal hormones, promotes increased reabsorption of sodium and loss of potassium from the renal tubules
Uses: Adrenal insufficiency, salt-losing adrenogenital syndrome
Dosage and routes:
• *Adult:* By mouth 0.05−0.3 mg daily
Available forms include: Tablets 0.1 mg
Side effects/adverse reactions:
INTEG: Acne, poor wound

healing, ecchymosis, petechiae, hirsutism, skin thinning, increased sweating, flushing
CNS: Depression, headache, mood changes, vertigo, convulsions, raised intracranial pressure, paraesthesia
CV: Hypertension, circulatory collapse, thrombophlebitis, embolism, tachycardia
HAEM: Thrombocytopenia
MS: Fractures, osteoporosis, weakness, proximal myopathy
GI: Diarrhoea, nausea, abdominal distention, GI haemorrhage, increased appetite, pancreatitis, ulcerative oesophagitis, peptic ulcer
EENT: Fungal infections, increased intraocular pressure, blurred vision, cataracts
ELECT: Sodium and fluid retention, hypokalaemia, hypokalaemic alkalosis
ENDO: Cushingoid states, menstrual irregularities, precipitation of diabetes mellitus, reduced adrenocortical stress response
METAB: Hyperglycaemia
SYST: Weight gain
Precautions: Psychosis, hypersensitivity, idiopathic thrombocytopenia, acute glomerulonephritis, amoebiasis, myasthenia gravis, exathematous disease, recent intestinal anastomoses, chronic nephritis, diuretic colitis, viral or fungal infection, peptic ulcer, metastatic cancer, osteoporosis, diverticulitis, hypertension, previous steroid myopathy, pregnancy, diabetes mellitus, glaucoma, seizure disorders, ulcerative colitis hypothyroidism, cirrhosis, congestive cardiac failure
Pharmacokinetics:
Rapid and complete absorption, plasma peak 1–2 hr, half-life 30 min, metabolised by liver, excreted in urine
Interactions/incompatibilities:

• Decreased action of this drug: cholestyramine, colestipol, barbiturates, rifampicin, phenytoin, carbamazepine
• Decreased effects of: anticonvulsants, antidiabetics, toxoids, vaccines, antihypertensives, diuretics
• Increased side effects: salicylates, indomethacin, amphotericin B, digitalis preparations, diuretics, carbenoxolone
Clinical assessment:
• Potassium, blood sugar, urine glucose while on long-term therapy; hypokalaemia and hyperglycaemia
Lab. test interferences:
False negative: Skin allergy tests
Treatment of overdose: Plenty of water by mouth. Monitor serum electrolytes; restrict and supplement intake accordingly
NURSING CONSIDERATIONS
Assess:
• Baseline weight
Administer:
• With food or milk to decrease GI symptoms
Perform/provide:
• Assistance with ambulation in patient with bone tissue disease to prevent fractures
• Assistance with other activities of living as required
Evaluate:
• Weight daily, notify clinician of weekly gain greater than 2 kg
• Temperature
• BP pulse 4 hrly, notify clinician if chest pain occurs
• Fluid balance, be alert for decreasing urinary output and increasing oedema
• Infection: increased temperature, WBC, even after withdrawal of medication; drug masks symptoms of infection
• Potassium depletion: paraesthesia, fatigue, nausea, vomiting, depression, polyuria, dysrhythmias, weakness

• Oedema, hypotension, cardiac symptoms
• Mental status: affect, mood, behavioural changes, aggression

Teach patient/family:
• That identity card as steroid user should be carried
• To notify clinician if therapeutic response decreases; dosage adjustment may be necessary
• That medication must not be stopped abruptly or adrenal crisis can result
• To avoid non-prescribed drugs: salicylates, alcohol in cough products, cold preparations unless directed by clinician
• All aspects of drug use, including Cushingoid symptoms
• Symptoms of adrenal insufficiency: nausea, anorexia, fatigue, dizziness, dyspnoea, weakness, joint pain

---

flumazenil

Anexate
Func. class.: Specific benzodiazepine antagonist
Chem. class.: Benzodiazepine analogue
Legal class.: POM

Action: Competes with benzodiazepines for receptors and reverses their anxiolytic and sedative effects
Uses: Reversal of benzodiazepine sedation in intensive care, after anaesthesia and short diagnostic procedures

Dosage and routes:
• Slow IV injection 200 mcg over 15 seconds, then 100 mcg at 1 min intervals if required (usual range 300−600 mcg; maximum total dose 1 mg or, in intensive care, 2 mg)
• IV infusion if drowsiness recurs after injection, 100−400 mcg/hr according to level of arousal

Available forms include: Injection, 100 mcg/ml 5 ml ampoule
Side effects/adverse reactions:
CNS: Over-rapid wakening leading to anxiety, fear, agitation; convulsions, symptoms of benzodiazepine withdrawal (anxiety attacks, tachycardia, sweating, dizziness) in long-term benzodiazepine users
GI: Nausea, vomiting
INTEG: Flushing
CV: Transient increase in heart rate, BP, in intensive care patients
Contraindications: Epileptics who have received prolonged benzodiazepine therapy, hypersensitivity to benzodiazepines
Precautions: Benzodiazepine dependence, anxiety, after major surgery ensure neuromuscular blockade is cleared before giving drug, avoid rapid administration; hepatic impairment, pregnancy, lactation
Pharmacokinetics: Metabolised in liver, half-life 50 min, excreted in urine as inactive metabolites
Interactions/incompatibilities:
• Decreased effects of: benzodiazepines, zopiclone
• May unmask toxic effects of drugs taken in overdose (e.g. tricyclic antidepressants)

NURSING CONSIDERATIONS
Assess:
• Ensure patient is not receiving Benzodiazepine therapy
• Baseline vital signs
Administer:
• Repeat doses may be necessary as drug is short acting
• IV very slowly or by continuous infusion
• Can be diluted in saline or dextrose
• Infusion solution must be discarded after 24 hr
Perform/provide:
• Continuous monitoring for 6 hr after a dose

• Respiratory rate and level of awareness; these may vary during treatment

Evaluate:

• Pulse, BP — tachycardia and hypertension may occur intensive care

• Avoid rapid administration

• For therapeutic action — reversal of sedative effects of benzodiazepines

• Need for repeat dose if drug effect is wearing off

Teach patient/family:

• Essential to avoid operating machinery or driving a vehicle for 24 hr

---

flunitrazepam

Rohypnol

Func. class.: Sedative hypnotic
Chem. class.: Benzodiazepine
Legal class.: CD Benz POM (~~NHS~~)

Action: Depresses CNS with sedative effect

Uses: Short-term treatment of insomnia

Dosage and routes:

• By mouth, 0.5−1 mg half an hour before bedtime; may be increased to 2 mg in severe insomnia; reduce starting dose to 0.5 mg and maximum to 1 mg in elderly patients

Available forms include: Tablets, 1 mg

Side effects/adverse reactions:

GI: GI upsets, jaundice
CVS: Hypotension, thromboembolic effects
HAEM: Blood dyscrasias (rare)
INTEG: Skin rashes
GU: Urinary retention
CNS: Drowsiness and lightheadedness the following day; ataxia, confusion, especially in elderly; headaches, vertigo, dependence, paradoxical aggression, excitement, unmasking of depression, changes in libido, visual disturbances

Contraindications: Acute pulmonary insufficiency, respiratory depression, porphyria, phobic or obsessional states, psychoses, hypersensitivity to benzodiazepines

Precautions: History of drug abuse or personality disorder; renal or hepatic impairment; pregnancy, lactation; reduce dose in elderly or debilitated patients; avoid prolonged use and abrupt withdrawal; where morning alertness important

Pharmacokinetics: Extensively metabolised in the liver; half-life 22 hr, excreted as metabolites in urine, 80% protein bound

Interactions/incompatibilities:

• Increased action of both drugs: alcohol, CNS depressants

• Increased toxicity of: antiepileptics

Treatment of overdose: Gastric lavage if performed promptly, supportive treatment, flumazenil may be used to antagonise

NURSING CONSIDERATIONS

Assess:

• Pulse and blood pressure

• All drugs patient is on for compatibility. (Elderly often hoard drugs)

Administer:

• Drug to be taken before retiring

• Use lowest dose possible to relieve symptoms

• Avoid long-term use

Perform/provide:

• Assist with mobility (mainly elderly)

Evaluate:

• Therapeutic response; decreased insomnia

• For suicidal tendencies which may be released in depressed patients

• Side effects, drowsiness, ataxia,

headaches, changes in libido and urinary retention
• Drug dependency if used long term

Teach patient/family:
• To use the lowest dose
• Not to discontinue medication without medical advice. Drug should be tapered off slowly
• Not to sleep during the day
• That suitable physical activity may aid sleep
• To avoid driving or hazardous activity if drowsiness occurs
• Not to drink coffee, take or do anything at night to interfere with sleep

---

fluocinolone acetonide

Synalar, Synalar 1 in 4 dilution, Synalar 1 in 10 dilution, Synalar C, Synalar N combination products
Func. class.: Potent topical corticosteroid
Chem. class.: Fluorinated corticosteroid
Legal class.: POM

Action: Reduces inflammation
Uses: Inflammatory skin disorders e.g. eczema, seborrhoeic dermatitis, psoriasis
Dosage and routes: Apply topical preparations sparingly, 2−3 times daily; reduce strength and frequency as condition responds
Available forms include: Cream, 0.025%, 0.00625%, 0.0025%, 0.025% with clioquinol 3%, 0.025% with neomycin sulphate 0.5%, all in water-miscible base; gel, 0.025% in water miscible base; ointment, 0.025%, 0.00625%
Side effects/adverse reactions:
INTEG: Spread and worsening of untreated infection, thinning of the skin, irreversible striae atrophicae, perioral dermatitis, acne at site of application, mild depigmentation, increased hair growth
ENDO: Suppression of hypothalamic-pituitary-adrenal axis producing growth retardation and suppressed plasma cortisol, Cushing's syndrome, reduced glucose tolerance
Contraindications: Untreated bacterial (except Synalar C/N), fungal (except Synalar C) or viral skin infections, napkin eruptions, perioral dermatitis
Precautions: Pregnancy, lactation, occlusive dressings
Clinical assessment:
• Prescribe for not more than 5 days for treatment of face or children
• Use for shortest possible time on smallest possible area

NURSING CONSIDERATIONS
Administer:
• Cleanse area thoroughly before application especially if occlusive dressing required
• Apply sparingly
• Use occlusive dressings with care (increase side effects, whilst increasing effect)
Observe:
• For local atrophic skin changes in long-term therapy: striae, thinning skin
• For systemic signs of adrenal suppression
Evaluate:
• Unfavourable reactions: cease treatment at once if these occur
• Therapeutic response: less inflammation, itching etc
Teach patient/family:
• To avoid drug contact with eyes
• To avoid sunlight on treated areas as burns may occur
• About proper use of cream
• About side effects
• That cream is not a cure but alleviates symptoms

fluorescein sodium

Fluorets, Minims Fluorescein Sodium
Func. class.: Diagnostic agent, opthalmic
Chem. class.: Fluorescent dye
Legal class.: POM

Action: Allows breaks in the corneal tissue to absorb dye and show up as bright green under cobalt blue light
Uses: Diagnostic aid in identifying foreign bodies, fitting hard contact lenses, fundus photography, tonometry, identifying corneal abrasions, retinal angiography
Dosage and routes:
• *Adult:* Instil 1 drop of eye drops, or wet strip with sterile water and touch conjunctiva or fornix, flush eye with irrigating solution
Available forms include: Eye drops 1%, 2%; impregnated paper strips 1 mg
Side effects/adverse reactions:
EENT: Stinging, burning, conjunctival redness
Contraindications: Hypersensitivity
Interactions/incompatibilities: None known
NURSING CONSIDERATIONS
Administer:
• Solution, encourage patient to close eyelids for 1 min if possible
Evaluate:
• Eye colour after application: defects are green under normal light or bright yellow under cobalt blue light
Teach patient/family:
• Solution may sting or burn

fluorometholone

FML
Func. class.: Ophthalmic anti-inflammatory
Chem. class.: Corticosteroid
Legal class.: POM

Action: Decreases inflammation, resulting in decreased pain, photophobia, hyperaemia, cellular infiltration
Uses: Steroid-responsive inflammation of conjunctiva, cornea and anterior globe
Dosage and routes:
• *Adult and child:* Instil 1–2 drops into conjunctival sac hrly for 2 days if needed then 2 to 4 times a day
Available forms include: Ophthalmic suspension 0.1%
Side effects/adverse reactions:
EENT: Increased intraocular pressure, poor corneal wound healing, increased possibility of corneal infections, glaucoma, cataract, optic nerve damage, decreased acuity, visual field defects, thinning of facial skin, striae, telangiectasia around eye
Contraindications: Hypersensitivity, acute superficial herpes simplex, fungal/viral diseases of the eye or conjunctiva, active diabetes mellitus, ocular tuberculosis, infections of the eye, soft contact lenses
Precautions: Corneal abrasions, glaucoma, thinning of the cornea/sclera, pregnancy
Interactions/incompatibilities: Soft contact lenses
Clinical assessment:
• Intraocular pressure and signs of fungal infection should be checked during prolonged therapy
NURSING CONSIDERATIONS
Administer:
• After shaking
Evaluate:

• Allergic reactions: redness, itching, swelling, lacrimation
• Therapeutic response: absence of swelling, redness, exudate
Teach patient/family:
• Instillation method: pressure on lacrimal sac for 1 min
• Not to share eye medications with others
• If both eyes being treated do not interchange right eye/left eye drops
• That soft contact lenses may not be used

---

fluorouracil (topical)

Efudix
Func. class.: Antineoplastic, antimetabolite
Chem. class.: Pyrimidine analogue
Legal class.: POM

Action: Inhibits synthesis of DNA, RNA in susceptible cells
Uses: Topical for malignant skin conditions including keratoses, superficial basal cell carcinoma, Bowen's disease
Dosage and routes:
• *Adult:* Topical, apply to affected area once or twice a day, under occlusive dressing if lesion malignant
Available forms include: Cream 5%
Side effects/adverse reactions:
INTEG: Erythema and irritation of healthy skin around lesions
Contraindications: Hypersensitivity, pregnancy, lactation
Pharmacokinetics: Systemic absorbtion normally negligible
NURSING CONSIDERATIONS
Administer:
• Gloves or applicator must be used; avoid spillage
Evaluate:
• Therapeutic response: decreased size of lesion

• Area of body involved for redness, swelling
• Check oral cavity daily for stomatitis; if present discontinue drug, indicates systemic absorption
Perform/provide:
• An occlusive dressing if required
• Thorough washing of hands after application
Teach patient/family:
• To apply with care; care with washing of skin
• To avoid application on normal skin or getting cream in eyes
• To wash hands after application
• To discontinue use if rash or irritation occurs
• Not to change application; use exactly as prescribed
• To avoid sunlight or use sunscreen, photosensitivity may occur
• Lesion will disappear in 1−2 months

---

fluorouracil (5-fluorouracil)

Fluoro-uracil
Func. class.: Antineoplastic, antimetabolite
Chem. class.: Pyrimidine analogue
Legal class.: POM

Action: Inhibits DNA synthesis; interferes with cell replication by competitively inhibiting thymidylate synthesis
Uses: Cancer of breast, colon, rectum, stomach, pancreas
Dosage and routes:
• *Adult:* By mouth 15 mg/kg daily for 6 days, then 15 mg/kg once weekly
• IV/intra-arterial toxicity highly schedule-dependent; doses very variable seek specialist advice
Available forms include: Capsules 250 mg; IV/intra-arterial injection

25 mg/ml. Injection may be given by mouth

Side effects/adverse reactions:

HAEM: Thrombocytopenia, leucopenia, myelosuppression, anaemia

GI: Anorexia, stomatitis, diarrhoea, nausea, vomiting, haemorrhage

CVS: Angina, ECG changes, myocardial infarction, spasm of vein used for infusion

EENT: Epistaxis, lacrimation, photophobia

INTEG: Rash, alopecia, fever

CNS: Lethargy, malaise, weakness confusion, headache, acute cerebellar syndrome, nystagmus

Contraindications: Hypersensitivity, myelosuppression, pregnancy, serious infections, lactation

Precautions: Renal disease, hepatic disease, bone marrow depression, cardiovascular disease, radiation, chemotherapy, probable carcinogen

Pharmacokinetics: Half-life 10–20 min, 20 hr terminal, metabolised in the liver, excreted in the urine, crosses blood-brain barrier, oral absorption erratic

Interactions/incompatibilities:

• Increased toxicity/therapeutic potency: radiation, other antineoplastics, calcium folinate, α-interferon

• Decreased effect: allopurinol

Clinical assessment:

• Full blood count, differential white cell count, platelet count weekly; withhold drug if WBC is less than 3500/mm^3 or platelet count is less than 100,000/mm^3. Cancer treatment centres may have different guidelines

Lab. test interferences:

Increase: Thyroxine and liothyronine

Treatment of overdose: Supportive

NURSING CONSIDERATIONS

Assess:

• Baseline temperature, pulse, respirations, BP

Administer:

• In accordance with local cytotoxic policy

• Other medications by oral route if possible; avoid IM, subcutaneous, IV routes to prevent infections

• Antiemetic 30–60 min before giving drug to prevent vomiting (if ordered)

• Topical or systemic analgesics for pain (as ordered)

• Transfusion for anaemia

• Antispasmodic for diarrhoea

Perform/provide:

• Strict asepsis, protective isolation if WBC levels are low

• Strict fluid balance — or daily weight to indicate fluid overload

• Rinsing of mouth 3 or 4 times a day with water, or prescribed mouth washes, brushing of teeth 2 or 3 times a day with soft brush or cotton-tipped applicators for stomatitis; use unwaxed dental floss

• Nutritious diet with iron, vitamin supplements as ordered

• Consider patient's likes/dislikes and preferences

• Offer smaller meals more often if desirable

Evaluate:

• Bleeding due to thrombocytopenia: haematuria, bruising or petechiae, mucosa or orifices 8 hrly

• Food preferences; list likes, dislikes

• Inflammation of mucosa, breaks in skin

• Buccal cavity 8 hrly for dryness due to stomatitis, sores or ulceration, white patches, oral pain, bleeding, dysphagia

• Symptoms indicating severe allergic reaction: rash, urticaria, itching, flushing

• GI symptoms: frequency of stools, cramping

• Acidosis, signs of dehydration: rapid respirations, poor skin turgour, decreased urine output, dry skin, restlessness, weakness

Teach patient/family:

• Why protective isolation precautions are necessary, only if indicated

• To report any complaints, side effects to the nurse or clinician

• To avoid foods with citric acid, hot or rough texture if stomatitis is present

• Avoid highly spiced or salty foods

• Good mouth care and to report stomatitis

---

fluoxetine ▼

Prozac

Func. class.: Antidepressant, serotonin reuptake inhibitor

Chem. class.: Phenylpropylamine derivative

Legal class.: POM

Action: Inhibits CNS neurone uptake of serotonin, but not of noradrenaline

Uses: Depression, bulimia nervosa

Dosage and routes:

• *Adult:* By mouth, depression 20 mg daily; bulimia 60 mg daily

Available forms include: Capsules 20 mg (as hydrochloride)

Side effects/adverse reactions:

CNS: Headache, nervousness, insomnia, drowsiness, anxiety, tremor, dizziness, fatigue, sedation, poor concentration, abnormal dreams, agitation, convulsions, apathy, euphoria, hallucinations, delusions, psychosis, dyskinesia

GI: Nausea, diarrhoea, dry mouth, anorexia, dyspepsia, constipation, cramps, vomiting, taste changes, pancreatitis

INTEG: Sweating, rash, pruritus, urticaria

RESP: Infection, pharyngitis, sinusitis, cough, dyspnoea, bronchitis, pulmonary inflammation/fibrosis

CV: Vasculitis, cerebral vascular accident

MS: Pain, arthritis, twitching

GU: Dysmenorrhoea, decreased libido, urinary frequency, urinary tract infection, amenorrhoea, cystitis, impotence

SYST: Asthenia, fever

ENDO: Hyperprolactinaemia

HAEM: Thrombocytopenia

ELECT: Hyponatraemia

Contraindications: Hypersensitivity, severe renal failure, unstable epilepsy, MAOIs within last 14 days

Precautions: Pregnancy, lactation, children, elderly, epilepsy, renal or hepatic impairment

Pharmacokinetics:

Period of onset: Peak 6−8 hr; metabolised in liver, excreted in urine; half-life 2−7 days, protein bound

Interactions/incompatibilities:

• Do not use MAOIs until at least 5 weeks after discontinuing fluoxetine, do not use fluoxetine for 14 days after discontinuing MAOIs

• Increased agitation: L-tryptophan

• Increased side effects: highly protein bound drugs (e.g. anticoagulants, hypoglycaemics), cyclic antidepressants, diazepam

• Changes in lithium levels

Clinical assessment:

• Perform ECG: flattening of the T wave, bundle branch block, atrioventricular block and dysrhythmias may occur in cardiac patients

Treatment of overdose: Gastric lavage, activated charcoal, then supportive measures

NURSING CONSIDERATIONS

Assess:
• Baseline observations including neutral status

Administer:
• Increase fluid intake and dietary fibre if constipation or urinary retention occur
• Give with food or milk to avoid gastric irritation
• Tablets may be crushed if the patient is unable to swallow them whole
• Give at bedtime if sedation occurs during the day: the entire dose may be taken before retiring although this regime may not be tolerated well by the elderly
• Provide frequent mouth care
• Store at room temperature: avoid freezing
• Supervise ambulant patients carefully once the drug has been administered, as drowsiness and dizziness occur
• Check to ensure that all capsules have been swallowed

Evaluate:
• Mental status: mood, affect, suicidal tendencies, increase in psychiatric symptomatology, depression, panic attacks
• Blood pressure lying and standing and pulse 4 hrly. If systolic blood pressure falls by 20 mmHg drug should be withheld and clinician informed. For patients with cardiovascular disease vital signs must be reported 4 hrly
• Weigh 4 times a week, as appetite may decrease
• Extrapyramidal symptoms in the elderly, indicated by rigidity, dystonia and akathisia
• Urinary retention, constipation
• Withdrawal symptoms: headache, nausea, vomiting, muscular pain and weakness; usually if drug is discontinued suddenly
• If alcohol is taken the drug must be withheld until the following morning

Teach patient/family:
• The drug may not be effective for 2−3 weeks
• Caution must be taken when driving or performing other activities requiring mental alertness as drowsiness, dizziness and blurred vision may develop
• The drug must not be discontinued suddenly after long-term treatment as this may result in nausea, headache and malaise
• Alcohol and other CNS depressants must be avoided
• The clinician must be informed if patient/client becomes pregnant or if pregnancy and breast-feeding are planned

flupenthixol

Depixol, Depixol-Conc, Fluanxol
Func. class.: Antipsychotic/neuroleptic
Chem. class.: Thioxanthene
Legal class.: POM

Action: Dopamine antagonist
Uses: Schizophrenia and related disorders (but not mania or psychomotor hyperactivity), depressive illness, short-term adjunctive treatment of severe anxiety

Dosage and routes:
Schizophrenia and related disorders
• *Adult:* By mouth, 3−9 mg daily adjusted according to response; maximum 18 mg daily
• Depot injection, deep IM, 20−40 mg repeated at intervals of 2−4 weeks, adjusted according to response; maximum 400 mg weekly
Depression
• *Adult:* By mouth, initially 1 mg in morning, increased after 1 week to 2 mg if necessary; maximum dose, 3 mg; elderly patients, half standard dose, maximum dose, 2 mg; daily doses above 2 mg

(1 mg in elderly) to be divided and second portion to be given before 4 pm

Available forms include: Tablets, 0.5, 1, 3 mg (as dihydrochloride) Injection (oily), 20 mg/ml, 100 mg/ml (both as decanoate)

Side effects/adverse reactions:

CNS: Reversible extrapyramidal symptoms, tardive dyskinesia, drowsiness, apathy, insomnia, nightmares, depression, agitation, aggression, restlessness, dizziness, headache, mental dulling, convulsions

HAEM: Agranulocytosis, leucopenia, leucocytosis, haemolytic anaemia

EENT: Dry mouth, nasal congestion, corneal and lens opacities, purple pigmentation of cornea, conjunctiva and retina, blurred vision

META: Menstrual disturbances, galactorrhoea, gynaecomastia, weight gain, hyperprolactinaemia, impaired thermoregulation

GI: Constipation, nausea, changes in liver function tests

GU: Difficulty with micturition, impotence, impaired ejaculation, urinary incontinence and frequency, changes in libido

INTEG: Rashes, purple pigmentation of skin, pain, nodule formation at injection site, photosensitisation

CV: Hypotension, tachycardia, arrhythmias, oedema, ECG changes

SYSTEM: Lupus erythematosus-like syndrome, jaundice, hypersensitivity, neuroleptic malignant syndrome

Contraindications: Porphyria, bone marrow depression, coma caused by CNS depressants, closed-angle glaucoma, hypersensitivity, excitation, agitation, mania, severe depression requiring hospitalisation or electroconvulsive therapy, pregnancy, lactation, hypersensitivity

Precautions: Cardiovascular or severe respiratory disease, renal or hepatic impairment, epilepsy, parkinsonism, phaeochromocytoma, hypothyroidism, myasthenia gravis, prostatic hypertrophy, history of jaundice or leucopenia; prescribe with caution in elderly particularly in very hot or cold weather, avoid abrupt withdrawal, senile state, alcohol withdrawal, brain damage

Pharmacokinetics: After depot injection, plasma concentrations maximal after 4–7 days; after oral administration, peak concentration within 3–8 hours. Metabolised in liver

Interactions/incompatibilities:

• Reduced effects of: antiepileptics, dopamine agonists (e.g. bromocriptine, levodopa, lysuride), adrenaline and other sympathomimetics, guanethidine, clonidine

• Increased anticholinergic effects: tricyclic antidepressants, anticholinergics

• Effects of the following possibly increased: digoxin, quinidine, diazoxide, neuromuscular blockers

Clinical assessment:

• Try test dose of injection before treatment as undesirable side effects are prolonged

• Titrate dose and dose interval according to individual response

• Perform blood counts if prolonged, unexpected fever

• Prescribe anticholinergic drugs if extrapyramidal symptoms are a problem

• Avoid abrupt withdrawal

• Short course/lowest dose possible

• Close supervision

• Monitor symptoms of tardive dyskinesia, diabetic control, concurrent anticoagulant treatment

Treatment of overdose:
• Gastric lavage following tablet ingestion
• Symptomatic and supportive therapy, treat extrapyramidal symptoms with anticholinergics

NURSING CONSIDERATIONS
Assess:
• Baseline pulse and BP
Administer:
After test dose is given
• With care as contact sensitisation may occur
• Ensure by aspiration before injecting, that drug not given intravascularly
• Not more than 2−3 ml oily injection at any one site
• Do not withdraw drug abruptly
Perform/provide:
• For extrapyramidal symptoms, give anticholinergic drugs as prescribed
• Boiled sweets, sips of water for dry mouth
Evaluate:
• Check to ensure patient swallowed tablets
• Patient may need help with walking and other tasks if blurred vision occurs
• Therapeutic response: improvement in schizophrenic state, depressed state etc
• For side effects
• BP−hypotension may occur
• Pulse−tachycardia and arrhythmias may occur

NB: Stop drug and inform clinician at once if signs of neuroleptic malignant syndrome occur (hyperthermia, fluctuating loss of consciousness, muscular rigidity, pallor, tachycardia, labile BP, sweating, urinary incontinence)

Teach patient/family:
• Rise slowly as fainting may occur
• To avoid alcohol
• To avoid driving and other activities requiring alertness until certain that drowsiness does not occur
• Check with clinician before taking non-prescribed preparations
• Side effects may include menstrual disturbances or impotence
• Not to discontinue the medication abruptly
• Report any side-effects to clinician

---

fluphenazine decanoate/fluphenazine HCl

Modecate
Func. class.: Antipsychotic/neuroleptic
Chem. class.: Phenothiazine derivative
Legal class.: POM

Action: Dopamine antagonist with α-adrenergic and cholinergic blocking action
Uses: Psychotic disorders, schizophrenia, short-term adjunct in severe anxiety
Dosage and routes:
Decanoate
• *Adult:* IM schizophrenia, paranoid psychosis initially 12.5 mg (6.25 mg in elderly) then 12.5−100 mg 2−5 weekly
HCl
• *Adult:* By mouth, severe anxiety 1−2 mg twice daily; psychoses 2.5−10 mg daily in 2−3 doses; maximum 20 mg daily (10 mg in elderly)
Available forms include: Hydrochloride tablets 1, 2.5, 5 mg; injection IM, decanoate 25, 100 mg/ml
Side effects/adverse reactions:
RESP: Laryngospasm, dyspnoea, respiratory depression
CNS: Extrapyramidal symptoms: pseudoparkinsonism, akathisia,

dystonia, tardive dyskinesia, drowsiness, headache, seizures

HAEM: Anaemia, leucopenia, leukocytosis, agranulocytosis

INTEG: Rash, dermatitis

EENT: Blurred vision, glaucoma, lens opacities

GI: Dry mouth, nausea, vomiting, anorexia, constipation, diarrhoea, jaundice, weight gain, changes in liver function tests

GU: Urinary retention, urinary frequency, enuresis, impotence, amenorrhoea, gynaecomastia

CV: Orthostatic hypotension, hypertension, cardiac arrest, ECG changes, tachycardia, oedema

SYST: Hyperthermia, hypothermia, neuroleptic malignant syndrome

Contraindications: Hypersensitivity, circulatory collapse, cerebral arteriosclerosis, coma, cardiac insufficiency, bone marrow depression, renal failure, severe depression, phaeochromocytoma, liver failure

Precautions: Pregnancy, lactation, seizure disorders, hypertension/ hypotension, hepatic disease, thyrotoxicosis, Parkinson's disease, narrow angle glaucoma, hypothyroidism, prostatic hypertrophy, myasthenia gravis, brain damage, alcohol withdrawal, severe respiratory disease, diabetes, epilepsy, very hot weather

Pharmacokinetics:

By mouth (HCl): Onset 1 hr, peak 2−4 hr, duration 6−8 hr

IM (Decanoate): Onset 1−3 days, peak 1−2 days, duration over 4 weeks, half-life 2.5−16 weeks. Metabolised by liver, excreted in urine (metabolites), enters breast milk

Interactions/incompatibilities:

• Enhanced CNS depression with: alcohol, hypnotics, strong analgesics, other CNS depressants

• Reduced effects of: anti-epileptics, dopamine agonists (e.g. bromocriptine, levodopa, pergolide, lysuride), adrenaline and other sympathomimetics, guanethidine, clonidine

• Increased anticholinergic effects: anticholinergics, tricyclic antidepressants

• Increased toxicity of: quinidine, digoxin, neuromuscular blocking agents, lithium, anticoagulants

• Decreased absorbtion (HCl): antacids

Clinical assessment:

• Prescribe drugs for extrapyramidal symptoms

• Blood counts if prolonged, unexplained fever

• Control of diabetes, symptoms of tardive dyskinesia, concurrent anticoagulant treatment

• Inspect for lens/corneal opacities during prolonged use

Treatment of overdose: Lavage, if orally ingested. Symptomatic treatment, treat extrapyramidal symptoms with antimuscarinics

NURSING CONSIDERATIONS

Administer:

• Withdraw treatment gradually

• Short course/lowest dose possible

• Under close supervision

• Not more than 2−3 ml injection at any one site

Perform/provide:

• Decreased noise input by dimming lights, avoiding loud noises

• Supervised ambulation until stabilised on medication; do not involve in strenuous exercise programme because fainting is possible; patient should not stand still for long periods of time

• Increased fluids to prevent constipation

• Frequent sips of water for dry mouth to encourage salivation

Evaluate:

• Swallowing of oral medication; check for hoarding or giving of

medication to other patients
• Skin turgor daily
• Constipation, urinary retention daily; if these occur, increase fibre, fluids in diet
• All side effects

Teach patient/family:
• That orthostatic hypotension occurs often, to rise from sitting or lying position gradually
• To avoid hot baths, hot showers, since hypotension may occur
• To avoid abrupt withdrawal of this drug or extrapyramidal symptoms may result; drug should be withdrawn slowly on graduated doses
• To avoid non-prescribed preparations (cough, hayfever, cold) unless approved by clinician since serious drug interactions may occur; avoid use with alcohol or CNS depressants; increased drowsiness may occur
• To use a sunscreen during sun exposure to prevent burns
• Regarding compliance with drug regimen
• About extrapyramidal symptoms and necessity for meticulous oral hygiene since oral candidiasis may occur
• To report sore throat, malaise, fever, bleeding, mouth sores; if these occur, full blood count should be performed and drug discontinued

---

flurandrenolone

Haelan, Haelan-C
Func. class.: Moderately potent topical corticosteroid
Chem. class.: Fluorinated corticosteroid
Legal class.: POM

Action: Reduces inflammation
Uses: 0.05% preparations, severe inflammatory skin disorders e.g.

eczema unresponsive to less potent corticosteroids; 0.0125% preparations, milder inflammatory skin disorders

Dosage and routes: Apply topical preparations, except tape, sparingly, 2–3 times daily; reduce strength and frequency as condition responds. Tape: Apply to lesions for 12–24 hr

Available forms include: Cream, 0.0125%, in water-miscible basis; 0.0125% with clioquinol 3%. Ointment, 0.0125%, in anhydrous greasy basis; 0.0125% with clioquinol 3%. Impregnated occlusive adhesive tape 4 mcg per cm^2

Side effects/adverse reactions:
INTEG: Spread and worsening of untreated infection; thinning of the skin; irreversible striae atrophicae; perioral dermatitis; acne at site of application; depigmentation; increased hair growth, telangiectasia
ENDO: Suppression of hypothalamic-pituitary-adrenal axis producing growth retardation and suppressed plasma cortisol, Cushing's syndrome, reduced glucose tolerance
CNS: Cranial hypertension in children

Contraindications: Untreated bacterial, fungal or viral skin infections, hypersensitivity to clioquinol (Haelan-C)
Precautions: Pregnancy, lactation, use with great care under occlusive dressings including nappies
Pharmacokinetics: Significant absorption can occur, especially under occlusive dressings

NURSING CONSIDERATIONS
Administer:
• Cleanse before applying drug
• Only to affected areas, avoid contact with eyes
• Apply cream to weeping lesions, ointment to scaly lesions
• Only to dermatoses, not to surrounding or infected areas

- Apply sparingly

Evaluate:
- Temperature if fever develops, discontinue drug
- Therapeutic response: absence of severe itching, patches on skin, flaking
- Systemic absorption: fever, infection, irritation

Teach patient/family:
- Apply sparingly to affected area only
- Avoid contact with eyes
- Avoid sunlight on skin, burns may occur

---

flurazepam HCl

Dalmane
Func. class.: Hypnotic/sedative
Chem. class.: Benzodiazepine
Legal class.: CD (Sch. 4) POM (NHS)

Action: Produces CNS depression at the limbic, thalamic, hypothalamic levels of CNS; may be mediated by neurotransmitter gamma aminobutyric (GABA); results are sedation, hypnosis, skeletal muscle relaxation anxiolytic action

Uses: Insomnia, short-term treatment

Dosage and routes:
- *Adult:* By mouth 15−30 mg at night
- *Geriatric:* By mouth 15 mg at night

Available forms include: Capsules 15, 30 mg

Side effects/adverse reactions:
HAEM: Leucopenia, granulocytopenia (rare)
CNS: Lethargy, drowsiness, daytime sedation, dizziness, confusion, lightheadedness, headache, anxiety, irritability, dependence potential, changes in libido, paradoxical aggression, excitement, unmasking of depression
GI: Nausea, vomiting, diarrhoea, heartburn, abdominal pain, constipation, bitter taste
CV: Chest pain, pulse changes
GU: Urinary retention

Contraindications: Hypersensitivity to benzodiazepines, acute pulmonary insufficiency, respiratory depression, intermittent porphyria

Precautions: Anaemia, hepatic disease, renal disease, suicidal individuals, drug abuse, elderly, psychosis, child, lactation, pregnancy, where morning alertness important

Pharmacokinetics:
Period of onset: Onset 15−45 min, duration 7−8 hr; metabolised by liver, excreted by kidneys (inactive/active metabolites), excreted in breast milk; half-life 47−100 hr, additional 100 hr for active metabolites

Interactions/incompatibilities:
- Increased effects of this drug: cimetidine
- Increased action of both drugs: alcohol, CNS depressants

Clinical assessment:
- Continued requirement for treatment

Lab. test interferences:
False increase: Urinary 17-hydroxycorticosteroids

Treatment of overdose: Lavage, activated charcoal, monitor electrolytes, vital signs, flumazenil may be used to antagonise

NURSING CONSIDERATIONS

Administer:
- After trying conservative measures for insomnia
- ½−1 hr before bedtime for sleeplessness
- On empty stomach for maximum effect but may be taken with food if GI symptoms occur

Perform/provide:

• Assistance with mobilisation after receiving dose
• Safety measure: cot sides, call-bell within easy reach
• Checking to see oral medication has been swallowed

Evaluate:
• Therapeutic response: ability to sleep at night, decreased amount of early morning awakening if taking drug for insomnia
• Mental status: mood, alertness, affect, memory (long, short)
• Type of sleep problem: falling asleep, staying asleep
• Effectiveness of treatment by sleep patterns

Teach patient/family:
• To avoid driving or other activities requiring alertness until drug is stabilised
• To avoid alcohol ingestion or CNS depressants; serious CNS depression may result
• Alternative measures to improve sleep: reading, exercise several hours before bedtime, warm bath, warm milk, TV, self-hypnosis, deep breathing
• That hangover is common in elderly

---

flurbiprofen

Froben
Func. class.: Non-steroidal anti-inflammatory drug
Chem. class.: Propionic acid derivative
Legal class.: POM

Action: Inhibits prostaglandin synthesis; possesses analgesic, anti-inflammatory, antipyretic properties
Uses: Rheumatoid arthritis, osteo-arthritis, ankylosing spondylitis
Dosage and routes:
• *Adult:* By mouth/per rectum 150–300 mg in divided doses daily; modified-release, 200 mg daily
Available forms include: Tablets 50, 100 mg; modified-release capsules 200 mg; suppositories 100 mg
Side effects/adverse reactions:
GI: Nausea, anorexia, vomiting, diarrhoea, cholestatic jaundice, peptic ulcer, dyspepsia, indigestion, glossitis, gastrointestinal bleeding, local irritation after rectal administration
CNS: Dizziness, drowsiness, myalgia, headache
CV: Peripheral oedema
INTEG: Rash, urticaria, angio-oedema, exfoliative dermatitis (rare), alopecia
GU: Nephrotoxicity: dysuria, haematuria, oliguria, azotaemia, cystitis, nocturia, renal insufficiency
HAEM: blood dyscrasias, bone marrow depression
EENT: Tinnitus, hearing loss, blurred vision
RESP: Dyspnoea, haemoptysis, bronchospasm, rhinitis, shortness of breath
Contraindications: Hypersensitivity, hypersensitivity to other NSAIDs agents, peptic ulceration, gastrointestinal haemorrhage, ulcerative colitis, asthma, avoid rectal administration in inflammatory disease of rectum and peri-anal area
Precautions: Pregnancy, lactation, children, bleeding disorders, GI disorders, cardiac disorders, severe renal disease, severe hepatic disease, hypertension, elderly
Pharmacokinetics:
Period of onset: Peak 1½ hr, half-life 6 hr, metabolised in liver, excreted in urine (metabolites), breast milk, 99% protein bound
Interactions/incompatibilities:
• May increase action of: anticoagulants, phenytoin, sulphonyl-urea hypoglycaemics

• Decreased effects of: β-blockers, frusemide
• Enhanced toxicity of: methotrexate, cyclosporin, lithium

Clinical assessment:
• Patient at high risk of peptic ulceration or GI bleeding
• Renal and hepatic function if impairment expected

Treatment of overdose:
Gastric lavage, supportive treatment, correct serum electrolytes

NURSING CONSIDERATIONS
Assess:
• Test hearing and eyesight before, during and after treatment

Administer:
• With food to reduce gastric irritation

Perform/provide:
• Store suppositories in a cool dry place between 2° and 25°C

Evaluate:
• Response to treatment indicated by decreased pain and joint stiffness, swollen joints and ability to move more easily
• Eye and ear problems: blurred vision, tinnitus may suggest toxicity
• Report any indigestion or black tarry stools

Teach patient/family:
• To inform clinician of blurred vision and tinnitus as these may suggest toxicity
• To avoid driving, operating machinery etc., if drowsiness or dizziness occur
• To report changes in urinary output, weight gain, oedema, fever and blood in urine as nephrotoxicity may occur
• The drug may not be fully effective until up to a month after start of treatment
• To store medication as above
• To take with food, milk or antacids to avoid gastric upset
• To avoid aspirin and alcohol
• To report any indigestion or black tarry stools

fluspirilene

Redeptin
Func. class.: Antipsychotic, neuroleptic
Chem. class.: Diphenylbutyl-piperidine
Legal class.: POM

Action: Dopamine antagonist
Uses: Maintenance treatment in schizophrenia and related psychoses

Dosage and routes:
• *Adults:* Deep IM injection 2 mg, increased by 2 mg at weekly intervals according to response; usual maintenance dose 2−8 mg weekly, maximum 20 mg weekly
• *Elderly:* A quarter to half the usual starting dose may be required
Available forms include: Injection 2 mg/ml; 1 ml, 3 ml ampoules, 6 ml vials (aqueous suspension)

Side effects/adverse reactions:
CVS: Hypotension, arrhythmias
INTEG: Pain, erythema, swelling, nodules at injection site, pallor, photosensitisation, rashes, sweating
CNS: Extrapyramidal symptoms, tardive dyskinesia, moderate sedative effects, drowsiness, apathy, depression, insomnia, restlessness, agitation, nightmares, blurred vision, headache
GI: Dry mouth, constipation, salivation, jaundice
GU: Difficulty with micturition, impotence
EENT: Nasal congestion
META: Hypothermia, pyrexia, menstrual disturbances, galactorrhoea, gynaecomastia, weight gain
SYST: Neuroleptic malignant syndrome

Contraindications: Coma caused by CNS depressants, hypersensitivity to this drug or other diphenybutylpiperidines, lactation
Precautions: Cardiovascular dis-

ease, renal or hepatic impairment, parkinsonism, epilepsy, prostatic hypertrophy, elderly, alcoholism, brain damage, lithium therapy

Pharmacokinetics: Duration of action 5–15 days. Maximum plasma concentrations within 4–8 hr after IM injection; half-life 3 weeks, metabolite excreted in urine

Interactions/incompatibilities:
• Reduced effects of: antiepileptics, dopamine agonists (e.g. bromocriptine, levodopa, lysuride, pergolide)
• Enhanced CNS depression with: alcohol, hypnotics, strong analgesics, other CNS depressants
• Possible enhanced toxicity of both drugs: lithium
• Enhanced hypotension with: anaesthetics
• Enhanced antimuscarinic side-effects with: tricyclic antidepressants

Clinical assessment:
• Caution, it masks nausea/vomiting of other conditions
• Monitor renal and hepatic function of impaired
• Monitor for signs of tardive dyskinesia during long-term therapy

Treatment of overdose: Symptomatic treatment, treat extrapyramidal symptoms with antimuscarinics

NURSING CONSIDERATIONS

Assess:
• Baseline BP (lying and standing), pulse, respiration and temperature

Administer:
• By deep IM injection; rotating sites
• Shake well before use

Perform/provide:
• Fluids/boiled sweets for dry mouth
• Local treatment for pain at site
• Safe environment: cot sides, help with mobilisation

• Fibre/fluids for constipation
• Sexual counselling as required

Evaluate:
• Subcutaneous nodules
• Restlessness, agitation, changes in sleep pattern
• Fluid balance
• Sweating, rashes and sore throats
• Fever, hypothermia
• Weight gain
• Mood and mental state

Teach patient/family:
• Warn about side effects such as nightmares, weight gain, blurred vision, sexual problems, menstrual cycle changes and nicturition difficulties
• To report fever, infection and sore throat and rashes
• To avoid the sun and use a sunscreen
• That drug may take several weeks to take effect
• Change position slowly to avoid dizziness
• Avoid hot baths
• May cause drowsiness, if affected do not drive or operate machinery. Take no alcohol or any other medicines unless specifically prescribed

---

flutamide ▼

Drogenil
Func. class.: Antiandrogen
Legal class.: POM

Action: Blocks androgen receptors at target tissues

Uses: Treatment of advanced prostatic carcinoma in which suppression of testosterone effects is indicated

Dosage and routes:
• *Adult:* By mouth 250 mg 3 times a day

Available forms include: Tablets 250 mg

Side effects/adverse reactions:

GI: Nausea, vomiting, diarrhoea, ulcer-like pain, heartburn, liver dysfunction, thirst

CNS: Increased appetite, anorexia, insomnia, tiredness, headache, dizziness, weakness, malaise, blurred vision, anxiety

CV: Oedema, lymphoedema

GU: Gynaecomastia and/or breast tenderness, galactorrhoea, decreased libido, reduced sperm counts

HAEM: Ecchymoses, haemolytic anaemia, macrocytic anaemia

RESP: Chest pain

INTEG: Pruritus, lupus-like syndrome, herpes zoster

Contraindications: Sensitivity to flutamide

Precautions: Cardiac disease, hepatic disease

Pharmacokinetics: Rapid and complete absorption after oral administration, with rapid metabolism to active metabolite. Half-life of both flutamide and major metabolite 5–6 hr

Interactions/incompatibilities:
• Increased effect of warfarin

Clinical assessment:
• Periodic liver function tests
• Monitor concurrent warfarin therapy closely

Treatment of overdose: Forced gastric emptying, supportive care

NURSING CONSIDERATIONS:

Perform/provide:
• All supporting measures for patient with cancer

Evaluate:
• Side effects

Teach patient/family:
• To report side-effects and any increasing symptoms

fluvoxamine maleate

Faverin

Func. class.: Antidepressant, serotonin uptake inhibitor

Legal class.: POM

Action: Selectively inhibits re-uptake of central neurotransmitter 5-HT with little effect on noradrenaline

Uses: Depressive illness

Dosage and routes:
• By mouth usually 100–200 mg daily; maximum daily dose 300 mg; doses over 100 mg must be divided

Available forms include: Tablets 50 mg, 100 mg

Side effects/adverse reactions:

GI: Nausea, vomiting, constipation, diarrhoea, raised liver enzyme levels

CNS: Headache, drowsiness, agitation, tremor, convulsions, dizziness, anxiety

CV: Bradycardia, hypotension, ECG changes

Contraindications: History of epilepsy, MAOIs within 2 weeks of starting treatment

Precautions: Renal or hepatic impairment, pregnancy, lactation

Pharmacokinetics: Onset of effect within 2 weeks; half-life is 15 hr, converted in liver to inactive metabolites which are excreted in urine. Completely absorbed orally, 80% protein bound

Interactions/incompatibilities:
• Increased effects of: alcohol
• Potentiation: nicoumalone, warfarin, MAOIs, propranolol, theophylline, phenytoin
• Effects possibly enhanced by: lithium, tryptophan

Clinical assessment:
• ECG if CV side effects occur
• Renal function if impairment suspected

- Liver function if impairment suspected
- Serum levels of oral anticoagulants, phenytoin, theophylline during concomitant therapy

Treatment of overdose: Gastric lavage and activated charcoal; symptomatic treatment

NURSING CONSIDERATIONS

Administer:
- In the evening
- Avoiding antacids/alkalis

Perform/provide:
- Fibre and fluids for constipation
- Small portions of favourite foods

Evaluate:
- Pulse 4 hrly
- Appetite or nausea
- Fits or neurological events
- Weight, improving sleep pattern, mental state and mood

Teach patient/family:
- To avoid alcohol
- That agitation may increase
- Tablet to be swallowed whole, not chewed
- Not to take indigestion medicines
- Not to drive or operate machinery if drowsy

---

folic acid

Lexpec

Func. class.: Vitamin B complex group

Chemical class.: Pteroylglutamic acid

Legal class.: POM

Action: Needed for erythropoiesis; increases RBC and platelet formation in megaloblastic anaemias

Uses: Megaloblastic or macrocytic anaemia caused by folic acid deficiency, liver disease, alcoholism, haemolysis

Dosage and routes:
- *Adult:* Initially 5 mg daily for 4 months then 5 mg a day to 5 mg week
- *Child:* Under 1 yr: 500 mcg/kg daily; over 1 yr as adult dose

Available forms include: Tablets 5 mg, syrup 2.5 mg/5 ml

Side effects/adverse reactions:

RESP: Bronchospasm

Contraindications: Hypersensitivity, should not be given alone in pernicious anaemia and other B_{12}-deficiency states because of the risk of subacute combined degeneration of the spinal cord; folate deficiency due to dihydrofolate reductase inhibitors

Pharmacokinetics:

Period of onset: Peak ½−1 hr, bound to plasma proteins, excreted in breast milk, methylated in liver, excreted in urine (small amounts)

Clinical assessment:
- Full blood count

NURSING CONSIDERATIONS

Assess:
- Drugs currently taken: alcohol, hydantoins, trimethoprim, these drugs may cause increased folic acid use by body

Evaluate:
- Therapeutic response: increased weight, oriented well-being, absence of fatigue

Teach patient/family:
- Take drug exactly as prescribed
- Notify clinician of side effects e.g. anorexia, occasionally nausea, abdominal distension and flatulence
- Correct dietary intake

folinic acid

Refolinon, Rescufolin, Calcium
Folinate, Calcium Leucovorin,
Lederfolin
Func. class.: Vitamin/folic acid
antagonist antidote
Chem. class.: Tetrahydrofolic acid
derivative
Legal class.: POM

Action: Converted to essential
cofactor tetrahydrofolate, cir-
cumventing enzyme inhibition by
drugs, prevents toxicity during
antineoplastic therapy by protecting normal cells. Modifies metabolism of 5-fluorouracil enhancing
its potency
Uses: Megaloblastic or macrocytic
anaemia caused by folic acid deficiency, overdose of folic acid
antagonist, methotrexate toxicity,
toxicity caused by pyrimethamine
or trimethoprim. Adjunct to 5-
fluorouracil treatment of cancer

Dosage and routes:
*Megaloblastic anaemia caused by
folate deficiency*
• *Adult:* 10−20 mg once a day
• *Child:* 0.25 mg/kg daily

*Prevention of toxicity after thera-
peutic doses of methotrexate*
• *Adult and child:* IM, IV infusion,
IV injection, by mouth up to
120 mg in divided doses over 12−
24 hr then 12−15 mg IM or 15 mg
by mouth 6-hrly for 48 hr. Prolonged and/or higher doses needed
after high doses of methotrexate
or when clearance impaired. Begin
8−24 hr after methotrexate infusion started

*Prevention of toxicity after metho-
trexate overdose*
• Immediate administration of an
equal or greater dose of folinic
acid

Potentiation of 5-fluorouracil

25−200 mg/m^2 immediately before
5-fluorouracil
Available forms include: Tablets
15 mg; injection IM/IV 3 mg/ml,
1, 2, 10 ml amps; powder for
injection 15, 30, 50, 100, 350 mg
Side effects/adverse reactions:
SYSTEM: Pyrexia
RESP: Wheezing
Contraindications: Pernicious
anaemia/megaloblastic anaemia
where vitamin B$_{12}$ is deficient
Pharmacokinetics: Not known
Interactions/incompatibilities:
• Nullifies effects of antineoplastic
folate antagonists e.g. methotrex-
ate if given simultaneously
• Increases effect of 5-fluorouracil
Clinical assessment:
• Methotrexate levels during
folinic acid rescue after high
methotrexate doses or where
impaired clearance anticipated
NURSING CONSIDERATIONS
Administer:
• After reconstituting with water
for injection
Perform/provide:
• Increase fluid intake if used to
treat folic acid inhibitor overdose
Evaluate:
• Therapeutic response: increased
weight, oriented well-being,
absence of fatigue
• Fluid balance, watch for nausea
and vomiting
• Respiratory status, especially
wheezing
• Drugs currently taken: alcohol,
hydantoins, trimethoprim may
cause increased folic acid use by
body
Teach patient/family:
• To take drug exactly as
prescribed
• To notify clinician of side effects
• To eat vitamin B-rich diet

fosfestrol tetrasodium

Honvan
Func. class.: Oestrogen pro-drug
Chem. class.: Salt of the oestrogen
stilboestrol
Legal class.: POM

Action: Produces stilboestrol when
activated by the enzyme acid
phosphatase, producing local
cytotoxic effect
Uses: All stages of prostatic carcinoma, including pain due to
metastases
Dosage and routes:
• By mouth 100−200 mg 3 times
daily, reducing to 100−300 mg
daily in divided doses; Slow IV
injection 552−1104 mg daily for at
least 5 days; maintenance dose
276 mg 1−4 times weekly
Available forms include: Tablets
100 mg; injection 55.2 mg/ml,
5-ml ampoule
Side effects/adverse reactions:
CNS: Dizziness, headache, migraine, depression
CV: Hypertension, thrombophlebitis, oedema, thromboembolism, CVA, pulmonary
embolism, myocardial infarction
GI: Nausea, vomiting, diarrhoea,
anorexia, pancreatitis, cramps,
constipation, increased appetite,
increased myopia, astigmatism
GU: Gynaecomastia, testicular
atrophy, impotence, feminisation
INTEG: Rash, urticaria, acne, oily
skin, seborrhoea, purpura,
chloasma
META: Folic acid deficiency,
hypercalcaemia, hyperglycaemia
MS: Perineal burning and discomfort, pain in bony metastases
Precautions: Hypertension gallbladder disease, congestive cardiac
failure, diabetes, poor cardiac reserve, fluid retention, depression,
history of cholestatic jaundice

Clinical assessment:
• Check cardiac functions
• Use only in specialist oncology
unit
• Analgesia if given IV for prostatic cancer
• IV administration should be
slow, with patient lying supine
• Diuretics if fluid retention
present
• Evaluate size of tumour, acid
phosphatase, level of side effects
Treatment of overdose: Gastric
lavage if swallowed. Supportive
treatment paying special attention
to electrolytes

NURSING CONSIDERATIONS
Assess:
• Fluid balance, BP and pulse

Administer:
• Orally, with food if required to
decrease nausea. Close links to a
oncology unit should be maintained
• Intravenously, slowly directly
into vein each day, with patient
supine. Special handling preparation, administration and disposal of syringe and needle is by
trained non-pregnant, staff wearing protective clothing
• Facilities for regular monitoring
of clinical, biochemical and haematological effects during and after
administration (IV)

Perform/provide:
• Suitable analgesic, antiemetics
and diuretics
• Diet suitable to enhance each
patient's good health
• Aid with mobility

Evaluate:
• Therapeutic response; destruction of malignant cell, decreased
malignant growth, and pain from
metastases
• Input and output of fluids, check
for retention
• Blood pressure and pulse especially during IV therapy
• Regular urinalysis

• Weigh before initial dose then at regular intervals
• Increased urinary function and patient's well being
• Maintain on lowest dose that will control disease
• Signs of feminising of men, impotence, enlarged breasts, testicular atrophy
• Perineal and bony metastatic pain after IV treatment
Teach patient/family:
• That addition of analgesia is available when required
• To understand body changes may occur, including breasts in men
• To report any body changes; including dizziness, pain, soreness, weight loss or gain, oedema, skin changes, jaundice

framycetin sulphate

Sofradex (with gramicidin and dexamethasone), Soframycin (with gramicidin)
Func. class.: Topical antibiotic
Chem. class.: Aminoglycoside
Legal class.: POM

Action: Impairs bacterial protein synthesis; bactericidal
Uses: Bacterial infection in otitis externa; bacterial skin infections
Dosage and routes:
• Eye drops: Instil 1−2 drops up to 6 times a day; eye oitnment: apply 2 or 3 times a day; ear drops: 2−3 drops 3 or 4 times a day
• Ear ointment: apply once or twice a day
• Impregnated dressing: directly to infected wound and covered
Available forms include: Eye/eardrops, eye ointment, 0.5%; cream, ointment 1.5%; impregnated paraffin gauze dressing 1%
Side effects/adverse reactions:

EENT: Local sensitivity, ototoxicity
Contraindications: Hypersensitivity to framycetin or other ingredients
Precautions: Perforated eardrum, short term use only or fungal infections may occur, contact lenses, pregnancy, lactation, sensitivity to other aminoglycoside antibiotics
Pharmacokinetics: Significant absorption possible during prolonged use
Clinical assessment:
• Avoid long-term use (fungal infection may occur)
• Systemic antibiotic may be required
• Check sensitivity to framycetin and neomycin
• Culture and sensitivity tests
NURSING CONSIDERATIONS
Assess:
• Check ear drum intact before use
Administer:
• After obtaining samples for culture and sensitivity
Perform/provide:
• Store in refrigerator (avoid freezing)
• Discard 4 weeks after opening
• Simple comfort e.g. warm cloth
• Ear hygiene
• Hearing tests if ototoxicity occurs
Evaluate:
• Hearing loss
• Discharge from ear
• Improvement in condition
Teach patient/family:
• Ear drop instillation and care of drugs
• Report hearing changes/local reactions
• To finish course

frusemide

Lasix, Aluzine, Diuresal, Dryptal, Frumax, Rusyde, many combination products
Func. class.: Loop diuretic
Chem. class.: Sulphonamide derivative
Legal class.: POM

Action: Acts on loop of Henle by increasing excretion of chloride, sodium

Uses: Pulmonary oedema, oedema in congestive cardiac failure, liver disease, renal disease, hypertension

Dosage and routes:
• *Adult:* By mouth 20−80 mg daily in the morning; IM/slow IV 20−50 mg, increased until desired response
• *Child:* By mouth 1−3 mg/kg daily; IM/slow IV 0.5−1.5 mg/kg to maximum of 20 mg daily
Oliguria
• By mouth: initially 250 mg daily increasing by increments of 250 mg every 4−6 hr if necessary to maximum single dose 2 g; IV infusion 0.25−1 g daily, rate not exceeding 4 mg/min
Available forms include: Tablets 20, 40, 500 mg; oral solution 1 mg/ml; injection IM, IV 10 mg/ml, 2 ml, 5 ml and 25 ml ampoules

Side effects/adverse reactions:
GU: Renal failure, glycosuria
ELECT: Hypokalaemia, hypochloraemic alkalosis, hypomagnesaemia, hyperuricaemia, hypocalcaemia, hyponatraemia
CNS: Headache, fatigue, weakness, vertigo, paraesthesia
GI: Nausea, diarrhoea, dry mouth, vomiting, anorexia, cramps, oral, gastric irritations
EENT: Loss of hearing, ear pain, tinnitus, blurred vision
INTEG: Rash, pruritus, purpura, Stevens-Johnson syndrome, sweating, photosensitivity, urticaria
MS: Cramps, gout, stiffness
ENDO: Hyperglycaemia
HAEM: Thrombocytopenia, agranulocytosis, leucopenia, anaemia
CV: Orthostatic hypotension

Contraindications: Hypersensitivity to sulphonamides, anuria, hypovolaemia, electrolyte depletion, precomatose states associated with liver cirrhosis

Precautions: Diabetes mellitus, dehydration, ascites, severe renal disease, pregnancy, lactation, prostatic hypertrophy

Pharmacokinetics:
By mouth: Onset 1 hr, peak 1−2 hr, duration 6−8 hr
IV: Onset 5 min, peak ½ hr, duration 2 hr
Excreted in urine, faeces, excreted in breast milk

Interactions/incompatibilities:
• Increased toxicity: digitalis, aminoglycoside antibiotics, cephalosporins, NSAIDs, antiarrhythmics, vancomycin, corticosteroids, carbenoxolone, cisplatin
• Decreased effects of: antidiabetics, pressor amines, mexiletine, tocainide, lignocaine (as antiarrhythmic)
• Increased action of: antihypertensives especially angiotensin converting enzyme inhibitors, tubocurarine, gallamine lithium, salicylates
• Increased orthostatic hypotension: alcohol, barbiturates, narcotics
• Decreased effect of frusemide: indomethacin and NSAIDs, phenytoin, aspirin, phenobarbitone, carbenoxolone

Clinical assessment:
• Electrolytes; potassium, sodium, chloride; include blood urea nitrogen, blood sugar, full blood count, serum creatinine, serum uric acid

Lab. test interferences:

Interfere: Glucose tolerance test
Treatment of overdose: Lavage if taken orally, monitor electrolytes, administer fluids and electrolytes

NURSING CONSIDERATIONS
Assess:
• Baseline BP, weight and fluid balance
• Initial effect of drug, increase or decrease dose, then reduce where possible to maintenance
• Glucose in urine if patient is diabetic
Administer:
• Orally in the morning to avoid interference with sleep if using drug as a diuretic
• Intravenous injection in emergency only, give slowly directly into vein. If larger doses are then required give by slow infusion and titrate according to response. Maximum dose and rate must be checked.
• IV route preferred to IM
• Potassium replacement if potassium is less than 3.0 mmol/l
• With food, if nausea occurs, absorption may be decreased slightly
Perform/provide:
• Drug increases urinary output; if patient is not able to move quickly ensure toilet facilities nearby
Evaluate:
• Improvement in oedema of feet, legs, sacral area daily if medication is being used in congestive cardiac failure
• Weight, fluid balance daily to determine fluid loss; effect of drug may be decreased if used daily
• Rate, depth, rhythm of respiration, effect of exertion
• BP lying, standing; postural hypotension may occur
• Improvement in CVP 8 hrly
• Signs of metabolic acidosis: drowsiness, restlessness
• Signs of hypokalaemia: postural hypotension, malaise, fatigue, tachycardia, leg cramps, weakness
• Rashes, temperature elevation, pruritis daily
• Confusion, especially in elderly
Teach patient/family:
• To increase fluid intake 2–3 litres daily unless contraindicated
• To rise slowly from lying or sitting position
• To inform clinician if experience muscle cramps, weakness, nausea, dizziness
• Take with food or milk for GI symptoms
• Take early in day to prevent nocturia

---

gallamine triethiodide

Flaxedil
Func. class.: Non-depolarising muscle relaxant
Legal class.: POM

Action: Inhibits transmission of nerve impulses by competing for cholinergic receptor sites, antagonising action of acetylcholine
Uses: Facilitation of endotracheal intubation, skeletal muscle relaxation during mechanical ventilation, surgery, or general anaesthesia
Dosage and routes:
• *Adult:* IV 80–120 mg then 20–40 mg as required. May be given IM if not suitable vein
• *Child:* IV 1.5 mg/kg
• *Neonate:* 600 mcg/kg
Available forms include: Injection IV 40 mg/ml
Side effects/adverse reactions:
CV: Bradycardia, tachycardia, decreased BP
RESP: Prolonged apnoea, bronchospasm, cyanosis, respiratory depression
EENT: Increased secretions

INTEG: Rash, flushing, pruritus, urticaria
GI: Decreased motility
Contraindications: Hypersensitivity, myasthenia gravis, shock, severe renal impairment (glomerular filtration rate less than 50 ml/min)
Precautions: Pregnancy, cardiac disease, children, electrolyte imbalances, dehydration, respiratory disease, renal disease
Pharmacokinetics:
IV: Onset 2 min, duration 20−60 min; half-life 2 min, 29 min (terminal), excreted in urine, faeces (metabolites)
Interactions/incompatibilities:
• Increased neuromuscular blockade: aminoglycosides, clindamycin, lincomycin, quinidine, local anaesthetics, polymyxin antibiotics, lithium, narcotic analgesics, thiazides, enflurane, isoflurane, halothane, diazepam, nifedipine, verapamil
• Reduced neuromuscular blockade: azathioprine
• Do not mix with barbiturates or pethidine in solution or syringe
Clinical assessment:
• For electrolyte imbalances (potassium, magnesium); may lead to increased action of this drug
• By anaesthetist to determine neuromuscular blockade
Treatment of overdose: Edrophonium or neostigmine, atropine, monitor vital signs; may require mechanical ventilation
NURSING CONSIDERATIONS
Assess:
• History of renal impairment, myasthenia gravis
• Electrolyte levels
• Vital signs (BP, pulse, respirations)
Administer:
• IV: 80−120 mg
• IM: by anaesthetist only if no vein available
• Not to be mixed with barbiturate
• By slow IV over 1−2 min (only by qualified person, usually an anaesthetist)
Perform/provide:
• Flush vein with saline before and after administration
• Reassurance if communication is difficult during recovery from neuromuscular blockade
Evaluate:
• Therapeutic response: level and dose of paralysis
• Vital signs especially tachycardia
• Allergic reactions: rash, fever, respiratory distress, pruritus; drug should be discontinued
Teach patient/family:
• That some muscle weakness present during recovery

---

ganciclovir

Cymevene
Func. class.: Antiviral
Chem. class.: Guanine derivative
Legal class.: POM

Action: Phosphorylated to active form within infected cell; inhibits viral DNA replication
Uses: Life-threatening or sight-threatening cytomegalovirus in immunocompromised patients
Dosage and routes: IV infusion over 1 hr, initially 5 mg/kg every 12 hr for 14−21 days; patients at risk of relapse, maintenance dose 6 mg/kg daily for 5 days per week or 5 mg/kg every day. Treatment should be based on individual response and toxicity
Available forms include: IV infusion powder for reconstitution, 500 mg vial
Side effects/adverse reactions:
HAEM: Thrombocytopenia, neutropenia, anaemia, eosinophilia, raised blood urea nitrogen or serum creatinine

GU: Impaired fertility, incontinence, anuria, haematuria
GI: Abdominal pain, bloating, anorexia, constipation, diarrhoea, haemorrhage, melaena
INTEG: Rashes, local reactions at infusion site, alopecia, pruritus
EENT: Sore throat, epistaxis
META: Abnormal liver function tests, acidosis, decreased glucose, potassium and sodium levels
CV: Syncope, hypotension, tachycardia, hypertension, haemorrhage, generalised oedema, arrhythmias, chest pain, cardiac arrest, myocardial infarction, phlebitis, paraesthesia
CNS: Headache, dizziness, anxiety, drowsiness, coma, confusion, hallucinations, ataxia, deafness, retinal detachment
SYSTEM: Sepsis, fever, malaise, facial oedema
MS: Arthralgia, myalgia, muscular twitching
RESP: Asthma, cough, dyspnoea
Contraindications: Pregnancy, lactation within 72 hr, abnormally low neutrophil counts, hypersensitivity to ganciclovir or acyclovir, neonatal or congenital cytomegalovirus
Precautions: Haematological toxicity, renal impairment, history of exposure to radiation or to drugs toxic to bone marrow, potential carcinogen, vesicant, prevent conception for 90 days after treatment (men and women)
Pharmacokinetics: Half-life 3 hr; eliminated in urine
Interactions/incompatibilities:
• Increase toxicity: cotrimoxazole, pentamidine, dapsone, flucytosine, zidovudine, amphotericin
• Increased risk of seizures when administered with this drug: imipenem-cilastatin
Clinical assessment:
• Renal function; dose adjusted in renal impairment
• Blood counts every 1−2 days for decreasing granulocytes; if Hb is too low, may require blood transfusion or drug to be withheld
• Liver function tests; serum electrolytes
Treatment of overdose: Consider haemodialysis
NURSING CONSIDERATIONS
Administer:
• By IV infusion slowly over 1 hr
• Wear gloves and safety goggles when reconstituting solution; toxic and a potential carcinogen
Evaluate:
• For facial oedema and a wide range of side effects
• For changes in physical condition
Teach patient/family:
• Drug is not a cure but will control symptoms
• To notify clinician of sore throat, epistaxis, malaise
• That serious drug interactions could occur if non-prescribed medications are taken
• That other drugs may be necessary to prevent any infections

gemeprost

Cervagem
Func. class.: Oxytoxic
Chem. class.: Prostaglandin E analogue
Legal class.: POM

Action: Softens and dilates the cervix, stimulates uterine contractions
Uses: Preparation of cervix prior to trans-cervical termination during first trimester of pregnancy; termination during second trimester
Dosage and routes: Vaginally, 1 mg 3 hr before surgery; therapeutic termination: 1 mg 3-hrly to a maximum of 5 pessaries; repeat

24 hr after first dose if necessary
Available forms include: Pessaries
1 mg
Side effects/adverse reactions:
GU: Vaginal bleeding, uterine
pain
GI: Nausea, vomiting, diarrhoea
CNS: Dizziness, headache
CV: Dyspnoea, chest pain,
palpitations
MS: Backache, muscle weakness
SYSTEM: Chills, pyrexia
INTEG: Flushing
Contraindications: Hypersensi-
tivity to prostaglandins
Precautions: Cervicitis, vaginitis,
cardiovascular insufficiency, ob-
structive airways disease, raised
intraocular pressure
Pharmacokinetics: Duration of
effect 12 hr; gastrointestinal side
effects and uterine pain greater
after 3 hr
Clinical assesment:
• Exclude pregnancy during
follow-up
NURSING CONSIDERATIONS
Assess:
• Respiratory rate, rhythm; notify
clinician of any irregularities
• Vaginal discharge — check for
irritation, itchiness
• Pain, type and location
Administer:
• High in vagina after bladder is
emptied
• Antiemetic/antidiarrhoeal
before giving drug if prescribed
Evaluate:
• For fever, chills; use tepid
sponge
Teach patient/family:
• To remain lying down for
10−15 min after insertion

gemfibrozil

Lopid
Func. class.: Hypolipidaemic
Chem. class.: Aryloxisobutyric
acid derivative
Legal class.: POM

Action: Decreases serum triglycerides, very low density lipoproteins
and low density lipoproteins and
increases high density lipoproteins-
cholesterol, inhibiting atherosclerosis
Uses: Primary prevention of
heart disease in men aged 40−55
with hyperlipidaemia and hyperlipidaemia types IIA, IIB, III, IV
and V where diet is insufficient
Dosage and routes:
• *Adult:* By mouth 1200 mg daily
in two doses; maximum 1500 mg
daily
Available forms include: Capsules
300 mg, tablets 600 mg
Side effects/adverse reactions:
GI: Nausea, vomiting, dyspepsia,
diarrhoea, increased liver enzymes, stomatitis, flatulence,
hepatomegaly, gastritis
INTEG: Rash, urticaria, pruritus,
dry hair and skin, alopecia
HAEM: Leucopenia, anaemia,
eosinophilia
CNS: Fatigue, weakness,
headache, dizziness
GU: Decreased libido, impotence
MS: Myalgias, arthralgias
Contraindications: Severe hepatic disease, severe renal disease, gallstones, alcoholism,
hypersensitivity
Precautions: Peptic ulcer, pregnancy, lactation, monitor serum
lipids
Pharmacokinetics:
By mouth: Peak 2−6 hr, plasma
protein binding greater than 90%,
half-life 6−25 hr, 70% excreted in
urine, metabolised in liver

Interactions/incompatibilities:
• May increase effect of suphonyl-ureas used with this drug
• May increase anticoagulant properties of oral anticoagulants
• Decreased effect: rifampicin

Clinical assessment:
• Hepatic function if patient is on long-term therapy
• For signs of vitamin A, D, K deficiency
• Annual eye examination

Treatment of overdose: Symptomatic support

NURSING CONSIDERATIONS

Assess:
• Alcohol intake of patient (should not be used if patient is alcoholic)
• Withdraw drug after 3 months if the response is inadequate

Administer:
• Drug with meals if GI symptoms occur
• After serum lipid and full blood count

Evaluate:
• Bowel pattern daily; increase fibre and water in diet if constipation develops
• Activity levels of patient

Teach patient/family:
• Symptoms of hypothrombinaemia: bleeding mucous membranes, dark tarry stools, petechiae; these symptoms should be reported immediately
• That compliance is needed since toxicity may result if doses are missed
• That other risk factors should be decreased: high fat diet, smoking, absence of exercise
• That non-prescribed preparations should be avoided unless directed by clinician
• Birth control should be practised while on this drug
• Report GU symptoms: decreased libido, impotence, dysuria, proteinuria, oliguria

gentamicin sulphate

Genticin, Cidomycin
Func. class.: Antibiotic
Chem. class.: Aminoglycoside
Legal class.: POM

Action: Interferes with protein synthesis in bacterial cell by binding to ribosomal subunit, causing misreading of genetic code; inaccurate peptide sequence forms in protein chain, causing bacterial death

Uses: Severe systemic infections of CNS, respiratory, GI, urinary tract, bone, skin, soft tissues caused by susceptible strains of Gram-negative organisms and some Gram-positive organisms, including *P. aeruginosa, Proteus* spp, *Klebsiella* spp, *Serratia* spp, *E. coli, Enterobacter* spp, *Acinetobacter* spp, *Citrobacter* spp, *Staphylococcus* spp

Dosage and routes:
Severe systemic infections
• *Adult:* IV, IM, IV infusion 2−5 mg/kg daily in divided doses 8 hrly
• *Adult:* Intrathecal 1−5 mg/day with IM 2−4 mg/kg daily in divided doses 8 hrly
• *Child:* Less than 2 weeks 3 mg/kg 12-hrly; 2 weeks−12 yr 2 mg/kg 8-hrly

Dental/respiratory procedures/GI/GU surgery (prophylaxis endocarditis)
• *Adult:* IM 1.5 mg/kg with amoxycillin immediately before induction

Available forms include: Injection (as sulphate) IM, IV 40 mg/ml; intrathecal 5 mg/ml

Side effects/adverse reactions:
GU: Oliguria, renal damage, azotaemia, renal failure
CNS: Confusion, depression, numbness, tremors, convulsions, muscle twitching, neurotoxicity

(mostly after intrathecal injection)
EENT: Ototoxicity, visual disturbances
HAEM: Agranulocytosis, thrombocytopenia, leucopenia, anaemia
MS: Neuromuscular blockade, respiratory paralysis
INTEG: Rash, burning, urticaria, photosensitivity, dermatitis
Contraindications: Pregnancy, myasthenia gravis, hypersensitivity
Precautions: Neonates, renal disease, hearing deficits, lactation, elderly
Pharmacokinetics:
IM: Onset rapid, peak 1−2 hr
IV: Onset immediate, peak 1−2 hr. Plasma half-life 1−2 hr; duration 6−8 hr, not metabolised, excreted unchanged in urine
Interactions/incompatibilities:
• Increased ototoxicity, neurotoxicity, nephrotoxicity: other aminoglycosides, amphotericin B, polymyxin, vancomycin, ethacrynic acid, frusemide, mannitol, cisplatin, cephalosporins
• Decreased effects of: parenteral penicillins, neostigmine, pyridostigmine
• Do not mix in solution or syringe: penicillins, amphotericin B, cephalosporins, erythromycin, heparin, sodium bicarbonate, chloramphenicol
• Increased effects: non-depolarising muscle relaxants (e.g. tubocurarine), biphosphonates
Clinical assessment:
• Renal function. Dose adjustment required in impairment
• Serum peak, drawn at 30−60 min after IV infusion or 60 min after IM injection, and trough level drawn just before next dose; dose adjustment required if peak outside range 5−10 mcg/ml or trough above 2 mcg/ml
• Duration of treatment, should not normally exceed 7 days
Treatment of overdose: Haemo-

dialysis, monitor serum levels of drug

NURSING CONSIDERATIONS
Assess:
• Culture and sensitivity to identify infecting organism
• Weight before treatment; calculation of dosage is usually done based on ideal body weight, but may be calculated on actual body weight
• Hearing aids
Administer:
After culture and sensitivity administer appropriate therapy as indicated
• IM injection in large muscle mass, rotate injection sites
• Drug in evenly spaced doses to maintain blood level
• Bicarbonate to alkalinise urine if ordered for urinary tract infection, as drug is most active in alkaline environment
Perform/provide:
• Adequate fluids of 2−3 litres daily unless contraindicated to prevent irritation of tubules
• Flush IV line with 0.9% sodium chloride or 5% glucose in distilled water after infusion
• Supervised ambulation, other safety measures for vestibular dysfunction
Evaluate:
• Fluid balance, urinalysis daily for proteinuria, cells, casts; report sudden change in urine output
• Vital signs during infusion, watch for hypotension, change in pulse
• IV site for thrombophlebitis including pain, redness, swelling half hourly: get site changed if necessary
• Urine pH if drug is used for urinary tract infection; urine should be kept alkaline
• Therapeutic effect: absence of fever, draining wounds, negative

culture and sensitivity after treatment

• Hearing during and after treatment and/or ringing in ears, vertigo

• Signs of dehydration: high specific gravity, decrease in skin turgor, dry mucous membranes, dark urine

• Overgrowth of infection including increased temperature, malaise, redness, pain, swelling, perineal itching, diarrhoea, stomatitis, change in cough or sputum

• Vestibular dysfunction: nausea, vomiting, dizziness, headache; drug should be discontinued if severe

• Injection sites for redness, swelling, abscesses; use warm compresses at site

Teach patient/family:

• To report headache, dizziness, symptoms of overgrowth of infection, renal impairment

• To report loss of hearing, ringing, roaring in ears or feeling of fullness in head

• About side effects

---

gentamicin sulphate (ophthalmic/otic)

Genticin, Cidomycin, Minims
Func. class.: Antibiotic
Chem. class.: Aminoglycoside
Legal class.: POM

Action: Interferes with protein synthesis in bacterial cell by binding to ribosomal subunit, causing misreading of genetic code; inaccurate peptide sequence forms in protein chain, causing bacterial death

Uses: Infection of external eye, ear

Dosage and routes:

• *Adult and child:* Instil 1 or 2 drops in the eye or 2 or 3 drops in the ear 4−8 hrly; apply ointment to conjunctival sac 2 to 4 times a day

Available forms include: Ointment 0.3%; solution 0.3%

Side effects/adverse reactions:

EENT: Poor corneal wound healing, temporary visual haze, overgrowth of non-susceptible organisms, irritation, burning, stinging, itching

Contraindications: Hypersensitivity, fungal and viral infections

Precautions: Antibiotic hypersensitivity

Interactions/incompatibilities: None known

NURSING CONSIDERATIONS

Administer:

• After washing hands, cleanse crusts or discharge from eye before application

• Patient may instil drug under nurse's supervision

Evaluate:

• Therapeutic response: absence of redness, inflammation, tearing

• Allergy: itching, lacrimation, redness, swelling

Teach patient/family:

• To use drug exactly as prescribed

• Not to use eye makeup, towels, washcloths, eye medication of others; re-infection may occur

• Each eye should be cleaned completely separately or infection/re-infection to both eyes may occur

• That drug container tip should not be touched to eye

• To report itching, increased redness, burning, stinging, swelling; drug should be discontinued

• That application may cause blurred vision

• Not to wear contact lenses during treatment

gentamicin sulphate (topical)

Cidomycin, Genticin
Func. class.: Antibiotic
Chem. class.: Aminoglycoside
Legal class.: POM

Action: Interferes with protein synthesis in bacterial cell by binding to ribosomal subunit, causing misreading of genetic code; inaccurate peptide sequence forms in protein chain, causing bacterial death

Uses: Skin infections

Dosage and routes:
• *Adult and child:* Topical rub into affected area 3−4 times daily
Available forms include: Cream, ointment 0.3%

Side effects/adverse reactions:
INTEG: Rash, urticaria, stinging, burning, photosensitivity, pruritus

Contraindications: Hypersensitivity

Precautions: Pregnancy, open, large wounds

Interactions/incompatibilities: None known

Clinical assessment:
• Avoid long-term use, produces skin sensitisation and bacterial resistance
• Consider the need for systemic treatment

NURSING CONSIDERATIONS

Administer:
• Enough medication to cover lesions completely
• After cleansing with soap, water before each application, dry well

Evaluate:
• Allergic reaction: burning, stinging, swelling, redness
• Therapeutic response: decrease in size, number of lesions

Teach patient/family:
• Rub well into skin if not painful
• To apply using gloves
• To avoid use of non-prescribed creams, ointments, lotions unless directed by clinician
• To wash hands thoroughly before and after each application
• To avoid direct sunlight or wear sunscreen to prevent burns
• Not to exceed stated dose

gestronol hexanoate

Depostat
Func. class.: Depot progestogen
Chem. class.: Progestogen
Legal class.: POM

Action: Arrests endometrial proliferation and reduces prostatic weight

Uses: Endometrial carcinoma, mild benign prostatic hyperplasia when patient is at risk from surgery

Dosage and routes:
Endometrial carcinoma
• IM injection 200−400 mg every 5−7 days
Prostatic hyperplasia
• IM 200 mg weekly, maximum dose 400 mg
Available forms include: Injection 100 mg/ml, 2 ml ampoule

Side effects/adverse reactions:
GU: Changes in libido, breast tenderness, irregular menstruation inhibition of spermatogenesis
GI: Disturbances
INTEG: Acne, urticaria, jaundice, pain at injection site
META: Weight gain, oedema
RESP: Exacerbation of asthma, cough, dyspnoea
CNS: Exacerbation of migraine, epilepsy
CV: Circulatory irregularities
SYST: Abnormal liver function tests

Contraindications: Undiagnosed vaginal bleeding, mammary carcinoma, pregnancy, history of pemphigoid gestationis

Precautions: Hepatic or renal disease, hypertension, cardiac disease, diabetes mellitus, lactation, epilepsy, migraine, asthma
Pharmacokinetics: Response in endometrial carcinoma may require 8–12 weeks, in prostatic hyperplasia 3 months
Interactions/incompatibilities:
• Increased plasma concentrations of: cyclosporin
Clinical assessment:
• Prescribe lowest effective dose
• Check liver function periodically in patients with chronic liver disease
NURSING CONSIDERATIONS
Assess:
• Baseline weight and fluid balance
• BP at beginning of treatment and periodically
Administer:
• Titrated dose
• By deep IM injection
• Rotate injection sites
• In one dose daily
Evaluate:
• For hypertension, cardiac symptoms
• Weight and fluid balance
• For any changes in mental state
• Therapeutic response: decreased abnormal bleeding
• Oedema—increase or decrease
Teach patient/family:
• About all aspects of drug usage
• To report suspected pregnancy
• To report any chest pain, vaginal bleeding, oedema, dark urine, clay-coloured stools, headaches, excessive weight gain or GI upsets

glibenclamide

Daonil, Euglucon, Semi-Daonil Calabren, Libanil, Malix, Diabetamide
Func. class.: Oral hypoglycaemic
Chem. class.: Sulphonylurea
Legal class.: POM

Action: Causes functioning β-cells in pancreas to release insulin, leading to drop in blood glucose levels; may have extrapancreatic action also; not effective if patient lacks functioning β-cells
Uses: Non-insulin dependent diabetes mellitus (type II) not controlled by diet alone
Dosage and routes:
• *Adult:* By mouth 5 mg initially, then increased to desired response
• *Elderly:* By mouth 2.5 mg initially, then increased to desired response
• Maximum 15 mg daily
Available forms include: Tablets 2.5, 5 mg
Side effects/adverse reactions:
META: Weight gain
CNS: Headache, weakness, paraesthesia
GI: Nausea, fullness, heartburn, hepatotoxicity, cholestatic jaundice
HAEM: Leucopenia, thrombocytopenia, agranulocytosis, aplastic anaemia, increased aspartate aminotransferase, alanine aminotransferase, alkaline phosphatase
INTEG: Rash, allergic reactions, pruritus, urticaria, eczema, photosensitivity, erythema
ENDO: Hypoglycaemia, inappropriate ADH secretion with hyponatraemia
Contraindications: Hypersensitivity to sulphonylureas, juvenile or brittle diabetes, severe renal disease, severe hepatic disease, ketosis, coma, impaired thyroid or adrenocortical function, preg-

nancy, acidosis, surgery, breast feeding

Precautions: Elderly, cardiac disease, severe hypoglycaemic reactions

Pharmacokinetics:

By mouth: Completely absorbed by GI route, onset 15−60 min, peak 2−8 hr, duration 10−24 hr; half-life 2−5 hr, metabolised in liver, excreted in urine, faeces (metabolites) 90%−95% is plasma protein bound

Interactions/incompatibilities:

• Effects increased by: MAOIs azapropazone, sulphinpyrazone, phenylbutazone, clofibrate, beza-fibrate, salicylates, sulphonamides, chloramphenicol, fenfluramine, tetracyclines, anti-coagulants, β-blockers, alcohol, fluconazole, miconazole

• Antagonised by: corticosteroids, oral contraceptives, thiazide diuretics, thyroid preparations, oestrogens, phenothiazines, rifampicin, frusemide, bumetan-ide, diazoxide, lithium, nifedipine

Treatment of overdose: Symptomatic treatment of hypoglycaemia with oral glucose or sucrose, or IV glucose, or glucagon 1 mg subcutaneous or IM

NURSING CONSIDERATIONS

Assess:

• Baseline weight

Administer:

• Drug 30 min before meals

Perform/provide:

• Blood and urine glucose levels during treatment to determine diabetes control

Evaluate:

• Therapeutic response: decrease in polyuria, polydipsia

• Hypoglycaemic/hyperglycaemic reaction that can occur soon after meals

Teach patient/family:

• To use a blood glucose test while on this drug *or* to test urine glu-cose levels with reagent strip approximately 2 hr after each meal

• The symptoms of hypo/hyperglycaemia, what to do about each

• That drug must be continued on daily basis; explain consequence of discontinuing drug

• To take drug in morning to prevent hypoglycaemic reactions at night

• To avoid non-prescribed medi-cations unless prescribed by a clinician

• That diabetes is a life-long illness, medication will not cure disease

• That all food included in diet plan must be eaten in order to prevent hypoglycaemia

• To carry Diabetic ID card in case of emergency

---

gliclazide

Diamicron
Func. class.: Oral hypoglycaemic
Chem. class.: Sulphonylurea
Legal class.: POM

Action: Increases insulin secretion in diabetes mellitus when some pancreatic β-cell activity is still present; also reduces platelet adhesion and aggregation and increases fibrinolytic activity

Uses: Non insulin dependent diabetes mellitus (type II) un-responsive to diet alone

Dosage and routes:

• *Adult:* By mouth initially 40−80 mg daily adjusted according to response; up to 160 mg may be given as single dose with breakfast, higher doses should be divided; maximum daily dose 320 mg

Available forms include: Tablets 80 mg

Side effects/adverse reactions:

CNS: Headache

GI: Disturbances, hepatic impairment, liver failure, jaundice
META: Weight gain
HAEM: Thrombocytopenia, agranulocytosis, aplastic anaemia
INTEG: Rash, pruritus, erythema, exfoliative dermatitis

Contraindications: Ketoacidosis, pregnancy, lactation, juvenile onset diabetes, surgery, hypersensitivity to sulphonylureas

Precautions: Elderly, concurrent illness, hepatic or renal impairment

Pharmacokinetics: Well absorbed orally; duration of action at least 12 hr; half-life 10−12 hr; excreted in urine as unchanged drug and metabolite

Interactions/incompatibilities:
• Effects increased by: alcohol, azapropazone, β-blockers, chloramphenicol, clofibrate, cotrimoxazole, MAOIs, miconazole, phenylbutazone, sulphinpyrazone, bezafibrate, fluconazole, tetracyclines, oral anticoagulants
• Antagonised by: rifampicin, bumetanide, corticosteroids, corticotrophin, diazoxide, frusemide, oral contraceptives, thiazides, lithium, nifedipine, corticosteroids, thiazide diuretics, oestrogens, thyroid hormones

Treatment of overdose: Gastric lavage and symptomatic treatment of hypoglycaemia including oral/IV glucose

NURSING CONSIDERATIONS
Assess:
• Baseline weight
Administer:
• Drug 30 min before meals or as a single dose before breakfast
Perform/provide:
• Blood and urine glucose levels during treatment to determine diabetes control
Evaluate:
• For symptoms of hyper- or hypoglycaemia

• Therapeutic response: decrease in polyuria, polydipsia
Teach patient/family:
• To check blood sugar levels regularly *or* to check and test urine for glucose regularly
• Symptoms of hypoglycaemia/hyperglycaemia and how to treat
• That drug must be taken regularly as prescribed
• To avoid non-prescribed medication unless approved by clinician
• That diabetes is a life-long illness; medication will not cure the disease
• That a diet should be followed and all food eaten to prevent hypoglycaemia
• To carry a Medic-Alert card
• That some weight gain is possible

---

glipizide

Glibenese, Minodiab
Func. class.: Oral hypoglycaemic
Chem. class.: Sulphonylurea
Legal class.: POM

Action: Causes functioning β-cells in pancreas to release insulin, leading to drop in blood glucose levels; not effective if patient lacks functioning β-cells

Uses: Non-insulin dependent diabetes mellitus (type II) not controlled by diet alone

Dosage and routes:
• *Adult:* By mouth 5 mg initially, then increased to desired response, maximum 40 mg daily. Doses up to 15 mg as a single dose before breakfast, larger doses divided
• *Elderly:* By mouth 2.5−5 mg initially, then increased to desired response

Available forms include: Tablets 2.5, 5 mg

Side effects/adverse reactions:

CNS: Headache, weakness, dizziness, drowsiness

GI: Hepatotoxicity, cholestatic jaundice, nausea, vomiting, diarrhoea, constipation, anorexia, increased aspartate aminotransferase, alanine aminotransferase, alkaline phosphatase

INTEG: Rash, allergic reactions, pruritus, urticaria, eczema, photosensitivity, erythema

ENDO: Hypoglycaemia

META: Weight gain

Contraindications: Hypersensitivity to sulphonylureas, juvenile or brittle diabetes, severe renal disease, severe hepatic disease thyroid disease, severe trauma, sepsis or surgery, acidosis, pregnancy, lactation

Precautions: Elderly, cardiac disease, renal impairment, hepatic impairment

Pharmacokinetics:

By mouth: Completely absorbed by GI route, onset 1−1½ hr, duration 10−24 hr, half-life 2−4 hr, metabolised in liver, excreted in urine, 90%−95% is plasma protein bound

Interactions/incompatibilities:

• Effects increased by: MAOIs, cimetidine, bezafibrate, clofibrate, tetracyclines, cotrimoxazole, salicylates, sulphonamides, chloramphenicol, oral anticoagulants, β-blockers, alcohol, azapropazone, sulphinpyrazone, phenylbutazone, fluconazole, miconazole

• Antagonised by: corticosteroids, oral contraceptives, thiazide diuretics, thyroid preparations, oestrogens, phenothiazines, rifampicin, frusemide, bumetanide, diazoxide, lithium, nifedipine

Treatment of overdose: Gastric lavage and supportive treatment for hypoglycaemia including oral/IV glucose

NURSING CONSIDERATIONS

Assess:

• Baseline weight

Administer:

• Drug 30 min before meals

Perform/provide:

• Blood and urine glucose levels during treatment to determine diabetes control

Evaluate:

• Therapeutic response: decrease in polyuria, polydipsia, polyphagia, alertness, absence of dizziness, stable gait

• Hypoglycaemic/hyperglycaemic reaction that can occur soon after meals

Teach patient/family:

• To use blood glucose test while on this drug, *or* to test urine glucose levels with reagent strip approximately 2 hr after each meal

• The symptoms of hypo/hyperglycaemia; what to do about each

• That medication must be continued on daily basis; explain consequence of discontinuing

• To take dose in morning to prevent hypoglycaemic reactions at night

• To avoid non-prescribed medications unless approved by clinician

• That diabetes is a life-long illness; medication will not cure disease

• That all food included in diet plan must be eaten in order to prevent hypoglycaemia

• To carry Diabetic ID card for emergency purposes

• To continue weight control, dietary restrictions, exercise, hygiene

gliquidone

Glurenorm

Func. class.: Oral hypoglycaemic
Chem. class.: Sulphonylurea
Legal class.: POM

Action: Causes functioning β-cells

in pancreas to release insulin, leading to drop in blood glucose levels; not effective if patient lacks functioning β-cells

Uses: Non-insulin dependent diabetes mellitus (type II) not controlled by diet alone

Dosage and routes: By mouth initially 15 mg daily before breakfast, adjusted to 45−60 mg daily in 2−3 divided doses; maximum single dose 60 mg; maximum daily dose 180 mg

Available forms include: Tablets 30 mg

Side effects/adverse reactions:

CNS: Headache

GI: Disturbances

META: Weight gain

HAEM: Thrombocytopenia, agranulocytosis, aplastic anaemia

SYSTEM: Sensitivity reactions in first 6−8 weeks of therapy

Contraindications: Ketoacidosis, pregnancy, lactation, juvenile onset diabetes, surgery, hypersensitivity to sulphonylureas, severe hepatic or renal impairment

Precautions: Renal impairment, elderly, concurrent illness

Pharmacokinetics: Onset of effect within 1 hour, duration of optimal effect 2−3 hr. Converted in liver to inactive metabolites, half-life 1.4 hr, 95% of dose excreted via bile

Interactions/incompatibilities:

• Effects increased by: alcohol, azapropazone, β-blockers, chloramphenicol, clofibrate, cotrimoxazole, MAOIs, miconazole, phenylbutazone, sulphinpyrazone cimetidine, salicylates, sulphonamides, fluconazole, bezafibrate, clofibrate, oral anticoagulants, tetracyclines

• Antagonised by: rifampicin, oestrogens, thyroid hormones, bumetanide, corticosteroids, corticotrophin, diazoxide, frusemide, oral contraceptives, thiazides, phenothiazines, lithium, nifedipine

• Potentiated by gliquidone: barbiturates, vasopressin, oral anticoagulants

Treatment of overdose:
Gastric lavage and supportive treatment for hypoglycaemia including oral/IV glucose

NURSING CONSIDERATIONS

Assess:

• Baseline weight

Administer:

• Drug 30 min before meals or as a single dose before breakfast

Perform/provide:

• Blood and urine glucose levels during treatment to determine diabetes control

Evaluate:

• Therapeutic response, decrease in polyuria, polydipsia, polyphagia

• Mental status, absence of giddiness, stable gait

• Hypoglycaemic/hyperglycaemic reactions that could occur

Teach patient/family:

• To check urine and test for glucose regularly *or* to check blood sugar levels regularly

• That some weight gain is possible

• Symptoms for hypoglycaemia/hyperglycaemia and how to treat

• That medication must be taken regularly as prescribed

• To avoid non-prescribed drugs unless directed by clinician

• That diabetes is a life-long illness, drug will not cure disease

• That a diet plan should be followed and all food eaten to prevent hypoglycaemia

• To carry a Medic-Alert card in case of emergency

glucagon

Glucagon Injection
Func. class.: Hyperglycaemic
Chem. class.: Polypeptide hormone
Legal class.: POM

Action: Increases plasma glucose concentration by mobilising glycogen stores from the liver; reduces intestinal motility

Uses: Acute hypoglycaemia; aid in diagnostic intestinal radiography and endoscopy; symptomatic treatment of β-blocker poisoning (unlicensed indication)

Dosage and routes:
Acute hypoglycaemia
• IM/IV/subcutaneous injection 0.5−1 unit, repeated after 20 min if necessary, followed if no response by intravenous glucose

Radiography
• IM 1−2 units, IV 0.2−2 units
Available forms include: Powder for reconstitution, 1 unit vial, 10 unit vial

Side effects/adverse reactions:
GI: Nausea, vomiting, diarrhoea
SYSTEM: Hypersensitivity reactions (rare)

Contraindications: Insulinoma, phaeochromocytoma, glucagonoma

Precautions: Ineffective in chronic hypoglycaemia, starvation, adrenal insufficiency, pregnancy

Pharmacokinetics: Onset of effect on intestine 1 min after IV injection, 5−10 min after IM. Duration of action 10−30 min. Half-life 3−6 min; inactivated in liver, kidney and plasma

Clinical assessment:
• Monitor blood glucose levels in hypoglycaemic patient until stable and asymptomatic

Treatment of overdose: Symptomatic including phentolamine in severe hypertension and potassium in hypokalaemia

NURSING CONSIDERATIONS

Assess:
• Baseline vital signs

Administer:
• Using aseptic technique

Evaluate:
• Therapeutic response: adequate blood and urine glucose, absence of ketones in urine
• Injection sites for redness, swelling
• Monitor vital signs 4-hrly
• Mental status, level of consciousness

Teach patient/family:
• Symptoms of hypoglycaemia
• Importance of taking correct medication and diet
• Supportive care
• To carry a Medic-Alert card if patient is known diabetic

glycerine

Func. class.: Laxative, hyperosmotic
Chem. class.: Trihydric alcohol
Legal class.: GSL

Action: Increases osmotic pressure, draws fluid into colon

Uses: Constipation

Dosage and routes:
• *Adult:* rectal suppository, 4 g
• *Child:* rectal suppository, 2 g
• *Infant:* rectal suppository, 1 g
Available forms include: 1, 2, 4 g rectal suppository

Contraindications: Hypersensitivity

NURSING CONSIDERATIONS

Assess:
• Bowel pattern
• Cause of constipation; identify whether fluids, or exercise is missing from lifestyle

Perform/provide:
• Storage in cool environment, do not freeze

• Moisten with water as necessary for ease of insertion

Evaluate:

• Cramping, rectal bleeding, nausea, vomiting; if these symptoms occur, discontinue use

• Therapeutic response

Teach patient/family:

• Not to use laxatives for long-term therapy; bowel tone will be lost

• That bowel movements do not always occur daily

• Do not use in presence of abdominal pain, nausea, vomiting

• Notify clinician if constipation unrelieved or if symptoms of electrolyte imbalance occur: muscle cramps, pain, weakness, dizziness

---

glyceryl trinitrate

GTN, Coro-Nitro, Nitrocine, Nitrolingual, Nitrocontin, Suscard, Sustac, Nitronal, Tridil Deponit, Percutol, Transiderm-Nitro, Glytrin

Func. class.: Coronary vasodilator

Chem. class.: Nitrate

Legal class.: Oral P, Injection POM

Action: Decreases preload, afterload, which is responsible for decreasing left ventricular end diastolic pressure, systemic vascular resistance

Uses: Chronic stable angina pectoris, prophylaxis of angina pain, left ventricular failure

Dosage and routes:

• *Adult:* Sublingual dissolve tablet under tongue when pain begins, if required 0.3−1 mg 2−3 hrly; tablets modified-release 2.6−6.4 mg 8−12 hrly on empty stomach; buccal tablets 2 mg as required for angina, 1−10 mg 3 times daily prophylactically; topical ointment 0.5−2 inches to skin surface every

3−4 hr; IV 10−25 mcg/min, then increase by 5−25 mcg/min until desired response, normal maximum 400 mcg/min; transdermal patch, apply a pad daily to a site free of hair

Available forms include: Buccal tablets 1, 2, 3, 5 mg; aerosol 0.4 mg/dose spray; tablets modified-release 2.6, 6.4 mg; injection 0.5, 1, 5 mg/ml; sublingual tablets, 0.3, 0.5, 0.6 mg; topical ointment 2%; transdermal patch 5, 10 mg/24 hr

Side effects/adverse reactions:

CV: Postural hypotension, tachycardia, collapse, hypotension, palpitations

GI: Nausea, vomiting

INTEG: Pallor, sweating, local irritation and erythema with topical preparations

CNS: Headache, flushing, dizziness, apprehension, restlessness

HAEM: Methaemoglobinaemia

Contraindications: Hypersensitivity to this drug or nitrites, anaemia, increased intracranial pressure, cerebral haemorrhage, acute myocardial infarction, pregnancy, lactation, uncorrected hypovolaemia, severe hypotension

Precautions: Postural hypotension, glaucoma, severe renal or hepatic dysfunction

Pharmacokinetics:

Modified-release: Onset 1 hr, peak 3−4 hr, duration 8−12 hr

By mouth: Onset 15−60 min, peak 1−1½ hr, duration 4−12 hr

Sublingual: Onset 1−3 min, duration 30 min

Transdermal: Onset ½−1 hr, duration 24 hr

IV: Onset immediate, duration variable

Transmucosal: Onset 3 min, duration 10−30 min

Metabolised by liver, excreted in urine

Interactions/incompatibilities:

• Increased effects of this drug: β-blockers, narcotics, tricyclics, diuretics, antihypertensives, major tranquillisers
• Decreased effects: sympathomimetics
• Increased bioavailability of: dihydroergotamine producing coronary vasoconstriction
• Incompatible with PVC infusion systems
• Increased effects of: opiates, anticholinergic effects of tricyclics
Treatment of overdose: Supportive, with bed elevation and vasoconstrictors to maintain blood pressure. IV methylene blue for methaemaglobinaemia. Gastric lavage after oral ingestion

NURSING CONSIDERATIONS
Assess:
• Baseline BP, pulse
Administer:
• IV — give via infusion pump. BP assessed hrly until stable. Sublingual or buccal glyceryl trinitrate is more effective than oral. Topical patch — allow minimum 2 hr break between reapplication of new patch within 24 hr period to avoid developing tolerance
Evaluate:
• BP, pulse, respirations during treatment
• Pain: duration, time started, activity being performed, character
• Tolerance if taken over long period of time
• Headache, lightheadedness, decreased BP, may indicate a need for decreased dosage
Teach patient/family:
• That drug may be taken before stressful activity: exercise, sexual activity
• That sublingual tablet may sting when drug comes in contact with mucous membranes
• To avoid hazardous activities if dizziness occurs

• Stress patient compliance with complete medical regimen
• To make position changes slowly to prevent fainting
• To store sublingual tablets in glass containers with foil-lined cap. Discard remainder after 8 weeks

---

glycopyrronium bromide

Robinul
Func. class.: Anticholinergic
Chem. class.: Quaternary ammonium compound
Legal class.: POM

Action: Competes with acetylcholine for muscarinic receptor sites in autonomic nervous system, relaxes intestinal smooth muscle, reduces secretions
Uses: Adjunct to anaesthesia, preventing excessive secretions and bradycardia; to prevent muscarinic effects when using cholinesterase inhibitors to terminate neuromuscular block
Dosage and routes:
• *Adult:* Pre- or intra-operatively 200−400 mcg IV or IM; reversal of non-depolarising block 10−15 mcg/kg with 50 mcg/kg neostigmine, both IV
• *Child:* Pre- or intra-operatively 4−8 mcg/kg IM or IV, maximum 200 mcg; reversal of non-depolarising block 10 mcg/kg with 50 mcg/kg neostigmine, both IV
Available forms include: Injection 200 mcg/ml, 1 ml and 3 ml ampoules
Side effects/adverse reactions:
CNS: Confusion, anxiety, restlessness, irritability, delusions, hallucinations, headache, sedation, depression, incoherence, dizziness
EENT: Blurred vision, photophobia, dilated pupils, difficulty swallowing

CV: Palpitations, tachycardia, postural hypotension
GI: Dryness of mouth, constipation, nausea, vomiting, abdominal distress, paralytic ileus
GU: Hesitancy, retention
Contraindications: Hypersensitivity
Precautions: Pregnancy, elderly, lactation, prostatic hypertrophy coronary artery disease, congestive heart failure, arrhythmias, hypertension, thyrotoxicosis, fever, narrow-angle glaucoma, paralytic ileus, pyloric stenosis, myasthenia gravis

Pharmacokinetics:
Subcutaneous/IM: Peak 30–45 min, duration 7 hr
IV: Peak 10–15 min, duration 4 hr
Excreted in urine, bile, faeces (unchanged)

Interactions/incompatibilities:
• Increased anticholinergic effect: alcohol, antihistamines, phenothiazines, amantadine
• Do not mix with diazepam, chloramphenicol, pentobarbitone, dimenhydrinate, methohexitone, thiopentone, pentazocine, sodium bicarbonate in syringe or solution
Treatment of overdose: Administration of IV neostigmine to reverse peripheral anticholinergic effects

NURSING CONSIDERATIONS
Assess:
• Use in patients with cardiac disease
Administer:
• As single bolus intravenously whilst anaesthetised
• Supportive measures during anaesthesia
• Mouth care after
Evaluate:
• Fluid balance; retention commonly causes decreased urinary output
• Increase in sympathetic activity
• Vital signs; observe for tachycardia and palpitations

Teach patient/family:
• That effects include dry mouth and palpitations

---

gonadorelin HCl

Relefact LH-RH, HRF, Fertiral, combination product
Func. class.: Gonadotrophin
Chem. class.: Synthetic luteinizing hormone-releasing hormone
Legal class.: POM

Action: Causes release of LH and FSH from pituitary gland
Uses: Evaluation of pituitary function; treatment of amenorrhoea and female infertility
Dosage and routes:
• *Adult:* Diagnostic, 100 mcg IV/subcutaneous; therapeutic 10–20 mcg subcutaneous/IV over 1 min every 90 mins for maximum 6 months
Available forms include: Powder for injection subcutaneous, IV 100, 500 mcg/vial; solutions for injection subcutaneous, IV 500 mcg/ml in 2 ml ampoule and 100 mcg/ml in 1 ml ampoule
Side effects/adverse reactions:
CNS: Dizziness, headache, flushing
GI: Nausea
INTEG: Inflammation at injection site
GU: Increased menstrual bleeding
Contraindications: Hypersensitivity, pregnancy, endometrial cyst, polycystic disease of the ovaries
Pharmacokinetics: Excreted by kidneys
Interactions/incompatibilities:
• Increased effects of this drug: levodopa, spironolactone
• Decreased effects of this drug: digoxin, phenothiazines, dopamine antagonists, sex steroids, corticosteroids

• Any interacting drugs will interfere with diagnostic use of this agent

NURSING CONSIDERATIONS
Assess:
• Test result: Levels of FSH and LH are measured and diagnosis is based on comparison with local laboratory normal ranges according to time of menstrual cycle
Administer:
• Do not dilute or administer with any additive
• Repeated doses may be necessary to elevate pituitary gonadotrophin reserve
Teach patient/family:
• Give advice related to infertility

---

goserelin

Zoladex
Func. class.: Hormone antagonist
Chem. class.: Gonadotrophin-releasing hormone analogue
Legal class.: POM

Action: Causes initial stimulation of LH release by the pituitary gland followed by a decrease in LH secretion and a reduction in the production of testosterone
Uses: Metastatic prostate cancer, suitable for hormone manipulation
Dosage and routes:
• As implant into anterior abdominal wall 3.6 mg every 28 days
Available forms include: Depot implant, 3.6 mg
Side effects/adverse reactions:
GU: During weeks 1−2 of treatment, increased tumour growth may occur causing ureteric obstruction
ENDO: Hot flushes, decrease in libido, rarely gynaecomastia
INTEG: Rashes, bruising at injection site
MS: Initial increase in bone pain

due to transient increase in plasma testosterone; tumour growth may cause spinal cord compression
Contraindications: Surgical removal of testes, tumours unresponsive to hormone manipulation, hypersensitivity
Precautions: Disease flare may require treatment with anti-androgen e.g. cyproterone acetate 300 mg daily, for 3 days before and 3 weeks after starting goserelin

NURSING CONSIDERATIONS
Perform/provide:
• Symptoms should be treated as necessary
• Storage in sealed packet in refrigerator
Evaluate:
• Bone pain; temporary increase may occur and symptoms should be treated
• Signs of spinal cord compression or renal impairment due to ureteric obstruction; these should be reported at once
• Bruising may occur at the injection site
Teach patient/family:
• Possible side effects and the need to report these at once

---

griseofulvin

Grisovin, Fulcin
Func. class.: Antifungal
Chem. class.: Penicillium griseofulvum derivative
Legal class.: POM

Action: Arrests fungal cell division at metaphase of development, binds to human keratin making it resistant to disease
Uses: Fungal infections of the skin, scalp, hair and nails when topical treatment is inappropriate or has failed
Dosage and routes:
• *Adult:* By mouth 500−1000 mg

daily in single or divided doses
• *Child:* By mouth 10 mg/kg daily
Available forms include: Tablets 125, 500 mg, suspension 125 mg/5 ml
Side effects/adverse reactions:
INTEG: Rash, urticaria, photosensitivity, lichen planus, angioneurotic oedema, exfoliative dermatitis
CNS: Headache, peripheral neuritis, paraesthesias, confusion, dizziness, fatigue, insomnia, psychosis
EENT: Blurred vision, oral candidiasis, taste alterations
GU: Proteinuria
GI: Nausea, vomiting, anorexia, diarrhoea, cramps, dry mouth, flatulence
HAEM: Leucopenia, granulocytopenia, neutropenia
Contraindications: Hypersensitivity, porphyria, severe hepatic disease, lupus erythematosus, pregnancy
Pharmacokinetics: By mouth: Peak 4 hr, half-life 9−24 hr, metabolised in liver, excreted in urine (inactive metabolites), faeces, perspiration
Interactions/incompatibilities:
• Tachycardia: alcohol
• Decreased action of this drug: barbiturates
• Increased effect of: alcohol
• Decreased action of: warfarin, oral anticoagulants, oral contraceptives
Treatment of overdose: Symptomatic treatment only
NURSING CONSIDERATIONS
Assess:
• Fluid balance
• For history of penicillin allergy; may be cross-sensitive to this drug
Administer:
• After meals otherwise absorption is likely to be inadequate
• Until 3 separate cultures are negative for infective organism
Evalute:
• For limited side effects; headaches, nausea, vomiting, photosensitivity
• Therapeutic response
Teach patient/family:
• That long-term therapy may be needed to clear infection (2 weeks to 15 months depending on organism)
• Good hygiene: handwashing technique, nail care, use of concomitant topical agents if prescribed
• Stress compliance even after symptoms regress
• To use sunscreen or avoid direct sunlight to prevent photosensitivity
• To notify clinician of sore throat, fever, skin rash
• To avoid alcohol (effects enhanced)
• Impairment of driving may occur

---

guaiphenesin

Many combination products
Func. class.: Expectorant
Legal class.: P, (~~NHS~~)

Action: Reported to decrease sputum viscosity which may increase removal of mucus
Uses: Cough
Dosage and routes:
• *Adult:* By mouth 100−400 mg every 4−6 hr in cough mixtures, not to exceed 1.2 g daily
• *Child:* By mouth 12 mg/kg daily in 6 divided doses
Available forms include: Variety of multi-ingredient cough syrups
Side effects/adverse reactions:
CNS: Drowsiness
GI: Nausea, anorexia, vomiting
Contraindications: Hypersensitivity, persistent cough

Treatment of overdose: Other ingredients in cough mixtures likely to present more hazard

NURSING CONSIDERATIONS

Perform/provide:
• Increased fluids/room humidification to liquefy secretions

Evaluate:
• Therapeutic response: absence of cough
• Cough: type, frequency, character including sputum

Teach patient/family:
• Avoid driving, other hazardous activities if drowsiness occurs (rare)
• Avoid smoking, smoke-filled room, perfumes, dust, environmental pollutants, cleansers

---

guanethidine monosulphate

Ismelin

Func. class.: Antihypertensive
Chem. class.: Anti-adrenergic agent
Legal class.: POM

Action: Inhibits noradrenaline release from postganglionic, adrenergic neurones, depleting noradrenaline stores in adrenergic nerve endings

Uses: Moderate to severe hypertension in conjunction with a diuretic or β-blocker; by injection to control hypertensive crises

Dosage and routes:
• *Adult:* By mouth initially 10 mg daily, increase by 10 mg at weekly intervals; usual daily dose 25−50 mg
• *Adult:* IM 10−20 mg, repeat after 3 hr if necessary
• *Child:* Not recommended

Available forms include: Tablets 10, 25 mg; IM injection 10 mg/ml

Side effects/adverse reactions:

CV: Orthostatic hypotension, dizziness, bradycardia, congestive cardiac failure, angina, heart block, oedema
CNS: Depression, fatigue, lethargy, paraesthesia, headache
GI: Nausea, vomiting, diarrhoea, constipation, dry mouth, weight gain, anorexia
INTEG: Dermatitis, loss of scalp hair
HAEM: Thrombocytopenia, leucopenia, anaemia
EENT: Nasal congestion, ptosis, blurred vision
GU: Ejaculation failure, impotence, nocturia, retention increased blood urea nitrogen
RESP: Dyspnoea
MS: Muscle weakness

Contraindications: Hypersensitivity, phaeochromocytoma, renal failure, congestive cardiac failure

Precautions: Renal, cardiac or cerebral insufficiency, pregnancy, lactation, peptic ulcer, asthma

Pharmacokinetics:
By mouth: 50% absorbed, therapeutic level: 1−3 weeks, half-life 5 days, partially metabolised by liver, excreted in urine, breast milk

Interactions/incompatibilities:
• Increased hypotension: diuretics, other antihypertensives, anaesthetics
• Do not use within 14 days of MAOIs: risk hypertensive crisis
• Increased orthostatic hypotension: alcohol
• Decreased hypotensive effect: tricyclic antidepressants, phenothiazines, oral contraceptives, haloperidol, pizotifen
• Sinus bradycardia with digitalis and anti-arrythmics
• Hypersensitivity to: adrenaline, amphetamine, mazindol, phenylpropanolamine and other sympathomimetics

Clinical assessment:
• Renal function studies in renal

impairment (blood urea nitrogen, creatinine)

Treatment of overdose:
Lavage, activated charcoal, vaso-pressors given cautiously, brady-cardia treated with atropine

NURSING CONSIDERATIONS

Assess:
• Fluid balance in renal disease patient
• BP

Evaluate:
• BP, pulse, watch for hypotension
• Daily weight — observe for peripheral oedema
• Symptoms of congestive cardiac failure, oedema, dyspnoea

Teach patient/family:
• To avoid driving if drowsiness occurs
• Not to discontinue drug abruptly
• Not to use non-prescribed products unless directed by clinician; cough, cold preparations
• To report bradycardia, dizziness, confusion, depression, fever, sore throat
• That impotence, gynaecomastia may occur, but are reversible
• To rise slowly to sitting or standing position to minimise postural hypotension
• That therapeutic effect may take 2–4 weeks

---

guanethidine (ophthalmic)

Ismelin, combination products
Func. class.: Anti-hypertensive, occular
Chem. class.: Anti-adrenergic agent
Legal class.: POM

Action: Lowers intra-occular pressure, probably by reducing production of aqueous humour and increasing outflow via trabecular network. Interferes with sympathetic neurotransmission

Uses: Treatment of primary open angle or secondary glaucoma; treatment of lid retraction following exopthalmos and endocrine imbalance

Dosage and routes:
Glaucoma
• Initially 1 drop twice daily. Normal maximum 2 drops twice daily
Lid retraction
• Initially 1 drop twice daily for at least 1 week, reducing thereafter to 1 drop daily or on alternate days
Available forms include: Eyedrops 5%, 1% (with adrenaline 0.2%), 3% (with adrenaline 0.5%)

Side effects/adverse reactions:
EENT: Irritation of the eye, conjunctival vasodilation, conjunctival fibrosis with secondary corneal changes, ptosis
CVS: Adrenaline-containing products only: tachycardia, extra-systoles, hypertension

Contraindications: Closed angle glaucoma, hypersensitivity

Precautions: Pregnancy, lactation. For adrenaline-containing products only: hypertension, cardio-vascular disease, thyrotoxicosis

Pharmacokinetics: Systemic absorption possible

Interactions/incompatibilities:
• Soft contact lenses should not be worn
• Systemic MAOIs may potentiate the effects of adrenaline-containing preparations

Clinical assessment:
• Reduction in intra-occular pressure/improvement in lid retraction
• Use minimum dose to produce therapeutic response
• 6 monthly eye examinations

NURSING CONSIDERATIONS

Assess:
• Use with caution in patients with hypertension, heart disease

Administer:

• One drop into the lower fornix of the appropriate eye
Evaluate:
• BP and pulse
Teach patient/family:
• To report severe smarting and redness of eye
• Do not discontinue use of drug without seeking advice from clinician

---

haloperidol/haloperidol decanoate

Dozic, Haldol, Serenace
Func. class.: Antipsychotic neuroleptic
Chem. class.: Butyrophenone
Legal class.: POM

Action: Depresses cerebral cortex, hypothalamus, limbic system; controls activity and aggression; blocks neurotransmission produced by dopamine at synapse; exhibits strong α-adrenergic, anticholinergic blocking action
Uses: Psychotic disorders including schizophrenia, mania, behavioural or mental problems e.g. aggression, violent or dangerously impulsive behaviour; persistent hiccup, Tourette syndrome, elderly restlessness and agitation, nausea and vomiting, severe anxiety
Dosage and routes:
• *Adult:* By mouth initially 1.5 mg to 20 mg daily in divided doses; may be increased slowly to 100 mg daily and 200 mg daily in severe cases; debilitated or elderly initially half the adult dose. IM: 2−30 mg then 5 mg hrly if necessary (4−8 hrly if satisfactory)
• *Child:* By mouth initially 25−50 mcg per kg daily, maximum 10 mg daily
• *Adolescents:* Initially as for

adults but to a maximum of 30 mg daily and 60 mg in severe cases
For specific indications seek specialist advice
Available forms include: Tablets 1.5, 5, 10, 20 mg; capsules 0.5 mg; oral liquid 1, 2 mg/ml; oral liquid concentrate 10 mg/ml; injection 5, 10 mg/ml; depot injection 50, 100 mg/ml (as decanoate)
Side effects/adverse reactions:
CNS: Extrapyramidal symptoms: parkinsonism, akathisia, dystonia, rigidity, tremor; tardive dyskinesia, drowsiness, headache, excitement, agitation, insomnia, neuroleptic malignant syndrome (NMS)
INTEG: Pigmentation, photosensitivity, rash, dermatitis
GI: Nausea, appetite loss, dyspepsia, weight loss, dry mouth, constipation
GU: Amenorrhoea, gynaecomastia, impotence, urinary retention
EENT: Blurred vision
CV: Hypotension, ventricular arrhythmias
HAEM: Agranulocytosis, transient leucopenia
ENDO: Galactorrhoea
Contraindications: Hypersensitivity, coma, Parkinson's disease, bone marrow depression, breast feeding
Precautions: Pregnancy, liver disease, renal disease, phaeochromocytoma, epilepsy (or conditions predisposing to epilepsy e.g. barbiturate, alcohol withdrawal, brain damage), cardiac disease, thyrotoxicosis, convulsions, hypotension
Pharmacokinetics:
By mouth: Onset erratic, peak 2−6 hr, half-life 24 hr
IM: Onset 15−30 min, peak 15−20 min, half-life 21 hr
IM (Decanoate): Peak 4−11 days, half-life 3 weeks

Metabolised by liver, excreted in urine, bile, crosses placenta, enters breast milk

Interactions/incompatibilities:
• Enhanced sedative effect: alcohol, anxiolytics, hypnotics, sedatives, strong analgesics
• Antagonise action of: adrenaline, other sympathomimetic agents, phenindione
• Increased risk of extrapyramidal symptoms, neurotoxicity: lithium
• Increased metabolism of haloperidol: rifampicin
• Interference with metabolism of: tricyclic antidepressants

Clinical assessment:
• Monitor response and side effects

Treatment of overdose: Gastric lavage or aspiration for oral ingestion, maintain airway, provide artificial ventilation if necessary. For hypotension do not use adrenaline; use a plasma expander and vasopressor agents e.g. noradrenaline

NURSING CONSIDERATIONS
Assess:
• Base line, vital signs, BP standing and lying
• Swallowing of oral medication; check for hoarding or giving of medication to other patients
• Fluid balance
• Urinalysis before and during prolonged therapy

Administer:
• Antimuscarinic agent, to be used if extrapyramidal symptoms occur
• IM injection into large muscle mass

Perform/provide:
• Decreased noise input by dimming lights, avoiding loud noises
• Supervised ambulation until stabilised on medication; do not involve in strenuous exercise programme because fainting is possible; patient should not stand still for long periods of time
• Increased fluids and fibre in diet to prevent constipation
• Sips of water for dry mouth

Evaluate:
• Therapeutic response: decrease in emotional excitement, hallucinations, delusions, paranoia, reorganisation of patterns of thought, speech
• Take pulse and respirations 4 hrly during initial treatment; report drops of 30 mmHg
• Affect, orientation, level of consciousness, reflexes, gait, coordination, sleep pattern disturbances
• Dizziness, faintness, palpitations, tachycardia on rising
• Extrapyramidal symptoms including akathisia (inability to sit still, no pattern to movements, tardive dyskinesia (bizarre movements of jaw, mouth, tongue, extremities), pseudoparkinsonism (rigidity, tremors, pill rolling, shuffling gait)
• Skin turgor daily
• Constipation, urinary retention daily; if these occur, increase bulk, water in diet

Teach patient/family:
• That postural hypotension occurs often, and to rise from sitting or lying position gradually
• To remain lying down after IM injection for at least 30 min
• To avoid hot baths, hot showers, since hypotension may occur
• To avoid abrupt withdrawal of this drug as relapse may result; drug should be withdrawn slowly
• To avoid non-prescribed preparations (cough, hayfever, cold) unless approved by clinician since serious drug interactions may occur; avoid use with alcohol or CNS depressants, increased drowsiness may occur

• To use a sunscreen during sun exposure to prevent burns
• Regarding compliance with drug regimen
• About extrapyramidal symptoms and necessity for meticulous oral hygiene since oral candidiasis may occur
• To report impaired vision, jaundice, tremors, muscle twitching
• Advise not to drive or operate machinery when treatment started or high doses used until CNS effects known

---

heparin calcium/heparin sodium

Monoparin,   Uniparin,   Hepsal,
Hep-flush,   Minihep,   Heplok
Multiparin,   Unihep,   Pump-Hep,
Calciparine
Func. class.: Anticoagulant
Legal class.: POM

Action: Prevents conversion of fibrinogen to fibrin

Uses: Treatment of arterial and venous thrombosis or embolism e.g. deep vein thrombosis, myocardial infarction, prevention of post-operative venous thrombosis, extra-corporeal circulation, blood transfusions, coronary thrombosis, pulmonary embolism, thrombophlebitis, fat embolism

Dosage and routes:
• *Adult:* IV 5000 units then continuous infusion 1000−2000 units/hr (approximately 14−28 units/kg/hr) or IV 5000−10,000 units every 4 hr; subcutaneous deep vein thrombosis prophylaxis 5000 units 2 hr before surgery then 8−12 hrly until ambulant. Deep vein thrombosis treatment 10,000−20,000 units every 12 hr or 250 units/kg every 12 hr. Seek specialist advice for further doses/indications

Available forms include: Many, IV heparin sodium 1000, 5000, 10,000, 25,000 units/ml. Subcutaneous heparin sodium or calcium 25,000 units/ml. Heparin sodium flushes 10,000 units/ml

Side effects/adverse reactions:
INTEG: Alopecia, local irritation at injection site
HAEM: Acute reversible thrombocytopenia, haemorrhage
MISC: Osteoporosis, hypersensitivity

Contraindications: Hypersensitivity, bleeding tendencies e.g. haemophilia, gastric or duodenal ulcer, severe hypotension

Precautions: Surgery of brain, spinal cord, eye or other sites where haemorrhage a risk. Impaired renal or hepatic function. Preservatives used in heparin preparations have been implicated in adverse effects. Use concentrated solutions if large quantities of heparin to be used. Heparin does not cross the placenta or appear in breast milk

Pharmacokinetics:
IV: Peak 5 min, duration 2−6 hr
Subcutaneous: Onset 20−60 min, duration 8−12 hr. Half-life 1½ hr, excreted in urine

Interactions/incompatibilities:
• Increased action: oral anticoagulants, salicylates, dihydroergotamine, digitalis, steroids, indomethacin, probenecid, dipyridamole
• Many incompatibilities reported with other drugs for parenteral administration e.g. ampicillin sodium, gentamicin, benzylpenicillin sodium, vancomycin hydochloride. Check with manufacturers data sheet and seek advice before administration

Clinical assesment:
• Determine activated partial thromboplastin time and partial prothrombin time daily

• Platelet count should be measured if treatment longer than 5 days. Stop immediately if thrombocytopenia
• Avoid all IM injections that may cause bleeding

Lab. test interferences:
• Inhibition of aminoglycoside estimations

Treatment of overdose:
• Withdraw heparin therapy
• Administer protamine sulphate

NURSING CONSIDERATIONS

Assess:
• Baseline BP

Administer:
• Using aseptic technique when administering by subcutaneous or IV routes
• Avoid rubbing of area to prevent bruising

Evaluate:
• Therapeutic response: decrease of deep vein thrombosis, i.e. pain in limb
• BP 4 hrly initially then twice daily
• Observe injection sites for inflammation
• Bleeding gums, petechiae, ecchymosis, black tarry stools, haematuria
• Fever, skin rash, urticaria
• For signs of hypertension

Teach patient/family:
• To avoid non-prescribed preparations that may cause serious drug interactions, e.g. aspirin
• Drug may be witheld during active bleeding (menstruation)
• To use soft-bristle toothbrush or cotton wool to avoid bleeding gums
• To carry a Medic-Alert ID identifying drug taken
• Stress importance of patient compliance with therapy
• On all aspects of adjustments: dosage, route, action, side effects, when to notify clinician
• To report any signs of bleeding: gums, under skin, urine, stools
• To avoid hazardous activities (football, hockey, skiing) or dangerous work

---

hepatitis B vaccine

Engerix B
Func. class.: Vaccine
Legal class.: POM

Action: Provides active immunity to hepatitis B

Uses: Prevention of hepatitis B infection

Dosage and routes:
• *Adult and child over 12 yr:* IM 1 ml, then 1 ml after 1 month, then 1 ml 6 months after initial dose. For more rapid immunisation third dose at 2 months and booster at 12 months
• *Neonates and child under 12:* IM 0.5 ml, then 0.5 ml after 1 month, then 0.5 ml 6 months after initial dose
• *Infants born to HBsAg positive mothers:* 3 doses 0.5 ml, 1st dose at birth with hepatitis B immunoglobulin
Available forms include: IM 20 mcg/ml injection

Side effects/adverse reactions:
INTEG: Soreness at injection site, urticaria, erythema, swelling, rashes, induration
CNS: Headache, dizziness, fever
GI: Nausea, vomiting, abdominal pain
MS: Arthralgia, myalgia

Contraindications: Hypersensitivity, severe febrile infections

Precautions: Renal dialysis, immunocompromised patients, pregnancy (unless definite risk of hepatitis B)
Vaccine may be ineffective if hepatitis B infection is present

Interactions/incompatibilities:
• Do not mix in same syringe as

other vaccines or inject at same site

Clinical assessment:

• Prepare for anaphylactic reaction and have injection of adrenaline 1:1000 available

NURSING CONSIDERATIONS

Administer:

• Subcutaneous route may be considered for haemophiliacs

• Only with adrenaline 1:1000 on unit to treat laryngospasm

• Administer in deltoid region or antero-lateral aspect of thigh but not gluteal region

• In major muscle mass

Evaluate:

• For skin reactions; rash, induration, urticaria

• For history of allergies, skin conditions (eczema, psoriasis, dermatitis), reactions to vaccinations

• For anaphylaxis: dyspnoea bronchospasm, tachycardia, collapse

Teach patient/family:

• That there could be local effects of soreness and redness at vaccination site

• That immunity is not immediate, require full course

---

hetastarch

Hespan

Func. class.: Plasma expander
Chem. class.: Synthetic polymer
Legal class.: POM

Action: Similar to human albumin, which expands plasma volume by colloidal osmotic pressure

Uses: To expand and maintain blood volume in shock due to burns, sepsis, and in blood loss, acute trauma, surgery, etc

Dosage and routes: IV infusion 500−1000 ml, total dose not to exceed 1500 ml a day. Consult specialist information such as data sheet compendium

Available forms include: IV infusion 6% solution in 0.9% sodium chloride

Side effects/adverse reactions:

HAEM: Decreased haematocrit, increased bleeding and coagulation times

INTEG: Urticaria and other skin reactions

RESP: Bronchospasm, wheezing

GI: Vomiting, salivary gland enlargement

SYST: Anaphylaxis

CNS: Headache

EENT: Periorbital oedema

MISC: Fever, muscular pains

Contraindications: Hypersensitivity, use in pregnancy (unless benefits outweigh risks)

Precautions: Renal disease, severe bleeding disorders, congestive cardiac failure, liver disease, children (no information available). Take blood samples for crossmatching before infusion (ideally)

Pharmacokinetics:

IV: Expands blood volume 1−2 times the amount infused, excreted in urine and faeces

Interactions/incompatibilities:

None known

NURSING CONSIDERATIONS

Assess:

• Baseline vital signs including CVP

• Fluid balance

Administer: See dosage and routes

Perform/provide:

• Storage at constant temperature below 25°C; discard unused portions

Evaluate:

• Vital signs: pulse, BP, respiratory rate CVP (5−30 min) observing for signs of fluid overload (hypertension and pulmonary oedema) and allergic reaction

• CVP during infusion

• Urine output every hr
• Clotting studies if a large transfusion given
• Symptoms of allergic reactions
• Tachycardia, hypotension
• For circulatory overload: increased pulse, respirations, shortness of breath, wheezing, chest tightness, chest pain
• For all side effects

---

hexachlorophane

Ster-Zac DC Skin Cleanser, Ster-Zac Powder
Func. class.: Disinfectant
Chem. class.: Polychlorinated phenol derivative
Legal class.: Skin cleanser POM, powder P

Action: Inhibits growth of Gram-positive bacteria and to much lesser extent Gram-negative
Uses: Surgical scrub, skin cleanser, neonatal staphylococcal cross-infection prevention, furunculosis, cord stumps of newborn, routine trunk application in midwifery
Dosage and routes:
Skin cleanser cream 3–5 ml to pre-moistened hands and wash for up to 3 min. Powder, neonatal staphylococcal cross-infection prevention: after cord ligature, dust cord, and axillas, perineum, groin, front of abdomen. Repeat after napkin changes until cord stump drops away and wound heals
Available forms include: Cream 3%; Powder 0.33%
Side effects/adverse reactions:
INTEG: Sensitivity, photosensitivity
Contraindications: Hypersensitivity, burns, badly damaged skin, pregnancy, mucous membranes, vaginally, under occlusive dressings, large areas of skin. To chil-

dren under 2 yr use on medical advice only
Precautions: Use on premature or low birth-weight infants, reserved for outbreaks of staphylococcal infections in nurseries
Clinical assessment:
• Monitor skin condition
NURSING CONSIDERATIONS
Administer:
• To body areas only; do not apply to face lips, mouth, eyes, mucous membrane, anus, meata
• Only to adults; repeated use may lead to systemic absorption
Evaluate:
• Area of body involved; irritation, rash, breaks, dryness, scales
• Effectiveness of wound care
Teach patient/family:
• To report itching, irritation, dizziness, headache, confusion; discontinue drug immediately

---

homatropine hydrobromide (ophthalmic)

Minims Homatropine Hydrobromide
Func. class.: Mydriatic
Chem. class.: Synthetic alkaloid
Legal class.: POM

Action: Blocks response of iris sphincter muscle, muscle of accommodation of ciliary body to cholinergic simulation, resulting in dilatation, paralysis of accommodation
Uses: As a mydriatic and cycloplegic; uveitis
Dosage and routes:
• *Adult and child:* Instil 1 or 2 drops repeat in 5–10 min for refraction; uveitis 1 or 2 drops 2 to 3 times daily
Available forms include: Eyedrops,

solution 1%, 2%. Minims 2% and intended as single use

Side effects/adverse reactions:

EENT: Increased intraocular pressure, blurred vision, photophobia, irritation, oedema

INTEG: Contact dermatitis, rash, dry skin

CV: Bradycardia, tachycardia, palpitations, arrhythmias

CNS: Giddiness, ataxia, psychotic reactions

GI: Dry mouth, constipation, abdominal distension

Contraindications: Hypersensitivity, patients allergic to atropine, glaucoma or tendency to glaucoma (e.g. narrow anterior chamber angle), pregnancy, lactation

Precautions: Systemic reactions in young and very old. Due to visual disturbances after use caution patients against driving, etc., until vision is clear

Pharmacokinetics:

INSTIL: Peak ½−1 hr, duration 1−3 days

Interactions/incompatibilities:

Possible enhanced action by other drugs with antimuscarinic properties: some antihistamines, phenothiazines, tricyclic antidepressants, butyrophenones

Treatment of overdose: If systemic toxicity occurs provide supportive treatment

If ingested: emesis or gastric lavage

NURSING CONSIDERATIONS

Perform/provide:

• Cover eye with patch; danger of retinal damage due to excess light entering the eye

Evaluate:

• Monitor patient and report any systemic symptoms to clinician

• Therapeutic response: decrease in inflammation or cycloplegic refraction

• Eye pain, inform clinician, discontinue use

Teach patient/family:

• Teach patient to use clean swabs to wipe eye before and after, using different swabs for each treatment and each eye

• Do not touch dropper to eye

• Wait 5 min to use other drops

• To report change in vision, blurring or loss of sight, trouble breathing, sweating, flushing

• Not to engage in hazardous activities until able to see

• That blurred vision will decrease with repeated use of drug

---

hyaluronidase

Hyalase

Func. class.: Enzyme

Legal class.: POM

Action: Depolymerises the mucopolysaccharide hyaluronic acid which is a component of the 'tissue cement' of tissue space so reducing its viscosity. The tissue is rendered more permeable to injections

Uses: Increased tissue permeability to IM or subcutaneous injections; aids resorption of extravasated blood and excess fluids

Dosage and routes:

• *For tissue permeability:* Subcutaneous or IM injection, 1500 units with other drug or injected in site before drug; by subcutaneous infusion 1500 units before 500−1000 ml infusion

Available forms include: Injection, powder for reconstitution 1500 unit

Contraindications: Hypersensitivity; use at site of infections or malignancy, bites or stings; by intravenous route

NURSING CONSIDERATIONS

Administer:

• Immediately after mixing since solution is unstable

Evaluate:

• Therapeutic response: absence of swelling, pain after hypodermolysis

hydralazine HCl

Apresoline
Func. class.: Antihypertensive, direct-acting peripheral vasodilator
Chem. class.: Phthalazine
Legal class.: POM

Action: Vasodilatation through relaxation of arteriolar smooth muscle; reduction in blood pressure with reflex increases in cardiac function

Uses: Moderate to severe hypertension in addition to a β-blocker or thiazide diuretic; hypertensive crisis

Dosage and routes:
• *Adult:* By mouth 25 mg twice a day increasing to maximum of 50 mg twice a day. For higher doses see data sheet compendium. Injection, slow IV 5−10 mg over 20 min; repeated if necessary after 20−30 min; IV infusion initially 200−300 mcg/min then maintenance 50−150 mcg/min

Available forms include: Tablets 25, 50 mg; injection 20 mg

Side effects/adverse reactions:
CV: Tachycardia, palpitations, anginal symptoms, flushing, hypotension, oedema, heart failure
GI: Nausea, vomiting, and other disturbances
SYST: Lupus erythematosus-like syndrome
CNS: Headache, peripheral neuritis, dizziness, polyneuritis, paraesthesia
INTEG: Rashes
HAEM: Changes in blood count, anaemia, leucopenia, neutropenia, thrombocytopenia
GU: Proteinuria, haematuria, increased plasma creatinine, renal failure, urinary retention
EENT: Nasal congestion
MISC: Fever

Contraindications: Hypersensitivity to hydralazine or dihydralazine. Idiopathic systemic lupus erythematosus, severe tachycardia, high output heart failure, myocardial insufficiency due to mechanical obstruction, cor pulmonale, dissecting aortic aneurysm, porphyria

Precautions: Pregnancy, breast feeding, renal impairment and hepatic dysfunction — reduce dosage, coronary artery disease, cerebrovascular disease, low parenteral doses, possible over rapid BP reduction. Possible reaction impairment; patients should be warned of possible hazard driving or operating machinery

Pharmacokinetics:
By mouth: Onset 20−30 min, peak 1 hr, duration 2−4 hr
IM: Onset 5−10 min, peak 1 hr, duration 2−4 hr
IV: Onset 5−20 min, peak 10−80 min, duration 2−6 hr
Half-life 2−8 hr, metabolised by liver, less than 10% present in urine

Interactions/incompatibilities:
• Enhanced hypotensive effect: alcohol, anaesthetics, antidepressants, antipsychotics, anxiolytics, hypnotics, β-blockers, calcium channel blockers, diuretics, dopaminergics, muscle relaxants, nitrates, diazoxide
• Additive hypotensive effect: other antihypertensives
• Antagonise hypotensive effect: NSAIDs, corticosteroids, oestragens and combined oral contraceptives, carbenoxolone, use with caution: MAOIs

Clinical assessment:
• Monitor patient for side effects when treatment with hydralazine started

Treatment of overdose: Immediate gastric lavage and supportive measures. Activated charcoal may be used. If hypotension use a pressor agent (not adrenaline which causes tachycardia) to raise BP

NURSING CONSIDERATIONS

Assess:

• Baseline BP

Administer:

• Patient in recumbent position, keep in that position for 1 hr after administration

Perform/provide:

• BP, 5 min for 2 hr, then 1 hrly for 2 hr, then 4 hrly and jugular venous distension 4 hrly if administered parenterally

• Weight daily, fluid balance

Evaluate:

• Oedema in feet, legs daily

• Skin turgor, dryness of mucous membranes for hydration status

• Rales, dyspnoea, orthopnoea

• IV site for extravasation

• Fever, joint pain, tachycardia, palpitations, headache, nausea

• Mental status: affect, mood, behaviour, anxiety; check for personality changes

Teach patient/family:

• To take with food to increase bioavailability

• To avoid non-prescribed preparations unless approved by clinician

• To notify clinician if chest pain, severe fatigue, fever, muscle or joint pain occurs

---

hydroclorothiazide

HydroSaluric, Esidrex, many combination products

Func. class.: Thiazide diuretic
Chem. class.: Sulphonamide
Legal class.: POM

Action: Inhibits the reabsorption of sodium chloride and water probably at proximal tubules of kidney

Uses: Oedema of various causes e.g. congestive heart failure, renal dysfunction, hepatic conditions, premenstrual tension; hypertension; adjunct to other antihypertensive drugs

Dosage and routes:

• *Adults:* By mouth, oedema 25—100 mg once or twice daily reducing to maintenance of 25—50 mg alternate days; hypertension 25 mg daily increasing if necessary to 100 mg

Available forms include: Tablets 25, 50 mg

Side effects/adverse reactions:

CNS: Paraesthesia, headache, dizziness, vertigo

GI: Gastric irritation, vomiting, jaundice, pancreatitis nausea, anorexia, constipation, diarrhoea, cramps, salivary gland irritation

INTEG: Rash, photosensitivity, purpura

HAEM: Hyperglycaemia, hyperuricaemia, increased cholesterol, neutropenia, thrombocytopenia

ELECT: Hypokalaemia, hypomagnesaemia, hyponatraemia, hypercalcaemia, hypochloraemic alkalosis

CV: Hypotension, orthostatic hypotension

EENT: Yellow vision, blurred vision

GU: Impotence, interstitial nephritis, renal dysfunction, renal failure

SYST: Anaphylactic reactions

Contraindications: Hypersensitivity to thiazides or sulphonamides, severe renal and hepatic impairment, hypercalcaemia, Addison's disease, porphyria, lithium therapy, precoma associated with hepatic cirrhosis

Precautions: Hypokalaemia, renal and hepatic impairment, diabetes, gout, pregnancy, breast feeding, systemic lupus erythematosus

Monitor for signs of electrolyte imbalance

Pharmacokinetics:

By mouth: Onset 2 hr, peak 4 hr, duration 6—12 hr; excreted unchanged by kidneys, enters breast milk

Interactions/incompatibilities:

• Increased toxicity of: non-depolarising muscle relaxants, lithium, cardiac glycosides, tricyclic antidepressants, MAOIs

• Decreased effects of: antidiabetics, sex hormones

• Risk of hypercalcaemia: calcium salts

• Risk of hypokalaemia: corticosteroids, other diuretics, carbenoxolone

• Decreased effect of this drug: NSAIDs

• Electrolytes and renal function

Lab. test interferences:

Tests for parathyroid function

Treatment of overdose: Empty stomach by emesis or lavage, give symptomatic and supportive treatment

NURSING CONSIDERATIONS

Assess:

• Baseline BP, weight and fluid balance

• Rate, depth, rhythm of respiration, effect of exertion

• Glucose in urine if patient is diabetic

Administer:

• In morning to avoid interference with sleep if using drug as a diuretic

• Potassium replacement if potassium is less than 3.0 mmol/litre unless contraindicated

• With food, if nausea occurs, absorption may be decreased slightly

Evaluate:

• Fluid balance daily to determine fluid loss; effect of drug may be decreased if used daily

• Weight daily

• BP lying, standing; postural hypotension may occur

• Improvement in oedema of feet, legs, sacral area daily if medication is being used in heart failure

• Improvement in CVP and BP recordings

• Signs of metabolic acidosis: drowsiness, restlessness

• Signs of hypokalaemia: postural hypotension, malaise, fatigue, tachycardia, leg cramps, weakness

• Rashes, temperature elevation daily

• Confusion, especially in elderly; take safety precautions if needed

Teach patient/family:

• To increase fluid intake 2−3 litres daily unless contraindicated; to rise slowly from lying or sitting position

• To notify clinician of muscle weakness, cramps, nausea, dizziness

• Drug may be taken with food or milk

• That blood sugar may be increased in diabetics

• Take early in day to avoid nocturia

hydrocortisone acetate ophthalmic/otic

Combination products

Func. class.: Anti-inflammatory

Chem. class.: Synthetic corticosteroid

Legal class.: POM

Action: Anti-inflammatory by suppressing various components of the inflammatory reaction

Uses: Inflammation of the eye or ear

Dosage and routes:

• *Adult and child:* Instil 2 to 4 times a day

Available forms include: Ointment 0.5%, eye/ear drops 0.5%

Side effects/adverse reactions:

EENT: Itching, irritation

INTEG: Rash, urticaria

Contraindications: Hypersensitivity, perforated eardrum, bacterial, fungal or viral infection of the eye, corneal ulceration, glaucoma

NURSING CONSIDERATIONS
Administer:
• After removing impacted cerumen by irrigation of ear if necessary
• Drops or ointment directly into inflamed eye/ear
• Without contact of dropper to inflamed area

Perform/provide:
• Suitable analgesics if required

Evaluate:
• Therapeutic response: decreased pain, soreness and inflammation
• For redness, swelling, fever, pain in ear, which indicates infection

Teach patient/family:
• To instil after washing hands well, without touching dropper to ear/eye
• That balance may be impaired and dizziness occur
• Not to drive or operate machinery if dizziness occurs
• That two containers of hydrocortisone are required if both eyes/ears are inflammed. Containers marked 'left' and 'right' to be used only on that corresponding side
• To contact the clinician if redness, swelling, fever, pain in ear occurs

---

hydrocortisone/ hydrocortisone acetate/ hydrocortisone butyrate

Dioderm, Efcortelan, Mildison, Hydrocortistab, Locoid, Hydrocortisyl, many combination products
Func. class.: Topical corticosteroid
Chem. class.: Natural non-fluorinated, glucocorticoid
Legal class.: POM; unless in products specifically licensed as P

Action: Possesses antipruritic, anti-inflammatory actions, mildly potent (base and acetate), potent (butyrate)

Uses: Mild inflammatory skin conditions including the following: eczema, contact dermatitis, seborrhoeic dermatitis, intertrigo, insect bites, psoriasis

Dosage and routes:
• *Adult and child:* Apply sparingly 2−3 times a day

Available forms include: Hydrocortisone−ointment 0.5%, 1%, 2.5%; cream 0.1%, 0.125%, 0.5%, 1%, 2.5%; lotion 1%; acetate−cream 0.1%, 0.125%, 0.5%, 1%, 2.5%; butyrate−ointment 0.1%; cream 0.1%; acetate−cream 0.125%, 0.5%, 1%, 2.5% (many others)

Side effects/adverse reactions:
INTEG: Hypopigmentation, subcutaneous atrophy, acne, spread and worsening of untreated infection, striae, allergic contact dermatitis, thinning of skin, increasing hair growth

Contraindications: Hypersensitivity to corticosteroids, fungal, bacterial, or viral infections

Precautions: Pregnancy, lactation, prolonged administration in infants and children, extreme caution in dermatoses of infancy e.g. napkin eruption, use on face

NURSING CONSIDERATIONS
Assess:
• Skin area to be covered

Administer:
• Apply wearing gloves. Wash hands well before and after application
• Only to dermatoses; do not use on weeping, denuded, or infected area
• Only to affected areas; avoid eyes

Perform/provide:
• Cleansing before application of drug

• Treatment for a few days after area has cleared

Evaluate:

• Temperature; if fever develops, drug should be discontinued
• Extent of skin affected and any changes in condition
• Allergic reaction
• Hypopigmentation
• Therapeutic response: absence of severe itching, patches on skin, flaking

Teach patient/family:

• To avoid sunlight on affected area; burns may occur
• Not to use other non-prescribed products unless directed by clinician

---

hydrocortisone/ hydrocortisone acetate/ hydrocortisone sodium phosphate/ hydrocortisone sodium succinate

Colifoam, Corlan, Efcortelan Soluble, Efcortesol, Hydrocortistab, Hydrocortone, Solu-cortef

Func. class.: Corticosteroid,
Chem. class.: Glucocorticoid, short-acting
Legal class.: POM

Action: Decreases inflammation by suppression of migration of polymorphonuclear leucocytes, fibroblasts, reversal of increased capillary permeability and lysosomal stabilisation

Uses: Severe inflammation including status asthmaticus, acute allergic reactions, anaphylactic drug reactions; shock, acute adrenal insufficiency, joint conditions including tennis elbow, ulcerative colitis, severe erythema multiforme, systemic lupus erythematosus

Dosage and routes:

Adrenal insufficiency/inflammation shock

• *Adult:* IM, IV infusion, slow IV 100−500 mg (succinate or phosphate) repeated 3−4 times in 24 hr as needed
• *Child under 1 yr:* IV 25 mg; 1−5 yr: IV 50 mg; 6−12 yr: IV 100 mg repeated 3−4 times in 24 hr as needed

Colitis

• *Adult:* Aerosol one application nightly for 2−3 weeks then alternate days; suppository 25 mg night and morning and after a bowel movement

Joints

• *Adult:* Injection intra-articular, peri-articular 5−50 mg (acetate) according to joint; no more than 3 injections in 24 hr
• *Child:* 5−30 mg daily in divided doses

Replacement

• *Adult:* By mouth 20−30 mg daily in divided doses
• *Child:* 10−30 mg in divided doses

Available forms include: Tablets 10, 20 mg; phosphate injection 100 mg/ml; succinate injection 100 mg/vial; acetate injection 25 mg/ml; aerosol 10%; 25 mg suppository

Side effects/adverse reactions:

INTEG: Acne, poor wound healing, bruising, striae, telangiectasia, atrophy
CNS: Depression, psychological dependance, insomnia, euphoria, aggravation of schizophrenia
CV: Thromboembolism, sodium and water retention, hypertension, potassium loss
HAEM: Leucocytosis
MS: Fractures, osteoporosis, proximal myopathy, tendon rupture, avascular osteonecrosis
GI: Nausea, abdominal distension, increased appetite, peptic ulceration with perforation and haemorrhage, dyspepsia, oesophageal

ulceration, oesophageal candidiasis, acute pancreatitis

EENT: Increased intra-ocular pressure, glaucoma, exacerbation of ophthalmic viral or fungal disease, exophthalmos, corneal or scleral thinning, papilloedema

ENDO: Growth suppression in children and adolescents, suppression or hypothalomopituitary-adrenal axis, menstrual irregularity and amenorrhoea, weight gain, Cushingoid features, hirsutism, negative nitrogen balance, increased carbohydrate tolerance with increased requirement for antidiabetic therapy

MISC: Recurrence of dormant tuberculosis, opportunist infection

Contraindications: Hypersensitivity, do not inject into tendons, immunisation procedures, systemic infection unless specific anti-infective therapy is employed

Precautions: Pregnancy, lactation, diabetes mellitus, osteoporosis, glaucoma (or family history of glaucoma), peptic ulcer, congestive heart failure, epilepsy, psychosis or severe psychoneuroses, history of tuberculosis, hypertension, previous steroid myopathy, symptoms of infection suppressed, renal insufficiency

Pharmacokinetics:

By mouth: Onset 1−2 hr, peak 1 hr, duration 1−1½ days

IM/IV: Onset 20 min, peak 4−8 hr, duration 1−1½ days

Rectal: Onset 3−5 days

Metabolised by liver, excreted in urine (17-hydroxycorticosteroids, 17-ketosteroids)

Interactions/incompatibilities:

• Decreased action of this drug: barbiturates, carbamazepine, phenytoin, primidone, rifampicin, ephedrine, anticoagulants

• Decreased effects of: Cholecystographic X-ray media, salicylates, anticoagulants, hypoglycaemic

agents, anti-hypertensives, diuretics, anticholinesterases

• Increased risk of hypokalaemia: acetazolamide, loop diuretics, thiazides, carbenoxolone, β_2-sympathomimetics, amphotericin

Clinical assessment:

• Potassium, blood sugar, urine glucose while on long-term therapy; hypokalaemia, hypertension, mental changes, gastric discomfort, hyperglycaemia

• Plasma cortisol levels during long-term therapy (normal level: 138−635 nmol/litre when drawn at 8 a.m.)

NURSING CONSIDERATIONS

Assess:

• Baseline weight and BP

Administer:

• Orally with food or milk to decrease GI symptoms

• Shake suspension (parenteral)

• Titrated dose, use lowest effective dose

• IM injection deeply in large mass, rotate sites, avoid deltoid, use large bore needle

• In one dose in morning to prevent adrenal suppression, avoid subcutaneous administration, damage may be done to tissue

Perform/provide:

• Weight daily or twice weekly if stable

• Assistance with mobility in patient with bone tissue disease to prevent fractures

Evaluate:

• Fluid balance ratio, be alert for decreasing urinary output and increasing oedema

• Therapeutic response: ease of respirations, decreased inflammation

• Infection: increased temperature, WBC, even after withdrawal of medication; drug masks symptoms of infection

• Potassium depletion: paraesthesia, fatigue, nausea, vomiting,

depression, polyuria, dysrhythmias, weakness
• Oedema, hypotension, cardiac symptoms
• Mental status: affect, mood, behavioural changes, aggression, weight gain

Teach patient/family:
• That ID as steroid user should be carried
• To notify clinician if therapeutic response decreases; dosage adjustment may be needed
• Not to discontinue this medication abruptly or adrenal crisis can result
• To avoid non-prescribed products: salicylates, alcohol in cough products, cold preparations unless directed by clinician
• Teach patient all aspects of drug use, including Cushingoid symptoms
• Symptoms of adrenal insufficiency: nausea, anorexia, fatigue, dizziness, dyspnoea, weakness, joint pain

---

hydrocortisone butyrate

Locoid, combination product
Func. class.: Potent topical corticosteroid
Chem. class.: Non-fluorinated corticosteroid
Legal class.: POM

Action: Reduces inflammation
Uses: Severe inflammatory skin disorders e.g. eczema in patients unresponsive to less potent corticosteroids, psoriasis, etc.
Dosage and routes: Topically, apply thinly 2−4 times a day, reduce as condition responds
Available forms include: Cream, lipocream, ointment, scalp lotion, all 0.1%
Side effects/adverse reactions:

INTEG: Spread and worsening of untreated infection; thinning of the skin; irreversible striae atrophicae; perioral dermatitis; acne at site of application; mild depigmentation and vellus hair; increased hair growth
Contraindications: Untreated bacterial, fungal or viral skin infections
Precautions: Pregnancy and breast feeding (inadequate safety information), long term use, use with occlusion—restrict limited areas, rebound relapses in psoriasis following development of tolerance

NURSING CONSIDERATIONS
Administer:
• To clean, dry skin
• Apply sparingly to affected area only
Evaluate:
• Effect of drug—improving skin rash
• For localised side effects—rash may be worse to begin with, thinning of skin, hair growth
• For systemic reactions (usually only with long term treatment over large skin areas)—hypertension, water and sodium retention, signs of diabetes and adrenal suppression. Notify clinician at once
Teach patient/family:
• To avoid drug contact with eyes
• To apply sparingly to affected areas only
• Not to use for other skin eruptions
• To inform clinician of any side effects
• Check with G.P. before taking any other medications
• Withhold treatment and notify clinician if rash appears worse

hydrogen peroxide

Func. class.: Disinfectant
Chem. class.: Oxidising drug
Legal class.: Solution GSL

Action: Bactericidal
Uses: Skin disinfection, wound and ulcer cleaning and deodourising, mouthwash
Dosage and routes:
• *Adult and child:* Solution use as required
Available forms include: Solution 3%, 6%, 27% and 30% (dilute before use)
Side effects/adverse reactions:
INTEG: 'Irritating' burns
EENT: Use as mouthwash—reversible hypertrophy of papillae of tongue
Contraindications: Hypersensitivity, closed wounds
Precautions: Large or deep wounds, normal skin, bleaches fabric and clothing
Pharmacokinetics: Effective to end of bubbling (oxygen release)
NURSING CONSIDERATIONS
Assess:
• Appropriateness of agent as part of wound management/mouth care
• Patient's ability to avoid ingestion by swallowing if used as mouthwash
Administer:
• Only if no evidence that effeverscence can enter blood stream (i.e. not in deep wounds) in order to avoid air/gas embolus
• Diluted, as prescribed
• With care, onto sloughing area of wound avoiding healthy tissue where possible
• Irrigate with normal saline after application
• A as diluted mouth gargle for stomatitis
Evaluate:
• Effectiveness of wound cleansing by absence of sloughly material and evidence of tissue granulation—change to other non-desloughing agent at such time
• As mouthwash, oral condition improved, again change to a different preparation
Teach patient/family:
• Technique of administration
• Importance of medical review
• Other aspects to influence oral hygiene if appropriate
• To avoid swallowing

hydroxocobalamin (vitamin B$_{12}$)

Neo-cytamen, ~~NHS~~ Cobalin-H
Func. class.: Vitamin
Chem. class.: Fat-soluble vitamin
Legal class.: POM

Action: Needed for adequate nerve functioning, protein and carbohydrate metabolism, normal growth, RBC development
Uses: Vitamin B$_{12}$ deficiency, pernicious anaemia, vitamin B$_{12}$ malabsorption syndrome, tobacco amblyopia, Leber's optic atrophy, subacute combined degeneration of the spinal cord
Dosage and routes:
• *Adult and child:* IM 250—1000 mcg at intervals of 2—3 days for 5 doses; maintenance 1 mg every month. See data sheet for further information
Available forms include: Injection 1 mg
Side effects/adverse reactions:
CNS: Dizziness, hot flushes
INTEG: Itching, exanthema, acneform/bullous eruptions
MISC: Anaphylaxis, chills, fever
GI: Nausea
Contraindications: Hypersensitivity, megaloblastic anaemia of pregnancy
Precautions: Give only after estab-

lishing diagnosis; investigate folate metabolism if megaloblastic anaemia fails to respond; hypokalaemia

Pharmacokinetics: Stored in liver, kidneys, stomach; 50%–90% excreted in urine, breast milk

Interactions/incompatibilities:

• Decreased effect of this drug: chloramphenicol, oral contraceptives

• Increased absorption: prednisone

Clinical assessment:

• Full blood count for increase in reticulocyte count during first week of therapy, then increase in RBC and Hb

• Initial therapy: monitor patient for hypersensitivity reactions

Lab. test interferences: B_{12} assays by microbiological techniques invalidated by anti-metabolites and most antibiotics

Treatment of overdose:

Discontinue drug

NURSING CONSIDERATIONS

Assess:

• Potassium levels during beginning treatment

• Full blood count for increased reticulocyte count during 1st week of therapy

Evaluate:

• Therapeutic response: decreased anorexia, dyspnoea on excretion, palpitations, paraesthesia, psychosis, visual disturbances

• Nutritional status: should include good sources of vitamin B_{12}

• For pulmonary oedema, or worsening of congestive cardiac failure in cardiac patients

Teach patient/family:

• That treatment must continue for life if diagnosis is pernicious anaemia

• About taking a well balanced diet

• That itching skin eruptions must be reported to clinician immediately

hydroxychloroquine sulphate

Plaquenil
Func. class.: Antirheumatic
Chem. class.: 4-aminoquinoline derivative
Legal class.: POM

Action: Mode of action in rheumatism uncertain; may modify disease process

Uses: Rheumatoid arthritis, systemic and discoid lupus erythematosus, dermatological conditions sunlight related

Dosage and routes:

Rheumatoid arthritis, systemic lupus erythematosus

• *Adult:* By mouth initially 400 mg daily in divided doses reduced to 200–400 mg daily maintenance, maximum 6.5 mg/kg daily

• *Children:* Up to 6.5 mg/kg daily

Available forms include: Tablets 200 mg

Side effects/adverse reactions:

INTEG: Rashes, pigmentary changes, hair bleaching and loss, pruritus, skin eruptions

CNS: Headache, nervousness, emotional upsets, psychotic episodes

EENT: Visual disturbances, irreversible retinal damage, corneal opacities, photophobia, vertigo, tinnitus, deafness, difficulty focusing

GI: Nausea, vomiting, anorexia, diarrhoea, cramps

HAEM: Thrombocytopenia, agranulocytosis, aplastic anaemia

CV: Hypotension, ECG changes

Contraindications: Hypersensitivity, pregnancy, maculopathy

Precautions: Renal and hepatic impairment, porphyria, psoriasis, neurological disorders, severe gastrointestinal disorders, G6PD deficiency, elderly, visual defects, blood disorders. Ophthalmological examination before starting treatment. Possible visual accommodation impairment initially, warn patients against driving or operating machinery

Pharmacokinetics:

By mouth: Peak 1–2 hr, half-life 3–5 days, metabolised in liver, excreted in urine, faeces, breast milk

Interactions/incompatibilities:

• Decreased absorption of this drug: antacids

• Increased plasma concentration of this drug: cimetidine

• Increased plasma concentration of: digoxin

Treatment of overdose: Evacuate stomach by gastric lavage or emesis; further inhibit absorption with charcoal. Administer parenteral diazepam to reverse chloroquine cardiotoxicity. Prepare to give respiratory support and treatment for shock with fluids and if necessary plasma expanders. In severe cases consider using dopamine

NURSING CONSIDERATIONS

Administer:

• With or after meals at same time each day to maintain drug level

Perform/provide:

• Storage injection should be kept in cool environment

Teach patient/family:

• To use sunglasses in bright sunlight to decrease photophobia

• To report hearing, visual problems, fever, fatigue, bruising, bleeding, which may indicate blood dyscrasias

• To take with food to reduce upset stomach and mark bitter taste

• Other side-effects: nausea, diarrhoea, loss of appetite, skin rashes, lightening and thinning of hair

• Skin irritation in sunlight

• Importance of eye testing

• Allow 4 hr between taking indigestion medicine and hydrochloroquine

hydroxyprogesterone hexanoate

Proluton Depot

Func. class.: Progestogen hormone

Legal class.: POM

Action: Replaces progesterone in deficiency to maintain pregnancy

Uses: Habitual abortion associated with progesterone deficiency

Dosage and routes:

• *Adult:* IM 250–500 mg weekly during first half of pregnancy

Available forms include: Injection IM 250, 500 mg ampoules

Side effects/adverse reactions:

CNS: Depression

CV: Oedema

GI: Disturbances, cholestatic jaundice

INTEG: Acne, urticaria, allergic skin rashes

GU: Breast discomfort, gynaecomastia, irregular menstrual cycles, menstrual bleeding

MISC: Weight gain, changes in libido

Contraindications: History of pemphigoid gestationis, existing or previous liver tumours, undiagnosed vaginal bleeding, mammary carcinoma, missed or incomplete abortion, past severe arterial disease or current high risk, porphyria

Precautions: Hypertension, asthma, cardiovascular, renal or hepatic impairment, diabetes mellitus, depression, breast feeding, epilepsy, migraine

Pharmacokinetics:

IM: Half-life 5 min, excreted in urine, faeces, metabolised in liver

Clinical assessment:

• Liver function tests: alanine aminotransferase, aspartate aminotransferase, bilirubin, periodically during long-term therapy

NURSING CONSIDERATIONS
Assess:
- Baseline and fluid balance
- Weight
- BP at beginning of treatment and periodically

Administer:
- Oil solution deeply in large muscle mass (IM), rotate sites
- In one dose in the morning

Evaluate:
- Therapeutic response
- Oedema, hypertension, cardiac symptoms, jaundice
- Mental status: affect, mood, behavioural changes, depression
- Weight gain
- Fluid balance

Teach patient/family:
- All aspects of drug usage, including Cushingoid symptoms
- To report any side effects
- Explain full expected effects of drug

---

hydroxyurea

Hydrea
Func. class.: Antineoplastic
Chem. class.: Synthetic urea analogue
Legal class.: POM

Action: Acts by inhibiting DNA synthesis without interfering with RNA or protein synthesis; incorporates thymidine into DNA, causing direct damage to DNA strands

Uses: Chronic myeloid leukaemia, cancer of the cervix (with radiotherapy)

Dosage and routes:
- *Adult:* By mouth continuous regimen 20–30 mg/kg daily or intermittent regimen 80 mg/kg every third day. See data sheet compendium for further information

Available forms include: Capsules 500 mg

Side effects/adverse reactions:
HAEM: Leucopenia, anaemia, thrombocytopenia
GI: Nausea, vomiting, anorexia, diarrhoea, stomatitis, constipation, abdominal pain
GU: Increased blood urea nitrogen, uric acid and creatinine, renal function impairment, dysuria
INTEG: Rash, alopecia, erythema
CNS: Headache, drowsiness, dizziness, disorientation, hallucinations, convulsions

Contraindications: Hypersensitivity, marked thrombocytopenia, leucopenia, severe anaemia

Precautions: Renal dysfunction, pregnancy, elderly, increase in myelosuppressive activity with previous or ongoing cytotoxic treatment or radiotherapy. Monitor blood, bone marrow, renal and liver function, uric acid. Correct anaemia before therapy

Pharmacokinetics: Readily absorbed when taken orally, peak level in 2 hr, degraded in liver, excreted in urine, almost totally eliminated in 24 hr; readily crosses blood-brain barrier

Interactions/incompatibilities:
- Increased toxicity: other cytotoxic drugs

Clinical assessment:
- Liver function tests before, during therapy: bilirubin, alkaline phosphatase, aspartate aminotransferase, alanine aminotransferase, lactic dehydrogenase; as needed or monthly
- Other medications by oral route if possible

Treatment of overdose: Gastric lavage, supportive therapy short term. Long term monitor haemopoietic system with blood transfusion if necessary

NURSING CONSIDERATIONS
Administer:

• Anti-emetic 30−60 min before giving drug to prevent vomiting (severe in high doses)
• Transfusion for anaemia
• Antibiotics for prophylaxis of infection if indicated
• Topical or systemic analgesics for pain

Perform/provide:
• Nutritious diet with iron, vitamin supplements as ordered
• Strict oral hygiene 4 times a day

Evaluate:
• Fluid balance ratio, report fall in urine output to less than 30 ml/hr
• Monitor temperature 4 hrly; fever may indicate beginning infection
• Bleeding: haematuria, bruising or petechiae, mucosa or orifices 8 hrly
• Level of drowsiness which may occur after taking medication
• Buccal cavity 8 hrly for dryness, sores or ulceration, white patches, oral pain, bleeding, dysphagia
• Neurotoxicity: headaches, hallucinations, convulsions, dizziness
• Symptoms indicating severe allergic reaction: rash, urticaria, itching, flushing
• Inflammation of mucosa, breaks in skin
• Food preferences; list likes, dislikes
• Effects of alopecia on body image, discuss feelings about body changes

Teach patient/family:
• To report any complaints, side effects to nurse or clinician
• That hair may be lost during treatment, and wig or hair piece may be available on the NHS; tell patient that new hair may be different in colour, texture
• To avoid foods with citric acid, hot or rough texture if stomatitis is present
• To report stomatitis: any bleeding, white spots, ulcerations in the mouth; tell patient to examine mouth daily, report symptoms
• Contraceptive measures are recommended during therapy
• To drink 2 litres of fluid
• Notify clinician of fever, chills, sore throat, nausea, vomiting, anorexia, diarrhoea, bleeding, bruising; may indicate blood dyscrasias
• About side effects and benefits

---

hydroxyzine HCl

Atarax
Func. class.: Anti-anxiety; antihistamine
Chem. class.: Piperazine derivative
Legal class.: POM

Action: Depresses subcortical levels of CNS, including limbic system, reticular formation; competitive antagonist at H_1 receptors

Uses: Adjunct in treatment of anxiety, pruritus

Dosage and routes:
Anxiety
• *Adult:* Only 50−100 mg 4 times a day
Pruritus
• *Adult:* 25 mg at night initially and increasing to 25 mg 3 to 4 times daily if necessary
• *Child 6 months to 6 yr:* 5−15 mg daily increasing to 50 mg daily if necessary in divided doses; over 6 yr 15−25 mg increasing to 50−100 mg daily if necessary in divided doses

Available forms include: Tablets 10, 25 mg; syrup 10 mg/5 ml

Side effects/adverse reactions:
CNS: Dizziness, drowsiness, confusion, headache, tremor, convulsions, stimulation
GI: Gastrointestinal disturbances, dry mouth
INTEG: Rash, photosensitivity reactions

CV: ECG abnormalities
EENT: Blurred vision
Contraindications: Hypersensitivity, early pregnancy, lactation
Precautions: Impaired renal function, hepatic disease. May impair mental alertness or physical coordination, warn patients against driving or operating machinery if affected
Pharmacokinetics:
By mouth: Onset 15−30 min, duration 4−6 hr, half-life 3 hr
Interactions/incompatibilities:
• Increased CNS depressant effect: alcohol, barbiturates, other anxiolytics, hypnotics
Lab. test interferences:
False increase: estimation of urinary 17-hydroxycorticosteroids
Treatment of overdose: Induction of vomiting in conscious patients and gastric lavage, supportive care. If hypotension, control with intravenous fluids and noradrenaline or metaraminol

NURSING CONSIDERATIONS
Assess:
• Baseline BP (lying, standing), pulse
Administer:
• With food or milk for GI symptoms
• Crushed if patient is unable to swallow medication whole
• Frequent sips of water for dry mouth
Perform/provide:
• Assistance with mobility during beginning therapy, since drowsiness/dizziness occurs
• Safety measures, including cot sides
• Checking to see oral medication has been swallowed
Evaluate:
• Mental status: mood, alertness, affect
• Physical dependency and withdrawal symptoms: headache, nausea, vomiting, muscle pain, weakness after long-term use
• Increased sedation
Teach patient/family:
• Not to be used for everyday stress or used longer than 4 months
• Avoid non-prescribed preparations (cold, cough, hay fever) unless approved by clinician
• To avoid driving, activities that require alertness
• To avoid alcohol ingestion, or other psychotropic medications
• Not to discontinue medication quickly after long-term use
• To rise slowly or fainting may occur

---

hyoscine hydrobromide (transdermal)

Scopoderm TTS
Func. class.: Anti-emetic, anticholinergic
Chem. class.: Belladonna alkaloid
Legal class.: POM

Action: Competitive antagonist of acetylcholine and other parasympathomimetic agents. Action in preventing motion sickness in central nervous system unknown
Uses: Prevention of symptoms of motion sickness
Dosage and routes:
• *Adults and child over 10 yr:* Patch applied behind ear 5−6 hr before travel
Available forms include: Self adhesive patch (transdermal drug delivery system). Average drug absorbed over 72 hr 500 mcg
Side effects/adverse reactions:
CNS: Drowsiness, dizziness, restlessness, disorientation, confusion, visual hallucinations, memory and concentration impairment
EENT: Dilated pupils, visual disturbances
GI: Dry mouth
GU: Urine retention

Contraindications: Hypersensitivity, glaucoma

Precautions: Pyloric stenosis, bladder outflow obstruction, intestinal obstruction, elderly, impaired hepatic or renal function, pregnancy, lactation, epilepsy

Pharmacokinetics:

Patch: Onset 15−30 min, duration 72 hr

Interactions/incompatibilities:

• Increased antimuscarinic effects with: antidepressants, antihistamines, antipsychotics, use with caution with CNS acting drugs including alcohol

Treatment of overdose: Remove patch; give physostigmine by slow IV injection 1−4 mg (children 0.5 mg). Repeat if necessary. See further information in data sheet compendium

NURSING CONSIDERATIONS

Teach patient/family:

• Caution patients against driving or operating machinery. Side effects may last up to 24 hr after removing patch

• To wash, dry hands before applying to surface behind ear

• Apply at least 3 hr before traveling

• Change patch every 72 hr

• To wash hands after handling

• To wash application site after removing

• Report blurred vision, severe dizziness, drowsiness occurs; discontinue use

• To read label of all non-prescribed medications; if any hyoscine is found in product, avoid use

• Use only one patch at a time

---

hyoscine-N-butylbromide/hyoscine hydrobromide

Buscopan, combination product

Func. class.: Anticholinergic

Chem. class.: Belladonna alkaloid

Legal class.: POM

Action: Inhibits acetylcholine at receptor sites in autonomic nervous system, which controls secretions, acts on dopamine receptors in CNS, which decrease involuntary movements

Uses: Gastrointestinal antispasmodic, reduction of secretions before surgery, amnesia, motion sickness

Dosage and routes:

Antispasmodic

• *Adult:* By mouth (butylbromide) 20 mg 4 times a day

• *Child 6−12 yr:* 10 mg 3 times a day

Acute spasm

• IV or IV injection (butylbromide) 20 mg repeated after half an hour if necessary

Premedication

• *Adult:* Subcutaneous or IM injection (hydrobromide) 200−600 mcg half an hour to one hour before anaesthesia

• *Child:* 15 mcg per kg.

Usually given with papaveretum

Available forms include: Tablets (butylbromide) 10 mg; injection (butylbromide) 20 mg/ml, 1 ml ampoules; injection (hydrobromide) 400 mcg/ml, 1 ml, 600 mcg/ml, 1 ml

Side effects/adverse reactions:

CNS: Confusion, depression, psychotic reactions

EENT: Blurred vision, photophobia, dilated pupils, difficulty swallowing, increased ocular pressure

CV: Palpitations, bradycardia, tachycardia, arrhythmias
GI: Dry mouth, constipation, abdominal distension
GU: Urine retention
INTEG: Dry skin, rash
Contraindications: Hypersensitivity, glaucoma or tendency to glaucoma (e.g. narrow anterior chamber angle)
Precautions: Pregnancy, lactation, elderly, tachycardia, prostatic hypertrophy, urinary retention, paralytic ileus, pyloric stenosis, cardiac insufficiency, ulcerative colitis, gastro-oesophageal reflux
Pharmacokinetics:
By mouth: Peak 1 hr, duration 6 hr
Subcutaneous/IM: Peak 30−45 min, duration 7 hr
IV: Peak 10−15 min, duration 4 hr
Excreted in urine, bile, faeces (unchanged)
Interactions/incompatibilities:
• Possible enhanced action by other drugs with antimuscarinic properties: some antihistamines, phenothiazines, tricyclic antidepressants, butyrophenones
Treatment of overdose: Orally ingested: emesis or gastric lavage. If systemic toxicity use parasympathetic agents as necessary e.g. pilocarpine or neostigmine
NURSING CONSIDERATIONS
Assess:
• Baseline fluid balance and pulse
Administer:
• Orally at bedtime to avoid daytime drowsiness in patient with parkinsonism
Perform/provide:
• Storage at room temperature in light-resistant containers
• Frequent drinks, mouthwashes to relieve dry mouth
Evaluate:
• Therapeutic response
• Parkinsonism, extrapyramidal symptoms: shuffling gait, muscle rigidity, involuntary movements

• Urinary fluid balance retention
• Constipation; increase fluids, bulk, exercise if this occurs
• For tolerance over long-term therapy; dose may need to be increased or changed
Teach patient/family:
• Not to discontinue this drug abruptly; to taper off over 1 week
• To avoid driving or other hazardous activities; drowsiness may occur
• To avoid non-prescribed medication: cough, cold preparations with alcohol, antihistamines unless advised by clinician

---

hyoscine hydrobromide (ophthalmic)

Func. class.: Mydriatic
Chem. class.: Synthetic alkaloid
Legal class.: POM

Action: Blocks response of iris sphincter muscle, muscle of accommodation of ciliary body to cholinergic stimulation, resulting in dilatation, paralysis of accommodation
Uses: Uveitis, iritis, cycloplegic refraction
Dosage and routes:
• *Adult:* Instil 1−2 drops before refraction or 1−2 drops 1−3 times a day for iritis or uveitis
• *Child:* Instil 1 drop before refraction
Available forms include: Eyedrops 0.25%
Side effects/adverse reactions:
EENT: Increased intraocular pressure, blurred vision, photophobia, irritation, oedema
INTEG: Contact dermatitis, rash, dry skin
CV: Bradycardia, tachycardia, palpitations, arrhythmias
CNS: Giddiness, staggering, psychotic reactions

GI: Dry mouth, constipation, abdominal distension

Contraindications: Hypersensitivity, glaucoma or tendency to glaucoma (e.g. narrow anterior chamber angle)

Precautions: Systemic reactions in young and very old, pregnancy, lactation

Pharmacokinetics:

INSTIL: Peak 20−30 min, duration 3−7 days

Interactions/incompatibilities:

• Possible enhanced action by other drugs with antimuscarinic properties: some antihistamines, phenothiazines, tricyclic antidepressants, butyrophenones

Treatment of overdose: If systemic toxicity occurs provide supportive treatment

If ingested: emesis or gastric lavage

NURSING CONSIDERATIONS

Administer:

• Without contact of dropper to eye

Perform/provide:

• Mark container with date of opening and discard weekly if used in hospital ward, but daily if used in outpatients or casualty departments

• In operating theatres previously unopened containers should be used for each patient. Post-operative patient should always use separate contain even in outpatients

Evaluate:

• Therapeutic response: dilation of pupil, paralysis of muscles causing inability to contract pupil, decreased inflammation

• Eye pain, discontinue and inform the clinician

Teach patient/family:

• To install after washing hands well without touching dropper to eye

• To administer correctly never exceed dosage to avoid absorption into whole circulatory system

• To notify clinician if dry mouth, increased pulse, trouble breathing, sweating, flushing occur. Discontinue immediately

• That blurred vision is temporary and will decrease with repeated use

• Not to drive or use machinery until sight has returned to normal

• Wait 5 min before using other drops

---

ibuprofen

Apsifen, Arthrofen, Lidifen, Ebufac, Ibular, Rimafen, Motrin, Brufen, Fenbid, Junifen, many other proprietary brands available

Func. class.: Non-steroidal anti-inflammatory agent

Chem. class.: Propionic acid derivative

Legal class.: POM, but P if labelled for specific dosage and indications

Action: Inhibits prostaglandin synthesis by decreasing enzyme needed for biosynthesis; possesses analgesic, anti-inflammatory, antipyretic properties

Uses: As an analgesic and anti-inflammatory in rheumatoid arthritis, juvenile arthritis, ankylosing spondylitis, osteoarthritis, other musculoskeletal disorders — capsulitis, tendinitis, etc., soft tissue injuries. As an analgesic in dysmenorrhoea, dental pain, migraine, post-operative pain

Dosage and routes:

• *Adult:* 1200−1800 mg daily in 3−4 doses; maximum 2400 mg per day; maintenance 600−1200 mg daily

• *Child:* 20 mg/kg daily in divided doses; juvenile arthritis up to 40 mg/kg daily. Not recommended for children less than 7 kg

Available forms include: Tablets 200, 400, 600 mg; syrup 100 mg/5 ml; sachets 600 mg

Side effects/adverse reactions:

GI: Nausea, diarrhoea, gastrointestinal discomfort, bleeding, ulceration, dyspepsia

CNS: Dizziness, headache, nervousness, depression, drowsiness, insomnia

INTEG: Rash, pruritus

GU: Nephrotoxicity, haematuria, oliguria

HAEM: Blood dyscrasias—agranulocytosis, thrombocytopenia

EENT: Tinnitus, blurred vision

Contraindications: Asthma, severe renal disease, severe hepatic disease, peptic ulceration, hypersensitivity to NSAIDs

Precautions: Pregnancy, lactation, children, cardiac disorders, bleeding disorders

Pharmacokinetics:

By mouth: Peak 1−2 hr, half-life 2−4 hr, metabolised in liver (inactive metabolites), excreted in urine (inactive metabolites)

Interactions/incompatibilities:

• May increase action of: oral anti-coagulants, thiazide diuretics, lithium

Treatment of overdose: Gastric lavage, correction of plasma electrolytes and symptomatic relief

NURSING CONSIDERATIONS

Administer:

• With food or milk to decrease GI symptoms

Evaluate:

• Therapeutic response: decreased pain, stiffness in joints, decreased swelling in joints, ability to move more easily

• For eye, ear problems: blurred vision, tinnitus; may indicate toxicity

Teach patient/family:

• To report any wheeziness or breathlessness, rash, unresolved indigestion or black tarry stools

• To report blurred vision, ringing, roaring in ears; may indicate toxicity

• To avoid driving, other hazardous activities if dizziness, drowsiness occurs

• To report change in urine pattern, increased weight, oedema, increased pain in joints, fever, blood in urine; indicate nephrotoxicity

• That therapeutic effects may take up to 1 month

• To avoid alcohol, salicylates; bleeding may occur

idarubicin HCl ▼

Zavedos

Func. class.: Antineoplastic

Chem. class.: Anthracycline antibiotic

Legal class.: POM

Action: Interferes with DNA topoisomerase II activity, thus causing cell death

Uses: Acute non-lymphocytic leukaemia in adults, for remission induction in untreated patients or relapsed or refactory patients; acute lymphocytic leukaemia as second line treatment in adults and children. May be used in combination chemotherapy regimes

Dosage and routes:

Consult specialist for tailored regimen

Acute non-lymphocytic leukaemia

• *Adults:* IV 12 mg/m^2 daily for 3 days with cytarabine or 8 mg/m^2 daily for 5 days as single agent or in combination

Acute lymphocytic leukaemia

• *Adults:* IV 12 mg/m^2 daily for 3 days

• *Child:* IV 10 mg/m^2 daily for 3 days

Available forms include: IV infusion
5, 10 mg

Side effects/adverse reactions:

GI: Nausea, vomiting, mucositis,
oesophagitis, diarrhoea

CV: Cardiac toxicity: congestive
heart failure, acute arrhythmias

INTEG: Reversible alopecia, skin
rash, irritation

CNS: Fever, chills

HAEM: Severe myelosuppression,
elevation of liver enzymes and
bilirubin

GU: Red coloured urine

Contraindications: Severe renal
and hepatic impairment; uncontrolled infections; breast feeding.
Pregnancy should be avoided

Precautions: Pre-existing heart
disease and previous therapy with
anthracyclines in high cumulative
doses are co-factors for increased
risk of idarubicin cardiac toxicity.
Monitor cardiac function, monitor
blood (to include granulocytes, red
cells, platelets and uric acid), renal
and hepatic function; systemic
infection — control prior to
therapy, extravasation

Pharmacokinetics:

IV: Half-life 15−18 hr

Interactions/incompatibilities:

• Increased toxicity: other cytotoxic drugs

• Do not mix with heparin or other
drugs

Clinical assessment:

• Blood counts, liver function tests

• ECG for cardiotoxicity

Treatment of overdose: Supportive
treatment for acute myocardial
toxicity and myelosupression

NURSING CONSIDERATIONS

Assess:

• Baseline fluid balance prior to
therapy and monitor strict fluid
balance during therapy

• Careful haematological monitoring is required to check for
myelosuppression

• Potentially fatal congestive heart
failure, acute life-threatening
arrhythmias or other cardiomyo-
pathies may occur during therapy
or several weeks after therapy

Administer:

• For reconstitution the contents
of the 5 mg vial should be dissolved
in 5 ml water for injections and
10 mg vial 10 ml

• Administer for 5−10 minutes
via tubing of a freely running IV
infusion of sodium chloride 0.9%

• The dosage administered must
take account of the haematological
status of the patient and dosages
of concurrent cytotoxics

Evaluate:

• Liver and kidney function:
should be evaluated before and
during treatment; uric acid levels
should be monitored because of a
risk of hyperuricaemia

• Systemic infection: should be
controlled before starting therapy

• Extravasation: can cause severe
local tissue necrosis

Teach patient/family:

• Idarubicin may give urine a red
colour for 1 or 2 days; patients
should be advised that this is no
cause for alarm

---

idoxuridine

Herpid, Kerecid, Virudox, Idoxene

Func. class.: Antiviral

Chem. class.: Pyrimidine
nucleoside

Legal class.: POM

Action: Arrests replication of
DNA viruses

Uses: Cutaneous or ocular infection by herpes simplex and
other DNA viruses sensitive to
idoxuridine

Dosage and routes:

Eye

• *Adult and child:* Drops, apply
hourly during day and 2-hrly at

night; ointment, 4-hrly. Max. period of treatment 21 days

Skin

• *Adult:* Apply to lesions 6-hrly for 3−4 days; severe lesions, use 40% solution. Not recommended in children under 12 yr

Available forms include: Eye: drops 0.1%, ointment 0.5%

Skin: dimethyl sulphoxide, solution 5%, 40%

Side effects/adverse reactions:

EENT: Poor corneal wound healing, temporary visual haze, oedema, itching, occlusion of lacrymal puncta

INTEG: Stinging, taste changes, over usage may lead to maceration of skin

Contraindications: Hypersensitivity, pregnancy, demographia

Interactions/incompatibilities:

• Do not use boric acid with this drug

NURSING CONSIDERATIONS

Administer:

• Use gloves to avoid re-infecting other areas, especially face, genitalia

• Cleanse crusts or discharge from eye before application

Perform/provide:

• Storage at room temperature. Do not refrigerate

Evaluate:

• Therapeutic response: absence of redness, inflammation, tearing

• Allergy: itching, lacrimation, redness, swelling

Teach patient/family:

• To use drug exactly as prescribed

• Not to use eye makeup, towels, washcloths, eye medication of others; reinfection may occur

• That drug container tip should not be touched to eye

• To report itching, increased redness, burning, stinging, swelling; drug should be discontinued

• That drug may cause blurred vision when ointment is applied

• Skin preparations can damage some synthetic materials e.g. artificial silk, terylene, avoid contact

---

ifosfamide

Mitoxana

Func. class.: Antineoplastic alkylating agent

Chem. class.: Nitrogen mustard derivative

Legal class.: POM

Action: Alkylates DNA, RNA; inhibits enzymes that allow synthesis in proteins; is also responsible for cross linking DNA strands

Uses: Chronic lymphocytic leukaemia, lymphomas, solid tumours

Dosage and routes:

Ifosfamide must be given with mesna: see manufacturer's data sheet

• *Adult:* IV 8−10 g/m² over 5 days repeated every 2−4 weeks or 5−6 g/m² (maximum 10 g) over 24 hr as infusion repeated every 3−4 weeks. Usual number of courses 4, maximum 7 (6 by 24-hr infusion)

• *Children:* IV 5-day regime only

Available forms include: Injection powder for reconstitution 500 mg vial, 1 g vial, 2 g vial

Side effects/adverse reactions:

CV: ECG changes, tachycardia, cardiotoxicity

HAEM: Leucopenia, thrombocytopenia, anaemia

GU: Haemorrhagic cystitis, sterility, haematuria, nephrotoxicity, glycosuria, proteinuria, aminoaciduria, renal rickets

INTEG: Alopecia, dermatitis

GI: Disturbances, diarrhoea, nausea, vomiting, hepatitis

RESP: Fibrosis

CNS: Confusion, lethargy, tonic-clonic spasms, depression of consciousness, motor unrest, emotional lability, disorientation,

EEG changes, aggression, echoalia

SYST: Allergy, immunosuppression

Contraindications: Hypersensitivity, bone marrow aplasia, myelosuppression, pregnancy, lactation, active infection including urinary tract infections, renal impairment, acute urothelial toxicity, hepatic impairment

Precautions: Contraception for both partners, elderly, debilitated, diabetes mellitus, evidence of myelosuppression, recent radiotherapy or chemotherapy, previous treatment with platinum compounds, nephrectomy

Pharmacokinetics: Converted in liver to active metabolites; excreted in urine

Interactions/incompatibilities:
• Enhanced effects of: Warfarin and other anticoagulants

Clinical assessment:
• Full blood count, differential and platelet count weekly; withhold drug if WBC less than 4000 and platelets less than 75,000
• Pulmonary function tests: chest X-ray before and during treatment
• Renal function tests: blood urea, serum uric acid, urine creatinine clearance
• Liver function tests: bilirubin, aspartate aminotransferase, alanine aminotransferase, lactic dehydrogenase

Treatment of overdose: Recognised with 24 hr, or possibly 48 hr, administer IV mesna
Administer broad spectrum antibiotic, whole blood transfusion as necessary. See data sheet compendium for further information

NURSING CONSIDERATIONS

Assess:
• Food preferences; list likes and dislikes

Administer:
• Anti-emetic 30−60 min before giving drug to prevent vomiting
• Allopurinol or sodium bicarbonate to maintain uric acid levels
• Antibiotics for prophylaxis of infection
• Analgesics for pain
• By slow IV infusion using appropriate size needle

Perform/provide:
• Ensure mesna given as prescribed
• Test all urine for blood (early signs of haemorrhage in cystitis)
• Strict aseptic technique only when indicated. Protective isolation if WBC count is low
• Good skin care
• Physiotherapy and deep breathing exercises
• Increased fluid intake to 2−3 litre/day and strict fluid balance chart
• Sensible diet that can be tolerated

Evaluate:
• For any bleeding (haematuria, gums)
• For dyspnoea, chest pain, unproductive cough
• Effects on body image (i.e. alopecia)
• Abdominal pain, fever, nausea, vomiting, diarrhoea
• Oedema in feet, joint pain
• Symptoms indicating allergic reaction
• Tachypnoea, ECG changes

Teach patient/family:
• Of protective isolation precautions
• To report any complaints or side effects to clinician
• That impotence or amenorrhoea may occur
• To report any changes in breathing or coughing
• To report any change in colour of stool or urine
• To report any bleeding, white spots or ulceration in the mouth. Check daily

imipenem with cilastatin

Primaxin
Func. class.: Antibiotic, broad spectrum
Chem. class.: Thienamycin β-lactam antibiotic with specific enzyme inhibitor
Legal class.: POM

Action: Inhibits bacterial cell wall synthesis; stable to bacterial beta-lactamase and bactericidal. Cilastatin blocks metabolism of imipenem in kidney

Uses: Aerobic, anaerobic Gram-negative or Gram-positive infections

Dosage and routes: Doses are in terms of imipenem
• *Adult:* IV infusion 1−2 g daily in 3−4 divided doses; less sensitive organisms up to 50 mg/kg daily, maximum 4 g daily
• *Child:* IV infusion over 3 months 60 mg/kg daily in 4 divided doses, maximum 2 g daily
• *Adult:* IM injection 500−750 mg 12 hrly. Gonococcal urethritis or cervicitis, single dose of 500 mg
For further dosage information see manufacturer's data sheet

Available forms include: IV infusion powder for reconstitution 250 mg imipenem/250 mg cilastatin, 60 ml vial; 500 mg imipenem/500 mg cilastatin, 120 ml vial. IM injection powder for reconstitution 500 mg imipenem/500 mg cilastatin, 15 ml vial

Side effects/adverse reactions:
GI: Nausea, vomiting, diarrhoea, pseudomembraneous colitis, taste disturbances
CNS: Convulsions, confusion, mental disturbances, myoclonic activity
HAEM: Increased liver enzymes and bilirubin, thrombophlebitis, neutropenia, eosinophilia, thrombocytopenia, positive direct Coombs' test
INTEG: Rash, urticaria, pruritus, erythema, local pain and induration
SYST: Pyrexia, anaphylaxis, abnormal liver function tests
GU: Elevated serum creatinine and blood urea, red discoloration of urine in children, oliguria, anuria, polyuria, acute renal failure

Contraindications: Hypersensitivity to imipenem or cilastatin, lactation, pregnancy (unless risk benefit outweighs risk)

Precautions: Hypersensitivity to penicillins, cephalosporins and other β-lactam antibiotics, history of gastrointestinal disease particularly colitis, renal impairment (reduce dosage), epilepsy and other CNS disorders

Pharmacokinetics: Cilastatin inhibits renal degradation of imipenem; excreted in urine largely as unchanged drug

Interactions/incompatibilities:
• Plasma levels of cilastatin increased by: probenecid

Clinical assessment:
• Liver function tests: aspartate aminotransferase, alanine aminotransferase
• Blood studies: Hb, haematocrit, prothrombin time, WBC, RBC
• Renal function tests: urine for blood and protein
• Culture and sensitivity to identify infecting organisms
• Monitor side effects

NURSING CONSIDERATIONS
Assess:
• Fluid balance
• Bowel pattern
• Respiratory state; tightness or wheeziness in chest
Administer:
• After culture and sensitivity has been taken
• By IV infusion

Perform/provide:
• Equipment for resuscitation in case of severe reaction
• Adequate fluid intake
Evaluate:
• Fluid balance; report any haematuria to clinician
• Mental state for signs of confusion
• Local reaction to injection site
• Any skin eruptions, signs of allergy
• Therapeutic effect; absence of fever
• Bowel pattern
Teach patient/family:
• Culture to be taken when course completed
• To report sore throat/fever — could indicate further infection
• To inform clinician if diarrhoea persists
• To carry a Medic Alert card if allergic to penicillins

---

imipramine HCl

Tofranil
Func. class.: Antidepressant, tricyclic
Chem. class.: Dibenzazepine — tertiary amine
Legal class.: POM

Action: Blocks reuptake of noradrenaline and serotonin into nerve endings, increasing action of noradrenaline and serotonin in nerve cells
Uses: Depression, nocturnal enuresis in children
Dosage and routes:
• *Adult:* By mouth 75 mg daily in divided doses, may increase gradually to 200 mg, up to 150 mg may be given as a single dose at bed time
• *Child:* Nocturnal enuresis by mouth 7 yr: 25 mg at night, 8– 11 yr: 25–50 mg at night, over 11 yr 50–75 mg at night, maximum duration 3 months (including gradual withdrawal)
Available forms include: Tablets 10, 25 mg; syrup 25 mg/5 ml
Side effects/adverse reactions:
HAEM: Agranulocytosis, thrombocytopenia, eosinophilia, leucopenia
CNS: Dizziness, drowsiness, confusion, headache, anxiety, tremors, weakness, insomnia, nightmares, increased psychiatric symptoms, paraesthesia, epileptic seizures
GI: Diarrhoea, dry mouth, nausea, vomiting, paralytic ileus, increased appetite, cramps, epigastric distress, jaundice, hepatitis, stomatitis
GU: Retention, acute renal failure
INTEG: Rash, urticaria, sweating, pruritus, photosensitivity, hair loss
CV: Orthostatic hypotension, ECG changes, tachycardia, hypertension, palpitations
EENT: Blurred vision, tinnitus, mydriasis, glaucoma
ENDO: Weight gain, disturbances of libido, galactorrhoea, hyper- or hypoglycaemia, occasional weight loss
Contraindications: Hypersensitivity to tricyclic antidepressants, recent myocardial infarction, urine retention, narrow angle glaucoma, child under 6 yr, heart block, arrhythmias, severe liver disease, mania
Precautions: Suicidal patients, severe depression, increased intraocular pressure, cardiac disease, hepatic disease, hyperthyroidism, electroshock therapy, elective surgery, elderly, pregnancy, convulsive disorders, prostatic hypertrophy
Pharmacokinetics:
By mouth: Steady state 2–5 days; metabolised by liver, excreted in

faeces, excreted in breast milk, half-life 6−20 hr

Interactions/incompatibilities:
• Decreased effects of: guanethidine, debrisoquine, clonidine, indirect acting sympathomimetics (ephedrine), antiepileptics
• Increased effects of: direct acting sympathomimetics (adrenaline), alcohol, barbiturates, benzodiazepines, CNS depressants, antihistamines
• Increased concentration by: methylphenidate, neuroleptics, diltiazem, verapamil, cimetidine
• Hyperpyretic crisis, convulsions, hypertensive episode: MAOIs (avoid imipramine for 3 weeks after stopping MAOI)

Clinical assessment:
• Blood studies: full blood count
• Hepatic studies: aspartate aminotransferase, alanine aminotransferase, bilirubin
• ECG for flattening of T wave, bundle branch block, atrioventricular block, dysrhythmias in cardiac patients

Lab. test interferences:
Increase: Serum bilirubin, alkaline phosphatase, blood glucose
Decrease: 5-hydroxyindoleacetic acid, vanillylmandelic acid, urinary catecholamines
Treatment of overdose: ECG monitoring, induce emesis, lavage, activated charcoal, administer anticonvulsant if necessary

NURSING CONSIDERATIONS

Assess:
• Baseline BP (lying, standing), pulse, weight

Administer:
• With food or milk for GI symptoms
• Dosage at bedtime if oversedation occurs during day; may take entire dose at bed time; elderly may not tolerate once daily dosing
• Mouthwashes, or frequent sips of water for dry mouth

Perform/provide:
• Assistance with mobilisation during beginning therapy since drowsiness/dizziness occurs
• Safety measures including cot sides primarily in elderly

Evaluate:
• Take vital signs 4 hrly in patients with cardiovascular disease
• Weight weekly, appetite may increase with drug
• Mental status: mood, alertness, affect, suicidal tendencies, increase in psychiatric symptoms: depression, panic
• Urinary retention, constipation; constipation is more likely to occur in children; increase fluids, fibre indiet
• Withdrawal symptoms: headache, nausea, vomiting, muscle pain, weakness; do not usually occur unless drug was discontinued abruptly
• Alcohol consumption; if alcohol is consumed, hold dose until morning

Teach patient/family:
• That therapeutic effects may take 2−3 weeks
• Use caution in driving or other activities requiring alertness because of drowsiness, dizziness, blurred vision
• To avoid alcohol ingestion, other CNS depressants
• Not to discontinue medication quickly after long-term use, may cause nausea, headache, malaise
• To wear sunscreen or large hat since photosensitivity occurs

immunoglobulin, human

Sandoglobulin, Gammabulin, Gamimune-N, Endobulin, Kabiglobulin, Venoglobulin
Func. class.: Antibodies, serum
Chem. class.: IgG
Legal class.: POM

Action: Provides passive immunity
Uses: Agammaglobulinaemia, hepatitis A exposure, measles exposure, measles vaccine complications, purpura, rubella exposure, chicken-pox exposure, idiopathic thrombocytopenic purpura, Kawasaki syndrome
Dosage and routes: See specialist literature for advice on doses
Side effects/adverse reactions:
INTEG: Pain at injection site, rash, pruritus
MS: Arthralgia
SYST: Lymphadenopathy, anaphylaxis, fever, chills
CNS: Headache, fatigue, malaise
GI: Abdominal pain, hepatitis
Contraindications: Hypersensitivity
Interactions/incompatibilities:
• Diminished immune response: live virus vaccines (except yellow fever). Do not administer live virus vaccines 3 weeks before or 3 months after this drug
NURSING CONSIDERATIONS
Assess:
• Active or suspected infection
• Weigh before treatment
Administer:
• IM to large muscle site. 3 ml or less in site
• Within six weeks of exposure to hepatitis A
• Repeat doses as directed
Provide:
• Adrenaline 1:1000 and resuscitative equipment nearby
• Store in refrigerator, following manufacturer's recommendations
Teach patient/family:
• That passive immunity is temporary

indapamide

Natrilix
Func. class.: Diuretic
Chem. class.: Indoline
Legal class.: POM

Action: Acts on proximal section of distal renal tubule by inhibiting reabsorption of sodium; may act by direct vasodilation caused by blocking of calcium channel
Uses: Hypertension
Dosage and routes:
• *Adult:* By mouth 2.5 mg daily in the morning
Available forms include: Tablets 2.5 mg
Side effects/adverse reactions:
GU: Impotence
ELECT: Metabolic alkalosis, hyperuricaemia, hypokalaemia, hyperglycaemia
CNS: Headache, dizziness, fatigue, weakness, paraesthesia
GI: Nausea, diarrhoea, dry mouth, dyspepsia, anorexia, constipation
EENT: Reversible acute myopia
INTEG: Rash, pruritus, photosensitivity
CV: Orthostatic hypotension
Contraindications: Recent CVA, severe hepatic failure, sulphonamide hypersensitivity
Precautions: Hypokalaemia, dehydration, ascites, hepatic disease, severe renal disease, pregnancy, breast feeding
Pharmacokinetics:
By mouth: Onset 1−2 hr, peak 2 hr, duration up to 36 hr; excreted in urine, faeces, half-life 14−18 hr
Interactions/incompatibilities:
• Increased hypokalaemia: carbenoxolone, diuretics, steroids
• Increased blood levels of: lithium

Clinical assessment:
• Electrolytes: potassium, sodium, include serum urea, serum creatinine

Treatment of overdose: Lavage if taken orally, monitor electrolytes, administer IV fluids

NURSING CONSIDERATIONS

Assess:
• Baseline BP, weight
• Rate, depth, rhythm of respiration, effect of exertion

Administer:
• In morning to avoid interference with sleep
• With food, if nausea occurs, absorption may be decreased slightly

Evaluate:
• Weight daily, fluid balance daily to determine fluid loss; effect of drug may be decreased if used daily
• BP lying, standing; postural hypotension may occur
• Improvement in oedema of feet, legs, sacral area daily if medication is being used in congestive cardiac failure
• Improvement in CVP and BP recordings
• Signs of metabolic alkalosis
• Signs of hyperkalaemia
• Rashes, temperature elevation 6-hrly
• Confusion, especially in elderly; take safety precautions if needed
• Hydration: skin turgor, thirst, dry mucous membranes

Teach patient/family:
• To increase fluid intake 2–3 litres daily unless contraindicated; to rise slowly from lying or sitting position
• Adverse reactions: muscle cramps, weakness, nausea, dizziness
• Take with food or milk for GI symptoms
• Take early in day to prevent nocturia

indomethacin

Flexin-Continus, Indocid, Indocid-R, Indomax 75 SR, Indolar SR, Indomod, Rheumacin LA, Slo-Indo
Func. class.: Non-steroidal anti-inflammatory agent
Chem. class.: Propionic acid derivative
Legal class.: POM

Action: Inhibits prostaglandin synthesis by decreasing enzyme needed for biosynthesis; possesses analgesic, anti-inflammatory, antipyretic properties

Uses: Pain and moderate to severe inflammation in rheumatic disease and other acute musculoskeletal disorders; acute gout, dysmenorrhoea

Dosage and routes:
• *Adult:* By mouth, arthritis 50–200 mg daily in divided doses; dysmenorrhoea, up to 75 mg daily; by rectum, 100 mg once or twice a day; modified-release 75 mg daily, may increase to 75 mg twice a day

Available forms include: Capsules 25, 50 mg; capsules modified-release 75 mg; suspension 25 mg/5 ml; suppository 100 mg

Side effects/adverse reactions:
GI: Nausea, anorexia, vomiting, diarrhoea, jaundice, cholestatic hepatitis, constipation, flatulence, cramps, dry mouth, ulceration, bleeding
CNS: Dizziness, drowsiness, fatigue, tremors, confusion, insomnia, anxiety, depression, headache
CV: Tachycardia, peripheral oedema, palpitations, dysrhythmias, hypertension, hypotension, chest pain
INTEG: Purpura, rash, pruritus, sweating
GU: Nephrotoxicity, haematuria, proteinuria, interstitial nephritis, nephrotic syndrome

META: Hyperkalaemia, hyperglycaemia
HAEM: Anaemia, inhibition of platelet aggregation
EENT: Tinnitus, hearing loss, eye changes

Contraindications: Hypersensitivity, asthmatic attacks with aspirin or other NSAIDs, active peptic ulcer, nasal polyps associated with angioneurotic oedema, history of gastrointestinal lesions, suppositories in patients with proctitis or rectal bleeding

Precautions: Pregnancy, lactation, children, bleeding disorders, cardiac disorders, hypersensitivity to other NSAIDs psychiatric disorders, epilepsy, parkinsonism, renal or hepatic disorders

Pharmacokinetics:
By mouth: Onset 1−2 hr, peak 3 hr, duration 4−6 hr; metabolised in liver, kidneys, excreted in urine, bile, faeces, excreted in breast milk

Interactions/incompatibilities:
• May increase action of: coumarin, sulphonamides, methotrexate
• Increased toxicity: diflunisal, lithium, potassium-sparing diuretics, angiotensin converting enzyme inhibitors, probenecid
• Reduced efficacy: diuretics, antihypertensives

Clinical assessment:
• Renal function tests, liver, blood studies: serum urea, creatinine, aspartate aminotransferase, alanine aminotransferase, Hb, before treatment, periodically thereafter
• Audiometric, ophthalmic exam before, during, after treatment

NURSING CONSIDERATIONS
Administer:
• With food or milk to decrease GI symptoms

Evaluate:
• Therapeutic response: decreased pain, stiffness in joints, decreased swelling in joints, ability to move more easily
• For eye, ear problems: blurred vision, tinnitus; may indicate toxicity

Teach patient/family:
• To report blurred vision, ringing, roaring in ears; may indicate toxicity
• To avoid driving, other hazardous activities if dizziness, drowsiness occurs
• To report change in urine pattern, increased weight, oedema, increased pain in joints, fever, blood in urine; indicate nephrotoxicity
• To report any wheeziness or shortness of breath
• That therapeutic effects may take up to 1 month
• To avoid alcohol, salicylates; bleeding may occur
• To report any related indigestion or black tarry stools (may indicate bleeding)
• Teach patient/relative how to administer suppositories

---

indoramin

Baratol, Doralese
Func. class.: Selective postsynaptic α_1-receptor antagonist
Chem. class.: Substituted benzamide
Legal class.: POM

Action: Decreases peripheral resistance by vasodilatation; reduces urinary outflow obstruction

Uses: Baratol: hypertension, usually in conjunction with β-blocker or thiazide, Doralese: management of urinary outflow obstruction in benign prostatic hypertrophy

Dosage and routes:
Hypertension
• By mouth initially 25 mg twice

daily increased by 25−50 mg daily at intervals of 2 weeks; maximum dose 200 mg daily in 2−3 divided doses

Outflow obstruction
• By mouth 20 mg twice daily increased by 20 mg increments every 2 weeks to maximum of 100 mg daily in divided doses

Available forms include: Tablets 20, 25, 50 mg

Side effects/adverse reactions:
CNS: Sedation, dizziness, depression, extrapyramidal effects, drowsiness
EENT: Dry mouth, nasal congestion
GU: Failure of ejaculation
META: Weight gain
Contraindications: Established heart failure, treatment with MAOIs
Precautions: Incipient heart failure, hepatic or renal impairment, pregnancy, lactation, Parkinson's disease, epilepsy, history of depression, elderly (reduce dosage)
Pharmacokinetics: Half-life 5 hr; metabolised in liver and excreted in urine and faeces as metabolites, some of which may be active
Interactions/incompatibilities:
• Do not use concurrently with: MAOIs
Treatment of overdose: Gastric lavage, assisted ventilation and circulatory support, diazepam for convulsions, monitor temperature for hypothermia
NURSING CONSIDERATIONS
Assess:
• Baseline BP and pulse
• Weight and fluid balance
Administer:
• Tablet whole; should not be chewed or crushed
Perform:
• Store in airtight container
Evaluate:
• BP 4-hrly

• Feet and legs daily for oedema
• Skin turgor − dryness of mucous membranes for hydration status
• For dyspnoea and jugular vein distension
Teach patient/family:
• Effects increased by: alcohol
• That fainting occasionally occurs after first dose; do not drive or operate machinery for 4 hr after first dose
• To report any side effects

---

influenza virus vaccine, trivalent A & B (surface antigen/split virion)

Fluvirin, Influvac, MFV-ject, Fluzone
Func. class.: Vaccine
Legal class.: POM

Action: Active immunisation against influenza
Uses: Prevention of influenza
Dosage and routes:
• *Adult and child over 13 yr:* IM, deep subcutaneous 0.5 ml in 1 dose
• *Child 4−13 yr:* IM 0.5 ml, repeat in 1 month
• *Child 6 months−3 yr:* IM 0.25 ml, repeat in 1 month (Fluzone)
Available forms include: Injection IM, subcutaneous
Side effects/adverse reactions:
CNS: Fever
INTEG: Urticaria, induration, erythema
SYST: Anaphylaxis, malaise
MS: Myalgia
Contraindications: Hypersensitivity, active infection, chicken or egg allergy
Precautions: Immunosuppression, pregnancy, polymyxin sensitivity
NURSING CONSIDERATIONS
Assess:
• Active or suspected infections
• History of allergies, skin

conditions, reactions to vaccines
• History of allergy to chicken, eggs, feathers
Administer:
• Intramuscular or deep subcutaneous after bringing preparation to room temperature
Provide:
• Adrenaline 1:1000 and resuscitative equipment nearby
• Store in light proof container at 2−10°C (check brand used)
Evaluate:
• For anaphylaxis: dyspnoea tachycardia, profuse sweating, collapse
• Redness and soreness at injection site
• Headache, pyrexia, malaise
Teach patient/family:
• That immunity is not long term

---

inosine pranobex

Imunovir
Func. class.: Antiviral and immunomodulator
Chem. class.: Inosine with dimepranol and acedoben
Legal class.: POM

Action: Modifies cell-mediated immune mechanisms; mild antiviral action
Uses: Mucocutaneous herpes simplex type I or II, adjunctive treatment of genital warts
Dosage and routes:
Herpes simplex
• By mouth 1 g 4 times daily for 7−14 days
Genital warts
• By mouth 1 g 3 times daily for 14−28 days
Available forms include: Tablets 500 mg
Side effects/adverse reactions:
HAEM: Increased serum uric acid
GU: Increased urinary uric acid

Contraindications: Renal impairment
Precautions: History of gout or hyperuricaemia, renal impairment, lactation
Pharmacokinetics: Inosine component converted to uric acid and excreted in urine; remainder metabolised in liver and excreted in urine
Clinical assessment:
• Renal function tests
• Blood serum uric acid
NURSING CONSIDERATIONS
Assess:
• Fluid balance
Evaluate:
• Skin for rashes, urticaria
• Therapeutic response: absence of itchiness, decrease in number and size of lesions
Teach patient/family:
• That drug may be taken orally before infection occurs; should be taken when itching or pain occurs, usually before eruptions
• In genital herpes, sexual partner may also require treatment and/or be at risk from infection
• Advisability of refraining from intimate sexual contact during acute episode of genital herpes
• To report sore throat or fever
• That drug must be taken regularly for the time prescribed to be effective
• To notify clinician of any urinary symptoms

---

insulin, isophane

Hypurin Isophane, Insulatard, Humulin I, Protaphane
Func. class.: Antidiabetic
Chem. class.: Exogenous unmodified insulin
Legal class.: P

Action: Decreases blood sugar

Uses: Diabetes mellitus (intermediate acting therapy)

Dosage and routes:
• *Adult:* Subcutaneous dosage individualised by blood, urine glucose, do not give IV

Available forms include: Subcutaneous injection 100 units/ml

Side effects/adverse reactions:
CNS: Headache, lethargy, tremors, weakness, fatigue, delirium, sweating
CV: Tachycardia, palpitations
EENT: Blurred vision
GI: Hunger, nausea
META: Hypoglycaemia
INTEG: Flushing, rash, urticaria, warmth
SYST: Anaphylaxis

Contraindications: Hypersensitivity, hypoglycaemia

Interactions/incompatibilities:
• Increased hypoglycaemia: alcohol, β-blockers, oral hypoglycaemics, MAOIs, octreotide
• Hyperglycaemia: thiazides, thyroid hormones, oral contraceptives, corticosteroids, lithium, diazoxide, loop diuretics

Pharmacokinetics:
Subcutaneous: Onset 2 hr, peak 4−12 hr, duration up to 24 hr

Clinical assessment:
• Fasting blood glucose (3.3−5.6 mmol/litre)

Treatment of overdose: Glucose by mouth if conscious or glucose 50% IV if comatose, glucagon 1 mg IM, subcutaneous or IV if glucose not convenient

NURSING CONSIDERATIONS

Perform/provide:
• Store bottle in use at room temperature for less than 1 month; refrigerate all other supply; do not use discoloured or cloudy solution
• Rotation of injection sites: abdomen, thighs, upper arm, buttocks

Evaluate:
• Therapeutic response: decrease in polyuria, polydipsia, polyphagia, clear sensorium, absence of dizziness, stable gait
• Hypoglycaemic/hyperglycaemic reaction that can occur soon after meals

Teach patient/family:
• Dosage, route, mixing instructions, dietary advice
• Effects of diet and exercise on blood glucose
• To carry dextrasol or lump sugar to treat hypoglycaemia
• That drug does not cure diabetes, but controls symptoms
• That blurred vision occurs, not to change corrective lens until vision is stabilised 1−2 months
• To carry Medic Alert or Diabetic Card
• Hypoglycaemia reaction: headache, tremors, fatigue, weakness, sweating, visual disturbances
• Symptoms of ketoacidosis: nausea, thirst, polyuria, dry mouth, dry flushed skin, acetone breath, drowsiness
• Blood glucose testing, make sure patient is able to determine glucose, test urine for ketones if blood sugar is high
• To avoid non-prescribed medicines unless approved by clinician
• To consult clinician in cases of colds/flu as this could necessitate altering dosage

---

insulin, biphasic isophane

Mixtard 30/70, Actraphane 30/70, Initard 50/50, Humulin M1, Humulin M2, Humulin M3, Humulin M4
Func. class.: Antidiabetic
Chem. class.: Exogenous unmodified insulin
Legal class.: P

Action: Decreases blood sugar
Uses: Diabetes mellitus (intermediate acting therapy)

Dosage and routes:
• *Adult:* Subcutaneous individualised dose, do not give IV
Available forms include: Subcutaneous injection 100 units/ml

Side effects/adverse reactions:
CNS: Headache, lethargy, tremors, weakness, fatigue, delirium, sweating
CV: Tachycardia, palpitations
EENT: Blurred vision
GI: Hunger, nausea
META: Hypoglycaemia
INTEG: Flushing, rash, urticaria, warmth, lipodystrophy, pruritus, erythema
SYST: Anaphylaxis

Contraindications: Hypersensitivity, hypoglycaemia

Pharmacokinetics:
Subcutaneous: Onset 2 hr, peak 4−12 hr, duration up to 24 hr

Interactions/incompatibilities:
• Increased hypoglycaemia: alcohol, β-blockers, oral hypoglycaemics, MAOIs, octreotide
• Hyperglycaemia: thiazides, thyroid hormones, oral contraceptives, corticosteroids, lithium, diazoxide, loop diuretics

Clinical assessment:
• Fasting blood glucose (3.3−5.6 mmol/litre)

Treatment of overdose: Glucose by mouth if conscious or glucose 50% IV if comatose, glucagon 1 mg IM, subcutaneous, IV if glucose not available

NURSING CONSIDERATIONS
Perform/provide:
• Store bottle in use at room temperature for less than 1 month; refrigerate all other supply; do not use discoloured or cloudy solution
• Rotation of injection sites: abdomen, thighs, upper arm, buttocks, keep record of sites

Evaluate:
• Therapeutic response: decrease in polyuria, polydipsia, alertness

• Hypoglycaemic/hyperglycaemic reaction that can occur

Teach patient/family:
• Dosage, route, mixing instructions, any dietary advice, disease process
• Effect of diet and exercise on blood glucose
• To carry dextrasol or lump sugar to treat hypoglycaemia
• That drug does not cure diabetes, but controls symptoms
• That blurred vision occurs, not to change corrective lens until vision is stabilised 1−2 months
• To carry Medic Alert ID or Diabetic card
• Hypoglycaemia reaction: headache, tremors, fatigue, weakness, sweating, visual disturbances
• Symptoms of ketoacidosis: nausea, thirst, polyuria, dry mouth, dry flushed skin, acetone breath, drowsiness
• Blood glucose testing, make sure patient is able to determine glucose, test urine for ketones if blood sugar is high
• The pregnant patient to use glucose oxidase reagents
• To avoid non-prescribed drugs unless directed by clinician

---

insulin, protamine zinc suspension

Hypurin Protamine Zinc
Func. class.: Antidiabetic
Chem. class.: Exogenous unmodified insulin
Legal class.: P

Action: Decreases blood sugar
Uses: Diabetes mellitus (long-acting therapy)
Dosage and routes:
• *Adult:* Subcutaneous individualised dose, do not give IV

Available forms include: Subcutaneous 100 units/ml

Side effects/adverse reactions:

CNS: Headache, lethargy, tremors, weakness, fatigue, delirium, sweating

CV: Tachycardia, palpitations

EENT: Blurred vision

GI: Hunger, nausea

META: Hypoglycaemia

INTEG: Flushing, rash, urticaria warmth, lipodystrophy, pruritus, erythema

SYST: Anaphylaxis

Contraindications: Hypersensitivity, hypoglycaemia

Pharmacokinetics:

Subcutaneous: Onset 4−8 hr, peak 14−20 hr, duration 24−36 hr

Interactions/incompatibilities:

• Increased hypoglycaemia: alcohol, β-blockers, oral hypoglycaemics, MAOIs, octreotide

• Hyperglycaemia: thiazides, thyroid hormones, oral contraceptives, corticosteroids, lithium, diazoxide, loop diuretics

Clinical assessment:

• Fasting blood glucose (3.3−5.6 mmol/litre)

Treatment of overdose: Glucose by mouth if conscious or glucose 50% IV if comatose, glucagon 1 mg IM, subcutaneous or IV

NURSING CONSIDERATIONS

Perform/provide:

• Store bottle in use at room temperature for less than 1 month; refrigerate all other supply; do not use discoloured or cloudy solution

• Rotation of injection sites: abdomen, upper back, thighs, upper arm, buttocks; keep record of sites

Evaluate:

• Therapeutic response: decrease in polyuria, polydipsia, alertness

• Hypoglycaemic/hyperglycaemic reaction that can occur

Teach patient/family:

• Dosage, route, mixing instructions, if any diet restrictions, disease process

• Effect of diet and exercise on blood glucose

• To carry dextrasol or lump sugar to treat hypoglycaemia

• That drug does not cure diabetes, but controls symptoms

• That blurred vision occurs, not to change corrective lens until vision is stabilised 1−2 months

• To carry Medic Alert ID as diabetic

• Hypoglycaemia reaction: headache, tremors, fatigue, weakness, sweating and visual disturbances

• Symptoms of ketoacidosis: nausea, thirst, polyuria, dry mouth, dry flushed skin, acetone breath, drowsiness

• Blood glucose testing; make sure patient is able to determine glucose

• The pregnant patient to use glucose oxidase reagents

• To avoid non-prescribed drugs unless directed by clinician

• Test urine for ketones if blood sugar is high

insulin, soluble (insulin injection, neutral insulin)

Hypurin Neutral, Velosulin Velosulin Cartridge, Human Actrapid, Human Actrapid Penfill, Human Velosulin, Humulin S, Pur-In Neutral

Func. class.: Antidiabetic

Chem. class.: Exogenous unmodified insulin

Legal class.: P

Action: Decreases blood sugar, increases blood pyruvate, lactate, decreases phosphate, potassium

Uses: Diabetes mellitus, diabetic ketoacidosis

Dosage and routes:
• *Adult:* Subcutaneous, IM, IV injection or IV infusion according to patients requirements
Available forms include: IV/IM/subcutaneous injection, 100 units/ml

Side effects/adverse reactions:
META: Insulin resistance
INTEG: Flushing, rash, urticaria, warmth, lipodystrophy at injection site
SYST: Hypersensitivity

Contraindications: Hypersensitivity, hypoglycaemia

Pharmacokinetics:
Subcutaneous: Onset 30−60 min, peak 2−3 hr, duration 5−7 hr, half-life 4 hr
IV: Onset 10−30 min, peak 30−60 min, duration 1−2 hr, half-life 3−5 min
Metabolised by liver, muscle, kidneys, excreted in urine

Interactions/incompatibilities:
• Increased hypoglycaemia, alcohol, β-blockers, oral hypoglycaemics, clofibrate
• Hyperglycaemia: thiazides, triamterene, phenothiazines, phenytoin, oral contraceptives, lithium
• Mask signs/symptoms of hypoglycaemia: β-blocker

Clinical assessment:
• Fasting glucose test
• Increased doses if tolerance occurs
• Human insulin to those allergic to beef or pork
• IV after diluting with 0.9% sodium chloride injection

Treatment of overdose: 10%−50% glucose by mouth if conscious or IV if comatose, or glucagon 1 mg by subcutaneous injection

NURSING CONSIDERATIONS

Administer:
• 10−30 min before meals, so peak action coincides with peak sugar level

Perform/provide:
• Check blood sugar levels before meals and bedtime
• Storage in a refrigerator between 2°−8°C, do not use discoloured, or cloudy solution
• Rotation of injection sites: abdomen, upper back, thighs, upper arm, buttocks; keep record of sites

Evaluate:
• Therapeutic response: decrease in polyuria, polydipsia, and blood sugar levels within normal range 4−9 mmol/litre
• Hypoglycaemic/hyperglycaemic reaction that can occur soon after meals in newly diagnosed diabetic

Teach patient/family:
• To keep insulin, equipment available at all times
• Dosage, route, mixing instructions, disease process
• To carry glucose sweets, sugar lumps, to treat hypoglycaemia
• Advise insulin action in association with diet and exercise
• That drug does not cure diabetes, but controls symptoms
• If blurred vision occurs, not to change corrective lens until vision is stabilised 1−2 months
• To carry Diabetic or other Medical Identity Card
• Hypoglycaemia reaction: headache, tremors, fatigue, weakness, sweating
• Symptoms of ketoacidosis: nausea, thirst, polyuria, dry mouth, dry, flushed skin, acetone breath, drowsiness
• Home blood glucose monitoring and how to interpret results
• To test urine for ketones if blood sugar is greater than 17
• To avoid non-prescribed drugs unless directed by clinician

insulin zinc suspension

Hypurin Lente, Lentard MC, Human Monotard, Humulin Lente
Func. class.: Antidiabetic
Chem. class.: Exogenous unmodified insulin
Legal class.: P

Action: Decreases blood sugar

Uses: Diabetes mellitus (long-acting therapy)

Dosage and routes:
• *Adult:* Subcutaneous individualised; do not give IV

Available forms include: Subcutaneous injection 100 units/ml

Side effects/adverse reactions:
CNS: Headache, lethargy, tremors, weakness, fatigue, delirium, sweating
CV: Tachycardia, palpitations
EENT: Blurred vision
GI: Hunger, nausea
META: Hypoglycaemia
INTEG: Flushing, rash, urticaria, warmth, lipodystrophy, erythema, pruritus
SYST: Anaphylaxis

Contraindications: Hypersensitivity, hypoglycaemia

Pharmacokinetics:
Subcutaneous: Onset 4 hr, duration up to 36 hr

Interactions/incompatibilities:
• Increased hypoglycaemia: alcohol, β-blockers, oral hypoglycaemics, MAOIs, octreotide
• Hyperglycaemia: thiazides, thyroid hormones, oral contraceptives, corticosteroids, lithium, diazoxide, loop diuretics

Clinical assessment:
• Fasting blood glucose (3.3–5.6 mmol/litre)

Treatment of overdose: Glucose by mouth if conscious or glucose 50% IV if comatose, glucagon 1 mg IM, subcutaneous, IV

NURSING CONSIDERATIONS

Perform/provide:
• Store bottle in use at room temperature for less than 1 month; refrigerate all other supply; do not use discoloured or cloudy solution
• Rotation of injection sites: abdomen, thighs, upper arm, buttocks

Evaluate:
• Therapeutic response: decrease in polyuria, polydipsia, alertness
• Hypoglycaemic/hyperglycaemic reaction that can occur

Teach patient/family:
• Dosage, route, mixing instructions, dietary advice, disease process
• Effects of diet and exercise on blood glucose
• To carry dextrasol or lump sugar to treat hypoglycaemia
• That drug does not cure diabetes, but controls symptoms
• That blurred vision occurs, not to change corrective lens until vision is stabilised 1–2 months
• To carry Medic Alert ID as diabetic
• Hypoglycaemia reaction: headache, tremors, fatigue, weakness
• Symptoms of ketoacidosis: nausea, thirst, polyuria, dry mouth, dry flushed skin, acetone breath, drowsiness
• Blood glucose testing; make sure patient is able to determine glucose
• To avoid non-prescribed drugs unless directed by clinician

insulin, zinc suspension crystalline

Human Ultratard (long acting),
Humulin Zn (intermediate acting)
Func. class.: Antidiabetic
Chem. class.: Exogenous unmodified insulin
Legal class.: P

Action: Decreases blood sugar
Uses: Diabetes mellitus
Dosage and routes:
• *Adult:* Subcutaneous individualised; do not give IV
Available forms include: Subcutaneous injection 100 units/ml
Side effects/adverse reactions:
CNS: Headache, lethargy, tremors, weakness, fatigue, delirium, sweating
CV: Tachycardia, palpitations
EENT: Blurred vision
GI: Hunger, nausea
META: Hypoglycaemia
INTEG: Flushing, rash, urticaria, warmth, lipoatrophy, lipohypertrophy, erythema, pruritus
SYST: Anaphylaxis
Contraindications: Hypersensitivity, hypoglycaemia
Pharmacokinetics:
Subcutaneous: Onset 4−8 hr, peak 16−18 hr, duration 24−36 hr
Interactions/incompatibilities:
• Increased hypoglycaemia: alcohol, β-blockers, oral hypoglycaemics, MAOIs, octreotide
• Hyperglycaemia: thiazides, thyroid hormones, oral contraceptives, corticosteroids, lithium, diazoxide, loop diuretics
Clinical assessment:
• Fasting blood glucose (3.3−5.6 mmol/litre)
Treatment of overdose: Glucose by mouth if conscious or glucose 50% IV if comatose, glucagon 1 mg IM, IV, subcutaneous

NURSING CONSIDERATIONS
Perform/provide:
• Store bottle in use at room temperature for less than 1 month; refrigerate all other supply; do not use discoloured or cloudy solution
• Rotation of injection sites: abdomen, thighs, upper arm, buttocks
Evaluate:
• Therapeutic response: decrease in polyuria, polydipsia, alertness
• Hypoglycaemic/hyperglycaemic reaction that can occur
Teach patient/family:
• Dosage, route, mixing instructions, dietary advice, disease process
• Effects of diet and exercise on blood glucose
• To carry dextrasol or lump sugar to treat hypoglycaemia
• That drug does not cure diabetes, but controls symptoms
• That blurred vision occurs, not to change corrective lens until vision is stabilised 1−2 months
• To carry Medic Alert ID as diabetic
• Hypoglycaemia reaction: headache, tremors, fatigue, weakness, sweating, visual disturbances
• Symptoms of ketoacidosis: nausea, thirst, polyuria, dry mouth, dry flushed skin, acetone breath, drowsiness
• Blood glucose testing, make sure patient is able to determine glucose test urine for ketones if blood sugar is high
• To avoid non-prescription drugs unless directed by clinician

insulin, zinc suspension amorphous

Semitard MC
Func. class.: Antidiabetic
Chem. class.: Exogenous unmodified insulin
Legal class.: P

Action: Decreases blood sugar
Uses: Diabetes mellitus (intermediate-acting therapy)
Dosage and routes:
• *Adult:* Subcutaneous individualised; do not give IV
Available forms include: Subcutaneous injection 100 units/ml
Side effects/adverse reactions:
CNS: Headache, lethargy, tremors, weakness, fatigue, delirium, sweating
CV: Tachycardia, palpitations
EENT: Blurred vision
GI: Hunger, nausea
META: Hypoglycaemia
INTEG: Flushing, rash, urticaria, warmth, lipoatrophy, lipohypertrophy, erythema, pruritus
SYST: Anaphylaxis
Contraindications: Hypersensitivity, hypoglycaemia
Pharmacokinetics:
Subcutaneous: Onset 2 hr, peak 4−12 hr, duration up to 24 hr
Interactions/incompatibilities:
• Increased hypoglycaemia: alcohol, β-blockers, oral hypoglycaemics, MAOIs, octreotide
• Hyperglycaemia: thiazides, thyroid hormones, oral contraceptives, corticosteroids, lithium, diazoxide, loop diuretics
Clinical assessment:
• Fasting blood glucose (3.3−5.6 mmol/litre)
Treatment of overdose: Glucose by mouth if conscious or glucose 50% IV if comatose, glucagon 1 mg IM, IV, subcutaneous

NURSING CONSIDERATIONS
Perform/provide:
• Store bottle in use at room temperature for less than 1 month; refrigerate all other supply; do not use discoloured or cloudy solution
• Rotation of injection sites: abdomen, thighs, upper arm, buttocks
Evaluate:
• Therapeutic response: decrease in polyuria, polydipsia, alertness
• Hypoglycaemic/hyperglycaemic reaction that can occur
Teach patient/family:
• Dosage, route, mixing instructions, dietary advice
• Effects of diet and exercise on blood glucose
• To carry dextrasol or lump sugar to treat hypoglycaemia
• That drug does not cure diabetes, but controls symptoms
• That blurred vision occurs, not to change corrective lens until vision is stabilised 1−2 months
• To carry Medic Alert ID as diabetic
• Hypoglycaemia reaction: headache, tremors, fatigue, weakness, sweating, visual disturbances
• Symptoms of ketoacidosis: nausea, thirst, polyuria, dry mouth, dry flushed skin, acetone breath, drowsiness
• Blood glucose testing, make sure patient is able to determine glucose, test urine for ketones if blood sugar is high
• The pregnant patient to use glucose oxidase reagents
• To avoid non-prescribed drugs unless directed by clinician

ipecacuanha emetic mixture, paediatric

Func. class.: Emetic
Chem. class.: Alkaloids
Legal class.: P

Action: Acts on chemoreceptor trigger zone to induce vomiting, irritates gastric mucosa
Uses: In poisoning to induce vomiting
Dosage and routes:
• *Adult:* By mouth 30 ml, then 200−300 ml water
• *Child 6−18 months:* By mouth 10 ml, then 100−200 water
• *Child over 18 months:* By mouth 15 ml, then 100−200 ml water; may repeat dose if needed once after 20 min
Available forms include: Mixture, prepared from ipecacuanha liquid extract
Side effects/adverse reactions:
CNS: Depression, convulsions, coma
GI: Bloody diarrhoea, mucosal damage
RESP: Inhalation of vomitus
CV: Circulatory failure, atrial fibrillation, fatal myocarditis, dysrhythmias
Contraindications: Hypersensitivity, unconscious/semiconscious, depressed gag reflex, poisoning with petroleum or corrosive products with low systemic toxicity, convulsions, low risk of toxicity for ingested product, late presentation
Precautions: Lactation, pregnancy
Pharmacokinetics:
By mouth: Onset 15−30 min
Interactions/incompatibilities:
• Decreased effect of ipecacuanha: activated charcoal
Clinical assessment:
• Type of poisoning; do not administer if petroleum products or caustic substances have been ingested; contact Poisons Centre
NURSING CONSIDERATIONS
Assess:
• Vital signs, BP; check patients with cardiac disease more often
Administer:
• Then bounce child to increase emetic effect
• Activated charcoal if this drug doesn't work; may begin lavage after 10−15 min
Evaluate:
• Respiratory status before, during, after administration of emetic; check rate, rhythm, character; respiratory depression can occur rapidly with elderly or debilitated patients
• Response − satisfactory quantity of vomit

ipratropium bromide

Atrovent, Atrovent Forte, combination product
Func. class.: Anticholinergic bronchodilator
Chem. class.: Synthetic quaternary ammonium compound
Legal class.: POM

Action: Inhibits interaction of acetylcholine at receptor sites on the bronchial smooth muscle, resulting in bronchodilation
Uses: Bronchodilation in obstructive airways disease
Dosage and routes:
• *Adult:* 2 inhalations (40 mcg) 3−4 times daily, sometimes up to 4 puffs during early treatment
• *Child up to 6 yr:* 1 inhalation 3 times daily; 6−12 yr 1−2 inhalations 3 times daily
• *Adult:* Nebulised 100−500 mcg up to 4 times a day
• *Child:* Nebulised 100−500 mcg up to 3 times a day
Available forms include: Aerosol

inhaler 20 mcg/puff, 40 mcg/puff; nebuliser solution 250 mcg, 500 mcg vials

Side effects/adverse reactions:
GI: Constipation
EENT: Dry mouth, blurred vision
Contraindications: Hypersensitivity to this drug or atropine
Precautions: Pregnancy, lactation, glaucoma, prostatic hypertrophy
Pharmacokinetics: Negligible amounts absorbed from the lungs, half-life of swallowed drug 3−4 hr

NURSING CONSIDERATIONS

Assess:
• For bronchoconstriction; if severe, drug may need to be changed

Administer:
• With salbutamol in the same nebuliser if indicated

Perform/provide:
• Frequent drinks, sugarless gum to relieve dry mouth

Evaluate:
• Therapeutic response: ability to breathe adequately − assessed by use of peak flows
• For tolerance over long-term therapy; dose may need to be increased or changed

Teach patient/family:
• Use inhaler/nebuliser according to prescribed number of inhalations/24 hr, or overdose may occur
• It is a preventative treatment rather than for the control of bronchospasm
• How to use inhaler aerosol or nebuliser equipment

iron dextran

Imferon
Func. class.: Haematinic
Chem. class.: Ferric hydroxide complexed with dextran
Legal class.: POM

Action: Iron dextran is removed from the plasma and split into its components. The iron binds to protein to form iron transfer molecules and is used to replenish haemoglobin and depleted iron stores

Dosage and routes:
• *Adult and child:* The dose is calculated according to weight (W, kg) and haemoglobin level (H, g/dl): Dose volume =
Men $[0.0476 \times W \times (14.8 - H)] + 14.0$ ml
Women $[0.0476 \times W \times (14.8 - H)] + 6.0$ ml
Child up to 15 yr $[0.0476 \times W \times (14.8 - H)]$ ml
• Test dose (Undiluted IV injection): IV 0.5 ml in 4−5 ml blood; observe for at least 30 min before giving full dose; give full dose slowly at no more than 1 ml/min
• IM by Z track technique not exceeding the following volumes.
• *Infant less than 5 kg:* 0.5 ml
• *Child more than 9 kg:* 1.0 ml
• *Adult:* 2.0−5.0 ml
The total dose is given as a series of injections, usually daily
• IV total dose infusion at no more than 5 drops/min for first 10 min then increased gradually to maximum 45−60 drops/min

Available forms include: Injection IM/IV 50 mg/ml (elemental iron)

Side effects/adverse reactions:
CNS: Headache, paraesthesia, dizziness, shivering, weakness
GI: Nausea, vomiting, abdominal pain

INTEG: Rash, pruritus, urticaria, sweating, chills, brown skin discolouration at injection site (IM), necrosis, sterile abscesses (IM), phlebitis (IV)
CV: Chest pain, shock, hypotension, tachycardia
RESP: Dyspnoea
SYST: Anaphylaxis, fever
Contraindications: Hypersensitivity, first trimester of pregnancy, asthma if given intravenously, acute infections, kidney disease
Precautions: Renal disease, rheumatoid arthritis (IV), infants less than 4 months, hepatic disease, infection, history of allergy

Pharmacokinetics:
IM: Excreted in faeces, urine, bile, breast milk

Interactions/incompatibilities:
• Not to mix with other drugs in syringe
• Increased toxicity: oral iron — do not use together

Clinical assessment:
• Blood studies: haematocrit, Hb, reticulocytes, bilirubin before treatment, at least monthly

Lab. test interferences:
False increase: Serum bilirubin
False decrease: Serum calcium
False positive: ^{99m}Tc diphosphate bone scan, iron test (large doses over 2 ml)

NURSING CONSIDERATIONS
Assess:
• Baseline BP and pulse
• Cause of iron loss or anaemia including salicylates, sulphonamides
• Nutritional status; amount of iron in diet (meat, dark green leafy vegetables, dried beans, dried fruits, eggs)
Administer:
• IV: only after test dose 1:1000 given by clinician
• Via volume controlled infusion pump

• Remainder of dose only 1 hr after test dose
• IM deeply into the upper quadrant of buttock, using Z-track method and a large gauge 2–3 inch needle; ensure needle is long enough to place injection deep in muscle
Perform/provide:
• Adrenaline in case of anaphylactic reaction
• Easily seen bed position
• All care as for a blood transfusion; potentially as dangerous
• Recumbent position for 30 min after injection
• Storage at room temperature in cool environment
Evaluate:
• BP and pulse every 15 min during first hr of infusion; 30 min during second hr; hrly thereafter during infusion
• Allergy: anaphylaxis, rash, pruritus, fever, chills
• Cardiac status: chest pain, hypotension, tachycardia
Teach patient/family:
• That iron poisoning may occur if increased beyond recommended level
• Good dietary advice

---

isocarboxazid
Marplan
Func. class.: Antidepressant, MAOI
Chem. class.: Hydrazine
Legal class.: POM

Action: Increases concentrations of endogenous adrenaline noradrenaline, serotonin, dopamine in storage sites in CNS by inhibition of monoamine oxidase; increased concentration reduces depression
Uses: Depression
Dosage and routes:

- *Adult:* By mouth initially 30 mg daily in divided doses, if no improvement after 4 weeks 60 mg daily may be tried for no longer than 6 weeks, reduce dose to lowest effective dose when condition improves (usually 10–20 mg)

Available forms include: Tablets 10 mg

Side effects/adverse reactions:

HAEM: Anaemia, purpura, granulocytopenia

CNS: Dizziness, drowsiness, confusion, headache, anxiety, tremors, weakness, hyperreflexia, mania, insomnia, fatigue

GI: Constipation, dry mouth, nausea, vomiting, anorexia, diarrhoea, weight gain

GU: Change in libido, frequency

INTEG: Rash, flushing, increased perspiration, jaundice

CV: Orthostatic hypotension, hypertension, dysrhythmias, hypertensive crisis, peripheral oedema

EENT: Blurred vision

ENDO: SIADH-like syndrome

Contraindications: Hypersensitivity to MAOIs, hypertension congestive cardiac failure, hepatic disease, phaeochromocytoma, severe cardiac disease, cerebrovascular disease, lactation

Precautions: Suicidal patients, convulsive disorders, severe depression, schizophrenia, hyperactivity, diabetes mellitus, pregnancy, renal disease, agitation, blood dyscrasias, elderly

Pharmacokinetics:

By mouth: Duration up to 2 weeks; metabolised by liver, excreted by kidneys

Interactions/incompatibilities:

- Increased pressor effects: indirect acting sympathomimetics (ephedrine), amphetamines
- Increased effects of: direct acting sympathomimetics (adrenaline), local anaesthetics, hypoglycaemic agents, antihypertensives, anticholinergic drugs, alcohol, barbiturates, benzodiazepines, CNS depressants, phenothiazines, diuretics
- Hyperpyretic crisis, convulsions, hypertensive episode: tricyclic antidepressants, tyramine-containing foods, amphetamines, phenylpropanolamine, ephedrine, fenfluramine, dopamine, levodopa, pethidine (and possibly other narcotics)

Clinical assessment:

- Blood studies: full blood count, leucocytes, cardiac enzymes if patient is receiving long-term therapy
- Liver function tests: aspartate aminotransferase, alanine aminotransferase, bilirubin, hepatotoxicity may occur

Treatment of overdose: Lavage, activated charcoal, vital signs, diazepam IV for convulsions, phentolamine for severe hypertension, hydrocortisone for severe shock

NURSING CONSIDERATIONS

Assess:

- Baseline BP (lying, standing), pulse

Administer:

- Increased fluids, fibre in diet if constipation, urinary retention occur
- With food or milk for GI symptoms
- Crushed if patient is unable to swallow medication whole
- Dosage at bedtime if oversedation occurs during day
- Frequent sips of water for dry mouth

Perform/provide:

- Assistance with mobility during beginning therapy since drowsiness/dizziness occurs
- Safety measures including cotsides, with good explanation to patient

Evaluate:
• BP; if systolic drops 20 mmHg notify clinician
• Toxicity: increased headache, palpitation; discontinue drug immediately; prodromal signs of hypertensive crisis
• Mental status: mood, alertness, affect, memory (long, short), increase in pyschiatric symptoms
• Urinary retention, constipation, GI disturbance, oedema
• Weight weekly
• Withdrawal symptoms: headache, nausea, vomiting, muscle pain weakness

Teach patient/family:
• That therapeutic effects may take 1–4 weeks
• To avoid driving or other activities requiring alertness
• To avoid alcohol ingestion, CNS depressants or non-prescribed medications: for colds, hay fever, cough
• Not to discontinue medication quickly after long-term use
• To avoid high tyramine foods: mature cheese, sour cream, beer, wine, pickled products, liver, raisins, bananas, figs, avocados, meat tenderisers, chocolate, yogurt; increased caffeine
• Report headache, palpitation, neck stiffness
• To carry Medical Identity Card detailing drug therapy

---

isoniazid

Rimifon, combination products
Func. class.: Antitubercular, antibiotic
Chem. class.: Isonicotinic acid hydrazide
Legal class.: POM

Action: Interference with bacterial cell metabolism, leading to rupture of cell wall

Uses: Treatment, prophylaxis of tuberculosis in combination with other drugs, tuberculous meningitis

Dosage and routes:
Treatment
• *Adult:* By mouth/IM/IV 300 mg once a day or 15 mg/kg 3 times a week for potentially non-compliant patients
• *Child:* By mouth/IM/IV 10 mg/kg (maximum 300 mg) daily or 15 mg/kg 3 times a week

Tuberculous meningitis
• No generally accepted regimen: consult specialist literature

Prevention
• *Adult:* By mouth 300 mg once daily as single dose for 12 months
• *Child and infants:* By mouth 5–10 mg/kg daily in single or divided doses for 12 months (maximum 300 mg daily)

Available forms include: Tablets 50, 100 mg; injection 25 mg/ml; elixir 50 mg/5 ml

Side effects/adverse reactions:
MS: Peripheral neuropathy
SYST: Systemic lupus erythematosus-like syndrome, hepatitis, hyperglycaemia
INTEG: Dermatitis
CNS: Tremors, convulsions, confusion, psychosis
EENT: Optic neuritis

Contraindications: Hypersensitivity, drug-induced liver disease, porphyria

Precautions: Pregnancy, hepatic disease, epilepsy, alcoholism, lactation, renal disease, diabetic retinopathy, cataracts, ocular defects, child under 13 yr, history of psychosis

Pharmacokinetics:
By mouth: Peak 1–2 hr
IM: Peak 45–60 min
Metabolised in liver, excreted in urine (metabolites), excreted in breast milk

Interactions/incompatibilities:

- Reduced absorption: antacids
- Increased toxicity of: carbamazepine, phenytoin, primidone, ethosuximide, diazepam, theophylline
- Increased CNS toxicity with: cycloserine

Clinical assessment:
- Temperature, if less than 38.5° drug should be reduced
- Liver function tests each week: alanine aminotransferase, aspartate aminotransferase, bilirubin
- Renal status: before, every month, serum urea, creatinine, output, specific gravity, urinalysis
- Resistance to therapy if inadequate therapeutic response

NURSING CONSIDERATIONS
Administer:
- With meals to decrease GI symptoms
- Anti-emetic if vomiting occurs
- With other antitubercular drugs for effective treatment
- With pyridoxine to reduce risk of peripheral neuropathy

Evaluate:
- Mental status often: affect, mood, behavioural changes; psychosis may occur
- For signs and symptoms of peripheral neuropathy, i.e. tingline or loss of sensation in extremeties
- Hepatic status: decreased appetite, jaundice, dark urine, fatigue

Teach patient/family:
- That compliance with dosage schedule, length is necessary
- That scheduled appointments must be kept or relapse may occur
- Avoid alcohol while taking drug
- Prescribed pyridoxine should also be taken

isoprenaline HCl/ isoprenaline sulphate

Medihaler-Iso, Saventrine, Min-I-Jet, Isoprenaline, combination product
Func. class.: Adrenergic agonist
Chem. class.: Catecholamine
Legal class.: POM

Action: Causes increased contractility and heart rate by acting on β-receptors in heart, also causes peripheral vasodilatation by acting on β-receptors in blood vessel walls

Uses: Heart block, severe bradycardia, asthma, bronchitis

Dosage and routes:
- *Oral dosage:* 90 mg—840 g daily in divided doses, ranging from 2-hrly to 8-hrly administration

Asthma, bronchospasm
- *Adult:* Inhalation 1—3 puffs, may repeat after 30 min, maintenance 1—2 puffs 4—8 times daily

Heart block
- *Adult and child:* Infusion IV 0.5—10 mcg/min

Severe bradycardia
- *Adult and child:* 1—4 mcg/min

Shock
- *Adult and child:* IV 0.5—10 mcg/min, intracardiac 100 mcg in 10 ml water

Available forms include: Aerosol 80, 400 mcg inhalation; tablets 30 mg; injection 20 mcg/ml, 1 mg/ml

Side effects/adverse reactions:
CNS: Tremors, anxiety, headache, dizziness, sweating
CV: Palpitations, tachycardia, hypertension, cardiac arrest
GI: Nausea, diarrhoea

Contraindications: Hypersensitivity to sympathomimetics, acute coronary disease, ventricular fibrillation, tachycardia

Precautions: Pregnancy, cardiac

disorders, hyperthyroidism, diabetes mellitus, hypertension
Pharmacokinetics:
Inhalation: Onset rapid; duration 1−2 hr
Metabolised in liver, lungs, GI tract, excreted in urine as unchanged drug and metabolites
Interactions/incompatibilities:
• Increased effects of both drugs: other sympathomimetics
• Increased risk of: arrhythmias with: halothane
Treatment of overdose: Symptomatic care, administer β-blocker (but not in asthmatics), monitor heart rhythm
NURSING CONSIDERATIONS
Assess:
• BP, pulse prior to administration
• Fluid balance; check for urinary retention, frequency, hesitancy
Perform/provide:
• Storage at room temperature, do not use discoloured solutions
• Continuous cardiac monitoring during IV administration, preferably on a cardiac unit if given for arrhythmias
• BP ½−1 hrly
• Fluid balance
Evaluate:
• For paraesthesia and coldness of extremities, peripheral blood flow may decrease
• Injection site: tissue sloughing
• Therapeutic response: increased BP and heart rate
• Tachycardias − inform clinician immediately
Teach patient/family:
• Use of inhaler
• To avoid getting aerosol in eyes
• To wash inhaler in warm water and dry daily

isosorbide dinitrate

Sorbitrate, Cedocard, Isoket, Isordil, Soni-slo, Sorbichew, Sorbid SA, Vascardin
Func. class.: Antianginal
Chem. class.: Nitrate
Legal class.: P, injection POM

Action: Decreases preload, afterload, which is responsible for decreasing left ventricular end diastolic pressure, systemic vascular resistance
Uses: Chronic stable angina pectoris, prophylaxis of angina pain left ventricular failure
Dosage and routes:
Angina
• By mouth 30−120 mg daily in divided doses; sublingual 5−10 mg, may repeat 2−3 hrly
Left ventricular failure
• By mouth 40−160 mg maximum 240 mg daily in divided doses; IV infusion 2−10 mg/hr
Available forms include: Capsules modified-release 20, 40 mg; tablets 5, 10, 20, 40 mg; chewable tablets 5 mg; tablets modified-release 20, 40 mg; sublingual tablets 5 mg; IV infusion 1 mg/ml, 0.5 mg/ml
Side effects/adverse reactions:
CV: Postural hypotension, tachycardia
INTEG: Pallor, sweating, rash
CNS: Headache, flushing, dizziness, weakness
Contraindications: Hypersensitivity to this drug or nitrates, anaemia, increased intracranial pressure, cerebral haemorrhage, acute myocardial infarction, head trauma, closed-angle glaucoma
Precautions: Postural hypotension, pregnancy, lactation
Pharmacokinetics:
Modified-release: Duration 6−12 hr

By mouth: Onset 15−30 min, duration 4−6 hr
Sublingual: Onset 2−5 min, duration 1−2 hr
Chewable tablets: Onset 3 min, duration ½−3 hr
Metabolised by liver, excreted in urine as metabolites (80%−100%), which are also active vasodilators

Interactions/incompatibilities:
• Increased effects: β-blockers, narcotics, tricyclics, diuretics, antihypertensives
• Decreased effects: sympathomimetics, anticholinergics (sublingual preps only)

NURSING CONSIDERATIONS
Assess:
• BP ½−1 hrly, pulse in IV use, respirations when beginning therapy
• If used IV to treat heart failure, assess oedema, shortness of breath and fluid balance

Administer:
• With full glass of water on empty stomach (oral tablet)
• Clinician may consider oral administration in the morning and at lunch time to attempt to reduce tolerance (day time angina) and lunch and evening to reduce nocturnal angina
• IV rate is usually titrated to treat unstable angina within the limits of the patient's blood pressure
• IV administration: incompatible with PVC or wide bore IV tubes as the drug is absorbed into the plastic and may be up to 30% less effective
• Ideally administered via 50 ml syringe pump or in a poly fusor or glass container

Evaluate:
• Pain: duration, time started, activity being performed, character
• Headache, lightheadedness, decreased BP; may indicate a need for decreased dosage

Teach patient/family:
• That drug may be taken before stressful activity (exercise, sexual activity)
• That sublingual administration may sting when drug comes in contact with mucous membranes
• To avoid hazardous activities if dizziness occurs
• Stress patient compliance with complete medical regimen
• To make position changes slowly to prevent fainting
• That analgesia (such as paracetamol) may help headaches if taken at the same time as drug (unless otherwise contraindicated)
• Headaches often lessen after the initial first days of treatment
• Inform clinician of any episodes of angina. An ECG may be performed if pain lasts over 20 mins

---

isotretinoin

Roaccutane
Func. class.: Anti-acne, systemic
Chem. class.: Retinoic acid isomer, vitamin A derivative
Legal class.: POM

Action: Decreases size and activity of sebaceous glands
Uses: Cystic and conglobate acne and severe acne unresponsive to other treatment
Dosage and routes:
• *Adult:* By mouth initially 0.5 mg/kg daily for 4 weeks, continue for 8−12 weeks if improvement is seen; if little response increase to 1 mg/kg daily for 8−12 weeks; if intolerant reduce to 0.1−0.2 mg/kg daily
Available forms include: Capsules 5, 20 mg
Side effects/adverse reactions:
INTEG: Dry skin, pruritus, cheilosis, joint and muscle pain, hair loss, photosensitivity, urticarian bruising, hirsutism, sweating

MS: Myalgia, arthralgia
CV: Chest pain
ENDO: Raised serum triglycerides and cholesterol, hyperglycaemia, hyperuricaemia
GI: Nausea, vomiting, anorexia, increased liver enzymes, jaundice, hepatitis, inflammatory bowel disease
EENT: Eye irritation, conjunctivitis, epistaxis, dry nose, mouth, contact lens intolerance, papilloedema, optic neuritis, cataracts, decreased night vision, photophobia, blurred vision, hearing deficiency
HAEM: Thrombocytopenia, thrombocytosis, neutropaenia, anaemia
CNS: Lethargy, fatigue, headache, drowsiness, benign intracranial hypertension, depression, seizures
Contraindications: Hypersensitivity, hepatic or renal impairment, inflamed skin, pregnancy, lactation, hypervitaminosis A, hyperlipidaemia
Precautions: Diabetes, photosensitivity
Pharmacokinetics:
By mouth: Peak 1–4 hr, half-life 10–20 hr; metabolised in liver, excreted in urine, faeces. Bioavailability is enhanced by taking with meals
Interactions/incompatibilities:
• Additive toxic effects: vitamin A, do not take more than the recommended dietary allowance
• Benign intracranial hypertension: increased risk with tetracyclines
• Increased triglyceride levels: alcohol
Clinical assessment:
• Triglyceride levels, aspartate aminotransferase, alanine aminotransferase, alkaline phosphatase; before, during treatment (monthly)
Treatment of overdose: Gastric

lavage, supportive measures
NURSING CONSIDERATIONS
Assess:
• Urinalysis weekly for protein, blood
• Blood glucose in diabetics, periodically
Administer:
• Whole, do not crush; give with meals
Evaluate:
• Therapeutic response: decrease in size and number of lesions
• Area of body involved, what helps or aggravates condition
• Pseudotumour cerebri: headache, vomiting, nausea, visual disturbance; discontinue drug
Teach patient/family:
• To avoid sunlight or wear sunscreen since photosensitivity may occur
• That an increase in acne may occur during initial treatment; decrease in 4–6 weeks
• Not to take vitamin A supplements, to take drug with meals
• Regarding package insert
• Not to crush capsules
• Minimise or eliminate alcohol consumption
• Not to take if pregnancy suspected. Reliable contraceptive measures must be taken in women of childbearing potential for at least 4 weeks before, during and at least 4 weeks after stopping treatment

isoxsuprine HCl

Duvadilan
Func. class.: Peripheral vasodilator β₂-adrenoreceptor stimulant
Chem. class.: Nylidrin related agent
Legal class.: POM

Action: Adrenergic agonist acts directly on vascular smooth muscle; causes uterine relaxation

Uses: Uncomplicated premature labour

Dosage and routes:

• *Adult:* By intravenous infusion, initially 200−300 mcg/min gradually increased to 500 mcg/min until labour is arrested; subsequently by IM injection, 10 mg every 3 hr for 24 hr, then every 4−6 hr for 48 hr

Available forms include: Injection IM/IV 5 mg/ml

Sides effects/adverse reactions:

CV: Hypotension, tachycardia, palpitations, chest pain

CNS: Dizziness, weakness, tremors, anxiety

GI: Nausea, vomiting, abdominal pain, distention

INTEG: Severe rash, flushing

Contraindications: Hypersensitivity, recent arterial haemorrhage, heart disease, premature detachment of placenta, severe anaemia, infection

Precautions: Tachycardia

Interactions/incompatibilities:

• Increased incidence of tachycardia with atropine

NURSING CONSIDERATIONS

Assess:

• Baseline pulse, BP lying and standing

Evaluate:

• BP lying, standing; orthostatic hypotension is common

• Therapeutic response

• Maternal pulse rate

• Foetal heart rate; may cause hypotension in foetus

• Dilation of cervix

Teach patient/family:

• To report palpitations, flushing if severe

• To avoid changes in temperature; extremities should be kept warm to promote better circulation

itraconazole

Sporanox

Func. class.: Antifungal

Chem. class.: Triazole

Legal class.: POM

Action: Impairs the synthesis of ergosterol in fungal cell membranes

Uses: Vulvovaginal candidiasis, oropharyngeal candidiasis, pityriasis versicolor and other dermatophyte infections

Dosage and routes:

Vulvovaginal candidiasis

• *Adult:* By mouth 200 mg twice daily for 1 day

Pityriasis versicolor

• *Adult:* By mouth 200 mg daily for 7 days

Oropharyngeal candidiasis

• *Adult:* By mouth 100 mg daily for 15 days (or 200 mg daily for 15 days in AIDS and neutropenic patients)

Tinea corporis and tinea cruris

• *Adult:* By mouth 100 mg daily for 15 days

Tinea pedis and tinea manuum

• *Adult:* By mouth 100 mg daily for 30 days

Maximum period of treatment 30 days

• *Children and elderly:* Not recommended

Available forms include: Capsules 100 mg

Side effects/adverse reactions:

CNS: Headache

GI: Abdominal pain, nausea, dyspepsia

Contraindications: Pregnancy, contraception must be used during and for 1 month after treatment

Interactions:

• Reduced blood levels of itraconazole with: rifampicin, phenytoin

• Possible reduction in absorption

of itraconazole with: H_2 blockers, antacids

NURSING CONSIDERATIONS
Administer:
• 15−30 min before a meal. When a additional dose is required to control night time symptoms, the tablet should be taken at bedtime
Teach patient/family:
• Not to take non-prescribed antacids (reduce absorption)
• History of liver disease, liver toxicity with other drug therapy, lactation

---

kanamycin sulphate

Kannasyn
Func. class.: Antibiotic
Chem. class.: Aminoglycoside
Legal class.: POM

Action: Interferes with protein synthesis in bacterial cell by binding to ribosomal subunit, causing inaccurate peptide sequence to form in protein chain, causing bacterial death
Uses: Serious infections due to susceptible Gram-negative organisms which have proved resistant to other antibiotics; also certain staphylococcal infections due to multi-resistant strains and gonorrhoea
Dosage and routes:
Severe systemic infections
• *Adult and child:* IV infusion 15−30 mg/kg in 2−3 doses in concentration 2.5 mg/ml at rate of 3−4 ml/min
• *Adult:* IM acute infections 1 g daily in 2−4 doses maximum 6 days (not more than 10 g total dose), chronic infection, 3−4 g a week an alternate days, maximum 50 g total dose
• *Child:* IM acute infections 15 mg/kg daily in 2−4 doses for not more than 6 days

Available forms include: Injection IM, IV 1 g powder
Side effects/adverse reactions:
GU: Haematuria, renal damage, azootaemia, renal failure, nephrotoxicity
EENT: Ototoxicity, deafness, vestibular damage
INTEG: Rash, burning, urticaria, local intolerance and haematoma at IM injection site, photosensitivity, dermatitis
Contraindications: Hypersensitivity, pregnancy, lactation
Precautions: Neonates, myasthenia gravis, hearing deficits, renal disease
Pharmacokinetics:
IM: Onset rapid, peak 1 hr
IV: Onset immediate, peak 1−2 hr
Plasma half-life 3 hr; not metabolised, excreted unchanged in urine
Interactions/incompatibilities:
• Increased ototoxicity, neurotoxicity, nephrotoxicity: other aminoglycosides, amphotericin B, polymyxin, vancomycin, ethacrynic acid, frusemide, mannitol, cisplatin, cephalosporins
Clinical assessment:
• Weight before treatment; calculation of dosage is usually done based on ideal body weight, but may be calculated on actual body weight
• Serum peak, drawn at 30−60 min after IV infusion or 60 min after IM injection; trough level drawn just before next dose; peak levels should be less than 30 mcg/ml; trough levels should be less than 10 mcg/ml
• Renal impairment by measuring creatinine clearance, blood urea nitrogen, serum creatinine; adjust doses according to blood levels
• Deafness by audiometric testing, ringing, roaring in ears, vertigo; assess hearing before, during, after treatment

• Culture and sensitivity before starting treatment to identify infecting organism
• Vestibular dysfunction: nausea, vomiting, dizziness, headache; drug should be discontinued if severe
Treatment of overdose: Haemodialysis or peritoneal dialysis, monitor serum levels of drug
NURSING CONSIDERATIONS
Assess:
• Culture and sensitivity before treatment
• Weight before treatment
• Regular blood level studies, to monitor serum peak
Administer:
• IM injection in large muscle mass, rotate injection sites
• Drug in evenly spaced doses to maintain blood level
• Bicarbonate to alkalinise urine if ordered in treating urinary tract infection, as drug is most active in alkaline environment
• Intravenously: slow infusion at 3–4 ml/min (2.5 mg/ml). Close observation during infusion
• Blood level studies, repeated 30–60 min after infusion
Perform/provide:
• Adequate fluids of 2–3 litres daily unless contraindicated to prevent irritation of tubules
• Supervised mobilisation, other safety measures with vestibular dysfunction
Evaluate:
• Therapeutic effect: absence of inflammation, redness, fever, draining wounds, lesions
• Input and output of fluids; report haematuria and signs of renal impairment. Special care and treatment for patients with known renal disease
• Urinalysis if drug used for urinary tract infection
• Vestibular damage, tinnitus followed by affected hearing

• Overgrowth of infection: increased temperature, malaise, redness, pain, swelling, perineal itching, diarrhoea, stomatitis, change in cough, sputum
• Injection sites for redness, swelling, rash, haematoma, usually transient
• Effects of any other drug therapy
Teach patient/family:
• To report headaches, tinnitus loss of hearing immediately
• Not to drive or use machinery if dizziness occurs
• To report sore throat, fever malaise, pain, change in cough, sputum and urine indicate superimposed infection

---

kaolin, pectin

Kaopectate
Func. class.: Antidiarrhoeal
Chem. class.: Hydrated aluminium silicate
Legal class.: GSL

Action: Increases solidity of stool
Uses: Diarrhoea
Dosage and routes:
• *Adult:* By mouth 10–30 ml 4-hrly
• *Child 1–5 yr:* By mouth 10 ml 4-hrly by mouth
• *Child 1 yr:* By mouth 5 ml 4-hrly
Available forms include: Suspension Kaolin 1.03 g/5 ml
Side effects/adverse reactions: None known
Contraindications: Intestinal obstruction
Interactions/incompatibilities: May reduce absorption of other drugs from GI tract
NURSING CONSIDERATIONS
Assess:
• Stool consistency and frequency
• Dehydration (especially children)
Administer:

- For 48 hr only
- Increased fluids or oral rehydration solutions

Evaluate:
- Therapeutic response: decreased diarrhoea
- Bowel pattern before; for rebound constipation
- Dehydration in children

Teach patient/family:
- Not to exceed recommended dose
- To shake well before administration

---

ketamine HCl

Ketalar

Func. class.: Anaesthetic, general
Chem. class.: Phencyclidine derivative
Legal class.: POM

Action: Acts on limbic system, cortex to provide anaesthesia

Uses: Short anaesthesia for diagnostic/surgical procedures; induction agent

Dosage and routes:
- *Adult and child:* Pre-op: IV 2 mg/kg, IM 10 mg/kg
- Induction: IV 1−4.5 mg/kg IM 6.5−13 mg/kg
- Maintenance: ½-full induction dose as required, if used with other anaesthetics, dose may be reduced

Available forms include: Injection IM, IV 10 mg/ml (20 ml), 50 mg/ml (10 ml), 100 mg/ml (5 ml)

Side effects/adverse reactions:
CNS: Hallucinations, confusion, delirium, tremors, polyneuropathy, fasciculations, pseudoconvulsions
CV: Increased B/P, hypotension, bradycardia, increased pulse, arrhythmia
EENT: Diplopia, salivation, small increase in intraocular pressure, nystagmus

INTEG: Rash, pain at injection site
RESP: Apnoea, respiratory depression, laryngospasm

Contraindications: Hypersensitivity, CVA, increased intracranial pressure, severe hypertension, cardiac decompensation, preeclampsia, eclampsia

Precautions: Pregnancy, seizure disorders, psychiatric disorders, alcoholism

Pharmacokinetics:
IV: Peak 30 sec, duration 5−10 min
IM: Peak 3−4 min, duration 12−25 min

Interactions/incompatibilities:
- Increased action of this drug: narcotics, barbiturates
- Do not mix with barbiturates in solution or syringe, chemically incompatible

NURSING CONSIDERATIONS
Administer:
- Only with emergency trolley, resuscitation equipment nearby
- IV slowly only over 60 seconds
- Narcotic, or diazepam to control recovery symptoms

Perform/provide:
- Quiet environment for recovery to decrease psychotic symptoms

Evaluate:
- Therapeutic response: maintenance of anaesthesia
- Vital signs every 10 min during IV administration, half hrly after IM dose
- Hallucinations, delusions, separation from environment
- Extrapyramidal reactions: dystonia, motor restlessness
- Increasing heart rate or decreasing BP, notify clinician at once

ketoconazole

Nizoral
Func. class.: Antifungal
Chem. class.: Imidazole derivative
Legal class.: POM

Action: Alters cell membranes and interferes with fungal enzyme systems

Uses: Systemic candidiasis, chronic mucocandidiasis, severe candiduria, coccidioidomycosis, histoplasmosis, paracoccidioidomycosis, chronic unresponsive vaginal candidiasis, fungal infections of the skin or fingernails which have not responded to other treatment, prophylaxis of mycotic infections in the immunosuppressed

Dosage and routes:
• *Adult:* By mouth 200 mg once daily usually for 14 days may increase to 400 mg once daily if needed; take with food
• *Child:* By mouth 50−100 mg once daily (3 mg/kg daily)
Chronic vaginal candidiasis
• 400 mg once daily for 5 days, prophylaxis 200 mg daily
Available forms include: Tablets 200 mg; suspension 100 mg/5 ml
Side effects/adverse reactions:
GU: Gynaecomastia
INTEG: Pruritus, rash, dermatitis, purpura, urticaria
CNS: Headache
SYST: Anaphylaxis, angiooedema
GI: Nausea, vomiting, diarrhoea, cramps, abdominal pain, constipation, flatulence, hepatotoxicity
HAEM: Thrombocytopenia
Contraindications: Hypersensitivity, pregnancy, hepatic disease
Pharmacokinetics:
By mouth: Peak 1−2 hr, half-life 8 hr, metabolised in liver, excreted mainly in bile, faeces, some in urine; requires acid pH for absorption, distributed poorly to CSF, highly protein bound

Interactions/incompatibilities:
• Hepatotoxicity: other hepatotoxic drugs
• Increased concentration of cyclosporin, phenytoin
• Decreased ketoconazole action: antacids, H_2-receptor antagonists (anticholinergics, antihistamines), rifampicin, phenytoin
• Increased anticoagulant effect: coumarin anticoagulants
• Decreased concentration of: rifampicin

Clinical assessment:
• Liver studies (alanine aminotransferase, aspartate aminotransferase, bilirubin) if on long-term therapy

NURSING CONSIDERATIONS

Assess:
• Temperature, blood pressure, pulse and respiration
• Fluid balance

Administer:
• In the presence of acid products only; do not use alkaline products or antacids within 2 hr of drug; may give coffee, tea, acidic fruit juices
• With food to decrease GI symptoms

Evaluate:
• Therapeutic response: decreased fever, malaise, rash, negative culture and sensitivity for infecting organism
• For allergic reaction: rash, photosensitivity, urticaria, dermatitis
• For hepatotoxicity: nausea, vomiting, jaundice, clay-coloured stools, fatigue

Teach patient/family:
• That long-term therapy may be needed to clear infection (1 week−6 months depending on infection)
• To avoid antacids, non-

prescribed drugs, alkaline products
• Stress patient compliance with drug regimen
• To notify clinician if GI symptoms, signs of liver dysfunction (fatigue, nausea, anorexia, vomiting, dark urine, pale stools)

---

ketoprofen

Orudis, Alrheumat, Oruvail
Func. class.: Non-steroidal anti-inflammatory agent
Chem. class.: Propionic acid derivative
Legal class.: POM

Action: Inhibits prostaglandin synthesis by decreasing enzyme needed for biosynthesis; possesses analgesic, anti-inflammatory, antipyretic properties

Uses: Rheumatoid arthritis, osteoarthritis, ankylosing spondylitis, acute articular and periarticular disorders, fibrositis, cervical spondylitis, low back pain, painful musculoskeletal conditions, dysmenorrhoea (not suppositories), acute gout, control of pain and inflammation following orthopaedic surgery

Dosage and routes:
• *Adult:* By mouth 100−200 mg daily in divided doses; modified-release 100−200 mg daily, rectal 100 mg at night, IM 50−100 mg 4 hrly to a maximum of 200 mg in 24 hr. IM treatment should not exceed 3 days

Available forms include: Capsules 50, 100 mg; capsules modified-release 100, 200 mg; suppository 100 mg, IM injection 100 mg/2 ml

Side effects/adverse reactions:
GI: Nausea, anorexia, vomiting, diarrhoea, jaundice, cholestatic hepatitis, constipation, flatulence, cramps, dry mouth, peptic ulcer, indigestion
CNS: Dizziness, drowsiness, fatigue, tremors, confusion, insomnia, anxiety, depression, vertigo, headache
CV: Tachycardia, peripheral oedema, palpitations, dysrhythmias, anaphylaxis
INTEG: Purpura, rash, pruritus, sweating
GU: Nephrotoxicity: dysuria, haematuria, oliguria, azotaemia
HAEM: Thrombocytopenia
EENT: Tinnitus, hearing loss, blurred vision
RESP: Bronchospasm

Contraindications: Hypersensitivity, active peptic ulceration, hypersensitivity to other NSAIDs, severe renal dysfunction

Precautions: Pregnancy, lactation, children, bleeding disorders, GI disorders, cardiac disorders, renal disease, hepatic disease, asthma, allergic disorders

Pharmacokinetics:
By mouth: Peak ½−1 hr, half-life 2−3 hr, modified-release: peak 6−8 hr, half-life 8 hr metabolised in liver, excreted in urine (metabolites), and faeces

Interactions/incompatibilities:
• May increase action of: coumarins, sulphonamides, methotrexate
• Excretion delayed by: probenicid

NURSING CONSIDERATIONS
Administer:
• With food to decrease GI symptoms
Evaluate:
• Therapeutic response: decreased pain, stiffness in joints, decreased swelling in joints, ability to move more easily
• For eye, ear problems: blurred vision, tinnitus; may indicate toxicity
Teach patient/family:

• To report blurred vision, ringing, roaring in ears; may indicate toxicity
• To report change in urine pattern, increased weight, oedema, increased pain in joints, fever, blood in urine; indicate nephrotoxicity
• To report unresolved indigestion or black tarry stools
• To avoid driving, other hazardous activities if dizziness, drowsiness occurs
• That therapeutic effects may take up to 1 month

---

ketotifen

Zatiden
Func. class.: Anti-asthmatic/anti-allergic agents
Chem. class.: Thiophenone
Legal class.: POM

Action: Thought to prevent release of pharmacological mediators of bronchospasm by stabilising mast-cell membranes, also shows properties of antihistamines
Uses: Prophylaxis of asthma, relief of allergy including rhinitis and conjunctivitis
Dosage and routes:
• *Adult:* By mouth 1−2 mg twice daily with food
• *Child over 2 yr:* By mouth 1 mg twice daily with food
Initial treatment in readily sedated patients: 0.5−1 mg at night for first few days
Available forms include: Tablets 1 mg; capsules 1 mg; elixir 1 mg/5 ml
Side effects/adverse reactions:
CNS: Sedation, dizziness
EENT: Dry mouth
Contraindications: Should not be taken with oral antidiabetic drugs pregnancy, lactation

Precautions: Warn patient of drowsiness effect, alcohol. Continue any pre-existing anti-asthma treatment for at least 2 weeks after starting ketotifen
Interactions/incompatibilities:
• Reversible thrombocytopenia with: oral antidiabetics
• Enhanced sedative effect with: alcohol, other antimuscarinic drugs
Treatment of overdose: Elimination of drug by gastric lavage or emesis is recommended. General supportive treatment
NURSING CONSIDERATIONS
Perform/provide:
• Mouthwashes to relieve dry mouth
• Frequent rest periods to reduce drowsiness
Evaluate:
• Therapeutic effects or respiratory status
Teach patient/family:
• Not to drive or operate machinery
• To continue all other anti-asthma treatment for at least 2 weeks
• To continue regular usage as prescribed

---

labetalol

Trandate, Labrocol
Func. class.: Antihypertensive, nonselective α-, β-adrenergic receptor blocker
Chem. class.: Substituted benzamide
Legal class.: POM

Action: Produces falls in BP without reflex tachycardia or significant reduction in heart rate through mixture of α-blocking, β-blocking effects; elevated plasma renins are reduced

Uses: Mild-severe hypertension, hypertensive crisis, controlled hypotension during surgery

Dosage and routes:

Hypertension

• *Adult:* By mouth 100 mg twice a day, increased by 100 mg twice a day at intervals of 14 days to maximum of 800 mg twice a day, further increases to a maximum of 2.4 g daily should be split into 3–4 daily doses. More rapid dose escalation in severe hypertension possible in hospital

Hypertensive crisis

• *Adult:* IV bolus, 50 mg over 1 min, may repeat after 5 min, not to exceed 200 mg

• *IV infusion*, 2 mg/min; usual range 50–200 mg

Hypertension of pregnancy

• *IV infusion*, 20 mg/hr doubled every 30 min if needed, usual maximum 160 mg/hr

Following infarction

• *IV infusion*, 15 mg/hr gradually increased to maximum 120 mg/hr

Available forms include: Tablets 50, 100, 200, 400 mg; injection IV 5 mg/ml

Side effects/adverse reactions:

CV: Orthostatic hypotension, bradycardia, atrioventricular block, ankle oedema

CNS: Dizziness, mental changes, drowsiness, fatigue, headache, depression, tremor, nightmares, paraesthesia, lethargy

GI: Nausea, vomiting, diarrhoea, liver damage, epigastric pain

INTEG: Rash, urticaria, pruritus, sweating, lichenoid rash

EENT: Tinnitus, visual changes, burning eyes, nasal congestion

GU: Impotence, dysuria, ejaculatory failure, retention

RESP: Bronchospasm, dyspnoea

SYST: Allergic reactions: angio-edema, lupus-like syndrome, fever

Contraindications: Hypersensitivity, cardiogenic shock, heart block (2nd, 3rd degree), severe bradycardia, untreated congestive cardiac failure

Precautions: Pregnancy, lactation, diabetes mellitus, hyperthyroidism, chronic obstructive airways disease, well compensated heart failure

Pharmacokinetics:

By mouth: Well absorbed, extensive first-pass metabolism, peak plasma levels 1–2 hr

IV: Peak 5 min

Half-life 2–8 hr, metabolised by liver (metabolites inactive), excreted in urine, bile, excreted in breast milk

Interactions/incompatibilities:

• Increased hypotension: diuretics, other antihypertensives, halothane and other anaesthetics, cimetidine

• Decreased effects: sympathomimetics, theophylline

• Increased risk of hypoglycaemia: insulin, oral hypoglycaemics

• Increased risk of cardiotoxicity: amiodarone, diltiazem, nifedipine, verapamil, cardiac glycosides

• Increased risk of tremor with: tricyclic antidepressants

Lab. test interferences:

False increase: urinary catecholamines

Treatment of overdose: Lavage, IV atropine for bradycardia, nebulised β_2-agonist for bronchospasm; cardiac glycoside, O_2, diuretic for cardiac failure; noradrenaline for circulatory collapse. Keep patient supine, legs raised

NURSING CONSIDERATIONS

Assess:

• Baseline vital signs

Administer:

• By mouth, before meals, tablet may be crushed or swallowed whole

• Notify clinician of any significant changes in BP and pulse after oral administration

• Consider cardiac monitoring during IV administration
• BP and pulse every 15 min for 1 hr during IV administration
• IV, keep patient on bed rest for 3−6 hrs

Perform/provide:
• Storage in dry area at room temperature, do not freeze

Evaluate:
• Therapeutic response: decreased BP after 1−2 weeks
• Fluid balance, weight daily
• BP, pulse 4 hrly; note rate, rhythm, quality
• Signs of heart failure: evaluate daily for increased weight, ankle oedema, shortness of breath

Teach patient/family:
• Not to discontinue drug unless instructed by clinician
• Not to use non-prescribed drugs containing α-adrenergic stimulants (nasal decongestants, cold preparations) unless directed by clinician
• To report dizziness, confusion, depression, fever and impotence
• To avoid hazardous activities if dizziness is present
• To report: difficult breathing, especially on exertion or when lying down, night cough, swelling of extremities
• Rise slowly to sitting or standing position to minimise postural hypotension

lactulose

~~NHS~~ Duphalac
Func. class.: Laxative
Chem. class.: Disaccharide
Legal class.: P (only prescribable generically on NHS)

Action: Increases osmotic pressure within colon after bacterial degradation, stimulates peristalsis. Prevents formation and absorption of ammonia in colon

Uses: Constipation, hepatic encephalopathy/coma

Dosage and routes:
Constipation
• *Adult:* By mouth 15 ml twice daily adjusted to patient needs
• *Child under 1 yr:* By mouth 2.5 ml twice a day; 1−5 yr 5 ml twice a day; 6−12 yr 10 ml twice a day. Reduce dose gradually according to needs
Regular dosing essential − takes up to 48 hr to work
Encephalopathy
• *Adult:* By mouth 30−50 ml 3 times a day, adjusted to produce 2−3 soft stools daily

Available forms include: Oral solution 3.35 g/5 ml

Side effects/adverse reactions:
GI: Nausea, vomiting, cramps, diarrhoea, flatulence
MISC: Electrolyte imbalances if used excessively

Contraindications: Hypersensitivity, galactosaemia, intestinal obstruction

Precautions: Lactose intolerance

Pharmacokinetics: Metabolised in intestine

NURSING CONSIDERATIONS

Assess:
• Fluid balance
• Cause of constipation; identify whether fluids, bulk, or exercise is missing from diet or lifestyle

Perform/provide:
• Increase fluids to 2 litres daily

Evaluate:
• Therapeutic response
• Cramping, rectal bleeding, nausea, vomiting; if these symptoms occur, drug should be discontinued
• Clearing of confusion, lethargy, restlessness, irritability

Teach patient/family:
• That instant relief should not be expected

• That medication takes up to 48 hr to take effect

• Not to use laxatives for long-term therapy; bowel tone will be lost

• About changes in diet and lifestyle to relieve constipation

---

lanatoside C

Cedilanid

Func. class.: Antidysrhythmic, cardiac glycoside

Chem. class.: Digitalis preparation

Legal class.: POM

Action: Acts by influx of calcium ions from extracellular to intracellular cytoplasm; increases cardiac contractility and cardiac output

Uses: Congestive heart failure, atrial fibrillation, atrial flutter, atrial tachycardia

Dosage and routes:

• *Adult:* By mouth slow digitalisation 1.5−2 mg daily for 3−5 days; maintenance 0.25−1 mg daily

• *Child:* Seek specialist advice

Available forms include: Tablets 250 mcg

Side effects/adverse reactions:

CV: Arrhythmias, heart block, bradycardia

CNS: Headache, drowsiness, apathy, confusion, fatigue, depression, hallucinations

GI: Anorexia, nausea, vomiting, abdominal pain, diarrhoea

INTEG: Pruritus, urticaria, macular rashes

EENT: Blurred vision, yellow green halos, photophobia, diplopia

ENDO: Gynaecomastia

Contraindications: Complete atrioventricular block and 2nd degree atrioventricular block (especially 2:1), excessive sinus bradycardia, supraventricular arrythmias caused by Wolff-Parkinson-White syndrome

Precautions: Recent myocardial infarction; hypothyroidism; elderly patients (reduce dose), pregnancy, electrolyte disturbance (especially hypokalaemia), renal insufficiency

Pharmacokinetics: Poorly absorbed from GI tract, 20% of dose inactivated daily. Duration of action is 3−6 days. Mostly converted to digoxin and excreted in urine

Interactions/incompatibilities:

• Drugs increasing risk of hypokalaemia and lanatoside toxicity: diuretics, amphotericin B, corticosteroids, lithium, carbenoxolone

• Increased lanatoside blood levels: quinidine, verapamil, diltiazem, nicardipine, amiodarone, possibly other calcium antagonists, prazosin, erythromycin, tetracyclines, quinine

• Decreased lanatoside blood levels: anticholinergics, neomycin, sulphasalazine, certain cytotoxics, cholestyramine, colestipol

• Increased risk of cardiotoxicity: β-blockers, verapamil, suxamethonium, IV calcium

Clinical assessment

• Renal function tests: urea, creatinine before treatment; if change/toxicity suspected

• Serum electrolytes especially potassium before treatment; if change/toxicity suspected

• Monitor plasma levels of digoxin (therapeutic level 1.5−3.0 mcg/litre) once therapy stabilised; if toxicity suspected

Treatment of overdose: Gastric lavage if ingestion recent, correct any hypokalaemia, treat arrhythmias with non-cardiac glycoside drugs, consider administration of digoxin specific antibody fragments, monitor ECG continuously
NURSING CONSIDERATIONS

Assess:
- Baseline vital signs
- Apical pulse for 1 min before each dose: if greater than 60 withhold drug, take again in 1 hr; if still greater than 60, call clinician and withhold drug
- Fluid balance, weight daily

Administer:
- Orally using the lowest effective dose
- Potassium supplements if prescribed for potassium levels less than 3.0 mmol/litre

Evaluate:
- Visual changes headache
- Cardiac status, apical pulse, character, rate, rhythm
- Therapeutic response, decreased weight, oedema, pulse, respiration and increased urine output

Teach patient/family:
- Not to discontinue drug abruptly
- To report symptoms of toxicity, oedema
- To only take other medication on clinician's advice
- To take own pulse and contact clinician if it falls below 60
- Not to take antacid at the same time

---

levobunolol HCl (ophthalmic)

Betagan
Func. class.: Antihypotensive, ocular
Chem. class.: Non-selective β-blocker
Legal class.: POM

Action: Non-selective β-adrenergic agent
Uses: Reduction of intra-ocular pressure in chronic open-angle glaucoma and ocular hypertension
Dosage and routes:
- *Adult:* One drop in the affected eye(s) once or twice a day
- *Children:* Not recommended
Available forms include: Solution 0.5%
Side effects/adverse reactions:
EENT: Transient burning or stinging on instillation, blepharo-conjunctivitis and iridocyclitis
CV: Bradycardia, hypotension
INTEG: Urticaria, pruritus
RESP: Dyspnoea, asthma
CNS: Headache, lethargy, transient ataxia, dizziness
Contraindications: Bronchial asthma, history of bronchial asthma, chronic obstructive pulmonary disease, sinus bradycardia, second or third degree atrioventricular block, cardiac failure, cardiogenic shock, hypersensitivity to any component, soft contact lenses
Precautions: Pregnancy, breast-feeding
Pharmacokinetics: Onset of action within 1 hr, peak 2−8 hr, duration 24 hr. Significant systemic absorption possible; metabolised in liver, excreted in urine, half-life 6−7 hr
Interactions/incompatibilities:
- Should be used with caution in patients on oral β-blocking drugs (additive effects)

NURSING CONSIDERATIONS

Assess:
- History of asthma, bronchospasm or wheeziness
- Diabetic status

Administer:
- With appropriate support in case of bronchospasm

Evaluate:
- For side effects including transitory dryness of eyes

Teach patient/family:
- Should not be used in patients wearing hydrophilic (soft) contact lenses
- Full clinical response may take several weeks

levodopa

Brocadopa, Larodopa
Func. class.: Antiparkinsonism agent
Chem. class.: Phenylalanine derivative
Legal class.: POM

Action: Decarboxylation to dopamine, which increases dopamine levels in brain

Uses: Parkinsonism

Dosage and routes:
• *Adult:* By mouth 125−500 mg daily divided 2 to 5 times a day with meals, may increase by 0.5−1 g every 3−7 days, depending upon response, not normally to exceed 8 g daily. Non-hospitalised patients may require slower dose elevation and smaller dosage increments

Available forms include: Capsules 125, 250, 500 mg; tablets 500 mg

Side effects/adverse reactions:
HAEM: Haemolytic anaemia, transient leucopenia/thrombocytopenia
CNS: Choreiform involuntary movements, fatigue, headache, anxiety, twitching, numbness, weakness, confusion, agitation, insomnia, nightmares, psychosis, hallucination, hypomania, depression, dizziness, peripheral neuropathy
GI: Nausea, vomiting, anorexia, abdominal distress, bitter taste, transient rises in liver enzymes, GI bleeding
INTEG: Sweating, alopecia, flushing
CV: Orthostatic hypotension, tachycardia, hypertension, palpitation, arrhythmias
MISC: Reddish colouration of urine and other body fluids

Contraindications: Concurrent use of MAOIs (except selegiline), hypersensitivity, closed-angle glaucoma, history of or active malignant melanoma, psychosis, drug-induced parkinsonism

Precautions: Renal disease, cardiovascular disease, hepatic disease, peptic ulcer, diabetes, pregnancy

Pharmacokinetics:
By mouth: Peak 1−3 hr, metabolised in gut, liver, kidney, excreted in urine (metabolites), plasma half-life 45−65 min

Interactions/incompatibilities:
• Hypertensive crisis: MAOIs (except selegiline) or within 21 days of stopping
• Dysrhythmias: cyclopropane, halogenated hydrocarbon anaesthetics
• Increased effects of: guanethidine, methyldopa, other antihypertensives
• Decreased effects of: antipsychotics
• Effects of levodopa reduced by: benzodiazepines, pyridoxine, iron, metoclopramide

Clinical assessment:
• Adjust dosage depending on patient response
• Hepatic, haematological, renal, cardiovascular, psychiatric surveillance during prolonged therapy
• Prescribe domperidone for nausea

Lab. test interferences:
False positive: Urine ketones, urine glucose
False negative: Urine glucose (glucose oxidase)

Treatment of overdose: Gastric lavage, ECG monitoring, supportive treatment

NURSING CONSIDERATIONS

Administer:
• Drug to be given until patient is starved (before surgery)
• With meals; limit protein taken with drug

Perform/provide:

• Assistance with ambulation, during beginning of therapy
• Testing for diabetes mellitus, acromegaly if on long-term therapy

Evaluate:
• Mental status: affect, mood, behavioural changes, depression
• Assess suicidal tendencies
• Therapeutic response: decrease in involuntary movements, increased, increase mood

Teach patient/family:
• To change positions slowly to prevent orthostatic hypotension
• To report side effects: twitching, eye spasms; indicate overdose
• To use drug exactly as prescribed; if drug is discontinued abruptly, parkinsonian crisis may occur
• That urine, sweat may darken
• To avoid vitamin B_6 preparations, and vitamin-fortified foods containing B_6; these foods can reverse effects of levodopa

---

lignocaine HCl

Xylocard, Min-I-Jet, Select-A-Jet
Func. class.: Anti-arrhythmic
Chem. class.: Aminoacyl amide
Legal class.: POM

Action: Increases electrical stimulation threshold of ventrical, HIS Purkinje system, by stabilising cardiac membrane

Uses: Ventricular tachycardia, extrasystole, and arrhythmias especially after myocardial infarction

Dosage and routes:
• *Adult:* IV bolus 50−100 mg over 2 min, repeated once or twice after 5−10 min if necessary, not to exceed 300 mg in 1 hr; follow by IV infusion 2−4 mg/min

Available forms include: Injection 10, 20 mg/ml; injections for dilution 1, 2 g syringes equivalent to 200 mg/ml lignocaine; infusion solution 1, 2 mg/ml

Side effects/adverse reactions:
CNS: Headache, dizziness, drowsiness, paraesthesia, tremor, convulsions, unconsciousness
EENT: Tinnitus, blurred vision
CV: Hypotension, bradycardia, heart block, cardiac arrest
RESP: Dyspnoea, respiratory depression

Contraindications: Hypersensitivity to amides, atrioventricular block, other severe cardiac conduction disturbances and decompensation not dependant on treatable tachyarrhythmias, porphyria

Precautions: Renal disease, liver disease, congestive cardiac failure, hypokalaemia; solutions containing 200 mg/ml are for dilution before use

Pharmacokinetics:
IV: Onset 2 min, duration 20 min Half-life 8 min, 1−2 hr (terminal), metabolised in liver, excreted in urine

Interactions/incompatibilities:
• Increased effects of lignocaine: cimetidine, phenytoin, propranolol, quinidine and other anti-arrhythmics

Clinical assessment:
• ECG

Treatment of overdose: Supportive symptomatic care; temporary pacing may be required for atrioventricular block

NURSING CONSIDERATIONS

Assess:
• BP, pulse, ECG

Administer:
• Intravenously: bolus injection over 2 min directly into vein; effects can be observed within minutes, if necessary injection can be repeated at 5−10 min intervals once or twice
• Infusion at a rate of about 2−4 mg/min

Evaluate:
• Hypotension and bradycardia; may lead to cardiac arrest
• Cardiac rate, respiration: rate, rhythm, character, continuously
• Respiratory status: rate, rhythm, sound, watch for respiratory depression
• CNS effects: dizziness, confusion, loss of consciousness, paraesthaesia, convulsions; drug should be discontinued
• Lung fields, bilateral rales may occur in congestive cardiac failure patient
• Increased respiration, increased pulse; drug should be discontinued

---

lignocaine/lignocaine HCl (topical)

Xylocaine
Func. class.: Topical anaesthetic
Chem. class.: Aminoacyl amide
Legal class.: P

Action: Inhibits nerve impulses from sensory nerves, by stabilising neuronal membrane
Uses: Surface anaesthesia of skin, mucous membranes during examination, catheterisation, intubation or endoscopy; minor burns and abrasions of skin; local symptomatic relief of pain
Dosage and routes:
• *Adult:* Instilled into urethra up to 40 ml gel; topical application, up to 35 g ointment in 24 hr, or up to 7.5 ml topical solution or 20 activations of topical spray as a single dose
Available forms include: Gel 2% (hydrochloride); ointment 5%; metered spray 10% (10 mg/activation); topical solution 4% (hydrochloride)
Side effects/adverse reactions:
INTEG: Allergy, sensitisation

SYST: CNS stimulation, CV depression due to excessive absorption
Contraindications: Hypersensitivity
Precautions: Pregnancy, application to large areas or to denuded skin or in sepsis (risk of systemic absorption)

NURSING CONSIDERATIONS
Assess:
• For pre-existing infection (anaesthetic may be ineffective)
Administer:
• Using sterile dressing technique
• Topically to area for surface anaesthesia using gloves, swab, nozzle or spray
• Instil into urethra through nozzle applicator before catheterisation
• To dirty skin abrasions (children's knees and hands) before scrubbing clean
Evaluate:
• Therapeutic response: absence of local pain, decreased sensitivity during examination and catheterisation
• Allergy: sensitisation, redness swelling
Teach patient/family:
• How to apply
• Not to use on large areas or excessively as absorption into whole circulatory system occurs
• To report any signs of sensitivity

---

lignocaine HCl (local)

Lignostab, Xylocaine, Lignostab A
Func. class.: Anaesthetic, local
Chem. class.: Aminoacyl amide
Legal class.: POM

Action: Inhibits nerve impulses from sensory nerves by stabilising neuronal membrane
Uses: Peripheral nerve block, infiltration anaesthesia, caudal,

epidural, spinal anaesthesia, dental procedures

Dosage and routes:
Varies depending on route of anaesthesia; by injection usual maximum 200 mg given alone or 500 mg when given with adrenaline *Available forms include:* Injection 0.5% 1%, 1.5%, 2%, injection with adrenaline 0.5%, 1%, 2%

Side effects/adverse reactions:
CNS: Anxiety, dizziness, convulsions, loss of consciousness, drowsiness, tremors
CV: Myocardial depression, cardiac arrest, dysrhythmias, bradycardia, hypotension
EENT: Blurred vision, tinnitus
INTEG: Rash, urticaria, allergic reactions, oedema
RESP: Respiratory arrest, anaphylaxis

Contraindications: Hypersensitivity, hypovolaemia, heartblock, porphyria

Precautions: Elderly, debilitated, epilepsy, impaired cardiac conduction, impaired respiratory function, impaired hepatic function, bradycardia, pregnancy; facilities for resuscitation should be available; solutions containing adrenaline should not be used in appendages (vasoconstriction may impair blood supply)

Pharmacokinetics:
Onset 4−17 min, duration 3−6 hr; metabolised by liver, excreted in urine (metabolites)

Interactions/incompatibilities:
• Possibly increased systemic effects of lignocaine: cimetidine anti-arrhythmics, propranolol
• Possible interaction with adrenaline containing solutions: general anaesthetics, MAOIs, tricyclic anti-depressants

Treatment of overdose: Supportive symptomatic care

NURSING CONSIDERATIONS
Assess:
• For pre-existing local infection (anaesthesia may be ineffective)
• BP, pulse respiration

Administer:
• As appropriate for procedure to be undertaken. Wide range of uses e.g. subcutaneous for sutures, spinal infiltration
• Smallest dose producing required effect

Perform/provide:
• Resuscitation equipment
• Discard part-used units

Evaluate:
• Therapeutic response: anaesthetic level for procedure
• Allergic reactions; rash urticaria, oedema
• Fetal heart during labour
• Any changes in patient's speech, level of consciousness, complaints of dizziness during therapy
• Patient continuously during major use

Teach patient/family
• To seek medical help if dizziness, convulsions, drowsiness, breathing difficulties occur (up to 6 hr after therapy)

lignocaine and prilocaine (topical)

Emla
Func. class.: Anaesthetic, topical, local
Chem. class.: Aminoacyl amide
Legal class.: POM

Action: Inhibits conduction of nerve impulses from sensory nerves
Uses: Topical anaesthetic for skin anaesthesia, and genital mucosa to facilitate removal of warts in adults
Dosage and routes:
Skin
Adult and child over 1 year: Minor topical procedures 2 g Emla for

minimum 60 mins, maximum 5 hr; larger areas, $1.5-3$ g/10 cm^2 minimum 2 hr, maximum 5 hr

Genital mucosa

Adult: Up to 10 g for $5-10$ min prior to procedure

Available forms include: Cream 5%

Side effects/adverse reactions:

EENT: Swelling, burning, stinging, tissue necrosis, irritation

INTEG: Rash, urticaria, oedema

HAEM: Prilocaine has been known to cause methaemoglobinaemia when given parenterally

Contraindications: Hypersensitivity, secondary bacterial infections, infants

Precautions: Sepsis of affected area, pregnancy

Pharmacokinetics:

Topical: Peak $2-5$ min, duration ½-1 hr

NURSING CONSIDERATIONS

Administer:

• For surface anaesthesia, not to wounds

• Using spatula provided

• Thickly, under occlusive dressing at least 1 hr before venepuncture (except for infants)

• $5-10$ min before removal of genital warts

• Avoiding use near eyes

Perform/provide:

• Storage at room temperature in airtight container

Evaluate:

• For therapeutic response

• For redness, swelling

Teach patient/family:

• Not to apply cream to mucous membrane (except for genital warts in adults)

lincomycin HCl

Lincocin

Func. class.: Antibiotic

Chem. class.: Lincosamide derivative

Legal class.: POM

Action: Binds to 50S subunit of bacterial ribosomes, suppresses protein synthesis

Uses: Serious infections caused by susceptible Gram-positive cocci or anaerobes, especially joint and bone infections, intra-abdominal sepsis

Dosage and routes:

• *Adult:* By mouth 500 mg every $6-8$ hr; IM 600 mg every $12-24$ hr; slow IV 600 mg every $8-12$ hr, dilute in at least 250 ml glucose 5% or sodium chloride 0.9% and infused over not less than 1 hr

• *Child over 1 month:* By mouth $30-60$ mg/kg daily in divided doses; IM, slow IV $10-20$ mg/kg daily in divided doses

Available forms include: Capsules 500 mg; injection 300 mg/ml

Side effects/adverse reactions:

CV: Hypotension (rapid IV)

HAEM: Leucopenia, eosinophilia, agranulocytosis, thrombocytopenia

GI: Nausea, vomiting, abdominal pain, tenesmus, diarrhoea, *pseudomembranous colitis*, increased asparatate aminotransferase, alanine aminotransferase, bilirubin, alkaline phosphatase, jaundice

INTEG: Rash, urticaria, pruritus, erythema multiforme

Contraindications: Hypersensitivity, sensitivity to clindamycin, diarrhoeal states

Precautions: Renal disease, liver

disease; to be reserved for serious infections due to risk of antibiotic associated colitis

Pharmacokinetics:
By mouth: Peak 45 min, duration 6 hr
IM: Peak 3 hr, duration 8–12 hr Half-life 5.4 ± 1 hr, metabolised in liver, excreted in urine, bile, faeces as active, inactive metabolites, excreted in breast milk. Does not cross blood/brain barrier in therapeutically effective quantities

Interactions/incompatibilities:
• Increased neuromuscular blockade: non-depolarising muscle relaxants
• Decreased action of: neostigmine, pyridostigmine
• Decreased absorption of lincomycin: kaolin

Treatment of overdose: Supportive symptomatic care

NURSING CONSIDERATIONS

Assess:
• Allergies before treatment, reaction of each medication; note allergies on chart; notify all people giving drugs
• Any patient with compromised renal system; drug is excreted slowly in poor renal system function; toxicity may occur rapidly
• Culture and sensitivity before drug therapy
• Drug level in impaired hepatic, renal systems
• BP, pulse in patient receiving drug parenterally

Administer:
• IV by infusion only; do not administer bolus dose
• IM deep injection
• Orally with at least 200 ml water

Perform/provide:
• Adequate intake of fluids (2 litres daily) during diarrhoea episodes

Evaluate:
• Urinalysis for impaired renal function
• Therapeutic response: decreased temperature, negative culture and sensitivity
• Bowel pattern before, during treatment
• Skin eruptions, itching, dermatitis
• Respiratory status: rate, character, wheezing, tightness in chest

Teach patient/family:
• To take oral drug with full glass of water; may be taken with food if GI symptoms occur
• Aspects of drug therapy: need to complete entire course of medication to ensure organism death (10–14 days); culture may be taken after completed course of medication
• To report sore throat, fever, fatigue; could indicate superimposed infection
• That drug must be taken in equal intervals around clock to maintain blood levels
• To notify clinician or nurse of diarrhoea

---

lindane (gamma benzene hexachloride)

Quellada
Func. class.: Scabicide
Chem. class.: Chlorinated hydrocarbon (synthetic)
Legal class.: P

Action: Stimulates nervous system of arthropods, resulting in seizures, death of organism
Uses: Scabies, lice (body/head/pubic), nits
Dosage and routes:
Scabies

• Apply to skin surfaces excluding face and scalp, wash off after 24 hr; reapply after 7 days if needed

Lice

• Apply shampoo to dry hair, leave for 4 min, add water to form lather, rinse and dry

Available forms include: Lotion 1%, shampoo 1%

Side effects/adverse reactions:

INTEG: Irritation

CNS: Tremors, convulsions, stimulation, dizziness (ingestion or systemic absorption)

Contraindications: Hypersensitivity, pregnancy, young children, patients with known seizure disorders, broken or infected skin, low body weight

Precautions: Avoid contact with eyes and mucous membranes; no more than 2 applications/course

Pharmacokinetics: Stored in body fat, metabolised in liver, excreted in urine, faeces

Interactions/incompatibilities:

• Simultaneous application of creams, ointments, or oils may enhance absorption

NURSING CONSIDERATIONS

Assess:

• Signs of infection: scabies between toes and fingers, tracking, blisters, irritation

• Lice, nits, itching inflamed skin patches

Administer:

• To body areas, scalp only; do not apply to face, lips, mouth, eyes, any mucous membrane, anus, or meatus

• Topical corticosteroids as ordered to decrease contact dermatitis

• Lotions of menthol or phenol to control itching

• Topical antibiotics for infection

Perform/provide:

• Isolation until areas on skin, scalp have cleared and treatment is completed

• Removal of nits by using a fine-tooth comb rinsed in vinegar after treatment

Evaluate:

• Area of body involved, including crusts, nits, brownish trails on skin, itching papules in skin folds

Teach patient/family:

• To wash all inhabitants' clothing, using insecticide; preventive treatment may be required of all persons living in same house, using lotion or shampoo to decrease spread of infection

• That itching may continue for 4−6 weeks

• That drug must be reapplied if accidently washed off or treatment will be ineffective

• Do not apply to face

• Treat sexual contact simultaneously

---

liothyronine sodium (T₃)

Tri-iodothyronine injection, Tertroxin

Func. class.: Thyroid hormone

Chem. class.: Levoisomer of triiodothyronine

Legal class.: POM

Action: Increases metabolic rates, increases cardiac output, O_2 consumption, body temperature, blood volume, growth, development at cellular level

Uses: Severe hypothyroid states

Dosage and routes:

• *Adult:* By mouth 10−20 mcg daily increased gradually to 60 mcg daily in divided doses

• *Child:* Adult dose reduced in proportion to body weight

• *Elderly:* Initial dose 5 mcg daily, increased gradually as necessary

Hypothyroid coma

• IV 5−20 mcg by slow injection repeated every 4−12 hr if necessary

Available forms include: Tablets 20 mcg, injection 20 mcg
Side effects/adverse reactions:
INTEG: Sweating, flushing
CNS: Restlessness, excitability, tremors, headache
CV: Tachycardia, palpitations, angina, arrhythmias, heart failure (overdose)
GI: Vomiting, diarrhoea
MISC: Weight loss, heat intolerance
MS: Muscle cramp, weakness
Precautions: Cardiovascular disorders, elderly, adrenal insufficiency (give corticosteroids first)
Pharmacokinetics:
By mouth: Peak 12−48 hr, half-life 1−2 days
Interactions/incompatibilities:
• Decreased absorption of liothyronine: colestipol, cholestyramine
• Increased effects of: anticoagulants, tricyclic antidepressants
Clinical assessment:
• Thyroid function tests
NURSING CONSIDERATIONS
Assess:
• BP, pulse before each dose
• Fluid balance
Administer:
• In morning if possible as a single dose to decrease sleeplessness
• At same time each day to maintain drug level
Perform/provide:
• Removal of medication 4 weeks before radioactive iodine uptake test
Evaluate:
• Therapeutic response: absence of depression
• Increased weight loss, diuresis, pulse, appetite
• Absence of constipation, peripheral oedema, cold intolerance, pale, cool dry skin, brittle nails, alopecia, coarse hair, menorrhagia, night blindness, paraesthesia, syncope, stupor, coma, carotenaemia skin, rosy cheeks
• Increased nervousness, excitability, irritability, which may indicate too high dose of medication, usually after 1−3 weeks of treatment
• Cardiac status: angina, palpitation, chest pain, change in vital signs−seek medical advice
Teach patient/family:
• Hair loss will occur in child, but is temporary
• Report excitability, irritability, anxiety, which indicates overdose
• That hypothyroid child will show almost immediate behaviour/personality change
• That treatment drug is not to be taken to reduce weight
• To avoid non-prescribed medication containing iodine, read labels
• To avoid iodine in food; salt-iodinized, soya beans, tofu, turnips, some seafood, some breads

liquid paraffin

Petrolagar, combination product
Func. class.: Laxative
Chem. class.: Petroleum hydrocarbon
Legal class.: P

Action: Eases passage of stool by lubricating and softening
Uses: Constipation
Dosage and routes:
• *Adult:* By mouth 10−30 ml as needed
Available forms include: Oil emulsion
Side effects/adverse reactions:
GI: Nausea, anal seepage of paraffin and consequent irritation
RESP: Lipoid pneumonia
MISC: Granulomatous reactions caused by absorption (especially from emulsion)

Contraindications: Hypersensitivity, children under 3 yr abdominal pain, nausea/vomiting, prolonged use
Pharmacokinetics: Excreted in faeces
Interactions/incompatibilities:
• May decrease absorption of: fat-soluble vitamins
NURSING CONSIDERATIONS
Administer:
• Alone for better absorption; not within 1 hr of other drugs or within 1 hr of antacids, milk, or cimetidine
• In morning or evening (oral dose)
Evaluate:
• Therapeutic response: decrease in constipation
• Cause of constipation; identify whether fluids, bulk, or exercise is missing from patient's diet and lifestyle
• Nausea, vomiting; if these symptoms occur, drug should be discontinued
Teach patient/family:
• Not to use laxatives for long-term therapy; bowel tone will be lost
• That normal bowel movements do not always occur daily
• Not to use in presence of abdominal pain, nausea, vomiting
• Notify clinician if constipation unrelieved or if symptoms of electrolyte imbalance occur: muscle cramps, pain, weakness, dizziness
• Avoid prolonged use

---

lisinopril

Zestril, Carace, combination products
Func. class.: Angiotensin converting enzyme (ACE) inhibitor
Chem. class.: Lysine analogue of enalaprilat
Legal class.: POM

Action: Inhibits angiotensin converting enzyme, preventing conversion of angiotensin I to angiotensin II
Uses: Hypertension, congestive heart failure
Dosage and routes:
Hypertension
• *Adult:* By mouth initially 2.5 mg daily; maintenance 10–20 mg daily, maximum 40 mg daily
Congestive heart failure
• *Adult:* Initially 2.5 mg daily under hospital supervision, adjusted according to response within the range 5–20 mg daily
Available forms include: Tablets 2.5, 5, 10, 20 mg
Side effects/adverse reactions:
CVS: Hypotension, chest pain, palpitations
GI: Nausea, diarrhoea
GU: Renal insufficiency, impotence
INTEG: Rash, angioedema
CNS: Dizziness, headache, fatigue, asthenia
RESP: Cough, possible airways obstruction due to angioedema
Contraindications: Hypersensitivity, pregnancy, aortic stenosis, cor pulmonale or outflow tract obstruction, known or suspected renovascular disease
Precautions: Lactation, renal disease, peripheral vascular or cerebrovascular disease, ischaemic heart disease, congestive heart failure, volume depletion
Pharmacokinetics: Peak 6–8 hr, excreted unchanged in urine

Interactions/incompatibilities:
• Increased hypotensive effect: diuretics, other antihypertensives, alcohol, anaesthetics, antidepressants, anxiolytics, baclofen, levodopa, phenothiazines
• Decreased hypotensive effects when used with: NSAIDs, carbenoxolone, corticosteroids, oestrogens, oral contraceptives
• Increased potassium levels: potassium salt substitutes, potassium-sparing diuretics, potassium supplements
• Possibly increased toxicity: NSAIDs, lithium

Clinical assessment:
• Assess renal function before and during therapy

Treatment of overdose: Supportive symptomatic care

NURSING CONSIDERATIONS
Assess:
• Establish baseline fluid balance and assessment of renal function and electrolytes

Administer:
• Preferably at night to avoid possible postural hypotension
• Under medical supervision at start of treatment

Evaluate:
• Blood pressure and pulse 4 hrly when established drug dosage
• Hrly observations on instigation of drug; marked hypotension may occur
• For postural hypotension
• Hypertensive control to gauge maintenance dose
• Daily weight (often given with diuretictherapy)
• Control of symptoms of congestive cardiac failure — oedema dyspnoea and productive cough

Perform/provide:
• Bed rest at start of drug therapy
• Safe environment if postural hypotension occurs

Teach patient/family:
• Seek medical advice if symptoms recur
• To avoid sudden ceasation of therapy
• Possible side-effect — care on rising/standing up; headaches, fatigue are common
• General advice to manage symptoms of cardiac failure

---

lithium carbonate

Camcolit, Liskonum Phasal, Priadel
Func. class.: Antimanic
Chem. class.: Alkali metal ion salt
Legal class.: POM

Action: May alter sodium, potassium ion transport across cell membrane biogenic amines of noradrenaline, serotonin in CNS areas involved in emotional responses

Uses: Mania, prevention of manic depressive illness or recurrent depression

Dosage and routes:
• *Adult:* By mouth initially 0.4–2 g daily, adjusted to maintain plasma levels at 0.4–1.0 mmol lithium/litre 12 hr after a dose; concentrations in the lower end of the range are required in the elderly or during maintenance therapy

Available forms include: Tablets 250 mg; tablets modified-release 200, 300, 400, 450 mg

Side effects/adverse reactions:
CNS: Headache, drowsiness, dizziness, tremors, ataxia, cognitive impairment, slurred speech, incoordination, hyperreflexia, psychosis, confusion, stupor, memory loss, clonic movements; convulsions, coma (severe overdosage)
GI: Anorexia, nausea, vomiting, diarrhoea
GU: Polyuria, polydipsia, oedema,

renal impairment (long-term)
CV: Hypotension, ECG changes, arrhythmias, circulatory collapse
INTEG: Acne, rash, exacerbation of psoriasis
HAEM: Leucocytosis
EENT: Tinnitus, blurred vision
ENDO: Hypothyroidism, hyperparathyroidism
MS: Muscle weakness
MISC: Weight gain, antinuclear antibody formation

Contraindications: Renal disease, cardiovascular disease, untreated hypothyroidism, sodium imbalance, dehydration, debilitation, children, intercurrent infection

Precautions: Elderly, pregnancy (avoid if possible), breast feeding (avoid), myasthenia, disturbances of salt/fluid balance (e.g. vomiting, diarrhoea, excessive sweating), surgery
• Different preparations vary in bioavailability: a change in preparation requires monitoring and stabilisation as for initiation of therapy

Pharmacokinetics:
By mouth: Onset rapid, peak ½–4 hr, half-life 7–36 hr depending on age; crosses blood-brain barrier, excreted in urine, enters breast milk, well absorbed by oral method

Interactions/incompatibilities:
• Increased plasma lithium concentration: NSAIDs, angiotensin converting enzyme inhibitors, diuretics, tetracycline
• Decreased plasma-lithium concentration: sodium bicarbonate, acetazolamide, aminophylline
• Increased toxicity: antidepressants, anti-epileptics, diltiazem, methyldopa, metoclopramide, metronidazole, sumatriptan, verapamil
• Possibly decreased effects of: antidiabetics, diuretics, neostigmine, pyridostigmine

• Possibly increased effects of: muscle relaxants

Clinical assessment:
• Monitor plasma lithium weekly initially and for one month after stable dosage achieved, then every 1–3 months
• Monitor cardiac, renal, and thyroid function periodically

Treatment of overdose: Supportive symptomatic care; forced diuresis with an osmotic diuretic or sodium lactate or bicarbonate infusion, or dialysis for severe intoxication

NURSING CONSIDERATIONS

Assess:
• Baseline weight
• Sodium intake; decreased sodium intake with decreased fluid intake may lead to lithium retention; increased sodium and fluids may decrease lithium retention

Administer:
• With meals to avoid GI upset; do not crush modified-release preps, do not administer with hot drinks
• Adequate fluids (2–3 litres daily) to prevent dehydration during initial treatment, 1–2 litres daily during maintenance

Evaluate:
• Observe for CNS changes
• Signs of oedema

Teach patient/family:
• Symptoms of minor toxicity: vomiting, diarrhoea, poor coordination, fine motor tremors, weakness, lassitude; major toxicity: coarse tremors, severe thirst, tinnitus, dilute urine
• Action, dosage, side effects; when to notify clinician
• To monitor urine specific gravity
• That contraception is necessary since lithium may harm fetus
• Not to operate machinery until lithium levels are stable
• Maintain adequate fluid intake avoid dietary changes

lofepramine

Gamanil

Func. class.: Antidepressant
Chem. class.: Tricyclic
Legal class.: POM

Action: Block reuptake of biogenic amines from nerve endings in CNS; action in depression not fully understood

Uses: Depressive illness

Dosage and routes:

• *Adult:* By mouth, 140−210 mg daily in divided doses

Available forms include: Tablets, 70 mg (as hydrochloride)

Side effects/adverse reactions:

HAEM: Agranulocytosis, leucopenia, eosinophilia, purpura, thrombocytopenia

CNS: Headache, agitation, paraesthesia, tremor, confusion, hypomania, convulsions, dizziness, drowsiness

META: Blood sugar and weight changes

GI: Nausea, dry mouth, constipation

GU: Difficulty with micturition, changes in sexual function

INTEG: Sweating, rashes

CV: Postural hypotension, tachycardia, syncope

Contraindications: Hypersensitivity, recent myocardial infarction, arrhythmias, heart block, mania, porphyria, pregnancy and lactation (unless compelling medical reason), severe renal or hepatic impairment

Precautions: Diabetes, cardiac disease, epilepsy, renal or hepatic impairment, thyroid disease, psychoses, urinary retention; avoid abrupt cessation of therapy; caution in anaesthesia, narrow angle glaucoma, prostatic hypertrophy, elderly

Pharmacokinetics: Absorbed from GI tract, extensively demethylated during first pass metabolism in liver to primary metabolite desipramine

Interactions/incompatibilities:

• Concurrent administration with or within 2 weeks of cessation of treatment with MAOIs should be avoided

• Increased toxicity: alcohol, anaesthetic agents, antihypertensives, antihistamines, antimuscarinics, anxiolytics, diuretics, oral contraceptives, phenothiazines, sympathomimetics

• Increased effects of lofepramine: cimetidine, diltiazem, disulfiram, verapamil

• Decreased effects of lofepramine: antiepileptics, oral contraceptives

• Decreased effects of: adrenergic neurone blockers, antiepileptics, clonidine, sublingual nitrates

Treatment of overdose: Supportive symptomatic care

NURSING CONSIDERATIONS

Assess:

• All drugs patient is on for compatibility

• Pulse and blood pressure

Administer:

• Orally as directed

• Laxatives if necessary

Perform/provide:

• Store at room temperature in own packaging to protect from light and moisture

• Frequent drinks to prevent a dry mouth

• Diet high in fibre to alleviate constipation

Evaluate:

• Therapeutic response; decreased depression

• Most side effects are mild and transient, agitation, dizziness, postual hypotention, tachycardic sweating

Teach patient/family:

• To take high fibre/bulk diet

- That alcohol should be avoided
- That therapeutic effect may take up to 2 weeks
- Not to discontinue medication without medical advice. Drug should be tapered off slowly
- To take other medication only if directed by clinician. The effect of lofepramine is increased and decreased by several drugs and also effect other drugs

---

lomustine

CCNU
Func. class.: Antineoplastic alkylating agent
Chem. class.: Nitrosourea
Legal class.: POM

Action: Alkylates DNA, RNA; inhibits enzymes that allow synthesis of amino acids in proteins; also responsible for cross-linking DNA strands

Uses: Hodgkin's disease resistant to conventional therapy, other lymphomas, melanomas, multiple myeloma; brain, lung, bladder, kidney, gastrointestinal tract, breast, cervix tumours

Dosage and routes:
- *Adult:* By mouth 120–130 mg/m^2 as a single dose every 6 weeks. Do not give repeat dose unless WBC is above 4000/mm^3, platelet count above 100,000/mm^3
- *Children:* Only under exceptional circumstances and expert supervision. Dose as for adults

Available forms include: Capsules 10, 40 mg

Side effects/adverse reactions:
HAEM: Thrombocytopenia, leucopenia, anaemia, possibility of permanent marrow damage with prolonged use
GI: Nausea, vomiting, anorexia, stomatitis, raised liver enzymes
INTEG: Loss of scalp hair
CNS: Confusion, lethargy

Contraindications: Hypersensitivity, severe bone marrow depression, pregnancy, breast feeding, failure to respond to other nitrosoureas

Precautions: Radiation therapy

Pharmacokinetics: Metabolised in liver, excreted in urine; half-life 16–48 hr, 50% protein bound, crosses blood-brain barrier, appears in breast milk. Maximal bone marrow depression 4–6 weeks post dose, may last several weeks

Interactions/incompatibilities:
- Increased metabolism of this drug: phenobarbitone

Clinical assessment:
- Full blood count, differential, platelet count weekly; withhold drug if WBC is below 4000 or platelet count is below 100,000
- Liver function tests before, and monthly during therapy

Treatment of overdose: Supportive, no specific antidote. Blood products or filgrastim for marrow suppression

NURSING CONSIDERATIONS

Assess:
- Baseline temperature
- Fluid balance

Administer:
- Medications preferably by oral route unless central or Hickman line is available
- Anti-emetic 30–60 min before giving drug to prevent vomiting
- Antibiotics for prophylaxis of infection only if indicated
- By slow IV infusion using appropriate gauge needle
- Avoid IM subcutaneous or IV routes for other drugs to reduce the risk of infection
- Topical or systemic analgesics for pain
- Local or systemic drugs for infection if appropriate

Perform/provide:

- Strict medical asepsis, protective isolation if WBC levels are low
- Special skin care
- Increase fluid intake to 2−3 litres daily to prevent urate deposits, calculi formation
- Strict oral hygiene

Evaluate:
- Bleeding: haematuria, bruising or petechiae, mucosa or orifices 8 hrly
- Dyspnoea, rales, unproductive cough, chest pain, tachypnoea
- Food preferences; list likes, dislikes
- Inflammation of mucosa, breaks in skin
- Buccal cavity 8 hrly for dryness, sores or ulceration, white patches, oral pain, bleeding, dysphagia
- Symptoms indicating severe allergic reaction: rash, pruritus, urticaria, purpuric skin lesions, itching, flushing

Teach patient/family:
- Of protective isolation precautions if indicated
- To report any complaints or side effects to nurse or clinician
- To report any changes in breathing or coughing
- To avoid foods with citric acid, hot or rough texture
- To report any bleeding, white spots or ulcerations in mouth to clinician; tell patient to examine mouth daily

---

loperamide HCl

Arret, Diocalm Ultra, Imodium
Func. class.: Antidiarrhoeal
Chem. class.: Piperidine derivative
Legal class.: P, POM

Action: Direct action on intestinal muscles to decrease GI peristalsis
Uses: Diarrhoea
Dosage and routes:
Acute diarrhoea

- *Adult:* By mouth 4 mg, then 2 mg after each loose stool, not to exceed 16 mg daily for up to 5 days
- *Child 4 to 8 yr:* By mouth 1 mg 4 times daily for up to 3 days
- *Child 9−12 yr:* By mouth 2 mg 4 times a day for up to 5 days

Chronic diarrhoea
- *Adult:* By mouth 4−8 mg daily in divided doses initially, adjust according to response

Available forms include: Capsules 2 mg; liquid 1 mg/5 ml
Side effects/adverse reactions:
CNS: Dizziness, drowsiness, fatigue
GI: Abdominal cramps, dry mouth, bloating, ileus
INTEG: Rash, urticaria
Contraindications: Hypersensitivity, severe ulcerative colitis, pseudomembranous colitis abdominal distension, ileus, constipation
Precautions: Pregnancy, lactation, children, liver disease, dehydration, dysentery
Pharmacokinetics:
By mouth: Onset ½−1 hr, duration 4−5 hr, half-life 7−14 hr; metabolised in liver, excreted in faeces as unchanged drug, small amount in urine
Clinical assessment:
- Electrolytes if on long-term therapy (K, Na, CI)

NURSING CONSIDERATIONS
Assess:
- Fluid balance
- Diet

Administer:
- Orally in capsule and liquid forms
- Discontinue if acute diarrhoea persists longer than 5 days in adults and 3 days in a child, and seek further medical advise. Seek advice earlier if necessary

Perform/provide:
- Store a dilution of syrup for up to 2 weeks at 20°C

• Diet that does not cause increased peristalsis or irritation. Especially in chronic, long-term use

Evaluate:
• Therapeutic response; decreased diarrhoea
• Input and output of fluid especially in children. Observe for dehydration
• Bowel patterns before; rebound constipation
• Dehydration, especially children and elderly
• Potentially more serious condition — continuous diarrhoea, abdominal cramps distention
• Side effects urticaria, rash

Teach patient/family:
• That overuse will cause constipation
• To seek medical advice if children appear 'ill'
• To wash, dry gently and use a suitable cream on sore bottoms

---

loprazolam

Func. class.: Sedative, hypnotic
Chem. class.: Benzodiazepine
Legal class.: CD (Sch 4) POM

Action: Depresses CNS with sedative effect
Uses: Short-term treatment of insomnia
Dosage and routes:
• *Adult:* By mouth, 1 mg at bedtime; may be increased to 1.5–2 mg in severe insomnia; maximum dose in elderly or debilitated patients, 1 mg
Available forms include: Tablets, 1 mg
Side effects/adverse reactions:
CNS: Drowsiness, headaches, dizziness, and lightheadness the following day; ataxia, confusion, especially in elderly; amnesia;

dependence; rarely excitement, depression, aggression
GI: Nausea, jaundice
GU: Urinary retention, changes in libido
INTEG: Rash
HAEM: Blood dyscrasias
CV: Hypotension
EENT: Blurred vision
Contraindications: Acute pulmonary insufficiency, respiratory depression, phobic or obsessional states, chronic psychosis, mental depression, myasthenia gravis, hypersensitivity to benzodiazepines
Precautions: History of alcohol or drug abuse or personality disorder; cerebrovascular disease, renal or hepatic impairment; pregnancy, lactation; reduce dose in elderly or debilitated patients; avoid prolonged use and abrupt withdrawal
Pharmacokinetics: Absorbed from GI, metabolised to desmethyldiazepam, half-life reported as 7 to 15 hr

Interactions/incompatibilities:
• Enhanced CNS effects: alcohol, anaesthetics, opioid analgesics, antidepressants, antihistamines, α-blockers, antipsychotics, baclofen, cimetidine
• Possibly enhanced effects of: antihypertensives
• Possibly reduced effects of: levodopa

NURSING CONSIDERATIONS
Assess:
• Pulse and blood pressure
• All drugs patient is taking for compatibility

Administer:
• Orally at bedtime

Evaluate:
• Therapeutic response; decreased insomia
• Side effects, particularly drowsiness, dizziness, headache, ataxia, nausea the following morning
• For suicidal tendencies which

may be released in depressed patients
• Drug dependency if used long term

Teach patient/family:
• That treatment is for a few weeks only
• Not to take alcohol
• To take other medication only if directed by clinician (enhances effect of several drugs and alcohol)
• Not to discontinue medication without medical advice. Drug should be tapered off slowly
• To avoid driving or use of machinery if drowsiness or dizziness occurs
• Not to sleep during the day
• That suitable physical activity may enhance sleep pattern
• Not to drink coffee, take or do anything at night to interfere with sleep

---

lorazepam

NHS Ativan
Func. class.: Hypnotic, Anxiolytic
Chem. class.: Benzodiazepine
Legal class.: CD (Sch 4) POM

Action: Depresses subcortical levels of CNS, including limbic system and reticular formation
Uses: Anxiety, insomnia in psychiatric or organic disorders, premedication, status epilepticus
Dosage and routes:
Anxiety
• *Adult:* By mouth 1–4 mg daily in divided doses, not to exceed 10 mg daily; IM/IV 0.025–0.03 mg/kg every 6 hr if necessary
• *Elderly:* By mouth 1–2 mg daily
Insomnia
• *Adult:* By mouth 1–2 mg at bedtime
Premedication
• *Adult:* By mouth 1–4 mg; IM/IV 0.05 mg/kg

• *Child over 5 yr:* By mouth 0.5–2.5 mg
Status epilepticus
• *Adult:* IV 4 mg
• *Child:* IV 2 mg
Available forms include: Injection 4 mg/ml; tablets 1, 2.5 mg
Side effects/adverse reactions:
CNS: Dizziness, drowsiness, confusion, headache, hangover, restlessness, ataxia, depression, sleep disturbances, hallucinations
GI: Nausea, vomiting
INTEG: Rash
CV: Hypertension, hypotension
EENT: Blurred vision, diplopia
HAEM: Blood dyscrasias
Contraindications: Hypersensitivity to benzodiazepines, acute pulmonary insufficiency, respiratory depression, phobic or obsessional states, chronic psychosis, mental depression
Precautions: History of alcohol or drug abuse or personality disorder; cerebrovascular disease, renal or hepatic impairment; pregnancy; lactation; reduce dose in elderly or debilitated patients; avoid prolonged use and abrupt withdrawal
Pharmacokinetics:
By mouth: Peak 1–3 hr, duration 3–6 hr, metabolised by liver, excreted by kidneys, breast milk, half-life 12 hr
Interactions/incompatibilities:
• Enhanced CNS effects: alcohol, anaesthetics, opioid analgesics, antidepressants, antihistamines, α-blockers, antipsychotics, baclofen, cimetidine
• Possibly enhanced effects of: antihypertensives
• Possibly reduced effects of: levodopa
NURSING CONSIDERATIONS
Assess:
• Weight
Administer:
• Orally
• Intramuscular injection after

diluting with equal volume of sodium chloride 0.9% or water for injection
• Intravenous directly into vein or through 3-way tap in giving set

Perform/provide:
• Store injections in refrigerator 0−4°C protect from light
• Assist with mobility
• Safety measures; e.g. side rails

Evaluate:
• Drug dependency if used long term
• Blood pressure and pulse, also respiration if IM or IV administration

Teach patient/family:
• That treatment should be for short-term use only
• To take other medication only if directed by clinician (enhances effect of several drugs and alcohol)
• Not to take alcohol
• Not to discontinue medication without medical advice. Drug should be tapered off slowly
• To avoid driving or hazardous activities if dizziness or drowsiness occurs
• That suitable physical activity may aid sleep
• To seek psychiatric help if necessary

---

lormetazepam

Func. class.: Sedative-hypnotic
Chem. class.: Benzodiazepine
Legal class.: CD (Sch 4) POM

Action: Depresses CNS with sedative effect

Uses: Short treatment of insomnia

Dosage and routes:
• *Adult:* By mouth, 0.5−1.5 mg at bedtime; reduce dose to 0.5 mg in elderly patients

Available forms include: Tablets, 0.5, 1 mg

Side effects/adverse reactions:
CNS: Drowsiness, headache, dizziness and lightheadness the following day; ataxia, confusion, especially in elderly; amnesia; dependence; rarely excitement, aggression or uncovering suicidal tendencies
GI: Nausea, jaundice
GU: Urinary retention, changes in libido
CVS: Hypotension
INTEG: Rash
HAEM: Blood dyscrasias
EENT: Blurred vision

Contraindications: Acute pulmonary insufficiency, hypersensitivity to benzodiazepines, myasthenia gravis, respiratory depression, phobic or obsessional states, chronic psychosis, mental depression

Precautions: History of alcohol or drug abuse or personality disorder; cerebrovascular disease, renal or hepatic impairment; pregnancy, lactation; reduce dose in elderly or debilitated patients; avoid prolonged use and abrupt withdrawal

Pharmacokinetics: Rapidly absorbed from GI tract, metabolised to inactive glucuronide, half-life reported as 11 hr

Interactions/incompatibilities:
• Enhanced CNS effects: alcohol, anaesthetics, opioid analgesics, antidepressants, antihistamines, α-blockers, antipsychotics, baclofen, cimetidine
• Possibly enhanced effects of: antihypertensives
• Possibly reduced effects of: levodopa

NURSING CONSIDERATIONS

Assess:
• Pulse and blood pressure
• All drugs patient is taking for compatibility

Administer:
• Orally at bedtime

Evaluate:

- Therapeutic response
- Side effects, particularly drowsiness, headache, ataxia, nausea the following morning
- For suicidal tendencies which may be released in depressed patients
- Drug dependency if used long term

Teach patient/family:
- That treatment is for a few weeks only
- Avoid alcohol
- To take other medication only if by clinician. Enhanced effect of several drugs and alcohol
- To avoid driving or use of machinery if drowsiness or dizziness occurs
- Not to discontinue medication without medical advice. Drug should be tapered off slightly
- Not to sleep during the day
- That suitable physical activity may enhance sleep pattern
- Not to drink coffee, take or do anything at night that may interfere with sleep

---

loxapine

Loxapac
Func. class.: Antipsychotic
Chem. class.: Dibenzoxazepine
Legal class.: POM

Uses: Treatment of acute and chronic psychotic states

Dosage and routes:
- *Adult:* By mouth initially 20–50 mg daily in 2 divided doses, then increased over 7–10 days to 60–100 mg daily in 2 to 4 doses, until control achieved. Maximum 250 mg daily. Maintenance doses should be adjusted to the needs of the patient

Available forms include: Capsules 10, 25, 50 mg (as succinate)

Side effects/adverse reactions:
CNS: Dizziness, drowsiness, faintness, headache, staggering gait, muscle twitching, weakness, paraesthesia, confusional states, extrapyramidal reactions, akathisia, tardive dyskinesia, neuroleptic malignant syndrome
INTEG: Dermatitis, oedema, pruritus, seborrhoea, flushing
CV: Tachycardia, hypotension, hypertension, syncope
GI: Nausea, vomiting, constipation
EENT: Dry mouth, nasal congestion, blurred vision (anticholinergic effects)
RESP: Dyspnoea
MISC: Weight gain or loss, ptosis, hyperpyrexia, abnormal thirst

Contraindications: Comatose or semi-comatose patients, severe drug-induced depressed states, hypersensitivity, children, porphyria

Precautions: Convulsive disorders, cardiovascular disease, pregnancy, glaucoma, urinary retention; antiemetic effect of this drug may mask signs of overdosage of toxic drugs and obscure conditions such as intestinal obstruction, brain tumour

Interactions/incompatibilities:
- Increased anticholinergic effect: anticholinergic antiparkinsonian agents, other anticholinergic drugs (tricyclic antidepressants, antihistamines, other antipsychotics)
- Increased CNS depression: alcohol, anxiolytics and hypnotics, opioid analgesics
- Possibly increased effects of: antihypertensives
- Possibly decreased effects of: anti-epileptics

Treatment of overdose: Gastric lavage and general supportive measures

NURSING CONSIDERATIONS:
Administer:

• Ensuring dose is swallowed
Evaluate:
• Therapeutic effect
• For anti-emetic effect masking other conditions
• For extra pyramidal symptoms
Teach/patient/family:
• About side effects including extra-pyramidal symptoms and skin reaction
• Of need to take medication as prescribed (doses may be adjusted)

lypressin

Syntopressin
Func. class.: Pituitary hormone
Chem. class.: Lysine vasopressin
Legal class.: POM

Action: Promotes reabsorption of water by action on renal tubular epithelium, smooth muscles causing constriction with a vaso-pressor effect
Uses: Pituitary diabetes insipidus
Dosage and routes:
• *Adult:* Intranasal 2.5−5 units in one or both nostrils 3−7 times daily
Available forms include: Nasal spray 50 units/ml
Side effects/adverse reactions:
EENT: Nasal irritation, congestion, mucosal ulceration
GI: Nausea, abdominal pain, urge to defaecate
CV: Increased BP
Contraindications: Coronary heart disease, anaesthesia with halothane or cyclopropane
Precautions: Pregnancy, arteriosclerosis, peripheral vascular disease, hypertension, epilepsy, heart failure, asthma, migraine, renal failure
Pharmacokinetics:
Intranasal: Onset 1 hr duration 3−8 hr, half-life 15 min: metabolised in liver, kidneys, excreted in urine

Interactions/incompatibilities:
• Possibly enhanced effect of lypressin: carbamazepine, chlorpromamide, clofibrate
• Possibly decreased effect of lypressin: lithium
NURSING CONSIDERATIONS
Assess:
• Baseline weight
• Fluid balance
Evaluate:
• Therapeutic response: absence of severe thirst, decreased urine output, osmolality
• Weight daily, check for oedema in extremities, if water retention is severe, diuretic may be prescribed
• Water intoxication: lethargy, behavioural changes, disorientation, neuromuscular excitability
Teach patient/family:
• To clear nasal passages before using drug, not to inhale spray
• Use nasal spray within one month of opening
• To carry drug at all times
• All aspects of drug: action, side effects, dose, when to notify clinician

lysuride maleate ▼

Revanil
Func. class.: Dopamine agonist
Chem. class.: Ergot alkaloid derivative
Legal class.: POM

Action: Direct stimulation of surviving dopamine receptor
Uses: Parkinsonism
Dosage and routes:
• *Adult:* By mouth initially 200 mcg with food at bedtime, gradually increasing at weekly intervals by 200 mcg daily to a maximum of 5 mg daily in divided doses with food
Available forms include: Tablets 200 mcg

Side effects/adverse reactions:
CV: Hypotension, Raynaud's syndrome
GI: Nausea, vomiting, abdominal pain, constipation
CNS: Dizziness, headache, drowsiness, lethargy, malaise, psychotic reactions, hallucinations
INTEG: Transient exanthemata
Contraindications: Severe disturbances of peripheral circulation, coronary insufficiency, porphyria
Precautions: Pituitary tumour, pregnancy, history of psychosis
Interactions/incompatibilities
• Possibly reduced effects of both drugs: antipsychotics
NURSING CONSIDERATIONS
Assess:
• Blood pressure before, during and after treatment
Administer:
• Orally following the dosage regime for suitable gradual introduction
• Commence at bedtime and increase dosage until equal day and night time dosages are established
• With food to prevent nausea and vomiting
Evaluate:
• Therapeutic response: decreased dyskinesia, slow movement and excressive salivation
Teach patient/family:
• To stand up slowly to prevent postural hypotension
• That alcohol should not be taken, decreases effect of lysuride maleate
• Not to drive or operate machinery if dizziness occurs
• It may be necessary to use additional contraception if oral contraception is used or if female is of child bearing age

magaldrate (aluminum magnesium complex)

Dynese
Func. class.: Antacid
Chem. class.: Aluminium/ magnesium hydroxide
Legal class.: GSL

Action: Neutralises gastric acidity
Uses: Antacid
Dosage and routes:
• *Adult:* By mouth suspension 800−1600 mg (5−10 ml) after meals and at bedtime or as required
• *Child:* 400−800 mg (2.5−5 ml) after meals, at bedtime or as required
Available forms include: Suspension 800 mg/5 ml
Side effects/adverse reactions:
GI: Constipation, diarrhoea
META: Hypermagnesaemia
Contraindications: Hypersensitivity, hypophosphataemia, renal failure, GI obstruction, porphyria, hypermagnesaemia
Precautions: Renal disease
Pharmacokinetics:
By mouth: Duration 60 min, little absorption, excreted in urine
Interactions/incompatibilities:
• Decreased absorption of: iron salts, phenothiazines, phenytoin, tetracyclines, 4-quinolone antibiotics, rifampicin, isoniazid, pivampicillin, azithromycin, itraconazole, ketoconazole, dipyridamole, bisphosphonates, penicillamine
NURSING CONSIDERATIONS
Administer:
• Between meals
• After shaking suspension
• Laxatives or stool softeners if constipation occurs
Evaluate:
• Therapeutic response: absence of pain, decreased acidity

• Constipation: increase bulk in diet if needed

Teach patient/family:

• The need to eat small regular meals to reduce acidity

---

magnesium carbonate

Func. class.: Antacid
Chem. class.: Magnesium product
Legal class.: GSL (some combinations P or POM) many proprietories NHS

Action: Neutralises gastric acidity
Uses: Hyperacidity, constipation
Dosage and routes:
Antacid

• *Adult:* By mouth 250−500 mg after meals and at bedtime or as required

Laxative

• *Adult:* By mouth 2−5 g
Available forms include: Suspensions, combined preparations
Side effects/adverse reactions:
GI: Diarrhoea, flatulence, cramps, belching
META: Hypermagnesaemia
Contraindications: Hypersensitivity, hypophosphataemia, renal failure, porphyria, intestinal obstruction, hypermagnesaemia
Precautions: Severe renal disease, diarrhoea
Pharmacokinetics:
By mouth: Little absorption, excreted in urine
Interaction/incompatibilities:

• Decreased absorption of: iron salts, phenothiazines, phenytoin, tetracyclines, 4-quinolone antibiotics, rifampicin, isoniazid, pivampicillin, azithromycin, itraconazole, ketoconazole, dipyridamole, bisphosphonates, penicillamine
NURSING CONSIDERATIONS
Assess:

• Dietary habits
Evaluate:

• Attacks of diarrhoea. (Aluminium hydroxide may be prescribed instead)

• Therapeutic response: absence of pain, decreased acidity, decreased constipation

Teach patient/family:

• Not to change antacids unless directed by clinician

• To increase bulk in diet to aid constipation

• Store in tightly covered container

---

magnesium hydroxide/ oxide

Milk of Magnesia, many combination products
Func. class.: Antacid
Chem. class.: Magnesium product
Legal class: GSL

Action: Neutralises gastric acidity
Uses: Antacid, laxative
Dosage and routes:

• *Adult:* By mouth 250 mg−1 g after meals and at bedtime or as required

Laxative

• *Adult:* By mouth 2−4 g
Available forms include: Mixture 550 mg/10 ml
Side effects/adverse reactions:
GI: Diarrhoea
META: Hypermagnesaemia
Contraindications: Hypersensitivity, hypophosphataemia, renal failure, porphyria, intestinal obstruction, hypermagnesaemia
Precautions: Severe renal disease, diarrhoea
Pharmacokinetics:
By mouth: Little absorption, excreted in urine
Interactions/incompatibilities:

• Decreased absorption of: iron salts, phenothiazines, phenytoin, tetracyclines, 4-quinolone antibiotics, rifampicin, isoniazid, piv-ampicillin, azithromycin, itracon-azole, ketoconazole, dipyridamole, bisphosphonates, penicillamine

NURSING CONSIDERATIONS

Assess:

• Cause of acidity or constipation

Administer:

• Aluminium antacids if diarrhoea occurs

Evaluate:

• Therapeutic response: absence of pain, decreased acidity

• Decreased constipation, charac-teristics of stools

Teach patient/family:

• Not to change antacids unless directed by clinician

• Not to take at the same time as antibiotics

• About dietary causes

---

magnesium salts

Citramag, Epsom Salts, Magnesium Sulphate, Magnesium Hydroxide Mixture, Milk of Magnesia, many combination products

Func. class.: Laxative, osmotic

Legal class.: GSL

Action: Increases osmotic press-ure, draws fluid into colon

Uses: Constipation, bowel prep-aration before surgery or examination

Dosage and routes:

• *Adult and child more than 6 yr:*

For bowel preparation:

By mouth, 5−10 g in a tumblerful of water (Magnesium Sulphate); By mouth, 17.7 g as effervescent powder in water at bedtime (Magnesium Citrate);

For constipation:

By mouth, 25 to 50 ml (Magnesium Hydroxide Mixture)

Available forms include: Powder (Magnesium Sulphate), effer-vescent powder (Magnesium Citrate), suspension (Magnesium Hydroxide)

Side effects/adverse reactions:

GI: Gastrointestinal irritation, colic

META: Electrolyte, fluid im-balances

Contraindications: Acute gastro-intestinal conditions

Precautions: Renal impairment (risk of hypermagnesaemia and systemic magnesium toxicity)

NURSING CONSIDERATIONS

Assess:

• Cause of constipation; identify whether fluids, bulk or exercise is missing from diet and lifestyle

• Fluid balance; check for decrease in urinary output

Administer:

• With a full glass of water

Evaluate:

• Therapeutic response: decreased constipation

• Cramping, rectal bleeding, nausea, vomiting; if these symp-toms occur, drug should be discontinued

• Magnesium toxicity: thirst, confusion, decrease in reflexes

Teach patient/family:

• Not to use laxatives for long-term therapy; bowel tone will be lost

• About changes in diet and lifestyle

---

magnesium trisilicate

Func. class.: Antacid

Chem. class.: Magnesium product

Legal class.: GSL

Action: Neutralises gastric acidity

Uses: Dyspepsia

Dosage and routes:

• *Adult:* By mouth 10 ml of mixture, 1−2 tablets (chewed) or 1−5 g of powder 3 times a day, with water

Available forms include: Powder, mixture, tablets, (all compound preparations)

Side effects/adverse reactions:

GI: Diarrhoea

Contraindications: Hypersensitivity to this drug, hypophosphataemia

Precautions: Severe renal disease

Pharmacokinetics:

By mouth: Little absorption

Interactions/incompatibilities:

• Decreased absorption of: tetracyclines, 4-quinolones, isoniazid, rifampicin, biphosphonates chloroquine, hydroxychloroquine, penicillamine, anticholinergics, chlordiazepoxide, cimetidine, corticosteroids, oral iron salts, phenothiazines, phenytoin, fat-soluble vitamins, itraconazole, ketoconazole, fosinopril

NURSING CONSIDERATIONS

Administer:

• Given on an empty stomach, effect lasts for about 40 min. If given 1 hr after meals, effects last for approximately 2 hr

Evaluate:

• Therapeutic response: absence of pain, decreased acidity

• Observe for loose stools. Change to aluminium antacid if diarrhoea occurs

Teach patient/family:

• Not to use non-prescribed antacids unless directed by clinician

---

mannitol

Min-I-Jet Mannitol
Func. class.: Osmotic diuretic
Chem. class.: Hexahydric alcohol
Legal class.: POM

Action: Acts by increasing osmolarity of glomerular filtrate, which raises osmotic pressure of fluid in renal tubules; there is a decrease in reabsorption of water, increase in urinary output

Uses: To promote systemic diuresis in cerebral oedema, decrease intra-ocular pressure, improve renal function in acute renal failure

Dosage and routes:

Oliguria, treatment, renal failure

• *Adult:* IV, 1–2 test doses of 200 mg/kg (50 ml of 25%) over 3–5 min, then 50–100 g daily (maximum 200 g daily) adjusted to maintain urine flow of 30–50 ml/hr

Intraocular pressure/intracranial pressure

• *Adult:* IV 1.5–2 g/kg of a 15%–25% solution over ½–1 hr

• *Children:* 1–2 g/kg of a 15–25% solution over ½–1 hr

Available forms include: Injection IV 10%, 20%, 25%

Side effects/adverse reactions:

GU: Marked diuresis, acute renal failure

CNS: Dizziness, headache, convulsions

GI: Nausea, vomiting, dry mouth, thirst

CV: Oedema, thrombophlebitis, hypotension, hypertension, tachycardia, angina-like chest pains, fever, chills

RESP: Pulmonary oedema

ELECT: Fluid and electrolyte imbalances, acidosis, dehydration

EENT: Blurred vision, decreased intra-ocular pressure

Contraindications: Hypersensitivity, anuria, severe pulmonary congestion, severe dehydration metabolic oedema

Precautions: Dehydration, pregnancy, severe renal disease (test dose of 200 mg/kg body-weight may be required), lactation

Pharmacokinetics:

IV: Onset 30–60 min for diuresis, ½–1 hr for intra-ocular pressure, 25 min for cerebrospinal fluid; duration 2–3 hr for diuresis, 4–6

hr for intra-ocular pressure, 3–8 hr for cerebrospinal fluid; excreted in urine

Interactions/incompatibilities:
• Incompatible with whole blood, in solution or syringe with any other drug or solution

Clinical assessment:
• Electrolytes: potassium, sodium, chloride; include blood urea nitrogen, full blood count, serum creatinine, blood pH, arterial blood gases

Treatment of overdose: Discontinue infusion, correct fluid, electrolyte imbalances, haemodialysis

NURSING CONSIDERATIONS

Assess:
• Rate, depth, rhythm of respiration, effect of exertion

Administer:
• IV in 15%−25% solutions slowly do not mix with blood in transfusion apparatus use in-line filter for solutions of 20−25%

Perform/provide:
• Storage at 20−30°C, storage below 20°C may cause deposition of crystals, if necessary, redissolve crystals by heating to 60°C, cool to blood heat before use

Evaluate:
• Improvement in oedema of feet, legs, sacral area daily if medication is being used in congestive cardiac failure
• Weight, fluid balance daily to determine fluid loss; effect of drug may be decreased if used daily
• BP lying, standing, postural hypotension may occur
• Improvement in CVP 8 hrly
• Signs of metabolic acidosis: drowsiness, restlessness
• Signs of hypokalaemia: postural hypotension, malaise, fatigue, tachycardia, leg cramps, weakness
• Rashes, temperature elevation daily
• Confusion, especially in elderly;

take safety precautions if needed
• Hydration including skin turgor, thirst, dry mucous membranes

Teach patient/family:
• To increase fluid intake 2−3 litres daily unless contraindicated; to rise slowly from lying or sitting position

---

maprotiline HCl

Ludiomil
Func. class.: Antidepressant
Chem. class.: Tetracyclic
Legal class.: POM

Action: Blocks reuptake of noradrenaline into nerve endings, increasing action of noradrenaline on nerve cells

Uses: Depression, especially where sedation is required. Use in children not recommended

Dosage and routes:
• *Adults:* By mouth, initially 25−75 mg daily in 3 divided doses or as a single dose at night. Increasing at intervals of 1−2 weeks to a maximum of 150 mg daily
• *Elderly:* By mouth, initially 30 mg daily in 3 divided doses or as a single dose at night, increasing at intervals of 1−2 weeks to a maximum of 75 mg daily

Available forms include: Tablets 10, 25, 50, 75 mg

Side effects/adverse reactions:
HAEM: Agranulocytosis, eosinophilia, leucopenia
CNS: Dizziness, drowsiness, confusion (in elderly), headache, anxiety, tremors, stimulation, weakness, behavioural disturbances (in children), nightmares, insomnia, hypomania, extrapyramidal symptoms (in elderly) (e.g. tremor, akathisia, myoclonus), ataxia, dysarthria, par-

aesthesia, increased psychiatric symptoms, convulsions

GI: Dry mouth, nausea, vomiting, paralytic ileus, increased appetite, weight gain, cramps, epigastric distress, jaundice, stomatitis, taste disturbance, constipation

META: Hyperglycaemia, breast enlargement, galactorrhoea

GU: Urinary retention, difficulty with micturition, acute renal failure, interference with sexual function

INTEG: Rash, urticaria, sweating, pruritus, photosensitivity, angioedema, purpura, oedema, alopecia

CV: Postural hypotension, arrhythmias, tachycardia, syncope, hypertension, palpitations, atrioventricular block

EENT: Blurred vision, tinnitus, mydriasis

Contraindications: Hypersensitivity, recent myocardial infarction, convulsive disorders, prostatic hypertrophy, urinary retention, should not be given concurrently or within 2 weeks of therapy with MAOIs, heart block, mania, narrow angle glaucoma, severe renal or liver disease

Precautions: Suicidal patients, cardiac disease, hyperthyroidism, concurrent treatment for hypothyroidism, electroconvulsive therapy, elective surgery, pregnancy, elderly

Pharmacokinetics:

By mouth: Onset 15−30 min, peak 8 hr, duration up to 3 weeks, steady state 6−10 days; metabolised by liver, excreted by kidneys, in faeces, half-life 27−58 hr (mean 43 hr)

Interactions/incompatibilities:

• Decreased effects of: guanethidine, clonidine

• Increased effects of: direct acting sympathomimetics, alcohol, barbiturates, benzodiazepines, CNS depressants, antihistamines, antihypertensives, phenytoin

• Hyperpyretic crisis, convulsions, hypertensive episode: MAOIs within 14 days

• Plasma levels increased by: neuroleptics and methylphenidate cimetidine

• Increased risk of arrhythmias and hypotension with anaesthesia

Clinical assessment:

• Blood studies: White blood cell count, leucocytes, differential, cardiac enzymes if patient is receiving long-term therapy

• Hepatic studies: aspartate aminotransferase, alanine aminotransferase, bilirubin, creatinine if impairment expected

• ECG for flattening of T wave, bundle branch block. Atrioventricular block, dysrhythmias in cardiac patients

Lab. test interferences:

Increase: Serum bilirubin, blood glucose, alkaline phosphatase

False increase: Urinary catecholamines

Decrease: Vanillylmandelic acid, 5-hydroxyindoleacetic acid

Treatment of overdose: ECG monitoring, induce emesis, lavage, activated charcoal, administer anticonvulsant. IV diazepam if convulsions occur. Treat hypotension and circulatory collapse with a plasma expander, reduced myocardial function with dopamine/dobutamine, correct metabolic acidosis

NURSING CONSIDERATIONS

Assess:

• Baseline BP, pulse and weight

Administer:

• Increased fluids and fibre in diet if urinary retention and/or constipation occur

• With food or milk for GI symptoms

• Dosage at bedtime if over-sedation occurs during day; patient may take entire dose at bedtime; elderly may not tolerate once daily dosing

• Chewing gum, boiled sweets or frequent sips of water for dry mouth

• Take with fruit juice, water, or milk to disguise taste

Perform/provide:
• Assistance with ambulation during beginning therapy since drowsiness/dizziness occurs

• Safety measures including side-rails primarily in elderly

• Checking to see oral medication swallowed

Evaluate:
• Pulse 4 hrly BP (lying, standing) if systolic BP drops 20 mmHg withhold drug, notify clinician; take vital signs 4 hrly in patients with cardiovascular disease

• Weight weekly; appetite may increase with drug

• Extrapyramidal symptoms primarily in elderly: rigidity, dystonia, motor restlessness

• Mental status: mood, alertness affect, suicidal tendencies, increase in psychiatric symptoms: depression, panic

• Urinary retention, constipation; constipation is more likely to occur in children

• Withdrawal symptoms: headache, nausea, vomiting, insomnia restlessness; do not usually occur unless drug was discontinued abruptly

• Alcohol consumption; if alcohol is consumed, withhold dose until morning

Teach patient/family:
• That therapeutic effects may take 2–3 weeks

• Caution in driving or other activities requiring alertness because of drowsiness, dizziness, blurred vision

• To avoid alcohol, other CNS depressants

• Not to discontinue medication quickly after long-term use, may cause nausea, headache, insomnia

• To take precautions since photosensitivity can occur

---

mazindol

Teronac

Func. class.: Appetite suppressant
Chem. class.: Imidazoisoindole derivative
Legal class.: CD (Sch 3) POM

Action: Centrally acting sympathomimetic. Increases release of noradrenaline and dopamine in cerebral cortex to reticular activating system

Uses: Obesity in conjunction with diet. Use in children and elderly not recommended

Dosage and routes:
• *Adult:* 2 mg 1 hr after breakfast for a maximum of 3 months. Discontinue if weight loss does not occur within 1 month or if weight loss ceases

Available forms include: Tablets 2 mg

Side effects/adverse reactions:
CNS: Hyperactivity, insomnia, restlessness, hallucinations, euphoria, dizziness, headache, stimulation, irritability, syncope, drowsiness, weakness, tremor
GI: Nausea, anorexia, dry mouth, diarrhoea, constipation
GU: Disturbances in sexual function, difficulty urinating
CV: Palpitations, tachycardia
INTEG: Urticaria, rash, pallor, shivering, sweating
Contraindications: Severe renal insufficiency, hypersensitivity to sympathomimetic amines, glaucoma, drug abuse, cardiac insuf-

ficiency, cardiac arrhythmias, severe hypertension, alcoholism, peptic ulcer, previous history of psychiatric illness, lactation, concurrent administration of MAOIs or adrenergic neurone blockers, pregnancy, severe hepatic disease

Precautions: Diabetes mellitus, hypertension, depression, prostatic hypertrophy, concurrent thyroid medication, hyperthyroidism, psychostimulants and antihypertensive agents, severe agitation, local anaesthesia with products containing sympathomimetics, cold remedies, coronary heart disease

Pharmacokinetics:
By mouth: Onset ½−1 hr, duration 8−15 hr, metabolised by liver, excreted by kidneys

Interactions/incompatibilities:
• Hypertensive crisis: MAOIs or within 28 days of MAOIs
• Increased effect of this drug: phenothiazines, haloperidol
• Decreased effects of this drug: barbiturates
• Decreased effects of: guanethidine, other antihypertensives
• Risk of hypertension: sympathomimetics including cold remedies

Treatment of overdose: Induce emesis and gastric lavage as appropriate. Treat excess CNS stimulation with chlorpromazine

NURSING CONSIDERATIONS

Assess:
• Baseline vital signs and weight

Administer:
• In order to avoid sleeplessness, do not give doses in the evening
• For obesity only if patient is on weight reduction programme including dietary changes, exercise; patient will develop tolerance, and weight loss will not occur without additional methods
• Chewing gum, frequent sips of water for dry mouth

Perform/provide:
• Checking that medication has been swallowed

Evaluate:
• Vital signs; BP since this drug may reverse antihypertensives; check patients with cardiac disease more often
• Mental status: mood, alertness affect, stimulation, insomnia, aggressiveness
• Physical dependency; should not be used for more than 4 to 8 weeks; dose should be discontinued gradually
• Withdrawal symptoms: headache, nausea, vomiting, muscle pain, weakness
• Drug dependence after long-term use
• NB. This can be a drug of abuse

Teach patient/family:
• To decrease caffeine consumption (coffee, tea, cola, chocolate), which may increase irritability, stimulation
• Avoid non-prescribed drugs unless approved by clinician
• To taper off drug over several weeks, or depression, increased sleeping, lethargy may ensue
• Drug dosage must not be increased
• To avoid alcohol
• To avoid hazardous activities until patient is stabilised on medication
• To rest as desired; patients will feel more tired at end of day

mebendazole

Vermox, Ovex
Func. class.: Anthelmintic
Chem. class.: Carbamate
Legal class.: POM/P

Action: Inhibits glucose, nutrient uptake, degeneration of cytoplasmic microtubules in the cell;

interferes with absorption, secretory function

Uses: Pinworms, roundworms, hookworms, whipworms, threadworms

Dosage and routes:
• *Adult and child over 2 yr:* For threadworm, by mouth 100 mg as a single dose. If re-infection occurs, give a second dose after 2 weeks. For whipworm by mouth: 100 mg twice a day for 3 days

Available forms include: Tablets, chewable 100 mg, syrup 100 mg/ 5 ml

Side effects/adverse reactions:
CNS: Dizziness, fever
GI: Transient diarrhoea, abdominal pain

Contraindications: Hypersensitivity, pregnancy

Pharmacokinetics:
By mouth: Peak ½−7 hr, excreted in faeces primarily (metabolites), small amount in urine (unchanged), highly bound to plasma proteins

Interactions/incompatibilities: None known

Treatment of overdose: Gastric lavage

NURSING CONSIDERATIONS

Assess:
• Stools during entire treatment; specimens must be sent to laboratory while still warm

Administer:
• May be crushed, chewed if unable to swallow whole
• By mouth after meals to avoid GI symptoms since absorption is not altered by food
• Second course after 3 weeks if needed; usually recommended

Evaluate:
• For therapeutic response: expulsion of worms and 3 negative stool cultures after completion of treatment
• For allergic reaction: rash (rare)
• For diarrhoea during expulsion

of worms; prevent contamination with faeces
• For infection in other family members since transmission from person to person is common

Teach patient/family:
• Proper hygiene after bowel movement including handwashing technique; tell patient to avoid putting fingers in mouth
• That infected person should sleep alone
• To change bed linen daily, wash self and clothing in hot water
• To clean toilet daily with disinfectant
• Need for compliance with dosage schedule, duration of treatment
• To wear shoes
• To wash all fruits and vegetables well before eating

---

mebeverine HCl

Colofac, Colven
Func. class.: Antispasmodic
Chem. class.: Butyl veratrate derivative
Legal class.: POM

Action: Relaxes intestinal smooth muscle, without affecting motility

Uses: Gastrointestinal disease characterised by smooth muscle spasm, irritable bowel syndrome

Dosage and routes:
• *Adults and children over 10:* By mouth 1 tablet or 15 ml liquid 3 times daily, 20 min before food
• *Adult and children over 12:* Granules: By mouth one sachet twice a day, half an hour before meals, increasing to 3 times a day if necessary

Available forms include: Tablet 135 mg; liquid 50 mg/5 ml, granules 135 mg (with ispaghula)

Side effects/adverse reactions: None serious

Contraindications: Children less than 10 yr. Sachets contain 6.1 mmol of sodium and are therefore contraindicated in severe renal and cardiovascular disease
Precautions: Paralytic ileus, pregnancy, porphyria

NURSING CONSIDERATIONS
Administer:
• Mix granules in 250 ml of cold water
• 30 min before food
Perform/provide:
• Increased fluids, fibre in diet, exercise to decrease constipation
Evaluate:
• Therapeutic response, absence of abdominal pain—nausea
• Decrease in constipation
Teach patient/family:
• That tablets should be swallowed, not chewed
• That bowel actions do not occur daily
• That tablets should not be taken if there is severe pain or vomiting

---

medroxyprogesterone acetate

Depo-Provera, Farlutal, Provera
Func. class.: Progestogen
Chem. class.: Progesterone derivative
Legal class.: POM

Action: Inhibits secretion of pituitary gonadotrophins, which prevents follicular maturation and ovulation, stimulates growth of mammary tissue, antineoplastic action against endometrial renal and breast cancer
Uses: Uterine bleeding (abnormal), secondary amenorrhoea, endometriosis, endometrial, prostate, renal cancer, postmenopausal, breast cancer, contraception

Dosage and routes:
Contraception
• By deep IM, 150 mg during first 5 days menstrual cycle or before 6th week post partum, repeat every 3 months
Secondary amenorrhoea
• *Adult:* By mouth 2.5—10 mg for 5—10 days from 16th day of menstrual cycle for 3 consecutive cycles
Breast cancer
• *Adult:* By mouth 400—1500 mg daily, increasing to 2000 mg daily. IM initially 500 mg—1000 mg daily for 28 days, then 500 mg twice weekly
Endometriosis
• *Adult:* By mouth 10 mg 3 times a day starting from the first day of menstrual cycle for 90 days. Deep IM injection 50 mg once a week or 100 mg every 2 weeks for 6 months or more
Prostatic cancer
• *Adult:* By mouth 100—500 mg daily. IM initially 500 mg twice weekly, maintenance 500 mg once a week
Endometrial/renal cancer
• *Adult:* By mouth 100—500 mg daily. IM 400—1000 mg weekly. Dose may be increased to 1000 mg daily. Once disease is stabilised maintenance may be as little as 400 mg each month
Dysfunctional uterine bleeding
• *Adult:* By mouth 2.5—10 mg daily for 5—10 days starting on 16th day of menstrual cycle for 2 cycles. IM 50 mg weekly
Available forms include: Tablets 5, 10, 100, 200, 250, 400 and 500 mg; oral suspension 80 mg in 1 ml; injection: 50, 150, 200 mg/ml
Side effects/adverse reactions:
CNS: Dizziness, migraine headache, nervousness, insomnia, depression, fatigue
CV: Thrombophlebitis, oedema, thromboembolism, stroke, pul-

monary embolism, myocardial infarction

GI: Nausea, vomiting, anorexia, cramps, increased weight, cholestatic jaundice

EENT: Diplopia, acute impairement of vision

GU: Amenorrhoea, cervical erosion, breakthrough bleeding, dysmenorrhoea, vaginal candidiasis, breast changes, galactorrhoea, gynaecomastia, testicular atropy, impotence, endometriosis, spontaneous abortion, transient infertility (up to 2 yr following continuous treatment)

INTEG: Rash, urticaria, acne, hirsutism, alopecia, oily skin, seborrhoea, purpura, melasma, photosensitivity, angioneurotic oedema

SYST: Anaphylaxis, hyperpyrexia, back pain

META: Hyperglycaemia, hypercalcaemia

Contraindications: Pregnancy, hypersensitivity, thromboembolic disorders, reproductive cancer, genital bleeding (abnormal, undiagnosed), hepatic disease, missed abortion

Precautions: Lactation, puerperium, hypertension, asthma, blood dyscrasias, gallbladder disease, hypercalcaemia, congestive cardiac failure, diabetes mellitus, bone disease, depression, migraine headache, convulsive disorders, renal disease, family history of cancer of breast or reproductive tract, undiagnosed abnormal uterine bleeding hormone dependent tumours

Pharmacokinetics:
By mouth: Plasma half-life 2 days, steady state reacted in 10 days, excreted in urine and faeces, metabolised in liver

Interactions/incompatibilities:
None known

Clinical assessment:

• Titrated dose, use lowest effective dose

Lab. test interferences: Gonadotrophin levels, plasma progesterone, testosterone (male), oestrogen (female), cortisol levels, urinary pregnanediol levels, glucose tolerance and metyrapone tests

NURSING CONSIDERATIONS
Assess:
• Baseline BP and fluid balance
Administer:
• Shake vigorously to disperse IM injection
• Solution deeply in large muscle mass (IM), rotate sites
• In one dose in morning
• With food or milk to decrease GI symptoms with oral dose
Evaluate:
• BP periodically
• Fluid balance; be alert for decreasing urinary output; increasing oedema
• Therapeutic response: decreased abnormal uterine bleeding, absence of amenorrhoea
• Oedema, hypertension, cardiac symptoms, jaundice
• Mental status: affect, mood, behavioural changes, depression
• Hypercalcaemia
Teach patient/family:
• Counsel patient on long-term nature of product if used as contraceptive
• To avoid sunlight or use sunscreen; photosensitivity can occur
• All aspects of drug usage, including Cushingoid symptoms
• To report breast lumps, vaginal bleeding, oedema, jaundice, dark urine, clay-coloured stools, dyspnoea, headache, blurred vision, abdominal pain, numbness or stiffness in legs, chest pain; male to report impotence or gynaecomastia
• To report suspected pregnancy

mefenamic acid

Ponstan
Func. class.: Non-steroidal anti-inflammatory drug
Chem. class.: Anthranilic acid derivative
Legal class.: POM

Action: Inhibits prostaglandin synthesis by inhibiting an enzyme needed for biosynthesis; possesses analgesic, anti-inflammatory, antipyretic properties

Uses: Mild to moderate pain, osteoarthritis, rheumatoid arthritis pyrexia, primary dysmenorrhoea, menorrhagia due to dysfunctional cause

Dosage and routes:
• *Adult and child more than 12 yr:* By mouth 500 mg, 3 times a day
• *Child less than 12 yr:* By mouth, 0−6 months 25 mg/kg daily in divided doses, 6 months−1 yr, 50 mg 8 hrly, 2 yr−4 yr 100 mg 8 hrly, 5 yr−8 yr 150 mg 8 hrly, 9 yr−12 yr 200 mg 8 hrly
Discontinue treatment in children after 7 days (except Still's disease)
Available forms include: Capsules 250 mg; dispersible tablets 250 mg; suspension 50 mg/ml; tablets 500 mg

Side effects/adverse reactions:
GI: Nausea, anorexia, vomiting, diarrhoea leading to proctocolitis (discontinue), jaundice, cholestatic hepatitis, discomfort, dyspepsia, peptic ulcer
CNS: Dizziness, drowsiness
INTEG: Rash (discontinue)
GU: Nephrotoxicity: glomerulonephritis, dysuria, haematuria, oliguria, uraemia, renal failure (elderly)
HAEM: Thrombocytopenia, haemolytic anaemia
EENT: Tinnitus, hearing loss, blurred vision
RESP: Bronchospasm

Contraindications: Hypersensitivity, asthma, severe renal disease, severe hepatic disease peptic/intestinal ulceration, inflammatory bowel disease

Precautions: Pregnancy, lactation, children, bleeding disorders, GI disorders, cardiac disorders, hypersensitivity to other NSAIDs, renal disease, concurrent use with other plasma protein binding drugs, elderly especially with dehydration or renal disease

Pharmacokinetics:
By mouth: Peak 2 hr, half-life 3−3½ hr; metabolised in liver, excreted in urine (metabolites), excreted in breast milk. Highly bound to plasma proteins

Interactions/incompatibilities:
• May increase action of: coumarin anticoagulants, phenytoin, sulphonamides
• May antagonise: antihypertensives due to fluid retention

Clinical assessment:
• Renal, liver, blood studies: blood urea nitrogen, creatinine, aspartate aminotransferase, alanine aminotransferase, Hb before treatment, periodically thereafter if problems anticipated
• Audiometric, ophthalmic exam during, treatment if problems develop

Treatment of overdose: Gastric lavage and activated charcoal, intensive supportive measures

NURSING CONSIDERATIONS

Administer:
• With or after food to decrease GI symptoms

Evaluate:
• Therapeutic response: decreased pain, stiffness, swelling in joints, ability to move more easily
• For eye, ear problems: blurred vision, tinnitus (may indicate toxicity)

Teach patient/family:

- To report blurred vision, or ringing, roaring in ears (may indicate toxicity)
- To avoid driving or other hazardous activities if dizziness or drowsiness occurs
- To report change in urine pattern, weight increase, oedema, pain increase in joints, fever, blood in urine (indicates nephrotoxicity)
- That therapeutic effects may take up to 1 month
- To take with food or milk
- To report any indigestion or black tarry stools

---

mefloquine ▼

Lariam
Func. class.: Antimalarial
Chem. class.: Quinine derivative
Legal class.: POM

Action: Is thought to work by damaging the malarial plasmodium membrane

Uses: Therapy and prophylaxis of malaria. The drug is especially indicated for therapy of *Plasmodium falciparum* malaria in which the pathogen has become resistant to other antimalarial agents. Mefloquine prophylaxis is particularly recommended for travellers to malarious regions in which multiple resistant *P. falciparum* strains occur

Dosage and routes:
Malaria prophylaxis
(for brief stays 1−3 weeks)
- *Adult and children over 45 kg:* By mouth 250 mg once weekly
- *Children:* By mouth under 15 kg weight, not recommended
- *Weight 15−19 kg:* One quarter of a tablet
- *Weight 20−30 kg:* One half of a tablet
- *Weight 31−45 kg:* Three quarters of a tablet

- Dose should be taken once a week, always on the same day for 6 weeks. First dose one week before departure
For prolonged stays (more than 3 weeks): As above for first 4 weeks then take further doses at 2 week intervals. First dose 1 week before arriving in endemic area
Malaria treatment
- *Non-immune adults and children 45−60 kg:* By mouth, 3 tablets followed by 2 tablets after 6−8 hr
- *Non-immune adults and children over 60 kg:* By mouth 3 tablets followed by 2 tablets after 6−8 hr and 1 tablet after a further 6−8 hr
- *Semi-immune patients living in malarious areas 45−60 kg:* By mouth a single dose of 3 tablets
- *Semi-immune patients living in malaria areas over 60 kg:* By mouth 3 tablets, followed by 1 tablet after 6−8 hr
- *Children under 45 kg irrespective of immune status*: By mouth a single dose of 25 mg/kg
Available forms include: Tablets 250 mg mefloquine (as hydrochloride)
Side effects/adverse reactions:
Mainly at higher doses
CNS: Dizziness, disturbed sense of balance, loss of appetite, headache, feeling of weakness, rare cases of depression, confusion, anxiety, hallucinations and paranoid reactions. In prophylaxis—occasional reports of psychological changes. If noticed the drug must be discontinued
GI: Nausea, vomiting, diarrhoea, abdominal pain, elevation of transaminases (rare)
CV: Bradycardia
INTEG: Rash, pruritus
Contraindications: Prophylactic use in pregnancy, breast feeding, renal insufficiency, severe impairment of liver function, or in patients with a history of psychi-

atric disturbances or convulsions

Precautions: Women of child-bearing potential should take reliable contraceptive precautions during use and for 3 months after the last dose

Pharmacokinetics:

By mouth: peak plasma level is reached within 2−12 hr. Average half-life is 21 days and excretion is primarily in bile and faeces

Interactions: Avoid concurrent use of quinine due to increased incidence of convulsions except in severe cases where 1−2 days of IV quinine may be necessary followed by mefloquine. Possible increased risk of bradycardia with β-blockers, digoxin, some calcium channel blockers

NURSING CONSIDERATIONS

Assess:

• Baseline observations. BP, temperature, pulse, respiration

Administer:

• Swallow tablets whole with plenty of liquid and preferably not on an empty stomach

Perform/provide:

• Observe for side-effects

Evaluate:

• Fluid balance, watch for nausea, vomiting, diarrhoea

• Vital signs: bradycardia may occur

• Psychological status

Teach patient/family:

• Driving and similar tasks requiring fine coordination are not recommended during and 2 weeks after malaria treatment. Caution with regard to driving in prophylactic use

• If psychological changes occur when mefloquine is used for prophylaxis the drug must be stopped

• Give advice on contraception for women of child-bearing potential

• To take medication on same day of every week when taking for prophylaxis

megestrol acetate

Megace
Func. class.: Antineoplastic
Chem. class.: Progestogen
Legal class.: POM

Action: Affects endometrium by antiluteinising effect; this is thought to bring about cell death

Uses: Hormone dependent, breast, endometrial cancer

Dosage and routes:

Breast cancer

• *Adult:* 160 mg daily as a single dose or in divided doses

Endmetrial cancer

• *Adult:* By mouth 40−320 mg daily in divided doses

Available forms include: Tablets 40, 160 mg

Side effects/adverse reactions:

GI: Nausea, vomiting, diarrhoea, abdominal cramps, increased appetite

GU: Gynaecomastia, fluid retention, hypercalcaemia, changes in libido

INTEG: Alopecia, rash, pruritus, urticaria, acne, weight gain

CNS: Mood swings, carpal tunnel syndrome

HAEM: Thrombophlebitis

Contraindications: Hypersensitivity, pregnancy, undiagnosed vaginal bleeding, missed abortion, previous severe arterial disease, prophyria

Precautions: Thrombophlebitis, diabetes, lactation, hypertension, hepatic, cardiac and renal disease

Interactions/incompatibilities: None known

Clinical assessment:

• Pulmonary function tests, chest X-ray films before, during therapy; chest film should be obtained every 2 weeks during treatment

• Serum calcium

NURSING CONSIDERATIONS

Assess:
• Vital signs, fluid balance before treatment is commenced
Administer:
• Antacid before oral agent, give drug after evening meal, before bedtime
• Anti-emetic 30–60 min before giving drug to prevent vomiting
• Antispasmodics as prescribed
Perform/provide:
• Increase fluid intake to 2–3 litres daily to prevent dehydration
• Nutritious diet with iron, vitamin supplements as ordered
• Limitation of calcium (dairy products)
Evaluate:
• Vital signs 4 hrly
• Dyspnoea, râles, unproductive cough, chest pain, tachypnoea, fatigue, increased pulse, pallor, lethargy
• Food preferences; list likes, dislikes
• Effects of alopecia on body image; discuss feelings about body changes
• Fluid balance
• Oedema in feet, joints, hands, ankles; oliguria
• Symptoms indicating severe allergic reaction; rash, pruritus, urticaria, purpuric skin lesions, itching, flushing
• Frequency of stools, characteristics: cramping, acidosis, signs of dehydration (rapid respirations, poor skin turgor, decreased urine output, dry skin, restlessness, weakness)
• Mood swings
• Nausea, vomiting, diarrhoea constipation, weakness, loss of muscle tone
Teach patient/family:
• To report any complaints or side effects to nurse or clinician
• That (for women) gynaecomastia can occur; reversible after discontinuing treatment

melphalan

Alkeran
Func. class.: Antineoplastic alkylating agent
Chem. class.: Nitrogen mustard
Legal class.: POM

Action: Alkylates DNA, RNA; inhibits enzymes that allow synthesis of amino acids in proteins; also responsible for cross-linking DNA strands
Uses: Multiple myeloma, advanced breast cancer, soft tissue sarcoma, malignant melanoma, polycythaemia vera, advanced ovarian adenocarcinoma
Dosage and routes:
NB. Many other schedules used, often in combination with other cytotoxics
Multiple myeloma
• *By mouth* 0.15 mg/kg body-weight daily in divided doses for 4 days with 40 mg prednisolone a day for 4 days. Repeat at intervals of 6 weeks for 12 months
Ovarian adenocarcinoma
• *By mouth* 0.2 mg/kg daily in 3 divided doses for 5 days. Repeat every 4–8 weeks provided the bone marrow has recovered
• IV Infusion 1 mg/kg over 8 hr every 4 weeks
Advanced breast carcinoma
• *By mouth* 0.2–0.3 mg/kg daily or 6 mg/m² body surface area for 4–6 days. Repeat every 3–6 weeks
Malignant melanoma and soft tissue sarcoma
• Seek specialist's advice
Polycythaemia vera
• To induce remission, by mouth 6–10 mg daily for 7–10 days. For maintenance, by mouth 2–4 mg daily
Available forms include: Tablets 2, 5 mg, injection 100 mg

Side effects/adverse reactions:
HAEM: Thrombocytopenia, neutropenia, haemolytic anaemia, leucopenia, leukaemia
GI: Nausea, vomiting, stomatitis, diarrhoea
GU: Amenorrhoea, hyperuricaemia
INTEG: Rash, urticaria, alopecia
RESP: Pulmonary fibrosis
Precautions: Lactation, pregnancy, radiation therapy, bone marrow depression, concurrent cytotoxic therapy, renal impairment (in moderate−severe disease reduce dose and adjust according to response)
Pharmacokinetics:
Oral absorption maybe variable. Metabolised in liver, excreted in urine, half-life 1½ hr, highly bound to plasma proteins
Interactions/incompatibilities:
• Increased toxicity: antineoplastics, radiation, cyclosporin. Avoid concurrent use of nalidixic acid
• Unstable in IV infusion fluids but may be given in sodium chloride 0.9%, at room temperature within 2 hr of reconstitution. Do not use dextrose
Clinical assessment:
• Full blood count, differential, platelet count weekly; withhold drug if WBC is less than 2000/mm³ or platelet count is less than 75,000/mm³. Other institutions may have own guidelines
• Renal function studies: blood urea nitrogen, serum uric acid, urine creatinine clearance before, during therapy
• Liver function tests before, during therapy (bilirubin, aspartate aminotransferase, alanine aminotransferase, lactic dehydrogenase) as needed or monthly
Treatment of overdose: Supportive; monitor blood counts, give infusion products, filgrastin as appropriate

NURSING CONSIDERATIONS
Assess:
• Baseline vital signs including fluid balance
Administer:
• In accordance with local cytotoxic policy
• Other medications by oral route if possible; avoid IV routes—via tricaman to prevent infections
• Antiemetic 30−60 min before giving drug to prevent vomiting
• Antibiotics for prophylaxis of infection if indicated
• IV is unstable in infusion (infuse within 30 min of it being made up) and infuse over 2 hr
Perform/provide:
• Strict medical asepsis, protective isolation if WBC levels are low
• Strict fluid balance chart
• Increase fluid intake to 2−3 litres a day to prevent urate deposits, calculi formation
• Rinsing of mouth 3 or 4 times a day with water and prescribed mouthwashes to prevent ulceration and infection; brushing of teeth 2 or 3 times a day with soft brush or cotton tipped applicators for stomatitis; use unwaxed dental floss
• Warm compresses at injection site for inflammation, if indicated
Evaluate:
• Fluid balance; report fall in urine output of 30 ml/hr
• Bleeding: haematuria, bruising, petechiae due to thrombocytopenia mucosa or orifices 8 hrly
• IV site for extravasation and pain; if leakage stop infusion
• Food preferences; list likes, dislikes
• Yellowing of skin, sclera, dark urine, clay-coloured stools, itchy skin, abdominal pain, fever, diarrhoea
• Inflammation of mucosa, breaks in skin
• Buccal cavity 8 hrly for dryness,

meningococcal vaccine BP **411**

due to stomatitis and potential fungal infections, sores, ulceration, white patches, oral pain, bleeding, dysphagia
• Symptoms indicating severe allergic reaction: rash, pruritus, urticaria, purpuric skin lesions, itching, flushing
Teach patient/family:
• Of protective isolation precautions due to neutropenia
• To report any complaints or side effects to nurse or clinician
• That sterility, amenorrhoea can occur; reversible after discontinuing treatment
• That hair may be lost during treatment; a wig or hairpiece is available on NHS prescription; new hair may be different in colour, texture
• Good mouthcare and to report any bleeding, white spots, or ulcerations in mouth to clinician; tell patient to examine mouth daily

meningococcal vaccine BP (groups A & C polysaccharides)

AC VAX, Mengivac (A + C)
Func. class.: Vaccine
Legal class.: POM

Action: Active immunisation
Uses: Immunisation against meningococcal meningitis caused by group A and group C meningococci
Dosage and routes:
• *Adults and children aged 2 months and over:* Deep subcutaneous injection 0.5 ml of reconstituted vaccine
Available forms include: Subcutaneous injection 50 mcg of group A polysaccharide and 50 mcg of group C polysaccharide in 0.5 ml
Side effects/adverse reactions:

INTEG: Erythema, slight induration and tenderness or pain at the site of injection
CNS: Febrile reactions, chills
Contraindications: Hypersensitivity, febrile conditions
Precautions: If administered to patients on immunosuppressive therapy, the vaccine may not induce an effective response. It should not be given in pregnancy unless there is a definite risk from groups A and C meningococcal disease. The Menigivac brand is not recommended in children under 18 months (except in an epidemic) because of an alleged transient response to serogroup C and increased incidence of side effects
NURSING CONSIDERATIONS
Assess:
• Infection; vaccination must be delayed if acute infection
Administer:
• The vaccine must not be given intravenously under any circumstances
• The vaccine should be reconstituted with the diluent supplied by adding the entire contents of the diluent vial to the vaccine vial. As with all vaccinations a solution of 1:1000 adrenaline should be available for injection should an anaphylactic reaction occur; additionally follow local protocols
Perform/provide:
• Store between 2°C and 8°C. The reconstituted vaccine should be used immediately, and certainly within 1 hr
Teach patient/family:
• That low grade fever, irritability and fatigue may occasionally occur in the first 72 hr following vaccination

menotrophin

Pergonal, Humegon
Func. class.: Gonadotrophin
Chem. class.: Human follicle stimulating hormone (FSH); human luteinising hormone (LH)
Legal class.: POM

Action: In women increases follicular growth, maturation; in men, when given with HCG, stimulates spermatogenesis
Uses: Infertility in amenorrhoeic anovulatory women, women undergoing *in vitro* fertilisation, hypogonadotrophic hypogonadism in men
Dosage and routes:
Amenorrhoeic anovulatory women
• By IM injection, either a total of 3−5 ampoules given as 3 equal doses on alternate days, followed by up to 10,000 units of HCG 1 week after first injection or; by IM injection 1−2 ampoules each day, followed by up to 10,000 units HCG 24−48 hr after last injection. Both regimens should be adjusted at weekly intervals to gain best response
In vitro fertilisation and associated techniques
• 100 mg of clomiphene by mouth on days 2−6 followed by IM injection of 2−3 ampoules of menotrophin starting on day 5. Adjust dose according to response. A dose of up to 10,000 units of HCG is administered 24−48 hr after the last menotrophin injection or; by IM injection 2−3 ampoules of menotrophin daily from day 2−3 of cycle. Adjust dose according to response. A dose of up to 10,000 HCH is administered 24−48 hr after the last menotrophin injection
Hypogonadotrophic hypogonadism in men

• By IM injection 1 ampoule 3 times a week, with 2000 units HCG twice a week for at least 4 months
Available forms include: Powder for injection 75 units FSH/75 units LH, 150 units FSH/150 units LH
Side effects/adverse reactions:
CNS: Fever
CV: Hypovolaemia
GI: Nausea, vomiting, diarrhoea, abdominal pain and distension
GU: Ovarian enlargement, ovarian hyperstimulation, multiple births, ascites, pleural effusion
INTEG: Joint pain
Contraindications: Hypothyroidism, adrenal deficiency, hyperprolactinaemia, pituitary tumour unless these conditions have been treated. Ovarian dysgenesis, absent uterus, premature menopause
Treatment of overdose: The acute toxicity of menotrophin has been shown to be very low. However, too high a dosage for more than one day may lead to hyperstimulation of the ovaries

NURSING CONSIDERATIONS
Assess:
• Weight on alternate days
Administer:
• After reconstituting with 1−2 ml sterile saline injection; use immediately
Evaluate:
• Rapid weight gain
• Ovarian enlargement, abdominal distention/pain; report symptoms immediately
Teach patient/family:
• That multiple births are possible, pregnancy usually occurs in 4−6 weeks after start of treatment
• To keep appointment during treatment every other day for 2 weeks
• That daily intercourse is necessary from day preceding adminis-

tration of gonadotrophin until ovulation occurs

---

meptazinol, meptazinol hydrochloride

Meptid
Func. class.: Analgesic
Chem. class.: Partial opiod agonist
Legal class.: POM

Action: Acts on opiod receptors in CNS, stimulation of mu or kappa receptors produces analgesic effects

Uses: Moderate to severe pain, including postoperative pain, obstetric pain, renal colic

Dosage and routes:
• *Adults:* By mouth, 200 mg 3−6 hrly; IM injection, 75−100 mg 2−4 hrly, but for obstetric analgesia, 100−150 mg (approximately 2 mg/kg) 2−4 hrly
• Slow IV injection, 50−100 mg 2−4 hrly

Available forms include: Tablets, 200 mg; injection, 100 mg (as base)/ml

Side effects/adverse reactions:
CNS: Drowsiness, alteration of pupillary responses, dizziness, headache
GI: Nausea, vertigo, vomiting, dyspepsia, abdominal pain, diarrhoea
GU: Diarrhoea
INTEG: Pain and tissue at injection site, sweating
SYST: Tolerance, dependence

Contraindications: Not for use in patients with head injury as it may raise CSF pressure and mask symptoms

Precautions: Myocardial infarction, pregnancy (other than labour), severe respiratory depression, asthma, hepatic or renal impairment, head injury, elevated intracranial pressure

Pharmacokinetics: Onset within 15 min, duration of action 2 to 7 hr. Tablets subject to first pass hepatic metabolism and metabolites are excreted in the urine.

Interactions/incompatibilities:
• Delays absorption of: mexiletine may potentiate other CNS depressants
• Injection, should not be mixed with other drugs in the same syringe or infusion

Treatment of overdose:
• Resuscitate if necessary
• Gastric lavage if taken orally
• Naloxone if respiratory depression is evident
• Supportive therapy

NURSING CONSIDERATIONS

Assess:
• Pain and appropriate analgesia

Administer:
• As directed but before patient is in great pain
• An anti-emetic if vomiting occurs
• Do not mix injection in same syringe as other drugs
• If given intravenously, flush system with saline before and after administration

Evaluate:
• For side effects — nausea, vomiting, diarrhoea, constipation, sweating, abdominal pain, dyspepsia, rash, drowsiness
• For withdrawal symptoms when drug is stopped
• Therapeutic effect — diminished pain

Teach patient/family:
• Dizziness may occur so avoid any task requiring alertness (e.g. driving) until sure they are not affected
• Check with clinician before taking any other drugs

mercaptopurine (6-MP)

Puri-Nethol
Func. class.: Antineoplastic, antimetabolite
Chem. class.: Purine analogue
Legal class.: POM

Action: Inhibits purine metabolism by blocking inosinic acid conversion to adenine, which is responsible for DNA, RNA synthesis
Uses: Chronic granulocytic leukaemia, acute lymphoblastic leukaemia, acute myelogenous leukaemia
Dosage and routes:
• *Adult and child:* By mouth 2.5 mg/kg daily. Adjusted to the needs of the individual patient. Reduce dose if renal or hepatic function is reduced
Available forms include: Tablets 50 mg
Side effects/adverse reactions:
CNS: Fever, headache, weakness
HAEM: Thrombocytopenia, leucopenia, myelosuppression, anaemia
GI: Nausea, vomiting, anorexia, oral ulceration, hepatotoxicity (with high doses), jaundice
GU: Renal failure, hyperuricaemia, hyperuricosuria
INTEG: Rash
Precautions: Patients with prior drug resistance, leucopenia, thrombocytopenia, anaemia, pregnancy. Renal or hepatic disease
Pharmacokinetics: Incompletely absorbed when taken orally, metabolised in liver, excreted in urine
Interactions/incompatibilities:
• Increased toxicity: radiation or other antineoplastics
• Potentiated by: allopurinol (quarter mercaptopurine dose)
• Effects of warfarin reduced by mercaptopurine

Clinical assessment:
• Full blood count, differential, platelet count weekly; withhold drug if WBC is less than 3500 or platelet count is less than 100,000; drug should be discontinued
• Renal function studies: blood urea nitrogen, serum uric acid, urine creatinine clearance, electrolytes before, during therapy
• Liver function tests before, during therapy: bilirubin, alkaline phosphatase, aspartate aminotransferase, alanine aminotransferase, weekly during beginning therapy
Treatment of overdose: Supportive measures and blood transfusion if required
NURSING CONSIDERATIONS
Administer:
• Allopurinol or sodium bicarbonate to maintain uric acid levels, alkalinisation of urine
• Antibiotics for prophylaxis of infection
• Topical or systemic analgesics for pain
• Transfusion for anaemia
• Antacid before oral agent; give drug after evening meal before bedtime
• Anti-emetic 30−60 min before giving drug to prevent vomiting
• Mild nausea likely only with higher doses
Perform/provide:
• Increase fluid intake to 2−3 litres daily to prevent urate deposits, calculi formation, unless contraindicated
• Observe for signs of stomatitis and encourage oral hygiene four times a day
Evaluate:
• Monitor temperature 4 hrly, when indicated; fever may indicate beginning infection
• Effects of alopecia on body image; discuss feelings about body changes

• Inflammation of mucosa, breaks in skin
• Buccal cavity 8 hrly for dryness, sores, ulceration, white patches, oral pain, bleeding, dysphagia
• Symptoms indicating severe allergic reaction: rash, urticaria, itching, flushing

Teach patient/family:
• To report any complaints, side effects to nurse or clinician
• To avoid foods with citric acid, hot or rough texture if stomatitis is present
• To report stomatitis: any bleeding, white spots, ulcerations in mouth; tell patient to examine mouth daily, report symptoms
• Teach good oral hygiene
• Contraceptive measures are recommended during therapy
• To drink 10−12 glasses of fluid daily
• Notify clinician of fever, chills, sore throat, nausea, vomiting, anorexia, diarrhoea, bleeding, bruising, which may indicate blood dyscrasias

---

mesalazine

Asacol, Pentasa
Func. class.: Anti-inflammatory
Chem. class.: Salicylate
Legal class.: POM

Action: May diminish inflammation by inhibiting prostaglandin production in colon
Uses: Maintenance or remission of ulcerative colitis
Dosage and routes:
Acute disease
• *Adult:* By mouth 2400 mg daily in divided doses
• Rectally 750−1500 mg daily in divided doses (last dose at bedtime) or a 1 g enema once daily at night
Maintenance

• *Adult:* By mouth 1200−2400 mg daily in divided doses
• Rectally 750−1500 mg daily in divided doses as above
Available forms include: Tablets 400 mg; enema 1 g/100 ml; suppositories 250, 500 mg
Side effects/adverse reactions:
GI: Cramps, gas, nausea, diarrhoea, abdominal pain, pancreatitis, exacerbation of colitis, hepatitis
CNS: Headache
HAEM: Leucopenia, neutropenia, thrombocytopenia
GU: Nephritis, nephrotic syndrome, renal failure
Contraindications: Hypersensitivity to salicylates, severe renal impairment, (glomerular filtration rate less than 20 ml/min), children under 2 yr
Precautions: Renal disease, pregnancy, lactation, children, elderly
Pharmacokinetics:
Absorbed from colon; excreted rapidly by the kidney mainly as metabolite

NURSING CONSIDERATIONS
Evaluate:
• Response to treatment: absence of pain, bleeding from the gastrointestinal tract and decrease in diarrhoea
• Signs of gastrointestinal irritation indicated by cramp, flatulence, nausea, diarrhoea, rectal discomfort. If severe the drug must be discontinued
Teach patient/family:
• To inform clinician of gastrointestinal symptoms
• Advice on diet

mesna

Uromitexan

Func. class.: Urothelial anti-toxicity agent

Chem. class.: Sulphydryl containing compound

Legal class.: POM

Action: Reacts with acrolein (metabolite of cyclophosphamide and ifosamide) in urinary tract to reduce urothelial toxicity

Uses: In conjunction with cyclophosphamide or ifosamide to prevent urothelial toxicity

Dosage and routes:

• When cytotoxic given as IV bolus: 20% of cytotoxic dose w/w given simultaneously over 15–30 min then repeat after 4 and 8 hr. Dose can be increased to 4 doses of 40% w/w of cytotoxic dose given at 3 hrly intervals (larger dose recommended in children, previous urothelial toxicity, pelvic irradiation)

• When ifosfamide is given as 24 hr infusion, give an initial 20% w/w of cytotoxic dose as a bolus then 100% w/w of cytotoxic dose over 24 hr, then a further 60% w/w of cytotoxic dose over 12 hr (or for the last 12 hr, 3 doses of 20% w/w of cytotoxic dose given at 28, 32 and 36 hr)

• Orally, 40% w/w of cytotoxic dose is given with the infusion or as it stops and repeated after 4–8 hr

Available forms include: Injection 100 mg/ml, 4 ml, 10 ml ampoules; contents of ampoule can be taken by mouth in fruit juice

Side effects/adverse reactions: (Difficult to distinguish from cytotoxic therapy)

CNS: Headache, depression, irritability

GI: Nausea, vomiting, colic, diarrhoea

SYST: Fatigue, limb pains

INTEG: Rash

Contraindications: None known

Pharmacokinetics: Excreted in urine, inactivates toxic metabolite of cyclophosphamide or ifosfamide

Clinical assessment:

• Full blood count, differential, platelet count weekly

• Renal function tests, blood urea, electrolytes

Lab. test interferences: Mesna causes a false positive for urinary ketones test, producing a red-violet colour which fades rapidly on addition of glacial acetic acid

NURSING CONSIDERATIONS

Administer:

• Orally, drug should be taken immediately the ampoule is opened, in a soft drink (orange juice)

• Anti-emetic 30–60 mins before drug

• Slow IV infusion using appropriate size needle

Perform/provide:

• Reconstituted solution should be destroyed after 24 hr

• Plenty of fluids in diet—fluid intake 2–3 litres daily

• Frequent mouthwashes

Evaluate:

• Fluid balance, test urine for blood and protein. Report fall in urine output below 30 ml/hr

• Raised temperature; may indicate infection

• For any bleeding, haematuria; report to clinician

• For oedema in feet, joint pain, abdominal pain

• For all side effects

Teach patient/family:

• Of protective isolation precaution

• To report any complaints of side effects

- To report any bleeding
- To report any urinary symptoms

---

mesterolone

Pro-Viron
Func. class.: Male sex hormone
Chem. class.: Synthetic androgen
Legal class.: POM

Action: Supplements endogenous androgen production
Uses: Androgen deficiency, male infertility
Dosage and routes:
Androgen deficiency
- By mouth 25 mg 3−4 times daily for several months; maintenance dose 50−75 mg daily in divided doses
Male infertility
- 100 mg daily for several months
Available forms include: Tablets 25 mg
Side effects/adverse reactions:
GU: Prostatism in elderly, priapism
META: Oedema, weight gain
GI: Benign and in rare cases malignant liver tumours leading to isolated cases of life threatening intra-abdominal haemorrhage
Contraindications: Prostatic carcinoma, previous or existing liver tumours
Clinical assessment:
- Liver function tests, aspartate aminotransferase, alanine aminotransferase, bilirubin
Treatment of overdose: There have been no reports of ill effects from overdosage and treatment is generally unnecessary
NURSING CONSIDERATIONS
Assess:
- Baseline weight and BP
Perform/provide:
- Diet with increased protein; decrease salt if oedema occurs

- Regular examination of prostate during treatment
Evaluate:
- Regular examination of the prostate during treatment is advised
- Weight gain; notify clinician if gain is greater than 2.5 kg
- For oedema and hypertension
- Mental status—behavioural pattern
- For signs of impotence, testicular atrophy in males
- For symptoms of hypoglycaemia, lethargy, GI upsets
- Therapeutic response; may take several months
Teach patient/family:
- Drug needs to be combined with good diet, rest and exercise
- To notify clinician if therapeutic response decreases
- Teach patient all aspects of drug, including change in sex characteristics

---

metaraminol tartrate

Aramine
Func. class.: Sympathomimetic amine
Chem. class.: Substituted β-phenylethylamine
Legal class.: POM

Action: Both direct and indirect effects on sympathetic nerve terminals; inhibits GI, smooth muscle and vascular smooth muscle supplying skeletal muscle; cardiac excitatory effects; increases heart rate and force of heart muscle contraction
Uses: Acute hypotension
Dosage and routes:
Hypotension
- *Adult:* IV Infusion: 15−100 mg in 500 ml Dextrose 5% or sodium chloride 0.9%. Adjust rate according to response every 10 min

Grave emergency
• *Adult:* IV bolus 0.5−5 ´mg, then IV infusion of 15−100 mg/500 ml solution, adjusting dose every 10 min

Available forms include: Injection IV, 10 mg/ml

Side effects/adverse reactions:
CV: Palpitations, sinus or ventricular tachycardia, hypotension, ectopic beats, angina, circulatory collapse
INTEG: Necrosis, tissue sloughing with extravasation, abscess
RESP: Respiratory collapse, pulmonary oedema

Contraindications: Hypersensitivity

Precautions: Pregnancy, lactation, cardiac disease, history of malaria, treatment with digoxin, arterial embolism, peripheral vascular disease, hypertension, thyroid disease, diabetes mellitus, cirrhosis, concurrent use with cyclopropane or halothane anaesthesia

Pharmacokinetics:
IV: Onset 1−2 min duration 20 min−1 hr

Interactions/incompatibilities:
• Dysrhythmias: general anaesthetics
• Decreased action of this drug: other β-blockers
• Increased BP: oxytocics
• Increased pressor effect: tricyclic antidepressant, MAOIs
• Incompatible with alkaline solutions: sodium bicarbonate
• Concurrent use with cyclopropane or halothone unless clinical circumstance demands

Treatment of overdose: Administer an α-blocker, then noradrenaline for severe hypotension

NURSING CONSIDERATIONS

Assess:
• Baseline vital signs
• Fluid balance

Administer:
• Parenteral IV dose slowly, after reconstituting with 500 ml of dextrose 5% or 0.9% sodium chloride
• Plasma expanders for hypovolaemia if ordered

Perform/provide:
• Keep drug refrigerated
• Do not use discoloured solutions
• Continuous monitoring of vital signs (preferably with patient in ICU)

Evaluate:
• ECG during administration continuously, if BP increases, drug is decreased
• BP and pulse every 5 min after parenteral route
• CVP during infusion if possible
• For paraesthesia and coldness of extremities, peripheral blood flow may decrease
• Injection site for tissue sloughing
• Therapeutic response: increased BP with stabilisation

Teach patient/family:
• Reason for drug administration

---

metformin HCl

Glucophage, Orabet
Func. class.: Hypoglycaemic agent
Chem. class.: Biguanide
Legal class.: POM

Action: Uptake of glucose from gastrointestinal tract delayed; increases peripheral utilization of glucose; decreases gluconeogenesis

Uses: Non-insulin dependent diabetes; as an adjuvant in insulin dependent diabetic patients who are poorly controlled

Dosage and routes:
• By mouth 500 mg 8-hrly or 850 mg 12-hrly with or after food; maximum dose 3 g daily in divided doses

Available forms include: Tablets 500, 850 mg

Side effects/adverse reactions:
GI: Anorexia, nausea, vomiting,

decreased absorption of vitamin B_{12}, diarrhoea
METAB: Lactic acidosis
Contraindications: Condition associated with hypoxaemia, pulmonary insufficiency, incidence of or predisposition towards lactic acidosis; renal or hepatic failure, cardiac failure or recent myocardial infarction severe infection or trauma, dehydration, alcoholism; pregnancy, lactation. Children, hypersensitivity, diabetic coma and ketoacidosis, elderly with renal impairment
Pharmacokinetics: Control may be achieved after several days but full effects may not be seen for up to 2 weeks. Excreted unchanged in urine
Interactions/incompatibilities:
• Enhanced hypoglycaemic effect: alcohol, β-blockers, MAOIs, bezafibrate, clofibrate, cimetidine, lithium
• Antagonise hypoglycaemic effect: diazoxide, corticosteroids, diuretics, oral contraceptives
Clinical assessment:
• Monitor for hyperglycaemia or hypoglycaemia
• Monitor renal function, estimate B_{12} levels annually.
Treatment of overdose: Supportive measures with particular attention to correct metabolic disturbances and fluid loss
NURSING CONSIDERATIONS
Administer:
• With or after food
Evaluate:
• For signs of hyperglycaemic reaction
• Therapeutic response; decrease in polyuria, polydipsia, polyphagia
Teach patient/family:
• To check blood sugar regularly whilst taking the drug OR
• To check urine for sugar
• The symptoms of hyperglycaemia and how to respond to this

• That the drug should be taken regularly as prescribed
• To avoid non-prescribed medications unless approved by a clinician
• That diabetes is a life-long illness and that drug will not cure disease
• To carry a Medic Alert card for emergency purposes

---

methadone HCl

Physeptone
Func. class.: Opioid analgesic
Chem. class.: Synthetic opioid
Legal class.: CD (Sch 2) POM

Action: Inhibits ascending pain pathways in CNS, increases pain threshold, alters pain perception
Uses: Severe pain, narcotic withdrawal
Dosage and routes:
Pain
• *Adult:* By mouth, subcutaneous, IM, 5−10 mg 6−8 hrly and adjusted depending on response
Narcotic withdrawal
• *Adult:* By mouth doses in range 15−20 mg (higher in some patients to 40 mg) daily and reduce gradually
Available forms include: Injection subcutaneous, IM 10 mg/ml; tablets 5 mg; linctus 2 mg/5 ml; mixture 1 mg/ml
Side effects/adverse reactions:
CNS: Drowsiness, dizziness, euphoria, confusion, changes of mood, hallucinations
GI: Nausea, vomiting, constipation
GU: Difficulty with micturition, dysuria
INTEG: Urticaria, pruritus, flushing
EENT: Miosis
CV: Hypotension, bradycardia, palpitations
RESP: Respiratory depression

Contraindications: Hypersensitivity, respiratory depression, obstructive airways disease, obstetric use, concurrent administration with MAOIs or within 2 weeks of their discontinuation, raised intracranial pressure, head injuries

Precautions: Addiction, pregnancy, breast feeding, hepatic disease, asthma, obstructive bowel disorders, hypotension, hypothyroidism, myasthenia gravis; reduce dosage in renal impairment, elderly, debilitated

Pharmacokinetics:
By mouth: Onset 30–60 min, duration 6–8 hr
Subcutaneous/IM: Onset 10–20 min, peak 1 hr, duration 6–8 hr, cumulative 22–48 hr
Metabolised by liver, excreted by kidneys, excreted in breast milk, half-life 15–25 hr

Interactions/incompatibilities:
• Effects may be increased with other CNS depressants: alcohol, narcotics, sedative/hypnotics, antipsychotics, skeletal muscle relaxants
• Concurrent use of MAOIs

Treatment of overdose: Naloxone IV repeated every 5–10 min; elimination rate by kidney increased by acidification of urine.
N.B: lavage, dialysis and CNS stimulation are contraindicated

NURSING CONSIDERATIONS

Assess:
• Pain levels
• Vital signs

Administer:
• With anti-emetic if nausea, vomiting occur
• When pain is beginning to return; determine dosage interval by patient response

Perform/provide:
• Storage according to CD regulations and local procedures
• Assistance with mobility

Evaluate:
• Therapeutic response: decrease in pain
• Fluid balance check for decreasing output; may indicate urinary retention
• CNS changes: dizziness, drowsiness, hallucinations, euphoria, level of consciousness, pupil reaction
• Allergic reactions: rash, urticaria
• Respiratory dysfunction: respiratory depression, character, rate, rhythm; notify clinician if respirations are less than 12/min
• Need for pain medication, physical dependence

Teach patient/family:
• To report any symptoms of CNS changes, allergic reactions
• That physical dependency may result when used for extended periods of time
• Withdrawal symptoms may occur: nausea, vomiting, cramps, fever, faintness, anorexia
• To report increase in pain
• Abstain from narcotic drug abuse whilst undergoing methadone withdrawal regimen

methenamine hippurate

Hiprex
Func. class.: Antibiotic, urinary tract
Chem. class.: Methenamine mandelic acid
Legal class.: P

Action: In acid urine it is hydrolysed to formaldehyde which has antimicrobial activity; bacteriostatic
Uses: Treatment and prophylaxis against urinary tract infections caused by a wide range of Gram-positive and Gram-negative organisms including *Escherichia coli,*

Aerobacter aerogenes, Pseudomonas spp, some strains of *Proteus* spp

Dosage and routes:
• *Adult:* By mouth 1 g twice a day; may be increased in patients with catheter to 1 g 3 times a day
• *Child 6−12 yr:* 500 mg twice daily

Available forms include: Tablets 1 g

Side effects/adverse reactions:
INTEG: Rash
GI: Nausea, vomiting, diarrhoea and other disturbances
GU: Bladder irritation, painful and frequent micturation, haematuria, proteinuria

Contraindications: Severe dehydration, severe renal impairment, metabolic acidosis

Precautions: Renal insufficiency, pregnancy

Pharmacokinetics:
By mouth: Excreted in urine, half-life 4 hr

Interactions/incompatibilities:
• Insoluble precipitate in urine: (crystalluria): sulphonamides
• Urine alkalinising agents: potassium litrate, acetazolamide

Clinical assessment:
• Culture and sensitivity before treatment, after completion
• Check that urine pH is less than 5.5
• Up to 12 g of vitamin C if needed to acidify urine; cranberry, prune juice may be used

Lab. test interferences: Estimations for catacholamines, 17-hydroxycorticosteroids, oestrogens in urine

Treatment of overdose: Treat vomiting with an anti-emetic, haematuria by drinking copious amounts of water. Treat bladder symptoms by drinking copious amounts of water and 2−3 teaspoonfuls of bicarbonate of soda

NURSING CONSIDERATIONS
Assess:
• Fluid balance, urine pH less than 5.5 is ideal

Administer:
• After mid-stream urine or other samples are obtained for culture and sensitivity

Perform/provide:
• Give vitamin C or juices such as cranberry or prune to achieve desired urine activity
• Limited intake of alkaline foods or drugs: milk, dairy products, peanuts, vegetables, alkaline anti-acids, sodium bicarbonate

Evaluate:
• Therapeutic response: decreased pain, frequency, urgency, negative culture and sensitivity, absence of infection
• Allergy: fever, flushing, rash, urticaria, pruritus

Teach patient/family:
• Keep urine acidic by eating food that acidifies urine (meats, eggs, fish, gelatin products, prunes, plums, cranberries)
• Fluids must be increased to 3 litres daily to avoid crystallisation in kidneys
• Complete full course of drug therapy; take drug at evenly spaced intervals around clock for best results

methicillin sodium

Celbenin
Func. class.: Antibiotic, broad-spectrum
Chem. class.: Penicillinase resistant penicillin
Legal class.: POM

Action: Interferes with cell wall replication of susceptible organisms; osmotically unstable cell wall swells, bursts from osmotic pressure

Uses: Infections caused by β-lactamase producing staphylococci

Dosage and routes:
• *Adult:* IM or IV injection (over 3−4 min) 1 g 4−6 hrly; may also be given by IV infusion. Dosage may be increased in severe infections
• *Child under 2 yr:* Quarter adult dose; 2−10 yr half adult dose
Available forms include: Powder for injection 1 g

Side effects/adverse reactions:
HAEM: Bone marrow depression, leucopenia, agranulocytosis, anaemia, increased bleeding time, defective platelet function
GI: Upsets including diarrhoea and nausea, glossitis
MISC: Allergic reactions, anaphylatic shock

Contraindications: Penicillin hypersensitivity

Precautions: Pregnancy, lactation, history of allergy, renal impairment

Pharmacokinetics:
IM: Peak ½−1 hr, duration 4 hr
IV: Peak 15 min, duration 2 hr
Metabolised in liver, excreted in urine, bile, breast milk

Interactions/incompatibilities:
• Reduced excretion of methicillin: probenecid

Clinical assessment:
• Renal studies: urinalysis, protein, blood
• Culture and sensitivity before drug therapy; drug may be taken as soon as culture is taken
• Scratch test to assess allergy; usually done when penicillin is only drug of choice

Treatment of overdose: Symptomatic treatment in the unlikely event

NURSING CONSIDERATIONS
Assess:
• Bowel pattern
• Any patient with compromised renal system since drug is excreted slowly in poor renal system function; toxicity may occur rapidly

Administer:
• Drug after culture and sensitivity has been completed

Perform/provide:
• Adequate fluid intake 2 litres daily during diarrhoea episodes

Evaluate:
• Therapeutic effectiveness: absence of fever, draining wounds
• Bowel pattern before, during treatment
• Fluid balance; report haematuria, oliguria since penicillin in high doses is nephrotoxic
• Monitor for skin rash and report if seen. Treatment should be stopped
• Respiratory status: rate, character, wheezing, tightness in chest
• Allergies before initiation of treatment, reaction of each medication; highlight allergies on Nursing Care Plan

Teach patient/family:
• Culture may be taken after completed course of medication
• To report sore throat, fever, fatigue; could indicate superimposed infection
• To wear or carry Medic Alert identify if allergic to penicillins
• To notify nurse or clinician of diarrhoea

---

methixene HCl

Tremonil
Func. class.: Antiparkinsonism agent
Chem. class.: Antimuscarinic
Legal class.: POM

Action: Corrects central relative cholinergic excess thought to occur in parkinsonism as a result of dopamine deficiency

Uses: Parkinsonism, drug-induced extrapyramidal symptoms, senile tremor

Dosage and routes:
• By mouth 2.5 mg 3 times daily increased gradually; maintenance dose 15−60 mg daily in divided doses, 15−30 mg daily in divided doses for elderly
Available forms include: Tablets 5 mg
Side effects/adverse reactions:
CNS: Dizziness, nervousness, excitability, confusion, psychiatric disturbances
CV: Tachycardia
GU: Urinary retention
GI: Disturbances, dry mouth, constipation
EENT: Transient visual disturbances
Contraindications: Prostatic hypertrophy, urinary retention, narrow angle glaucoma, cardiac arrythmias, intestinal hypotonia, alcoholism, myasthenia gravis, intoxication with analgesics, hypnotics, psychotropics, alcohol, pyloric stenosis, paralytic ileus
Precautions: Hepatic or renal impairment, cardiovascular disease, initial autonomic disturbances, avoid sudden discontinuation of drug, drug liable to abuse
Pharmacokinetics: Absorbed from GI tract, excreted in urine partly unchanged and partly as isomeric sulphoxides or their metabolites
Interactions/incompatibilities:
• Increased antimuscarinic effects: drugs with antimuscarinic properties including disopyramide, anti-depressants, antihistamines, phenothiazines, amantadine, domperidone, metoclopramide
Treatment of overdose: Gastric lavage and supportive measures, giving fluids freely. Peripheral symptoms may be relieved by neostigmine
NURSING CONSIDERATIONS
Administer:
• With or after meals to prevent GI upsets

• At bedtime to avoid daytime drowsiness in patient with parkinsonism
Perform/provide:
• Frequent fluids, mouthwashes to relieve dry mouth
Evaluate:
• For extrapyramidial symptoms, shuffling gait, muscle rigidity, involuntary movements
• Fluid balance: retention commonly causes decreased urinary output
• For urinary hesitancy, retention
• For constipation − increase fluids, bulk, exercise
• For tolerance over long-term therapy − dose may need to be changed
• Mental status: affect, mood, CNS depression; if mental symptoms worsen during initial treatment, inform clinician
Teach patient/family:
• Not to discontinue drug abruptly
• To avoid driving or other hazardous activities; drowsiness may occur
• To avoid non-prescribed medications, alcohol, antihistamines, unless approved by clinician

---

methocarbamol

Robaxin 750, Robaxin Injectable, combination product
Func. class.: Skeletal muscle relaxant
Chem. class.: Carbamate derivative
Legal class.: POM

Action: CNS depressant; action may be from sedative effects; precise mechanism of action is unknown
Uses: Pain due to spasm in musculoskeletal conditions or trauma, tetanus management
Dosage and routes:

• *Adult:* By mouth 1.5 g 4 times daily but may be effective in reduced dosage, 750 mg 3 times daily
• *Elderly:* Half adult dose or less
• *Adult:* IV injection or infusion 1−3 g daily for maximum of 3 days; slow IV injection maximum rate 300 mg/min. By infusion in dextrose 5% or sodium chloride 0.9% 1 g not diluted to more than 250 ml
Available forms include: Tablets 750 mg; injection IV 1 g/10 ml
Side effects/adverse reactions:
CNS: Dizziness, drowsiness, tremor, lassitude, light-headedness, restlessness, anxiety, confusion, convulsions, vertigo, headache, syncope
GI: Nausea, vomiting, metallic taste
INTEG: Allergic rash, urticaria, flushing
EENT: Blurred vision
CV: Hypotension, bradycardia, angioedema
SYST: Anaphylaxis
Contraindications: Hypersensitivity, coma or pre-coma states, brain damage, epilepsy, myaesthenia gravis, use in children, pregnancy, lactation
Precautions: Renal disease, hepatic disease. May cause drowsiness−warn patients not to drive or operate machinery until affects known
Pharmacokinetics:
By mouth: Onset ½ hr, peak 1−2 hr, half-life 1−2 hr, metabolised in liver, excreted in urine (unchanged)
Interactions/incompatibilities:
• Increased CNS depression: alcohol, barbiturates
• Potentiation of effects: anorectics, antimuscarinics, some psychotropic agents

Clinical assessment:
• Monitor response and side effects
Lab. test interferences:
False positive: possibly in test for raised 5-hydroxyindoleacetic acid
Treatment of overdose: Gastric lavage with supportive measures; continue for 24 hr
NURSING CONSIDERATIONS
Administer:
• IV: by slow injection, or infusion
• (Oral dose) with meals for GI symptoms
Evaluate:
• Therapeutic response: decreased pain, spasticity (short-term acting drug)
• Allergic reactions: rash, fever, respiratory distress
• Severe weakness, numbness in extremities
• Psychological dependency: increased need for medication, more frequent requests for medication, increased pain
• CNS depression: dizziness, drowsiness, psychiatric symptoms
Teach patient/family:
• Not to discontinue medication quickly; insomnia, nausea, headache, spasticity, tachycardia will occur; drug should be tapered off over 1−2 weeks
• Not to take with alcohol, other CNS depressants
• To avoid changes to lifestyle whilst taking this drug
• To avoid hazardous activities if drowsiness, dizziness occurs; avoid driving, operating machinery
• To avoid using non-prescribed drugs: cough preparations, antihistamines, unless directed by clinician

methohexitone sodium

Brietal Sodium
Func. class.: Anaesthetic, general
Chem. class.: Barbiturate
Legal class.: POM

Action: Acts in reticular-activating system to produce anaesthesia

Uses: Rapid very short acting anaesthetic agent for induction and maintenance of anaesthesia in short procedures, used with other agents for more prolonged anaesthesia

Dosage and routes:
Induction
• *Adult:* IV 1% solution, 50–120 mg given at a rate of 10 mg in 5 seconds according to response
• *Child:* 1 mg/kg
Maintenance
• *IV:* 20–40 mg every 4–7 min of a 1% solution

Available forms include: Injection IV 100, 500 mg powder for reconstitution

Side effects/adverse reactions:
RESP: Transitory apnoea, respiratory depression, respiratory arrest, bronchospasm, sneezing, cough
CNS: Headache, persistent drowsiness
CV: Circulatory depression, cardiac arrest, hypotension, tachycardia
GI: Salivation, nausea, hiccup
INTEG: Shivering, thrombophlebitis, pain at injection site
MS: Skeletal muscle hyperactivity
MISC: Acute allergic reactions

Contraindications: Hypersensitivity to barbiturates, porphyria, epilepsy, status asthmaticus

Precautions: Cardiovascular disease, renal disease, liver disease, impaired respiratory function, impaired endocrine function, debilitated patients. Pregnancy, lactation, labour and delivery

Pharmacokinetics:
IV: Onset 30–40 sec; half-life 11.5 hr

Interactions/incompatibilities:
• Increased action: CNS depressants
• Decreased action: coumarin anticoagulants, endogenous steroids
• Increased occurrence of abnormal muscle movements: cyclizine, some phenothiazines
• Not to be mixed with acid solutions including: atropine sulphate, tubocurarine, succinylcholine
• Do not mix with solutions containing bacteriostats
• Do not allow contact with silicon treated components of syringes, etc.

Clinical assessment:
• Monitor and report level of anaesthesia during post-operative period

Treatment of overdose: Life-support measures as required

NURSING CONSIDERATIONS

Assess:
• Baseline vital signs
• Level of orientation before administration

Administer:
• Slowly, after preparation with sodium chloride solution of 0.9% or 5% dextrose as a 1% solution of methohexitone
• With resuscitative equipment nearby
• IV slowly only under direction of anaesthetist

Evaluate:
• Extravasation, if it occurs use nitroprusside or chloroprocaine to decrease pain, increase circulation
• Dysrhythmias or myocardial depression
• Level of respiratory excitability immediately after administration
• Vital signs for dysrhythmias, myocardial depression or hypotension

methotrexate/ methotrexate sodium

Methotrexate (Lederle), Maxtrex
Func. class.: Antineoplastic-antimetabolite
Chem. class.: Folic acid antagonist
Legal class.: POM

Action: Inhibits dihydrofolate reductase that reduces folic acid, which is needed for nucleic acid synthesis in reproducing cells

Uses: Choriocarcinoma and other trophoblastic tumours, childhood acute lymphoblastic leukaemia, meningeal leukaemia in children, non-Hodgkin's lymphoma, breast cancer, osteogenic sarcoma, bronchogenic sarcoma, head and neck cancer, bladder carcinoma, psoriasis

Dosage and route:
Cancer chemotherapy
Seek specialist advice for doses and regimens
Psoriasis
• *Adult:* By mouth 10−25 mg weekly
Available forms include: Tablets 2.5, 10 mg; injection solutions 2.5, 5, 25, 50, 100, 200, 500 mg, 1, 5 g; injection powder for reconstitution 500 mg

Side effects/adverse reactions:
HAEM: Bone marrow depression, leucopenia, thrombocytopenia, anaemia
GI: Nausea, vomiting, diarrhoea, ulcerative stomatitis, hepatic cirrhosis, acute liver atrophy, intestinal perforation, haemorrhagic enteritis
GU: Renal failure, severe nephropathy, suppression of ovarian and testicular function
INTEG: Rash, alopecia, photosensitivity, vasculitis, ulceration
EENT: Blurred vision
CNS: Headache, drowsiness,
ataxia, transient paresis, dementia, major convulsions

Contraindications: Serious leucopenia, thrombocytopenia, anaemia, severe renal or hepatic impairment, pregnancy, porphyria

Precautions: Lactation, haematological depression, renal impairment, ulceration of gastrointestinal tract, diarrhoea, debility, very young, elderly

Pharmacokinetics:
By mouth: Readily absorbed when taken orally, peak 1−4 hr
IV/IM: Peak ½−2 hr
Not metabolised, excreted in urine (unchanged), crosses blood-brain barrier, 50% plasma protein bound

Interactions/incompatibilities:
• Increased toxicity: aspirin and other salicylates, sulphonamides, diuretics, hypoglycaemic agents, diphenylhydantoin, chloramphenicol, tetracyclines, NSAIDs, cotrimoxazole, trimethoprim, phenytoin, tetretinate, probenecid
• Concurrent administration of: live vaccines
• Decreased effects of this drug: folic acid supplements

Clinical assessment:
• Full blood count prior to treatment and 10 days post treatment. Do not give next dose whilst patient neutropenic
• Renal function studies before/during treatment when impairment suspected or high dose therapy being given
• Liver function tests before and during therapy if severe impairment anticipated; liver biopsy should be done before start of therapy (psoriasis patients)
• Sodium bicarbonate to maintain urine pH above 7 during excretion phase after medium-high dose (greater than 100 mg/m^2 approximately) therapy

Treatment of overdose: IM, IV or orally calcium leucovorin at a dose equal or higher than overdose and administered within 1 hr, further doses if required

Supporting therapy of blood transfusion and renal dialysis if necessary

NURSING CONSIDERATIONS

Assess:

• Baseline vital signs

Administer:

• According to local cytotoxic policy

• Reconstitution to be performed by trained personnel

• Reconstituted and diluted solutions stable for 24 hr

• Should not be mixed with other IV drugs

• Other medications by oral route if possible; avoid IM, subcutaneous, IV routes to prevent infections

• Antacid before oral agent; give drug after evening meal before bedtime

• Anti-emetic 30−60 min before giving drug to prevent vomiting

• Give with food if taken orally

Perform/provide:

• Strict medical asepsis and protective isolation if WBC levels are low

• Liquid diet: carbonated beverage, dry toast, plain biscuits may be added when patient is not nauseated or vomiting

• Increased fluid intake to 2−3 litres daily to prevent urate deposits, calculi formation, unless contraindicated

• Diet low in purines: avoid offal meats (kidney, liver), dried beans, peas to maintain alkaline urine

• Rinsing of mouth 3 or 4 times a day with water, hydrogen peroxide; brushing of teeth 2 or 3 times a day with soft brush or cotton-tipped applicators for stomatitis; use unwaxed dental floss

• Nutritious diet with iron, vitamin supplements

Evaluate:

• Fluid balance; report fall in urine output to less than 30 ml/hr

• Bleeding: haematuria, bruising or petechiae, mucosa or orifices 8 hrly

• Food preferences; list likes, dislikes

• Effects of alopecia on body image; discuss feelings about body changes

• Hepatotoxicity: yellowing of skin, sclera, dark urine, clay-coloured stools, pruritus, abdominal pain, fever, diarrhoea

• Buccal cavity 8 hrly for dryness, sores, ulceration, white patches, oral pain, bleeding, dysphagia

• Symptoms indicating severe allergic reaction: rash, urticaria, itching, flushing

Teach patient/family:

• Why protective isolation precautions are needed

• To report any complaints, side effects to nurse or clinician: black tarry stools, chills, fever, sore throat, bleeding, bruising, cough, shortness of breath, dark or bloody urine

• That hair may be lost during treatment and wig or hairpiece is available on NHS prescription; tell patient that new hair may be different in colour, texture (alopecia is rare)

• To avoid foods with citric acid, hot or rough texture if stomatitis is present

• To report stomatitis: any bleeding, white spots, ulcerations in mouth; tell patient to examine mouth daily, report symptoms to nurse

• Contraceptive measures are recommended during therapy for at least 8 weeks following cessation of therapy

• To drink 10−12 glasses of fluid daily

• To avoid alcohol, salicylates

• Importance of regular blood tests

---

methotrimeprazine

Nozinan
Func. class.: Sedative-hypnotic
Chem. class.: Aliphatic propylamine-phenothiazine derivative
Legal class.: POM

Action: Depresses cerebral cortex, hypothalamus, limbic system; blocks neurotransmission produced by dopamine at synapse; exhibits strong α-adrenergic, anticholinergic blocking action

Uses: Terminal care-severe pain (with restlessness, distress, or vomiting), sedation, schizophrenia

Dosage and routes:

Terminal illness

• *Adult:* 12.5−50 mg orally 4−8 hrly; IM injection 12.5−25 mg; IV injection 12.5−25 mg (after dilution with equal volume of sodium chloride 0.9%) every 6−8 hr (severe agitation up to 50 mg); continuous subcutaneous infusion 25−200 mg daily diluted with sodium chloride 0.9%

Schizophrenia

• *Adult:* (Ambulant) 25−50 mg daily orally in 3 divided doses and increased as necessary. Bed-patients 100−200 mg daily orally in 3 divided doses increased as necessary to 1 g daily

Available forms include: Injection (hydrochloride) 25 mg/ml, tablets (maleate) 25 mg

Side effects/adverse reactions:

HAEM: Agranulocytosis, leucopenia, haemolytic anaemia, jaundice

CNS: Weakness, drowsiness, apathy, nightmares, insomnia, depression, agitation, extrapyramidal symptoms

GI: Dry mouth, constipation
INTEG: Sensitisation, rashes
EENT: Nasal congestion, blurred vision
CV: Hypotension, tachycardia, arrhythmias, ECG changes

Contraindications: Hypersensitivity, pregnancy (safety not established), coma, severe cardiac, renal and hepatic disease

Precautions: Postural hypotension (especially patients over 50 and elderly), children (maximum daily dose 40 mg, average for 10 yr old 15−20 mg daily), cardiac, renal and hepatic disease

Pharmacokinetics:

By mouth: Onset 20−30 min, peak 1−2 hr, duration 4 hr; metabolised by liver, excreted by kidneys and in faeces, excreted in breast milk

Interactions/incompatibilities:

• Increased sedation: alcohol, anxiolytics, hypnotics
• Enhanced hypotensive effect: anaesthetics, antihypertensives, calcium-channel blockers
• Avoid simultaneous administration of prochlorperazine and desferrioxamine

Treatment of overdose: Gastric lavage if within 6 hr, give activated charcoal, supportive care. See data sheet for further information

NURSING CONSIDERATIONS

Assess:

• Baseline vital signs

Administer:

• IM injection in deep large muscle mass to prevent tissue sloughing, rotate sites
• Lowest dose, then gradually increase; lower doses are required after general anaesthesia
• Subcutaneous infusion in terminally ill patient adjusted to provide optimum relief

Perform/provide:

• Bedrest for several hours after

injection if orthostatic hypotension occurs

• Safety measure: siderails, night-light, callbell within easy reach
• Assistance with ambulation for 6 hr after injection

Evaluate:

• Decreasing BP with increased pulse that may occur 10−30 min after injection
• Effect on uterine contractions, foetal heart tones if using for labour
• Therapeutic response: decrease in pain, grimacing, absence of change in vital signs, ability to cough and breathe deeply after surgery
• For extra-pyramidal signs

Teach patient/family:

• Drug may impair mental alertness or physical co-ordination, warn patients against driving or operating machinery if affected

---

methoxamine HCl

Vasoxine
Func. class.: Vasoconstrictor
Chem. class.: Sympathomimetic
Legal class.: POM

Action: Constricts peripheral blood vessels causing transient rise in BP

Uses: Hypotension in anaesthesia

Dosage and routes:

• *Adults:* IM injection 5−20 mg, slow IV injection 5−10 mg at rate of 1 mg/min
• *Child:* IM injection 250 mcg/kg body weight, IV injection 80 mcg/kg body weight

Available forms include: Injection 20 mg/ml, 1 ml ampoule

Side effects/adverse reactions:

CV: Hypertension, bradycardia
GI: Projectile vomiting
CNS: Headache
INTEG: Feeling cold, other skin sensations
GU: Desire to micturate
MISC: Sensation of fullness in neck and chest

Contraindications: Severe coronary or cardiovascular disease, pre-existent severe hypertension

Precautions: Hyperthyroidism, pregnancy, second dose to be injected only when first has ceased to act, make repeated arterial pressure measurements

Pharmacokinetics: Acts 1 or 2 min after IV injection and about 15−20 min after IM injection, in the latter case duration of action is 1½ hr

Interactions/incompatibilities:

• Increased response to drug: MAOIs, tricyclic antidepressants, β−blockers, other sympathomimetic agents, some appetite suppressants and amphetamine-like psychostimulants

Treatment of overdose: Administer phentolamine 5 mg IV if blood pressure does not return to normal after an appropriate time; repeat as necessary

NURSING CONSIDERATIONS

Assess:

• Baseline vital signs

Administer:

• Parenteral (IV) dose slowly according to clinician's instructions

Evaluate:

• Fluid balance—notify clinician if output less than 30 ml/hr
• ECG during administration; if BP increases, drug is decreased
• BP and pulse every 5 min after parenteral route
• CVP during infusion if possible
• For paraesthesiae and coldness of extremities, peripheral blood flow may decrease
• Therapeutic response: increased BP with stabilisation

Teach patient/family:

• The reason for drug administration

---

methyclothiazide

Enduron
Func. class.: Thiazide diuretic
Chem. class.: Sulphonamide derivative
Legal class.: POM

Action: Acts on distal tubule by increasing excretion of water, sodium, chloride, potassium

Uses: Oedema, hypertension

Dosage and routes:
• *Adult:* By mouth 2.5−5 mg daily, if necessary increased to 10 mg daily

Available forms include: Tablets 5 mg

Side effects/adverse reactions:
GU: Glycosuria, impotence
CNS: Dizziness, headache, weakness, paraesthesia
GI: Nausea, vomiting, anorexia, constipation, diarrhoea, pancreatitis
HAEM: Increased plasma cholesterol thrombocytopenia, agranulocytosis, aplastic anaemia, leucopenia, neutropenia
INTEG: Purpura, rash, photosensitivity
CV: Hypotension
ELECT: Hyperglycaemia, hyperuricaemia, hypokalaemia, hypomagnesaemia, hyponatraemia, hypercalcaemia, hypochloraemic alkalosis

Contraindications: Hypersensitivity to thiazides or sulphonamides, severe renal or hepatic disease, Addison's disease, hypercalcaemia, lithium therapy, porphyria

Precautions: May cause hypokalaemia, renal and hepatic impairment, pregnancy, lactation, diabetes, gout, electrolyte imbalance in elderly

Pharmacokinetics:
By mouth: Onset 2 hr, peak 6 hr, duration greater than 24 hr; excreted unchanged by kidneys, enters breast milk

Interactions/incompatibilities:
• Increased toxicity of: lithium, digitalis
• Decreased effects of: antidiabetics
• Decreased absorption of thiazides: cholestyramine, colestipol
• Risk of hypercalcaemia: calcium salts
• Increased risk of hypokalaemia: corticosteroids

Clinical assessment:
• Electrolytes; potassium, sodium, chloride, calcium
• Blood lipid analysis

Treatment of overdose: Recent ingestion: gastric lavage or emesis, supportive measures

NURSING CONSIDERATIONS

Assess:
• Baseline vital signs including BP standing/lying
• Weight
• Rate, depth, rhythm of respiration, effect of exertion
• Glucose in urine if patient is diabetic

Administer:
• In morning to avoid interference with sleep if using drug as a diuretic
• With food, if nausea occurs, absorption may be decreased slightly

Perform/provide:
• Daily blood sugar estimations
• Daily weighing, fluid balance

Evaluate:
• BP lying, standing, postural hypotension may occur early in use
• Improvement in oedema of feet, legs, sacral area daily if medication is being used in congestive cardiac failure

- Improvement in CVP 8 hrly
- Signs of metabolic acidosis: drowsiness, restlessness
- Signs of hypokalaemia: postural hypotension, malaise, fatigue, tachycardia, leg cramps, weakness
- Rashes, temperature elevation daily
- Confusion, especially in elderly; take safety precautions if needed

Teach patient/family:
- To increase fluid intake 2−3 litres daily unless contraindicated. To rise slowly from lying or sitting position
- To notify clinician of muscle weakness, cramps, nausea, dizziness
- Drug may be taken with food or milk
- That blood sugar may be increased in diabetics, urine or blood should be tested daily
- Take early in day to avoid nocturia

---

methylcellulose

Celevac, Nilstim
Func. class.: Laxative, bulk
Chem. class.: Hydrophilic, semi-synthetic cellulose derivative
Legal class.: GSL

Action: Attracts water, expands in intestine to increase peristalsis; also absorbs excess water in stool; decreases diarrhoea

Uses: Constipation, colostomy/ileostomy control, diverticular disease, diarrhoea, appetite control

Dosage and routes:
- By mouth: 3−6 tablets twice a day; take with a minimum of 300 ml water in constipation; minimise water intake 30 min before and after dose in colostomy/ileostomy control and diarrhoea and take with minimum of liquid
- 3 tablets 30 min before meals with 300 ml warm water in appetite control, repeated between meals if necessary

Available forms include: Tablets 500 mg. Mixture is available: 900 mg/10 ml
Dose: 5−15 ml, 3 times daily in tumblerful of water after meals−maintenance 5−15 ml daily
Also Nilstin-Tabs 400 mg
Dose: 2 tablets, chewed or crushed, with tumblerful of liquid 15 min before main meal or when hungry

Side effects/adverse reactions:
GI: Flatulence, abdominal distension, intestinal obstruction
Contraindications: Intestinal obstruction, faecal impaction, hypersensitivity, colonic atony
Precautions: Diarrhoea due to a pathological cause e.g. infective bowel disease
Pharmacokinetics:
By mouth: Onset 12−24 hr, peak 1−3 days
Treatment of overdose: Gastric lavage if necessary; rectal washout if obstruction develops

NURSING CONSIDERATIONS
Assess:
- Cause of constipation; identify whether fluids, bulk, or exercise is missing from lifestyle
- Fluid balance to identify fluid loss

Administer:
- Alone for better absorption (especially colostomy/ileostomy) do not take within 1 hr of other drugs or within 1 hr of antacids, milk, or cimetidine
- In morning or early evening (oral dose); should not be taken before going to bed
- 1−2 litres of fluid daily

Evaluate:
- Therapeutic response: decrease in constipation
- Cramping, rectal bleeding, nausea, vomiting; if these symp-

toms occur, drug should be discontinued

Teach patient/family:
- That normal bowel movements do not always occur daily
- Not to use if abdominal pain, nausea, vomiting occur
- Notify clinician if constipation unrelieved or if symptoms of electrolyte imbalance occur: muscle cramps, pain, weakness, dizziness
- That preparations swell in contact with liquid; carefully swallow with water and do not take immediately before going to bed
- About diet

---

methyldopa/ methyldopate HCl

Aldomet, Dopamet, combination product
Func. class.: Antihypertensive
Chem. class.: Centrally acting adrenergic inhibitor
Legal class.: POM

Action: Stimulates central α-adrenergic receptors or acts as false transmitter, resulting in reduction of arterial pressure
Uses: Hypertension in conjunction with a diuretic; hypotensive crisis
Dosage and route:
- *Adult:* By mouth 250 mg 2 or 3 times daily, then adjusted every 2 days as required, maximum daily dose 3 g. IV 250−500 mg in 100 ml dextrose 5% over 30−60 min, 6 hrly; not to exceed 1 g 6 hrly
- *Children:* By mouth 10 mg/kg daily is 2−4 divided doses; maximum daily dose 65 mg/kg or 3 g daily whichever less. IV 20−40 mg/kg/day in divided doses every 6 hr; maximum daily dose 65 mg/kg or 3 g daily whichever less

- *Elderly:* By mouth 125 mg twice a day initially, adjusted as required; maximum daily dose 2 g
Available forms include: Tablets (methyldopa) 125, 250, 500 mg; oral suspension (methyldopa) 250 mg 5 ml; injection IV (methyldopate HCl) 50 mg/ml

Side effects/adverse reactions:
GI: Nausea, vomiting, diarrhoea, constipation, hepatic dysfunction, distension, flatus, colitis, dry mouth, pancreatitis, sore or black tongue, sialadenitis, liver disorders
CV: Bradycardia, myocarditis, orthostatic hypotension, angina, oedema, weight gain, prolonged carotid sinus
CNS: Sedation, weakness, dizziness, headache, depression, psychosis, parkinsonism, paraesthesia, bell's palsy, involuntary choreoathetotic movement, impaired mental acuity, nightmares
INTEG: Eczema, lichenoid eruption, toxic epidermal necrolysis
GU: Decreased libido, impotence, failure to ejaculate
MISC: Allergic reactions
HAEM: Positive Coombs' test, bone marrow depression, leucopenia, thrombocytopenia, haemolytic anaemia, granulocytopenia
EENT: Nasal congestion
Contraindications: Hypersensitivity, active hepatic disease, history of depression, phaeochromocytoma, porphyria
Precautions: Pregnancy, lactation, Coombs' test, renal disease (reduce initial dose), severe cardiac disease
Pharmacokinetics:
By mouth: Peak 2−4 hr, duration 12−24 hr
IV: Peak 2 hr, duration 10−16 hr Metabolised by liver, excreted in urine
Interactions/incompatibilities:
- Reduced antihypertensive effect

with: phenothiazines, sympathomimetics, tricyclic antidepressants, MAOIs, NSAIDs, corticosteroids, oestrogens and combined oral contraceptives
• Enhanced hypotensive effect: anaesthetics, alcohol, other antihypertensives, antipsychotics, anxiolytics, hypnotics, β-blockers, calcium channel blockers, levodopa, nitrates
• Increased lithium toxicity

Clinical assessment:
• Blood counts
• Renal studies: protein, blood urea nitrogen, creatinine, watch for increased levels, may indicate nephrotic syndrome
• Baselines in renal, liver function tests before therapy begins
• Potassium levels, although hyperkalaemia rarely occurs

Lab. test interferences:
Positive direct Coombs' test in up to 20% of patients. Urinary uric acid measurement by phosphotungstate method, serum creatinine by alkaline picrate method, aspartate aminotransferase (SGOT) by colourimetric method, estimation of urinary catacholamines by fluorescent measurements

Treatment of overdose: Gastric lavage or emesis. Symptomatic treatment. Drug is dialysable

NURSING CONSIDERATIONS

Assess:
• BP prior to treatment as baseline

Evaluate:
• Therapeutic response: decrease in BP
• Allergic reaction: rash, fever, pruritus, urticaria; refer to medical staff if any reactions occur
• Symptoms of congestive cardiac failure: oedema, dyspnoea, BP
• Renal symptoms: polyuria, oliguria, frequency

Teach patient/family:
• To take 1 hr before meals

• Not to discontinue drug abruptly or withdrawal symptoms may occur: anxiety, increased BP, headache, insomnia, increased pulse, tremors, nausea, sweating
• Not to use non-prescribed (cough, cold, allergy) products unless directed by clinician
• Stress compliance with medication regime even if feeling better
• To rise slowly to sitting or standing position to minimise risk of postural hypotension
• Notify clinician if mouth sores, sore throat, fever, swelling of hands or feet, irregular heartbeat or chest pain, oedema occur
• Excessive perspiration, dehydration, vomiting and diarrhoea may lead to fall in BP; consult clinician if these occur
• Dizziness, fainting, lightheadedness may occur during first few days of therapy
• May cause skin rash or impaired perspiration

---

methylphenobarbitone

Prominal
Func. class.: Anticonvulsant
Chem. class.: Barbiturate
Legal class.: CD (Sch 4) POM

Action: Depresses the activity of the CNS
Uses: Generalised tonic-clonic (grand mal) seizures, partial (focal) seizures
Dosage and routes:
• *Adult:* By mouth 100−600 mg daily
• *Children:* 5−15 mg/kg daily in divided doses
Available forms include: Tablets 30, 60, 200 mg
Side effects/adverse reactions:
HAEM: Megaloblastic anaemia, hypoprothrombinaemia (neonates exposed to drug)

CNS: Drowsiness, ataxia, lethargy, mental depression, paradoxical excitement, confusion, restlessness, dependence
INTEG: Maculopapular rash, photosensitivity, fixed drug eruptions, exfoliative dermatitis, erythema multiform, toxic epidermal necrolysis
CV: Hypotension
RESP: Respiratory depression
GU: Acute interstitial nephritis
MISC: Arthritis, hepatitis
GI: Stomatitis
Contraindications: Hypersensitivity, porphyria, debilitated, severe renal or hepatic disease, senility, drug abuse, children
Precautions: Impaired renal or hepatic function, respiratory depression, pregnancy, lactation
Pharmacokinetics:
By mouth: Onset 20−60 min, duration 6−8 hr
Metabolised by liver, excreted by kidneys, half-life 34 hr
Interactions/incompatibilities:
• Increased effects: CNS depressants, other anti-epileptics
• Reduced effects of: disopyramide, quinidine, chloramphenicol, metronidazole, nicoumalone, warfarin, tricyclic antidepressants, griseofulvin, calcium channel blockers, digitoxin, corticosteroids, cyclosporin, oral contraceptives, theophylline, thyroxine
Treatment of overdose: Recent ingestion (4 hr): gastric lavage and aspiration; supportive therapy with attention particularly to cardiovascular, respiratory and renal function, and electrolyte balance
NURSING CONSIDERATIONS
Administer:
• With food to reduce GI symptoms
Evaluate:
• Mental status: mood, alertness, affect, memory (long, short)
• Respiratory depression: respiration less than 10/min, shallow
• Blood dyscrasias: fever, sore throat, bruising, rash, jaundice
Teach patient/family:
• All aspects of drug usage: action, side effects, dose, when to notify clinician
• To avoid alcohol
Teach patient/family:
• Drug may cause drowsiness, caution against driving or operating machinery if affected

methylprednisolone, methylprednisolone acetate, methylprednisolone sodium succinate

Medrone, Solu-Medrone, Depot-Medrone
Func. class.: Corticosteroid
Chem. class.: Glucocorticoid
Legal class.: POM

Action: Decreases inflammation by suppression of migration of polymorphonuclear leucocytes, fibroblasts, reversal of increased capillary permeability and lysosomal stabilisation
Uses: Suppression of severe inflammatory and allergic disorders including severe erythema multiform, anaphylaxis, bronchial asthma, ulcerative colitis, etc.; cerebral oedema, shock
Dosage and routes:
• *Adult:* By mouth, usual range 2−40 mg in 3 or 4 equally divided doses
• *Child:* By mouth, dose is based on clinical response
• *Adults and child:* IM/IV doses in range 10 mg to 1 g
• For specific indication seek further information in the BNF

and manufacturer's data sheet

Available forms include: Tablets 2, 4, 16 mg; injection IV (sodium succinate) 40 mg, 125 mg, 500 mg, 1 g, 2 g; depot injection IM (acetate) 40 mg/ml ampoules 1 ml, 2 ml, 3 ml

Side effects/adverse reactions:

INTEG: Acne, poor wound healing, bruising, striae

CNS: Depression, mood changes, euphoria, insomnia, convulsions, dependance

CV: Cardiovascular collapse (rapid administration), embolism, hypertension, congestive heart failure

HAEM: Leucocytosis

METAB: Primary and secondary adrenal insufficiency

MS: Fractures, osteoporosis, proximal myopathy, avascular osteonecrosis, tendon rupture

GI: Nausea, increased appetite, dyspepsia, peptic ulceration, abdominal distension, haemorrhage, pancreatitis, oesophageal ulceration and candidiasis

EENT: Increased intra-ocular pressure, glaucoma, exacerbation of viral disease

Contraindications: Hypersensitivity, systemic fungal infections, immunisation procedures

Precautions: Pregnancy, lactation, children, masking of signs of infection, tuberculosis, non-specific ulcerative colitis, prolonged use, hypokalaemia, osteoporosis, increased susceptibility to infections, diabetes, glaucoma, epilepsy, chronic psychotic reactions, congestive cardiac failure, myasthenia gravis, renal insufficiency, thrombophlebitis, hypertension, active or latent peptic ulcer, diverticulitis, ocular herpes simplex, fresh intestinal anastomoses,

Doses must be reduced slowly

Pharmacokinetics:

By mouth: Peak 1–2 hr

IM: Peak 4–8 days

Interactions/incompatibilities:

• Decreased effect of this drug: rifampicin, carbamazepine, phenobarbitone, phenytoin, primidone

• Decreased effects of: antidiabetics, antihypertensions, diuretics

• Increased risk of hypokalaemia with: acetazolamide, loop diuretics, thiazides, carbenoxolone

Clinical assessment:

• Potassium, blood sugar, urine glucose while on long-term therapy; hypokalaemia and hyperglycaemia

• Plasma cortisol levels during long-term therapy (normal level: 138–635 nmol/litre when drawn at 8 a.m.

• Titrated dose, use lowest effective dose

Lab. test interferences:

False negative: Skin allergy tests

NURSING CONSIDERATIONS

Assess:

• Baseline weight, BP, pulse, fluid balance

Administer:

• Tablets with food or milk to decrease GI symptoms

• Suspension; after shaking (parenteral)

• IM injection deeply in large mass, rotate sites, avoid deltoid, sub-cutaneous route, use 19G needle

• In one dose in morning to prevent adrenal suppression

Perform/provide:

• Assistance with ambulation in patient with bone tissue disease to prevent fractures

Evaluate:

• Fluid balance, be alert for decreasing urinary output and increasing oedema

• Therapeutic response: ease of respirations, decreased inflammation

• Weight gain daily; notify if weekly gain is greater than 2.5 kg

• Infection: increased temperature, WBC, even after withdrawal of medication; drug masks symptoms of infection
• Potassium depletion: paraesthesia, fatigue, nausea, vomiting, depression, polyuria, dysrhythmias, weakness
• Hypotension, cardiac symptoms, chest pain
• Mental status: affect, mood, behavioural changes, aggression

Teach patient/family:
• That steroid card must be carried at all times
• To notify clinician of any side effects or if therapeutic response decreases; dosage adjustment may be needed
• Not to discontinue this medication abruptly or adrenal crisis can result
• To avoid non-prescribed drugs: salicylates, alcohol in cough products, cold preparations unless directed by clinician
• Teach patient all aspects of drug use, including Cushingoid symptoms
• Symptoms of adrenal insufficiency: nausea, anorexia, fatigue, dizziness, dyspnoea, weakness, joint pain

---

methysergide maleate

Deseril
Func. class.: Adrenergic blocker
Chem. class: Ergot derivative
Legal class.: POM

Action: Potent serotonin antagonist in CNS; potentiates the effects of vasoconstrictor stimuli and inhibits pain-facilitating and permeability-increasing actions of serotonin

Uses: Prophylactic treatment of cluster headache, other vascular headaches, migraine, diarrhoea in Carcinoid syndrome

Dosage and routes:
• *Adult:* By mouth 1 mg at bedtime increased over 2 weeks to 1 or 2 mg 2 to 3 times daily with food.
Carcinoid syndrome
• *Adult:* By mouth 12−20 mg daily
Available forms include: Tablets 1 mg

Side effects/adverse reactions:
CNS: Dizziness, insomnia, psychic reactions, drowsiness, euphoria, confusion, ataxia, weakness, hallucinations
GI: Nausea, vomiting, heartburn, abdominal discomfort
MS: Leg cramps, joint and muscle pains
INTEG: Rashes, loss of scalp hair, eruptions
MISC: Retroperitoneal fibrosis, fibrosis in other areas
CV: Postural hypotension, tachycardia, vascular reactions including arterial spasm

Contraindications: Collagen disease, pregnancy, lactation, peripheral vascular disorders, pulmonary and cardiovascular disease, urinary tract disorders, cachetic or septic conditions, phlebitis or cellulitis of lower extremities, severe hypertension, impaired hepatic or renal function

Precautions: History of peptic ulceration, abrupt withdrawal, regular clinical supervision, concomitant use of ergotamine

Pharmacokinetics:
By mouth: Half-life 10 hr, metabolised by liver, excreted in urine (metabolites/unchanged drug)

Interactions/incompatibilities:
• Enhanced vasoconstriction: vasoconstrictors or vasopressors

Treatment of overdose: Aspiration or gastric lavage, supportive measures

NURSING CONSIDERATIONS
Assess:

• Baseline weight

Administer:

• Use requires hospital supervision

• At beginning of headache, dose must be titrated to patient response

• Give with meals or after meals to avoid GI symptoms

• Continuous therapy should not exceed 6 months. Drug free period of 1 month required before recommence

Perform/provide:

• Storage in dark area; do not use discoloured solutions

• Quiet, calm environment with decreased stimulation for noise, bright light, or excessive talking

Evaluate:

• Weight daily, check for peripheral oedema in feet, legs

• Withdraw treatment for reassessment after 6 months

• Therapeutic response: decrease in frequency, severity of headache

• For stress level, activity, recreation, coping mechanisms of patient

• Neurological status: level of consciousness, blurring vision, nausea, vomiting, tingling in extremities that occur preceding headache

Teach patient/family:

• Not to use non-prescribed drugs, serious drug interactions may occur

• To maintain dose at approved level, not to increase even if drug does not relieve headache

• To report side effects: increased vasoconstriction starting with cold extremities, then paraesthesia, weakness

• That an increase in headaches may occur when this drug is discontinued after long-term use

• Report at once: dyspnoea, paraesthesia, urinary problems, pain in abdomen, chest, back, legs

metipranolol (ophthalmic)

Minims Metipranolol, Glauline

Func. class.: Antihypertensive, ocular

Chem. class.: β-blocker

Legal class.: POM

Action: Reduces intra-ocular pressure, probably by reducing the rate of production of aqueous humour

Uses: Primary open-angle glaucoma, secondary glaucoma

Dosage and routes:

• *Adults, elderly:* Eye drops, one drop twice daily. Initially 0.1%, 0.3% if control not achieved

Available forms include: Eyedrops 0.1%, 0.3% 5 ml; unit dose 0.1%, 0.3% and 0.6%

Side effects/adverse reactions:

EENT: Eye irritation — burning, stinging, blurred vision, transitory dry eyes, allergic blepharoconjunctivitis, superficial keratitis, anterior uveitis

CV: Bradycardia, hypotension

RESP: Bronchospasm, dyspnoea, respiratory failure

CNS: Weakness, fatigue, headache, ataxia

INTEG: Rash, oedema

Contraindications: Bradycardia, heart block, heart failure, asthma, obstructive airways disease, hypersensitivity, pregnancy (unless benefits outweigh hazard)

Precautions: Breast feeding, patients wearing soft contact lenses, diabetic control monitored, cardiac disease

Interactions/incompatibilities: Additive effect: other β-blockers — oral administration

Treatment of overdose: Flush immediately with water or saline

NURSING CONSIDERATIONS

Teach patient/family:

• To report change in vision, with blurring or loss of sight
• Method of instillation; not to touch dropper to eye
• That long-term therapy could be required
• That blurred vision will decrease with continued use of the drug

---

metoclopramide

Maxolon, Gastrobid, Gastromax, Primperan, combination products
Func. class.: Anti-emetic
Chem. class.: Central dopamine receptor agonist
Legal class.: POM

Action: Enhances response of tissue to acetylcholine in upper GI tract, which causes contraction of gastric muscle, relaxes pyloric, duodenal segments, increases peristalsis. Selective action on the chemoreceptor trigger zone by inhibiting central dopamine receptors. Decreases sensitivity of visceral afferent nerves to the vomiting centre

Uses: Digestive disorders, relief of symptoms of heatburn, sickness, dyspepsia, flatulence, milk regurgitation and pain associated with gastro-duodenal dysfunction; nausea and vomiting associated with gastrointestinal disorders, treatment with cytotoxics or radiotherapy, migraine; post-operative conditions such as gastric hypotonia, diagnostic procedures

Dosage and routes:
Nausea/vomiting
• *Adult:* By mouth IV/IM 10 mg (5–10 mg in young adults) 3 times a day
• *Child:* By mouth IV/IM
• *Up to 1 yr:* 1 mg twice a day
• *1–2 yr:* 1 mg 2 or 3 times a day
• *3–5 yr:* 2 mg 2 or 3 times a day
• *6–9 yr:* 2.5 mg twice a day
• *10–14 yr:* 5 mg twice a day
Delayed gastric emptying
• *Adult:* By mouth 10 mg 30 min acute migraine, before meals for 2–8 weeks
Gastroesophageal reflux
• *Adult:* By mouth 10–15 mg 4 times a day 30 min before meals
Nausea vomiing—(cytotoxics)
• Up to 2 mg/kg every 2 hr for 5 doses 30 min before chemotherapy
• IV infusion. Seek specialist advice
Radiological examination
• IM/IV 10–20 mg 5–10 min prior to exam

Available forms include: Tablets 10 mg; syrup 5 mg/5 ml; injection IV 5 mg/ml; tablets modified-release 15 mg; capsules modified-release 30 mg. Paediatric liquid 1 mg/ml

Side effects/adverse reactions:
CNS: Drowsiness, restlessness, depression, extrapyramidal reactions of dystonic type, tardive dyskinesia
MS: Increased muscle tone
GI: Diarrhoea, constipation
GU: Galactorrhoea or related disorders, hyperprolactinaemia
CV: Hypotension

Contraindications: Hypersensitivity to metoclopramide, first trimester of pregnancy, patients under 20 except for intractable vomiting of known cause e.g. radiotherapy and cytotoxic therapy, pre-medication for surgical procedures; porphyria

Precautions: Renal or hepatic impairment (reduce dose), pregnancy, lactation, hypertensive response in phaeochromocytoma, masking of underlying disorder e.g. cerebral irritation, do not use for 3–4 days after gastrointestinal surgery

Pharmacokinetics:

IV: Onset 1−3 min, duration 1−2 hr

By mouth: Onset ½−1 hr, duration 1−2 hr

IM: Onset 10−15 min, duration 1−2 hr

Metabolised by liver, excreted in urine, half-life 4 hr

Interactions/incompatibilities:
• Increased absorption (and enhanced effect) of: aspirin, paracetamol
• Decreased action of this drug: opioid analgesics, antimuscarinics
• Increased risk of extrapyramidal effects: ranwolfia alkaloids, anti-psychotics, lithium, tetrabenazine
• Increased sedation: CNS depressants
• Antagonism of hypoprolactinaemic effect of bromocriptine
• Increased plasma level: levodopa

Lab. test interferences:
Increase: Prolactin

Treatment of overdose: Gastric lavage with supportive measures; dystonic symptoms, treat in severe cases with anticholinergic drugs

NURSING CONSIDERATIONS

Administer:
• ½−1 hr before meals for better absorption
• IV infusion and injection slowly
• IV preparations can be mixed with morphine/diamorphine and some cytotoxics under certain conditions: consult data sheet

Perform/provide:
• Frequent sips of water for dryness of mouth
• Discard open ampoules
• Measure paediatric doses accurately with pipette

Evaluate:
• Therapeutic response: absence of nausea, vomiting, anorexia, fullness; extrapyradical effect
• For side effects
• GI complaints: nausea, vomiting, anorexia, constipation

Teach patient/family:
• Avoid driving or other hazardous activities until patient is stabilised on this medication
• Avoid alcohol or other CNS depressants that will enhance sedating properties of this drug
• Accurate dosage
• Report side effects especially extrapyramidal side-effects

---

metolazone

Metenix 5, Xuret
Func. class.: Diuretic
Chem. class.: Thiazide-like; quinazoline derivative
Legal class.: POM

Action: Acts on distal tubule by increasing excretion of water, sodium, chloride, potassium

Uses: Mild and moderate hypertension cardiac, renal and hepatic oedema, ascites or toxaemia of pregnancy

Dosage and routes:

Oedema
• *Adult:* By mouth 5−10 mg daily, as single dose. Maximum 80 mg/24 h

Hypertension
• *Adult:* By mouth 5 mg daily as a single morning dose for 3−4 weaks then maintenance 5 mg on alternate days

Available forms include: Tablets 5, 10 mg. 500 mcg available only as Xuret brand

Side effects/adverse reactions:
GU: Uraemia, glycosuria
CNS: Anxiety, headache, dizziness, fatigue, weakness
GI: Nausea, vomiting, anorexia, abdominal discomfort, cramps, pancreatitis
INTEG: Rash, urticaria, fever, chills

META: Latent diabetes, hyper-uricaemia, azotaemia. Rarely clinical gout

HAEM: Leucopenia

CV: Orthostatic hypotension, tachycardia, chest pain

ELECT: Hypokalaemia, hypercalcaemia, hyponataemia, hypochloraemia, hypomagnasemia on prolonged use

Contraindications: Hypersensitivity to metolazone, anuria, electrolyte deficiency states, coma or precomatose states associated with liver cirrhosis

Precautions: Hypokalaemia, diabetes, gout, pregnancy, breast feeding, renal and hepatic impairment

Pharmacokinetics:

By mouth: Onset 1 hr, peak 2 hr, duration 12−24 hr; excreted unchanged by kidneys, enters breast milk, half-life 8 hr

Interactions/incompatibilities:
• Increased toxicity of: cardiac glycosides
• Increased risk of hypokalaemia: corticosteroids
• Decreased effects of: antidiabetics, insulin
• Decreased doses of non-diuretic antihypertensive agents may be needed
• Profound diuresis with: loop diuretics

Clinical assessment:
• Electrolytes: potassium, sodium, chloride; include blood urea nitrogen, blood sugar, serum creatinine

Treatment of overdose: Danger of dehydration and electrolyte depletion. Treatment should be aimed at fluid replacement and correction of electrolyte imbalance

NURSING CONSIDERATIONS

Assess:
• Baseline weight, fluid balance
• Rate, depth, rhythm of respiration, effect of exertion

• Glucose in urine if patient is diabetic

Administer:
• In morning to avoid interference with sleep if using drug as a diuretic
• Potassium replacement if potassium is less than 3.0 mmol/litre, unless contraindicated
• With food if nausea occurs; absorption may be decreased slightly

Evaluate:
• Weight, fluid balance daily to determine fluid loss; effect of drug may be decreased if used daily
• BP lying, standing; postural hypotension may occur
• Improvement in oedema of feet, legs, sacral area daily if medication is being used in congestive cardiac failure
• Improvement in CVP and BP recordings
• Signs of metabolic acidosis: drowsiness, restlessness
• Signs of hypokalaemia: postural hypotension, malaise, fatigue, tachycardia, leg cramps, weakness
• Rashes, temperature elevation daily
• Confusion, especially in elderly; take safety precautions if needed

Teach patient/family:
• To increase fluid intake 2−3 litres daily unless contraindicated. To rise slowly from lying or sitting position
• To notify clinician of muscle weakness, cramps, nausea, dizziness, loss of appetite
• Drug may be taken with food or milk
• That blood sugar may be increased in diabetics
• Take early in day to avoid nocturia

metoprolol tartrate

Betaloc, Arbralene, Betaloc SA
Lopresor SR, Lopresor, combination
products
Func. class.: Antihypertensive
Chem. class.: β₁-blocker
Legal class.: POM

Action: Produces falls in BP without reflex tachycardia or significant reduction in heart rate through β-blocking effects; elevated plasma renins are reduced; blocks β₂-adrenergic receptors in bronchial, vascular smooth muscle only at high doses (decreases rate of sino-atrial node)

Uses: Mild to moderate hypertension, acute myocardial infarction to reduce cardiovascular mortality, angina pectoris, adjunct in treatment of hyperthyroidism, prophylaxis of migraine, cardiac arrhythmias

Dosage and routes:
Hypertension
• *Adult:* By mouth twice a day starting dose 50 or mg, increase by 100 mg daily at weekly intervals, to give up to 200−450 mg given as a single or twice daily dose
Angina
• *Adult:* By mouth 50−100 mg 2 or 3 times a day
Arrhythmias
• *Adult:* By mouth 50 mg 2 or 3 times a day up to 300 mg once a day in divided doses
• Following treatment of acute arrhythmia with metoprolol injection, metoprolol tablets should be initiated 4−6 hr late, initial oral dose should not exceed 50 mg 3 times daily
Migraine prophylaxis
• *Adult:* By mouth 100−200 mg in divided doses daily
Myocardial infarction
• *Adult:* (Early treatment within 12 hr) IV injection 5 mg every 2 min to maximum of 15 mg total then 50 mg by mouth 15 min after last injection and every 6 hr for 48 hr; patients who cannot tolerate the full IV dose should be given half the suggested oral dose. Maintenance by mouth 100 mg twice a day given in divided dose

Available forms include: Tablets 50, 100 mg modified-release 200 mg; injection IV 1 mg/ml

Side effects/adverse reactions:
CV: Bradycardia, postural hypotension, heart failure, palpitations, cardiac arrhythmias, Raynaud's phenomenon, peripheral oedema and precordial pain. Isolated reports of cardiac conduction abnormalities, gangrene in patients with pre-existing severe peripheral circulating disorders
CNS: Sleep disturbances, dizziness, paraesthesia, personality changes, depression, anxiety, headaches, fatigue, lassitude
GI: Nausea, vomiting, abdominal pain, diarrhoea, constipation, dry mouth, abnormal liver function tests
INTEG: Rash, alopecia, urticaria, increased sweating, photosensitivity
HAEM: Thrombocytopenia
EENT: Dry irritated eyes, conjunctivities, vision disturbance, tinnitus
RESP: Bronchospasm, dyspnoea, wheezing, rhinitis
META: Weight gain, muscle cramps

Contraindications: Atrioventricular block, uncontrolled heart failure, severe bradycardia, sick sinus syndrome, cardiogenic shock, severe peripheral arterial disease, hypersensitivity to β-blockers, asthma or history of obstructive airway disease, myocardial infarction complicated by significant bradycardia, first degree heart block, systolic hypotension (less than 100 mmHg), severe heart failure

Precautions: May aggravate bradycardia, peripheral arterial circulatory disorders and anaphylactic shock. Should be withdrawn gradually over 10 days, diminishing doses to 25 mg a day for the last 6 days, patients should be monitored. Reversible obstructive airways disease. Labile and insulin dependant diabetes; hypoglycaemic therapy may need alteration. Bioavailability may be increased in liver cirrhosis. α-blocker should be given concomitantly in ₊phaeochromocytoma. Pregnancy, lactation. Warn anaesthetist if patient on β-blocker therapy. Diabetes mellitus

Pharmacokinetics:

By mouth: Peak 1.5−2 hr, duration 13−19 hr; half-life 3−4 hr, metabolised in liver (metabolites), exhibits genetic polymorphism, i.e. fast and poor metabolisers, excreted in urine, enters breast milk, no significant β-blocking effects in the neonate if mother on normal doses

Interactions/incompatibilities:

• Increased blood pressure with: adrenaline
• Increased hypotension, bradycardia: reserpine, hydralazine, methyldopa, prazosin, antichlolinergics
• Should not be given with: verapamil
• Decreased antihypertensive effects: indomethacin, sympathomimetics
• Increased hypoglycaemic effects: insulin
• Decreased bronchodilatation: theophyllines

Treatment of overdose: Lavage, IV atropine for bradycardia, IV theophylline for bronchospasm, digitalis, O_2, diuretic for cardiac failure, haemodialysis, hypotension administer vasopressor (dopamine or dobutamine)

NURSING CONSIDERATIONS

Assess:

• Baseline weight
• BP, pulse: note rate, rhythm, quality
• Respiratory rate−note any wheeze

Administer:

• By mouth before meals or bedtime; tablet may be crushed or swallowed whole
• ECG, directly when giving IV during initial treatment
• Reduced dosage in hepatic dysfunction
• IV, keep patient recumbent for 3 hr

Perform/provide:

• Regular peak flow readings if any previous chest disease or the patient complains of tight, wheezy chest

Evaluate:

• Therapeutic response: decreased BP after 1−2 weeks
• Weight increase
• May affect libido and/or potency
• For signs of heart failure, such as ankle oedema

Teach patient/family:

• Take with or immediately after meals
• Not to discontinue drug abruptly, taper over 2 weeks, may cause precipitate angina
• Not to use non-prescribed drugs containing α-adrenergic stimulants, (nasal decongestants, cold preparations) unless directed by clinician
• To report bradycardia, dizziness, confusion, depression, fever, sore throat, shortness of breath to clinician
• To take pulse at home, advise when to notify clinician
• To avoid alcohol, smoking
• Limit sodium intake
• To comply with weight control,

dietary adjustments, modified exercise programme
• To avoid hazardous activities if dizziness is present
• To report symptoms of congestive cardiac failure: difficult breathing, especially on exertion or when lying down, night cough, swelling of extremities
• Take medication at bedtime to maintain effect of orthostatic hypotension
• Wear support hose to minimise effects of orthostatic hypotension

---

metronidazole/metronidazole HCl

Elyzol, Flagyl S, Flagyl, Flagyl Compak, Metrolyl, Vaginyl, Zadstat
Func. class.: Antibiotic
Chem. class.: Nitroimidazole derivative
Legal class.: POM

Action: Direct-acting amoebicide/trichomonacide binds, degrades DNA inside, outside organism. High activity against anaerobic bacteria and protozoa

Uses: Intestinal and extraintestinal amoebiasis, including symptomless cyst passers, amoebic abscess, trichomoniasis, prevention and treatment of bacterial vaginitis, bacterial anaerobic infections, giardiasis, acute ulcerative gingivitis, acute dental infections, leg ulcers and pressure sores

Dosage and routes:
Anaerobic infections (usually treated for 7 days)
• *Adult:* By mouth 800 mg initially then 400 mg 8 hrly; by rectum 1 g 8 hrly for 3 days, then 1 g 12 hrly; by IV infusion 500 mg/kg 8 hrly
• *Child:* Any route 7.5 mg/kg 8 hrly
Leg ulcers and pressure sores
• By mouth 400 mg 8 hrly for 7 days

Bacterial vaginosis
• By mouth 400 mg twice daily for 7 days, or 2 g as single dose
Acute ulcerative gingivitis
• *Adult:* By mouth 200 g 8 hrly for 3 days
• *Child:* 1−3 yr 50 mg 8 hrly for 3 days, 3−7 yr 100 mg 12 hrly, 7−10 yr 100 mg 8 hrly
Acute dental infections
• By mouth 200 mg 8 hrly for 3−7 days
Surgical prophylaxis
• *Adult:* By mouth 400 mg 8 hrly during 24 hr before surgery followed by postoperative IV or rectal administration until able to take tablets
• *Child:* 7.5 mg/kg 8 hrly
• *IV:* 500 mg, shortly before surgery, repeat 8 hrly, start oral therapy 400 mg 8 hrly as soon as feasible
• *Child:* 7.5 mg/kg 8 hrly
• *Rectal: Adult:* 1 g 8 hrly
• *Child:* One half or one quarter 500 mg suppository 8 hrly
Trichomoniasis
• By mouth 200 mg 8 hrly or 400 mg 12 hrly for 7 days or 800 mg in morning and 1200 mg at night for 2 days or 2 g as single dose
• *Child:* 7−10 yr 100 mg 8 hrly for 7 days, 3−7 yr 100 mg 12 hrly for 7 days, 1−3 yr 50 mg 8 hrly for 7 days
Protozoal infections
See specialist texts
Available forms include: Tablets 200, 400 mg; film coated tablets 200, 400 mg; IV infusion 5 mg/ml; IV injection 5 mg/ml; suppositories 500 mg, 1 g; suspension 200 mg/(as benzoate)/5 ml
Side effects/adverse reactions:
HAEM: Leucopenia, anaphylaxis
INTEG: Rash, pruritus, urticaria
CNS: Headache, dizziness, ataxia,

drowsiness, peripheral neuropathy, incoordination, transient epileptiform seizures
EENT: Dry mouth, unpleasant taste, furry tongue, angioedema
GI: Nausea, vomiting, gastrointestinal disturbance
GU: Darkening of urine
Contraindications: Hypersensitivity
Precautions: Persistent gonococci infection after trichomonal treatment, metabolites retained in renal failure, significance unknown; both active drug and metabolites removed by dialysis. Dose reduction not required in renal failure. No routine dose reduction required in patients undergoing intermittent peritoneal dialysis or continuous ambulatory peritoneal dialysis. Impairment or clearance in hepatic disease. Dose reduction to one third given once daily to patients with hepatic encephalopathy. Active disease of the CNS other than brain abscess
Pharmacokinetics:
By mouth: Peak 20 min−3 hr, half-life 5−11 hr, excreted mainly in urine as metabolites
Interactions/incompatibilities:
• Disulfiram-like reaction: alcohol
• May increase action: warfarin
• May increase plasma level of: lithium. Lithium treatment should be tapered or withdrawn before concomitant treatment
• Psychosis: disulfiram
• Decreased action of this drug: phenobarbitone
Clinical assessment:
• Regular clinical and laboratory monitoring if drug given for more than 10 days
• Plasma concentration of lithium, creatinine and electrolytes should be monitored in patients given metronidazole and lithium together
Lab. test interferences:
Decrease: Aspartate aminotransferase alanine aminotransferase

NURSING CONSIDERATIONS
Assess:
• Fluid balance, stools for number, frequency, character
Administer:
• Suspension should be taken at least an hour before food
• Tablets, after meals, to avoid GI symptoms, metallic taste
• Other routes as indicated in pharmacological section
Evaluate:
• Stools during entire treatment; should be clear at end of therapy, for 1 yr before patient is considered cured (amoebiasis)
• Neurotoxicity: peripheral neuropathy, seizures, dizziness, incoordination, pruritus, joint pains; may be discontinued
• Ophthalmic examination during, after therapy; visual problems occur often
• Allergic reaction: fever, rash, itching, chills; drug should be discontinued if these occur
• Superimposed infection: fever, monilial growth, fatigue, malaise
• Renal and reproductive dysfunction: dysuria, polyuria, impotence, dyspareunia, decreased libido
Teach patient/family:
• Urine may turn dark reddish brown
• Proper hygiene after bowel movements: hand-washing technique
• Need for compliance with dosage schedule, duration of treatment
• To use condoms if treatment for trichomoniasis or cross contamination may occur
• Treatment of both partners is necessary
• To avoid alcohol (because disulfiram-like reaction will occur even with the smallest amounts of alcohol)

metyrapone

Metopirone
Func. class.: Competitive 11 β-hydroxylation inhibitor
Chem. class.:
Legal class.: POM

Action: Inhibits biosynthesis of cortisol (and to a lesser extent aldosterone) production leading to increased production of ACTH

Uses: Assessment of anterior pituitary function; Cushing's syndrome; resistant oedema due to increased aldosterone secretion in cirrhosis, nephrosis, congestive cardiac failure

Dosage and routes:

Assessment of pituitary function
• *Adult:* By mouth 750 mg 4-hrly for 6 doses
• *Child:* By mouth 15 mg/kg 4-hrly for 6 doses; minimum single dose 250 mg

Management of Cushing's syndrome
• *Adult:* By mouth: 250 mg−6 g daily tailored to cortisol production; use only under specialist advice

Oedema
• *Adult:* By mouth: 2.5−4.5 g daily in divided doses (with glucocorticoids)

Available forms include: Capsules 250 mg

Side effects/adverse reactions:
CNS: Dizziness, headache
CV: Hypotension
GI: Nausea, vomiting
INTEG: Allergic reactions

Contraindications: Pregnancy, lactation, hypersensitivity, adrenocortical insufficiency

Precautions: Patients with liver cirrhosis may show delayed response to metyrapone because of liver damage delaying cortisol metabolism. In thyroid hypofunction, urinary steroid levels may rise very slowly or not at all in response to metyrapone

Pharmacokinetics: Rapidly absorbed and eliminated from plasma. Peak plasma levels occur after 1 hr, following a dose of 750 mg, plasma levels average 3.7 mcg/ml decreasing to a mean value of 0.5 mcg/ml after 4 hr. Half-life is 20−26 min

Lab. test interferences: Anticonvulsants, antidepressants, neuroleptics, hormones affecting the hypothalamo-pituitary axis and antithyroid agents may affect the metyrapone diagnostic test

Treatment of overdose: Gastric lavage, forced emesis. Administer a large dose of hydrocortisone together with IV sodium chloride 0.9% and glucose. Repeat as necessary according to patient's clinical condition

NURSING CONSIDERATIONS

Assess:
• Baseline weight and BP

Administer:
• With meals and/or milk to prevent GI symptoms

Perform/provide:
• Fluid balance; weight daily

Evaluate:
• Standing/sitting BP to detect postural hypotension following treatment
• Additional symptom support as fatigue, heart failure, muscle weakness, may all be established resulting from disease

Teach patient/family:
• That capsules should be taken with milk or after food
• To change position slowly to prevent hypotension
• To use contraceptives to prevent pregnancy
• That therapeutic effect may take 2 months
• To avoid hazardous activity if dizziness occurs

• Supplemental information concerning management of Cushing's Syndrome symptoms

---

mexiletine HCl

Mexitil
Func. class.: Anti-arrhythmic
Chem. class.: Lignocaine analogue
Legal class.: POM

Action: Depresses maximum rate of depolarisation with little or no modification of resting potentials or duration of action potentials
Uses: Ventricular tachycardia, ventricular dysrhythmias during cardiac surgery, myocardial infarction or ischaemic heart disease. Ventricular arrhythmias indured by digitalis and other drugs. *Not* of proven value in arrhythmias in pre-excitation syndromes
Dosage and routes:
• *Adult:* IV injection 100−250 mg at 25 mg/min with ECG monitoring followed by IV infusion of 250 mg as a 0.1% solution over 1 hr, 125 mg/h for 2 hr, then 500 mcg/min; by mouth maintenance dose 200−250 mg, 3−4 times daily. Modified-release, one capsule twice daily
Available forms include: Capsules 50, 200; modified-release 360 mg; injection 250 mg/10 ml
Side effects/adverse reactions:
Mainly related to blood concentration
CNS: Headache, dizziness, lightheadedness, drowsiness, confusion, dizziness, incoordination, dysarthria, ataxia, tremor, paraesthesia, convulsions, psychiatric disorder
EENT: Blurred vision, nystagmus, diplopia
GI: Nausea, vomiting, indigestion, constipation, diarrhoea, abdominal pain, dry mouth, unpleasant taste, hiccups, jaundice
CV: Hypotension, bradycardia, atrial fibrillation, palpitation, conduction defects, exacerbation of arrhythmias and torsade de pointes
MS: Arthralgia
INTEG: Rash
SYST: Fever
HAEM: Thrombocytopenia, appearance of positive but symptomless antinuclear factor titres
Contraindications: Hypersensitivity to mexiletine, cardiogenic shock, high degree atrioventricular block unless a pacemaker is *in situ*
Precautions: Pregnancy, lactation, myocardial infarction results in prolonged absorption half-life mexiletine. Plasma elimination half-life prolonged in moderate to severe hepatic disease and where creatinine clearance in less than 10 ml/min
Pharmacokinetics:
By mouth: Peak 1 hr; half-life 12 hr, metabolised by liver, excreted by kidneys, small proportion of unchanged drug
Interactions/incompatibilities:
• Oral therapy: drugs which delay absorption rate e.g. opiates may reduce peak plasma concentration. Rate of absorption but not bioavailability may be delayed
• Drugs inducing hepatic mixed function oxidase system may lower levels of plasma mexiletine
• Drugs acidifying or alkalinising the urine may enhance or reduce rate of drug elimination
• Concomitant IV therapy with other local anaesthetic type agents e.g. lignocaine/procanamaide is not recommended. This has not been seen as a problem with oral mexiletine
Clinical assessment:
• ECG and BP monitoring should be carried out during treatment

• Blood levels (therapeutic level 0.75 mcg/ml)
• Electrolytes potassium, sodium, chloride
Treatment of overdose: Gastric lavage where appropriate. Transfer to intensive/coronary care unit for cardiopulmonary support. Arrhythmias: treat appropriately. Diazepan may be useful for convulsions

NURSING CONSIDERATIONS
Assess:
• Baseline vital signs
• Fluid balance, ECG
Administer:
• IV infusion rate using infusion pump, run at less than 4 mg/min
Perform/provide:
• Continuous cardiac monitoring during intravenous administration, preferably in a coronary care/cardiac unit
Evaluate:
• Malignant hyperthermia: tachypnoea, tachycardia, changes in BP, increased temperature
• BP continuously for fluctuations
• Cardiac rate, respiration: rate, rhythm, character, continuously
• Respiratory status: rate, rhythm, watch for respiratory depression
• CNS effects: dizziness, confusion, psychosis, paraesthesia, convulsions; inform medical staff if these occur
• Record any arrhythmias to medical staff. Infusions may need to be discontinued immediately if arrhythmias are life threatening
Teach patient/family:
• To take medication as prescribed
• That medication is a treatment rather than a cure
• Mexiletine can cause hiccups indigestion and dry mouth

mianserin HCl

Bolvidon, Norval
Func. class.: Antidepressant
Chem. class.: Tetracyclic
Legal class.: POM

Action: Blocks presynaptic α-adrenoceptors and increases turnover of brain noradrenaline
Uses: Depressive illness, particularly where sedation is required
Dosage and routes:
• *Adult:* By mouth, initially 30−40 mg daily, in divided doses or preferably as single dose at bedtime, increased gradually as necessary; maximum initial dose in elderly 30 mg; usual dose range 30−90 mg
Available forms include: Tablets 10, 20, 30 mg
Side effects/adverse reactions:
HAEM: Agranulocytosis, leucopenia, eosinophilia, purpura, aplastic anaemia, thrombocytopenia, jaundice
CNS: Sedation, blurred vision, confusion, hypomania, convulsions, dizziness, tremor, behavioural disturbances
GI: Nausea, dry mouth, constipation
INTEG: Sweating, rashes, breast disorders
CV: Arrhythmias, postural hypotension, oedema
MS: Arthritis, arthralgia, polyarthropathy
SYST: Influenza-like syndrome
Contraindications: Recent myocardial infarction or heart block
Precautions: Diabetes, cardiac disease, epilepsy, pregnancy, hepatic impairment, symptoms of prostatic hypertrophy; psychoses, urinary retention; avoid abrupt cessation of therapy; caution in anaesthesia, elderly, suicidal patients, renal disease, narrow angle glaucoma

Pharmacokinetics: Readily absorbed. Bioavailability reduced to 70% by first pass hepatic metabolism. Metabolised to desmethylmianserin and 8-hydroxymianserin which are active. Excreted in urine as metabolites either free or conjugated. Same also in faeces. Biphasic half-life, duration of terminal phase in 6–39 hr. Effect may not be seen for 2–4 weeks

Interactions/incompatibilities:
• Hypertensive crises: MAOIs
• Increased effect: alcohol
• Possible side effects: phenytoin (monitor plasma levels), antihypertensives (monitor BP), anticoagulants (monitor prothrombin time)

Clinical assessment:
• Blood tests: Full blood count, every 4 weeks during first 3 months of treatment. Monitor and if fever, sore throat or other signs of infection develop, stop treatment. Obtain full blood count
• ECG for flattening of T-wave, bundle branch block, atrioventricular block, dysrhythmias in cardiac patients

Treatment of overdose: Empty stomach by lavage. Treat symptomatically

NURSING CONSIDERATIONS

Assess:
• BP (lying, standing), pulse
• Weight

Administer:
• With food or milk for GI symptoms
• Dosage at bedtime if oversedation occurs during the day. May take entire dose at bedtime, elderly may not tolerate more than once a day dosing
• Add to fruit juice, water or milk to disguise taste

Perform/provide:
• Check to see oral medication swallowed
• Mouthwashes or frequent sips of water for dry mouth
• Increased fluids, fibre in diet if constipation, urinary retention occur
• Assistance with walking during beginning of therapy since drowsiness/dizziness occurs
• Safety measures, including cot sides, primarily in elderly; reason for using such measures should be fully explained to patient

Evaluate:
• BP (lying, standing) and pulse 4-hrly; if systolic BP drops 20 mmHg withhold drug and notify clinician
• Vital signs 4-hrly in patients with cardiovascular disease
• Weight gain; appetite may increase with drug
• Mental status, alertness, affect, sleeping pattern, drowsiness, dizziness
• For signs of physical dependence: withdrawal symptoms; nausea, vomiting, headache, muscle pain, weakness after long-term use
• For urinary retention, constipation; more likely to occur in younger people
• For alcohol consumption; if alcohol is consumed, hold dose until morning
• For signs of suicidal tendencies
• Therapeutic response, decreased anxiety, restlessness, sleeplessness

Teach patient/family:
• That therapeutic effects may take 2–4 weeks
• To avoid driving, activities that require alertness, since drowsiness may occur
• To avoid alcohol or other psychotropic medications
• Not to discontinue medication quickly after long-term use

miconazole

Daktarin
Func. class.: Antifungal
Chem. class.: Imidazole
Legal class.: POM; 15 g oral gel P

Action: Interferes with fungal DNA replication

Uses: Coccidioidomycosis, candidiasis, cryptococcosis, blastomycosis, paracoccidioides, chronic mucocutaneous candidiasis, systemic fungal intertain and of ovophorynx, gastrointestinal tract and suprainfections due to Gram-positive bacteria. IV used for severe infections only

Dosage and routes:
• *Adult:* IV infusion in 250−500 ml fluid 600 mg 8 hrly
• *Child:* IV infusion maximum 15 mg/kg 8 hrly up to 40 mg/kg daily
• *Adult:* By mouth, gel 5−10 ml after food 6 hrly
• *Child under 2 yr:* By mouth, gel 2.5 ml twice a day; 2−6 yr 5 ml twice a day; over 6 yr 5 ml 4 times a day
• *Adult:* By mouth, tablets 250 mg 6 hrly for 10 days or up to 2 days after symptoms clear

Available forms include: Injection IV 10 mg/ml, for dilution and use as infusion over at lean 30 min; tablets 250 mg; oral gel 2%

Side effects/adverse reactions:
CV: Tachycardia, dysrhythmias (rapid IV)
INTEG: Pruritus, rash, fever, flushing, anaphylaxis, urticaria, phlebitis
CNS: Drowsiness, headache
GI: Nausea, vomiting, anorexia, diarrhoea, cramps
HAEM: Decreased haematocrit, thrombocytopenia, hyperlipidaemia

Contraindications: Hypersensitivity, due to polyethoxylated castor oil in IV preparation

Precautions: Rapid IV may cause arrhythmias

Pharmacokinetics:
IV: Terminal half-life 24 hr, metabolised in liver to inactive metabolites, excreted in urine, 50% of oral dose may be excreted unchanged in faeces. Over 90% protein binding

Interactions/incompatibilities:
• Increased action of: anticoagulants anti-epileptics, hypoglycaemic drugs
• Antagonism of *in vitro* miconazole activity by: amphotericin

Clinical assessment:
• Cardiac system: BP, pulse, ECG; watch for increasing pulse, cardiac dysrhythmias; drug should be discontinued if these occur
• Blood studies: haemoglobin, haematocrit, serum sodium, lipids

Treatment of overdose: Tablets: gastric lavage, followed by a purgative and supportive treatment

NURSING CONSIDERATIONS

Administer:
• After culture and sensitivity is obtained to identify causative organism
• Anti-emetic for nausea and vomiting as ordered
• After test dose of 200 mg is given; watch for allergic reactions
• IV after diluting with dextrose 5%, 0.9% sodium chloride if hyponatraemia has occurred

Evaluate:
• For phlebitis, pruritus; may need IV antihistamine; continue unless reaction is severe
• Allergic reaction after test dose; have adrenaline available
• Therapeutic response: decreased fever, malaise, rash, negative culture and sensitivity for infecting organism

Teach patient/family:

- That long-term therapy may be required to clear infection (1 week−1 month)
- Proper hygiene: handwashing techniques, nail care
- Avoid contact with eyes, nose

---

miconazole nitrate

Daktarin, Gyno-Daktarin, combination product
Func. class.: Antifungal
Chem. class.: Synthetic miconazole
Legal class.: POM

Action: Interferes with fungal DNA replication
Uses: *Tinea pedis*, *tinea cruris*, *tinea corporis*, *tinea versicolor*, vaginal or vulvae *Candida albicans* and superinfection due to susceptible Gram-positive bacteria, intertigo, candida nappy rash, paronychia, erythrasma, fungal infection of the outer ear, nail infections, fungal skin infections
Dosage and routes:
Cream 2%
- *Adult and child:* Apply twice daily continuing for 10 days after lesions have healed; nail infections, apply daily under occlusive dressing
Powder
- *Adult and child:* Apply twice daily to skin lesions, separately or with cream, may also be dusted on clothing in contact with affected area
Not recommended for nail and hair infections
Intravaginal
- *Adult:* Cream 2%: insert two 5 g applicatorfuls nightly for 7 nights, use cream topically to anogenital area twice daily
- *Adult:* Pessary 100 mg: insert 2 pessaries for 7 nights
- *Adult:* Tampons 100 mg: insert 1 tampon night and morning for 5 days
- *Adult:* Ovule 1.2 g: insert 1 ovule at night as single dose
Available forms include: Cream 2%; vaginal tampon 100 mg; powder, spray powder 0.16%; vaginal cream 2%; pessary 100 mg; vaginal ovule 1200 mg
Side effects/adverse reactions:
GU: Vulvovaginal burning, itching
Contraindications: Hypersensitivity
Precautions: Child less than 2 yr, pregnancy
Interactions/incompatibilities:
- Vaginal contraceptive diaphragms
Treatment of overdose: Appropriate method of gastric emptying may be used
NURSING CONSIDERATIONS
Administer:
- After cleansing with soap, water before each application, dry well
- 1 filled applicator or 1 tablet/ovule deep-intravaginally each night; 1 tampon to be inserted night and morning for 5 days as directed
- Enough medication to cover lesions completely
- Powder/spray can be used in socks/clothing in contact with affected areas
Evaluate:
- Allergic reaction: burning, stinging, swelling, redness
- Therapeutic response: decrease in size, number of lesions
Teach patient/family:
- To avoid use of non-prescribed creams, ointments, lotions unless directed
- To wash hands before, after each application
- To avoid contact with eyes
- That intravaginal preparations damage latex condoms and diaphragms
- That cream should be applied

daily to the partner's penis to prevent re-infection in vaginal, vulval infection

---

midazolam

Hypnovel
Func. class.: Anaesthetic induction agent, sedative
Chem. class.: Benzodiazepine, short-acting
Legal class.: POM

Action: Depresses subcortical levels in CNS; may act on limbic system, reticular formation; may potentiate aminobutyric acid (GABA) by binding to specific benzodiazepine receptors

Uses: Induction of general anaesthesia, sedation for diagnostic endoscopic procedures, intubation, dental surgery

Dosage and routes:

Intravenous sedation
• *Adults:* Slow IV injection over 30 seconds 2 mg followed after 2 min by increments of 0.5−1 mg if necessary. Usual range 2.5−7.5 mg
• *Elderly:* Slow IV injection over 30 seconds initially 1−2 mg, increasing as above to a maximum of 1−1.5 mg
If opiates are being used for analgesia reduce initial doses by 50%

Induction of anaesthesia
• *Adults:* IM injection 70−100 mcg/kg 30−60 min preoperatively. Usual dose is 5 mg
• *Elderly:* IM injection as above but 2.5 mg may be adequate
• *Adults:* Slow IV injection, following opiate pre-medication 200 mcg/kg. Increase to 300 mcg/kg if no pre-medication has been given
• *Elderly:* Slow IV injection, following opiate pre-medication 100 mcg/kg. Increase to 200 mcg/kg if no pre-medication has been given
• *Child over 7 yr:* Slow IV injection 150 mcg/kg
Available forms include: Injection 2.5 mg/ml, 5 mg/ml (as hydrochloride)

Side effects/adverse reactions:
CNS: Retrograde amnesia, euphoria, confusion, headache, anxiety, insomnia, slurred speech, paraesthesia, disinhibition
RESP: Respiratory depression
CV: Hypotension, reduced cardiac output, stroke volume, systemic vascular resistance
EENT: Vertigo, visual disturbances
GI: Nausea, vomiting, increased salivation
INTEG: Pain, swelling at injection site, thrombophlebitis

Contraindications: 3rd trimester of pregnancy, hypersensitivity to benzodiazepines, respiratory depression, acute pulmonary insufficiency

Precautions: Impaired renal or hepatic function, elderly, myasthenia gravis, 1st and 2nd trimester of pregnancy, lactation, concurrent CNS depressants pulmonary insufficiency, personality disorders

Pharmacokinetics:
IM: Onset 15 min, peak ½−1 hr
IV: Onset 3−5 min, onset of anaesthesia 1½−2½ min, protein binding 97%, half-life 2 hr, metabolised in liver, metabolites excreted in urine, crosses placenta, blood−brain barrier

Interactions/incompatibilities:
• Prolonged respiratory depression: other CNS depressants, alcohol, barbiturates
• Increased hypnotic effect: fentanyl, narcotic agonists, analgesics, droperidol

NURSING CONSIDERATIONS
Assess:

- Vital signs
- Baseline level of consciousness

Administer:

- IM or IV at onset of anaesthesia (duration 1½−2½ min) or as continuous infusion

Perform/provide:

- Respiratory ventilation equipment if required

Evaluate:

- Degree of respiratory depression due to muscle relaxation
- Response to administration of induction agent/sedative
- Ensure patient is sedated as well as paralysed
- Ensure patient remains on bed resting until drug effects have worn off
- Injection site for signs of inflammation

Teach patient/family:

- To avoid driving and other activities requiring mental alertness until drowsiness and weakness subside
- If receiving drug by continuous infusion, some muscle weakness may be experienced

---

milrinone ▼

Primacor
Func. class.: Vasodilator
Legal class.: POM

Action: Selective inhibitor of peak III phosphodiesterase isoenzyme in cardiac and vascular muscle. Positive inotrope and vasodilator with little chronotropic activity; also improves left ventricular diastolic relaxation

Uses: Short-term treatment of severe congestive heart failure unresponsive to conventional maintenance therapy

Dosage and routes:

- *Adult:* Slow IV loading dose of 50 mcg/kg administered over 10 min followed by maintenance infusion of 0.5 mcg/kg/min. Maintenance dosage may be titrated between 0.375−0.75 mcg/kg/min to a maximum haemodynamic effect. Total dose should not exceed 1.13 mg/kg daily. Reduce dose in renal impairment

Available forms include: IV Injection 10 mg/10 ml

Side effects/adverse reactions:

CNS: Headache, tremor

CV: Supraventricular and ventricular arrhythmias, hypotension, angina

META: Hypokalaemia, thrombocytopenia

Contraindications: Hypersensitivity, immediately after acute myocardial infarction, severe obstructive aortic or pulmonary valvular disease, hypertrophic subaortic stenosis, pregnancy, lactation

Precautions: Supraventricular and ventricular arrhythmias, non-sustained ventricular tachycardias. May increase ventricular response rate in patients with uncontrolled atrial flutter/fibrillation; digitalisation or treatment with other agents to prolong atrioventricular node conduction time should be considered prior to milrinone therapy. Administer cautiously if prior diuretic therapy is suspected of causing a significant decrease in cardiac filling pressure. Improvement in cardiac output with resultant diuresis may necessitate a reduction in the dose of diuretic Fluid and electrolyte balance should be carefully monitored. Impaired renal function.

Pharmacokinetics: In congestive heart failure volume of distribution is approximately 0.4 litre/kg, half-life is approximately 2.3 hr and clearance is 0.13 litre/kg/hr. Milrinone is approximately 70%

bound to plasma proteins and primarily excreted in the urine

Interactions/incompatibilities:
• Precipitation occurs if parenteral milrinone is mixed with: frusemide, bumetanide, sodium bicarbonate

NURSING CONSIDERATIONS:
Assess:
• Baseline vital signs including fluid balance
Administer:
• By slow IV infusion, seek specialist advice
Perform/provide:
• Continuous monitoring preferably on intensive therapy unit or coronary care unit
Evaluate:
• Therapeutic response
• The usual period is 48 to 72 hr, but some patients have been maintained for up to 5 days
• Cardiovascular parameters, electrolytes and renal function should be monitored closely during the infusion

---

minocycline HCl

Minocin, Minocin MR
Func. class.: Antibiotic, broad spectrum
Chem. class.: Tetracycline
Legal class.: POM

Action: Inhibits protein synthesis, phosphorylation in micro-organisms by binding to 30S ribosomal sub-units, reversibly binding to 50S ribosomal subunits

Uses: Syphilis, gonorrhoea, lymphogranuloma venereum, staphylococci meningococcal carriers

Dosage and routes:
Routine use
• *Adult and child over 12 yr:* By mouth 100 mg 12 hrly or 50 mg 6 hrly

Gonorrhoea
• *Adult:* By mouth a single dose of 200 mg followed by 100 mg every 12 hr for at least 4 days in males. Females may require prolonged treatment
Acne
• *Adult:* By mouth 50 mg twice a day, modified release capsule 100 mg daily
Prophylaxis of asymptomatic meningococcal carriers
• *Adult:* By mouth 100 mg twice daily for 5 days followed by rifampicin

Available forms include: Tablets 50, 100 mg, modified release capsule 100 mg

Side effects/adverse reactions:
CNS: Headache, dizziness and vertigo, raised intracranial pressure
HAEM: Eosinophilia, neutropenia, thrombocytopenia, haemolytic anaemia
EENT: Decreased calcification of deciduous teeth
GI: Nausea, vomiting, diarrhoea, pseudomembranous colitis
CV: Pericarditis
INTEG: Rash, urticaria, photosensitivity, increased pigmentation, exfoliative dermatitis, pruritus
SYST: Angioneurotic oedema, Stevens-Johnson syndrome, anaphylaxis

Contraindications: Hypersensitivity to tetracyclines, children under 12 yr, systemic lupus erythematosus, complete renal failure
Precautions: Renal disease, hepatic disease, lactation, pregnancy
Pharmacokinetics:
By mouth: Half-life 11−17 hr; excreted in faeces, excreted in breast milk, 55%−88% protein bound

Interactions/incompatibilities:
• Decreased effect of this drug; antacids, large amounts of dairy products, alkali products,

(less significant than other tetracyclines), iron, calcium, magnesium salts, sucralfate, bismute chelate
- Increased effect: anticoagulants
- Decreased effect: penicillins
- Nephrotoxicity: methoxyflurane

Clinical assessment:
- Blood studies: prothrombin time, full blood count, aspartate aminotransferase, alanine aminotransferase, blood urea nitrogen, creatinine

NURSING CONSIDERATIONS
Assess:
- Culture and sensitivity before treatment
- Bowel pattern
- Fluid balance

Administer:
- Orally; dose and length of treatment appropriate for disease, e.g. Gonorrhoea, bolus; streptococcal infection, 10 days
- Not suitable for young children

Evaluate:
- Therapeutic response, absence of fever, lesions, redness, inflammation
- Negative culture and sensitivity
- Effect of any other drug therapy, e.g. increased action of anticoagulants
- Decreased drug action due to antacids
- Side effects nausea, diarrhoea, dizziness vertigo, rash, urticaria, photosensitivity overgrowth resistant glossitis, stomatitis vaginitis

Teach patient/family:
- To avoid large amounts of dairy products — decrease drug effect
- To take at evenly spaced intervals, always to complete course
- Report sore throat, fever, malaise, pain, could indicate superimposed infection
- Do not take alcohol
- Not to drive or use machinery if dizziness occurs during treatment
- To eat regular small amount of yoghurt if stomatitis occurs (small, white ulcers on mucous membrane)

---

minoxidil
Loniten, Regaine
Func. class.: Antihypertensive
Chem. class.: Vasodilator — peripheral
Legal class.: POM

Action: Directly relaxes arteriolar smooth muscle, causing vasodilatation
Uses: Severe hypertension not responsive to other therapy; topically to treat alopecia
Dosage and routes:
Hypertension
- *Adult and child over 12 yr:* By mouth initially 5 mg once a day, increasing to 10 mg then by 10 mg every 3 days if necessary. Maximum daily dose 100 mg. Minoxidil should be used in conjunction with a diuretic to avoid excess water retention and a β-blocker to prevent increased heart rate
- *Child under 12 yr:* Initially 0.2 mg/kg daily; increasing by 0.1–0.2 mg/kg every 3 days if necessary. Maximum daily dose 1.0 mg/kg
Alopecia
- *Adult:* Apply 1 ml topically, rub into scalp twice daily
Available forms include: Tablets 2.5, 5, 10 mg; topical solution 2%
Side effects/adverse reactions:
CV: Severe rebound hypertension, tachycardia, angina, increased T wave, congestive cardiac failure, pulmonary oedema, sodium, water retention, peripheral, oedema
CNS: Dizziness, headache
GI: Nausea, vomiting
GU: Gynaecomastia, breast tenderness, increased blood urea nitrogen and creatinine
INTEG: Rash, hypertrichosis

Contraindications: Acute myocardial infarction, dissecting aortic aneurysm, hypersensitivity, phaeochromocytoma

Precautions: Pregnancy, lactation, children, renal disease, congestive cardiac failure, elderly, pericardial effusion

Pharmacokinetics:

By mouth: Onset 30 min, peak 2−3 hr, duration 75 hr; half-life 4.2 hr, metabolised in liver, metabolites, excreted in urine, faeces.

Interactions/incompatibilities:

• Concurrent use with quanethidine may cause orthostatic hypotension

Clinical assessments:

• Electrolytes: potassium, sodium chloride, CO_2

• Renal function studies: catecholamines, blood urea nitrogen, creatinine

• Hepatic function studies: aspartate aminotransferase, alanine aminotransferase, alkaline phosphatase

Treatment of overdose: Administer sodium chloride 0.9%. Phenylephrine, angiotensin II, vasopressor, dopamine may reverse hypotension may be used if inadequate perfusion of a vital organ is evident

NURSING CONSIDERATIONS

Assess:

• Fluid balance

• Baseline weight

• Weigh before and during treatment

• Blood pressure and pulse ECG before and during treatment

Administer:

• Topically to scalp for alopecia

• Orally with food, following the dosage regimen for suitable gradual introduction until optimum blood pressure control is achieved

• With a diuretic to control salt and water retention; with a beta andronegic blocking agent

Evaluate:

• Therapeutic decreased and controlled blood pressure

• Increased hair growth for alopecia

• ECG alterations. Most changes are transient (increased T wave)

• Angina, peripheral oedema, increased heart rate

• Growth of body hair

• Input and output of fluids, check for fluid retention — oedema

• Report weight gains of 1.5 kg or more weekly

• Nausea and dizziness

• Breast tenderness, rash

Teach patient/family:

• That increased body hair will reverse when treatment finished

• Not to discontinue medication without medical advice. Drug should be tapered off slowly

• To avoid driving or hazardous activity if dizziness occurs

• To report pitting oedema, dizziness, weight gain more than 2.2 kg, shortness of breath, bruising or bleeding

---

misoprostol

Cytotec, combination product

Func. class.: Antiulcer and gastroprotective agent

Chem. class.: Prostaglandin E_1 analogue

Legal class.: POM

Action: Inhibits gastric acid secretion, protects gastroduodenal mucosa; increases bicarbonate, mucus production

Uses: Prophylaxis and healing of gastric and duodenal ulcers including those induced by NSAIDs

Dosage and routes:

• *Adult:* Healing, 800 mcg daily in 2−4 divided doses for 4−8 weeks

• Prophylaxis, 400−800 mcg daily in 2−4 divided doses

Available forms include: Tablets
200 mcg
Side effects/adverse reactions:
GI: Diarrhoea, nausea, vomiting
flatulence, dyspepsia, abdominal
pain
GU: Menorrhagia, abnormal
vaginal bleeding
CNS: Dizziness
SYST: Rashes
Contraindications: Hypersensitivity, pregnancy, lactation,
women of child-bearing age unless
effective contraceptive measures
are ensured
Precautions: Cerebrovascular
disease, hypertension, coronary
artery disease, severe peripheral
vascular disease
Pharmacokinetics:
By mouth: Peak 30 min, half-life is
20–40 min, plasma steady state
achieved within 2 days, excreted in
urine
Treatment of overdose: General
supportive measures
NURSING CONSIDERATIONS
Assess:
• Fluid balance, blood urea
nitrogen, creatinine
Evaluate:
• Response to treatment indicated
by absence of pain and gastrointestinal symptoms
Teach patient/family:
• Black pepper, caffeine, alcohol,
spices and very hot or cold food
are best avoided
• Not to take non-prescription
medicines for coughs and colds,
antacids and aspirin
• Pregnancy should be avoided
while taking drug as it can cause
miscarriage. If pregnancy is suspected the drug should be discontinued and the clinician informed
• Advise appropriate contraceptive methods

mitomycin

Mitomycin-C, Kyowa
Func. class.: Antineoplastic,
antibiotic
Legal class.: POM

Action: Inhibits DNA synthesis,
primarily; appears to cause cross-
linking of DNA
Uses: Pancreas, breast, stomach
cancer; adenocarcinoma of lung;
skin, bladder, rectal and other
cancers
Dosage and routes:
• *Adult:* IV 5–10 mg/m² every
3–6 weeks. A variety of other
schedules have been used. As a
bladder instillation in bladder
cancer, 10–40 mg in 20–40 ml
water 1–3 times a week for 10–20
doses; doses of 4–10 mg administered to a similar schedule have
been used to prevent recurrent
bladder tumours
Available forms include: Injection
IV 2, 10, 20 mg
Side effects/adverse reactions:
HAEM: Thrombocytopenia, leucopenia, anaemia, toxicity cumulative
GI: Nausea, vomiting, anorexia,
stomatitis, hepatotoxicity, diarrhoea
GU: Renal failure, oedema,
fibrosis of bladder following
instillation
INTEG: Rash, alopecia, severe
necrosis following extravasation
RESP: Fibrosis, pulmonary infiltrate, dyspnoea
CNS: Fever, paraesthesia
EENT: Blurred vision
Contraindications: Hypersensi-
tivity, pregnancy, breast feeding
Precautions: Renal disease, bone
marrow depression
Pharmacokinetics:
IV: Half-life approximately 17
min, metabolised in liver, 10%

excreted in urine (unchanged). Blood count nadir around 4 weeks post treatment

Interactions/incompatibilities:
• Increased toxicity: other antineoplastics or radiation

Clinical assessment:
• Full blood count, differential, platelet count prior to treatment and at nadir; withhold drug if patient excessively myelosuppressed
• Renal function studies: before, during therapy
• Liver function tests before, during therapy

Treatment of overdose: Supportive, no specific antidote, blood products or filgrastim for marrow suppression

NURSING CONSIDERATIONS

Administer:
• Following cytotoxic policy (vesicant drug)
• Reconstitution to be performed by qualified personnel in designated area
• Slow IV infusion using 21-, 23-, 25-gauge needle; check for extravasation
• Extravasation, skin, or eye contact: infiltrate or wash area with sodium bicarbonate 8.4%
• Other medication by oral route if possible; avoid IM, subcutaneous, IV routes to prevent infections only if thrombocytopenic
• Anti-emetic 30−60 min before giving drug to prevent vomiting

Perform/provide:
• Strict medical asepsis, protective isolation if WBC levels are low
• Strict oral hygiene 4 times a day
• Warm compresses at injection site for inflammation; check for extravasation

Evaluate:
• Bleeding: haematuria, bruising, petechiae, mucosa or orifices 8 hrly
• Dyspnoea, rales, unproductive cough, chest pain, tachypnola

fatigue, increaed pulse, pallor, lethargy
• Food preferences; list likes, dislikes
• Effects of alopecia on body image; discuss feelings about body changes
• Oedema in feet, joint, stomach pain, shaking
• Inflammation of mucosa, breaks in skin
• Buccal cavity 8 hrly for dryness, sores, ulceration, white patches, oral pain, bleeding, dysphagia
• Local irritation, pain, burning at injection site
• GI symptoms: frequency of stools, cramping
• Acidosis, signs of dehydration: rapid respirations, poor skin turgor, decreased urine output, dry skin, restlessness, weakness

Teach patient/family:
• Why protective isolation precautions are necessary
• To report any complaints, side effects to nurse or clinician
• That hair may be lost during treatment and wig or hairpiece is available on NHS; tell patient that new hair may be different in colour, texture
• To avoid foods with citric acid, hot or rough texture
• To report any bleeding, white spots, ulcerations in mouth; tell patient to examine mouth daily

mitozantrone

Novantrone
Func. class.: Antineoplastic agent
Chem. class.: Synthetic anthracenedione derivative
Legal class.: POM

Action: Binds to DNA, cytocidal effect on both proliferating and nonproliferating cells suggesting lack of cell cycle phase specificity

Uses: Acute non-lymphocytic leukaemia (adult), advanced breast cancer, non-Hodgkin's lymphoma, palliation of non-resectable primary hepatocellular carcinoma

Dosage and routes:

• *Adult:* Breast cancer, non-Hodgkin's lymphoma, hepatoma: single agent, IV 12–14 mg/m^2 repeated at 21-day intervals; adjusted according to WBC and platelet count; combination therapy, reduce dose by 2–4 mg/m^2 according to regime. Acute non-lymphocytic leukaemia relapse, IV 12 mg/m^2 daily on 5 consecutive days as single agent, or IV 10–12 mg/m^2 on 2–3 consecutive days with cytosine arabinoside

Available forms include: Injection 2 mg/ml (as hydrochloride)

Side effects/adverse reactions:

GI: Nausea, vomiting, diarrhoea, anorexia, mucositis, hepatotoxicity, gastrointestinal bleeding

HAEM: Thrombocytopenia, leucopenia, anaemia

INTEG: Rash, necrosis at injection site, dermatitis, thrombophlebitis at injection site, alopecia

CV: congestive cardiac failure, cardiomyopathy, dysrhythmias

MISC: Fever

RESP: Dyspnoea

EENT: Transient blue colouration of sclerae

CNS: Fatigue, weakness

GU: Transient blue-green coloration of urine, amenorrhoea

Contraindications: Hypersensitivity, pregnancy, breast feeding

Precautions: Myelosuppression, cardiac disease, children, renal, severe hepatic disease

Pharmacokinetics: Highly bound to plasma proteins, metabolised in liver, excreted via renal, hepatobiliary systems; elimination half-life 5–18 days. WBC nadir 10 days post-dosing

Interactions/incompatibilities:

• Do not mix with: heparin, precipitate will form

• Increased bone marrow depression given with: other cytotoxics, radiotherapy

Clinical assessment:

• Perform full blood count, differential WBC pre-treatment and 10 days post-treatment

• Regular assessment of cardiac function in patients with pre-existing cardiac disease or after cumulative dose greater than 160 mg/m^2

Treatment of overdose: Supportive, no specific antidote, blood products or filgrastim for marrow suppression

NURSING CONSIDERATION

Administer:

• In accordance with local policy for cytotoxics

• Other medications by oral route if possible; avoid injections to prevent infection

• Anti-emetic 30–60 min before mitozantrone to prevent vomiting

• By intravenous injection slowly, via appropriate gauge needle, checking for extravasation

• Following dilution, to at least 50 ml in any of the following intravenous infusions: sodium chloride 0.9%, glucose 5%, or sodium chloride 0.18% and glucose 4%

Perform/provide:

• Care to avoid contact of mitozantrone with the skin, mucous membranes, or eyes

• Strict oral hygiene 4 times a day

Evaluate:

• Bleeding e.g. haematuria, melaena, bruising and petechiae. Observe mucosal surfaces for bleeding 8 hrly

• Be aware of food preferences

• Observe for signs of jaundice e.g. yellowing of skin and sclera,

dark urine, clay-coloured stools, itching, abdominal pain, fever, diarrhoea
• Acidosis and signs of dehydration indicated by heightened respiratory rate, poor skin elasticity, decreased urinary output, restlessness or weakness

Teach patient/family:
• Mitozantrone may impart a blue-green coloration to the urine for 24 hr after administration
• Blue coloration of the sclerae may be seen very rarely and is reversible
• Patients and their partners should be advised to avoid conception for at least 1−6 months after cessation of therapy
• All side effects must be reported to clinician or nurse
• Hot foods and those which are coarse or contain citric acid are best avoided
• To report bleeding, mouth ulceration and white patches (indicative of *Candida*) to the clinician or nurse at once. The patient should examine his/her mouth at least once a day

---

morphine sulphate

MST Continus SRM-Rhotard, Oramorph, Sevredol, combination products
Func. class.: Narcotic analgesic
Chem. class.: Opioid
Legal class.: CD (Sch 2) POM

Action: Inhibits ascending pain pathways in CNS, increases pain threshold, alters pain perception. Acts of CNS opiate receptors
Uses: Severe pain
Dosage and routes:
• *Adult:* Subcutaneous/IM 4−15 mg 4 hrly as needed; By mouth 30−60 mg 4 hrly as needed; modi-fied-release 8−12 hrly; rectal 30−60 mg 4 hrly as needed; IV 4−10 mg diluted in 4−5 ml of water for injection, over 5 min
Myocardial infarction
• Slow IV 10 mg followed by 5−10 mg if required
Acute pulmonary oedema
• Slow IV 5−10 mg
Chronic pain
• *Adult:* By mouth, subcutaneous/IM injection 5−20 mg 4 hrly; rectally, 15−30 mg 4 hrly
• *Child:* By mouth, subcutaneous or IM injection; up to 1 month 150 mcg/kg, 1−12 months 200 mcg/kg 1−5 yr 2.5−5 mg, 6−12 yr 5−10 mg. Doses should be repeated 4 hrly
• Modified-release tablets: By mouth, take previous daily oral morphine requirement, divide by two and give this dose 12 hrly. Alternatively in adults start with 30 mg twice daily and increase with increments of 25−50%
Available forms include: Injection subcutaneous, IM, IV 10, 15, 30 mg/ml; oral solution 10 mg/5 ml, 100 mg/5 ml, 8.4 mg/ml; oral tablets 10, 20 mg; rectal suppository 15, 30 mg; modified-release tablets 10, 30, 60, 100, 200 mg
Side effects/adverse reactions:
CNS: Drowsiness, confusion, hallucinations, sedation, euphoria, alteration of pupillary responses
GI: Nausea, vomiting, anorexia, constipation, cramps, dry mouth
SYST: Tolerance, dependence
INTEG: Urticaria, flushing, pruritus, sweating, pain at site of injection
EENT: Miosis
GU: Retention
CV: Palpitations, bradycardia, hypotension
RESP: Respiratory depression, cough suppression
META: Hypothermia
Contraindications: Hypersensi-

tivity, paralytic ileus, respiratory depression, head injury, raised intracranial pressure, within 21 days of taking MAOIs

Precautions: Addictive personality, pregnancy, lactation, myocardial infarction (acute), severe heart disease, respiratory depression, hepatic disease, renal disease, obstructive airways disease, elderly (dosage reduction), hypothyroidism

Pharmacokinetics:

By mouth: Onset variable, peak variable, duration variable

Subcutaneous: Onset 15−30 min, peak 50−90 min

IV: Peak 20 min

Metabolised by liver, excreted by kidneys, excreted in breast milk, half-life 2½−3 hr

Interactions/incompatibilities:

• Effects may be increased with: other CNS depressants, alcohol, narcotics, sedative/hypnotics, antipsychotics, skeletal muscle relaxants, cimetidine

• Absorption of mexiletine may be delayed by opiates and cisapride action may be antagonised

Treatment of overdose: Naloxone 0.4−2 mg IV at 2 to 3 min intervals up to 10 mg, O_2, IV fluids, vasopressors; gastric lavage

NURSING CONSIDERATIONS

Assess:

• When pain is beginning to return; determine dosage interval by patient response

Administer:

• With anti-emetic if nausea, vomiting occur

• Before pain becomes severe

Perform/provide:

• Assistance with ambulation

• Safety measures: siderails, night light, call bell within easy reach

• Fluids and fibre if constipated

Evaluate:

• Therapeutic response: decrease in pain

• Fluid balance, check for decreasing output; may indicate urinary retention

• CNS changes: drowsiness, hallucinations, euphoria, level of consciousness, pupil reaction

• Allergic reactions: urticaria

• Respirations: respiratory depression, character, rate, rhythm; notify clinician if respirations are less than 12/min

• Need for additional analgesia, physical dependence

Teach patient/family:

• To report any symptoms of CNS changes, allergic reactions

• That dependency may result if dose taken is more than that needed to relieve pain

• Withdrawal symptoms may occur if high dose reduced too quickly: nausea, vomiting, cramps, fever, faintness, anorexia

• Importance of secure storage for controlled drug−social implications, risk to adults and children

---

mupirocin

Bactroban, Bactroban Nasal

Func. class.: Antibiotic, topical
Chem. class.: Pseudomonic acid
Legal class.: POM

Action: Inhibits bacterial protein synthesis by binding to specific protein complex, shows no cross resistance to most antibiotics

Uses: Bacterial skin infection, elimination of nasal carriage of *Staphylococcus aureus* including methicillin-resistant *Staphylococcus aureus* (MRSA)

Dosage and routes:

• Apply small amount to affected area 3 times a day for up to 10 days. Intranasal apply to arterior part of each nostril 2−3 times daily for 5−7 days. Gently press sides of nose together to spread ointment

Available forms include: Ointment 2% (20 mg/g); nasal ointment 2%
Side effects/adverse reactions:
INTEG: Burning, stinging, itching
Contraindications: Hypersensitivity to mupirocin, polyethylene glycols
Precautions: Pregnancy, lactation, moderate to severe renal impairment

NURSING CONSIDERATIONS

Assess:
• Affected area for persistent infection (indicated by increase in size of the lesions or an increase in their number)

Administer:
• After samples have been sent for culture and sensitivity
• Cover with gauze after application if indicated

Perform/provide:
• In presence of MRSA, patient should be barrier nursed with strict hygiene control of staff to avoid further spread of infection
• Regular swabs to determine evidence of continuing infection
• Follow local policy for MRSA infection
• Wash hands after applying ointment and wear gloves
• In hospital children should be nursed in isolation (2–5 days)

Evaluate:
• Response to treatment: reduction in size and number of lesions

Teach patient/family:
• Hands must be washed after applying ointment
• Child's fingernails must be trimmed to prevent scratching
• Irritation and worsening of condition must be reported to clinician or health visitor

mustine HCl

Func. class.: Antineoplastic alkylating agent
Chem. class.: Nitrogen mustard
Legal class.: POM

Action: Alkylates DNA, RNA; also responsible for cross-linking DNA strands
Uses: Principally Hodgkin's disease. Occasionally other cancers; topically in mycosis fungoides
Dosage and routes:
• *Adult:* IV 0.4 mg/kg as a single dose or 0.1 mg/kg as a course of 4 daily injections. Reconstituted in sodium chloride 0.9% or water for injections. Topical (in mycosis fungoides) as a 0.02% solution in sodium chloride 0.9%
Available forms include: 10 mg; Powder for injection
Side effects/adverse reactions:
After injection
EENT: Tinnitus, hearing loss
HAEM: Thrombocytopenia, leucopenia, agranulocytosis, anaemia
GI: Nausea, vomiting, diarrhoea, stomatitis, weight loss
CNS: Headache, dizziness, drowsiness
INTEG: Alopecia, pruritus
GU: Amenorrhoea, reduced spermatogenesis
SYST: Fever
After topical use
INTEG: Contact dermatitis, rash, alopecia
Contraindications: Pregnancy, severe leucopenia, thrombocytopenia or anaemia and coexistent or suspected granuloma, breast feeding
Precautions: Vesicant, only ever give systemically by IV injection, avoid extravasation. If extravasation occurs seek specialist advice
• Irritant to skin and mucous membranes, accidental contami-

nation requires irrigation or washing with large amounts of water — seek medical advice

Pharmacokinetics: Metabolised in liver, excreted in urine. Disappears from blood in 10 min

Interactions/incompatibilities:
• Increased toxicity: antineoplastics, radiation
• Rapidly unstable in alkaline solution

Clinical assessment:
• Full blood count, differential, before treatment and at nadir 10 days post-treatment. Withhold treatment if WBC below limits set in the treatment unit
• Anti-emetic 30−60 min before giving drug to prevent vomiting

Treatment of overdose: Sodium thiosulphate infusion 64 mg per mg mustine will neutralise mustine if given *immediately* afterwards, otherwise treatment is supportive

NURSING CONSIDERATIONS

Assess:
• Baseline temperature and fluid balance

Administer:
• With extreme care; vesicant and irritant
• In accordance with local cytotoxic policy
• Other medications by oral route; if possible avoid IM, subcutaneous, IV routes to prevent infections
• Slow IV injection using 21-, 23-, 25-gauge needle, with Luer' locks
• As bolus well flushed in with sodium chloride 0.9%; taking care to avoid extravasation

Perform/provide:
• Trained personnel should reconstitute drug in designated area
• Strict medical asepsis, protective isolation if WBC levels are low
• Special skin care
• Increase fluid intake to 2−3 litres daily to prevent urate deposits, calculi formation
• Strict oral hygiene 4 times a day with prescribed mouthwashes
• Warm compresses at injection site for inflammation

Evaluate:
• Bleeding: haematuria, bruising or petechiae, mucosa or orifices 8 hrly
• For extravasation; infusion should be stopped if local pain experienced
• Food preferences; list likes, dislikes
• Yellowing of skin, sclera, dark urine, clay-coloured stools, itchy skin, abdominal pain, fever, diarrhoea
• Effects of alopecia on body image; discuss feelings about body changes
• Inflammation of mucosa, breaks in skin
• Buccal cavity 8 hrly for dryness, sores, ulceration, white patches, oral pain, bleeding, dysphagia
• Local irritation, pain, burning, discoloration at injection site
• Symptoms indicating severe allergic reaction: rash, pruritus, urticaria, purpuric skin lesions, itching, flushing

Teach patient/family:
• Of protective isolation precautions
• To report any complaints or side effects to nurse or clinician
• That sterility, amenorrhoea can occur; reversible after discontinuing treatment
• That hair may be lost during treatment; a wig or hairpiece is available on NHS prescription; new hair may be different in colour, texture
• To avoid foods with citric acid, hot or rough texture
• To report any bleeding, white spots, or ulcerations in mouth to clinician; tell patient to examine mouth daily

nabilone

Cesamet
Func. class.: Anti-emetic
Chem. class.: Synthetic canni-binoid
Legal class.: POM

Action: Inhibition of vomiting control mechanism in the medulla oblongata

Uses: Nausea and vomiting caused by cytotoxic drugs, unresponsive to conventional anti-emetics

Dosage and routes:

• *Adult over 18 yr:* By mouth, 1 mg twice daily, increased if necessary to 2 mg twice daily, throughout each cycle of cytotoxic therapy and, if necessary, for 48 hr after last dose of each cycle; maximum 6 mg daily

• First dose taken the night before initiation of cytotoxic therapy, 2nd dose 1−3 hr before the first dose of cytotoxic drug

Available forms includes: Capsules 1 mg

Side effects/adverse reactions:

CNS: Drowsiness, confusion, disorientation, euphoria, psychosis, depression, hallucinations, lapses in concentration, decreased co-ordination, headache, blurred vision, tremors

CV: Postural hypotension, tachycardia

GI: Dry mouth, decreased appetite, abdominal cramps

Contraindications: Known allergy to cannabinoid agents, severe liver dysfunction and when nausea and vomiting causes from any cause other than cancer chemotherapy

Precautions: History of psychosis, pregnancy, lactation, elderly, heart disease, hypotension

Pharmacokinetics: Absorbed from the GI tract, undergoes metabolism possible to active metabolite, excreted predominately by biliary route. Half-life is 2 hr

Interactions/incompatibilities:

• Increased effects of: CNS depressants, including alcohol and narcotic analgesics

Treatment of overdose: Symptomatic and supportive therapy. Anticipate psychotic episodes, including hallucinations and anxiety reactions. Consider administration of a neuroleptic agent or activated charcoal to decrease absorption from GI tract

• Maintain airway
• Maintain body temperature
• Assess conscious state

NURSING CONSIDERATIONS

Assess:

• Baseline BP: lying and standing
• Pulse

Administer:

• For 24 hr after end of chemotherapy if necessary

Perform/provide:

• Boiled sweets, frequent sips of water for dry mouth

Evaluate:

• For neurological side effects including drowsiness, confusion, disorientation: may require assistance with ambulation

• Therapeutic effect: reduction of nausea and vomiting

• For postural hypotension and tachycardia

Teach patient/family:

• Rise slowly as fainting may occur
• Not to perform potentially hazardous tasks since mental and physical abilities may be impaired
• Avoid alcohol
• Deep breathing to assist in control of nausea

nabumetone

Relifex
Func. class.: Non-steroidal anti-inflammatory drug
Chem. class.: Butanone
Legal class.: POM

Action: Prostaglandin synthesis inhibitor. Has both analgesic and anti-inflammatory effects

Uses: Osteoarthritis, rheumatoid arthritis

Dosage and routes:
• By mouth 1 g at night; in severe conditions 0.5−1 g in morning as well, elderly patients 0.5−1 g daily

Available forms include: Tablets 500 mg; suspension 500 mg in 5 ml

Side effects/adverse reactions:
GI: Nausea, diarrhoea, constipation, dyspepsia, flatulence, abdominal pain
CNS: Headache, dizziness, vertigo, sedation
INTEG: Rashes, pruritus

Contraindications: Active peptic ulceration, severe hepatic impairment, hypersensitivity, pregnancy and lactation

Precautions: Elderly patients, history of peptic ulceration, allergic disorders, asthma, renal impairment, aspirin hypersensitivity

Pharmacokinetics: Absorbed from GI tract and rapidly metabolised in liver to principal active metabolite, 6-methoxy-2-naphthylacetic acid, which has a plasma half-life of 12−36 hr

Interactions/incompatibilities:
• Increased risk of side effects: anticoagulants, antihypertensives, anticonvulsants, sulphonylurea hypoglycaemics, cardiac glycosides, diuretics

Clinical assessment:
• Renal function tests: blood urea, creatinine, before treatment and periodically thereafter if problem anticipated

Treatment of overdose: No specific antidote. Treatment with gastric lavage, activated charcoal using up to 60 g orally in divided doses

NURSING CONSIDERATIONS

Administer:
• With or after food to decrease GI symptoms

Evaluate:
• Therapeutic response: decreased pain, stiffness, swelling in joints, ability to move more easily

Teach patient/family:
• To avoid driving or other hazardous activities if dizziness or drowsiness occurs
• To report change in urine pattern, weight increase, oedema, pain increase in joints, fever, blood in urine (indicates nephrotoxicity)
• That therapeutic effects may take up to 1 month
• To take with food or milk
• To report any indigestion or black tarry stools

nadolol

Corgard, combination product
Func. class.: Antihypertensive, anti-anginal
Chem. class.: β-adrenergic receptor blocking drugs
Legal class.: POM

Action: Long-acting, nonselective β-adrenergic receptor blocking agent; mechanism is similar to propranolol

Uses: Chronic stable angina pectoris, mild to moderate hypertension prophylaxis of migraine, arrhythmias, thyrotoxicosis

Dosage and routes:
Angina
• *Adult:* By mouth 40 mg daily increased at weekly intervals to 160 mg daily

Hypertension
- *Adult:* By mouth 80 mg daily increased at weekly intervals to maximum 240 mg daily

Arrhythmias
- *Adult:* By mouth 40 mg daily increased to 160 mg daily; reduce to 40 mg daily if bradycardia occurs

Migraine prophylaxis
- *Adult:* By mouth 40 mg daily increased at weekly intervals usually 80−160 mg daily

Thyrotoxicosis
- *Adult:* By mouth 80−160 mg daily

Available forms include: Tablets 40, 80 mg

Side effects/adverse reactions:
RESP: Respiratory dysfunction
CV: Bradycardia, hypotension
CNS: Fatigue, lightheadedness, paraesthesia, depression, insomnia
GI: Nausea, vomiting, diarrhoea, colitis, constipation, cramps, dry mouth
INTEG: Rash, pruritus, fever, cold extremities, alopecia

Contraindications: Cardiac failure, cardiogenic shock, 2nd or 3rd degree heart block, obstructive airways disease, asthma, sinus bradycardia, congestive cardiac failure

Precautions: Diabetes mellitus, pregnancy, renal disease, lactation, congestive cardiac failure, hyperthyroidism, chronic obstructive airways disease, angina, hepatic disease

Pharmacokinetics:
By mouth: Onset variable, peak 3−4 hr, duration 17−24 hr; half-life 16−20 hr, not metabolised, excreted in urine (unchanged), bile, breast milk

Interactions/incompatibilities:
- Increased effects: alcohol, anaesthetics, anti-arrhythmics, antidiabetics, antihypertensives, calcium channel blockers, cardiac glycosides, corticosteroids, diuretics

- Decreased effects: analgesics, sympathomimetics, MAOIs

Clinical assessment:
- Fluid balance; creatinine clearance if kidney damage is diagnosed

Treatment of overdose: Excessive bradycardia treated with atropine; if no response isoprenaline given with caution. Cardiac failure with digitalisation and diuretics. Glucagon may be useful. Hypotension managed with adrenaline. Bronchospasm counteracted with isoprenaline and aminophylline. May be removed from circulation by haemodialysis

NURSING CONSIDERATIONS

Assess:
- Baseline vital signs

Evaluate:
- Therapeutic response (dependant on dose)
- Reduction in hypertension
- Relief of angina
- Reduced arrhythmias
- Respiratory status, may cause bronchospasm
- Heart rate — bradycardia, heart block
- Observe for increased cardiac failure (oedema, weight gain, dyspnoea)
- Reduced doses required with renal failure
- Control of migraine
- Relief from thyrotoxic symptoms

Teach patient/family:
- May cause cold extremities, fatigue, sleep disturbances

---

naftidrofuryl oxalate

Praxilene, Praxilene Forte
Func. class.: Vasodilator
Legal class.: POM

Action: Potent spasmolytic; exerts a direct effect on intracellular metabolism increasing ATP levels and decreasing lactic acid levels in ischaemic conditions

Uses: Cerebral and peripheral vascular disease, intermittent claudication, night cramps, Raynaud's syndrome

Dosage and routes:

Cerebral vascular disease

• By mouth 100 mg 3 times daily

Peripheral vascular disease

• By mouth 100–200 mg 3 times daily; IV or intra-arterial infusion 200 mg in dextrose 5% or sodium chloride 0.9% over at least 90 min twice daily

Available forms include: Capsules 100 mg; injection 20 mg/ml, 10 ml ampoule

Side effects/adverse reactions:

GU: Nausea, epigastric pain

INTEG: Rash

Contraindications: Parenteral administration in atrioventricular block, bolus injection, hypersensitivity

Precautions: Pregnancy, lactation, severe cardiac insufficiency, renal, hepatic disease

Interactions: β-Blockers, antiarrhythmic drugs, incompatible with solutions containing calcium ions

Treatment of overdose: Depression of cardiac conduction may require isoprenaline, convulsions may be managed by diazepam

NURSING CONSIDERATIONS

Assess:

• Baseline BP and pulse

Administer:

• With meals to reduce GI upsets

Evaluate:

• Therapeutic response: increased temperature in extremities, orientation, long- and short-term memory

• BP, pulse during treatment until stable

• Record BP lying and standing — postural hypotension is common

Teach patient/family:

• That medication may need to be taken continuously, therapeutic response may not be seen for 2–3 months

• That it is necessary to stop smoking to prevent excessive vasoconstriction

• Dizziness may occur

• To make positional changes slowly, or fainting may occur

• To discontinue drug, notify clinician if rash develops

• To report palpitations, flushing if severe

• To avoid changes in temperature; extremities should be kept warm to promote better circulation

---

nalbuphine HCl

Nubain

Func. class.: Narcotic analgesic

Chem. class.: Partial opiate agonist

Legal class.: POM

Action: Inhibits ascending pain pathways in CNS, increases pain threshold, alters pain perception

Uses: Moderate to severe pain, peri-operative analgesia

Dosage and routes:

• *Adult:* Subcutaneous/IM/IV 10–20 mg every 3–6 hr as required

• *Child:* 300 mcg/kg repeated once or twice as necessary

Myocardial infarction, suspected

• *Adult:* Slow IV 10–20 mg repeated after 30 min if necessary

Premedication

• *Adult:* Subcutaneous/IM/IV 100–200 mcg/kg

Induction

• *Adult:* IV 0.3–1 mg/kg over 10–15 min

Intra-operative analgesia

• *Adult:* IV 250–500 mcg/kg at 30 min intervals

Available forms include: Injection

subcutaneous, IM, IV 10 mg/ml
1 ml, 2 ml
Side effects/adverse reactions:
CNS: Dizziness, confusion, head-
ache, sedation, speech difficulty
GI: Nausea, vomiting
INTEG: Urticaria, flushing
EENT: Blurred vision
CV: Tachycardia, bradycardia,
change in BP
RESP: Respiratory depression
Contraindications: Hypersensi-
tivity, addiction (opioid), in-
creased intracranial pressure
Precautions: Addictive person-
ality, pregnancy, lactation, respir-
atory depression, hepatic disease,
renal disease, asthma
Pharmacokinetics:
Subcutaneous/IM/IV: Duration
3–6 hr; metabolised by liver, ex-
creted by kidneys, half-life 5 hr
Interactions/incompatibilities:
• Effects may be increased with
other CNS depressants: alcohol,
narcotics, sedative/hypnotics,
antipsychotics
Treatment of overdose: Naloxone
IV, O_2, IV fluids, vasopressors
NURSING CONSIDERATIONS
Assess:
• Baseline vital signs, pupil size
and reaction
• Fluid balance
• When pain is beginning to re-
turn; determine dosage interval by
patient response
Administer:
• With anti-emetic if nausea,
vomiting occur
Perform/provide:
• Storage in CD cupboard
• Assistance with ambulation
• Safety measures: siderails, night
light, call-bell within easy reach
Evaluate:
• Therapeutic response: decrease
in pain
• CNS changes: drowsiness, hal-
lucinations, euphoria, level of con-
sciousness, pupil reaction

• Allergic reactions: rash, urticaria
• Respirations: respiratory depression, character, rate, rhythm;
notify clinician if respirations are
less than 12/min
• Therapeutic response
Teach patient/family:
• To report any symptoms of CNS
changes, allergic reactions
• That physical dependency may
result when used for extended
periods of time
• Withdrawal symptoms may
occur: nausea, vomiting, cramps,
fever, faintness, anorexia
• Importance of safe storage; risk
to children

---

nalidixic acid

Negram, Mictral, Uriben
Func. class.: Antibiotic, urinary
tract
Chem. class.: 4-Quinolone
Legal class.: POM

Action: Appears to inhibit DNA
polymerisation, primary target
being single-stranded DNA pre-
cursors in late stages of chromo-
somal replication
Uses: Urinary tract infections
Dosage and routes:
• *Adult:* By mouth 1 g 4 times a
day for 7 days reduced to 500 mg
every 6 hr in long-term treatment.
Granules, 660 mg in water 3 times
daily for 3 days
• *Child over 3 months:* By mouth
50 mg/kg daily in 4 divided doses;
30 mg/kg daily for long-term
treatment
Available forms include: Tablets
500 mg; suspension 300 mg/5 ml,
granules 660 mg/4.1 g sachet
Side effects/adverse reactions:
INTEG: Pruritus, rash, urticaria,
photosensitivity, angioedema,
arthralgia

CNS: Dizziness, headache, drowsiness, convulsions, weakness
GI: Nausea, vomiting, abdominal pain, diarrhoea
EENT: Sensitivity to light, blurred vision, change in colour perception
Contraindications: Hypersensitivity, 1st trimester of pregnancy, lactation, liver disease, liver failure, infants less than 3 months epilepsy, CNS lesions, porphyria
Precautions: Elderly, renal disease, hepatic disease, G6PD deficiency
Pharmacokinetics:
By mouth: Peak 1−2 hr, metabolised in liver, excreted in urine (unchanged conjugates)
Interactions/incompatibilities:
• Increased effects of: oral anticoagulants
• Decreased effects of: antacids, iron supplements
Clinical assessment:
• Blood count for patients on chronic therapy
• Renal, hepatic function
Lab. test interferences:
False positive: Urinary glucose
False increase: 17-hydroxycorticosteroids, vanillylmandelic acid
NURSING CONSIDERATIONS
Assess:
• Fluid balance
Administer:
• After mid-stream urine is obtained for culture and sensitivity
Perform/provide:
• 2 litre fluid daily ensures that urinary pH is greater than 5.5
• Limited intake of alkaline foods, drugs: milk, dairy products, peanuts, vegetables, alkaline antacids, sodium bicarbonate
• Protect drug from freezing
Evaluate:
• CNS symptoms: insomnia, vertigo, headache, drowsiness, convulsions
• Allergy: fever, flushing, rash, urticaria, pruritus
• For photosensitivity
Teach patient/family:
• That photosensitivity occurs; that patient should avoid sunlight or use sunscreen to prevent burns
• Instruct patient to protect suspension from freezing, shake well before taking
• May cause drowsiness; advise patient not to drive or operate machinery while on medication and to seek help for walking if affected
• Instruct patients with diabetes that Clinitest may prove false positive for glucose

---

naloxone HCl

Narcan, Narcan Neonatal
Func. class.: Narcotic antagonist
Chem. class.: Thebaine derivative
Legal class.: POM

Action: Competes with opioids at opioid receptor sites
Uses: Opioid-induced respiratory depression including pentazocine, dextropropoxyphene
Dosage and routes:
Opioid-induced respiratory depression
• *Adult:* IV/subcutaneous/IM 0.8−2 mg; repeat every 2−3 min, if required to maximum 10 mg (IV route faster onset)
• *Child:* 100 mcg/kg; then 100 mcg/kg if no response
Postoperative respiratory depression
• *Adult:* IV 0.1−0.2 mg every 2 min as required. Further doses by IM injection after 1−2 hr if required
• *Child:* IV 10 mcg/kg, then 0.1 mg/kg if no response. If IV route not possible may be given by IM or subcutaneous route in divided doses

• *Neonate:* IV/subcutaneous/IM 10 mcg/kg repeated every 2−3 min or 200 mcg (60 mcg/kg) IM at birth (onset on action slower)

Available forms include: Injection IV, IM, subcutaneous 20 mcg/ml, 0.4 mg/ml, 1 mg/ml

Side effects/adverse reactions:
GI: Nausea, vomiting

Contraindications: Hypersensitivity

Precautions: Pregnancy, opiate dependence (may precipitate acute withdrawal symptoms), cardiac irritability

Pharmacokinetics:
Metabolised by liver, excreted by kidneys, excreted in breast milk, half-life 1−3½ hr

NURSING CONSIDERATIONS

Assess:
• Baseline vital signs and neurological status
• Level of consciousness and respiratory rate to determine whether complete or partial reversal of opiate is required

Administer:
• IV, IM or subcutaneously
• Can be diluted in 0.9% sodium chloride or in 5% dextrose

Evaluate:
• Signs of withdrawal in drug-dependent individuals
• Therapeutic effect
• Cardiac status: tachycardia, hypertension
• Respiratory dysfunction: respiratory depression, character, rate, rhythm; if respirations are less than 10/min, respiratory stimulant should be administered

nandrolone decanoate/ nandrolone phenylpropionate

Deca-Durabolin,   Deca-Durabolin 100, Durabolin

Func. class.: Androgenic anabolic steroid

Chem. class.: Halogenated testosterone derivative

Legal class.: POM

Action: Increases weight by building body tissue, increases potassium, phosphorus, chloride, nitrogen levels, increases bone development

Uses: Osteoporosis in postmenopausal women; aplastic anaemia

Dosage and routes:
Post-menopausal women
• Deep IM 50 mg every 3 weeks (decanoate). Deep IM 50 mg weekly (phenylpropionate)

Aplastic anaemia
• Deep IM 50−150 mg weekly (decanoate)

Available forms include: Phenylpropionate injection IM 25, 50 mg/ml; decanoate injection IM 25, 50, 100 mg/ml

Side effects/adverse reactions:
INTEG: Acneiform lesions, oily hair, acne vulgaris, hirsutism
MS: Premature epiphyseal closure
GU: Amenorrhoea, increased libido, inhibition of spermatogenesis, sodium and water retention, decreased breast size, clitoral hypertrophy
GI: Occasionally abnormal liver function tests
EENT: Voice deepening, hoarseness
ENDO: Abnormal glucose tolerance test

Contraindications: Known or suspected carcinoma of the prostate or mammary carcinoma in the male

Precautions: Diabetes mellitus, CV disease, liver dysfunction, skeletal metastases, renal dysfunction, hypertension, epilepsy, migraine

Pharmacokinetics:

IM: Metabolised in liver, excreted in urine, excreted in the breast milk

Interactions/incompatibilities:

• Increased effects of: oral anti-diabetics
• Increased prothrombin urine: anticoagulants
• Decreased effects of: insulin

Clinical assessment:

• Electrolytes: potassium, sodium, chloride calcium; cholesterol
• Liver function studies: alanine aminotransferase, aspartate aminotransferase, bilirubin

NURSING CONSIDERATIONS

Assess:

• Baseline weight, and BP

Administer:

• By deep IM injection

Perform/provide:

• Diet with increased calories, protein; decrease sodium if oedema occurs

Evaluate:

• Weight daily, notify clinician if weekly weight gain is greater than 2.5 kg
• Fluid balance; be alert for decreasing urinary output, increasing oedema
• Growth rate in children since growth rate may be uneven (linear/bone growth) when used for extended periods of time
• Therapeutic response: increased appetite, increased stamina
• Oedema, hypertension, cardiac symptoms, jaundice
• Mental status: affect, mood, behavioural changes, aggression
• Signs of masculinisation in female: increased libido, deepening of voice (sometimes irreversible), male: gynaecomastia, impotence, testicular atrophy
• Hypoglycaemia in diabetics; since oral anticoagulant action is decreased
• Acne, hirustism

Teach patient/family:

• Drug needs to be combined with complete health plan: diet, rest, exercise
• To notify clinician if therapeutic response decreases
• Not to discontinue medication abruptly
• All aspects of drug usage; drug can be abused by athletes
• Females to report menstrual irregularities
• That long-term use may be necessary

---

naproxen/naproxen sodium

Naprosyn Nycopren, Synflex

Func. class.: Non-steroidal anti-inflammatory drug

Chem. class.: Propionic acid derivative

Legal class.: POM

Action: Inhibits prostaglandin synthesis by decreasing an enzyme needed for biosynthesis; possesses analgesic, anti-inflammatory, antipyretic properties

Uses: Mild to moderate pain, osteoarthritis, rheumatoid arthritis (including juvenile arthritis), acute gout, other musculoskeletal disorders

Dosage and routes:

• *Adult:* By mouth 500 mg−1 g daily in 2 divided doses, or 1 g once daily (base); 550 mg, then 275 mg every 6−8 hr as needed, not to exceed 1375 mg (sodium). Rectal route 500 mg at bedtime

Available forms include: Tablets 250, 275, 500 mg, granules 500 mg/sachet, suspension 125 mg/5 ml, suppositories 500 mg

Side effects/adverse reactions:

GI: Nausea, vomiting, cholestatic jaundice; ulcerative stomatitis, peptic ulcer, colitis, bleeding

CNS: Insomnia, headache, inability to concentrate, vertigo

CV: Peripheral oedema

INTEG: Purpura, rash, pruritus, sweating, vasculitis

GU: Nephrotoxicity: haematuria

HAEM: Blood dyscrasias

EENT: Tinnitus, hearing loss, blurred vision

Contraindications: Hypersensitivity, asthma, severe renal disease, severe hepatic disease, peptic ulcer

Precautions: Pregnancy, lactation, children, bleeding disorders, GI disorders, cardiac disorders, hypersensitivity to other NSAIDs

Pharmacokinetics:

By mouth: Peak 2 hr, half-life 3–3½ hr; metabolised in liver, excreted in urine (metabolites), excreted in breast milk

Interactions/incompatibilities:

• May increase action of: coumarin, phenytoin, sulphonamides when used with this drug

• Decreased antihypertensive effect of: propranolol and other β-blockers

• Increased blood levels of: lithium

• Increased levels of this drug: probenecid

• Enhanced toxicity of: methotrexate

Clinical assessment:

• Renal, liver, blood studies: blood urea nitrogen, creatinine, aspartate aminotransferase, alanine aminotransferase, Hb before treatment, periodically thereafter if problems anticipated

Lab. test interereferences:

Discontinue therapy 48 hr prior to adrenal function tests. May affect tests for urinary 5-hydroxyindole-acetic acid

Treatment of overdose: Gastric lavage and supportive measures; administer activated charcoal; haemodialysis may be appropriate in a patient with renal failure

NURSING CONSIDERATIONS

Administer:

• With or after food to decrease GI symptoms

Evaluate:

• Therapeutic response: decreased pain, stiffness, swelling in joints, ability to move more easily

• For eye, ear problems: blurred vision, tinnitus (may indicate toxicity)

Teach patient/family:

• To report blurred vision, ringing, roaring in ears (may indicate toxicity)

• To avoid driving or other hazardous activities if dizziness or drowsiness occurs

• To report change in urine pattern, weight increase, oedema, pain increase in joints, fever, blood in urine (indicates nephrotoxicity)

• That therapeutic effects may take up to 1 month

• To take with food or milk

• To report indigestion or black tarry stools

---

nedocromil sodium

Tilade

Func. class.: Anti-asthmatic
Chem. class.: Quinoline
Legal class.: POM

Action: Thought to prevent release of pharmacological mediators of bronchospasm by stabilising mast-cell membranes

Uses: Prophylaxis of reversible obstructive airways disease

Dosage and routes:
• Inhale 2 puffs (4 mg) twice daily increased to 2 puffs 6 hrly if necessary
Available forms include: Aerosol inhalation, 2 mg/dose
Side effects/adverse reactions:
CNS: Headache
GI: Nausea
EENT: Bitter taste in mouth
Contraindications: Children under 12 yr
Precautions: Pregnancy, lactation
Pharmacokinetics: After inhalation nedocromil is deposited in the lungs, absorbed and excreted unchanged in bile and urine. Drug deposited in oropharynx is swallowed and poorly absorbed from GI tract. Drug does not accumulate on long-term dosing and is not retained in any tissues
NURSING CONSIDERATIONS
Administer:
• By inhalation
Perform/provide:
• Gargle, sip of water to decrease irritation in throat
Evaluate:
• Respiratory status, respiratory rate, rhythm characteristics, cough, wheezing, dyspnoea
Teach patient/family:
• To clear mucus before using
• Proper inhalation technique: exhale, use inhaler, inhale deeply, remove, hold breath, exhale, repeat until all of the drug is inhaled
• That therapeutic effect may take up to 4 weeks
• Regular use is necessary
• Not effective during asthma attack

nefopam HCl

Acupan
Func. class.: Analgesic
Chem. class.: Benzoxazocine
Legal class.: POM

Action: Not established
Uses: Relief of acute and chronic pain
Dosage and routes:
• By mouth initially 60 mg 3 times daily adjusted according to response; usual range 30−90 mg 3 times daily
• IM injection 20 mg 6-hrly
Available forms include: Tablets 30 mg; injection 20 mg/ml, 1 ml ampoule
Side effects/adverse reactions:
CNS: Nervousness, insomnia, drowsiness, blurred vision, headache
GI: Nausea, dry mouth, vomiting
CV: Tachycardia
INTEG: Sweating
GU: Urinary retention, may colour urine pink
Contraindications: Convulsive disorders, myocardial infarction, patients receiving MAOIs
Precautions: Renal or liver disease, glaucoma, urinary retention. Administer IM injection with patient lying down. Reduced dosage for elderly
Pharmacokinetics: Onset of effect after IM injection is 15−20 min, peak effect within 1½ hr. 60 mg oral is equivalent to 20 mg IM
Interactions:
• Tricyclic antidepressants, MAOIs
Tests/investigations: Renal and liver function tests if impairment suspected
Treatment of overdose: Gastric lavage and supportive measures. Administer activated charcoal
NURSING CONSIDERATIONS

Assess:
• Location, duration and severity of pain
Administer:
• With food to decrease GI symptoms
Perform/provide:
• Mouthwashes to relieve mouth dryness
Evaluate:
• Therapeutic response: decreased pain, stiffness, swelling in joints, ability to move more easily
• For eye, ear problems: blurred vision, tinnitus (may indicate toxicity)
• Urinary output
Teach patient/family:
• To report blurred vision, ringing, roaring in ears (may indicate toxicity)
• To avoid driving or other hazardous activities if dizziness or drowsiness occurs
• To report change in urine pattern, weight increase, oedema, pain increase in joints, fever, blood in urine (indicates nephrotoxicity)
• That therapeutic effects may take up to 1 month

---

neomycin sulphate

Mycifradin, Nivemycin
Func. class.: Antibiotic
Chem. class.: Aminoglycoside
Legal class.: POM

Action: Interferes with protein synthesis in bacterial cell by binding to ribosomal subunit causing inaccurate peptide sequence to form in protein chain, causing bacterial death
Uses: Hepatic coma. Pre-operatively to sterilise bowel
Dosage and routes: By mouth
Pre-operative bowel sterilisation
• *Adult:* 1 g every 1 hr for 4 doses, then 4 hrly for 2 or 3 days

• *Child more than 12 yr:* 1 g 4 hrly for 2–3 days
• *Child 6–12 yr:* 250–500 mg 4 hrly for 2–3 days
• *Child 1–5 yr:* 10–20 ml 4 hrly for 2–3 days
• *Child less than 1 yr*: 2.5–10 ml 4 hrly for 2–3 days
Hepatic coma
• *Adults:* 4–12 g daily in divided doses for 5–7 days
• *Child:* 50–100 mg/kg daily in divided doses
Available forms include: Tablets 500 mg; elixir 100 mg/5 ml
Side effects/adverse reactions:
GU: Nephrotoxicity
CNS: Confusion, nystagmus, paraesthesia, disorientation
EENT: Ototoxicity
HAEM: Haemolytic anaemia, blood dyscrasias
GI: Nausea, vomiting, diarrhoea, increased salivation, stomatitis, increased alanine aminotransferase, aspartate aminotransferase, bilirubin
CV: Hypotension, myocarditis
INTEG: Dermatitis, pruritus, drug fever, anaphylaxis
Contraindications: Bowel obstruction, hypersensitivity
Precautions: Neonates, hepatic coma (minimum period of administration), renal disease, pregnancy, hearing deficits, lactation, neuromuscular disorders
Pharmacokinetics: Only about 3% absorbed orally, but accumulation to toxic levels can occur especially in renal impairment. Excreted unchanged by kidneys, half-life 2 hr
Interactions/incompatibilities:
• Increased ototoxicity, neurotoxicity, nephrotoxicity: other aminoglycosides, amphotericin B, polymyxin, vancomycin, cyclosporin, cisplatin, cephalosporins, loop diuretics
• Increased effects: non-depolari-

sing muscle relaxants, oral anti-coagulants when given with oral neomycin
• Decreased effects of: oral digoxin, oral penicillin, oral contraceptives when given with oral neomycin

Treatment of overdose: Monitor renal and auditory function — if impaired dialysis indicated

NURSING CONSIDERATIONS

Assess:
• Weight before treatment; calculation of dosage is usually done based on ideal body weight, but may be calculated on actual body weight

Administer:
• After specimens taken for culture and sensitivity

Perform/provide:
• Adequate fluids of 2–3 litres daily unless contraindicated to prevent irritation of tubules
• Supervised ambulation, other safety measures for patients with vestibular dysfunction

Evaluate:
• Fluid balance, urinalysis daily for proteinuria, cells, casts; report sudden change in urine output
• Urine pH if drug is used for urinary tract infection; urine should be kept alkaline
• When given in hepatic coma, or as pre-operative bowel preparation ensure that bowel motions take place
• Therapeutic effect: absence of fever, draining wounds, negative culture and sensitivity after treatment
• Renal impairment by securing urine for creatinine clearance testing, blood urea nitrogen, serum creatinine; lower dosage should be given in renal impairment (creatinine clearance less than 80 ml/min)
• Deafness by audiometric testing, ringing, roaring in ears, vertigo;

assess hearing before, during, after treatment
• Dehydration: high specific gravity, decrease in skin turgor, dry mucous membranes, dark urine
• Vestibular dysfunction: nausea, vomiting, dizziness, headache; drug should be discontinued if severe

Teach patient/family:
• To report headache, dizziness, symptoms of overgrowth of infection, renal impairment
• To report loss of hearing, ringing, roaring in ears or a feeling of fullness in head

---

neomycin sulphate (ophthalmic/otic)

Minims, Neomycin sulphate, many combination products
Func. class.: Antibiotic
Chemical class.: Aminoglycoside
Legal class.: POM

Action: Inhibits protein synthesis in susceptible micro-organisms

Uses: Eye/ear infection (external)

Dosage and routes:
• *Adult and child:* Instil 2–4 drops 3 or 4 times a day into affected eye or ear. Eye ointment apply to eye one or more times daily

Available forms include: Single use Minims eye drops 0.5%, 0.5 ml. Many combination preparations of ear/eye drops/ointment

Side effects/adverse reactions:
EENT: Itching, irritation in ear/eye
INTEG: Rash

Contraindications: Hypersensitivity, perforated eardrum, glaucoma, avoid prolonged use

NURSING CONSIDERATIONS

Evaluate:
• Therapeutic response: decreased pain, reduced inflammation of the eye

• For redness, swelling, fever, pain in ear/eye, which indicates superimposed infection
Teach patient/family:
• Method of instillation using aseptic technique, including not touching dropper to ear/eye
• That dizziness may occur after instillation into ears

neomycin sulphate (topical)

Many combination products
Func. class.: Antibiotic
Chemical class.: Aminoglycoside
Legal class.: POM

Action: Interferes with bacterial protein synthesis
Uses: Skin infections
Dosage and routes:
• *Adult and child:* Topical apply to affected area 2 or 3 times a day
Available forms include: Combinations in cream, ointment, dusting powder, powder spray, spray application
Side effects/adverse reactions:
INTEG: Rash, urticaria, scaling, redness
Contraindications: Hypersensitivity, large areas, deafness, avoid prolonged usage, broken skin
Precautions: Pregnancy, lactation
Interactions/incompatibilities: None known
NURSING CONSIDERATIONS
Administer:
• After cleansing with soap, water before each application, dry well
• Enough medication to cover lesions completely
Evaluate:
• Allergic reaction: burning, stinging, swelling, redness
• Therapeutic response: decrease in size, number of lesions
Teach patient/family:

• To wash hands before, after each application
• To apply using gloves to prevent further infection
• To avoid use of non-prescribed creams, ointments, lotions unless directed by clinician

neostigmine bromide/ neostigmine methylsulphate

Prostigmin, combination product
Func. class.: Anticholinesterase
Chem. class.: Quaternary compound
Legal class.: POM

Action: Inhibits destruction of acetylcholine, which increases concentration at sites where acetylcholine is released; this facilitates transmission of impulses across myoneural junction
Uses: Myasthenia gravis, neuromuscular blocking agent antagonist, bladder distention, paralytic ileus
Dosage and routes:
Myasthenia gravis
• *Adult:* By mouth 15−30 mg at intervals throughout the day. Total daily dose usually 5−20 tablets (higher doses may be needed); IM/subcutaneous injection 1−2.5 mg at intervals throughout the day, usual daily dose 5−20 mg
• *Child up to 6 yr:* By mouth, initially 7.5 mg
• *Child 6−12 yr:* By mouth initially 15 mg, usual total daily dose 15−90 mg
• *Child:* IM/subcutaneous injection 200−500 mcg as required
• *Neonate:* By mouth 1−5 mg every 4 hr, half an hour before feeds; IM/subcutaneous injection 50−250 mcg every 4 hr

Tubocurarine antagonist
- *Adult:* Slow IV 0.05−0.07 mg/kg, may repeat if required, give 0.02−0.03 mg/kg atropine with or before this drug

Other indications
- *Adult:* IM/subcutaneous injection 0.5−2.5 mg or 1−2 tablets orally 4−6 hrly depending on condition
- *Child:* 2.5−15 mg orally or IM/subcutaneous injection 0.125−1 mg 4−6 hrly depending on condition

Available forms include: Tablets (bromide) 15 mg; injection IM, subcutaneous, IV (methylsulphate) 2.5 mg/ml

Side effects/adverse reactions:
GI: Nausea, diarrhoea, vomiting, cramps, increased salivation

Contraindications: Obstruction of intestine, urinary system, pregnancy, hypersensitivity, lactation

Precautions: Seizure disorders, bronchial asthma, coronary occlusion, vagotonia, peptic ulcer, bradycardia, parkinsonism, hypotension

Pharmacokinetics:
By mouth: Onset 2−4 hr, duration 2½−4 hr
IM/IV/subcutaneous: Onset 10−30 min, duration 2½−4 hr
Metabolised in liver, excreted in urine

Interactions/incompatibilities:
- Decreased action of: gallamine, metocurine, pancuronium, tubocurarine, atropine
- Increased action of: decamethonium, suxamethonium
- Decreased action of this drug: aminoglycosides, anaesthetics, β-blockers, lithium, procainamide, quinidine

Treatment of overdose: Artificial ventilation initiated if respiratory depression is severe. Atropine IV 1−2 mg antidote to muscarinic effects

NURSING CONSIDERATIONS
Assess:
- Baseline vital signs
Administer:
- On empty stomach for better absorption but with milk to avoid GT symptoms
- May be given with atropine to minimise muscarinic effects
Perform/provide:
- Storage at room temperature
Evaluate:
- Therapeutic response: increased muscle strength, hand grasp, improved gait, absence of laboured breathing (if severe)
- Vital signs, respiration 4 hrly; more frequently if given to reverse anaesthetic paralysis
- Fluid balance; check for urinary retention or incontinence
- Bradycardia, hypotension, bronchospasm, headache, dizziness, convulsions, respiratory depression; drug should be discontinued if toxicity occurs
Teach patient/family:
- That drug is not a cure, it only relieves symptoms
- All aspects of drug: action, side effects, dose, when to notify clinician
- To wear Medic Alert ID specifying Myasthenia Gravis and drugs

---

netilmicin sulphate

Netillin
Func. class.: Antibiotic
Chem. class.: Aminoglycoside
Legal class.: POM

Action: Interferes with protein synthesis in bacterial cell by binding to ribosomal subunit, causing inaccurate peptide sequence to form in protein chain, causing bacterial death

Uses: Severe systemic infections of

CNS, respiratory, GI, urinary tract, bone, skin, soft tissues, bacteraemia, septicaemia caused by *P. aeruginosa, E. coli, Enterobacter, Acinetobacter, Providencia, Citrobacter, Staphylococcus* spp, *K. pneumoniae, P. mirabilis, Serratia* spp plus all Gram-negative infections resistant to gentamicin

Dosage and routes:
Normal renal function
• *Adult and child over 12 yr:* IM/IV 4−6 mg/kg daily as a single daily dose or in divided doses 8−12 hrly, severe infections up to 7.5 mg/kg daily in divided doses every 8 hr
• *Child and infants 6 weeks−12 yr:* IM/IV 6.0−7.5 mg/kg daily in divided doses 8−12 hrly
• *Neonate over 1 week:* IM/IV 7.5−9.0 mg/kg daily in divided doses 8 hrly
• *Neonates under 1 week:* IM/IV 6 mg/kg daily in divided doses 12 hrly
• IV injection must be given over 3−5 minutes or by intravenous infusion
• Adjust dose in renal impairment and according to blood drug level
Available forms include: Injection IM, IV 10, 50, 100 mg/ml

Side effects/adverse reactions:
GU: Adverse renal effects, generally mild in nature
CNS: Dizziness, headache, paraesthesia, vertigo
EENT: Ototoxicity, deafness, visual disturbances, tinnitus, roaring in the ears
GI: Vomiting, malaise, diarrhoea
CV: Hypotension, myocarditis, tachycardia
INTEG: Rash
Contraindications: Hypersensitivity
Precautions: Neonates, renal disease, pregnancy, children less than 12 yr, lactation, myasthenia gravis, hearing deficit

Pharmacokinetics:
IM: Onset rapid, peak 1−2 hr
IV: Onset immediate, peak 1−2 hr
Plasma half-life 2−3 hr, not metabolised, excreted unchanged in urine
Interactions/incompatibilities:
• Increased ototoxicity, neurotoxicity, nephrotoxicity: other aminoglycosides, amphotericin B, polymyxin, vancomycin, frusemide, mannitol, cisplatin, cephalosporins
• Do not mix in solution or syringe: carbenicillin, ticarcillin, amphotericin B, cephalothin, erythromycin, heparin
• Increased effects: non-depolarising muscle relaxants
Clinical assessment:
• Serum peak, drawn at 60 min after IV infusion or 60 min after IM injection (peak 5−12 mg/litre); trough level drawn just before next dose (trough less than 2 mg/litre). Higher peak acceptable in once daily dosing
Lab. test interferences:
Increase: Blood sugar, alkaline phosphatase, aspartate aminotransferase, alanine aminotransferase, prothrombin time
Decrease: Hb, WBC, platelets
Treatment of overdose: Haemodialysis, monitor serum levels of drug
NURSING CONSIDERATIONS
Assess:
• Baseline vital signs
• Weight before treatment; calculation of dosage is usually done based on ideal body weight, but may be calculated on actual body weight
• Fluid balance
• Ensure "peak and trough" levels are seen before administering second 24 hr prescribed regime
Administer:
• After samples have been sent for culture and sensitivity

- IM injection in large muscle mass, rotate injection sites
- IV as 3−5 min bolus or, more safely as an infusion over 30 min
- Drug in evenly spaced doses to maintain blood level

Perform/provide:
- Adequate fluids of 2−3 litre daily unless contraindicated to prevent irritation of tubules
- Flushing of IV line with sodium chloride 0.9% or dextrose 5% after infusion
- Supervised mobilisation, other safety measures for patients with vestibular dysfunction

Evaluate:
- Vital signs during infusion, watch for hypotension, change in pulse
- IV site for thrombophlebitis including pain, redness, swelling every 30 min, change site if needed; apply warm compresses to discontinued site
- Therapeutic effect: absence of fever, draining wounds, negative culture and sensitivity after treatment
- Daily fluid balance, urinalysis for proteinuria, cells, casts; report sudden change in urinary output
- Dehydration: high specific gravity, decrease in skin turgor, dry mucous membranes, dark urine
- Renal impairment by securing urine for creatinine clearance testing, blood urea nitrogen, serum creatinine; a lower dosage should be given in renal impairment (creatinine clearance less than 100 ml/min)
- Deafness by audiometric testing, ringing, roaring in ears, vertigo; assess hearing before, during, after treatment
- Secondary infection: increased temperature, malaise, redness, pain, swelling, perineal itching, diarrhoea, stomatitis, change in cough or sputum
- Vestibular dysfunction: nausea, vomiting, dizziness, headache; drug should be discontinued if severe

Teach patient/family:
- To report headache, dizziness, symptoms of overgrowth of infection, renal impairment
- To report loss of hearing, ringing, roaring in ears or feeling of fullness in head

---

nicardipine

Cardene
Func. class.: Antihypertensive, antianginal
Chem. class.: Calcium-channel blockers
Legal class.: POM

Action: Inhibits calcium ion influx across cell membrane during cardiac depolarisation; produces relaxation of coronary vascular smooth muscle, peripheral vascular smooth muscle

Uses: Chronic stable angina pectoris, mild to moderate hypertension

Dosage and routes:
Angina
- *Adult:* By mouth 20 mg 3 times a day initially, may increase after 3 days (range 20−40 mg 3 times a day)

Hypertension
- *Adult:* By mouth 20 mg 3 times a day initially, then increase after 3 days; if controlled on 20−30 mg 3 times daily can be given 30−40 mg twice daily

Available forms include: Capsules 20, 30 mg (as hydrochloride)

Side effects/adverse reactions:
CV: Dysrythmia, oedema, atrio-

ventricular block, ventricular tachycardia, hypotension, palpitations, myocardial infarction, intracranial haemorrhage
GI: Nausea, vomiting, diarrhoea, gastric upset, constipation, hepatitis, salivation
GU: Polyuria, acute renal failure
INTEG: Rash, pruritus, urticaria
CNS: Headache, drowsiness, dizziness, depression, paraesthesia, somnolence
Contraindications: Pregnancy, lactation, advanced aortic stenosis, hypersensitivity
Precautions: Congestive cardiac failure, hypotension, hepatic impairment, children, renal disease, elderly
Pharmacokinetics:
By mouth: Onset 10 min, peak 1−2 hr, half-life 2−5 hr; metabolised by liver, excreted in urine (98% as metabolites)
Interactions/incompatibilities:
• Increased effects of: digitalis, neuromuscular blocking agents, cyclosporin
• Increased effects of nicardipine: cimetidine
Lab. test interferences:
Transient elevation of liver function tests, glucose, serum bilirubin, blood urea nitrogen and creatinine. Triiodothyronine, thyroxine and TSH may also be affected abnormally
NURSING CONSIDERATIONS
Assess:
• Baseline vital signs, ECG
Evaluate:
• Response to treatment: decrease in pain from angina, fall in blood pressure
• Cardiac function: blood pressure, pulse, respirations, ECG daily
• For side effects
Teach patient/family:
• To avoid non-prescription

medicines unless directed by clinician
• Emphasise the importance of every aspect of treatment: diet, exercise, reduction in stress and smoking as well as taking drug
• Clinician must be informed of palpitations, shortness of breath, swollen feet and hands, pronounced dizziness, constipation, nausea

niclosamide

Yomesan
Func. class.: Anthelmintic
Chem. class.: Salicylamilide derivative
Legal class.: P

Action: Inhibits synthesis in mitochondria; leads to destruction in intestine where worm may be digested, removed in faeces; not effective for ova or larval stage
Uses: Regular, dwarf tapeworms
Dosage and routes:
Taenia solium
• *Adult:* By mouth 2 g as a single dose after a light breakfast, followed by a purgative after 2 hr
• *Child up to 2 yr:* By mouth 500 mg
• *Child 2−6 yr:* By mouth 1 g
T. saginata and Diphyllobothrium latcum
• As for *T. solium*, but half the dose may be taken after breakfast and the remainder 1 hr later followed by a purgative after a further 2 hr
Hymenolepsis nana
• *Adult:* 2 g on first day, then 1 g daily for 6 days
• *Child up to 2 yr:* By mouth quarter adult dose
• *Child 2−6 yr:* By mouth half adult dose

Available forms include: Tablets, chewable 500 mg
Side effects/adverse reactions:
INTEG: Pruritus
CNS: Dizziness
GI: Nausea, vomiting, abdominal pain
Contraindications: Hypersensitivity
Precautions: Child under 2 yr, pregnancy, lactation
Treatment of overdose: Enemas, laxatives; do not induce vomiting

NURSING CONSIDERATIONS
Assess:
• Stools during entire treatment, 1, 3 months after treatment; specimens must be sent to laboratory while still warm. Gloves must be worn when handling any stools
Administer:
• May be crushed and washed down with water, mixed with water if unable to swallow whole
• Laxatives if constipated; not necessary for drug to work, but will assist expulsion of worm
• After breakfast, tablet must be chewed, and then swallowed
Perform/provide:
• Storage in original packaging
Evaluate:
• Therapeutic response; expulsion of worms, 3 negative stool cultures after completion of treatment
• For allergic reaction: rash
• For diarrhoea during expulsion of worms
• For infection in other family members since infection from person to person is common
Teach patient/family:
• Proper hygiene after bowel movement including handwashing technique; tell patient to avoid putting fingers in mouth
• That infected person should sleep alone
• That bed linen should be changed daily and washed in hot water
• Bed clothes should not be shaken

• To clean toilet daily with disinfectant
• Need for compliance with dosage schedule, duration of treatment
• To drink fruit juice to remove mucous that intestinal tapeworms burrow in, aids in expulsion of worms (dwarf tapeworms only)
• To avoid alcohol
• To wash all fresh fruit and vegetables

nicotinamide

Func. class.: B vitamin
Chem. class.: Pyridine derivative
Legal class.: GSL

Action: Necessary for conversion of fats, protein, carbohydrates by oxidation reduction. Deficiency causes pellagra
Uses: Prophylactic, vitamin B deficiency
Dosage and routes:
Prophylactic
• *Adult:* By mouth 15−30 mg daily
Vitamin B deficiency
• *Adult:* By mouth usually 60−120 mg, but up to 920 mg daily by IV infusion (as high potency vitamins B and C injection) in Wernicke's encephalopathy and Korsakoff's psychosis
Available forms include: Tablets 50 mg; many combination products: tablets, capsules, injections
Side effects/adverse reactions:
Unlikely in therapeutic doses, though anaphylactic reactions possible with vitamins B and C injection IV
Contraindications: Hypersensitivity
Pharmacokinetics: Well absorbed orally, metabolised in liver, small amounts excreted unchanged in urine

Treatment of overdose: Unlikely to be of clinical significance
NURSING CONSIDERATIONS
Assess:
• Baseline vital signs
• Ability of patient to manage own medication
Administer:
• IV, slowly (over 10 min); IM into large muscle mass; when oral intake is inadequate or impossible orally
Perform/provide:
• Equipment and drugs to deal with anaphylaxis
Evaluate:
• For allergic reactions during or shortly after IV or IM administration
• That tablets are taken
• Therapeutic response
Teach patient/family:
• Reason for medication
• Other supporting mechanisms (in chronic alcoholism)

nicotine resin complex

Nicorette, (NHS) Nicotinelle TTS
Func. class.: Smoking deterrent
Chem. class.: Cholinergic
Legal class.: POM/P (depending upon strength)

Action: Increase catecholamine release from adrenal medulla by stimulating receptors in CNS
Uses: Nicotine substitution as an aid to smoking cessation
Dosage and routes:
• *Adult:* Gum, 1 piece 2 mg or 4 mg chewed for ½ hr as required to abstain from smoking, maximum 15 4-mg pieces daily; Patch, apply one patch of required size for 24 hr and remove. Allow several days break before applying next patch (at different site). Consult manufacturer's literature for full dosage instructions for patch and gum
Available forms include: Chewing gum 2, 4 mg; Patch 17.5 mg, 35 mg, 52.5 mg
Side effects/adverse reactions:
EENT: Jaw ache, irritation in buccal cavity, excessive salivation
CNS: Dizziness, headache
GI: Nausea, indigestion
INTEG: At site of patch, skin reactions have included erythema, pruritus, blisters, burning/pinching sensations
MISC: Hiccup
Contraindications: Hypersensitivity, pregnancy
Precautions: Gastritis, peptic ulcer, angina, coronary artery disease
Pharmacokinetics: Metabolised in liver, excreted in urine, half-life 2−3 hr, all available nicotine is released from gum after 30 min chewing. Patch: 1−2 hr for nicotine passage into plasma. Plateau plasma concentrations at 8−10 hr after application
Treatment of overdose: Gastric lavage with wide bore tube, activated charcoal, supportive care
NURSING CONSIDERATIONS
Assess:
• Number of cigarettes smoked and dependence
• Local skin reaction due to patch application
Evaluate:
• Adverse reaction: irritation of buccal cavity, dislike of taste, jaw ache
• Therapeutic response: decrease in urge to smoke, decreased need for gum after 3−6 months
Teach patient/family:
• To chew gum slowly for 30 min to promote buccal absorption of the drug; do not chew over 45 min
• Not to exceed the recommended dose
• To begin drug withdrawal after

3 months use; not to exceed 6 months
• All aspects of drug; give package insert to patient
• That gum will not stick to dentures, dental appliances
• That gum is as toxic as cigarette; it is to be used only as an aid to smoking cessation
• Not to use during pregnancy; birth defects may occur

nicotinic acid

Func. class.: Hypolipidaemic
Chem. class.: Pyridine derivative
Legal class.: P

Action: B vitamin with actions of nicotinamide, though seldom used in deficiency because of side effects; high doses decrease serum lipids
Uses: Hyperlipidaemias, has also been used in peripheral vascular disease
Dosage and routes:
Adjunct in hyperlipidaemia
• *Adult:* By mouth 300–600 mg daily in 3 divided doses after meals, may be increased to 6 g daily over 2–4 weeks
Available forms include: Tablets 50 mg; many combination products
Side effects/adverse reactions:
CNS: Headache, dizziness, faintness
GI: Nausea, vomiting, anorexia, flatulence, jaundice, diarrhoea, peptic ulcer, abdominal cramps
GU: Hyperuricaemia, glycosuria
CV: Postural hypotension, pounding in head
EENT: Blurred vision, ptosis
INTEG: Flushing, dry skin, rash, hyperpigmentation, pruritus
SYST: Sensation of heat
METAB: Decreased glucose tolerance

Contraindications: Hypersensitivity, pregnancy, lactation
Precautions: Glaucoma, cardiovascular disease, diabetes mellitus, gout, history of peptic ulceration, impaired liver function
Pharmacokinetics:
By mouth: Peak 30–70 min, half-life 45 min, metabolised in liver, 30% excreted unchanged in urine (more after high doses)

NURSING CONSIDERATIONS
Assess:
• Blood glucose before and during treatment
Administer:
• With meals for GI symptoms
Evaluate:
• Therapeutic response: decreased lipids, warm extremities, absence of numbness in extremities
• Nutritional status
• Liver dysfunction: clay coloured stools, itching, dark urine, jaundice
• CNS symptoms: headache, paraesthesias, blurred vision
Teach patient/family:
• To remain recumbent if postural hypotension occurs
• To abstain from alcohol if drug is prescribed for hyperlipidaemia
• To avoid sunlight if skin lesions are present
• To take a diet rich in liver, yeast, legumes, lean poultry, offal

nicoumalone

Sinthrome
Func. class.: Anticoagulant
Chem. class.: Coumarin analogue
Legal class.: POM

Action: Interferes with blood clotting. Antagonises effects of vitamin K-dependent coagulation factors

Uses: Deep vein thrombosis, pulmonary embolism, transient ischaemic attacks, prophylaxis of embolism with prosthetic heart valves, rheumatic

Dosage and routes:

• *Adult:* By mouth 8–12 mg on day 1; 4–8 mg on day 2; maintenance dose usually 1–8 mg daily according to individual requirements

Available forms include: Tablets 1, 4 mg

Side effects/adverse reactions:

CNS: Fever

GI: Loss of appetite, nausea, vomiting

HAEM: Haemorrhage

INTEG: Reversible alopecia, dermatitis, urticaria, haemorrhagic skin necrosis

Contraindications: Severe hypertension, pericarditis, pericardial effusion, subacute endocarditis, severe hepatic or renal disease, increased fibrinolytic activity following surgery on lung, prostate, and uterus, peptic ulcer, pregnancy, hypersensitivity, haemorrhagic diathesis, blood dyscrasias, pre- and post-surgery on CNS or eyes. Haemorrhage in GI, urogenital or respiratory tracts, cardiovascular system

Precautions: Hepatic or renal disease, lactation (give infant vitamin K), thyrotoxicosis, tumours, infection, inflammation, severe heart failure, elderly, other IM injections

Pharmacokinetics: Rapidly absorbed, at least 60% of dose is available systemically. Peak plasma concentration after 1–3 hr. Over 98% bound to plasma protein. Extensively metabolised, in liver and excreted in faeces and urine. Plasma half-life is 8–11 hr

Interactions/incompatibilities:

• May be inhibited by: aminoglutethimide, barbiturates, carbamazepine, dichloralphenazone, griseofulvin, oral contraceptives, phenytoin, primidone, rifampicin, vitamin K, cholestyramine, thiazide diuretics

• May be potentiated by: alcohol, allopurinol, amiodarone, anabolic steroids, androgens, anti-arrhythmics, azapropazone, aztreonam, bezafibrate, cephamandole, chloral hydrate, chloramphenicol, cimetidine, clofibrate, co-trimoxazole, danazol, azithromycin, ciprofloxacin, dextropropoxyphene, enoximone, diflunisal, disulfiram, erythromycin, ethacrynic acid, glucagon, heparin, fluvoxamine, ifosfamide, oral hypoglycaemics paroxetine, omeprazole, flurbiprofen, fluconazole, itraconazole, gemfibrozil, ketoconazole, latamoxef, mefenamic acid, metronidazole, miconazole, nalidixic acid, neomycin, norfloxacin, flutamide, influenza vaccine, phenylbutazone, phenytoin, piroxicam, quinidine, propafenone, proguanil, simvastatin, rowachol, sulindac, sulphinpyrazone, sulphonamides, tamoxifen, tetracyclines, thyroxine, tolmetin, trimethoprim

• Increased prothrombin time: broad-spectrum antibiotics

• Increased risk of bleeding due to antiplatelet effect: aspirin, dipyridamole

Clinical assessment:

• Blood tests (Hb, platelets, occult blood in stools) 3 monthly

• Prothrombin time daily until stabilised

Lab. test interferences:

Increase: Triiodothyronine uptake

Decrease: Uric acid

Treatment of overdose: If patient's thromboplastin time was normal at time of overdosage, reduce drug absorption by emesis or gastric lavage combined with activated charcoal or fast-acting laxative.

Vitamin K may antagonise nicoumalone in 3–5 hr. Moderate haemorrhage: give vitamin K by mouth 2–5 mg, severe cases require 1–10 mg by very slow IV injection. In life-threatening haemorrhage give fresh frozen plasma or whole blood

NURSING CONSIDERATIONS
Assess:
• BP
Administer:
• At the same time each day to maintain steady blood levels
• Alone — do not give with food
• Avoid all IM injections that may cause bleeding
Evaluate:
• For signs of hypertension
• Therapeutic response: decrease in deep vein thrombosis
• Any signs of bleeding, e.g. black stools, haematuria
Teach patient/family:
• To take drug at same time every day
• To avoid non-prescribed medications unless directed by clinician
• Urine may be discoloured
• To report any signs of bleeding to the clinician

---

nifedipine

Adalat, Adalat Retard, Adalat LA, Adalat IC, Corceten, Angiopine, Calcilat, combination products
Func. class.: Antihypertensive, antianginal; calcium channel blocker
Chem. class.: Dihydropyridine
Legal class.: POM

Action: Inhibits calcium ion flux across cell membranes relaxing arterial smooth muscle both in the coronary and peripheral circulation

Uses: Prophylaxis and treatment of angina, treatment of Raynaud's phenomenon, and hypertension
Dosage and routes:
• *Capsules:* By mouth 5–20 mg 3 times daily taken with a little fluid with or after food. Where an immediate effect is required, capsules may be bitten open, and the liquid retained in the mouth
• *Modified-release tablets:* Adalat Retard, by mouth 10–40 mg twice daily; Adalat LA, 30 mg daily increasing to a maximum of 90 mg daily
• *Modified-release capsules:* Corceten, by mouth 20 mg twice daily increasing to 40 mg twice daily
• *Coronary injection:* 150–200 mcg in coronary catheter over 90–120 seconds, do not exceed total of 6 200-mcg injections in 3 hr
Available forms include: Capsules 5, 10 mg; tablets modified-release 10, 20, 30, 60 mg; capsules modified-release 20 mg; coronary injection 100 mcg/ml 2 ml ampoule
Side effects/adverse reactions:
CV: Oedema, tachycardia, hypotension, palpitations, ischaemic pain
GI: Nausea, gastric upset, gingival hyperplasia
INTEG: Rash, pruritus, flushing
CNS: Headache, fatigue, drowsiness, dizziness, anxiety, depression, paraesthesia
Contraindications: Hypersensitivity, GI obstruction, oesophageal obstruction, lactation, severe hypotension, cardiogenic shock
Precautions: Congestive cardiac failure, hypotension, hypovolaemia, hepatic impairment, children, renal disease, diabetes mellitus, pregnancy
Pharmacokinetics:
By mouth: Capsules onset 10 min, peak 30 min, tablets duration 6–12 hr, half-life 4 hr; 90% protein bound, metabolised by

liver, excreted in urine (98% as metabolites)

Interactions/incompatibilities:
• Effects of nifedipine may be potentiated by: cimetidine
• Increased effects of: hypoglycaemia, levodopa, quinidine
• Decreased effects: noradrenaline, isoprenaline, digitoxin

Treatment of overdose: Gastric lavage and charcoal instillation have been used. Calcium gluconate may be helpful with IV atropine for bradycardia

NURSING CONSIDERATIONS

Assess:
• Baseline vital signs and ECG; blood sugar (glucose) levels

Administer:
• Sublingually; break capsule

Perform/provide:
• Ensure capsule breaks and content is absorbed in the mouth

Evaluate:
• Therapeutic response: decreased anginal pain
• Improvement in temperature of digits

Teach patient/family:
• How to take pulse before taking drug; record or graph should be kept
• To avoid hazardous activities until stabilised on drug or dizziness is no longer a problem
• To limit caffeine consumption (coffee, tea, chocolate)
• To avoid non-prescribed drugs unless directed by clinician
• Stress patient compliance to all areas of medical regimen, diet, exercise, stress reduction, drug therapy
• To report side effects; headaches, dizziness, paraesthesia

nimodipine

Nimotop
Func. class.: Cerebral vasodilator
Chem. class.: Calcium channel blocker
Legal class.: POM

Action: Interferes with inward displacement of calcium ions through the slow channels of active smooth muscle cell membranes resulting in relaxation

Uses: Treatment and prevention of ischaemic neurological deficits caused by arterial spasm following subarachnoid haemorrhage

Dosage and routes:
Prophylactic
• *Adult:* By mouth, 60 mg 4-hrly for 21 days
Therapeutic
• *Adult:* IV infusion via central catheter; initially 1 mg/hr, increased after 2 hr to 2 mg/hr provided no severe decrease in BP has occurred; in patients with unstable BP or weighing less than 70 kg initially 500 mcg/hr. Treatment to start as soon as possible and continue for 5−14 days; if surgery performed while treatment is in progress, continue for at least 5 days after

Available forms include: IV infusion, 200 mcg/ml; tablets 30 mg

Side effects/adverse reactions:
CV: Hypotension, variation in heart rate
CNS: Headache
GI: Disturbances, nausea, transient increase in liver enzymes during infusion
SYST: Feeling of warmth
INTEG: Flushing

Precautions: Cerebral oedema, raised intracranial pressure, impaired renal function, pregnancy

Pharmacokinetics: 50% absorbed orally, extensive first-pass metabolism. Metabolised in liver, plasma half-life 1−6 hr; 95% protein bound

Interactions/incompatibilities:
• Nimodipine potentiates: other hypotensives, avoid co-administration with calcium channel blockers/β-blockers if possible
• Increased risk of nephrotoxicity with: nephrotoxic drugs
• Incompatible with: PVC infusion materials

Clinical assessment:
• BP
• Renal function in patients with impairment or on nephrotoxic drugs

Treatment of overdose: Gastric lavage and activated charcoal after oral ingestion/stop IV infusion. Monitor BP, give dopamine or noradrenaline if very low

NURSING CONSIDERATIONS

Assess:
• Baseline vital signs and weight (if possible)

Administer:
• By intravenous infusion via central catheter
• Orally in tablet form

Evaluate:
• Therapeutic response
• Vital signs

Perform/provide:
• Full neurological observations
• Use of PVC apparatus should be avoided

---

nitrofurantoin

Furandantin, Macrodantin
Func. class.: Antibiotic
Chem. class.: Synthetic nitrofurantoin derivative
Legal class.: POM

Action: Unclear but may involve interference with a number of bacterial enzymes

Uses: Urinary tract infection, pyelitis

Dosage and routes:
Acute infection
• *Adults:* By mouth 50 mg 4 times a day for 7 days, increased to 100 mg 4 times a day in severe infection
• *Child over 1 month:* By mouth 3 mg/kg daily in 4 divided doses for 7 days

Surgical prophylaxis
• *Adults:* By mouth 50 mg 4 times a day on the day of procedure and for another 3 days

Long term suppressive treatment
• *Adults:* By mouth 50−100 mg daily
• *Child over 1 month:* By mouth 1 mg/kg daily as a single dose

Available forms include: Capsules 50, 100 mg; tablets 50, 100 mg; suspension 25 mg/5ml

Side effects/adverse reactions:
INTEG: Pruritus, rash, urticaria, angioedema, alopecia, erythema multiforme, exfoliative dermatitis, arthralgia
CNS: Dizziness, headache, drowsiness, vertigo, nystagmus, asthenia
RESP: Acute and subacute pulmonary reactions (fever, chills, cough, chest pain, dyspnoea, pulmonary infiltration and consolidation, pleural effusion), chronic pulmonary reactions (malaise, dyspnoea on exertion, cough, altered pulmonary function)
HAEM: Agranulocytosis, leucopenia, granulocylopenia, haemolytic anaemia, anaemia, thrombocytopenia, megaloblastic anaemia, eosinophilia, aplastic anaemia
GI: Nausea, vomiting, abdominal pain, diarrhoea, cholestatic jaundice, chronic active hepatitis, pancreatitis

Contraindications: Hypersensitivity, severe renal disease (creatinine clearance less than 60 ml/min), infants under 1 month

Precautions: Pregnancy, lactation, G6PD deficiency, anaemia, diabetes mellitus, electrolyte imbalance, vitamin B_{12} or folate deficiency, pulmonary disease, hepatic impairment, neurological disorders, allergic diathesis

Interactions:
• Effects of nitrofurantoin increased by: probenecid
• Effects of nitrofurantoin antagonised by: nalidixic acid, quinolones
• Absorption of nitrofurantoin decreased by: magnesium trisilicate

Treatment of overdose: Induction of emesis or gastric lavage, maintain a high fluid intake. Nitrofurantoin can be haemodialysed

NURSING CONSIDERATIONS

Assess:
• Fluid balance, urine pH less than 5.5 is ideal for urinary tract infection

Administer:
• After clean-catch urine is obtained for culture and sensitivity
• As two daily doses if urine output is high or if patient has diabetes (medical decision)
• 2 litres fluid in 24 hr

Perform provide:
• Limited intake of alkaline foods or drugs: milk, dairy products, peanuts, vegetables, alkaline antacids, sodium bicarbonate

Evaluate:
• CNS symptoms: insomnia, vertigo, headache, drowsiness, convulsions
• Allergy: fever, flushing, rash, urticaria, pruritus

Teach patient/family:
• Take medication with food to decrease GI irritation
• Instruct patient to protect suspension from freezing and shake well before taking

• May cause drowsiness; instruct patient to seek aid in walking and other activities; advise patient not to drive or operate machinery while on medication
• Instruct patients with diabetes that Clinitest may prove false-positive for glucose; Clinistix or Labstix should be used
• Urine may be coloured dark yellow or brown whilst receiving drug

---

nizatidine

Axid
Func. class.: H_2-receptor antagonist
Legal class.: POM

Action: Blocks H_2 receptors thereby reducing gastric acid output

Uses: Benign gastric and duodenal ulceration, prevention of duodenal ulcer recurrence, symptomatic relief of gastro-oesophageal reflux

Dosage and routes:
Gastric and duodenal ulcer disease
• *Adult:* By mouth 300 mg at night or 150 mg twice daily for 4–8 weeks; maintenance 150 mg at night for up to 1 yr
Gastro-oesophageal reflux
• *Adult:* By mouth, 150–300 mg twice daily for up to 12 weeks
Available forms include: Capsules 150, 300 mg

Side effects/adverse reactions:
CNS: Headache, somnolence, confusion, abnormal dreams
ENDO: Gynaecomastia
HAEM: Thrombocytopenia, eosinophilia
INTEG: Pruritus, sweating, urticaria, exfoliative dermatitis
MS: Myalgia
RESP: Bronchospasm, laryngeal oedema
METAB: Hyperuricaemia

GI: Elevated liver enzymes, hepatitis, jaundice, nausea
Contraindications: Hypersensitivity
Precautions: Renal or hepatic impairment (reduce dose in renal impairment), pregnancy, lactation
Pharmacokinetics: Partially metabolised by the liver and principally excreted by the kidney, plasma half-life 1.5 hr, 70% absorbed orally, small amount (0.1% of plasma concentration) enters breast milk, 35% bound to plasma proteins
Clinical assessment:
• Renal function tests: if impairment anticipated
Treatment of overdose: Symptomatic and supportive therapy is recommended. Activated charcoal, emesis or lavage may reduce absorption
NURSING CONSIDERATIONS
Assess:
• Gastric pH (greater than 5 should be maintained)
• Fluid balance
Administer:
• With meals for prolonged drug effect
• Antacids 1 hr before or 1 hr after drug
Evaluate:
• Mental status, confusion, dizziness, depression, anxiety, weakness, tremors, psychosis, diarrhoea, jaundice, report immediately
• For GI symptoms; nausea, vomiting, diarrhoea, cramps
Teach patient/family:
• That occasionally gynaecomastia, impotence may occur but are reversible
• Avoid driving or other hazardous activities until patient is stabilised
• To avoid black pepper, caffeine, alcohol, harsh spices, extremes in temperature of food
• To avoid non-prescribed preparations; aspirin, cough, cold preparations

noradrenaline injection

Levophed Levophed Special
Func. class.: Adrenergic
Chem. class.: Catecholamine
Legal class.: POM

Action: Causes increased contractility and heart rate by acting on β-receptors in heart; also, acts on α-receptors, causing vasoconstriction in blood vessels; when larger doses are administered, causes vasodilatation in renal, intracerebral, coronary blood vessels
Uses: Acute hypotension
Dosage and routes:
• *Adult:* IV infusion 8−12 mcg/min titrated to BP
Levophed special
• *Adult:* IV or intracardiac at once 0.5−0.75 ml
Available forms include: Injection IV 200 mcg, 2 mg/ml
Side effects/adverse reactions:
CNS: Headache
CV: Palpitations, tachycardia, hypertension, ectopic beats, angina
GI: Nausea, vomiting
INTEG: Necrosis, tissue sloughing with extravasation, gangrene
Contraindications: Hypersensitivity, ventricular fibrillation, tachydysrhythmias, phaeochromocytoma
Precautions: Pregnancy, lactation, arterial embolism, peripheral vascular disease
Pharmacokinetics:
IV: Onset 1−2 min, metabolised in liver, excreted in urine (inactive metabolites)
Interactions/incompatibilities:
• Do not use within 2 weeks of MAOIs or hypertensive crisis may result

- Dysrhythmias: general anaesthetics, cardiac sensitising agents
- Decreased action of this drug: other β-blockers
- Increased BP: oxytocics
- Increased pressor effect: tricyclic antidepressant, MAOIs
- Incompatible with alkaline solutions: sodium bicarbonate, frusemide injection, phenytoin

Clinical assessment:
- ECG during administration continuously, if BP increases, drug is decreased
- CVP during infusion if possible

Administer:
- Plasma expanders for hypovolaemia
- Using 2 bottle set up so drug may be discontinued while IV is still running

Treatment of overdose: Administer phentolamine with care

NURSING CONSIDERATIONS

Assess:
- Baseline vital signs and ECG
- Fluid balance

Perform/provide:
- Dilute with dextrose 5% if necessary in preference to other infusion solutions
- Storage of reconstituted solution if refrigerated for no longer than 24 hr
- Do not use discoloured solutions
- Protect from light
- Continuous monitoring of vital signs (patient preferably in ICU)

Evaluate:
- For paraesthesia and coldness of extremities, peripheral blood flow may decrease: doppler monitoring
- Injection site: tissue sloughing; if this occurs, administer phentolamine mixed with normal saline
- Therapeutic response: increased BP with stabilisation

Teach patient/family:
- Reason for drug administration

norethisterone acetate/enanthate

Micronor, Noristerat, Primolut-N, Utovlan, Noriday, Menzon, SH420, many combination products

Func. class.: Progestogen
Chem. class.: Progesterone derivative
Legal class.: POM

Action: Inhibits secretion of pituitary gonadotrophin, which prevents follicular maturation and ovulation

Uses: Menorrhagia, premenstrual syndrome, amenorrhea, endometriosis, progestogen-only contraception, also component of several oestrogen/progestogen oral contraceptives, inoperable breast cancer

Dosage and routes:

Menorrhagia, premenstrual tension
- *Adult:* By mouth 5 mg 2−3 times daily from the 19th−26th day of the cycle

Dysmenorrhoea
- *Adult:* By mouth 5 mg 3 times daily for 20 days, starting from the 5th day of the cycle for 3−4 cycles

Dysfunctional uterine bleeding
- *Adult:* By mouth 5 mg 3 times daily for 10 days

Prophylaxis
- 5 mg twice daily on the 19th to 26th days of cycle

Progestogen-only contraception
- *Adult:* By mouth 350 mcg (1 tablet) daily continuously. IM injection 200 mg within the first 5 days of menstrual cycle. Effects last for 8 weeks and injection may be repeated once

Endometriosis
- *Adult:* By mouth initially 10 mg daily, increasing to 30 mg daily if necessary. Duration of treatment, 6 months

Inoperable breast cancer
• *Adult:* By mouth 10 mg (as acetate) 3 times a day for 6 weeks, then increase to 20 mg 3 times a day if necessary

Available forms include: Tablets 350 mcg, 5 mg; tablets 10 mg (as acetate), injection 200 mg/ml (as enanthate)

Side effects/adverse reactions:

CNS: Dizziness, headache, migraine, depression, fatigue, exacerbation of epilepsy

CV: Hypotension, thrombophlebitis, oedema, thromboembolism, stroke, pulmonary embolism, myocardial infarction

GI: Nausea, vomiting, anorexia, cramps, weight gain, cholestatic jaundice

EENT: Diplopia

GU: Amenorrhoea, cervical erosion, breakthrough bleeding, dysmenorrhoea, vaginal candidiasis, breast changes, (gynaecomastia, testicular atrophy, impotence), endometriosis, chloasma, spontaneous abortion

INTEG: Hirsutism, acne, photosensitivity

META: Hyperglycaemia, malignant and benign hepatic tumours, hypercholesterolaemia

Contraindications: Breast cancer, or hormone dependant neoplasia, hypersensitivity, thrombophlebitis, thromboembolic disorders, reproductive cancer, genital bleeding (abnormal, undiagnosed), pregnancy, history of idiopathic jaundice, severe pruritus or herpes gestationis during pregnancy, Dubin–Johnson or Rotor syndromes

Precautions: Lactation, hypertension, asthma, congestive cardiac failure, myocardial infarction, diabetes mellitus, bone disease, depression, migraine headache, convulsive disorders, hepatic disease, renal disease, family history of breast or reproductive tract cancer, amenorrhoea, fluid retention

Pharmacokinetics:

By mouth: Duration 24 hr, excreted in urine, faeces, metabolised in liver

Interactions/incompatibilities:
• Efficacy of norethisterone may be reduced by: rifampicin, barbiturates, phenytoin, ampicillin, tetracycline, griseofulvin

NURSING CONSIDERATIONS

Assess:
• Baseline weight
• BP at beginning of treatment and periodically thereafter

Administer:
• Titrated dose, use lowest effective dose
• Solution deeply in large muscle mass (IM), rotate sites
• In one dose in morning
• With food or milk to decrease GI symptoms

Evaluate:
• Therapeutic response: decreased abnormal uterine bleeding, absence of amenorrhea
• For potential side-effects regularly

Teach patient/family:
• To avoid sunlight or use sunscreen, photosensitivity can occur
• All aspects of drug usage, including cushingoid symptoms
• To report side-effects, e.g. breast lumps, vaginal bleeding, oedema, jaundice, dark urine, clay-coloured stools, dyspnoea, headache, blurred vision, abdominal pain, numbness or stiffness in legs, chest pain; male to report impotence or gynaecomastia
• To report suspected pregnancy promptly

norgestrel (levonorgestrel)

Cyclo-Progynova, Prempack C (all with oestrodiol)
Func. class.: Progestogen
Chem. class.: Progesterone derivative
Legal class.: POM

Action: Inhibits secretion of pituitary gonadotrophins, which prevents follicular maturation and ovulation

Uses: In combined preparations for menopausal symptoms

Dosage and routes:
• *Adult:* By mouth 1 tablet daily for 10 days of cycle

Side effects/adverse reactions:
CNS: Dizziness, headache, migraine, depression, fatigue, anxiety
CV: Hypotension, thrombophlebitis, oedema, thromboembolism, stroke, pulmonary embolism, myocardial infarction, cardiac symptoms
GI: Nausea, vomiting, anorexia, cramps, increased weight and appetite, cholestatic jaundice, dyspesia
Available forms include: Tablets 500 mcg (with 1 mg or 2 mg oestradiol), 150 mcg
EENT: Diplopia
GU: Amenorrhoea, cervical erosion, breakthrough bleeding, dysmenorrhoea, vaginal candidiasis, breast changes, endometriosis, spontaneous abortion, altered libido
INTEG: Rash, acne, hirsutism, photosensitivity, leg pain and swelling
META: Hyperglycaemia
Contraindications: Breast cancer, hypersensitivity, thromboembolic disorders, hormone dependent cancer, genital bleeding (ab-normal, undiagnosed), cerebral haemorrhage, pregnancy, severe hepatic disease, liver tumour, history of idiopathic jaundice or pruritus in pregnancy, Dubin–Johnson or Rotor syndrome, sickle-cell anaemia, congenital disturbance of lipid metabolism, history of herpes gestationis, endometriosis, severe diabetes with vascular changes

Precautions: Lactation, hypertension, asthma, blood dyscrasias, gallbladder disease, congestive cardiac failure diabetes mellitus, bone disease, depression, migraine headache, convulsive disorders, hepatic disease, renal disease, family history of breast or porphyria, otosclerosis, reproductive tract cancer, multiple sclerosis, epilepsy, thyrotoxicosis

Pharmacokinetics:
By mouth: Duration 24 hr, excreted in urine and faeces, metabolised in liver

Clinical assessment:
• Liver function studies, aspartate aminotransferase, alanine aminotransferase, bilirubin, periodically during long-term therapy
• Use lowest effective dose

NURSING CONSIDERATIONS
Assess:
• Baseline BP, weight
Evaluate:
• Weight gain
• Alterations in BP
• Therapeutic response: decreased abnormal uterine bleeding, resumption of menses
• Oedema, hypertension, cardiac symptoms, jaundice
• Mental status: anxiety levels, mood, behavioural changes, depression
• Hypercalcaemia
Teach patient/family:
• Photosensitivity can occur rarely
• All aspects of drug usage, including Cushingoid symptoms

- To report side effects
- To report suspected pregnancy
- To monitor blood sugar, if diabetic
- Importance of taking tablets as prescribed

---

nortriptyline HCl

Aventyl, Allegron, combination products
Func. class.: Antidepressant, tricyclic
Chem. class.: Dibenzocyclo-heptene — secondary amine
Legal class.: POM

Action: Blocks reuptake of nor-adrenaline, serotonin into nerve endings, increasing action of nor-adrenaline, serotonin in nerve cells
Uses: Endogenous depression, nocturnal enuresis
Dosage and routes:
- *Adults:* By mouth 25 mg 3 to 4 times daily, increased to a maximum of 150 mg daily
- *Elderly and child over 12 yr:* By mouth 30−50 mg daily in divided doses
Nocturnal enuresis
- *Child:* By mouth 6−7 yr (20−25 kg) 10 mg at night, 8−11 yr (25−35 kg) 10−20 mg at night, over 11 yr (35−54 kg) 25−35 mg at night. Treatment should be for a maximum of 3 months
Available forms include: Capsules 10, 25, 75 mg; tablets 10, 25 mg
Side effects/adverse reactions:
HAEM: Agranulocytosis, thrombocytopenia, eosinophilia, leucopenia, purpura
CNS: Dizziness, drowsiness, confusion, headache, anxiety, hallucinations, disorientation, delusions, restlessness, agitation, panic, hypomania, tremors, stimulation, weakness, insomnia, nightmares, extrapyramidal symptoms (elderly), increased psychiatric symptoms, numbness, tingling, paraesthesia of extremeties, ataxia, peripheral neuropathy, seizures, EEG changes
GI: Constipation, dry mouth, nausea, vomiting, paralytic ileus, taste disturbance, weight gain or loss, parotid swelling, increased appetite, cramps, epigastric distress, jaundice, hepatitis, stomatitis, gingivitis, black tongue
GU: Retention, acute renal failure, urinary frequency, nocturia
INTEG: Rash, urticaria, sweating, pruritus, photosensitivity
CV: Orthostatic hypotension, ECG changes, tachycardia, hypertension, myocardial infarction, arrhythmias, heart block, stroke
EENT: Blurred vision, tinnitus, mydriasis
META: Breast enlargement, galactorrhoea, altered libido, altered blood glucose levels, inappropriate secretion of antidiuretic hormone
Contraindications: Hypersensitivity to tricyclic antidepressants, heart block, cardiac arrhythmias, recent myocardial infarction, convulsive disorders, severe liver disease, mania, children under 6 yr, lactation
Precautions: Suicidal patients, schizophrenia, severe depression, increased intra-ocular pressure, narrow-angle glaucoma, urinary retention, cardiac disease, hepatic disease, hyperthyroidism, electroshock therapy, elective surgery, pregnancy, cardiovascular disease, epilepsy
Pharmacokinetics:
By mouth: Steady state 4−19 days; metabolised by liver, excreted by kidneys, excreted in breast milk, half-life 18−28 hr
Interactions/incompatibilities:
- Decreased effects of: guanethidine, clonidine
- Increased effects of: direct acting

sympathomimetics, adrenaline, alcohol, barbiturates, benzodiazepines, CNS depressants
• Hyperpyretic crisis, convulsions, hypertensive episode: MAOIs or within 2 weeks of their administration
• Effects of nortriptyline may be reduced by: barbiturates
• Effects of nortriptyline may be potentiated by: cimetidine, fluoxetine
Treatment of overdose: ECG and electrolyte monitoring, induce emesis, lavage, activated charcoal, administer anti-arrhythmics or anticonvulsants if necessary
NURSING CONSIDERATIONS
Assess:
• BP (lying, standing), pulse
• Vital signs 4-hrly in patients with cardiovascular disease
• Weight
• Mental status; mood, affect, depression, panic
Administer:
• Increased fluids, bulk in diet if constipation, urinary retention occur
• With food or milk for GI symptoms
• Dosage at bedtime if over-sedation occurs during day; may take entire dose at bedtime; elderly may not tolerate once day dosing
• Mouthwashes, or frequent sips of water for dry mouth
• Mix with fruit juice, water, or milk to disguise taste
Perform/provide:
• BP; if systolic drops 20 mmHg inform clinician and withhold drug
• Assistance with ambulation during beginning therapy since drowsiness/dizziness occurs
• Safety measures including side-rails primarily in elderly
• Checking to see oral medication swallowed
Evaluate:
• Extrapyramidal symptoms

primarily in elderly: rigidity, dystonia, motor restlessness alertness
• Mental status: mood, affect, suicidal tendencies, increase in psychiatric symptoms: depression, panic
• Urinary retention, constipation; constipation is more likely to occur in children
• Withdrawal symptoms: headache, nausea, vomiting, muscle pain, weakness; do not usually occur unless drug was discontinued abruptly
• Alcohol consumption; if alcohol is consumed, hold dose until morning
Teach patient/family:
• That therapeutic effects may take 2−3 weeks
• Use caution in driving or other activities requiring alertness because of drowsiness, dizziness, blurred vision
• To avoid alcohol other CNS depressants
• Not to discontinue medication quickly after long-term use, may cause nausea, headache, malaise
• To wear sunscreen or large hat since photosensitivity occurs

noxythiolin

Noxyflex S
Func. class.: Antibacterial/Antifungal
Chem. class.: Thiourea derivative
Legal class.: POM

Action: Destroys most fungal and bacterial pathogens partly by slow release of formaldehyde into solution
Uses: Bladder infections, peritonitis, treatment of other infected body cavities
Dosage and routes:
Seek specialist advice

for further details of dosage routes and methods of administration

Bladder infections
• Instil 100 ml of 2.5% solution twice daily (2–3 times weekly for prophylaxis)

Intraperitoneal use
• Instil 200 ml of 2.5% solution prior to closure or at time of catheter insertion, thereafter 100 ml of 2.5% solution twice daily via umbilical catheter
• Should not exceed a daily dose of 10 g for accumulative installations or continuous irrigation regimens

Available forms include: Powder for reconstitution 2.5 g in 20-ml vial

Side effects/adverse reactions:
GU: Burning sensation on application to bladder

Precautions: Requires aseptic technique during preparation, not a substitute for appropriate systemic antibacterial/antifungal therapy

NURSING CONSIDERATIONS
Assess:
• Fluid balance, odour and concentration of urine
• Temperature daily

Administer:
• After samples have been sent for culture and sensitivity
• Reconstituted solution into bladder only using aseptic technique
• Local anaesthetic may be desirable for certain procedures

Evaluate:
• For bladder irritation: frequency of micturation, urinary output
• For decrease in fever

Teach patient/family:
• The importance of using an aseptic technique
• The importance of fluid intake—2 litre/day
• To report any haematuria, or burning sensation in bladder

---

nystatin (oral)

Nystan, Nystatin-Dome
Func. class.: Antifungal
Chem. class.: Amphoteric polyene macrolide
Legal class.: POM

Action: Binds to sterols in cell membrane of fungi, allowing intracellular components to leak

Uses: Oral, intestinal infections caused by *Candida* spp

Dosage and routes:
Oral infection
• *Adult, children:* 100,000 units as suspension or pastille 4 times a day after meals

GI infection
• *Adult:* By mouth 500,000–1,000,000 units 4 times a day
• *Child:* By mouth 100,000 units 4 times a day

Available forms include: Tablets 500,000 units; pastilles 100,000 units; suspension 100,000 units/ml

Side effects/adverse reactions:
GI: Nausea, vomiting, diarrhoea

Contraindications: Hypersensitivity

Pharmacokinetics:
By mouth: Negligible absorption, excreted in faeces

Treatment of overdose: Absorption negligible, no systemic toxicity

NURSING CONSIDERATIONS
Administer:
• After samples have been sent for culture and sensitivity
• Oral suspension dose by placing ½ in each cheek, retain for as long as possible, then swallow
• Topical dose after cleansing area; mouth may be swabbed

Evaluate:
• For allergic reaction: rash, urticaria; drug may need to be discontinued
• For predisposing factors, antibiotic therapy, pregnancy, diabetes mellitus

Teach patient/family:
• That long-term therapy may be required to clear infection; to complete entire course of medication
• Good oral hygiene

---

nystatin (topical)

Nystan, many combination products
Func. class.: Antifungal
Chem. class.: Amphoteric polyene macrolide
Legal class.: POM

Action: Binds sterols in fungal cell membrane, which increases permeability, causing leaking of cell contents

Uses: Cutaneous and vulvovaginal candidiasis

Dosage and routes:
Topical
• *Adult and child:* Topical apply to affected area 2−4 times a day continuing at least 7 days after lesions heal
Vaginal
• Vaginally 100,000−200,000 units as pessaries or vaginal cream each night for at least 14 nights. Apply gel or cream to anogenital area 2−4 times a day for vulval infection
Available forms include: Cream, gel, ointment (all 100,000 units/g); vaginal pessaries 100,000 units; vaginal cream 100,000 units/application

Side effects/adverse reactions:
INTEG: Rash, urticaria, stinging, burning

Contraindications: Hypersensitivity

Precautions: Pregnancy

Interactions/incompatibilities:
• Vaginal cream damages condoms and contraceptive diaphragms

NURSING CONSIDERATIONS
Administer:
• After samples have been taken for culture and sensitivity
• After cleansing with soap, water before each application, dry well
• Enough medication to cover lesions completely
• Vaginal tablets by inserting high into vagina

Evaluate:
• Allergic reaction: burning, stinging, swelling, redness
• Therapeutic response: decrease in size, number of lesions, decreased itching, white patches on vulvae

Teach patient/family:
• Wash hands before, after each application
• To avoid use of non-prescribed creams, ointments, lotions in area of treatment unless directed by clinician
• To apply with glove to prevent further infection
• Avoid sexual contact during treatment of vaginal infection to minimise reinfection
• That relief from itching should occur after 24−72 hr

---

octreotide

Sandostatin
Func. class.: Somatostatin analogue
Chem. class.: Peptide
Legal class.: POM

Action: Inhibits secretion of peptides of the gastroenteropancreatic endocrine system and of growth hormone. Synthetic analogue of somatostatin with a longer duration of action

Uses: Relief of symptoms associated with gastroenteropancreatic endocrine tumours, carcinoid tumours with features of the carcinoid syndrome, VIPomas, and glucagonomas

Dosage and routes:
Gastroenteropancreatic endocrine tumours
• *Adult:* Subcutaneous (or IV if rapid response needed) initially 50 mcg once or twice daily gradually increased up to 200 mcg 3 times a day if needed. Exceptionally, higher doses may be required. Maintenance doses are variable
Acromegaly
• Subcutaneous 100−200 mcg 3 times daily
Available forms include: Injection subcutaneous octreotide (as acetate) 50 mcg/ml, 100 mcg/ml, 500 mcg/ml, 1 ml ampoules; 200 mcg/ml, 5 ml vial

Side effects/adverse reactions:
GI: Anorexia, nausea, vomiting, abdominal pain, diarrhoea, steatorrhoea, bloating, flatulence, formation of gallstones, liver enzyme abnormalities, hepatitis
INTEG: Pain, stinging, burning at injection site with redness and swelling
ENDO: Impaired postprandial glucose tolerance, rarely persistent hyperglycaemia

Contraindications: Hypersensitivity, pregnancy, lactation

Precautions: Sudden escape of gastroenteropancreatic endocrine tumours from symptomatic control may occur infrequently. Diabetics may show reduced hypoglycaemic requirements, increased depth and duration of hypoglycaemia in insulinoma

Pharmacokinetics: Metabolised in the liver. Plasma half-life 90−120 min

Interactions/incompatibilities:
• Alters requirements for insulin/oral hypoglycaemics in diabetics

Clinical assessment:
• Monitor hypoglycaemic control closely in diabetics
• Ultrasonic examination of the gall bladder is recommended prior to and at 6−12 month intervals during therapy
• Monitor thyroid function during long-term therapy

NURSING CONSIDERATIONS

Assess:
• Thyroid function during long term therapy
• Gall bladder by ultra sonic examination before and six monthly during therapy
• Electrolytes
• Input and output of fluids
• Blood sugar levels
• Weight

Administer:
• Intravenously for rapid response in carcinoid crises
• Dilute with normal saline for bolus injection or short-term therapy
• Subcutaneously following the dosage regime for suitable gradual introduction
• Injections should be given with solution at room temp
• Avoid multiple injections at short intervals at the same site
• In carcinoid tumour, discontinue if there is no beneficial effect within 1 week

Perform/provide:
• For prolonged storage ampoules should be stored between 2 and 8°C. For day-to-day use store at room temperature for up to 2 weeks

Evaluate:
• Therapeutic response, improved symptoms, quality of life, electrolyte abnormalities; reduced excretions and diarrhoea
• Weight gain
• Fluctuation of blood glucose
• Local skin reactions pain, stinging, redness and swelling
• Flatulence, bloating, signs of jaundice

Teach patient/family:
• That insulin or oral hypogly-

caemic drugs may be reduced for diabetics
• That drug needs to be combined with complete health plan: diet, rest exercise
• To notify clinician if it is any yellowing in skin, clay coloured stool, dark urine

---

oestradiol/oestradiol valerate

Estraderm TTS, Climaval Progynova
Func. class.: Oestrogen
Chem. class.: Nonsteroidal synthetic oestrogen
Legal class.: POM

Action: Necessary for adequate functioning of female reproductive system; affects release of pituitary gonadotropins, inhibits ovulation, adequate calcium use in bone structures
Uses: Menopause, primary amenorrhoea, atrophic vaginitis
Dosage and routes:
Menopause/hypogonadism/casttration/ovarian failure
• *Adult:* By mouth 1 mg daily for 3 weeks of each cycle. Increase to 2 mg daily if necessary
• *Adult:* Implant 25−100 mg every 4−8 months with cyclical progesteron on 10−13 days of each cycle if uterus intact
• Transderm patch, menopausal symptoms (not oesteoporosis prophylaxis) initially one 50 mcg patch applied twice a week. Adjust dose according to response. Maximum dose 100 mcg daily. Progestrogen essential (unless hysterectomy) on last 12 days of cycle
Available forms include: Tablets 1, 2 mg; implants 25, 50, 100 mg; patch 25, 50, 100 mcg 24 hr

Side effects/adverse reactions:
CNS: Dizziness, headache, migraine, depression, vertigo
CV: Thrombophlebitis, oedema, thromboembolism, stroke, pulmonary embolism, myocardial infarction, hypertension, palpitations
GI: Nausea, vomiting, diarrhoea, anorexia, pancreatitis, cramps, dyspepsia, flatulence, constipation, increased appetite, abdominal pain, increased weight, cholestatic jaundice
EENT: Contact lens intolerance, increased myopia, astigmatism
GU: Amenorrhoea, cervical erosion, breakthrough bleeding, dysmenorrhoea, vaginal candidiasis, breast changes
INTEG: Rash, urticaria, acne, chloasma, hirsutism, melasma, erythema nodosum
META: Hyperglycaemia, sodium and water retention
Contraindications: Breast cancer, hyperlipoproteinaemia, thromboembolic disorders, oestrogen-dependent neoplasms, cholestatic jaundice, history of jaundice or herpes gestationis, pregnancy, Dubin−Johnson syndrome, Rotor syndrome, moderate to severe sickle cell anaemia, genital bleeding (abnormal, undiagnosed), pregnancy porphyria, congestive cardiac failure, severe hepatic disease or renal disease, endometriosis
Precautions: Asthma, blood dyscrasias, gallbladder disease, diabetes mellitus, bone disease, multiple sclerosis, depression, migraine headache, severe varicose veins, chloasma, convulsive disorders, family history of cancer of breast or reproductive tract, hypertension, cholelithiasis
Pharmacokinetics:
By mouth: Degraded in liver, excreted in urine

Transdermal: Onset 4 hr, duration up to 4 days

Interactions/incompatibilities:
• Decreased action of: anticoagulants, oral hypoglycaemics and insulins
• Toxicity: tricyclic antidepressants
• Decreased action of this drug: anticonvulsants, barbiturates, phenylbutazone, rifampicin
• Increased action of: corticosteroids

Clinical assessment:
• Liver function studies, including aspartate aminotransferase, alanine aminotransferase, bilirubin, alkaline phosphatase

Lab. test interferences:
Increase: Thyroxine, thyroxine-binding globulin (TBG)
Decrease: Triiodothyronine resin uptake test

NURSING CONSIDERATIONS

Assess:
• Baseline weight and BP before therapy and regularly during the course

Administer:
• Titrated dose, use lowest effective dose
• Implant should be inserted subcutaneously into an area where there is little or no movement or blood supply e.g. buttock, lower abdominal wall
• Insert implant using a trocar and cannular under local anaesthetic; could insert in wound at time of laparotomy
• With food or milk to decrease GI symptoms (oral)
• Patch to be applied to clean, dry,. unbroken skin on trunk below waistline; not to be applied on or near breasts

Evaluate:
• Urinary glucose in patient with diabetes, increased urine glucose may occur
• Weight daily, notify clinician of weekly weight gain greater than 2.5 kg; if increase, diuretic may be ordered
• BP 4 hrly watch for increase caused by water and sodium retention
• For decreasing urinary output and increasing oedema
• Therapeutic response: absence of breast engorgement, reversal of menopausal symptoms
• Oedema, hypertension, cardiac symptoms, jaundice
• Mental status: affect, mood, behavioural changes, aggression

Teach patient/family:
• Weight weekly, report gain greater than 2.5 kg
• Warn contact lense wearers that vision may alter slightly; allow time to settle before seeking opticians advice
• Avoid sunlight or wear sunscreen; burns may occur
• Patch should be removed after 3−4 days and replaced with fresh patch on slightly different site

---

oestriol

Ovestin, combination products
Func. class.: Oestrogen
Chem. class.: Female sex hormone
Legal class.: POM

Action: Enables female reproductive system to function adequately; affects release of pituitary gonadotrophins; inhibits ovulation

Uses: GU symptoms associated with oestrogen deficiency states; infertility associated with poor cervical penetration

Dosage and routes:
GU symptoms
• *Adult:* By mouth, 0.5−3 mg daily as single dose for up to 1 month then 0.5−1 mg daily until epithelial

integrity is restored (short-term use only)

Infertility
• *Adult:* By mouth, 0.25−1 mg daily as single dose on days 6−15 of menstrual cycle (with regular monitoring)

Available forms include: Tablets 0.25 mg (250 mcg)

Side effects/adverse reactions:
HAEM: Changes in liver function
CNS: Depression, headache
GU: Endometrial carcinoma in postmenopausal women treated with unopposed oestrogen therapy. For patients with intact uterus, progestogen should be administered cyclically. Withdrawal bleeding (rarely)
GI: Nausea, vomiting
META: Weight gain, breast tenderness and enlargement, sodium retention with oedema
INTEG: Jaundice, chloasma, rashes

Contraindications: Oestrogen-dependent carcinoma, history of thromboembolism, hepatic impairment, sickle-cell anaemia, undiagnosed vaginal bleeding, pregnancy, severe hypertension

Precautions: Diabetes mellitus, epilepsy, hypertension, migraine, cardiac or renal disease, history of jaundice, wearing of contact lenses, lactation. Prolonged treatment, endometriosis, fibrocystic mastopathy, hyperlipoproteinaemia, history of herpes gestationis, porphyria

Pharmacokinetics: Oestriol is short acting, due to short nuclear retention time in the target tissues, its low affinity for plasma protein and rapid metabolic clearance

Interactions/incompatibilities:
• Decreased effect: concurrent administration of liver enzyme inducing agents e.g. rifampicin, barbiturates, carbamazepine, phenytoin

Treatment of overdose: Symptomatic treatment only

NURSING CONSIDERATIONS
Assess:
• Baseline BP, weight, urinalysis (in diabetics)
Administer:
• Titrated dose
• With food or milk to avoid GI symptoms
Evaluate:
• Therapeutic response, absence of breast enlargement, reversal of menopause
• Mental changes—mood and behavioural patterns
• Oedema, hypertension, cardiac symptoms, jaundice, hyperglycaemia
• Fluid balance; observe urinary output and increasing oedema
• Glucose in urine; may increase in diabetic patients
Teach patient/family:
• To weigh weekly, report gain more than 2.5 kg
• To report breast lumps, vaginal bleeding, oedema, GI upsets, abdominal pain or numbness in joints

---

oestrogens, conjugated

Premarin, combination product
Func. class.: Oestrogen
Chem. class.: Equine and synthetic oestrogens
Legal class.: POM

Action: Oestrogens needed for adequate functioning of female reproductive system; it affects release of pituitary gonadotropins, inhibits ovulation, adequate calcium use in bone structures
Uses: Oestrogen replacement therapy in menopausal and postmenopausal women. Menopause, breast cancer, prostatic cancer, primary ovarian failure, osteopo-

rosis, atrophic vaginitis, Kraurosis vulvae. Unopposed oestrogen therapy in women following hysterectomy. In patients with intact uterus cyclical progestogen must be administered

Dosage and routes:

Menopause
• *Adult:* By mouth 1.25 mg daily 3 weeks on, 1 week off

Prostatic cancer
• *Adult:* By mouth 1.25−2.5 mg three times a day

Breast cancer
• *Adult:* By mouth 10 mg 3 times a day for 3 months or longer; palliative, for women who are at least 5 years post menopause

Primary ovarian failure/ osteoporosis
• *Adult:* By mouth 0.25−1.25 mg daily 3 weeks on, 1 week off

Atrophic vaginitis
• By mouth 0.625−1.25 cyclically daily; vaginal cream 1−2 g daily 3 weeks on, 1 week off

Available forms include: Tablets 0.625, 1.25, 2.5 mg; cream 0.625 mg/g

Side effects/adverse reactions:

CNS: Dizziness, headache, migraine, depression

CV: Hypotension, thrombophlebitis, oedema, thromboembolism, stroke, pulmonary embolism, myocardial infarction

GI: Nausea, vomiting, diarrhoea, anorexia, pancreatitis, cramps, constipation, increased appetite, increased weight, cholestatic jaundice

EENT: Contact lens intolerance, increased myopia, astigmatism

GU: Amenorrhoea, cervical erosion, breakthrough bleeding, dysmenorrhoea, vaginal candidiasis, breast changes, gynaecomastia, testicular atrophy, impotence

INTEG: Rash, urticaria, acne, hirsutism, alopecia, oily skin, seborrhoea, purpura, melasma

META: Folic acid deficiency, hypercalcaemia, hyperglycaemia, alters lipid profile in postmenopausal women

Contraindications: Thromboembolic disorders, oestrogen-dependent neoplasm, genital bleeding (abnormal, undiagnosed), pregnancy, active thromboembolic disease, acute liver disease severe cardiac, renal disease

Precautions: Hypertension, asthma, blood dyscrasias, gallbladder disease, congestive cardiac failure, diabetes mellitus, bone disease, depression, migraine headache, convulsive disorders, hepatic disease, renal disease, family history of cancer of breast or reproductive tract, long term treatment should be accompanied by administration of a progestogen

Pharmacokinetics:

By mouth, IV/IM: Degraded in liver, excreted in urine, excreted in breast milk

Interactions/incompatibilities:

• Decreased action of: anticoagulants, oral hypoglycaemics
• Toxicity: tricyclic antidepressants
• Decreased action of this drug: anticonvulsants, barbiturates, phenylbutazone, rifampicin
• Increased action of: corticosteroids

Clinical assessment:

• Liver function studies including aspartate aminotransferase alanine aminotransferase, bilirubin, alkaline phosphatase

NURSING CONSIDERATIONS

Assess:

• Baseline BP, weight, urinalysis (in diabetics)

Administer:

• Titrated dose, use lowest effective dose

• With food or milk to decrease GI symptoms by mouth
Evaluate:
• BP 4 hrly; watch for increase caused by water and sodium retention
• Fluid balance, be alert for decreasing urinary output and increasing oedema
• Therapeutic response: absence of breast engorgement, reversal of menopausal symptoms, or decrease in tumour size in prostatic cancer
• Oedema, hypertension, cardiac symptoms, jaundice, hypercalcaemia
• Mental status: affect, mood, behavioral changes, aggression
Teach patient/family:
• Weigh weekly, report gain greater than 2.5 kg
• Report any breakthrough bleeding, amenorrhoea; gynaecomastia, testicular atrophy (male)

---

olsalazine

Dipentum
Func. class.: Anti-inflammatory agent
Chem. class.: Salicylate derivative
Legal class.: POM

Action: Olsalazine is converted in the colon to 5-aminosalicylic acid which acts topically on the colonic mucosa
Uses: Treatment and maintenance of remission in acute mild ulcerative colitis
Dosage and routes:
Acute mild disease
• *Adult:* By mouth initially 1 g daily in divided doses increased up to a maximum of 3 g daily over 1 week. A single dose should not exceed 1 g
Remission maintenance

• *Adult and elderly:* By mouth 0.5 g twice a day
Available forms include: Capsules 250 mg
Side effects/adverse reactions:
GI: Diarrhoea, abdominal cramps, nausea, dyspepsia, reversible pancreatitis
INTEG: Rash
CNS: Headache
MS: Arthralgia
Contraindications: Hypersensitivity to salicylates, significant renal impairment, pregnancy, lactation
Pharmacokinetics: The systemic absorption of olsalazine is minimal
Treatment of overdose: Minimal systemic absorption, no specific antidote, treatment supportive
NURSING CONSIDERATIONS
Assess:
• Nutritional status, dietary habits
Administer:
• With or just after food
Evaluate:
• Therapeutic effect
• For side effects; diarrhoea and GI disturbance, rashes arthralgia
Teach patient/family:
• Importance of maintenance dose
• About diet, stress alleviation
• To report side effects

---

oral contraceptives, combined

Func. class.: Hormone
Chem. class.: Oestrogen/progestogen combinations
Legal class.: POM

Action: Prevents ovulation by suppressing follicle stimulating, luteinizing hormone
Uses: To prevent pregnancy, endometriosis, hypermenorrhoea

Dosage and routes:
• *Adult:* By mouth 1 tablet daily starting on day 1 of menstrual cycle
21 tablet packs
• 1 tablet daily for 21 days followed by a 7 day gap
28 tablet packs
• 1 tablet daily continuously
Triphasic/Biphasic
• 1 tablet daily as shown on package insert
Available forms include: Numerous brands
Side effects/adverse reactions:
GI: Nausea, vomiting, cramps, diarrhoea, bloating, constipation, change in appetite, cholestatic jaundice, weight gain, impairment of liver function, hepatic tumours
INTEG: Chloasma, melasma, acne, rash, urticaria, erythema, pruritus, hirsutism, photosensitivity
CV: Increased BP, thrombo-embolic conditions, fluid retention, oedema
ENDO: Decreased glucose tolerance
GU: Breakthrough bleeding, amenorrhoea, spotting, dysmenorrhoea, galactorrhoea, endo-cervical hyperplasia, vaginitis, cystitis-like syndrome, breast change, changes in libido
CNS: Depression, fatigue, dizziness, nervousness, anxiety, headache
EENT: Retinal thrombosis
HAEM: Increased fibrinogen, clotting factor
Contraindications: Pregnancy, lactation, reproductive cancer, history of thromboembolic disease, recurrent jaundice, porphyria, undiagnosed vaginal bleeding, history of pruritis of pregnancy or herpes gestationis, deterioration of otosclerosis, thrombophlebitis, myocardial infarction, hepatic tumours, hepatic disease, coronary artery disease, women over 40 yr,

hyperlipidaemia, severe or focal migraine, Dubin-Johnson and Rotor syndrome, mammary, endometrial or oestrogen dependent tumours
Precautions: Depression, hypertension, renal disease, seizure disorders, lupus erythematosus, multiple sclerosis, rheumatic disease, migraine headache, amenorrhoea, irregular menses, breast cancer (fibrocystic), gallbladder disease
Pharmacokinetics: Degraded in liver, excreted in urine
Interactions/incompatibilities:
• Decreased effectiveness of oral contraceptives: ampicillin, tetracycline, rifampicin, analgesics, carbamazepine, phenobarbitone, phenytoin, primidone, antihistamines, griseofulvin
• Decreased action of: oral anticoagulants, antidepressants, oral hypoglycaemics and insulins, antihypertensives
• Increased clotting: aminocaproic acid
• Increased plasma concentrations of: cyclosporin, theophylline
Clinical assessment:
• Glucose, thyroid function, liver function tests
Lab. test interferences:
Increase: Thyroid binding globulin, protein bound iodine, thyroxine, platelet aggregability, protein bound iodine
Decrease: Triiodothyronine, antithrombin
NURSING CONSIDERATIONS
Evaluate:
• Therapeutic response: absence of pregnancy, endometriosis, menorrhagia
• Reproductive changes: change in breasts, tumours, positive PAP smear; drug should be discontinued if changes occur
Teach patient/family:
• Detection of clots using Homan's

sign (dorsiflexion of foot causing pain in calf)

• To use sunscreen or avoid sunlight; photosensitivity can occur

• To take at same time each day to ensure equal drug level

• To report GI symptoms that occur after 4 months

• To use another birth control method during 1st week of oral contraceptive use

• To take another tablet as soon as possible if one is missed. If this is more than 12 hr late contraception may not work. Continue taking tablets but use additional precautions for 7 days. If these 7 days run beyond the end of the pack, start the new pack immediately the current one is finished

• That after drug is discontinued, pregnancy may not occur for several months

• To report abdominal pain, change in vision, shortness of breath, change in menstrual flow, spotting, breakthrough bleeding, breast lumps, swelling

• That continuing medical care is needed: PAP smear and gynaecologic examinations 6 monthly

---

orciprenaline sulphate

Alupent
Func. class.: Adrenergic
Chem. class.: Synthetic sympathomimate amine
Legal class.: POM

Action: Relaxes bronchial smooth muscle by direct action on β-adrenergic receptors

Uses: Bronchial asthma, bronchospasm

Dosage and routes:

• *Adult:* Inhalation, 1−2 puffs, may repeat if necessary after not less than 30 min, not to exceed 12 puffs daily

• *Child up to 6 yr:* 1 puff up to 4 times daily; 6−12 yr 1−2 puffs up to 4 times daily

• *Adult:* By mouth 20 mg 6−8 hrly

• *Child:* By mouth, up to 1 yr 5−10 mg 3 times daily; 1−3 yr 5−10 mg 4 times daily; 3−12 yr 40−60 mg daily in divided doses

Available forms include: Tablets, 20 mg; aerosol 750 mcg/metered inhalation; syrup 10 mg/5 ml;

Side effects/adverse reactions:
CNS: Tremors, anxiety, insomnia, headache, dizziness, stimulation
CV: Palpitations, tachycardia, hypertension, cardiac arrest
GI: Nausea

Contraindications: Hypersensitivity to sympathomimetics, thyrotoxicosis

Precautions: Pregnancy, cardiac disorders, diabetes mellitus, prostatic hypertrophy, hyperthyroidism, hypertension, elderly, MAOIs. Due to risk of arrhythmias and other side effects, more selective β$_2$-adrenoreceptor stimulants are preferred for routine therapy

Interactions/incompatibilities:

• Increased effects of both drugs: other sympathomimetics

• Decreased action: β-blockers

Clinical assessment:

• Respiratory function: vital capacity, forced expiratory volume, arterial blood gases

• Monitor serum potassium particularly if administered with xanthines

NURSING CONSIDERATIONS
Administer:

• In terms of numbers of inhalations at one time

• 2 hr before bedtime to avoid sleeplessness

Evaluate:

• Therapeutic response: absence of dyspnoea, wheezing

• Tolerance over long-term

therapy, dose may need to be increased or changed

Teach patient/family:
• Not to use non-prescribed drug, extra stimulation may occur
• Inhaler technique and advise on maximum number of inhalations in 24 hr
• Review package insert with patient
• To avoid getting aerosol in eyes
• To wash inhaler in warm water and dry daily
• On all aspects of drug; avoid smoking, smoke-filled rooms

---

orphenadrine citrate/ hydrochloride

Norflex, Biorphien, Disipal
Func. class.: Skeletal muscle relaxant, central acting
Chem. class.: Tertiary amine
Legal class.: POM

Action: Acts centrally on skeletal muscle to relax, inhibit muscle spasm

Uses: Parkinsonism, short-term relief of muscle spasm

Dosage and routes:
Parkinson's disease
• *Adult:* By mouth 150 mg daily in divided doses. Increase by 25–50 mg daily every 2–3 days if necessary. Maximum dosage is 400 mg daily

Short term relief of muscle spasm
• *Adult:* IM or IV injection 60 mg (given over 5 min if IV). Repeat after 12 hr

Available forms include: Tablets 50 mg, injection 30 mg/ml; solution 25 mg, 5 ml

Side effects/adverse reactions:
HAEM: Aplastic anaemia
CNS: Dizziness, weakness, fatigue, drowsiness, headache, disorientation, insomnia, stimulation, euphoria, hallucination, agitation, nervousness
EENT: Nasal congestion, blurred vision, increased intra-ocular pressure
CV: Hypotension, tachycardia
GI: Nausea, vomiting, constipation, dry mouth, numbness of the tongue and mouth, difficulty with micturition
GU: Urinary frequency, hesitancy
INTEG: Rash, pruritus, urticaria

Contraindications: Hypersensitivity, narrow-angle glaucoma, GI obstruction, myasthenia gravis, stenosing peptic ulcer, urinary retention, lactation, children under 12 yr, acute pulmonary insufficiency, prostatic hypertrophy, tardive dyskinesia

Precautions: Pregnancy, cardiac disease, chronic pulmonary insufficiency, elderly, tachycardia, hypertension, liver or kidney dysfunction

Interactions/incompatibilities:
• Increased CNS effects: coproxamol

Clinical assessment:
• Blood studies: full blood count, WBC, differential, blood dyscrasias may occur (rare)

Lab. test interference: Elevated triiodothyronine (Sephadex method)

Treatment of overdose: Gastric lavage, emetic and high enema. Cholinergic agents such as carbachol may be useful

NURSING CONSIDERATIONS
Assess:
• Blood studies before and periodically in long-term use. Check for anaemia and dyscrasis

Administer:
• Intravenous injection directly into vein over 5 min. Further doses at 12 hr intervals
• Intramuscular or intravenous injection
• Orally with meals if nausea

occurs. Increase dosage at recommended rate until optimum response with minimum side effects

Perform/provide:
• Help with mobility
• Frequent drink to prevent dry mouth

Evaluate:
• Therapeutic response: decreased rigidity, spasms
• Input and output of fluids, retention, frequency, hesitancy
• Side effects: nausea, dry mouth, numb tongue and mouth, visual disturbances, dizziness, micturition difficulties are usually transient or controlled by slight reduction in dosage
• Blood; plastic anaemia, rash, dyscrasis-rare

Teach patient/family:
• Not to discontinue medication without medical advice. Drug should be tapered off slowly
• To take other medication only if directed by clinician
• That alcohol should not be taken nor CNS depressants
• To avoid driving or use of machinery until therapy established

---

oxazepam

Func. class.: Anxiolytic
Chem. class.: Benzodiazepine
Legal class.: CD (Sch 4) POM

Action: Depresses subcortical levels of CNS, including limbic system and reticular formation
Uses: Anxiety (short-term use), alcohol withdrawal
Dosage and routes:
Moderate anxiety
• *Adult:* By mouth 15−30 mg 3 or 4 times a day
• *Elderly:* By mouth 10−20 mg 3 or 4 times a day

Insomnia associated with anxiety
• *Adult:* By mouth 15−25 mg one hour before bedtime. Maximum dose 50 mg
Available forms include: Tablets 10, 15 mg
Side effects/adverse reactions:
CNS: Dizziness, drowsiness, confusion, headache, anxiety, excitement, disorientation amnesia, ataxia, vertigo, syncope, lethargy, tremors, stimulation, fatigue, depression, insomnia, hallucinations, suicidal tendency, paradoxical aggression
GI: Constipation, dry mouth, nausea, vomiting, anorexia, diarrhoea, increased liver enzymes, jaundice
GU: Altered libido, urinary retention
HAEM: Blood dyscrasias, leucopenia
INTEG: Rash, dermatitis, itching
CV: Hypotension, oedema
EENT: Blurred vision
Contraindications: Hypersensitivity to benzodiazepines, narrow-angle glaucoma, psychosis, pregnancy, child under 18 yr, acute pulmonary insufficiency
Precautions: Elderly, debilitated, hepatic disease, renal disease, history of alcoholism or drug abuse, personality disorders, chronic pulmonary insufficiency, concurrent CNS depressants including alcohol, general anaesthesia, opiates, MAOIs, antidepressants
Pharmacokinetics:
By mouth: Peak 2−4 hr, metabolised by liver, excreted by kidneys, half-life 6−8 hr
Interactions/incompatibilities:
• Increased effects of this drug: CNS depressants, alcohol, cimetidine, disulfiram, omeprazole
• Increased effects of: alcohol, general anaesthetics, opioid analgesics, MAOIs, antihypertensives

Clinical assessment:
• Blood studies: Full blood count during long-term therapy, blood dyscrasias have occurred rarely
• Liver function tests; aspartate aminotransferase, alanine amino-transferase, bilirubin, creatinine, lactic dehydrogenase, alkaline phosphatase
Treatment of overdose: Lavage, vital signs, supportive care
NURSING CONSIDERATIONS
Assess:
• Baseline pulse; BP
Administer:
• With food or milk for GI symptoms
• Crushed if patient is unable to swallow medication whole
Perform/provide:
• Frequent sips of water for dry mouth
Evaluate:
• Pulse, BP for first 24 hr of treatment
• Lying and standing BP if indicated
• Therapeutic response: decreased anxiety, restlessness, insomnia
• Mental status: mood, alertness, affect, sleeping pattern, drowsiness, dizziness
• Physical dependency, with-drawal symptoms: headache, nausea, vomiting, muscle pain, weakness after long-term use
• Suicidal tendencies
Teach patient/family:
• That drug may be taken with food
• Not to be used for everyday stress or used longer than 4 months, unless directed by clinician
• Avoid non-prescribed prep-arations (cough, cold, hay fever) unless approved by physician
• To avoid driving, activities that require alertness, since drowsiness may occur
• To avoid alcohol or other psychotropic medications unless prescribed by clinician
• Not to discontinue medication abruptly after long-term use
• To stand up slowly or fainting may occur
• That drowsiness might worsen at beginning of treatment

---

oxidized cellulose

Oxycel, Surgicel
Func. class.: Haemostatic
Chem. class.: Cellulose product
Legal class.: GSL

Action: Forms gel acting as physical barrier to bleeding
Uses: Haemostasis in surgery, epistaxis
Dosage and routes:
• *Adult and child:* Topical, apply using sterile technique as needed, remove after bleeding stops, if possible, or leave in place if not
Available forms include: Knitted fabric, gauze or lint
Side effects/adverse reactions:
EENT: Sneezing and burning when used in the nose
INTEG: Burning, stinging at site of application
CNS: Headache when used in the nose
MISC: Inhibits epithelialisation
Contraindications: Hypersensi-tivity, large artery haemorrhage, oozing surfaces, implantation or packing in bone surgery, infected wounds
Interactions/incompatibilities:
• Application after silver nitrate or other escharotics inhibits absorption
• Inactivates thrombin
NURSING CONSIDERATIONS
Administer:
• Using sterile technique
• Dry, use only amount needed to control bleeding

• Loosely, remove excess before closure in surgery; irrigate first, then remove using sterile technique

Evaluate:
• Allergy: fever, rash, itching, burning, stinging
• Bleeding: mucous membranes, epistaxis, ecchymosis, petechiae, haematuria, haematemesis

Teach patient/family:
• To report any signs of bleeding: gums, under skin, urine, stools, emesis

---

oxprenolol HCl

Apsolox, Slow-Trasicor, Trasicor, combination product
Func. class.: Antihypertensive, antianginal
Chem. class.: β-adrenergic blocker, non cardioselective
Legal class.: POM

Action: Decreases preload, afterload, which is responsible for decreasing left ventricular end diastolic pressure, systemic vascular resistance
Uses: Angina, arrhythmias, hypertension, anxiety-induced tachycardia, hypertrophic obstructive cardiomyopathy, thyrotoxicosis
Dosage and routes:
Angina
• By mouth, 40−160 mg 3 times daily
Arrhythmias, anxiety-induced tachycardia, hypertrophic obstructive cardiomyopathy, thyroxicosis
• *Adults:* By mouth, initially 20−40 mg 3 times daily, increased as required, maximum dose 480 mg daily; modified-release, 160 mg once daily increased if necessary to a maximum of 480 mg
Hypertension
• By mouth, initially 80 mg twice daily increased at weekly intervals as needed; maximum dose 480 mg daily; modified-release, 160 mg once daily, increased to a maximum of 480 mg
Anxiety symptoms
• *Adults:* By mouth 40 mg twice daily. Increase to a maximum of 160 mg daily
Available forms include: Tablets 20, 40, 80, 160 mg; modified-release tablets 160 mg
Side effects/adverse reactions:
CNS: Dizziness, drowsiness, headache, insomnia, excitability
CV: Heart failure, bradycardia, atrioventricular conduction disorders, peripheral vasoconstriction, hypotension
EENT: Visual disturbances, keratoconjunctivitis, dry eyes
GI: Disturbances, dry mouth
GU: Loss of libido
RESP: Bronchospasm, dyspnoea
HAEM: Thrombocytopenia
INTEG: Cold extremities, rash
Interactions/incompatibilities:
• Effects of oxprenolol may be enhanced by: other antihypertensives, calcium antagonists, anti-arrhythmics, cimetidine, fluvoxamine, mefloquine, digoxin, diuretics
• Oxprenolol, may potentiate: alcohol, analgesia, antihistamines, tricyclic antidepressants, anti-arrhythmics of the quinidine type and amiodarone, insulin, oral anti-diabetic agents, chlorpromazine
• Effects of oxprenolol may be reduced by: indomethacin, rifampicin, corticosteroids, thyroxine, carbenoxolone, xamoterol
• Oxprenolol may reduce effects of: neostigmine, pyridostigmine, xamoterol
• Severe hypertension may occur with concurrent use of: sympathomimetics such as adrenaline, noradrenaline and also in cough and cold remedies
Contraindications: Uncontrolled

heart failure, 2nd or 3rd degree heart block, asthma, cardiogenic shock, marked bradycardia, hypersensitivity, sick-sinus syndrome, chloroform or ether anaesthesia

Precautions: Pregnancy, lactation, hepatic or renal impairment, avoid abrupt withdrawal in angina, chronic bronchitis, hypoglycaemia, insulin dependent or labile diabetes, thyrotoxic crisis, peripheral vascular disorders, uncontrolled cardiac failure, pulse rate less than 50 beats/min, alcoholism diabetic acidosis, emphysema, Raynaud's disease, phaeochromocytoma (unless treated with a α-adrenergic blocker)

Pharmacokinetics:
Almost completely absorbed from GI tract, subject to considerable first pass metabolism. Peak levels occur after 1−2 hr. Metabolised the liver and excreted in urine

Clinical assessment:
• Perform creatinine clearance if kidney damage is diagnosed

Lab. test interferences:
Increase: Serum potassium, serum uric acid, alanine aminotransferase, aspartate aminotransferase alkaline phosphatase, lactic dehydrogenase
Decrease: Blood glucose

Treatment of overdose: For sinus bradycardia and hypotension 10.5−2 mg atropine by slow 1V infusion followed by isoprenaline of 25 mcg IV if necessary. In cardiogenic shock 5−10 mg glucagon IV may be helpful. Salbutamol by inhalation or 4 mcg/kg slow IV injection can be given for bronchospasm

NURSING CONSIDERATIONS
Assess:
• Baseline BP, pulse, respirations and weight
• Fluid balance

• Pain: duration, time started, activity being performed
Administer:
• With full glass of water on empty stomach
Evaluate:
• Observe for postural hypotension
• Tolerance, if taken over a long period of time
• Therapeutic response, degree of palpitations, breathlessness, anxiety levels
• BP, heart and respiratory rates
Teach patient/family:
• That dose must be taken with a glass of water
• That drug should be taken before stressful activity or exercise
• That if taken sublingually, mucous membranes may sting
• To avoid hazardous activities if dizziness occurs
• Stress patient compliance with complete medical regime
• To make positional changes slowly to prevent fainting

---

oxycodone pectinate

Func. class.: Narcotic analgesic
Chem. class.: Opioid, semisynthetic derivative
Legal class.: CD (Sch 2) POM

Action: Inhibits ascending pain pathways in CNS, increases pain threshold, alters pain perception
Uses: Moderate to severe pain in terminal illness
Dosage and routes:
• *Adult:* Rectally 30−60 mg every 6−8 hr
Available forms include: Suppositories 30 mg (special order from Boots)
Side effects/adverse reaction:
CNS: Drowsiness, dizziness, confusion, sedation, euphoria

GI: Nausea, vomiting, anorexia, constipation, cramps
GU: Dysuria
INTEG: Rash, urticaria, flushing, diaphoresis, pruritus
EENT: Tinnitus, blurred vision, miosis, diplopia, dry mouth
CV: Palpitations, bradycardia, orthostatic hypotension
RESP: Respiratory depression
SYST: Hypothermia

Contraindications: Hypersensitivity
Precautions: Addictive personality, pregnancy, lactation, increased intracranial pressure, respiratory depression, hepatic disease, renal disease, hyperthyroidism, prostatic hypertrophy, myxoedema, adrenocortical insufficiency

Pharmacokinetics: Well absorbed from GI tract, metabolised in liver excreted in urine as metabolite and unchanged

Interactions/incompatibilities:
• Increased CNS depression with: alcohol, sedative/hypnotics, antipsychotics, skeletal muscle relaxants, other CNS depressants
• Serious hypertensive/hypotensive reactions with CNS excitation/depression with: MAOIs
• Antagonism of GI effects of: cisapride, metoclopramide, domperidone

Treatment of overdose: Naloxone IV, symptomatic treatment

NURSING CONSIDERATIONS
Assess:
• Pain levels
• Fluid balance
Administer:
• With anti-emetic if nausea, vomiting occur
• When pain is beginning to return; determine dosage interval by patient response
Perform/provide:
• Storage in CD cupboard
• All supportive measures
• Assistance with ambulation
• Safety measures: cot sides, night light, callbell within easy reach
Evaluate:
• Therapeutic response: decrease in pain
• CNS changes: dizziness, drowsiness, hallucinations, euphoria, level of consciousness, pupil reaction
• GI symptoms including constipation
• Respiratory rate and character
• Need for pain medication, physical dependence, other supportive care
Teach patient/family:
• To report any gross changes
• Withdrawal symptoms may occur; nausea, vomiting, cramps, fever, faintness, anorexia
• How to insert suppositories
• The need for secure storage

---

oxymetholone

Anapolon 50
Func. class.: Androgenic anabolic steroid
Chem. class.: Testosterone derivative
Legal class.: POM

Action: Increases weight by building body tissue, increases potassium, phosphorus, chloride, and nitrogen levels, increases bone development, stimulates erythropoiesis
Uses: Aplastic anaemia
Dosage and routes:
• *Adult:* By mouth 2−5 mg/kg daily, titrated to patient response, for at least 3 months
Available forms include: Tablets 50 mg
Side effects/adverse reactions:
INTEG: Acne, alopecia, hirsutism
CNS: Excitation, insomnia
MS: Cramps, premature skeletal maturation in children

CV: Congestive heart failure, oedema

GU: Amenorrhoea, vaginitis, virilisation, decreased libido, decreased breast size, clitoral enlargement, testicular atrophy, gynaecomastia

GI: Nausea, vomiting, diarrhoea, cholestatic jaundice

ENDO: Abnormal glucose tolerance test

Contraindications: Severe renal disease, porphyria, severe hepatic disease, hypersensitivity, pregnancy, lactation, hypercalcaemia, carcinoma of breast or prostrate in males

Precautions: Diabetes mellitus, cardiac, renal, or hepatic disease, prostatic hypertrophy, myocardial infarction, epilepsy, hypertension, migraine

Pharmacokinetics:

By mouth: Metabolised in liver, excreted in urine, excreted in breast milk

Interactions/incompatibilities:
• Adjustments in insulin, oral antidiabetic dosage
• Increased prothrombin time: anticoagulants
• Oedema: ACTH, adrenal steroids

Clinical assessment:
• Electrolytes: potassium, sodium, chloride, calcium; cholesterol
• Liver function studies: aspartate aminotransferase, alanine aminotransferase, bilirubin

Administer:
• Titrated dose, use lowest effective dose

Lab. test interferences:
Glucose tolerance, thyroid function

NURSING CONSIDERATIONS

Administer:
• With food to reduce GI symptoms

Perform/provide:
• Diet with increased calories and protein; decrease sodium if oedema occurs

NB. That drug is one of abuse by athletes

Evaluate:
• Weight daily, notify clinician if weekly weight gain is greater than 2.5 kg
• BP 4 hrly
• Fluid balance oedema, be alert for decreasing urinary output, increasing oedema
• Growth rate in children since growth rate may be uneven (linear/bone growth) when used for extended period; premature closure of epiphyses in children
• Oedema, hypertension, cardiac symptoms, jaundice
• Mental status: affect, mood, behavioural changes, aggression
• Signs of masculinisation in female: increased libido, deepening of voice, breast tissue, enlarged clitoris, menstrual irregularities; male: gynaecomastia, impotence, testicular atrophy
• Hypercalcaemia: lethargy, polyuria, polydipsia, nausea, vomiting, constipation; drug may need to be decreased
• Hypoglycaemia in diabetics, since oral anticoagulant action is decreased

Teach patient/family:
• Drug needs to be combined with complete health plan: diet, rest, exercise
• To notify clinician if therapeutic response decreases
• Not to discontinue this medication abruptly
• Teach patient all aspects of drug usage, including changes in sex characteristics
• Women to report menstrual irregularities
• That 1−3 month course is necessary for response in breast cancer
• That drug can be abused

oxyphenbutazone (ophthalmic)

Tanderil
Func. class.: Non-steroidal anti-inflammatory drug
Chem. class.: Pyrazolone derivative
Legal class.: POM

Action: Inhibits prostaglandin synthesis by inhibiting an enzyme needed for biosynthesis; possesses analgesic, anti-inflammatory, antipyretic properties
Uses: Local treatment of ocular inflammation
Dosage and routes:
• *Adult:* Apply to inner surface of lower eyelid, 2−5 times a day
Available forms include: Eye ointment 10%
Side effects/adverse reactions:
EENT: Oedema of eyelid, redness of conjunctiva
Contraindications: Hypersensitivity, pregnancy, lactation, infants under 6 months of age
Precautions: Glaucoma
NURSING CONSIDERATIONS
Administer:
• Use aseptic technique
• Use within 1 month of opening tube
Evaluate:
• For eye, ear problems; blurred vision, tinnitus (may indicate toxicity)
Teach patient/family:
• To report blurred vision, or ringing, roaring in ears (may indicate toxicity)

oxytetracycline HCl

Berkmycen, Imperacin, Unimycin, Terramycin
Func. class.: Antibiotic, broad spectrum
Chem. class.: Tetracycline
Legal class.: POM

Action: Inhibits protein synthesis, phosphorylation in micro-organisms by binding to 30S ribosomal subunits, reversibly binding to 50S ribosomal subunits
Uses: Syphilis, gonorrhoea, Lyme disease, leptospirosis, infections due to *Brucella*, *Chlamydia*, *Mycoplasma* and *Rickettsiae* spp, other sensitive bacterial infections, exacerbations of chronic bronchitis, acne vulgaris
Dosage and routes:
• *Adult:* By mouth 250−500 mg 6 hrly
• *Child over 8 yr:* By mouth 25−50 mg/kg daily in divided doses 6 hrly
Acne
• *Adult:* By mouth 250 mg 3 times a day for 1−4 weeks then 250 mg twice a day
Available forms include: Tablets 250 mg; capsules 250 mg; mixture 125 mg/5 ml
Side effects/adverse reactions:
CNS: Raised intracranial pressure, headache
HAEM: Neutropenia, thrombocytopenia, haemolytic anaemia
EENT: Discolouration and enamel defects in developing teeth, oral candidiasis
GI: Nausea, vomiting, hepatotoxicity, stomatitis, pseudomembranous colitis
CV: Pericarditis
GU: Increased blood urea nitrogen, polyuria, polydipsia, renal failure

INTEG: Rash, photosensitivity, exfoliative dermatitis
Contraindications: Hypersensitivity to tetracyclines, children under 8 yr, pregnancy (3rd trimester), renal disease
Precautions: Hepatic disease, lactation, pregnancy
Pharmacokinetics:
By mouth: Peak 2−4 hr, half-life 6−9 hr; excreted in urine, bile, faeces, 10%−40% protein bound
Interactions/incompatibilities:
• Impaired oxytetracycline absorption: antacids, sodium bicarbonate, dairy products, iron products, alkali products
• Increased effect: anticoagulants
• Decreased effect: penicillins
• Nephrotoxicity: methoxyflurane
Lab. test interferences:
False positive: Urine glucose with Clinistix
False increase: Urinary catecholamines
NURSING CONSIDERATIONS
Assess:
• Fluid balance
• Bowel patterns
Administer:
• After specimens have been sent for culture and sensitivity
• 2 hr before or after laxative or ferrous products, 3 hr after antacid
• Not to children under 8
Evaluate:
• Therapeutic response: decreased temperature, absence of lesions, negative culture and sensitivity
• Allergic reactions: rash, itching, pruritus, angioneurotic oedema
• Nausea, vomiting, diarrhoea; administer anti-emetic, antacids as ordered
• Overgrowth of infection: increased temperature, malaise, redness, pain, swelling, drainage, perineal itching, diarrhoea, changes in cough or sputum
Teach patient/family:
• To avoid sun exposure since

burns may occur; sunscreen does not seem to decrease photosensitivity
• If diabetic to avoid use of Clinistix, Diastix, for urine glucose testing
• That all prescribed medication must be taken unless advised otherwise by clinician
• To avoid milk products for a few hours before and after taking tablets

---

oxytocin, synthetic

Syntocinon, combination product
Func. class.: Oxytocic
Chem. class.: Synthetic Hormone
Legal class.: POM

Action: Directly acts on myofibrils producing uterine contraction, breast stimulation
Uses: Stimulation of labour, induction; missed or incomplete abortion; postpartum bleeding
Dosage and routes:
Stimulation of labour
• *Adult:* IV infusion, as solution containing 1 unit/litre in dextrose 5% or other suitable diluent, 1 to 3 milliunits/min increase gradually until contractions occur every 2 to 5 min; rate should not exceed 12 milliunits/min
Incomplete abortion
• *Adult:* IV infusion, as solution containing 10 to 20 units/500 ml of dextrose 5% or other suitable diluent, 10 to 30 drops/min, increased in strength by 10−20 units/500 ml every hour; should not exceed 100 units/500 ml
Available forms include: Injection IV 2 units/2 ml, 5 units/ml, 10 units/ml and 50 units/5 ml
Side effects/adverse reactions:
CNS: Headache, lethargy, coma,

and convulsions (water intoxication)
GI: Nausea, vomiting
CV: Hypertension, subarachnoid, haemorrhage
GU: Uterine rupture, uterine spasm
MISC: Fetal asphyxia, neonatal jaundice
Contraindications: Hypersensitivity, severe toxaemia, cephalopelvic disproportion, hypertonic uterine inertia, mechanical obstruction to delivery, failed trial labour, fetal distress, placenta praevia, predisposition to amniotic fluid embolism or uterine rupture
Precautions: Hypertension, multiple pregnancy, high parity, abnormal presentation, previous Caesarean section
Pharmacokinetics:
IV: Onset 1 min, duration 30 min, half-life 12−17 min
Interactions/incompatibilities:
• May cause hypertension when used with vasopressors
NURSING CONSIDERATIONS
Assess:
• Baseline vital signs for mother and baby (if appropriate)
Administer:
• Do not administer through same line as blood/plasma
• By IV infusion
• With resuscitation equipment and drugs at hand
• With continuous monitoring
Evaluate:
• Fluid balance
• Contraction, fetal heart trace, BP, pulse, respiration
• BP, pulse; watch for changes that may indicate haemorrhage
• Respiratory rate, rhythm, depth; notify clinician of abnormalities
• Length, duration of contraction; report contractions lasting over 1 min or absence of contractions
Teach patient/family:
• To report increased blood loss, abdominal cramps, increased temperature or foul-smelling lochia

---

pamidronate disodium ▼

Aredia
Func. class.: Parathyroid agent (calcium regulator)
Chem. class.: Biphosphonate
Legal class.: POM

Action: Potent inhibitor of bone resorption, exact mechanism of action not yet established
Uses: Tumour-induced hypercalcaemia
Dosage and routes:
• *Adult:* Slow IV infusion, 15 to 90 mg, according to plasma calcium concentration as single infusion or in divided doses over 2−4 days
Available forms include: IV infusion concentrate 15 mg/5 ml
Side effects/adverse reactions:
CNS: Convulsions (due to electrolyte disturbances)
HAEM: Transient lymphocytopenia
SYST: Mild transient rise in body temperature
Contraindications: Hypersensitivity
Precautions: Pregnancy, renal insufficiency
NURSING CONSIDERATIONS
Administer:
• After appropriate parenteral/oral rehydration
• Dilute ampoule contents in a calcium free infusion solution and infuse slowly depending on concentration
• Dosage is determined by the patient's initial calcium level
• Total dosage may be given as a single infusion or in divided doses
Evaluate:
• Serum calcium levels start to decrease 24 to 28 hr after drug administration and maximum lowering

can be expected after 4 to 5 days. If normocalcaemia is not achieved within this period, a further dose may be given
• Duration of response varies. Treatment can be repeated when hypercalcaemia recurs
• Do not give as a bolus injection since severe local reactions and thrombophlebitis may occur.
• Transient asymptomatic hypocalcaemia is not uncommon; symptomatic hypocalcaemia is rare
• In patients with severe renal insufficiency, it is recommended that the chosen dose be administered as multiple doses

Perform/provide:
• Store ampoules in a refrigerator
• Do not store the diluted infusion
• Do not mix with calcium containing infusion solutions

---

pancreatin

Cotazym, Creon, Nutrizym GR, Pancrease, Pancrex, Pancrex V
Func. class.: Digestant
Chem. class.: Pancreatic enzyme concentrate — porcine
Legal class.: P or GSL

Action: Pancreatic enzyme needed for proper pancreatic functioning
Uses: Exocrine pancreatic secretion insufficiency in cystic fibrosis, pancreatectomy, total gastrectomy, chronic pancreatitis
Dosage and routes:
• Mixed with food (contents of capsules, granules, powder) or swallowed whole (capsules, tablets), doses providing 160 to 3300 units of protease activity, 5000 to 56,000 units lipase activity, 3300 to 60,000 units amylase activity
• Adjust according to size, number and consistency of stool, so that patient thrives; extra allowance may be required for snacks between meals
Available forms include: Tablets, capsules, granules and powder, providing varying amounts of protease, lipase and amylase activity
Side effects/adverse reactions:
GI: Anal soreness
GU: Hyperuricosuria, hyperuricaemia
INTEG: Rash, hypersensitivity
EENT: Buccal soreness
Contraindications: Hypersensitivity to pig protein
Interactions/incompatibilities:
• Concurrent antacids may dissolve enteric coatings

NURSING CONSIDERATIONS
Assess:
• For allergy to pork
Administer:
• After antacid or cimetidine; decreased pH inactivates drug
• Whole, not to be crushed, chewed (enteric coated)
• Low fat diet to decrease GI symptoms
• With or immediately before or after food
Evaluate:
• Therapeutic effect; dose may be adjusted freely depending on stools
Teach patient/family:
• All aspects of enzyme including side effects

---

pancuronium bromide

Pavulon
Func. class.: Non-depolarising muscle relaxant
Chem. class.: Synthetic curariform
Legal class.: POM

Action: Inhibits transmission of nerve impulses by binding with cholinergic receptor sites, antagonizing action of acetylcholine

Uses: Facilitation of endotracheal intubation, skeletal muscle relaxation during mechanical ventilation, surgery, or general anaesthesia

Dosage and routes:

• *Adult surgery:* IV 50−80 mcg/kg or 80−100 mcg/kg. Incremental doses: 10−20 mcg/kg

• *Child surgery:* Initial dose 60−100 mcg/kg. Incremental doses, 10−20 mcg/kg

• *Neonatal surgery:* IV 30−40 mcg/kg. As neonates are sensitive incremental doses should be adjusted according to initial response

• *Intensive care adults:* IV 60 mcg/kg every 1½ hr or even less frequently

• Doses should be reduced if given after suxamethonium

Available forms include: Injection IV 2 mg/ml

Side effects/adverse reactions:

CV: Tachycardia, increased, decreased BP

RESP: Prolonged apnoea, bronchospasm (rare)

EENT: Increased secretions

MS: Weakness due to prolonged skeletal muscle relaxation

Contraindications: Hypersensitivity, use before suxamethonium

Precautions: Pregnancy, reduced dose in renal disease, altered circulation time, hypothermia, electrolyte imbalances, dehydration, neuromuscular disease, respiratory disease, liver disease, carcinomatosis, myasthenia gravis

Pharmacokinetics:

IV: Onset 30−45 sec, peak 1½−5 min; metabolised (small amounts), excreted in urine (unchanged), duration 45−60 mins

Interactions/incompatibilities:

• Increased neuromuscular blockade: general anaesthetics, narcotic analgesics, diazepam, other muscle relaxants; also aminoglycosides, some polypeptide antibiotics (azlocillin, clindomycin, lincomycin, mezlocillin, polymyxins), β-blockers, diuretics, glyceryl trinitrate, lithium, magnesium salts (parenteral), MAOIs, metronidazole, nifedipine, phenytoin, quinidine, verapamil

• Decreased effect: proprandol, neostigmine, pyridostigmine, endrophonium, noradrenaline, adrenaline, potassium, sodium, or calcium chloride, heparin, azathioprine, theophylline, previous corticosteroid therapy

• Arrhythmias: tricyclic antidepressants

Administer:

• Using nerve stimulator by anaesthetist to determine neuromuscular blockade

• Anticholinesterase to reverse neuromuscular blockade

• By qualified persons, usually an anaesthetist

Treatment of overdose: Endrophonium or neostigmine, atropine, monitor vital signs; maintain mechanical ventilation until spontaneous breathing restored

NURSING CONSIDERATIONS

Assess:

• Baseline vital signs (BP, pulse, respirations, airway)

Perform/provide:

• Reassurance if communication is difficult during recovery from neuromuscular blockade

Administer:

• As IV bolus or by continous infusion under direction of anaesthetist

• Always preceded by sedation

Evaluate:

• Therapeutic response: paralysis of jaw, eyelid, head, neck, rest of body

• Recovery: decreased paralysis of face, diaphragm, leg, arm, rest of body

- Allergic reactions: rash, fever, respiratory distress, pruritus; drug should be discontinued
- Vital signs
- Fluid balance, retention
- Degree of respiratory depression due to muscle relaxation
- Ensure that patient is sedated as well as paralysed
- Use nerve stimulator to determine degree of neuromuscular block

Teach patient/family:
- Discuss effects of the drug with patient
- Reassure that sedation precedes paralysis

---

papaveretum

Omnopon (mixed opium alkaloids), Papaveretum

Func. class.: Narcotic analgesic
Chem. class.: Hydrochlorides of opium alkaloids containing morphine, codeine, noscapine and papaverine. *Note* Omnopon preparations do not contain noscapine
Legal class.: CD (Sch 2) POM

Action: Exerts marked narcotic effect on CNS and on the periphery as an antispasmodic
Uses: Pre-operative sedation, analgesia during and after surgery, relief of severe chronic pain
Dosage and routes:
Acute pain
- *Adult:* Subcutaneous, IM injection, 10−20 mg (according to weight), slow IV injection 2.5−10 mg, repeated 4 hrly if necessary
- *Infant up to 1 month:* 150 mcg/kg
- *Infant 1−12 months:* 200 mcg/kg
- *Child 1−12 yr:* 200−300 mcg/kg; when given IV, dose is generally quarter to half corresponding subcutaneous/IM dose

Pre-operative sedation
- *Adult:* Subcutaneous, IM injection, 10−20 mg, 45−60 min before anaesthesia
- *Child:* Single doses as above

Available forms include: Injection, 10 mg/ml, 20 mg/ml, 20 mg with hyoscine hydrobromide 400 mcg/ml

Side effects/adverse reactions:
RESP: Respiratory depression, cough suppression, pulmonary oedema (overdosage)
CNS: Drowsiness, alteration of pupillary responses, hallucinations, mood changes, dependence, confusion, neonatal convulsions
CV: Bradycardia, palpitations, postural hypotension
GI: Nausea, vomiting, reduced motility, constipation, dry mouth
GU: Urinary retention
INTEG: Urticaria, pruritus
SYSTEM: Hypothermia
Contraindications: Respiratory depression, obstructive airway disease, coma, hypersensitivity, treatment with MAOIs in last 2 weeks. Noscapine in papaveretum containing preparations is contraindicated in women of child-bearing potential
Precautions: History of drug abuse, acute alcoholism, convulsive disorders, respiratory insufficiency, head injury, raised intracranial pressure; dosage may need to be reduced for elderly or debilitated patients. Pregnancy, lactation, severe renal or hepatic impairment, biliary tract disorders, hypothyroidism, adrenocortical insufficiency, shock, prostatic hypertrophy, supraventricular tachycardia
Interactions/incompatibilities:
- Actions may be potentiated by other CNS depressants, such

as anaesthetic agents, alcohol. MAOIs, phenothiazines

Treatment of overdose: Signs are similar to overdosage with morphine. Supportive care. Administer naloxone for reversal

NURSING CONSIDERATIONS

Assess:
- Respiratory rate, BP
- Fluid balance
- Pain control and appropriateness of analgesia

Administer:
- Before the patient is in severe pain for the best effect
- With anti-emetic if nausea, vomiting, occur

Perform/provide:
- Storage in CDA cupboard (hospital)

Evaluate:
- Therapeutic response; decrease in pains
- Respiratory rate and depth for signs of respiratory depression
- Pulse, BP for signs of cardio-vascular depression
- Other side effects—nausea, vomiting, constipation, urinary retention
- Dependence on drug. Increased dose may be indicated

Teach patient/family:
- Avoid alcohol whilst taking drug
- Advise patient not to mobilise unaided
- Check with clinician before taking other medications
- Need for secure storage

paracetamol

Alvedon, Calpol, Disprol, Panadol, many combination products

Func. class.: Non-opioid analgesic
Chem. class.: Nonsalicylate, para aminophenol derivative
Legal class.: P, GSL

Action: Inhibition of prostaglandin synthesis; antipyretic action results from inhibition of hypothalamic heat-regulating centre

Uses: Mild to moderate pain or fever

Dosage and routes:
- *Adult and child over 12 yr:* By mouth 0.5−1 g 4−6 hrly, maximum 4 g in 24 hr
- *Child 3 months−1yr:* By mouth 60−120 mg
- *1−5 yr:* By mouth, 120−250 mg; rectal, 125−250 mg
- *6−12 yr:* By mouth 250−500 mg Doses given 4−6 hrly, maximum 4 doses in 24 hr

Available forms include: Tablets 500 mg, elixir (oral solution) 120 mg/5 ml, mixture (oral suspension) 120 mg/5 ml, 250 mg/ 5 ml, suppositories 125 mg

Side effects/adverse reactions:
HAEM: Blood dyscrasias (rare)
GI: Overdosage may produce nausea, vomiting, abdominal pain; delayed, progressive, hepato-toxicity leading to death
GU: Papillary necrosis (long-term use), nephrotoxicity (overdosage)
INTEG: Rash, urticaria

Contraindications: Hypersensitivity

Precautions: Hepatic disease, renal disease, chronic alcoholism

Pharmacokinetics:
By mouth: Onset 10−30 min, peak ½−2 hr, duration 4−6 hr. Metabolised by liver, excreted by kidneys, half-life 1−4 hr

Interactions/incompatibilities:
- Increased effects of: anti-

coagulants, chloramphenicol
• Increased risk of neutropenia: zidovudine
• Decreased effects of this drug: cholestyramine, oral contraceptives, narcotics, anticholinergics, anticonvulsants
• Increased effect of this drug: metoclopramide
• Increased toxicity: barbiturates, alcohol, rifampicin, anticonvulsants

Treatment of overdose: Gastric lavage, administer prompt IV acetylcysteine or oral methionine; further treatment based on plasma paracetamol concentrations 4 hr or more after ingestion. Antidotes are generally ineffective more than 15 hr after overdose

NURSING CONSIDERATIONS
Assess:
• Fluid balance; decreasing output may indicate renal failure (long-term therapy)
Administer:
• With food or milk to decrease gastric symptoms
Evaluate:
• Therapeutic response: absence of pain, fever
• For rash, blood disorders, acute pancreatitis
• Renal dysfunction: decreased urine output
Teach patient/family:
• Not to exceed recommended dosage; acute poisoning may result
• To read label on other non-prescribed medicines; many contain paracetamol

---

paraldehyde

Func. class.: Hypnotic/Sedative; Anticonvulsant
Chem. class.: Cyclic ether
Legal class.: POM

Action: CNS depressant; exact mechanism of action is unknown
Uses: Refractory seizures, status epilepticus
Dosage and routes:
• *Adult:* Deep IM injection 5–10 ml, no more than; IV 5 ml at any site infusion (requires specialist experience), 4–5 ml diluted to 4% solution; rectal 5–10 ml, as 10% enema in sodium chloride 0.9%
• *Child:* Deep IM injection, rectal (as 10% enema in sodium chloride 0.9%)
• *up to 3 months:* 0.5 ml
• *3–6 months:* 1 ml
• *6–12 months:* 1.5 ml
• *1–2 yr:* 2 ml
• *3–5 yr:* 3–4 ml
• *6–12 yr:* 5–6 ml
Available forms include: Injection
Side effects/adverse reactions:
CNS: Drowsiness
GI: Foul breath, local irritation, hepatotoxicity (overdosage)
GU: Nephrotoxicity (overdosage)
INTEG: Rash
CV: Hypotension, collapse
MISC: Pain, sterile abscess after IM injection
RESP: Pulmonary oedema, pulmonary haemorrhage
Contraindications: Hypersensitivity, old or discoloured product (may contain glacial acetic acid and lead to severe corrosive poisoning); do not give rectally in colitis
Precautions: Asthma, hepatic disease, pulmonary disease; avoid contact with rubber and plastic (use glass syringe) injection near sciatic or other nerves may cause nerve damage
Interactions/incompatibilities:
• Enhanced effect of paraldehyde: alcohol, CNS depressants, general anaesthetics, disulfiram
NURSING CONSIDERATIONS
Assess:
• Baseline vital signs including temperature

Administer:
• Use glass syringe (drug affects plastic)
• IM injection in deep large muscle mass to prevent tissue sloughing
• After conservative measures have been tried for insomnia
• Rectal after diluting in 200 ml 0.9% sodium chloride for enema

Perform/provide:
• Ventilation of room (drug is excreted via lungs)

Evaluate:
• Mental status: mood, alertness, affect, memory (long, short)
• Respiratory dysfunction; respiratory depression, character, rate, rhythm; hold drug if respirations are more than 12/min or if pupils are dilated

Teach patient/family:
• That physical dependency may result when used for extended periods of time
• To avoid driving, other activities that require alertness
• Not to discontinue medication quickly after long-term use, taper over several weeks
• Dangers of misuse

---

penicillamine

Distamine, Pendramine
Func. class.: Antirheumatic
Chem. class.: Chelating agent
Legal class.: POM

Action: A chelating agent which aids the elimination from the body of certain heavy metal ions by forming stable soluble complexes which can be excreted via kidney
Uses: Severe active or progressive rheumatoid arthritis, cystinuria, chronic active hepatitis, Wilson's disease, copper or lead poisoning
Dosage and routes: By mouth
Rheumatoid arthritis
• *Adult:* Initial dose 125−250 mg daily before food, for 1 month, then increase dose by this amount every 4−12 weeks until remission occurs. Usual maintenance dosage 500−750 mg daily, but up to 1.5 g or more daily may be required
• *Elderly:* Initial dose 50−125 mg increased in similar increments to maximum 1 g daily
• *Child:* Initial dose 50 mg daily before food, for 1 month, then increase dose at 4 week intervals to maintenance dose of 15−20 mg/kg daily
Drug to be discontinued if no improvement within 1 year
Wilson's disease
• *Adults:* 1.5−2 g daily in divided doses before food, reduced to 0.75−1 g daily once disease is controlled. Do not continue dose of 2 g daily for more than 1 yr
• *Elderly:* 20 mg/kg/day in divided doses before food
• *Child:* Up to 20 mg/kg/day in divided doses. Minimum 500 mg/day
Cystinuria: dissolution of stones
• *Adults:* 1−3 g daily in divided doses 30 min before food − urine cystine levels of not more than 200 mg/litre should be maintained
Prevention of cystine stones:
• *Adult:* 0.5−1 g at bedtime. Maintain fluid intake above 3 litres daily
• *Elderly and children:* No dosage range established, use the minimum dose to maintain urinary cystine level below 200 mg/litre
Lead poisoning
• *Adults:* 1−2 g daily in divided doses before meals until total daily urinary lead is less than 0.5 mg daily
• *Elderly and child:* 20 mg/kg daily in divided doses before meals
Chronic active hepatitis
• *Adults:* (Maintenance only) − 500 mg daily in divided doses before meals increasing to 1.25 g daily over 3 months. Monitor disease

status with periodic liver function tests

Available forms include: Tablets 50, 125, 250 mg

Side effects/adverse reactions:

HAEM: Agranulocytosis, severe thrombocytopenia, leucopenia

GI: Nausea, anorexia, taste loss, mouth ulcers

GU: Proteinuria, nephrotic syndrome, haematuria (rare)

INTEG: Rashes, pruritus, epidermolysis bullosa, increased skin friability, Stevens-Johnson syndrome, pemphigus

MS: Muscle weakness, joint pain

SYSTEM: Fever, myasthenia, lupus erythematosus

Contraindications: Hypersensitivity, lupus erythematosus, agranulocytosis, thrombocytopenia

Precautions: Renal impairment, pregnancy, portal hypertension; withdraw if platelets or WBC count low

Pharmacokinetics: Absorbed from GI tract, peak concentration in 1 hr. Rapidly excreted in urine, traces in plasma after 48 hr due to protein binding

Interactions/incompatibilities:

• Concomitant nephrotoxic or myelosuppressant drugs such as gold, antimalarials, cytotoxics and immunosuppressants

• Phenylbutazone, iron salts should not be given within 2 hr of penicillamine

Clinical assessment:

• Attempt dose reduction if remission is achieved in treatment of rheumatoid arthritis

• Full blood count weekly or two weekly in first 8 weeks of therapy and after each increase in dose, or monthly during maintenance

• Periodic liver function tests in chronic active hepatitis

• Urinalysis weekly initially and after each dosage increase, monthly during maintenance

NURSING CONSIDERATIONS

Administer:

• 1 hr before food or at bed time for maximum absorption

• Do not give iron or other heavy metals within 2 hr

• Withhold drug and inform clinician if haematuria presents

Evaluate:

• Urine—test weekly for proteinuria and haematuria

• Urine measurement for signs of renal failure

• For signs of side effects—nausea and vomiting, anorexia, fever, rash, loss of taste. Treat these as appropriate

• Patient's response to drug—any improvement in condition

Teach patient/family:

• That improvement in their condition may not occur for 6–12 weeks

• To check with clinician before taking any other medication

• Serious side effects—any which occur must be reported at once

• May experience metallic taste which will disappear

• If rashes, nausea, loss of appetite, mouth ulcers occur these should be reported

• Teach patient to test own urine (if appropriate) for protein or have regular testing via the clinician

• To carry penicillamine record card

• Importance of 4 weekly blood testing

• The difference between penicillamine and penicillin

• Need to drink 3 litres daily

pentaerythritol tetranitrate

Cardiacap, Mycardol
Func. class.: Vasodilator, coronary
Chem. class.: Nitrate
Legal class.: P

Action: Decreases vascular resistance and venous return, thus decreasing left ventricular work
Uses: Chronic stable angina pectoris, prophylaxis of angina pain as an adjunct to glyceryl trinitrate
Dosage and routes:
• *Adult:* By mouth 60 mg 3 to 4 times a day before meals SUS REL 30 mg every 12 hr
Available forms include: Capsules modified release 30 mg; tablets 30 mg
Side effects/adverse reactions:
CV: Postural hypotension, tachycardia, syncope, cyanosis, methaemoglobinaemia
GI: Nausea, vomiting
INTEG: Pallor, sweating, rash
CNS: Headache, flushing, dizziness, lethargy, drowsiness
Contraindications: Hypersensitivity to this drug or other nitrates, anaemia, increased intracranial pressure due to head trauma or cerebral haemorrhage, acute myocardial infarction
Precautions: Pregnancy, closed-angle glaucoma, hypotension
Pharmacokinetics:
By mouth: Onset 20−60 min, peak 4−8 hr
Modified release: Duration 12 hr. Metabolised by liver, excreted in faeces and urine
Interactions/incompatibilities:
• Increased effects: alcohol, β-blockers, narcotics, tricyclics antidepressants, diuretics, antihypertensives, general anaesthetics
• Decreased effects: sympathomimetics, acetylcholine, histamine
NURSING CONSIDERATIONS
Assess:
• BP, pulse, respirations before beginning therapy
Administer:
• Orally before meals
Evaluate:
• Therapeutic response, stabilizing of angina pectoris
• Effect of any other drug therapy
• Pain — duration, character, activity being performed
• Headache, lethargy and nausea, if at commencement of treatment should be transient
• Side effects: toxicity — cyanosis, syncope, methaemoglobin-aernia, rash, servere headache fall in blood pressure, dizziness, palpitation
Perform/provide:
• Suitable physical activity to encourage healthier living
Teach patient/family:
• To give up smoking and encourage a healthy diet and physical activity
• To avoid driving and hazardous activities if dizziness occurs
• Not to drink alcohol
• To take other medication only if directed by clinician
• To report palpitations or vomiting immediately

pentamidine isethionate

Pentacarinat
Func. class.: Antiprotozoal
Chem. class.: Aromatic diamidine derivative
Legal class.: POM

Action: Interferes with DNA/RNA synthesis in protozoa

Uses: *Pneumocystis carinii* infections. Visceral leishmaniasis, cutaneous leishmaniasis, trypanosomiasis

Dosage and routes:

Pneumocystis carnii

• *Adult and child:* Slow IV infusion/deep IM injection 4 mg/kg daily for 2 weeks

• Inhalation, 600 mg daily via a suitable nebuliser system; for prophylaxis, 300 mg every 4 weeks

Visceral leishmaniasis

• Deep IM 3−4 mg/kg alternate days to maximum total of 10 injections. Repeat if required

Cutaneous leishmaniasis

• Deep IM 3−4 mg/kg, once or twice weekly

Trypanosomiasis

• Deep IM/slow IV infusion 4 mg/kg daily or alternate days to total of 7−10 injections

Available forms include: Injection 300 mg/vial; nebuliser solution 300 mg/bottle

Side effects/adverse reactions:

CV: Hypotension, cardiac arrhythmias, ventricular tachycardia, hypertension, syncope, flushing

HAEM: Anaemia, leucopenia, thrombocytopenia

INTEG: Sterile abscess, pain at injection site (IM); pruritus, urticaria, rash

GU: Acute renal failure, azotaemia

GI: Nausea, vomiting, taste disturbances, hepatic impairment, acute pancreatitis

CNS: Disorientation, hallucinations, dizziness

META: Hyperkalaemia, hypocalcaemia, hypoglycaemia, hyperglycaemia

RESP: Cough, bronchospasm, or pneumothorax (inhalation route)

Precautions: Blood dyscrasias, hepatic disease, renal disease (reduce dose), hyperglycaemia, hypoglycaemia, hypertension, hypotension, pregnancy, lactation

Pharmacokinetics: Elimination half-life about 6 hr (IV), 9 hr (IM); accumulates in liver, kidney. Small amounts excreted unchanged in urine. Half-life in lung fluid prolonged; about 5% of inhaled dose absorbed

Clinical assessment:

• Blood studies, fasting blood glucose (daily during therapy and periodically afterwards); full blood count, platelets (daily); serum calcium (weekly); serum electrolytes (daily)

• ECG for cardiac dysrhythmias

• Liver function tests: aspartate aminotransferase, alanine aminotransferase bilirubin, alkaline phosphatase

• Renal studies daily: urinalysis, blood urea nitrogen, creatinine

NURSING CONSIDERATIONS

Assess:

• Bowel pattern

• Fluid balance

• Allergies before treatment, reaction of each medication; place allergies on nursing care plan; notify all people giving drugs

Administer:

• Direct bolus injection should be avoided. Intramuscular injections should be deep and preferably given into the buttock

• Patients should be supine during parenteral administration

• Inhaled bronchodilators prior to nebulised solution

Perform/provide:

• Storage in refrigerator for reconstituted solution

Evaluate:

• Therapeutic response: decreased temperature, ability to breathe

• BP during administration and at intervals during treatment

• Bowel pattern during treatment

• Sterile abscess, pain at injection site

• Respiratory status: rate, character, wheezing, dyspnoea
• Fluid balance; report haematuria, oliguria
• Any patient with compromised renal system; drug is excreted slowly in poor renal system function; toxicity may occur rapidly
• Dizziness, confusion, hallucination

Teach patient/family:
• To report sore throat, fever, fatigue, could indicate superimposed infection

---

pentazocine HCl/ pentazocine lactate

Fortral
Func. class.: Narcotic analgesic
Chem. class.: Synthetic benzomorphan
Legal class.: CD (Sch 3) POM

Action: Inhibits ascending pain pathways in CNS, increases pain threshold, alters pain perception
Uses: Moderate to severe pain
Dosage and routes:
• *Adult:* By mouth, pentazocine HCl 50−100 mg 3−4 hrly as needed; IV/IM/subcutaneous injection, pentazocine 30−60 mg (as lactate) 3−4 hrly as needed, dose not to exceed 1 mg/kg (subcutaneous, IM) or 0.5 mg/kg (IV); rectal, pentazocine 50 mg (as lactate) up to 4 times daily
• *Child 1−6 yr:* IM/subcutaneous injection, pentazocine (as lactate) 1 mg/kg; IV, pentazocine (as lactate) 0.5 mg/kg
• *Child 6−12 yr:* By mouth, pentazocine HCl 25 mg 3−4 hrly as needed; IM/subcutaneous injection, pentazocine (as lactate) 1 mg/kg; IV, pentazocine (as lactate) 0.5 mg/kg

Available forms include: Injection, pentazocine (as lactate) 30 mg/ml; suppositories, pentazocine (as lactate) 50 mg; capsules, pentazocine HCl 50 mg; tablets, pentazocine HCl 25 mg

Side effects/adverse reactions:
CNS: Drowsiness, sleep disturbances, dizziness, confusion, headache, hallucinations, sedation, paraesthesia, mood changes, raised intracranial pressure, convulsions, coma (overdosage), dependence
GI: Nausea, vomiting, dry mouth, constipation
GU: Urinary retention, biliary spasm
INTEG: Sweating, flushing, pruritus, local damage at injection site
EENT: Visual disturbances
CV: Tachycardia, hypotension, transient hypertension
RESP: Respiratory depression
Contraindications: Hypersensitivity, dependence (narcotic), respiratory depression, raised intracranial pressure, head injury, hypertension, asthma, heart failure, porphyria
Precautions: Pregnancy, lactation, myocardial infarction (acute), hepatic disease, renal disease, phaeochromocytoma, hypothyroidism, adrenocortical insufficiency, prostatic hypertrophy, inflammatory or obstructive bowel disease

Pharmacokinetics:
By mouth, about 50% available, peak 1−3 hr
Subcutaneous/IM: Onset 15−30 min, peak 1−2 hr, duration 2−4 hr
IV: Onset 2−3 min, duration 4−6 hr
Metabolised by liver, excreted by kidneys

Interactions/incompatibilities:
• Effects may be increased with other CNS depressants: alcohol,

anaesthetics, sedative/hypnotics, antipsychotics
• Enhanced clearance in smokers (decreased effect)
• May decrease effects of other opioids (weak antagonist properties)
• Interacts with MAOIs (enhanced toxicity)

Treatment of overdose: Naloxone, gastric lavage, supportive care including anticonvulsants as required

NURSING CONSIDERATIONS

Assess:
• Fluid balance
• Respiratory function
• Pain control and appropriateness of analgesia

Administer:
• With anti-emetic if nausea, vomiting occur
• When pain is beginning to return; determine dosage interval by patient response

Perform/provide:
• Storage in CD cupboard (hospital)
• Assistance with ambulation, only after dose has taken effect in case of dizziness
• Safety measures: cot sides, night light, callbell within easy reach as necessary

Evaluate:
• Therapeutic response: decrease in pain
• CNS changes: dizziness, drowsiness, hallucinations, euphoria, level of consciousness, pupil reaction
• Decrease in urinary output: may indicate urinary retention
• Allergic reactions: rash, urticaria
• Respiratory dysfunction: respiratory depression, character, rate, rhythm; notify clinician if respirations are less than 12/min
• Need for pain medication, physical dependence

Teach patient/family:
• To report any symptoms of CNS changes, allergic reactions
• That physical dependency may result when used for extended periods of time
• Avoid potentially hazardous tasks until certain that dizziness does not occur
• Measures to reduce risk of constipation
• Withdrawal symptoms may occur: nausea, vomiting, cramps, fever, faintness, anorexia if drug is suddenly stopped after a long period
• Not to exceed prescribed dosage without consulting clinician

---

pericyazine

Neulactil
Func. class.: Antipsychotic
Chem. class.: Phenothiazine derivative (Group 2)
Legal class.: POM

Action: Depresses cerebral cortex, hypothalamus, limbic system, which controls aggression; blocks neurotransmission produced by dopamine at synapse; exhibits strong α-adrenergic, anticholinergic blocking action

Uses: Behavioural disturbances, schizophrenia and related psychotic disorders, short-term adjunctive treatment of severe anxiety, psychomotor agitation

Dosage and routes:
• *Adult:* By mouth 15−30 mg (elderly 5−10 mg) daily (anxiety, agitation); give in 2 unequal doses, taking the larger at bedtime; adjust according to response
• By mouth, 75 mg daily in divided doses (psychoses, severe illness); increase by 25 mg at weekly intervals; usual maintenance dose up to 300 mg daily
• *Child:* By mouth initially 0.5 mg

daily for child weighing 10 kg; increased by 1 mg for each additional 5 kg body weight up to maximum 10 mg daily; maintenance dose not to exceed twice initial dose

Available forms include: Tablets 2.5, 10, 25 mg; syrup 10 mg/5 ml

Side effects/adverse reactions:

CNS: Extrapyramidal symptoms, tardive dyskinesia, sedation, drowsiness, apathy, nightmares, insomnia, depression, agitation

CV: Arrhythmias, hypotension, ECG changes

HAEM: Agranulocytosis, leucopenia, haemolytic anaemia

GU: Difficulty with micturition, menstrual disturbances, impotence

ENDO: Galactorrhoea, gynaecomastia, weight gain

SYST: Neuroleptic malignant syndrome

INTEG: Pallor, photosensitisation, contact sensitization, rashes

EENT: Dry mouth, nasal congestion, blurred vision, corneal and lens opacities

GI: Constipation, jaundice

Contraindications: Coma caused by CNS depressants, bone marrow depression, closed-angle glaucoma, hypersensitivity

Precautions: Cardiovascular or cerebrovascular disease, respiratory disease, parkinsonism, epilepsy, phaeochromocytoma, renal or hepatic impairment, history of jaundice or leucopenia, myasthenia gravis, hypothyroidism, elderly patients, pregnancy, lactation, prostatic hypertrophy

Pharmacokinetics: None known

Interactions/incompatibilities:

• Effects may be increased with other CNS depressants: alcohol, sedative/hypnotics

• Increased antimuscarinic effect, possibly reduced antipsychotic effect with other antimuscarinic drugs

• Decreased absorption with antacids, antiparkinsonian agents, lithium

• Decreased effect of amphetamines, levodopa, clonidine, guanethidine, adrenaline, oral hypoglycaemics

• Possible encephalopathy with desferrioxamine

Clinical assessment:

• Periodic eye, skin examinations on long-term therapy

Treatment of overdose:

• Lavage, supportive care

Lab. test interferences:

False positive: Pregnancy tests

NURSING CONSIDERATIONS

Assess:

• Fluid balance

Administer:

• Antimuscarinic antiparkinsonian agent may be prescribed if extrapyramidal symptoms appear

Perform/provide:

• Urinalysis before and during prolonged therapy

• Supervised ambulation, until stabilised on medication, do not involve in strenuous exercise programme because fainting is possible; patient should not stand still for long periods of time

• Increased fluids to prevent constipation

• Sips of water, mouthwashes for dry mouth

Evaluate:

• For dizziness, faintness, palpitations, tachycardia on rising

• For extrapyramidal symptoms including akathisia (inability to sit still, no pattern to movement), tardive dyskinesia (bizarre movements of jaw, mouth, tongue, extremities), pseudoparkinsonism (rigidity, tremors, pill rolling, shuffling gait)

• For constipation, urinary retention daily; if these occur, increase bulk, water in diet

• Affect, orientation, level of consciousness, reflexes, gait, coordination, sleep pattern; report any disturbances to clinician

• Therapeutic response: decrease in emotional excitement, hallucinations, delusions, paranoia, reorganisation of patterns of thought, speech

Teach patient/family:

• That orthostatic hypotension occurs frequently, and to rise from sitting or lying position gradually

• To remain lying down after IM injection for at least 30 min

• To avoid hot baths, hot showers since hypotension may occur

• To avoid abrupt withdrawal of this drug, drugs should be withdrawn slowly

• To avoid non-prescribed medication (cough, hayfever, cold) unless approved by clinician, since serious drug interactions may occur; avoid use with alcohol or CNS depressants, increased drowsiness may occur

• To use sunscreen during sun exposure to prevent burns

• Importance of compliance with drug regimen

• To report sore throat, malaise, fever, bleeding, mouth sores; if these occur, full blood count should be done and drug discontinued

---

perindopril tert-butylamine

Conversyl
Func. class.: Antihypertensive
Chem. class.: Angiotensin-converting enzyme inhibitor
Legal class.: POM

Action: Inhibits the conversion of angiotensin I to vasoconstrictive angiotensin II and reduces degradation of vasodilatory bradykinin

Uses: Essential hypertension where standard therapy is ineffective or inappropriate; adjunct in heart failure

Dosage and routes:

Hypertension

• *Adult:* By mouth, initially, perindopril 2 mg/day as tert-butylamine salt increasing to maintenance dose of 4 to 8 mg/day which may be combined with diuretic therapy. Maximum daily dose 8 mg

• *Elderly:* Initiate under close supervision

Heart failure

• *Adult:* By mouth, initially perindopril 2 mg in the morning, under close hospital supervision, with a loop diuretic; increase if necessary to usual maintenance dose of 4 mg

Available forms include: Tablets perindopril 2 mg, 4 mg (as tert-butylamine salt)

Side effects/adverse reactions:

HAEM: Decreases in haemoglobin, red cells and platelets

CV: Hypotension (with initial doses, especially with concurrent diuretics)

CNS: Fatigue, asthenia, malaise, headache, mood and sleep disturbances

GU: Proteinuria, increased blood urea and creatinine

RESP: Cough

GI: Taste impairment, epigastric discomfort, nausea, abdominal pain

INTEG: Skin rashes, pruritus, flushing, angioneurotic oedema

Contraindications: Bilateral renal artery stenosis (risk of renal failure), hypersensitivity, pregnancy, lactation, or in women of childbearing potential unless protected by effective contraception

Precautions: Renal insufficiency (reduce dose), peripheral vascular disease, atherosclerosis

Pharmacokinetics: Perindopril acts

through its active metabolite perindoprilat, the other metabolites being inactive

Interactions/incompatibilities

• Increased hypotensive effect: diuretics and other antihypertensives, neuroleptics, tricyclic antidepressants, anaesthetics
• Increased plasma concentrations of: lithium, potassium

Clinical assessment:

• The doses should be titrated against blood pressure to achieve optimum control
• It is recommended that diuretic therapy is discontinued 3 days before starting treatment, if required, the diuretic should be reintroduced at the lowest dose
• Potassium sparing diuretics should be avoided or used with extreme caution
• Assess renal function before and during treatment where appropriate
• Combination of potassium supplements or potassium sparing diuretics with perindopril is not recommended
• The dose should be taken before a meal

NURSING CONSIDERATIONS

Assess:

• Renal and liver function tests before therapy and occasionally during treatment

Evaluate:

• Pulse and blood pressure regularly until therapeutic response obtained; lower blood pressure
• Oedema in feet and legs
• Input and output of fluids check for fluid retention
• Effect of any other medication
• Hypotension
• Symptoms of congestive cardiac failure

Teach patient/family:

• To take other medication only if directed by clinician
• To report oedema

• To avoid driving or use of machinery until therapy establish
• To report oliguria and any other renal changes

---

perphenazine

Fentazin, combination product
Func. class.: Antipsychotic
Chem. class.: Phenothiazine-piperidine
Legal class.: POM

Action: Depresses cerebral cortex, hypothalamus, limbic system, which control activity, aggression; blocks neurotransmission produced by dopamine at synapse; exhibits strong α-adrenergic, anticholinergic blocking action; as antiemetic inhibits medullary chemoreceptor trigger zone

Uses: Psychotic disorders, schizophrenia, short-term adjunctive treatment of severe anxiety, psychomotor agitation, nausea, vomiting

Dosage and routes:

Nausea/vomiting/hiccups/alcoholism

• *Adult and child over 14 yr:* By mouth initially 4 mg 3 times daily adjusted according to response to a maximum of 24 mg daily
• *Elderly:* By mouth quarter to half usual adult dose

Available forms include: Tablets 2, 4 mg

Side effects/adverse reactions:

CNS: Extrapyramidal symptoms especially dystonia, tardive dyskinesia; seizures, headache, drowsiness, confusion, sedation, agitation, insomnia, paradoxical excitement

HAEM: Anaemia, leucopenia, agranulocytosis

INTEG: Rash, photosensitivity

EENT: Blurred vision, dry mouth,

nasal congestion, corneal and lens opacities, retinopathy
GI: Constipation, jaundice
GU: Urinary retention, impotence, amenorrhoea
CV: Orthostatic hypotension, arrhythmias, ECG changes (prolongation of QT interval and T-wave changes), tachycardia
ENDO: Galactorrhoea, gynaecomastia, weight gain
SYST: Neuroleptic malignant syndrome, hypothermia

Contraindications: Hypersensitivity, blood dyscrasias, coma, child below 14 yr, bone marrow depression

Precautions: Pregnancy, lactation, renal failure, hypothyroidism, hepatic disease, arrhythmias, cardiac failure, coronary artery disease, severe respiratory disease, epilepsy, Parkinson's disease, myasthenia gravis, personal or family history of closed-angle glaucoma, phaeochromocytoma, prostatic hypertrophy, elderly patients, especially during extreme climatic conditions

Pharmacokinetics:
By mouth: Onset erratic, peak 2–4 hr
Metabolised by liver, excreted in urine, enters breast milk

Interactions/incompatibilities:
• Oversedation: other CNS depressants such as alcohol, analgesics, sedative/hypnotics
• Decreased absorption: antacids, tea, coffee (concurrent administration)
• Decreased effects of: lithium, levodopa, anticonvulsants, oral hypoglycaemics, adrenaline and other sympathomimetics, guanethidine, clonidine
• Increased effects of: quinidine, diazoxide, neuromuscular blockers, corticosteroids, digoxin
• Increased anticholinergic effects: anticholinergics

Lab. test interferences:
False positive: Pregnancy tests
Treatment of overdose: Lavage, supportive care

NURSING CONSIDERATIONS
Assess:
• Fluid balance
Administer:
• Orally, dose titrated to patient's requirements
Perform/provide:
• Urinalysis before and during prolonged therapy
• Supervised ambulation until stabilised on medication; do not involve in strenuous exercise programme because fainting is possible; patient should not stand still for long periods of time
• Increased fluids to prevent constipation
• Sips of water for dry mouth
Evaluate:
• Therapeutic response: decrease in emotional excitement, hallucinations, delusions, paranoia, reorganisation of patterns of thought, speech
• Affect, orientation, level of consciousness, reflexes, gait, coordination, sleep pattern disturbances
• Dizziness, faintness, palpitations, tachycardia on rising
• Extrapyramidal symptoms including motor restlessness (inability to sit still, no pattern to movements), tardive dyskinesia (bizarre movements of jaw, mouth, tongue, extremities), pseudoparkinsonism (rigidity, tremors, pill rolling, shuffling gait)
• Constipation, urinary retention daily; if these occur, increase bulk, water in diet
Teach patient/family:
• That postural hypotension occurs frequently, and to rise from sitting or lying position gradually
• To remain lying down after IM

injection for at least 30 min
• To avoid hot showers, or baths since hypotension may occur
• To avoid abrupt withdrawal of this drug, drugs should be withdrawn slowly
• To avoid non-prescribed preparations (cough, hayfever, cold) unless approved by clinician since serious drug interactions may occur; avoid use with alcohol or CNS depressants, increased drowsiness may occur
• To use a sunscreen during sun exposure to prevent burns
• Importance of compliance with drug regimen
• About necessity for meticulous oral hygiene since oral candidiasis may occur
• To report sore throat, malaise, fever, bleeding, mouth sores; if these occur, full blood count should be drawn and drug discontinued

---

pethidine HCl

Pethidine-Roche
Func. class.: Narcotic analgesic
Chem. class.: Opioid, phenylpiperidine derivative
Legal class.: CD (Sch 2) POM

Action: Inhibits ascending pain pathways in CNS, increases pain threshold, alters pain perception
Uses: Moderate to severe pain, peri-operative analgesia, obstetric analgesia
Dosage and routes:
Pain
• *Adult:* By mouth 50−150 mg every 4 hr as needed; subcutaneous/IM 25−100 mg every 4 hr as needed; IV 25−50 mg every 4 hr as needed
• *Child:* By mouth/subcutaneous/ IM 0.5−2 mg/kg every 4 hr as needed

Peri-operatively
• *Adult:* IM 25−100 mg 1 hr before surgery, IV 10−25 mg as needed (adjunct to nitrous oxide/oxygen)
• *Child:* IM 0.5−2 mg/kg 1 hr before surgery
Obstetric analgesia
• Subcutaneous/IM 50−100 mg, repeat after 1−3 hr as needed, maximum 400 mg in 24 hr
Available forms include: Injection 10 mg/ml, 50 mg/ml; tablets 50 mg
Side effects/adverse reactions:
CNS: Drowsiness, dizziness, confusion, headache, sedation, CNS stimulation, mood changes, convulsions, coma (overdosage), raised intracranial pressure, dependence
GI: Nausea, vomiting, dry mouth, constipation
GU: Urinary retention, biliary spasm
INTEG: Sweating, flushing, pruritus, local reaction at injection site
EENT: Visual disturbances
CV: Palpitations, bradycardia, hypotension
RESP: Respiratory depression
Contraindications: Hypersensitivity, coma, obstructive airways disease
Precautions: Dependence, pregnancy, lactation, head injury or increased intracranial pressure, adrenocortical insufficiency, biliary tract disorders, shock, respiratory depression, hepatic disease, renal disease, neonates, premature babies, hypothyroidism, prostatic hypertrophy, supraventricular tachycardia, elderly or debilitated, cancer, sickle cell disease
Pharmacokinetics:
By mouth: Onset 15 min, peak 1 hr, duration 2−4 hr
Subcutaneous/IM: Onset 10 min, peak 1 hr, duration 2−4 hr
IV: Onset 5 min, duration 2 hr
Metabolised by liver (to active/

inactive metabolites), excreted by kidneys, excreted in breast milk

Interactions/incompatibilities:
• Effects may be increased with other CNS depressants: alcohol, anaesthetics, narcotics, sedative/hypnotics, antipsychotics
• Interacts with MAOIs (enhanced toxicity)

Treatment of overdose: Naloxone, gastric lavage, supportive care including anticonvulsants as required

NURSING CONSIDERATIONS

Assess:
• Respiratory rate, BP
• Pain control and appropriateness of analgesia

Administer:
• With anti-emetic if nausea, vomiting occur
• When pain is beginning to return; determine dosage interval by patient response

Perform/provide:
• Storage in CD cupboard (hospital)

Evaluate:
• Therapeutic response: decrease in pain
• CNS changes: dizziness, drowsiness, hallucinations, level of consciousness, pupil reaction
• Allergic reactions: rash, urticaria
• Respiratory dysfunction: respiratory depression
• Side effects—nausea, vomiting, constipation urinary retention
• Need for pain medication, physical dependence, tolerance

Teach patient/family:
• To report any symptoms of CNS changes, allergic reactions
• Advise patient not to mobilise unsupervised
• Need for secure storage

phenazocine hydrobromide

Narphen
Func. class.: Narcotic analgesic
Chem. class.: Synthetic benzomorphan
Legal class.: CD (Sch 2) POM

Action: Inhibits ascending pain pathways in CNS, increases pain threshold, alters pain perception; considered to be less sedating than morphine

Uses: Severe pain

Dosage and routes:
• By mouth or sublingually, 5 mg 4–6 hrly when necessary; maximum single dose, 20 mg
Available forms include: Tablets 5 mg

Side effects/adverse reactions:
RESP: Respiratory depression, cough suppression
CV: Hypotension
CNS: Drowsiness, dizziness, dependence
GI: Nausea, reduced motility, constipation, vomiting, dry mouth
GU: Urinary retention
INTEG: Pruritus, sweating

Contraindications: Hypotension, myxoedema, respiratory depression, obstructive airways disease, coma, convulsive disorders, delirium tremens, alcoholism

Precautions: Labour (may cause neonatal respiratory depression), history of drug abuse, renal impairment, head injury, raised intracranial pressure; dosage may need to be reduced for elderly patients, in hepatic disease, or hypothyroidism

Pharmacokinetics: Onset within 20 min, duration 5–6 hr

Interactions/incompatibilities:
• MAOIs (increased toxicity)
• Enhanced effect with narcotic

analgesics, sedatives/hypnotics, anaesthetics

Treatment of overdose: Naloxone, supportive care

NURSING CONSIDERATIONS

Assess:
• Pain control and effectiveness of analgesia
• Respiratory function, baseline
• Blood pressure baseline
• Urinary output

Administer:
• Sublingually as prescribed
• Before or when pain recurs
• With anti-emetic if indicated

Perform/provide:
• Safe environment (potent analgesic). Patient not to mobilise until drug has taken effect as dizziness may occur
• Storage in CD cupboard (hospital)

Evaluate:
• CNS and respiratory function as drug is a respiratory depressant
• BP
• Urinary output for retention
• Effectiveness of pain control
• Tolerance and/or dependence

Teach patient/family:
• Not to exceed the prescribed dose without medical advice
• To report signs of CNS disturbance
• To avoid potentially hazardous tasks until drug has taken effect without dizziness occurring
• That physical dependence may result if taken for long periods and then stopped suddenly
• Need for safe storage

phenelzine sulphate

Nardil
Func. class.: Antidepressant (MAOI)
Chem. class.: Hydrazine
Legal class.: POM

Action: Increases concentrations of endogenous adrenaline, noradrenaline, serotonin, dopamine in storage sites in CNS by inhibition of monoamine oxidase; increased concentration reduces depression

Uses: Depression, especially where phobic symptoms are present, when uncontrolled by other means

Dosage and routes:
• *Adult:* By mouth 15 mg 3 times daily, may increase to 15 mg 4 times daily if necessary (up to 30 mg 3 times daily in hospital), reduced to lowest possible maintenance dose once response occurs

Available forms include: Tablets phenelzine 15 mg (as sulphate)

Side effects/adverse reactions:
HAEM: Blood dyscrasias
CNS: Dizziness, drowsiness, peripheral neuropathy, paraesthesia, headache, anxiety, tremors, weakness, euphoria, mania, insomnia, fatigue, convulsions
GI: Constipation, dry mouth, nausea, vomiting, increased appetite, weight gain, jaundice
GU: Micturition difficulty, impotence, delayed ejaculation
INTEG: Rash, sweating, purpura
CV: Orthostatic hypotension, arrhythmias, hypertensive crisis (interaction with drugs or food)
EENT: Blurred vision

Contraindications: Hypersensitivity to MAOIs, cerebrovascular disease, hepatic disease, phaeochromocytoma, children, concurrent use of tricyclic antidepressants

Precautions: Suicidal patients,

epilepsy, cardiovascular disease, blood dyscrasias, renal disease, diabetes mellitus, pregnancy, elderly or agitated patients

Pharmacokinetics: Metabolised by liver, excreted by kidneys

Interactions/incompatibilities:

• Increased pressor effects (hypertensive crisis): indirect acting sympathomimetics, dopamine, levodopa, amphetamines, anoectics, tyramine-containing foods

• Increased effects of: alcohol, barbiturates and other hypnotics, antimuscarinics, diuretics, antihypertensives, hypoglycaemics

• Hypotension, convulsions: tricyclic antidepressants, pethidine and other opioid analgesics (administer in reduced dose initially)

Treatment of overdose: Lavage, symptomatic care (IV fluids, hydrocortisone for hypotension, phentolamine for hypertension, chlorpromazine for restlessness)

NURSING CONSIDERATIONS

Assess:

• Baseline BP

Administer:

• Increased fluids, bulk in diet if constipation, urinary retention occur

• With food or milk or GI symptoms

• Dosage at bedtime if oversedation occurs during day

• Frequent sips of water for dry mouth

Perform/provide:

• Assistance with ambulation during beginning therapy since drowsiness/dizziness occurs

• Check patient compliance

Evaluate:

• BP (lying, standing), pulse; if systolic BP drops 20 mmHg notify clinician

• Toxicity: increased headache, palpitation, discontinue drug immediately; prodromal signs of hypertensive crisis

• Mental status: mood, alertness, affect, memory (long, short); increase in psychiatric symptoms

• Urinary retention, constipation, oedema, take weight weekly

• Withdrawal symptoms: headache, nausea, vomiting, muscle pain, weakness

Teach patient/family:

• That therapeutic effects may take 1−4 weeks

• To avoid driving or other activities requiring alertness

• Give patient MAOI warning card to be carried at all times

• To avoid alcohol ingestion, CNS depressants or non-prescribed drugs: cold, weight, hay fever, cough syrup

• Not to discontinue medication quickly after long-term use

• To avoid high tyramine foods: cheese, sour cream, beer, wine, pickled products, liver, raisins, bananas, figs, avocados, meat tenderisers, chocolate, yoghurt; bovril, caffeine containing products, oxo, marmite, broad beans, heavy red wines

• Report headache, palpitation, neck stiffness

---

phenobarbitone, phenobarbitone sodium

Gardenal Sodium

Func. class.: Anticonvulsant
Chem. class.: Barbiturate
Legal class.: CD (Sch 3) POM

Action: Decreases impulse transmission, increases seizure threshold at cerebral cortex level

Uses: All forms of epilepsy (except absence seizures), status epilepticus, febrile seizures in children

Dosage and routes:

Phenobarbitone and phenobarbitone sodium are given in the same doses

Seizures
• *Adult:* By mouth 60−180 mg daily at bedtime; IM/IV 50−200 mg repeated after 6 hr if necessary; maximum dose 600 mg daily
• *Child:* By mouth 5−8 mg/kg daily; IM 15 mg/kg, followed by therapy by mouth if necessary
Status epilepticus
• *Adult:* IV 400−800 mg
Available forms include: Elixir (phenobarbitone) 15 mg/5 ml; tablets (phenobarbitone) 15, 30, 60, 100 mg; tablets (phenobarbitone sodium) 30, 60 mg; injection (phenobarbitone sodium) 200 mg/ml

Side effects/adverse reactions:
HAEM: Folate deficiency, megaloblastic anaemia
CNS: Paradoxical stimulation drowsiness, sedation, lethargy, hangover, dependence, coma (overdosage)
GI: Nausea, vomiting
INTEG: Rash, urticaria, Stevens-Johnson syndrome, angioneurotic oedema, local pain at injection site
RESP: Respiratory depression (overdosage)

Contraindications: Hypersensitivity to barbiturates, porphyria
Precautions: Impaired renal or hepatic function (reduce dose), respiratory depression, elderly, debilitated, children, pregnancy, lactation

Pharmacokinetics:
By mouth: Onset 20−60 min, peak 8−12 hr, duration 6−10 hr, metabolised by liver, excreted by kidneys, excreted in breast milk, half-life 53−118 hr

Interactions/incompatibilities:
• Increased effects: CNS depressants, alcohol, chloramphenicol, valproic acid
• Decreased effects: antidepressants, antipsychotic agents
• Enhances hepatic metabolism and may decrease effects of: anticoagulants, tricyclic antidepressants, calcium channel blockers, corticosteroids, chloramphenicol, cyclosporin, oral contraceptives, griseofulvin, metronidazole, phenytoin

Clinical assessment:
• Therapeutic level 10−40 mg/litre
Treatment of overdose: Supportive care

NURSING CONSIDERATIONS
Assess:
• Mental status
Perform/provide:
• Regular assessment of respiratory status
Evaluate:
• Control of seizures
• Mental status: mood, alertness affect, memory (long, short)
• Respiratory depression
• Blood dyscrasias: fever, sore throat, bruising, rash, jaundice
Teach patient/family:
• All aspects of drug administration: action, dose, route; when to notify clinician
• Not to withdraw medication abruptly

---

phenoperidine HCl

Operidine
Func. class.: Narcotic analgesic
Chem. class.: Opioid phenyl-piperidine derivative
Legal class.: CD (Sch 2) POM

Action: Inhibits ascending pain pathways in CNS, increases pain threshold, alters pain perception
Uses: Enhancement of anaesthetics, analgesia during surgery; as respiratory depressant in prolonged assisted respiration
Dosage and routes:
With spontaneous respiration
• *Adult:* IV injection up to 1 mg,

then 0.5 mg every 40−60 min as required

• *Child:* IV injection 30−50 mcg/kg

With assisted ventilation

• *Adult:* IV injection 2−5 mg, then 1 mg as required

• *Child:* IV injection 100−150 mcg/kg

Available forms include: Injection 1 mg/ml

Side effects/adverse reactions:

RESP: Respiratory depression, cough suppression

CNS: Drowsiness

CV: Bradycardia

EENT: Visual disturbances

GI: Nausea, vomiting, reduced motility, constipation, jaundice

GU: Urinary retention

MS: Rigidity

SYST: Reduced tolerance, dependence

Contraindications: Hypersensitivity, obstructive airways disease, respiratory depression (if not ventilating mechanically)

Precautions: Hypothyroidism, hepatic impairment, dependence, pregnancy, renal disease, biliary tract disorders, adrenocortical insufficiency, shock, prostatic hypertrophy, supraventricular tachycardia, head injury, raised intraneonates, premature infants, elderly or debilitated patients

Pharmacokinetics: Metabolised in liver, excreted in urine

Interactions/incompatibilities:

• MAOIs (enhanced toxicity)

• Effects may be enhanced with other CNS depressants: alcohol, anaesthetics, narcotics, sedative/hypnotics, antipsychotics

Treatment of overdose: Naloxone, supportive care

NURSING CONSIDERATIONS

Assess:

• Baseline vital signs, pupil size and reaction

• Fluid balance

• When pain is starting to return

Administer:

• Before pain becomes severe

• With anti-emetic if nausea or vomiting occurs

Perform/provide:

• Storage in CD cupboard

• Assistance with walking; drowsiness, dizziness may occur

• Safety measures including cotsides if necessary

Evaluate:

• For CNS changes

• For respiratory changes; depression, rate, rhythm; notify clinician if respirations are under 12/min

• Therapeutic response; dependency

Teach patient/family:

• About all aspects of the drug

• That physical dependence may occur if drug is used for an extended period

• That withdrawal symptoms could occur if drug is discontinued abruptly

• Not to drive or engage in other hazardous activities if drowsiness/dizziness occur

• Secure storage

---

phenoxybenzamine HCl

Dibenyline

Func. class.: Antihypertensive

Chem. class.: α-Adrenergic blocker

Legal class.: POM

Action: α-Adrenergic blocker, which binds to α-adrenergic receptors, dilating peripheral blood vessels, lowers peripheral resistance, lowers blood pressure

Uses: Phaeochromocytoma

Dosage and routes:

• *Adult:* By mouth 10 mg daily, increase by 10 mg daily; usual range: 1−2 mg/kg daily in two doses, with concomitant β-blockade if required

Phaeochromocytoma hypertensive crisis and adjunct in severe shock:
• *Adult:* By IV infusion 1 mg/kg daily in 200 ml sodium chloride 0.9% over at least 2 hr; do not repeat within 24 hr

Available forms include: Capsules 10 mg, injection 50 mg/ml (hospital only)

Side effects/adverse reactions:

GI: Dry mouth, nausea, vomiting, diarrhoea

CV: Postural hypotension, tachycardia

CNS: Dizziness, drowsiness, sedation, lassitude

GU: Inhibition of ejaculation

EENT: Nasal congestion, miosis

Contraindications: Hypersensitivity, history of cerebrovascular accident, 3−4 weeks after myocardial infarction, porphyria

Precautions: Severe heart disease, congestive heart failure, cerebrovascular disease, renal damage, respiratory infection, elderly, pregnancy

Pharmacokinetics:

By mouth: Onset 2 hr, peak 4−6 hr, duration 3−4 days; half-life 24 hr, metabolised in liver, excreted in urine, bile

Interactions/incompatibilities:
• Hypotensive response: adrenaline, antihypertensives

Treatment of overdose: Supportive care (IV saline, noradrenaline, elevate legs)

NURSING CONSIDERATIONS

Assess:
• Weight before initial dose
• Pulse, blood pressure lying and standing before and regularly during treatment

Administer:
• IV infusion with intensive care facilities available
• Avoid contamination of hands

with injection solution due to risk of contact sensitivity
• Orally following dosage regime for suitable gradual introduction, until control of hypertension or postural hypotension occurs
• With food or milk if GI symptoms occur

Perform/provide:
• Frequent drinks to prevent a dry mouth

Evaluate:
• Effect of any other therapy
• Therapeutic response: decreased BP, increased peripheral pulses
• Nausea, vomiting, diarrhoea, dry mouth
• Postural hypotension, tachycardia
• Dizziness

Teach patient/family:
• Avoid alcohol
• To report dizziness, palpitations, fainting
• To change position slowly or fainting may occur
• To take drug exactly as prescribed
• To avoid driving and hazardous activities until treatment established
• To only take other medication if directed by clinician
• To give up smoking and encourage or healthy diet

---

phenoxymethylpenicillin potassium

Apsin VK, Distaquaine VK, Stabillin VK, V-Cil-K

Func. class.: Antibiotic, broad-spectrum

Chem. class.: Natural penicillin

Legal class.: POM

Action: Interferes with cell wall replication of susceptible organisms; osmotically unstable cell wall swells, bursts from osmotic pressure

Uses: Mild to moderate streptococcal, pneumococcal, staphylococcal, spirochaetal and other bacterial infections due to susceptible organisms; prophylaxis of rheumatic fever

Dosage and routes:
• *Adult:* By mouth 250−500 mg every 6 hr at least 30 min before meals
• *Child 6−12 yr:* By mouth 250 mg 6 hrly before meals
• *Child 1−5 yr:* 125 mg 6 hrly
• *Child up to 1 yr:* 62.5 mg 6 hrly before meals

Available forms include: Capsules 250 mg; tablets 250 mg; powder for oral suspension 62.5, 125, 250 mg/5 ml

Side effects/adverse reactions:
GI: Nausea, vomiting, diarrhoea, abdominal pain, glossitis
META: Hyperkalaemia
SYST: Hypersensitivity (anaphylaxis, rashes, urticaria, serum sickness, chills, fever, oedema, arthralgia, eosinophilia, angioedema)
MISC: Infection (overgrowth) with resistant organisms

Contraindications: Hypersensitivity to penicillins; severe acute infection (absorption may be inadequate), meningococcal or gonococcal infection

Precautions: History of significant allergies and/or asthma, impaired renal function

Pharmacokinetics:
By mouth: Absorption variable, incomplete; peak 30−60 min, duration 6−8 hr, half-life 30 min, metabolised in liver, excreted in urine

Interactions/incompatibilities:
• Decreased antimicrobial effectiveness of this drug: bacteriostatic agents such as tetracyclines, erythromycin; chloroquine, guar gum (decreased absorption)
• Increased penicillin concentrations when used with: probenecid

Clinical assessment:
• Culture organism and assess sensitivity before drug therapy; drug may be taken once culture sample is taken
• Consider patch test to assess allergy, if penicillin is only drug of choice

Lab. test interferences:
Decrease: Uric acid
False positive: Urine glucose, urine protein

Treatment of overdose: Activated charcoal plus sorbitol, symptomatic supportive care

NURSING CONSIDERATIONS
Assess:
• Bowel pattern
• Fluid balance
• Allergy status, history of allergies (asthma, hay fever)
• Any patient with compromised renal system since drug is excreted slowly in poor renal system function; toxicity may occur rapidly

Administer:
• On an empty stomach for best absorption
• After culture and sensitivity has been completed

Perform/provide:
• Adequate fluid intake (2 litres/day) during diarrhoea episodes
• Refrigerate after reconstituting oral elixir

Evaluate:
• Therapeutic effectiveness: absence of fever, draining wounds
• Bowel pattern before and during treatment
• Fluid balance; report haematuria, oliguria since penicillin in high doses is nephrotoxic
• Skin eruptions after administration of penicillin to 1 week after discontinuing drug

• Respiratory status: rate, character, wheezing, tightness in chest
• Allergies before initiation of treatment, reaction of each medication; highlight allergies on nursing care plan

Teach patient/family:
• Aspects of drug therapy, including need to complete entire course of medication to ensure organism death (10−14 days); culture may be taken after completed course
• To report sore throat, fever, fatigue; could indicate superimposed infection
• To wear or carry ID if allergic to penicillins
• To notify nurse of diarrhoea stools

---

phentermine

Duromine, Ionamin
Func. class.: Cerebral stimulant
Chem. class.: Sympathomimetic amine
Legal class.: CD (Sch 3) POM

Action: Increases release of noradrenaline, dopamine in CNS reduces appetite

Uses: Severe obesity

Dosage and routes:
• *Adult:* By mouth 15−30 mg daily before breakfast

Available forms include: Capsules (modified release) 15, 30 mg

Side effects/adverse reactions:
CNS: Hyperactivity, insomnia, restlessness, dizziness, nervousness
GI: Nausea, dry mouth, constipation, unpleasant taste, vomiting
GU: Impotence, change in libido, urinary frequency
CV: Palpitations, tachycardia, hypertension
INTEG: Urticaria, facial oedema
MISC: Risk of dependence

Contraindications: Hypersensitivity, hyperthyroidism, hypertension, glaucoma, sensitivity to sympathomimetics, history of psychiatric illness or drug abuse, porphyria

Precautions: Anxiety, cardiovascular disease, pregnancy, diabetes mellitus

Pharmacokinetics:
Modified release capsules: Duration 10−14 hr; metabolised by liver, excreted by kidneys

Interactions/incompatibilities:
• Risk of hypertensive crisis when given within 14 days of MAOIs
• Decrease effect of: antihypertensives
• Hypoglycaemic treatment may require adjustment in diabetics
• Diminished effect of sedatives

Clinical assessment:
• Discontinue if weight gain not achieved
• Limit therapy to 4−8 weeks

Treatment of overdose: Gastric lavage or emesis if ingestion within last 4 hr, activated charcoal, supportive treatment including diazepam for sedation if needed. Forced acid diuresis possible

NURSING CONSIDERATIONS

Assess:
• Vital signs, BP (drug may reverse antihypertensives). Check patients with cardiac disease more often
• Height and growth rate in children; growth rate may be decreased

Administer:
• At least 6 hr before sleeping
• For obesity only if patient is on weight reduction programme including dietary changes, exercise; patient will develop tolerance, and loss of weight will not occur without additional methods
• Frequent sips of water for dry mouth
• If drug is being given for obesity, 1 hr before meals

Perform/provide:
• Check to see oral medication has been swallowed
Evaluate:
• Mental status: mood, alertness, affect, stimulation, insomnia, aggressiveness
• For symptoms of abuse
• Physical dependency: should not be used for extended periods of time; dose should be discontinued gradually
• Withdrawal symptoms: headache, nausea, vomiting, muscle pain, weakness
• Drug tolerance after long-term use
Teach patient/family:
• Drug should not be increased if tolerance develops
• To decrease caffeine consumption (coffee, tea, cola, chocolate), which may increase irritability, stimulation
• Avoid non-prescribed preparations unless approved by clinician
• To taper off drug over several weeks, or depression, increased sleeping, lethargy may ensue
• To avoid alcohol ingestion
• To avoid hazardous activities including driving until patient is stabilised on medication
• To get needed rest; patients will feel more tired at end of day
• That drug is one of abuse

---

phentolamine mesylate

Rogitine
Func. class.: Antihypertensive
Chem. class.: α-Adrenergic blocker
Legal class.: POM

Action: α-Adrenergic blocker, binds to α-adrenergic receptors, dilating peripheral blood vessels, lowering peripheral resistances, lowering blood pressure
Uses: Cardiogenic shock, paroxysmal, hypertension, diagnostic test for phaeochromocytoma
Dosage and routes:
Cardiogenic shock
• IV 5−60 mg in 5% Dextrose or 0.9% sodium chloride at 0.2−2 mg/min, may be increased to 5 mg/min in first minute. Reduced rate if systolic pressure drops below 100 mm Hg
Paroxysmal hypertension
• IV/IM 5−10 mg once, repeat as required. Prior to surgical removal of phaeochromocytoma, administer 2 hr prior to surgery and repeat as necessary
Diagnostic test for phaeochromocytoma
• Establish basal BP then IV 5 mg (1−5 mg in children). Positive response is seen as a rapid fall in BP with quick return to basal levels. Maximum depressor effect occurs within 2 mins
Available forms include: Injection IM, IV 10 mg/ml
Side effects/adverse reactions:
GI: Dry mouth, nausea, vomiting, diarrhoea, abdominal pain
CV: Hypotension, tachycardia, angina, arrhythmias, myocardial infarction
CNS: Dizziness, weakness, anxiety
EENT: Nasal congestion
INTEG: Flushing, sweating
Contraindications: Hypersensitivity, hypotension
Precautions: Pregnancy, severe hypotension, lactation, myocardial infarction, coronary insufficiency, angina
Pharmacokinetics:
IV: Peak 2 min, duration 10−15 min
IM: Peak 15−20 min, duration 3−4 hr
Metabolised in liver, excreted in urine, plasma half life 19 min
Interactions/incompatibilities:

• May increase effects of anti-hypertensives
• Not to be mixed in solution or syringe with any drug
Clinical assessment:
• Monitor blood pressure
Treatment of overdose: Discontinue drug. Effects can be attenuated with noradrenaline if necessary

NURSING CONSIDERATIONS
Assess:
• Baseline vital signs including B/P lying, standing
Administer:
• Frequent mouth washes for dry mouth
• After having vasopressor nearby
• After discontinuing all medication for 24 hr if using for diagnostic purpose
Evaluate:
• Postural hypotension
• Cardiac system: pulse, ECG, B/P (lying, standing) 4 hourly
• Dryness of mucous membrane
• Oedema in feet, legs daily
Teach patient/family:
• That bedrest is required during treatment, and for 1 hr after

phenylbutazone
Butacote
Func. class.: Non-steroidal anti-inflammatory drug
Chem. class.: Pyrazolone derivative
Legal class: POM

Action: Inhibits prostaglandin synthesis by decreasing an enzyme needed for biosynthesis; possesses analgesic, anti-inflammatory anti-pyretic properties
Uses: Ankylosing spondylitis (hospitals only)
Dosage and routes:
• *Adult:* 200 mg 2 or 3 times a day

for 2 days, then reduce to the minimum effective, usually 100 mg, 2 or 3 times a day
Not for children under 14 yr
Available forms include: Tablets 100 mg
Side effects/adverse reactions:
GI: Nausea, dyspepsia, ulcerative stomatitis, vomiting, hepatitis, peptic ulcer, epigastric pain, bleeding
CNS: Headache
CV: Peripheral oedema due to sodium retention
INTEG: Purpura, rash, pruritus, Stevens-Johnson syndrome
GU: Nephritis
HAEM: Agranulocytosis, aplastic anaemia, thrombocytopenia, leucopenia
EENT: Blurred vision
META: Goitre
RESP: Acute pulmonary syndrome (rare)
Contraindications: Thyroid disease, history of peptic ulceration, GI haemorrhage, Sjögren's syndrome, asthma, hypersensitivity, blood dyscrasias, severe cardiac disease, severe renal disease, severe hepatic disease, last trimester of pregnancy, porphyria
Precautions: Lactation, children, bleeding disorders, history of dyspepsia, elderly (reduce dose), hypersensitivity to other NSAIDs, pregnancy
Pharmacokinetics:
By mouth: Peak 2 hr, half-life 3−3½ hr; metabolised in liver, excreted in urine (metabolites), excreted in breast milk
Interactions/incompatibilities:
• May increase action of anti-coagulants, antidiabetics, phenytoin, sulphonamides, methotrexate, lithium
• Reduced action of this drug: with concurrent hepatic microsomal enzyme inducers e.g. rifampicin, phenobarbitone

Clinical assessment:
• Renal, liver, blood studies: serum urea, creatinine, aspartate aminotransferase, alanine aminotransferase, Hb, before treatment, periodically thereafter
• If decrease in leucocyte and/or platelets or haematocrit observed, drug should be withdrawn

Treatment of overdose: Evacuation of the stomach and activated charcoal. If necessary, haemofiltration and supportive therapy

NURSING CONSIDERATIONS

Administer:
• With food to decrease GI symptoms
• Swallow whole

Evaluate:
• Therapeutic response: decreased pain, stiffness, swelling in joints, ability to move more easily
• For eye, ear problems: blurred vision, tinnitus (may indicate toxicity)
• Persistent indigestion

Teach patient/family:
• To report blurred vision or ringing, roaring in ears (may indicate toxicity)
• To avoid driving or other hazardous activities if dizziness or drowsiness occurs
• To report persistent indigestion or black tarry stools
• To take with food or milk
• To report change in urine pattern, weight increase, oedema, pain increase in joints, fever, blood in urine (indicates nephrotoxicity)
• To report bruising, fever, sore throat, rash, mouth ulceration
• That therapeutic effects may take up to 1 month

phenylephrine HCl

Func. class.: Adrenergic, direct acting
Chem. class.: Substituted phenylethylamine
Legal class.: POM

Action: Selective (α1) receptor agonist causing contraction of blood vessels
Uses: Acute hypotension
Dosage and routes:
Hypotension
• *Adult:* Subcutaneous IM 2−5 mg, IV 0.1−0.5 mg, may repeat after at least 15 min if necessary. Continuous IV infusion 30−60 mcg/minute according to response
Available forms include: Injection, IV, Subcutaneous, IM, 1% (10 mg/ml)
Side effects/adverse reactions:
CNS: Headache
CV: Palpitations, tachycardia, ectopic beats, angina, hypertension, reflex bradycardia
GI: Nausea, vomiting
INTEG: Necrosis, tissue, sloughing with extravasation, gangrene, skin tingling
Contraindications: Hypersensitivity, ventricular fibrillation, tachydysrhythmias, phaeochromocytoma, myocardial infarction, pregnancy, severe hypertension, hyperthyroidism
Precautions: Lactation, arterial embolism, peripheral vascular disease, angina pectoris, diabetes mellitus closed angle glaucoma
Pharmacokinetics:
IV: Duration 20−30 min
IM, subcutaneous: Duration 45−60 min
Interactions/incompatibilities:
• Reversal of effects of antihypertensives with potentially serious consequences

- Do not use within 2 weeks of MAOIs or hypertensive crisis may result
- Increased risk of cardiac arrhythmias when given with inhalation anaesthetics, quinidine, cardiac glycosides
- Decreased action of this drug: α-blockers
- Increased pressor effect when given with: tricyclic antidepressant
- Incompatible with alkaline solutions e.g. sodium bicarbonate

Clinical assessment:
- ECG during administration continuously; if BP increases, drug is decreased
- CVP during infusion if possible

Treatment of overdose: Administer phentolamine with care

NURSING CONSIDERATIONS
Assess:
- Baseline vital signs, CVP, ECG

Administer
- Plasma expanders for hypovolemia
- IV directly into vein, wait 15 min to repeat if necessary
- IV by infusion, 500 ml of dextrose 5% or normal saline at 30−60 mcg per minute, according to response

Evaluate:
- Input and output of fluids, check output hourly
- E.C.G continuously during administration; if blood pressure increases, drug is decreased
- Blood pressure and pulse at 5 min intervals after administration
- CVP during infusion
- Patients medication
- Side effects, palpitation, ectopic beats, tachycardia, angina hypertension, reflex bradycardia, nausea, vomiting
- Injection site: tissue sloughing, if this occurs administer phentolamine mixed with 0.9% sodium chloride

- For therapeutic response: increase BP with stabilization

Teach patient/family:
- The reason for drug administration
- To report pain, loss of sensation at injection site immediately

phenylephrine HCl (ophthalmic)

Minims phenylephrine, Isopto Frin
Func. class.: Mydriatic
Legal class.: P

Action: Blocks response of iris sphincter muscle, muscle of accommodation of ciliary body to cholinergic stimulation, resulting in dilation of pupil, paralysis of accommodation, causes vasoconstriction

Uses: Mydriasis, posterior synechia, redness due to minor eye irritation

Dosage and routes:
Mydriatic prior to examination
- *Adult:* Instil 1 drop of 10% solution
- *Elderly, child:* Instil 1 drop of 2.5% solution
Therapeutic mydriasis
- *Adult:* Instil 1 drop of 10% solution as necessary
Redness due to minor irritation
- *Adult and child:* 1 drop 0.12% solution up to 4 times a day

Available forms include: Solution 0.12, 2.5, 10%

Side effects/adverse reactions:
CV: Palpitations, tachycardia, hypertension, myocardial infarction
RESP: Bronchospasm
EENT: Blurred vision, stinging, photophobia

Contraindications: Hypersensitivity to sympathomimetic amines, narrow-angle glaucoma, dysrhythmias, cardiogenic shock

Precautions: Elderly, hypertension, diabetes mellitus, cerebral arteriosclerosis, pregnancy, contact lenses

Pharmacokinetics: Onset 1 hr, peak 4−8 hr, duration 12−24 hr

Interactions/incompatibilities:

• Reversal of effects of antihypertensives with potentially serious consequences

• Increased pressor effects when given with: tricyclic antidepressants

• May interact with systemic MAOIs, increasing risk of hypertensive reactions

• Increased risk of cardiac arrhythmias when given with: inhalation anaesthetics, quinidine, cardiac glycosides

Clinical assessment:

• Tonometer readings during long-term treatment

• Risk of systemic side-effects and drug interactions much smaller with 0.12% drops

Treatment of overdose: Supportive, injection of α-blocker e.g. phentolamine 5−10 mg IV may be useful

NURSING CONSIDERATIONS

Assess:

• BP, pulse, respirations

Evaluate:

• Allergic reaction: itching, oedema of eyelids, eye discharge; drug should be discontinued

Teach patient/family:

• To report pain or loss of sight, trouble breathing, sweating, flushing

• Method of instillation: into lower conjunctival sac. Keep eye closed for approx 1 min; use cotton wool ball to mop up excess, discourage rubbing the eye; do not touch dropper to eye

phenytoin sodium

Epanutin

Func. class.: Anticonvulsant
Chem. class.: Hydantoin
Legal class.: POM

Action: Inhibits spread of seizure activity in brain

Uses: All types of epilepsy except absence seizures, trigeminal neuralgia, arrhythmias

Dosage and routes:

Seizures

• *Adult:* IV loading dose of 10−15 mg/kg run at less than 50 mg/min; then 100 mg run at less than 50 mg/min every 6−8 hr. By mouth loading dose of 12−15 mg/kg in divided doses over 1 day may be given. Subsequent dosing adjusted according to response and blood levels of drug, normal range 200−500 mg/day. Single or divided doses. Dose adjustments at least 1 week apart

• *Child:* IV loading dose of 10−15 mg/kg run at less than 50 mg/min; then 4−8 mg/kg run at less than 50 mg/min, every 6−8 hr; by mouth loading dose of 12−15 mg/kg in divided doses over 1 day may be given. Subsequent dosing adjusted according to response on blood levels of drug, normal range 4−8 mg/kg/day in 2 or 3 divided doses. Dose adjustments at least 1 week apart

• *Neonate:* IV loading dose at 15−20 mg/kg at rate of 1−3 mg/kg/min. Oral absorption unreliable, subsequent treatment requires specialist knowledge supported by blood level monitoring

Neuritic pain

• *Adult:* By mouth 200−400 mg daily

Cardiac arrhythmias

• *Adult:* IV 3.5−5 mg/kg body

weight run at less than 50 mg/min. Repeat once if necessary

Available forms include: Suspension 30 mg/5 ml contains phenytoin base; 15 ml is equivalent to 100 mg phenytoin sodium tablet/capsule; tablets 50, 100 mg; injection 50 mg/ml; capsules 25 mg, 50, 100, 300 mg; chewable tablets 50 mg

Side effects/adverse reactions:

HAEM: Agranulocytosis, leucopenia, aplastic anaemia, lymphadenopathy, megaloblastic anaemia

CNS: Drowsiness, dizziness, insomnia, paraesthesias, aggression, headache, nystagmus, slurred speech, dyskinesias, ataxia

HAEM: Lymphadenopathy

GI: Nausea, vomiting, constipation, anorexia, weight loss, hepatitis, jaundice

GU: Nephritis, albuminuria, Peyronie's disease

INTEG: Rash, exfoliative dermatitis, hirsutism, gingival hyperplasmia acne

CV: Atrial and ventricular arrhythmias after IV use

MS: Muscle twitching, polyarthropathy

EENT: Blurred vision

ELECT: Hypocalcaemia

Contraindications: Hypersensitivity, porphyria IV — sinus bradycardia, AV block, Adams — Stokes syndrome

Precautions: Allergies, hepatic disease, serious renal disease, pregnancy

Pharmacokinetics:

By mouth: Absorption by mouth slow but nearly complete. Half life variable, about 22 hr, metabolised by liver, excreted by kidneys. About 90% protein bound, therapeutic plasma range 10 — 20 mg/litre

Interactions/incompatibilities:

• Decreased effects of phenytoin: alcohol (chronic use), antacids, rifampicin, folic acid, carbamazepine, sucralfate, tricyclic antidepressants, neuroleptics

• Increased effects of phenytoin: chloramphenicol, disulfiram, sulphonamides, cimetidine, phenylbutazone, isoniazid, dicoumarol, sulphinpyrazone, omeprazole, imidazole anti-fungals, amiodarone

• Increased or decreased effects of phenytoin: phenobarbitone, sodium valproate

• Effects increased or decreased by phenytoin: sodium valproate, phenytoin, warfarin

• Decreased effect of: corticosteroids, dicoumarol, doxycycline, oral contraceptives, quinidine, vitamin D, cyclosporin, disopyramide, mexiletine

• Do not mix injection with any other drug or infusion solution; risk of crystallisation

Clinical assessment:

• Serum phenytoin levels to adjust dosage initially and if problems develop

Treatment of overdose: Empty stomach if ingested in last 4 hr, then supportive measures

NURSING CONSIDERATIONS

Assess:

• Baseline vital signs, including ECG if given for cardiac arrhythmia

• Body weight

• Frequency of seizures

Administer:

• IV injection slowly into large vein through large gauge needle or catheter

• Flush injection through with sodium chloride 0.9% to avoid local irritation at site of injection

• IV infusion is not recommended. Seek specialist advice IM route should not be used

• Orally with 200 ml water with or after food

Evaluate:

• Mental status: mood, alertness,

effects memory (long-, short-term)
• Respiratory depression
• Blood dyscrasias: fever, sore throat, bruising, rash, jaundice
• Therapeutic response: reduction in number and severity of seizures
• Local inflammation at injection site
• Monitor ECG continuously during IV administration

Teach patient/family:
• All aspects of drug administration: route, action, dose, when to notify clinician
• Seek advice about ability to drive. Patient should be seizure free for 2 yr, or if subject to attacks only while asleep, have established a 3 yr period of asleep attacks without awake attacks
• Patients affected by drowsiness should not drive or operate machinery
• To carry a Medic Alert card detailing medication
• About side effects

phosphates (rectal)

Carbalax (Beogex), Fletchers' Phosphate Enema
Func. class.: Osmotic laxative
Legal class.: P

Action: Increases water absorption in colon by osmotic action
Uses: Constipation, bowel evacuation prior to abdominal procedures and surgery

Dosage and routes:
• *Adult:* 1 enema (128 ml), as required. 1 suppository, inserted 30 min before evacuation required, moisten with water before use
• *Children over 3 yr:* Enema only, reduced volume according to body weight
Available forms include: Enemas, suppositories

Side effects/adverse reactions:
GI: Nausea, cramps, diarrhoea, anal irritation (with prolonged use)
META: Electrolyte, fluid imbalances
Contraindications: Hypersensitivity, abdominal pain, nausea/vomiting, appendicitis, acute gastrointestinal conditions
Precautions: Intestinal obstruction
Pharmacokinetics: Excreted in faeces
Interactions/incompatibilities: None known
Clinical assessment:
• Electrolyte balance should be maintained during extend use

NURSING CONSIDERATIONS
Assess:
• Fluid balance to identify fluid loss
• Cause of constipation
Administer:
• At room temperature or warmed in warm water before use
• With patient lying on his/her left side
Evaluate:
• Therapeutic response
• Cramping, rectal bleeding, nausea, vomiting; seek medical advice if these occur
Teach patient/family:
• That normal bowel movements do not always occur daily
• That shortage of fluids, fibre and lack of exercise contribute to constipation
• Not to use laxatives for long-term therapy; bowel tone will be lost
• Do not use in presence of abdominal pain, nausea, vomiting
• Notify clinician if constipation unrelieved or if symptoms of electrolyte imbalance occur: muscle cramps, pain, weakness, dizziness
• That necrosis of bowel can occur with overuse

physostigmine sulphate (ophthalmic)

Func. class.: Miotic
Chem. class.: Cholinesterase inhibitor
Legal class.: POM

Action: Increases concentration of acetylcholine at cholinergic transmission sites, thus causing prolonged, exaggerated action; induces miosis, spasm of accommodation, fall in intraocular pressure by opening up drainage channels, aiding in aqueous humour drainage

Uses: Used in treatment of chronic simple glaucoma, usually with pilocarpine

Dosage and routes:
• *Adult and child:* Instil 1−2 drops of a 0.25% or 0.5% solution into conjunctival sac 2−6 times a day depending upon response
Available forms include: Drops 0.25%, 0.5%

Side effects/adverse reactions:
CNS: Convulsions, headache
CV: Hypotension, bradycardia, irregular pulse
GI: Nausea, vomiting, abdominal cramps
RESP: Bronchospasm, dyspnoea, pulmonary oedema
EENT: Blurred vision, conjunctivitis, allergic reactions, rhinorrhoea, salivation, brow pain, lacrimation, twitching of eyelids

Contraindications: Inflammatory disease of iris or ciliary body, soft contact lenses

Precautions: Epilepsy, parkinsonism, bradycardia, hypertension, obstructive airway disease

Clinical assessment:
• Awareness of possibility of systemic side effects

NURSING CONSIDERATIONS
Administer:

• Topically to conjunctival sac
• Only clear solutions, never pink or brown

Teach patient/family:
• To report change in vision, blurring or loss of sight, trouble breathing, sweating, flushing
• Method of instillation, not to touch dropper to eye
• That long-term therapy may be required
• That blurred vision will decrease with repeated use of drug
• That drug may be prescribed for bedtime use to prevent nocturnal rise in ocular tension
• That maximal effect of topical application is reached in 30 min, may last 12−36 hr
• To observe eyes for irritation, development of cataracts

phytomenadione (vitamin K₁)

Konakion
Func. class.: Fat-soluble vitamin
Legal class.: POM

Action: Needed for adequate blood clotting (Factors II, VII, IX, X)

Uses: Actual or threatened haemorrhage associated with low blood prothrombin, Factor VII. Coumarin anticoagulant overdose. Prevention/treatment of neonatal haemorrhage

Dosage and routes:
• *Adult: As an antidote to anticoagulant drugs*
• *Potentially fatal and severe haemorrhage:* IV 10−20 mg repeated if prothrombin time 3 hr post-dose shows inadequate response, maximum 40 mg in 24 hr, should be accompanied by whole blood/clotting factors
• *Less severe haemorrhage:* By mouth/IM 10 mg repeated if pro-

thrombin level 8-12 hr post-dose shows inadequate response. Maximum 40 mg in 24 hr

• *Dangerously lowered prothrombin without haemorrhage:* By mouth 5−10 mg as a single dose
• *Other indications:* 10−20 mg as required
• *Elderly:* Use dose towards bottom end of dose range
• *Children:* By mouth/IM/IV 5−10 mg
• *Neonates:* Prophylactic: IM 1 mg; therapeutic: IM 1 mg repeated 8 hrly if required
Available forms include: Tablets, chewable 10 mg, injection IV, IM 1 mg in 0.5 ml, 10 mg in 1 ml
Side effects/adverse reactions:
SYST: Anaphylactoid reactions after too rapid IV injection
INTEG: Rash, urticaria. Local cutaneous changes after repeated IM injection
Contraindications: Hypersensitivity
Precautions:
• Should only be given IV in life-threatening situations
• IV injections must be very slow
• Pregnancy
Pharmacokinetics: Onset of action up to 12 hr, duration several days−weeks
Interactions/incompatibilities:
• Decreased absorption of this drug: cholestyramine, mineral oil
• Decreased action of: oral anticoagulants
• Do not dilute injection
Clinical assessment:
• Prothrombin time during treatment
NURSING CONSIDERATIONS
Administer:
• IV: only in cases of severe haemorrhage or critical illness with hepatic dysfunction
• By slow infusion over 30 min
Evaluate:
• Therapeutic response: decreased bleeding tendencies, prothrombin time, clotting time
Perform/provide:
• Monitor ECG if given by infusion
Teach patient/family:
• Not to take other supplements, unless directed by clinician

---

pilocarpine HCl/ pilocarpine nitrate (ophthalmic)

Isopto Carpine, Sno-pilo, Ocusert, Minims Pilocarpine Nitrate
Func. class.: Miotic, direct-acting
Chem. class.: Cholinergic agonist
Legal class.: POM

Action: Directly acts on cholinergic receptor sites, induces miosis, spasm of accommodation, fall in intraocular pressure by opening up drainage channels causing outflow of aqueous humour
Uses: Treatment of chronic simple glaucoma and, prior to surgery treatment of acute (closed angle) glaucoma. Also used to produce miosis to counter effects of mydriatic and cycloplegic eye drops. Primary glaucoma, early stages of wide-angle glaucoma (less useful in advanced stages), chronic open-angle glaucoma, acute narrow-angle glaucoma before emergency surgery; also used to neutralise mydriatics used during eye exam; may be used alternately with mydriatics to break adhesions between iris and lens
Dosage and routes:
• *Adult:* Instil 1−2 drops every 4−8 hr, strength of drops and frequency adjusted to response; Ocusert 20/40 in conjunctival sac of eye once a week at bedtime
Available forms include: Drops 0.5, 1, 2, 3, 4%; modified release intra-

ocular delivery systems Ocusert
Pilo-20, Pilo-40
Side effects/adverse reactions:
CV: Hypertension, tachycardia
RESP: Bronchospasm
GI: Nausea, vomiting, abdominal
cramps, diarrhoea
EENT: Blurred vision, brow ache,
twitching of eyelids, eye pain with
change in focus, hypersalivation,
lens changes, retinal detachment
Contraindications: Acute iritis,
soft contact lenses, hyper-
sensitivity
Precautions: Bronchial asthma,
hypertension, pregnancy, breast
feeding
Interactions/incompatibilities:
• Ocusert products may increase
systemic absorption of autonomic
drugs e.g. adrenaline from the eye
NURSING CONSIDERATIONS
Administer:
• Topically to conjunctival sac
Perform/provide:
• Protect solution from light
• Store Ocusert systems between
2° and 8°C
• Atropine should be readily avail-
able as antidote
Teach patient/family:
• To report change in vision, blur-
ring or loss of sight, trouble
breathing, sweating, flushing
• To store in fridge
• Not to touch dropper to eye
• That long-term therapy may be
required
• That blurred vision will decrease
with repeated use of drug
• To discontinue use if local hyper-
sensitivity reaction occurs
• That acuity in dim light will be
reduced

pimozide

Orap
Func. class.: Antipsychotic/
neuroleptic
Chem. class.: Diphenylbutyl-
piperidine
Legal class.: POM

Action: Depresses cerebral
cortex, hypothalamus, and limbic
system, which control activity,
aggression; blocks neurotransmission produced by dopamine at
synapse by blocking CNS dopamine receptors
Uses: Acute and chronic schizophrenia, other psychoses, mania
and hypomania
Dosage and routes:
Schizophrenia
• *Adult and child over 12 yr:* In
acute phase by mouth 10 mg daily
increased gradually, if needed,
maximum 20 mg daily
• Prevention of relapse 2–20 mg
daily
*Monosymptomatic hypochondria,
other paranoid states*
• *Adult:* By mouth, 4 mg daily increased gradually, if needed to
16 mg daily
*Mania, hypomania, psychomotor
agitation*
• *Adult:* By mouth 10 mg daily,
increased gradually, if needed,
maximum 16 mg daily
• *Elderly:* Half normal starting
dose
Available forms include: Tablets 2,
4, 10 mg
Side effects/adverse reactions:
CNS: Extrapyramidal symptoms:
pseudoparkinsonism, akathisia,
dystonia; tardive dyskinesia,
drowsiness, headache, seizures,
anxiety, loss of libido, respiratory
depression
INTEG: Rash
EENT: Blurred vision, cataracts

GI: Dry mouth, nausea, vomiting, anorexia, constipation, diarrhoea, dyspepsia

GU: Impotence, amenorrhoea, gynaecomastia

CV: Orthostatic hypotension, hypertension, cardiac arrest, ECG changes, tachycardia

MISC: Neuroleptic malignant syndrome

Contraindications: History of cardiac arrhythmias, congenital prolongation of QT interval, severe CNS depression, breast feeding

Precautions: Pregnancy, epilepsy, parkinsonism, lactation, hepatic disease, cardiac disease, renal disease, alcohol withdrawal, brain damage, electrolyte disturbances

Pharmacokinetics:

By mouth: 50% absorbed, peak 6−8 hr, metabolised by liver, excreted in urine, half-life 50−55 hr

Interactions/incompatibilities:

• Decreased convulsive threshold: anticonvulsants

• Increased CNS depression: analgesics, sedatives, anxiolytics, alcohol

• Reduced effect of: bromocriptine, lysuride, pergolide, levodopa

• Increased cardiotoxicity with: phenothiazines, tricyclics, antidysrhythmics, other cardioactive drugs

Clinical assessment:

• Review need for treatment in those developing arrhythmias/ECG changes

• Those taking anticonvulsants for increased seizure activity

Treatment of overdose: Lavage if orally ingested; provide an airway; monitor ECG; *do not induce vomiting*; procyclidine treatment if extrapyramidal side effects severe; observe for at least 4 days

NURSING CONSIDERATIONS

Assess:

• Swallowing of oral medication; check for hoarding or giving of medication to other patients

• Fluid balance

• Baseline BP

• Urinalysis is recommended before and during prolonged therapy

Administer:

• Procyclidine agent, after securing order from clinician to be used if extrapyramidal systems occur

Perform/provide:

• ECG before starting treatment and at regular intervals if daily dose greater than 16 mg

• Supervised walking until stabilised on medication; do not involve in strenuous exercise programme because fainting is possible; patient should not stand still for long periods of time

• Increased fluids to prevent constipation

• Sips of water, mouthwashes or dry mouth

Evaluate:

• BP standing and lying; also pulse, respirations 4 hrly during initial treatment; report drops of 30 mmHg from baseline

• Dizziness, faintness, palpitations, tachycardia on rising

• Extrapyramidal symptoms including akathisia (inability to sit still, no pattern to movements), tardive dyskinesia (bizarre movements of the jaw, mouth, tongue, extremities), pseudoparkinsonism (rigidity, tremors, pill rolling, shuffling gait)

• Skin turgor daily

• Constipation, urinary retention daily; if these occur increase bulk, water in diet

Teach patient/family:

• That tardive dyskinesia may develop with chronic use

• Not to exceed prescribed dose

• That postural hypotension may

occur and to rise from sitting or lying position gradually

• To avoid hot baths or showers, since hypotension may occur

• To avoid abrupt withdrawal of this drug; drugs should be withdrawn slowly

• To avoid non-prescribed preparations (cough, hayfever, cold) unless approved by clinicians since serious drug interactions may occur; avoid use with alcohol or CNS depressants, increased drowsiness may occur

• To avoid hazardous activities if drowsiness or dizziness occurs

• Importance of compliance with drug regimen

• About necessity for meticulous oral hygiene since oral candidiasis may occur

• To report impaired vision, jaundice, tremors, muscle twitching

---

pindolol

Visken

Func. class.: Antihypertensive, antianginal

Chem. class.: Nonselective β-blocker

Legal class.: POM

Action: Competitively blocks stimulation of β-adrenergic receptor within vascular smooth muscle causing vasodilation and reduction in blood pressure. Cardiac β-blockade prevents excessive stimulation with increase in myocardial oxygen demand. Intrinsic sympathomimetic activity minimises myocardial depression

Uses: Mild to moderate hypertension, angina pectoris

Dosage and routes:

Hypertension

• *Adult:* By mouth, initially 10–15 mg daily adjusted according to response. Usual maintenance dose 15–30 mg daily, maximum 45 mg, given as a single breakfast time dose or divided

Angina Pectoris

• *Adult:* By mouth 2.5–5 mg 3 times

Available forms include: Tablets 5, 15 mg

Side effects/adverse reactions:

CV: Hypotension, bradycardia, congestive heart failure, oedema, chest pain, palpitation, claudication, tachycardia, cold extremities, AV block

CNS: Insomnia, dizziness, hallucinations, anxiety, fatigue, depression, headaches

GI: Nausea, vomiting, ischaemic colitis, diarrhoea, abdominal pain

INTEG: Rash, alopecia, pruritus, fever

HAEM: Agranulocytosis

EENT: Visual changes, dry burning eyes

RESP: Bronchospasm, dyspnoea

MS: Muscle fatigue

Contraindications: Hypersensitivity to β-blockers, cardiogenic shock, heart block (2nd, 3rd degree), sinus bradycardia, cardiac failure, severe renal impairment, obstructive pulmonary disease, cor pulmonale, prolonged fasting, metabolic acidosis

Precautions: Major surgery, pregnancy, lactation, diabetes mellitus, renal disease, thyroid disease, chronic obstructive air-ways disease, well compensated heart failure, coronary artery disease; do not give without α-blocker in phaeochromocytoma

Pharmacokinetics:

By mouth: Almost completely absorbed; peak 2–4 hr; half-life 3–4 hr, excreted 30%–45% unchanged, 60%–65% is metabolised by liver, excreted in breast milk

Interactions/incompatibilities:
• Increased hypotension, brady-cardia: reserpine, hydralazine, methyldopa, prazosin, nifedipine, verapamil, other antihypertensives
• Hypertensive reactions when given with: adrenaline, noradrena-line, sympathomimetics
• Increased hypoglycaemic effect: of antidiabetics (and masking of warning signs)
• Risk of heart block/failure with: diltiazem, nifedipine, verapamil amiodarone
• Increased myocardial depression: halothane, cyclopropane, tri-chloroethylene, ether, chloroform

Clinical assessment:
• Baseline renal, liver function tests before therapy begins if significant impairment suspected

Treatment of overdose: Lavage, IV atropine for bradycardia, IV theophylline for bronchospasm, digitalis, O_2, diuretic for cardiac failure, haemodialysis, hypoten-sion; administer vasopressor (iso-prenaline)

NURSING CONSIDERATIONS

Assess:
• Fluid balance, weight
• Apical/radial pulse before ad-ministration; notify clinician of any significant changes

Administer:
• Orally, before meals, at bed-time, tablet may be crushed or swallowed whole
• Reduced dosage in renal dysfunction

Perform/provide:
• Storage in dry area at room temperature

Evaluate:
• Therapeutic response: decreased BP after 1–2 weeks
• BP, pulse 4 hrly, note rate, rhythm, quality
• Peripheral oedema
• Weight daily

Teach patient/family:
• Take with or immediately after meals
• Not to discontinue drug ab-ruptly, taper over 2 weeks may cause precipitate angina
• Not to use non-prescribed pro-ducts containing α-adrenergic stimulants (nasal decongestants, non-prescribed cold preparations)
• To report bradycardia, dizziness, confusion, depression, fever, sore throat, shortness of breath to clinician
• To take pulse at home, advise when to notify clinician ·
• To avoid alcohol, smoking, sodium intake
• The importance of weight control, dietary adjustments, modified exercise programme
• To avoid hazardous activities if dizziness is present
• To report symptoms of con-gestive cardiac failure: difficult breathing, especially on exertion or when lying down, night cough, swelling of extremities

---

piperacillin sodium

Pipril

Func. class.: Antibiotic, broad-spectrum
Chem. class.: Semisynthetic penicillin
Legal class.: POM

Action: Bactericidal antibiotic, interferes with cell wall replication of susceptible organisms

Uses: Treatment of severe local/systemic infection where par-enteral therapy is indicated. Surgical prophylaxis, effective against Gram-positive cocci (*S. aureus, S. pyogenes, S. viridans, S. faecalis, S. bovis, S. pneu-moniae*); Gram-negative cocci (*N. gonorrhoeae, N. meningitidis*); anaerobes, (*C. perfringens,*

C. tetani, Bacteroides, Peptococcus spp); Gram-negative bacilli (*E. coli, Klebsiella* spp, *P. mirabilis, P. vulgaris, P. rehgesii, Enterobacter* spp, *Citrobacter* spp, *P. aeruginosa, Serratia* spp, *Acinetobacter* spp, *H. influenza*). Not effective against β-lactamase-producing *Staphylococcus* spp

Dosage and routes:
Systemic infections
• *Adult and child over 12 yr:* IM/IV 100−300 mg/kg in divided doses 4−6 hrly. Maximum single IM dose 2 g
• *Child: 2 months-12 yr:* IM/IV 100−300 mg/kg daily in 3 or 4 divided doses. Maximum single IM dose 0.5 g
• *Neonates and infants:* IM/IV 100−300 mg/kg daily in 2 divided doses
Prophylaxis of surgical infections
• *Adult:* IV/IM 2 g just before procedure, repeated at least twice at 4 or 6 hr intervals
Acute gonorrhoea
• *Adult:* IM 2 g single dose
Available forms include: Injection IM, IV 1, 2 g; IV infusion 4 g

Side effects/adverse reactions:
HAEM: Increased bleeding time, bone marrow depression
GI: Nausea, vomiting, diarrhoea, raised liver enzymes, abdominal pain, glossitis, colitis, cholestatic jaundice
GU: Haematuria, vaginitis, moniliasis, glomerulonephritis
CNS: Lethargy, twitching, coma, convulsions
SYST: Anaphylaxis
INTEG: Rash, pruritus, rarely exfoliative dermatitis
MISC: Thrombophlebitis and pain at injection site

Contraindications: Hypersensitivity to penicillins
Precautions: Pregnancy, hypersensitivity to cephalosporins, lactation, infectious mononucleosis, renal insufficiency (modify dose)

Pharmacokinetics:
IM: Peak 30−50 min
Half-life 0.7−1.33 hr, excreted in urine, bile, breast milk largely unchanged

Interactions/incompatibilities:
• Decreased antimicrobial effect of this drug: cefoxitin
• Increased penicillin concentrations: aspirin, probenecid
• Synergistic with aminoglycoside antibiotics (but incompatible *in vitro*)

Clinical assessment:
• Culture and sensitivity before drug therapy; drug may be given as soon as culture is taken

Lab. test interferences:
False positive: Urine glucose, tested with copper-reduction method (Clinitest)

Treatment of overdose: Supportive, drug may be removed by dialysis. Anticonvulsants such as diazepam or phenobarbitone may be appropriate

NURSING CONSIDERATIONS
Assess:
• Bowel pattern
• Fluid balance
• For penicillin sensitivity or previous allergy

Administer:
• After specimens sent for culture and sensitivity completed
• By slow bolus or, more usually, by infusion over ½ hr

Perform/provide:
• Resuscitation equipment if anaphylaxis should occur
• Adequate (2 litre) daily fluid intake

Evaluate:
• Therapeutic response: absence of fever, redness, inflammation, purulent drainage
• Fluid balance daily—bowel pattern daily for diarrhoea

- IV site for phlebitis or extravasation
- Urinalysis for haematuria

Teach patient/family:
- To notify nurse of diarrhoea/frequency of stools
- To report sore throat, fever, rashes

---

piperazine citrate
piperazine phosphate

Pripsen, Antepar
Func. class.: Anthelmintic
Legal class.: P

Action: Causes paralysis in worm, leading to expulsion

Uses: Pinworm, roundworm, threadworm

Dosage and routes (Recommendations vary with product):

Pinworm, threadworm
- *Adult:* Pripsen sachets: By mouth, one sachet, repeated after 14 days
- Antepar tablets: By mouth, 4 × 500 mg tablets daily for 7 days, repeated after 7 days if necessary
- *Child:* Pripsen sachets: By mouth, as a single dose, repeated after 14 days, 3 months−1 year, ⅓ sachet; 1−6 yr, ⅔ sachet; over 6 yr, 1 sachet.
- Antepar tablets: By mouth, a dose given daily for 7 days and repeated after 7 days if necessary, under 2 yr, 50−75 mg piperazine hydrate/kg body weight; 2−4 yr, 1½ tablets; 5−12 yr, 3 tablets

Roundworm
- *Adult:* Pripsen sachets: By mouth, one sachet, repeated after 14 days. Repeat at monthly intervals for up to 3 months if reinfection risk
- Antepar tablets: By mouth, 8 × 500 mg tablets as a single dose
- *Child:* Pripsen sachets: By mouth, as a single dose, repeated after 14 days, 3 months−1 year, ⅓ sachet; 1−6 yr, ⅔ sachet; over 6 yr, 1 sachet
- Antepar tablets: By mouth as a single dose, under 2 yr, 120 mg piperazine hydrate/kg body weight; 2−4 yr, 3 tablets; 5−6 yr, 4½ × 500 mg tablets; 6−10 yr, 6 × 500 mg tablets; over 10 yr, 8 × 500 mg tablets

Available forms include: Tablets 500 mg; Granules 4 g sachets

Side effects/adverse reactions:
HAEM: Haemolytic anaemia in glucose-6-phosphate dehydrogenase deficiency
INTEG: Rash, urticaria, photosensitivity
RESP: Bronchospasm
CNS: Dizziness, headache, paraesthesia, convulsions, drowsiness, ataxia
EENT: Blurred vision
GI: Nausea, vomiting, anorexia, diarrhoea, abdominal cramps
SYST: Fever, angioedema
MS: Muscle hypotonia, joint pain

Contraindications: Hypersensitivity, severe renal disease, hepatic disease, seizure disorders

Precautions: Severe malnutrition, pregnancy, chronic disorders of central nervous system

Pharmacokinetics:
Readily absorbed, excreted in urine partly as metabolites, half-life variable

Interactions/incompatibilities:
- May increase extrapyramidal symptoms when used with phenothiazines
- Effects reduced by pyrantel pamoate

Treatment of overdose: Gastric lavage. Supportive treatment including anticonvulsants if necessary

NURSING CONSIDERATIONS
Assess:
- Stools during entire treatment,

1, 3, months after treatment; specimens must be sent to lab while still warm

Administer:
• To be crushed or chewed
• Laxatives if constipated; not needed for drug to work
• Second course after 1 week off drug, if infection is severe

Evaluate:
• Nausea, vomiting
• Therapeutic response: expulsion of worms, 3 negative stool cultures after completion of treatment
• For allergic reaction: rash, itching, urticaria
• For infestation in other family members since transmission from person to person is common

Teach patient/family:
• Good hygiene: hand washing after bowel movement; avoid putting fingers in mouth; to take a daily bath or shower; to change bed linen daily
• That infested person should sleep alone
• To clean toilet daily with disinfectant
• Need for compliance with dosage schedule and duration of treatment
• That urine may turn orange or red
• To avoid hazardous activities since drowsiness occurs
• That seizures may recur in patient who is controlled on medication

---

pipothiazine palmitate

Piportil Depot
Func. class.: Neuroleptic
Chem. class.: Phenothiazine
Legal class.: POM

Action: Depresses cerebral cortex, hypothalamus, limbic system, which control activity; aggression; blocks neurotransmission pro-duced by dopamine at synapse; exhibits antagonism of α-adrenergic, cholinergic effects

Uses: Maintenance in schizophrenia and related psychoses

Dosage and routes: Deep IM injection into gluteal muscle; test dose 25 mg, then adjusted, according to response, in 25—50 mg increments every 4 weeks; usual maintenance range 50—100 mg every 4 weeks; maximum dose 200 mg every 4 weeks

Available forms include: Injection 50 mg/ml; 1-ml, 2-ml ampoules

Side effects/adverse reactions:
CVS: Hypotension, arrhythmias, atrioventricular block, ventricular tachycardia
HAEM: Agranulocytosis, leucopenia
INTEG: Pain, erythema, swelling, nodules at injection site, pallor, photosensitisation, contact sensitisation, rashes
CNS: Extrapyramidal symptoms, tardive dyskinesia, drowsiness, apathy, insomnia, depression, agitation, nightmares, blurred vision, tremor, rigidity, respiratory depression
GI: Dry mouth, constipation, obstructive jaundice
GU: Difficulty with micturition, impotence
EENT: Nasal congestion, ocular changes
MISC: Hypothermia, pyrexia, menstrual disturbances, galactorrhoea, gynaecomastia, weight gain, neuroleptic malignant syndrome

Contraindications: Coma, marked cerebral atherosclerosis, phaechromocytoma, renal or liver failure, severe cardiac insufficiency, hypersensitivity

Precautions: Cardiovascular disease, severe respiratory disease, renal or hepatic impairment, parkinsonism, epilepsy, acute infections, hypothyroidism, myasthenia gravis, leucopenia, history of jaundice, prostatic hypertrophy, elderly, alcohol withdrawal symptoms, brain damage, history of narrow angle glaucoma, thyrotoxicosis, pregnancy, lactation

Pharmacokinetics: Poorly understood

Interactions/incompatibilities:

• Increases CNS depression with: alcohol, barbiturates, other sedatives

• Increases the effects of: most antihypertensives, anticholinergic drugs including tricyclic antidepressants

• Decreased effects of: amphetamine, levodopa, bromocriptine, lysuride, pergolide, clonidine, guanethidine, adrenaline, hypoglycaemic drugs, anticonvulsants (lowered seizure threshold)

• Increased extrapyramidal effects with, and toxicity of, lithium

Clinical assessment:

• Administer small test dose to ensure patient does not experience undesirable side effects

• Adjust dosage and dosage interval to suit individual

• Adjust dosage of concurrently administered drugs if interaction occurs

• Immediate investigation of unexplained fever/infection

Treatment of overdose: Generalised vasodilation may occur, raising patient's legs may be sufficient, volume expanders may be required. Positive inotropic agents such as dopamine may be given for circulatory collapse if fluid replacement is insufficient. Anti-arrythmic agents (avoid lignocaine and long-acting types) may be required. Severe dystonic reactions respond to procyclidine (5−10 mg) or orphenadrine (20−40 mg) IM or IV. Convulsions treatment diazepam IV

NURSING CONSIDERATIONS

Assess:

• Baseline BP and pulse, weight

Administer:

• Deep IM preferably in gluteal region to avoid pain at injection site

• Not more than 2−3 ml of oily injection at any one site

Evaluate:

• Pulse; arrhythmias and tachycardia may occur

• BP: hypotension may occur

• For development of jaundice — withhold drug if this develops

Teach patient/family:

• Not to drink alcohol whilst taking drug

• To avoid exposure to direct sunlight as skin may be sensitive

• To stand up slowly to avoid orthostatic hypotension

• That weight gain is possible whilst using this drug

• Seek medical advice before taking any medications

---

pirbuterol

Exirel

Func. class.: Bronchodilator
Chem. class.: β-Adrenergic agonist
Legal class.: POM

Action: Causes bronchodilation by stimulating bronchial β-receptors

Uses: Asthma, bronchospasm associated with bronchitis and emphysema

Dosage and routes:

• *Adult and child over 12 yr:* Aerosol 1−2 puffs (0.2−0.4 mg) 3 or 4 times a day, may be increased to maximum 12 puffs a day. By mouth 10−15 mg 3 or 4 times a day

Available forms include: Capsules 10, 15 mg; aerosol delivers 0.2 mg pirbuterol (as acetate) per actuation

Side effects/adverse reactions:
CNS: Tremors, anxiety, insomnia, headache
EENT: Irritation of nose, throat with inhaler
CV: Palpitations, tachycardia, hypertension, angina, hypotension, dysrhythmias
MS: Muscle cramps
RESP: Bronchospasm, dyspnoea, coughing especially after inhalation
MISC: Hypokalaemia
Contraindications: Hypersensitivity to sympathomimetics, concurrent use of non-selective β-blocker
Precautions: Lactation, pregnancy, coronary artery disease, dysrhythmias, hyperthyroidism, children under 12 yr
Pharmacokinetics:
By mouth: onset 1 hr, peak 1−2 hr, duration 6 hr. Half-life 2 hr, excreted in urine as sulphate conjugate
Inhalation: Onset 5−10 min, peak 15−30 min, duration 5 hr, plasma levels undetectable
Interactions/incompatibilities:
• Increased risk of hypokalaemia with: theophylline, aminophylline, choline theophyllinate, steroids, diuretics, long-term laxatives
• Decreased action of pirbuterol: β-blockers
Clinical assessment:
• Monitor serum potassium in patients at risk of hypokalaemia
Treatment of overdose: Symptomatic and supportive. Cardioselective β-blockers may be useful (caution in patients with history of bronchospasm)
NURSING CONSIDERATIONS
Assess:
• Respiratory function: vital capacity, forced expiratory volume, arterial blood gases
Administer:
• After shaking inhaler: instruct patient to exhale, place mouthpiece in mouth, inhale slowly, hold breath, remove mouthpiece and exhale slowly
Perform/provide:
• Frequent mouthcare and drinks for dry mouth
Evaluate:
• Response to treatment: indicated by resolution of dyspnoea and wheezing during the hour following administration
• Improvement of peak expiratory flow rate
Teach patient/family:
• How to use inhaler. Ensure patient has read and understood the enclosed instructions
• To avoid getting aerosol in the eyes
• To wash and dry inhaler once daily
• Not to take non-prescription medicines as they may negate the effects of pirbuterol
• Provide information about all aspects of the drug and its administration: to avoid smoking and smokey atmospheres and exposure to respiratory infections

---

pirenzepine dihydrochloride

Gastrozepin
Func. class.: Selective antimuscarinic
Chem. class.: Dihydrobenzodiazepinone
Legal class.: POM

Action: Inhibits gastric acid and pepsin secretion
Uses: Gastric and duodenal ulceration
Dosage and routes:
• By mouth 50 mg twice daily 30 min before meals, increased if necessary to maximum of 150 mg

daily in 3 divided doses for 4–6 weeks; in resistant cases for up to 3 months

Available forms include: Tablets 50 mg

Side effects/adverse reactions:

GI: Dry mouth

EENT: Visual disturbances

HAEM: Agranulocytosis, thrombocytopenia

Contraindications: Hypersensitivity, prostate enlargement, organic pyloric stenosis, paralytic ileus, closed angle glaucoma, pregnancy

Precautions: Lactation, renal impairment

Pharmacokinetics: 25% absorbed orally (10–20% with food) mean half life of 12 hr, 90% excreted unchanged in faeces

Interactions/incompatibilities:

• Anticholinergic side effects may be enhanced by: atropine, antihistamines, butyrophenones, phenothiazines, tricyclic antidepressants

• Theoretical interaction with: MAOIs and sympathomimetics

Clinical assessment:

• Continue treatment for 4–6 weeks even when symptoms have subsided

Treatment of overdose: Symptomatic

NURSING CONSIDERATIONS

Administer:

• Give at least 30 min before meals, with liquid

Evaluate:

• For visual disturbances — patient may require assistance with activities

• Therapeutic response — lessening of symptoms

Teach patient/family:

• Consult clinician before taking non-prescribed medication

piroxicam

Feldene, Larapam, Pirozip

Func. class.: Non-steroidal anti-inflammatory drug

Chem. class.: Oxicam derivative

Legal class.: POM

Action: Inhibits prostaglandin synthesis by inhibiting an enzyme needed for biosynthesis; possesses analgesic, anti-inflammatory, antipyretic properties

Uses: Mild to moderate pain, osteoarthritis, rheumatoid arthritis

Dosage and routes:

• *Adult:* By mouth, per rectum in chronic conditions, normally 20 mg daily, occasionally 10 mg daily sufficient, maximum 30 mg daily. Acute gout: 40 mg daily for 5–7 days. Acute musculoskeletal disorders: 40 mg daily for 2 days, then 20 mg daily for 7–14 days. Daily doses may be divided

• *Child over 6 yr:* By mouth in juvenile chronic arthritis, body weight less than 15 kg, 5 mg daily; 16–25 kg, 10 mg daily; 26–45 kg, 15 mg daily; over 46 kg, 20 mg daily

Available forms include: Capsules 10, 20 mg; dispersible tablets 10, 20 mg; melt-in-mouth tablets 20 mg; suppositories 20 mg

Side effects/adverse reactions:

GI: Nausea, anorexia, vomiting, diarrhoea, jaundice, cholestatic hepatitis, constipation, flatulence, cramps, peptic ulcer, gastrointestinal bleeding. Local pain; irritation, tenesmus with suppositories

CNS: Dizziness, drowsiness, fatigue, confusion, insomnia, anxiety, depression

CV: Peripheral oedema, palpitations

INTEG: Purpura, rash, pruritus, alopecia, epidermal necrolysis

GU: Nephrotoxicity: raised serum creatinine and blood urea nitrogen
HAEM: Blood dyscrasias
EENT: Tinnitus, hearing loss, blurred vision
SYST: Hypersensitivity reactions: anaphylaxis, angiodema, serum sickness

Contraindications: Hypersensitivity, active or recurrent peptic ulceration. Suppositories only: inflammatory lesions of the rectum/anus, recent history of rectal/anal bleeding

Precautions: Pregnancy, lactation, children, bleeding disorders, upper GI disorders, cardiac disorders, hypersensitivity to other NSAIDs, renal disease, severe hepatic disease

Pharmacokinetics:
By mouth: Peak 2 hr, half-life 50 hr; metabolised in liver, excreted in urine (metabolites) excreted in breast milk, 99% protein bound

Interactions/incompatibilities:
• May increase action of oral anticoagulants, phenytoin, lithium, sulphonylurea hypoglycaemic agents, methotrexate

Clinical assessment:
• Monitor therapeutic response to, and blood levels of lithium, phenytoin during concurrent treatment
• Monitor therapeutic response to oral anticoagulants, sulphonylurea hypoglycaemics during concurrent therapy
• Opthalmic examination if visual problems develop
• Withdraw drug during methotrexate therapy

Treatment of overdose: Supportive and symptomatic. Activated charcoal may be useful

NURSING CONSIDERATIONS
Administer:
• With food to decrease GI symptoms

Evaluate:
• Therapeutic response: decreased pain, stiffness, swelling in joints, ability to move more easily
• For eye, ear problems: blurred vision, tinnitus (may indicate toxicity)

Teach patient/family:
• To report blurred vision or ringing, roaring in ears (may indicate toxicity)
• To avoid driving or other hazardous activities if dizziness or drowsiness occurs
• To take with food or milk
• To report change in urine pattern, weight increase, oedema, pain increase in joints, fever, blood in urine (indicates nephrotoxicity)
• That therapeutic effects may take up to 1 month
• Report any persistant indigestion or black tarry stools

---

piroxicam (topical)

Feldene Gel, Feldene Sports Gel
Func. class.: Nonsteroidal antiinflammatory
Chem. class.: Oxicam derivative
Legal class.: POM

Action: Inhibits prostaglandin synthesis by inhibiting an enzyme needed for biosynthesis; possesses analgesic, antiinflammatory properties

Uses: Topical application to superficial joints affected by osteoarthritis and musculoskeletal injuries

Dosage and routes:
• *Adult:* Massage approximately 1 g of Gel (3 cm strip) into the affected area 3−4 times a day

Side effects/adverse reactions:
INTEG: Erythema, rash, desquamation, pruritus
Systemic side-effects uncommon

and usually mild after topical use, but the following are possible:

GI: Nausea, anorexia, vomiting, diarrhoea, jaundice, cholestatic hepatitis, constipation, flatulence, cramps, peptic ulcer, gastrointestinal bleeding

CNS: Dizziness, drowsiness, fatigue, confusion, insomnia, anxiety, depression

CV: Peripheral oedema, palpitations

GU: Nephrotoxicity

HAEM: Blood dyscrasias

EENT: Tinnitus, hearing loss, blurred vision

Contraindications: Hypersensitivity to piroxicam or aspirin

Precautions: Pregnancy, breast feeding, hypersensitivity to other non-steroidal antiinflammatories. Do not use on open wounds, mucosal surfances, infected lesions, dermatoses

Pharmacokinetics: Rapid equilibration by gel with tissue under site of application. In chronic use plasma levels rise to approximately one-twentieth dose found after 20 mg orally

Interactions/incompatibilities: Unlikely to occur at low plasma levels achieved

NURSING CONSIDERATIONS

Evaluate:

• Therapeutic response

• Side effects

Teach patient/family:

• How to use the gel

• Not to apply it to open or infected wounds

• To discontinue use and report any side effects

pivampicillin

Pondocillin

Func. class.: Broad spectrum antibiotic

Chem. class.: Pivaloyloxy methyl ester of ampicillin

Legal class.: POM

Action: Ampicillin derivative, which is rapidly broken down in GI tract to ampicillin to increase bioavailability from oral dose, bactericidal antibotic

Uses: Urinary tract infections, acute and chronic bronchitis, invasive salmonellosis, gonorrhoea, ear, nose and throat infection, gynaecological infections. Skin and soft tissue infections

Dosage and routes:

• *Adult:* By mouth 500 mg every 12 hr, doubled in severe infections

• *Child up to 1 yr:* By mouth 40−60 mg/kg daily in divided doses; *1−5 yr:* 350−525 mg daily; *6−10 yr:* 525−700 mg daily

Gonorrhea

• 1.5−2 g as a single dose with 1 g of probenicid

Available forms include:

Tablets, 500 mg; suspension, 175 mg/5 ml when reconstituted with water; granules, 175 mg/sachet

Side effects/adverse reactions:

GI: Diarrhoea, Nausea, vomiting, flatulence

INTEG: Rashes, urticaria

CV: Angioedema

MS: Joint pains

SYST: Fever, anaphylactic shock

CNS: Dizziness

Contraindications: Penicillin hypersensitivity, porphyria, glandular fever

Precautions: History of allergy, renal or hepatic impairment, cephalosporin hypersensitivity.

Pregnancy, lactation, lymphatic leukaemia

Pharmacokinetics: Rapidly hydro-lysed to ampicillin by non-specific enzymes present in the serum, GI mucosa and other tissues. Plasma levels are 2−3 times higher than equimolar doses of ampicillin. Peak levels within 1 hr. Not affected by food, in GI tract

Interactions/incompatibilities: Reduced absorbtion with antacids

Treatment of overdose: Supportive measures

NURSING CONSIDERATIONS

Assess:
• Bowel pattern
• Fluid balance
• For penicillin hypersensitivity or allergy

Administer:
• After specimens have been sent for culture and sensitivity
• With food if needed for GI symptoms

Perform/provide:
• Resuscitation equipment if anaphylaxis occurs
• Adequate (2 litre) daily fluid intake

Evaluate:
• Therapeutic response: decreased fever, malaise, chills
• Daily fluid balance
• Bowel pattern daily; if severe diarrhoea occurs, report to clinician — may be discontinued

Teach patient/family:
• To complete antibiotic course as prescribed
• To report signs of rashes, joint pains, shortness of breath and other signs of sensitivity/anaphylaxis immediately

pivmecillinam

Selexid, Miraxid, Pondocillin Plus
Func. class.: Antibiotic, broad spectrum
Chem. class.: Pivaloyloxymethyl ester of mecillinam
Legal class.: POM

Action: Hydrolysed to mecillinam *in vivo*, interferes with biosynthesis of bacterial cell wall

Uses: Acute uncomplicated cystitis, chronic or recurrent bacteriuria, salmonellosis, alternative antibiotic in treatment of acute typhoid fever. Highly active against most Enterobacteriaceae; less active against Gram-positive organisms; *Ps. aeruginosa* and *Strep. faecalis* virtually resistant

Dosage and routes:
Cystitis
• *Adults:* 400 mg by mouth initially, then 200 mg 8 hrly for 3 days
Bacteriuria
• *Adults:* 400 mg every 6−8 hr
• *Child less than 40 kg:* 20−40 mg/kg in 3 or 4 divided doses
Salmonellosis
• *Adults:* 1.2−2.4 g daily for 14 days; 14−28 days for carriers
• *Child less than 40 kg:* 30−60 mg/kg daily in 3 or 4 divided doses
Available forms include: Tablets, 200 mg; suspension, granules 100 mg/sachet

Side effects/adverse reactions:
GI: Diarrhoea, nausea, vomiting, indigestion
INTEG: Rashes, urticaria
SYST: Anaphylactic shock

Contraindications: Penicillin and cephalosporin, hypersensitivity

Precautions: History of allergy, renal or hepatic impairment, pregnancy

Pharmacokinetics: Hydrolysed to mecillinam *in vivo*. Well absorbed from GI tract. Peak plasma concentrations of 5 mcg per ml have been achieved 1 to 2 hr after 400 mg dose. 50% of dose may be excreted as mecillinam in urine, mainly within 6 hr of a dose, serum half life is 1.2 hr

NURSING CONSIDERATIONS:
Assess:
• Baseline observations: temperature pulse and respiration
• Bacteriological screen: swabs, stool sample, etc
Administer:
• By mouth as directed i.e. before or with food for better absorbtion
• With copious fluids
• Concurrent administration of probenecid delays oral excretion of mecillinam, producing sustained serum levels
Perform/provide:
• Secure container and storage at room temperature
• Fluid balance chart
Evaluate:
• Therapeutic response, decrease in fever and symptoms
• Signs of anaphylaxis: rash, etc.
• Side effects of GI disturbance
Teach patient/family:
• To finish course of prescribed antibiotics
• Health education issues to avoid reoccurrence of symptoms
• Seek medical advice if symptoms/malaise reoccurs

---

pizotifen

Sanomigran
Func. class.: Antiserotonergic antihistamine with some antimuscarinic action
Legal class.: POM

Action: Prevents abnormal dilation of cranial blood vessels and sensitisation of surrounding pain receptors
Uses: Prophylaxis of vascular headache, including classical migraine, common migraine, cluster headache
Dosage and routes:
• *Adult:* By mouth 1.5 mg at night or 500 mcg 3 times daily adjusted for response; usual range 0.5–3 mg daily; maximum single dose 3 mg, maximum daily dose 6 mg
• *Child:* By mouth up to 1.5 mg/day; maximum single dose at night 1 mg
Available forms include: Tablets 500 mcg, 1.5 mg; elixir 250 mcg/5 ml
Side effects/adverse reactions:
CNS: Drowsiness, dizziness, stimulation in children
GI: Nausea
META: Weight gain
MS: Muscle pain
Precautions: Closed angle glaucoma, renal insufficiency, pregnancy, lactation, predisposition to urinary retention
Pharmacokinetics:
Readily absorbed from GI tract, metabolised with liver excreted as metabolites in urine
Interactions/incompatibilities:
• Increased sedation with: alcohol, antihistamines sedatives, hypnotics
• Decreased effect of: adrenergic neurone blocking antihypertensives
Treatment of overdose: Gastric lavage and diuresis. Severe hypotension should be corrected (caution: adrenaline may cause paradoxical effects). Convulsions managed with benzodiazepines or barbiturates
NURSING CONSIDERATIONS
Assess:
• Baseline weight
Administer:
• At beginning of headache; dose

must be titrated to patient response
• Give with meals or after meals to avoid GI symptoms

Provide:
• Quiet, calm environment with decreased stimulation from noise, bright light or excessive talking

Evaluate:
• Weight daily, check for peripheral oedema in feet, legs
• For stress level, activity, recreation, coping mechanisms of patient
• Neurological status, level of consciousness, blurring vision, nausea, vomiting, tingling in extremities that occur preceding headache
• Ingestion of tyramine foods (pickled products, beer, red wine, mature cheese), food additives, preservatives, colourings, artificial sweeteners, chocolate, caffeine; all/any may precipitate these types of headache
• Therapeutic response: decrease in frequency, severity of headache

Teach patient/family:
• Not to use non-prescribed medications, serious drug interactions may occur
• To maintain dose at approved level, not to increase even if drug does not relieve headache
• To report side effects; increased vasoconstriction, starting with cold extremities, then paraesthesia, weakness
• That an increase in headaches may occur when the drug is discontinued after long-term use
• Report at once: dyspnoea, paraesthesiae, urinary problems, pain in abdomen, chest, back, legs

plicamycin (mithramycin)

Mithracin
Func. class.: Antineoplastic antibiotic
Chem. class.: Crystalline aglycone
Legal class.: POM

Action: Inhibits DNA, RNA, protein synthesis; may lower serum calcium levels by blocking osteoclast response to parathyroid hormone

Uses: Refractory hypercalcaemia associated with a variety of neoplasms, specifically where standard therapeutic methods have failed

Dosage and routes:
• *Adult:* IV 25 mcg/kg/day for 3–4 days, repeat at intervals of 1 week. Frequency may be reduced for maintenance

Available forms include: Injection IV 2.5 mg

Side effects/adverse reactions:
META: Decreased serum phosphorus, potassium
HAEM: Haemorrhage, thrombocytopenia, WBC count, increased clotting time
GI: Nausea, vomiting, anorexia, diarrhoea, stomatitis, increased liver enzymes
GU: Increased serum urea, creatinine, proteinuria
INTEG: Rash, cellulitis, local irritation at injection site flushing
CNS: Drowsiness, weakness, lethargy, headache, depression
SYST: Fever

Contraindications: Hypersensitivity, thrombocytopenia, bone marrow depression, bleeding disorders, pregnancy, breast feeding

Precautions: Renal disease, hepatic disease, electrolyte imbalances

Pharmacokinetics: Crosses blood–brain barrier, excreted in urine; little known about pharmacokinetics

Interactions/incompatibilities:
• Increased toxicity: other anti-neoplastics or radiation

Clinical assessment:
• Full blood count, platelet count, prothrombin time, bleeding time before, regularly during and a few days after treatment
• Renal function: Monitor before, during treatment
• Liver function tests before, during therapy

Treatment of overdose: Supportive

NURSING CONSIDERATIONS

Administer:
• In accordance with local chemotherapy policy
• Antiemetics before chemotherapy
• Medications by oral route if possible; avoid IM, subcutaneous, IV routes to prevent infections
• Anti-emetic 30–60 min before giving drug to prevent vomiting
• Antibiotics for prophylaxis of infection
• Slow IV infusion using appropriate-gauge needle; check for extravasation
• Transfusion for anaemia
• Anti-spasmodic for GI symptoms
• Toxicity: facial flushing, epistaxis, increased prothrombin time, thrombocytopenia; drug should be discontinued

Perform/provide:
• Drug must not be handled by pregnant staff
• Staff to use protective garments/gloves/goggles
• Reconstitution in designated aseptic area
• Usage immediately after mixing
• Strict medical asepsis, protective isolation if WBC levels are low
• Observe oral mucosa for ulceration/breakdown. Encourage oral hygiene 4 times a day
• Warm compresses at injection site for inflammation; check for extravasation

Evaluate:
• Observe for diarrhoea and administer anti-diarrhoea drugs as required
• Bleeding: haematuria, bruising or petechiae, mucosa or orifices 8 hrly
• For signs of thrombocytopenia and depression of clotting factors 10 days after administration
• Food preferences; list likes, dislikes
• Inflammation of mucosa, breaks in skin
• Yellowing of skin, sclera, dark urine, clay-coloured stools, itchy skin, abdominal pain, fever, diarrhoea
• Buccal cavity 8 hrly for dryness, sores, ulceration, white patches, oral pain, bleeding, dysphagia
• Local irritation, pain, burning at injection site (vesicant drug)
• Frequency of stools, characteristics, cramping
• Temperature if indicated

Teach patient/family:
• Why protective isolation precautions are necessary in same cases
• To report any complaints or side effects to nurse or clinician
• To avoid foods with citric acid, hot or rough texture
• To report to clinician any bleeding, white spots, ulcerations in the mouth; tell patient to examine mouth daily
• To avoid driving or activities requiring alertness, drowsiness may occur
• To report leg cramps, tingling of fingertips, weakness; may indicate hypokalaemia
• Can cause metallic taste in mouth: encourage bland diet

pneumococcal vaccine

Pneumovax II
Func. class.: Polyvalent pneumo-
coccal vaccine
Chem. class.: Mixture of 23
purified polysaccharide capsular
antigens from serotypes of
Streptococcus pneumoniae
Legal class.: POM

Action: Promotes development of
antibody-mediated immunity
Uses: Individuals at particular risk
of contracting pneumococcal
disease, e.g. those who have
had a splenectomy
Dosage and routes: IM/subcu-
taneous injection 0.5 ml as single
dose
Available forms include: 0.5 ml
single-dose vial
Side effects/adverse reactions:
INTEG: Erythema, soreness,
induration at injection site
SYSTEM: Fever, anaphylactic
shock
HAEM: Relapse of idiopathic
thrombocytopenic purpura
NEURO: Possibly paraesthesias,
acute radiculopathy, Guillain-
Barré syndrome
Contraindications: Children less
than 2 yr, pregnancy, 10 days
before and during immunosuppressive therapy, Hodgkin's disease suffers with history of
extensive chemotherapy and/or
nodal irradiation, breast feeding,
hypersensitivity
Precautions: Cardiovascular or
respiratory disease, previously
immunised adult patients, children
immunised within last 3 yr
Clinical assessment:
• Mark patient notes clearly to
prevent revaccination
NURSING CONSIDERATIONS
Administer:
• After inspecting to ensure it is
clear, colourless and free from
suspended particles
• Undiluted
• IM or deep subcutaneous into
deltoid muscle or lateral aspect of
mid-thigh
• Do *not* inject intravascularly
Perform/provide:
• Refrigerated storage
• Adrenaline in case of anaphylaxis
Evaluate:
• For anaphylaxis
Teach patient/family:
• That local reaction (swelling,
redness at injection site) is com-
mon for 48 hr and mild fever may
occur
• No booster dose is required
• Protection will be afforded for
up to 5 yr
• They may still contract pneu-
monia since protection is against
only some of the serotypes

podophyllum resin

Posalfilin, Podophyllin Paint Com-
pound BP
Func. class.: Keratolytic
Chem. class.: Podophyllum de-
rivative
Legal class.: POM

Action: Arrests mitosis by binding to tubulin, protein subunit
of spindle microtubules; also
interferes with movements of
chromosomes
Uses: Venereal warts, keratoses,
multiple superficial, epitheliomatoses
Dosage and routes:
Warts
• *Adult:* Topical cover wart, cover
with wax paper, bandage for 4–
6 hr, wash, may repeat weekly if
needed
Keratoses/epitheliomatoses
• *Adult:* Topical apply daily with

applicator, let dry, remove tissue, may reapply if needed
Available forms include: Paint 15%
Side effects/adverse reactions:
HAEM: Thrombocytopenia, leucopenia
INTEG: Irritation of unaffected areas
CNS: Peripheral neuropathy, hallucination, confusion, dizziness, stupor, ataxia, hypotonin, convulsions, coma
GI: Nausea, vomiting, diarrhoea abdominal pain
Contraindications: Hypersensitivity, pregnancy facial warts
Interactions/incompatibilities:
• Necrosis of skin: when used with other keratolytic
NURSING CONSIDERATIONS
Assess:
• Platelets, full blood count if systemic absorption occurs
Administer:
• Only to affected area; protect surrounding normal skin
• Only to small areas or for short periods of time or absorption (systemic) may occur
Evaluate:
• Therapeutic response: decrease in size and amount of lesions
• Allergic reactions: irritation, redness, itching, stinging, burning; drug should be discontinued
• Blood dyscrasias if systemic absorption is suspected: decrease platelets
• Peripheral neuropathy; drug should be discontinued
Teach patient/family:
• That discomfort will begin after 12−24 hr, subside in 2−4 days
• Accurate and safe method of application

poliovirus vaccine, live, oral, trivalent

Func. class.: Vaccine
Legal class.: POM

Action: Produces specific antibodies for poliomyelitis
Uses: Prevention of polio
Dosage and routes: Consult manufacturer's data sheet
• *Adults:* (Unimmunised) one dose every 4 weeks for a total of three doses
• *Infants:* 1st dose at 2 months, 2nd and 3rd dose at intervals of 4 weeks
• *Reinforcement:* One dose at school entry, one further dose at school leaving
Available forms include: Oral vaccine 1 dose or 10 dose
Side effects/adverse reactions:
SYST: Paralysis
Contraindications: Hypersensitivity, active infection, allergy to any component of the vaccine, efficacy impaired if subject has diarrhoea or vomiting, immunosuppression
Precautions: Pregnancy
Interactions/incompatibilities:
• Do not use TB skin test within 6 weeks of vaccine
• Do not use within 3 months of transfusion of whole blood, plasma, or use with immune serum globulin
NURSING CONSIDERATIONS
Assess:
• Active or suspected infection, diarrhoea or vomiting
• History of allergies, especially hypersensitivity to penicillin or streptomycin
Administer:
• Orally; after shaking well, dose is dropped onto sugar cube. Usually primary course 3 doses then reinforcing doses

Perform/provide:
- Store vaccines at 2−6°C

Evaluate:
- For anaphylaxis; dyspnoea, bronchospasm, tachycardia, profuse sweating, collapse
- History of allergies, skin conditions reactions to vaccinations

Teach patient/family:
- That a reinforcing dose is needed by adults when exposure to disease is likely
- That there is a very slight risk of recipient paralysis from vaccination

---

polymyxin B sulphate

Aerosporin, Polybactrin
Func. class.: Antibiotic
Chem. class.: Polymyxin
Legal class.: POM

Action: Interferes with phospholipids, penetrates cell wall; changes occur immediately in bacterial membrane causing leakage of essential metabolites

Uses: Serious *PS. aeruginosa*, *E. aerogenes*, *K. pneumoniae*, *E. coli*, *H. influenzae* infections or when other antibiotics cannot be used

Dosage and routes:
- *Adult and child:* IV infusion 15,000−25,000 U/kg/day in divided doses every 12 hr, or as a continuous infusion. Total daily dosage must not exceed 2,000,000 units
- *Neonates:* A total of 15,000−45,000 U per kg bodyweight per day in low equally divided doses

Available forms include: Injection IV 500,000 U

Side effects/adverse reactions:
INTEG: Urticaria
CNS: Dizziness, weakness, paraesthesia
RESP: Paralysis
GU: Nephrotoxicity, azotemia, oliguria
SYST: Anaphylaxis

Contraindications: Hypersensitivity
Precautions: Pregnancy, renal impairment mysthenia gravis

Interactions/incompatibilities:
- Increased skeletal muscle relaxation: anesthetics, neuromuscular blockers (tubocurarine decamethonium, succinylcholine, gallamine)
- Increased nephrotoxicity, neurotoxicity: aminoglycosides, sodium citrate, parenteral quinine, parenteral quinidine, polypeptides, antibiotics with muscle relaxant properties
- Do not mix in solution or syringe with cephalothin sodium, chloramphenicol sodium succinate, chlorothiazide, heparin, penicillins, tetracyclines, cobalt, magnesium, iron, amphotericin B, nitrofurantoin, prednisolone

Clinical assessment:
- Monitor serum urea, creatinine
- Renal studies: urinalysis, protein, blood
- Culture and sensitivity before drug therapy; drug may be taken as soon as culture is taken; culture and sensitivity may be done after completion of therapy

Treatment of overdose: Withdraw drug, maintain airway, administer, adrenaline, aminophylline, O_2, IV corticosteroids

NURSING CONSIDERATIONS
Assess:
- Any patient with compromised renal system; drug is excreted slowly in poor renal system function; toxicity may occur rapidly

Administer:
- IV after reconstituting with 300−500 ml dextrose 5% given over 60−120 min
- After samples have been taken for culture and sensitivity

Perform/provide:

- Storage in dark area at room temperature
- Ensure resuscitation equipment and adrenaline nearby
- Adequate intake of fluids (2000 ml) during diarrhoea episodes

Evaluate:
- Fluid balance; report, oliguria
- Therapeutic response: absence of fever, purulent drainage, culture and sensitivity negative
- Skin eruptions, itching; drug should be discontinued
- Respiratory status: rate, character, dyspnoea, symptoms of neuromuscular blockade, tightness in chest; discontinue drug if these occur
- Allergies before initiation of treatment, reaction of each medication; note allergies on nursing care plan in bright red letters; notify all people giving drugs
- For flushing of face, dizziness, disorientation, weakness, paraesthesia, blurred vision, slurred speech, restlessness, irritability; indicate neurotoxicity

Teach patient/family:
- To report sore throat, fever, fatigue; could indicate superimposed infection

---

polynoxylin

Anaflex

Func. class.: Antifungal
Chem. class.: Condensation product of formaldehyde and urea
Legal class.: P

Action: May act by the release of formaldehyde
Uses: Antibacterial and antifungal for use in mild skin, aural and nasal infections
Dosage and routes:
- *Topical:* Apply once or twice daily

Available forms include: Cream 10%
Side effects/adverse reactions:
INTEG: Local reaction to any constituents of topical preparation
Contraindications: None

NURSING CONSIDERATIONS
Administer:
- Cleanse skin before application
Perform/provide:
- Storage of cream below 25°C
Evaluate:
- Therapeutic response
- Lesions diminished
Teach patient/family:
- To seek medical advice if sign of infection worsening; may require systemic therapy

---

polythiazide

Nephril

Func. class.: Thiazide diuretic
Chem. class.: Sulphonamide derivative
Legal class.: POM

Action: Acts on distal tubule by increasing excretion of water, sodium, chloride, potassium
Uses: Oedema, hypertension
Dosage and routes:
- *Adult:* By mouth 1−4 mg/day
Available forms include: Tablets 1 mg
Side effects/adverse reactions:
GU: Frequency, polyuria, glucosuria
CNS: Paraesthesia, headache, dizziness, weakness
GI: Nausea, vomiting, anorexia, constipation, diarrhoea, cramps, pancreatitis, GI irritation, jaundice
EENT: Xanthopsia
INTEG: Rash, urticaria, purpura, photosensitivity, fever, necrotising angiitis
META: Hyperglycaemia, hyperuricaemia

HAEM: Aplastic anaemia, leucopenia, agranulocytosis, thrombocytopenia

CV: Orthostatic hypotension

ELECT: Hypokalaemia, hyponatraemia, hypochloraemia

Contraindications: Hypersensitivity to thiazides or sulphonamides, anuria

Precautions: Hypokalaemia, renal electrolyte imbalance disease, pregnancy, hepatic disease, gout, chronic obstructive airways disease, lupus erythematosus, diabetes mellitus, breast feeding

Pharmacokinetics:

By mouth: Onset 2 hr, peak 6 hr, duration 24−48 hr; excreted unchanged by kidneys, enters breast milk, half-life 26 hr

Interactions/incompatibilities:

• Increased toxicity of: lithium, non-depolarising skeletal muscle relaxants, cardiac glycosides

• Decreased effects of: antidiabetics

• Decreased absorption of: thiazides: cholestyramine, colestipol

• Decreased hypotensive response: indomethacin

• Increased action of: quinidine

Clinical assessment:

• BP lying, standing; postural hypotension may occur

• Electrolytes: potassium, sodium, chloride; include serum urea, blood sugar, full blood count, serum creatinine, blood pH, arterial blood gases

• Potassium replacement if potassium is less than 3.0 mmol/litre

Lab. test interferences:

Increase: Bromsulphthalein retention, calcium, amylase

Decrease: Protein bound iodine, phenolsulphthalein

Treatment of overdose: Lavage if taken orally, monitor electrolytes, supportive therapy

NURSING CONSIDERATIONS

Assess:

• Rate, depth, rhythm of respiration, effect of exertion

• Glucose in urine if patient is diabetic

Administer:

• In morning to avoid interference with sleep if using drug as a diuretic

• With food, if nausea occurs; absorption may be decreased slightly

Evaluate:

• Weight, fluid balance daily to determine fluid loss; effect of drug may be decreased if used daily

• Improvement in oedema of feet, legs, sacral area daily if medication is being used in congestive cardiac failure

• Signs of metabolic acidosis: drowsiness, restlessness

• Signs of hypokalaemia: postural hypotension, malaise, fatigue, tachycardia, leg cramps, weakness

• Rashes, temperature elevation daily

• Confusion, especially in elderly; take safety precautions if needed

Teach patient/family:

• To increase fluid intake 2−3 litres/day unless contraindicated; to rise slowly from lying or sitting position

• To notify clinician of muscle weakness, cramps, nausea, dizziness

• Drug may be taken with food or milk

• That blood sugar may be increased in diabetics

• Take early in day to avoid nocturia

potassium bicarbonate/ potassium benzoate/ potassium chloride

Kay-Cee-L, Kloref, Kloref-S, Sando K, Leo-K, Nu-K, Slow-K, combination products

Func. class.: Electrolyte
Chem. class.: Potassium
Legal class.: P

Action: Necessary for adequate transmission of nerve impulses and cardiac contraction, renal function, intracellular ion maintenance

Uses: Prevention and treatment of hypokalaemia

Dosage and routes:

Potassium chloride

• *Adult:* Prevention of hypokalaemia: 25−50 mmols daily by mouth

• Treatment of hypokalaemia: 135−200 mmols daily by mouth

• *IV:* 20 mmols diluted to 500 ml, given over 2−3 hr. Repeat according to plasma levels

Available forms include: Many preparations; tablets, capsules, syrup, injections, infusion solutions

Side effects/adverse reactions:

CNS: Cardiac depression, arrhythmias, arrest, peaking T waves, lowered R and depressed RST, prolonged P-R interval, widened QRS complex

GI: Nausea, vomiting, cramps, pain, diarrhoea, oesophageal or small bowel ulceration

INTEG: Cold extremities

Contraindications: Renal disease (severe), severe haemolytic disease, Addison's disease, hyperkalaemia, acute dehydration, extensive tissue breakdown

Precautions: Cardiac disease, potassium sparing diuretic therapy, systemic acidosis

Interactions/incompatibilities:

• Hyperkalaemia, potassium sparing, diuretic, or other potassium products

Pharmacokinetics:

By mouth: Excreted by kidneys and in faeces

Clinical assessment:

• ECG for peaking T waves, lowered R, depressed RST, prolonged P-R interval, widening QRS complex, hyperkalaemia; drug should be reduced or discontinued

• Potassium level during treatment (3.5−5.0 mmol/litre normal level)

• Cardiac status: rate, rhythm, CVP, if being monitored directly

NURSING CONSIDERATIONS

Assess:

• Baseline fluid balance

• Urea and electrolyte levels

• Digoxin toxicity if indicated

Administer:

• Orally−in tablet form; IV− dilute 20 mmols in 500 ml dextrose or sodium chloride solution

• IV infusion slowly over 2−3 hr

• Do not mix with other drugs

• Avoiding peripheral lines

Perform/provide:

• Storage at room temperature

Evaluate:

• Therapeutic response: absence of fatigue, muscle weakness

• Degree of cardiac arrhythmias, ST elevation or depression

• Fluid balance, urinary output

Teach patient/family:

• To add potassium-rich foods to diet: bananas, orange juice, avocados; whole grains, broccoli, carrots, prunes, cocoa after this medication is discontinued

• To avoid non-prescribed products: antacids, salt substitutes, analgesics, vitamin preparations

• To report symptoms of hyperkalaemia (lethargy, confusion, diarrhoea, nausea, vomiting, fainting, decreased output) or continued hypokalaemia (fatigue, weakness, polyuria, polydipsia, cardiac changes)

potassium canrenoate

Spiroctan-M
Func. class.: Diuretic
Chem. class.: Potassium salt of canrenone
Legal class.: POM

Action: Competitive inhibition of aldosterone
Uses: Oedema associated with secondary aldosteronism, liver failure, chronic decompensated heart disease, diagnosis and treatment of primary hyper-aldosteronism
Dosage and routes: Slow IV injection/infusion 200−400 mg/day; up to 800 mg/day in exceptional cases
Available forms include: Injection 20 mg/ml, 10-ml ampoule
Side effects/adverse reactions:
META: Gynaecomastia (males), mastodynia
GI: Nausea, vomiting
CNS: Transient confusion syndrome (high doses)
INTEG: Pain, irritation at injection site
ELECT: Hyperkalaemia
Contraindications: Hyponatraemia, hyperkalaemia, renal failure, porphyria, Addison's disease, pregnancy, lactation
Precautions: Children
Pharmacokinetics: Diuresis normally commences within the first 24 hr, although long latent periods can be seen in refractory cases
Interactions/incompatibilities:
• Antagonism: anti-inflammatory analgesics, carbenoxolone, corticosteroids, corticotrophin
• Potentiation: Angiotension converting enzyme inhibitors

• Increased risk of renal failure: anti-inflammatory analgesics
Clinical assessment:
• Use only when treatment with other diuretic agents inadequate and when oral aldosterone antagonists cannot be used
• Adjust dosage to needs and response of individual
• Use for as short a time as possible
• Monitor electrolyte balance regularly in long-term use
• Prescribe anti-emetic for nausea and vomiting
• Full blood count, urine and electrolytes
Lab. test interferences:
Increase: Blood urea nitrogen
Treatment of overdose: Cease therapy, anti-emetics, potassium eliminating drug if hyperkalaemia
NURSING CONSIDERATIONS
Assess:
• Weight and fluid balance
Administer:
• Check visually for precipitation
• Do not add other drugs to injection solution
• Slowly over 2−3 mins to avoid pain and initiation at injection site
• Anti-emetics, as prescribed, for nausea and vomiting
Evaluate:
• Therapeutic response — fluid loss

potassium iodide

Aqueous Iodine, Oral Solution (Lugol's solution)
Func. class.: Thyroid hormone antagonist
Chem. class.: Iodine product
Legal class.: P

Action: Inhibits secretion of thyroid hormone, fosters colloid accumulation in thyroid follicles, decreases vascularity of gland
Uses: Preparation for thyroid-

ectomy, adjunct in thyrotoxic
crisis

Dosage and routes:

Thyrotoxic crisis

• *Adult and child:* By mouth 1 ml
in water 3 times daily after meals

Preparation for thyroidectomy

• *Adult and child:* By mouth
0.1−0.3 ml three times a day (well
diluted)

Available forms include: Solution
10%

Side effects/adverse reactions:

ENDO: Hypothyroidism, hyper-
thyroid adenoma

INTEG: Rash, urticaria, angioneurotic oedema, acne, mucosal
hemorrhage, fever

CNS: Headache

HAEM: Eosinophilia

GI: Nausea, diarrhoea, vomiting,
small bowel lesions, upper gastric
pain

MS: Arthralgia

EENT: Metallic taste, stomatitis,
salivation, periorbital oedema

Contraindications: Hypersensitivity to iodine, hyperkalaemia,
breast feeding

Precautions: Pregnancy, lactation,
children, prolonged therapy

Pharmacokinetics:

By mouth: Onset 24−48 hr, peak
10−15 days after continuous therapy, uptake by thyroid gland or
excreted in urine; crosses placenta

Interactions/incompatibilities:

• Lithium may add to hypothyroid
effect

Lab. test interferences:

Interferes: Urinary 17-hydroxy-
corticosteroids

NURSING CONSIDERATIONS

Assess:

• Baseline pulse, BP, temperature
daily

• Fluid balance

• Weight daily

Administer:

• Through straw to prevent tooth
discolouration

• With meals to decrease GI upset

• At same time each day, to maintain drug level

• Lowest dose that relieves
symptoms

Perform/provide:

• Fluids to 3−4 litres/day, unless
contraindicated

Evaluate:

• Therapeutic effect: weight
gain, decreased; pulse, puffy
hands, feet

• Overdose: peripheral oedema,
heat intolerance, diaphoresis,
palpitations, arrhythmias, severe
tachycardia, increased temperature, delirium, CNS irritability

• Hypersensitivity: rash, enlarged
cervical lymph nodes may indicate
drug needs to be discontinued

• Hypoprothrombinaemia: bleeding, petechiae, ecchymosis

• Clinical response: after 3 weeks
should include increased weight,
pulse; decreased thyroxine

Teach patient/family:

• To abstain from breast feeding
after delivery

• To take pulse daily

• To keep graph of weight, pulse,
mood

• Avoid non-prescribed drugs that
contain iodine

• That seafood, other iodine
products may be restricted

• Not to discontinue this medication abruptly; thyroid crisis may
occur

• That response may take several
months if thyroid is large

• Discontinue drug, notify clinician
if any of the following occur: fever,
rash, metallic taste, swelling of
throat, burning of mouth, throat,
sore gums, teeth, severe GI distress, enlargement of thyroid,
pinhead-sized spots or bruising

povidone-iodine

Disadine, Videne, Betadine, Savlon Dry
Func. class.: Antiseptic
Chem. class.: Iodophore
Legal class.: P

Action: Destroys a wide variety of microorganisms after local irrigation by germicidal action due to the release of iodine
Uses: Cleansing wounds, disinfection, pre-operative skin preparation
Dosage and routes:
• *Adult and child:* Use as required for anti-sepsis
Available forms include: Paint 10%, spray 5%, solution 10%, scrub 7.5%, gargle 1%, powder spray 0.5–2.5%, pessaries 200 mg, vaginal gel 10%; vaginal cleansing kit 10%; scalp and skin cleanser solution 7.5%; skin cleanser solution 4%; dusting powder 5%; dressing 10%
Side effects/adverse reactions:
INTEG: Irritation
Contraindications: Hypersensitivity to iodine, pregnancy (vaginal antiseptic), lactation, regular use in subjects with thyroid disorders, or on lithium therapy
Precautions: Extensive burns, broken skin
NURSING CONSIDERATIONS
Perform/provide:
• Consider patch testing for long term usage
Evaluate:
• Area of the body involved: irritation, rash, breaks, dryness, scales
Teach patient/family:
• To discontinue use if rash, irritation, or redness occurs and seek medical advice

pralidoxime mesylate

P2S, 2 PAM Chloride
Func. class.: Cholinesterase reactivator
Chem. class.: Quaternary ammonium oxide
Legal class.: POM

Action: Displaces enzymes at receptor site by reactivation of cholinesterase inhibited by phosphate esters
Uses: Organophosphate poisoning antidote as an adjunct to atropine
Dosage and routes:
Organophosphate poisoning
• *IM injection:* 1 g initially followed by 1–2 further doses if necessary
• *IV injection:* 1–2 g initially in 10–15 ml water for injections followed by a further 1–2 doses if necessary
• *IV infusion:* 1–2 g in 100 ml–0.9% saline over 15–30 mins. Usual most 12 g in 24 hr
• *Child:* 20–60 mg/kg as required
Available forms include: Injection IV 200 mg/ml (5 ml ampoule)
Side effects/adverse reactions:
CNS: Dizziness, headache, drowsiness, visual disturbances
GI: Nausea
MS: Weakness, muscle rigidity
CV: Tachycardia
RESP: Hyperventilation, laryngospasm
Contraindications: Hypersensitivity, inorganic phosphates, carbonates, organophosphates with anticholinesterase activity
Precautions: Myasthenia gravis, pregnancy, renal insufficiency
Pharmacokinetics:
IV: Peak 5–15 min
IM: Peak 10–20 min
Half-life 1½ hr, metabolised in liver, excreted in urine (unchanged)

NURSING CONSIDERATIONS
Assess:
• Baseline vital signs and fluid balance
Administer:
• Only with resuscitation equipment available
• As soon as possible after poisoning; within 4 hr
• IM into deep muscle; IV slowly, diluted with water, over 5–10 minutes
• Concurrent dose of atropine
Evaluate:
• BP, pulse, fluid balance; observe for decreased urinary output for 48–72 hr after poisoning to determine atropine toxicity from poisoning effects
• Airway, need for assistance with respiration
• Respiratory status: rate, rhythm, characteristics

---

prazosin HCl
Hypovase
Func. class.: Antihypertensive
Chem. class.: α-Adrenergic blocker, quinazoline derivative
Legal class.: POM

Action: Peripheral blood vessels are dilated, peripheral resistance lowered, reduction in blood pressure results from post-synaptic α-adrenergic receptors being blocked
Uses: Hypertension, refractory congestive heart failure, Raynaud's vasospasm. Benign prostatic hyperplasia
Dosage and routes:
• *Adult:* By mouth initially 500 mcg two or three times a day, increasing to 20 mg daily in divided doses if required, usual range 6–15 mg/day
• *Benign prostatic hypertrophy:* Initially 500 mcg twice daily, increasing to 2 mg twice daily, unless

required as antihypertensive therapy
Available forms include: Tablets 0.5, 1, 2, 5 mg
Side effects/adverse reactions:
CV: Palpitations, orthostatic hypotension, tachycardia, oedema
CNS: Dizziness, headache, drowsiness, anxiety, depression, vertigo, weakness, fatigue, hallucinations
GI: Nausea, vomiting, diarrhoea, constipation, abdominal pain, pancreatitis, liver junction abnormalities
GU: Urinary frequency, incontinence, impotence, priapism
EENT: Blurred vision, epistaxis, tinnitus, dry mouth, red sclera
INTEG: Rash, pruritus, alopecia, lichen planus, fever
Contraindications: Hypersensitivity
Precautions: Pregnancy, children under 12 yr, aortic and mitral valve stenosis, lactation
Pharmacokinetics:
By mouth: Onset 2 hr, peak 1–3 hr, duration 6–12 hr; half-life 2–4 hr, metabolised in liver, excreted via bile, faeces (over 90%), in urine (under 10%)
Interactions/incompatibilities:
• Increased hypotensive effects: β-blockers, calcium channel antagonists
Clinical assessment:
• Jugular venous distension 4 hrly
• Blood urea, uric acid if on long-term therapy
Treatment of overdose: Administer volume expanders or vasopressors, discontinue drug, place in supine position
NURSING CONSIDERATIONS
Assess:
• Baseline BP, fluid balance, weight
Administer:
• Whole, do not chew or crush tablets
Evaluate:
• BP pulse 4 hrly

- Weight daily, fluid balance
- Oedema in feet, legs daily
- Skin turgor, dryness of mucous membranes for hydration status
- Rales, dyspnoea, orthopnoea

Teach patient/family:
- Fainting occasionally occurs after initial dose

prednisolone/ prednisolone acetate/ prednisolone phosphate/ prednisolone steaglate

Deltacortril-Enteric, Deltastab, Precortisyl, Precortisyl-Forte, Prednesol, Sintisone, Predfoam, Predenema
Func. class.: Corticosteroid
Chem. class.: Glucocorticoid, immediate acting
Legal class.: POM

Action: Decreases inflammation by suppression of migration of polymorphonuclear leucocytes, fibroblasts, reversal to increase capillary permeability and lysosomal stabilization

Uses: Severe inflammation, immunosuppression, neoplasms

Dosage and routes:
- *Adult:* By mouth 5−60 mg daily as a single dose. IM (acetate) 25−100 mg once or twice weekly. Articular (acetate): 5−25 mg depending on size of joint (maximum 3 joints per day)
- *Rectal:* 20 mg once or twice daily for 2−4 weeks

Available forms include: Tablets 1, 5, 25 mg; tablets EC 2.5, 5 mg; tablets soluble, 5 mg (sodium phosphate) tablets (steaglate) 6.65 mg; injection, 25 mg/ml aqueous suspension (1 ml) acetate; enema (disodium phosphate) 20 mg, Foam Enema (metasul phobenzoate sodium) 20 mg

Side effects/adverse reactions:
INTEG: Acne, poor wound healing, ecchymosis, petechiae, hirsutism
CNS: Depression, headache, mood changes, insomnia
CV: Embolism, hypotension on rapid withdrawal
HAEM: Thrombocytopenia
MS: Fractures, osteoporosis, proximal myopathy, avascular osteonecrosis, tendon rupture
GI: Diarrhoea, nausea, abdominal distension, GI haemorrhage, increased appetite, pancreatitis, dyspepsia, peptic and esophageal ulceration, oesophageal candidiasis
EENT: Fungal infections, increased intraocular pressure, blurred vision
ELECT: Sodium and water retention, hypertension, hypokalaemic alkalosis
META: Suppression of hypothalamo-pituitary adrenal axis, growth retardation in children, menstrual irregularity, diabetogenic

Contraindications: Systemic injection, unless specific anti-injective therapy is employed

Precautions: Pregnancy, diabetes mellitus, glaucoma, osteoporosis, seizure disorders, ulcerative colitis, tuberculosis, hypertension, psychosis, peptic ulceration, previous steroid myopathy, children, ocular herpes simplex, family history of diabetes mellitus, family history of glaucoma

Pharmacokinetics:
By mouth: Peak 1−2 hr, duration 2 days
IM: Peak 3−45 hr

Interactions/incompatibilities:
- Decreased effects of: cholestyramine, colestipol, barbiturates, rifampicin, ephedrine, phenytoin, carbamazepine
- Decreased effects of: anticoagu-

lants, anticonvulsants, antidiabetics, diuretics
• Increased side effects: alcohol, salicylates, amphotericin B, digitalis preparations, non-steroidal anti-inflammatory drugs, live vaccines
• Increased effect of: salicylates
• Diuretics: may cause excessive potassium loss

Clinical assessment:
• Potassium, blood sugar, urine glucose while on long-term therapy; hypokalaemia and hyperglycaemia
• Plasma cortisol levels during long-term therapy (normal level: 138−635 nmol/litre when drawn at 8 AM)
• Titrated dose, use lowest effective dose
• Radiography: bone density on long-term therapy
• Fluid balance, be alert for decreasing urinary output and increasing oedema

Lab. test interferences:
Increase: Cholesterol, sodium, blood glucose, uric acid, calcium, urine glucose
Decrease: Calcium, potassium, thyroxine, triiodothyronine, thyroid ^{131}I uptake test, urine 17-hydroxycorticosteroids, 17-ketosteroids, protein bound iodine
False negative: Skin allergy tests

NURSING CONSIDERATIONS
Assess:
• Baseline BP, pulse and weight
Administer:
• IM injection deeply in large mass, rotate sites, avoid deltoid
• In one dose in AM to prevent adrenal suppression. Avoid SC administration; damage may be done to tissue
• After shaking suspension (parenteral)
• With food or milk to decrease GI symptoms
Perform/provide:
• Assistance with movement in patient with bone tissue disease to prevent fractures
• Weight gain more than 2.5 kilo (to be reported)
• For chest pain
• Therapeutic response: ease of respirations, decreased inflammation
• Infection: increased temperature, WBC, even after withdrawal of medication; drug masks symptoms of infection
• Potassium depletion: paraesthesias, fatigue, nausea, vomiting, depression, polyuria, arrhythmias, weakness
• Oedema, hypotension, cardiac symptoms
• Mental status: affect, mood, behavioural changes, aggression
Teach patient/family:
• That warning card, as steroid user should be carried
• To notify clinician if therapeutic response decreases; dosage adjustment may be needed
• Not to discontinue this medication abruptly or adrenal crisis can result
• To avoid non-prescribed products: salicylates, alcohol in cough products, cold preparations unless directed by clinician
• Teach patient all aspects of drug use, including Cushingoid symptoms
• Symptoms of adrenal insufficiency; nausea, anorexia, fatigue, dizziness, dyspnoea, weakness, joint pain
• Supplement verbal information with instruction leaflet

prednisolone acetate/ prednisolone sodium phosphate (ophthalmic, otic)

Minims, Pred Forte, Predsol, combination product
Func. class.: Anti-inflammatory, Corticosteroid
Chem. class.: Glucocorticoid, immediate acting
Legal class.: POM

Action: Decreases inflammation, resulting in decreases in pain, photophobia, cellular infiltration
Uses: Inflammation of eye, lids, conjunctiva, cornea, uveitis, iridocyclitis, allergic condition, burns, foreign bodies, inflammatory conditions of the ear
Dosage and routes:
• *Adult and child:* Eyes: Instil 1−2 drops into conjunctival sac every 1−2 hr until controlled, then reduce frequency
• Ears: 2−3 drops every 2−3 hr until controlled, then reduce frequency
Available forms include: Suspension 1%; solution 0.5%
Side effects/adverse reactions:
EENT: Increased intra-ocular pressure, poor corneal wound healing, increased possibility of corneal infections, glaucoma exacerbation, cataracts, thinning of the cornea
Contraindications: Hypersensitivity, acute superficial herpes simplex, fungal/viral diseases of eye or conjunctiva, ocular tuberculosis infections of the eye
Precautions: Corneal abrasions, glaucoma, soft contact lenses, administration to 'red eyes'
NURSING CONSIDERATIONS
Administer:
• After shaking suspension

Evaluate:
• Allergic reactions: redness, itching, swelling, lacrimation
• Therapeutic response: absence of swelling, redness, exudate
Teach patient/family:
• Instillation method
• Wash hands thoroughly before administrations
• Not to share eye medications with others
• Discard eye-drops after 28 days of opening − discarding unused product

prednisone

Decortisyl
Func. class.: Corticosteroid
Chem. class.: Glucocorticoid, immediate acting
Legal class.: POM

Action: Decreases inflammation by suppression of migration of polymorphonuclear leucocytes, fibroblasts, reversal to increase capillary permeability, and lysosomal stabilisation
Uses: Severe inflammation, immunosuppression, neoplasms, multiple sclerosis
Dosage and routes:
• *Adult:* By mouth 2.5−15 mg 2 to 4 times a day, then daily or alternate days maintenance
• *Child under 1 yr:* Not recommended; 1−7 yr: quarter to half adult dose; 7−12 yr: half to three quarters adult dose
Available forms include: Tablets 5 mg
Side effects/adverse reactions:
INTEG: Acne, poor wound healing, ecchymosis, petechiae, hirsuitism
CNS: Depression, headache, mood changes insomnia
CV: Hypotension on rapid withdrawal, embolism

HAEM: Thrombocytopenia
MS: Fractures, osteoporosis, proximal myopathy, avascular osteonecrosis, tendon rupture
GI: Diarrhoea, nausea, abdominal distention, GI haemorrhage, increased appetite, pancreatitis dyspepsia, peptic and oesophageal ulceration oesophageal candidiasis
EENT: Fungal infections, increased intraocular pressure, blurred vision
ELECT: Sodium and water retention, hypertension, hypokalaemic acidosis
META: Suppression of hypothalamo-pituitary adrenal axis, growth retardation in children, menstrual irregularities, diabetogenic

Contraindications: Systemic infection, unless specific anti-infective therapy is employed

Precautions: Pregnancy, diabetes mellitus, glaucoma, osteoporosis, seizure disorders, ulcerative colitis, tuberculosis, hypertension, psychosis, peptic ulceration, previous steroid myopathy children, ocular herpes simplex, family history of diabetes mellitus, family history of glaucoma

Pharmacokinetics:
By mouth: Peak 1−2 hr, duration 1−1½ days, half-life 3½−4 days

Interactions/incompatibilities:
• Decreased effects of: cholestyramine, colestipol, barbiturates, rifampicin, ephedrine, phenytoin, carbamazepine
• Decreased effects of: anticoagulants, anticonvulsants, antidiabetics, diuretics
• Increased side effects: alcohol, non-steroidal anti-inflammatory drugs, salicylates, amphotericin B, digitalis preparations, live vaccines
• Increased effects of: salicylates, oestrogens, indomethacin
• Diuretics may cause excessive potassium loss

Clinical assessment:
• Potassium, blood sugar, urine glucose while on long-term therapy; hypokalaemia and hyperglycaemia
• Plasma cortisol levels during long-term therapy (normal level: 138−635 nmol/litre when drawn at 8 AM)

Lab. test interferences:
Increase: Cholesterol, sodium, blood glucose, uric acid, calcium, urine glucose
Decrease: Calcium, potassium, thyroxine, triiodothyronine, thyroid ^{131}I uptake test, urine 17-hydroxycorticosteroids, 17-ketosteroids, protein bound iodine
False negative: Skin allergy tests

NURSING CONSIDERATIONS
Assess:
• Baseline BP, pulse and weight
• With food or milk to decrease GI symptoms
Administer:
• Titrate dose, use lowest effective dose
Perform/provide:
• Assistance with movement in patient with bone tissue disease to prevent fractures
Evaluate:
• Weight weekly, notify clinician of weekly gain over 2 kg
• BP 4 hrly, pulse, notify clinician if chest pain occurs
• Fluid balance, be alert for decreasing urinary output and increasing oedema
• Avoid use of surgical tape
• Daily urinalysis when on high dosage
• Radiography: bone density on long-term therapy
• Infection: increased temperature, WBC, even after withdrawal of medication; drug masks symptoms of infection

• Potassium depletion: paraesthesias, fatigue, nausea, vomiting, depression, polyuria, arrhythmias, weakness
• Oedema, hypotension, cardiac symptoms
• Mental status: affect, mood, behavioural changes, aggression
• Therapeutic response: ease of respirations, decreased inflammation

Teach patient/family:
• That warning card as steroid user should be carried
• To notify clinician if therapeutic response decreases; dosage adjustment may be needed
• Not to discontinue this medication abruptly or adrenal crisis can result
• To avoid non-prescribed products: salicylates, alcohol in cough products, cold preparations unless directed by clinician
• Teach patient all aspects of drug use, including Cushingoid symptoms
• Symptoms of adrenal insufficiency: nausea, anorexia, fatigue, dizziness, dyspnoea, weakness, joint pain
• That wounds will take longer to heal
• To avoid use of surgical tape

---

prilocaine HCl

Citanest, Citanest with Octapressin
Func. class.: Anaesthetic, local
Chem. class.: Aminoacylamide
Legal class.: POM

Action: Inhibits nerve impulses from sensory nerves, thereby producing anaesthesia
Uses: Infiltration, regional nerve block, spinal anaesthesia, regional IV analgesia, dental anaesthesia
Dosage and routes:
• Local injection, dose adjusted according to site of operation to maximum of 400 mg used alone or 600 mg if used with adrenaline or felypressin
Available forms include: Injection 1%, 10 mg/ml, 20 ml, 50 ml vials; injection 0.5%, 5 mg/ml 20 ml, 50 ml vials; injection 4%, 40 mg/ml, 2-ml cartridge with octopressin; injection 3%, 30 mg/ml, 2-ml cartridge and self-aspirating cartridge
Side effects/adverse reactions:
CV: Cardiac arrest, bradycardia, hypotension, myocardial depression
CNS: Agitation, euphoria, convulsions, dizziness, tremors, unconsciousness
RESP: Respiratory depression
INTEG: Cutaneous, lesion, urticaria, oedema, anaphylactic reactions
Contraindications: Hypersensitivity, anaemia, methaemoglobinaemia
Precautions: Impaired cardiac conduction, renal or hepatic impairment, epilepsy, elderly or debilitated patients, impaired respiratory function
Pharmacokinetics: Rapidly metabolised mainly in the liver and also the kidneys. Principal metabolite excreted in urine is *o*-tomidine Prelocains Crosses placenta during prolonged epidural anaesthesia producing methaemoglobinaemia in the foetus
Treatment of overdose: Maintain airway; administer O_2, vasopressor, IV fluids, anticonvulsants for seizures

NURSING CONSIDERATIONS
Assess:
• BP, pulse, respiration
Administer:
• With resuscitation equipment nearby
• Only drugs without preserv-

atives for epidural or caudal anaesthesia

Perform/provide:
• Use new solution, discard part-used units

Evaluate:
• Therapeutic response, anaesthesia necessary for procedure
• Allergic reactions, rash, urticaria, itching
• Cardiac status, ECG for arrhythmias, pulse, BP during treatment
• Foetal heart tones if drug is used during labour

---

primaquine phosphate

Func. class.: Antimalarial
Chem. class.: Synthetic 8-amino-quinolone
Legal class.: P

Action: Action is unknown; thought to destroy exoerythrocytic forms by gametocidal action, and inhibition of mitochondrial respiration

Uses: Malaria caused by *Plasmodium vivax*, *Plasmodium ovale*

Dosage and routes:
• *Adult:* By mouth 15 mg primaquine base daily for 10–14 days
• *Child:* 0.2–0.3 mg primaquine base per kg body weight daily for 10–14 days

Available forms include: Tablets 13.2 mg (7.5 mg base)

Side effects/adverse reactions:
GI: Nausea, vomiting, abdominal pain
HAEM: Haemolytic anemia, methaemoglobinaemia

Contraindications: Hypersensitivity, lupus erythematosus, rheumatoid arthritis, methaemoglobulinaemia, G6PD deficiency, pregnancy, lactation, concurrent with drugs that induce haemolysis or bone marrow depression

Pharmacokinetics:
By mouth: Metabolised by liver (metabolites), half-life 3.7–9.6 hr

Interactions/incompatibilities:
• Toxicity: mepacrine

Clinical assessment:
• Ophthalmic test if long-term treatment or drug dosage over 150 mg/day
• Liver studies every week: aspartate aminotransferase, alanine aminotransferase, bilirubin, if on long-term therapy
• Blood studies, full blood count, since blood dyscrasias occur

NURSING CONSIDERATIONS
Administer:
• Before or after meals at same time each day to maintain drug level

Evaluate:
• Therapeutic effect

Teach patient/family:
• To report any new symptoms

---

primidone

Mysoline
Func. class.: Anticonvulsant
Chem. class.: Barbiturate derivative
Legal class.: POM

Action: Raises seizure threshold: is converted to active drug phenobarbitone

Uses: Management of grand mal and psychomotor (temporal lobe), epilepsy, focal or Jacksonian seizures, petit mal, myoclonic jerks and akinetic attacks. Management of essential tremor

Dosage and routes:
Epilepsy
• *Adult and child over 9 yr:* By mouth, commence 125 mg daily at night increasing by 125 mg daily every 3 days until patient receiving daily 500 mg thereafter increasing by 250 mg tablet daily until re-

sponse obtained not to exceed 1.5 g/day usually in two equally divided doses

• *Child:* By mouth, under 2 yr, 250–500 mg daily; 2–5 yr, 500–750 mg daily; 6–9 yr 750–1000 mg daily. All daily doses usually divided into 2 equal portions, and adjusted according to tolerability, response

Essential tremor

• *Adult:* Starting dose 50 mg daily increased over 2–3 weeks according to toleration/response to maximum 750 mg daily in divided doses

Available forms include: Tablets, 250 mg; suspension 250 mg/5 ml

Side effects/adverse reactions:

HAEM: Thrombocytopenia, leucopenia, neutropenia, eosinophilia, megaloblastic anemia, lymphadenopathy, folic acid deficiency

CNS: Stimulation, drowsiness, dizziness, confusion, sedation, headache, flushing, hallucinations, coma, psychosis, ataxia

GI: Nausea, vomiting, anorexia

INTEG: Rash, oedema, lupus-like syndrome (rare)

EENT: Diplopia, nystagmus

GU: Impotence, polyuria

Contraindications: Hypersensitivity, porphyria

Precautions: Chronic obstructive airways disease, hepatic disease, renal disease, hyperactive children, lactation, pregnancy

Pharmacokinetics:

By mouth: Peak 4 hr, excreted by kidneys, excreted in breast milk, half-life 3–24 hr. Metabolised to active metabolites including phenobarbitone

Interactions/incompatibilities:

• Decreased effects: Tricyclic antidepressants and antipsychotics (lower seizure threshold)

• Effects reduced (accelerated metabolism): disopyramide, quinidine, chloramphenicol, doxycycline, metronidazole, coumarin anticoagulants, tricyclic antidepressants, clonazepam, phenytoin, phenobarbitone, griseofulvin, felodipine, isradipine, corticosteroids, cyclosporin, sex hormones including oral contraceptives, theophylline, thyroxine

• Enhanced CNS side-effects with other CNS depressants including alcohol

Clinical assessment:

• Drug level: therapeutic level of derived phenobarbitone 15–40 mg/litre

Treatment of overdose: Aspiration of stomach contents if recently ingested, no specific antidote, give supportive treatment

NURSING CONSIDERATIONS

Administer:

• Total daily dose best given in two divided doses

• Oral suspension requires special diluent for low doses

Evaluate:

• Mental status: mood, alertness, effect, memory (long-, short-term)

• Respiratory depression

• Blood dyscrasias: fever, sore throat, bruising, rash, jaundice

Teach patient/family:

• Emphasise necessity of taking drug at appropriate time and on a continuing basis

• All aspects of drug administration: action, route, dose, when to notify clinician

• About side effects

---

probenecid

Benemid

Func. class.: Uricosuric

Chem. class.: Sulphonamide derivative

Legal class.: POM

Action: Inhibits tubular reabsorption of urate, with increased excretion of uric acid, inhibits urinary excretion of β-lactam antibiotics

Uses: Treatment of hyperuricaemia in gout, gouty arthritis, adjunct to cephalosporin or penicillin treatment especially of gonorrhoea

Dosage and routes:
Gout/gouty arthritis
• *Adult:* By mouth 250 mg twice a day for 1 week, then 500 mg twice a day, increasing by 500 mg every 4 weeks if needed; not to exceed 2 g/day; maintenance: as long as patient is asymptomatic dosage may be reduced by 500 mg every 6 months to minimum effective dose

Adjunct in penicillin/cephalosporin treatment
• *Adult and child over 50 kg:* By mouth 500 mg four times a day
• *Child (over 2 yr) under 50 kg:* By mouth 25 mg/kg, then 40 mg/kg in divided doses four times a day

Gonorrhoea
• *Adult:* By mouth 1 g with oral ampicillin or IM ½ hr before procaine penicillin or cefoxitin

Available forms include: Tablets 0.5 g

Side effects/adverse reactions:
CNS: Drowsiness, headache, confusion, stimulation, dizziness, in overdose: EEG changes, convulsions
GU: Frequency, nephrotic syndrome. In gouty patients: haematuria, renal colic, urate stones
GI: Gastric irritation, nausea, vomiting, anorexia, hepatic necrosis, sore gums
INTEG: Rash, dermatitis, pruritus, flushing, alopecia
SYST: Fever, anaphylaxis
HAEM: Anaemia, haemolytic anaemia, leucopenia, aplastic anaemia
MISC: Exacerbation of gout

Contraindications: Hypersensitivity, severe hepatic disease, blood dyscrasias, severe renal disease, child under 2 yr, renal urate stones, porphyria, acute gout

Precautions: Pregnancy, lactation, peptic ulceration, low fluid intake

Pharmacokinetics:
By mouth: Peak 2−4 hr, duration 8 hr, half-life 8−10 hr; metabolised by liver, excreted in urine, 85−95% bound to plasma proteins

Interactions/incompatibilities:
• Increased blood levels of these drugs (significance uncertain): sulphonamides, dapsone, nalidixic acid, nitrofurantoin, acyclovir, PAS, indomethacin, ketoprofen, meclofamate, lorazepam rifampicin, naproxen, sodium iodothalamate and some other contrast media, β-lactam antibiotics, pantothenic acid
• Increased blood levels of these drugs, likely toxicity: methotrexate, sulphonylurea hypoglycaemics, zidovudine
• Decreased effect: salicylates, pyrazinamide

Clinical assessment:
• Uric acid levels within normal limits

Lab. test interferences:
False positive: Benedict's test
Decrease: Urinary 17-ketosteroids, phenolsulphthalein (PSP), sulphabromophthalein (BSP), *p*-aminohippuric acid (PAH)

Treatment of overdose: Induce emesis or gastric lavage. No specific antidote, treatment symptomatic including IV diazepam or short-acting barbiturate for CNS stimulation

NURSING CONSIDERATIONS
Assess:
• pH of urine
• Fluid balance
• Dietary intake
Administer:

• After food or with milk if GI symptoms occur
• With treatment for an acute attack if this develops
• With appropriate antibiotic
• After culture and sensitivity tests, including those for concurrent infections

Perform/provide:
• Low purine diet restricting: offal, anchovies, sardines, meat gravy, dried beans, meat extracts

Evaluate:
• Therapeutic response; resolution of infection
• Therapeutic result; dimunition of gout pain
• Recidivist tendencies
• Urinary pH and fluid balance regularly

Teach patient/family:
• To avoid non-prescribed preparations, particularly
• Necessity of taking entire course of medication as prescribed
• To drink at least 2 litres of fluid daily, avoiding alcohol
• To report side-effects, including GI pain, urinary symptoms
• That starting treatment may precipitate an acute attack
• Counselling about protection during sexual intercourse, contact tracing of partners if treating gonorrhoea

---

probucol

Lurselle

Func. class.: Hypolipidaemic
Chem. class.: Butylphenol derivative
Legal class.: POM

Action: Lowers elevated serum cholesterol, effect on triglycerides less consistent; underlying mechanisms unclear

Uses: Type IV hyperlipidaemia, Severe hypercholesterolemia dietary treatment unsuccessful

Dosage and routes:
• *Adult:* By mouth 500 mg twice daily with breakfast, supper

Available forms include: Tablets 250 mg

Side effects/adverse reactions:
GI: Nausea, vomiting, diarrhoea, constipation, anorexia, flatulence, abdominal pain
INTEG: Flushing, alopecia, sweating, hyperthermia
CV: Palpitations, arrhythmias, prolonged QT interval
EENT: Visual disturbances
CNS: Palpitations, paraesthesias
SYST: Hypersensitivity reactions including angioedema

Contraindications: Hypersensitivity
Precautions: Arrhythmias, myocardial damage, angina pectoris, pregnancy, lactation, children

Pharmacokinetics:
By mouth: Absorption low and variable, better with food; excreted in bile/faeces

Clinical assessment:
• ECG before treatment in patients with recent myocardial damage
• For signs of vitamin A, D, K deficiency

Evaluate:
• Therapeutic response: decreased triglycerides, cholesterol levels (hyperlipidaemia), diarrhoea, pruritus (excess bile area)

Lab. test interferences:
• *Increase:* Liver function studies, CPK, renal function studies, blood glucose

NURSING CONSIDERATIONS

Assess:
• Baseline BP and ECG
• Dietary habits and smoking status

Administer:
• Drug with meals
• Bowel pattern daily; increase

fibre, fluid, in diet to prevent constipation occurring

Teach patient/family:

• That compliance is needed since toxicity may result if doses are missed

• That risk factors should be decreased: high fat diet, smoking, alcohol consumption, absence of exercise

• That non-prescribed preparations should be avoided unless directed by clinician

• About side effects; nausea; belching

---

procainamide HCl

Procainamide Durules, Pronestyl
Func. class.: Antiarrhythmic (Class IA)
Chem. class.: Procaine analogue
Legal class.: POM

Action: Increases electrical stimulation threshold of ventricle, His Purkinje system, which stabilises cardiac membrane

Uses: Supraventricular tachyarrhythmias, ventricular arrhythmias, digitalis induced arrhythmias

Dosage and routes:

• *Adult:* By mouth is preferred, initially 50 mg/kg/day given as divided doses every 3−6 hr or 2−3 modified release 500 mg tablets 3 times a day, subsequently adjusted to maintain serum concentration within range 4−8 mcg/ml and maintain normal rhythm

• IV, by slow injection, rate not exceeding 50 mg/min, 100 mg, repeated at 5-min intervals, maximum 1 g

• IV, by infusion, 500−600 mg over 25−30 min, followed by maintenance at rate of 2−6 mg/min, transfer to oral therapy, 3−4 hr after end of infusion

Available forms include: Tablets 250 mg; tablets modified release 500 mg; injection IV 100 mg/ml

Side effects/adverse reactions:

CNS: Headache, dizziness, confusion, psychosis, depression

GI: Nausea, vomiting, anorexia, diarrhoea, bitter taste, hepatitis

CV: Hypotension, cardiovascular collapse, arrest cardiac arrhythmias

HAEM: Lupus-like syndrome, agranulocytosis, neutropenia, thrombocytopenia, haemolytic anaemia

INTEG: Rash, urticaria, oedema, flushing

SYST: Chills, fever, allergic reactions

MS: Joint and muscle pain, muscle weakness

Contraindications: Hypersensitivity, severe heart block, heart failure, hypotension

Precautions: Pregnancy, lactation, renal disease, liver disease, congestive heart failure, respiratory depression, elderly, myasthenia gravis, asthma, SLE

Pharmacokinetics

By mouth: Peak 1−2 hr, duration 3 hr (8 hr extended)

Half-life 3 hr, metabolised in liver to active metabolites, excreted unchanged by kidneys (60%) effective concentration is 4−8 mcg/ml, toxicity rare below 12 mcg/ml

Interactions/incompatibilities:

• Increased effects of neuromuscular blockers neostigmine, pyridostigmine, propranolol, muscle relaxants, antihypertensives

• Increased myocardial depression with other anti-arrhythmics

• Increased procainamide serum levels with amiodarone, cimetidine

• Trimethoprim, propranolol

• Decreased effects of: sulphonamide antibiotics

• Risk of neutropenia/Stevens−Johnson syndrome with captopril

Clinical assessment:

• ECG continuously during acute therapy to determine increased P-R or QRS segments; if these develop, discontinue immediately; watch for increased ventricular ectopic beats

• Plasma concentrations

• Monthly serological tests for antinuclear factors suggestive of lupus-like syndrome; stop treatment if they occur

• Full blood count if symptoms suggest agranulocytosis

Treatment of overdose: Induce vomiting/use gastric lavage or administer activated charcoal if recent oral ingestion. No specific antidote. Monitor ECG. Removable by haemodialysis. General supportive measures include sympathomimetic agents and fluid expansion for cardiovascular symptoms. Temporary ventricular pacing may be needed

NURSING CONSIDERATIONS
Assess:

• Blood gases

• Baseline vital signs

• Fluid balance, electrolytes (potassium, sodium chloride)

• BP and ECG continuously for fluctuations during IV use

Evaluate:

• Therapeutic response: re-establish normal sinus rhythm

• Check site daily for infiltration or extravasation

• Malignant hyperthermia: tachypnoea, tachycardia, changes in BP, increased temperature

• Cardiac rate, respiration: rate, rhythm, character, continuously

• Respiratory status: rate, rhythm, lung fields, watch for respiratory depression

• CNS effects: dizziness, confusion, psychosis, paraesthesia, convulsions; drug should be discontinued

• Lung fields, bilateral rales may occur in congestive heart failure patient

• Increased respiration, increased pulse; drug should be discontinued

---

procaine HCl

Func. class.: Local anaesthetic
Chem. class.: Ester
Legal class.: POM

Action: Competes with calcium for sites in nerve membrane that control sodium transport across cell membrane; decreases rise of depolarisation phase of action potential

Uses: Local anaesthesia by infiltration and regional routes

Dosage and routes:

• Injection up to 1 g (200 ml of 0.5% solution or 100 ml of 1%) with adrenaline 1 in 200,000

Available forms include: Injection 1%, 2%

Side effects/adverse reactions:

CNS: Anxiety, restlessness, convulsions, loss of consciousness, drowsiness, disorientation, tremors, shivering

CV: Myocardial depression, cardiac arrest, arrhythmias, bradycardia, hypotension, fetal bradycardia

GI: Nausea, vomiting

EENT: Blurred vision, tinnitus, pupil constriction

INTEG: Rash, urticaria, allergic reactions, oedema, burning, skin discolouration at injection site, pallor, sweating

RESP: Status asthmaticus, respiratory arrest, anaphylaxis

Contraindications: Hypersensitivity, severe liver disease

Precautions: Elderly

Pharmacokinetics:
Onset 2–5 min, duration 1 hr; metabolised by plasma cholin-

esterases, liver, excreted in urine (metabolites)

Interactions/incompatibilities:
• Arrhythmias: adrenaline, halothane, enflurane

Treatment of overdose: Airway, O_2, vasopressor, IV fluids, anticonvulsants for seizures

NURSING CONSIDERATIONS

Assess:
• Baseline BP, pulse, respiration before treatment

Administer:
• Only drugs that are not cloudy, do not contain precipitate
• Only with resuscitation equipment nearby
• Only drugs without preservatives for epidural or caudal anaesthesia

Evaluate:
• Therapeutic response: anaesthesia necessary for procedure
• Allergic reactions: rash, urticaria, itching
• Cardiac status: ECG for arrhythmias, pulse, BP during anaesthesia
• Fetal heart tones if drug is to be used during labour

Teach patient/family:
• Effect of injection

---

procarbazine HCl

Natulan
Func. class.: Antineoplastic
Chem. class.: Methylhydrazine derivative
Legal class.: POM

Action: Inhibits DNA, RNA, protein synthesis; has multiple sites of action

Uses: Hodgkin's disease, cancers resistant to other therapy

Dosage and routes:
• *Adult:* By mouth usually in combination with other drugs at a dose of 100 mg/m²/day for 10–14 days repeated 4–6 weekly. As a single agent 50 mg/day increased over 6 days to 250–300 mg/day in divided doses, reducing once maximal response achieved to 50–150 mg daily in divided doses. Continue to cumulative total of at least 6 g
• *Child:* By mouth 50 mg/day for 7 days, then 100 mg/m² until desired response, leucopenia, or thrombocytopenia occurs

Available forms include: Capsules 58.3 mg (50 mg base)

Side effects/adverse reactions:
HAEM: Thrombocytopenia, anaemia, leucopenia, bleeding disorders
GI: Nausea, vomiting, anorexia, diarrhoea, constipation, dry mouth, stomatitis, impaired liver function
EENT: Retinal haemorrhage, papiloedema
INTEG: Rash, pruritus, alopecia, hyperpigmentation
CNS: Headache, insomnia, confusion, coma pain, chills, fever, sweating, paraesthesias, drowsiness, anxiety, tremor, convulsions
RESP: Cough, pneumonitis
CVS: Tachycardia, hypotension

Contraindications: Hypersensitivity, severe bone marrow depression, severe hepatic/renal damage, pregnancy, breast feeding

Precautions: Renal disease, hepatic disease, radiation therapy, phaeochromocytoma, epilepsy, elderly, cardiovascular disease

Pharmacokinetics: Half-life 1 hr; concentrates in liver, kidney, skin; metabolised in liver, excreted in urine; WBC nadir 2–3 weeks postdose

Interactions/incompatibilities:
• Increased CNS depression given with: barbiturates, antihistamines, narcotics, phenothiazines
• Disulfiram-like reaction: ethyl alcohol
• Procarbazine is weak mono-MAOI; low risk of hypertension

with: tricyclic antidepressants, narcotic analgesics; tyramine-rich foods, guanethidine, levodopa, reserpine, amphetamines and other sympathomimetics

• Hypertension: guanethidine, levodopa, methyldopa, reserpine

Clinical assessment:

• Full blood count, differential, platelet count weekly during treatment and until nadir blood counts have been passed; withhold drug if myelosuppression is excessive

• Renal function studies: before, during therapy

• Liver function tests before, during therapy

Treatment of overdose: Gastric lavage, supportive treatment, no specific antidotes, regular blood counts, blood products and/or filgrastim to treat myelosuppression

NURSING CONSIDERATIONS

Administer:

• In accordance with local cytotoxic policy

• Other medications by oral route if possible; avoid IM, SC, IV routes to prevent infection

• Antispasmodics for GI symptoms

• Anti-emetic 30−60 min before giving drug to prevent vomiting

• Antibiotics for prophylaxis of infection

• Topical or systemic analgesics for pain

Perform/provide:

• Strict medical asepsis and protection isolation if WBC levels are low

• Liquid diet: carbonated drinks, jelly; dry toast, plain biscuits may be added if patient is not nauseated or vomiting

• Storage in tight, light-resistant container in cool environment

Evaluate:

• Toxicity: facial flushing, epistaxis, thrombocytopenia; drug should be discontinued

• Bleeding: haematuria, bruising or petechiae, mucosa or orifices 8 hrly

• Skin rashes: drug should be discontinued

• Food preferences; list likes, dislikes

• Effects of alopecia on body image; discuss feelings about body changes

• Inflammation of mucosa, breaks in skin

• Yellowing of skin, sclera, dark urine, clay-coloured stools, itchy skin, abdominal pain, fever, diarrhoea

• Oral mucosa regularly for dryness, sores or ulceration, white patches, oral pain, dysphagia

• Local irritation, pain, burning at injection site

• GI symptoms: frequency of stools, cramping

• Acidosis, signs of dehydration: rapid respirations, poor skin turgor, decreased urine output, dry skin, restlessness, weakness

Teach patient/family:

• Why protective isolation precautions are necessary

• To report any complaints, side effects to nurse or clinician: cough, shortness of breath, fever, chills, sore throat, bleeding, bruising, vomiting blood, black tarry stools

• MAOI drug, avoid foods such as marmite, cheese, alcohol

• That hair may be lost during treatment and wig or hairpiece may be available in the NHS; tell patient that new hair may be different in colour, texture

• To avoid foods with citric acid, hot or rough texture

• To report any bleeding, white spots, ulcerations in mouth to physician; tell patient to examine mouth daily

• To avoid driving or activities requiring alertness; drowsiness may occur

- That contraceptive measures are recommended during therapy
- Avoid ingestion of alcohol, tyramine-containing foods; cold, hayfever, or weight-reducing products may cause serious drug interactions

prochlorperazine mesylate/ prochlorperazine maleate

Buccastem, Vertigon, Stemetil, Stemetil Eff
Func. class.: Anti-emetic
Chem. class.: Phenothiazine, piperazine derivative
Legal class.: POM

Action: Acts centrally by blocking chemoreceptor trigger zone, which in turn acts on vomiting centre
Uses: Nausea, vomiting, Ménière's syndrome, psychoses
Dosage and routes:
Postoperative nausea/vomiting
- *Adult:* IM 12.5 mg 1−2 hr before anaesthesia; may repeat in 30 min; followed by oral medication after 6 hr as needed
Severe nausea/vomiting, Ménière's, labyrinthitis, anxiety
- *Adult:* By mouth 5−10 mg three or four times a day; modified release capsule 15 mg once or twice daily. Rectal 25 mg twice or three times a day; IM 12.5 mg followed by oral medication; buccal 3−6 mg twice a day
Schizophrenia, other psychoses
- IM 12.5−25 mg 2−3 times daily or rectal 25 mg 2−3 times daily until oral treatment possible. Oral starting dose 25 mg/day in divided doses increased at 4−7 day intervals until satisfactory to response obtained, usually 75−100 mg/day in divided doses

- *Child over 10 kg:* By mouth only, 250 mcg/kg two or three times a day
Available forms include: IM injection 12.5 mg/ml; tablets 5, 25 mg; modified release capsules 10, 15 mg; syrup 5 mg/5 ml, suppository 5 mg, 25 mg; buccal tablets 3 mg; effervescent granules 5 mg sachets
Side effects/adverse reactions:
CNS: Depression, restlessness, tremor, dystonia, dyskinesia, tardive dyskinesia, drowsiness, dizziness
GI: Nausea, vomiting, anorexia, dry mouth, diarrhoea, constipation, weight loss, metallic taste, cramps, jaundice
CV: Circulatory failure, hypotension, cardiac arrhythmias
RESP: Respiratory depression
HAEM: Leucopenia, agranulocytosis
EENT: Ocular changes, nasal congestion
INTEG: Skin rashes, photosensitivity, contact dermatitis greyish-mauve skin colouration
SYST: Neuroleptic malignant syndrome, hypothermia
ENDO: Gynaecomastia, galactorrhoea, amenorrhoea, impotence
GU: Urinary retention
Contraindications: Hypersensitivity to phenothiazines, coma, seizure, encephalopathy, pregnancy, breast feeding, phaeochromocytoma
Precautions: Children under 2 yr, elderly, renal dysfunction, epilepsy, Parkinsonism, hypothyroidism, myasthenia gravis, prostate hypertrophy, narrow angle glaucoma, liver disease, phaechromocytoma, blood dyscrasias, bone marrow depression
Pharmacokinetics:
By mouth: Onset 30−40 min, duration 3−4 hr. Onset 30−40 min, duration 10−12 hr

Rectal: Onset 60 min, duration 3–4 hr

IM: Onset 10–20 min, duration 12 hr, metabolised by liver, excreted by kidneys, excreted in breast milk

Interactions/incompatibilities:
• Decreased effects: antacids, lithium, anti-cholinergic agents (antipsychotic effects)
• Increased anticholinergic action: anticholinergics, tricyclic antidepressants
• Do not mix with other drugs in syringe or solution
• Increased CNS depression given with: barbiturates, alcohol, other sedatives
• Increased hypotension with anaesthetics
• Risk of arrhythmias with antiarrhythmics
• Effects increased: antihypertensives especially α-adrenoceptor blockers
• Effects reduced: amphetamine, levodopa, bromocriptine, lysuride, pergolide, clonidine, guanethidine, adrenaline, anticonvulsants
• Encephalopathy when administered with desferrioxamine

Clinical assessment:
• Carry out immediate haematological investigation if signs of unexplained infection/fever

Treatment of overdose: Gastric lavage and activated charcoal if within 6 hr of oral ingestion, no specific antidote, treatment supportive; volume expansion and inotropes in circulatory collapse, maintain normal body temperature, treat dystonias with anticholinergic

NURSING CONSIDERATIONS

Assess:
• Vital signs, BP; check patients with cardiac disease more often

Administer:
• IM deep injection in large muscle mass; withdraw to avoid IV administration
• Reduce dose to minimum and use for minimum time
• Stop treatment if jaundice develops

Evaluate:
• Therapeutic response: absence of nausea, vomiting
• Respiratory status before, during, after administration of emetic; check rate, rhythm, character; respiratory depression can occur rapidly with elderly or debilitated patients

Teach patient/family:
• Avoid hazardous activities, activities requiring alertness; dizziness may occur

---

procyclidine HCl

Kemadrin Arpicolin
Func. class.: Anticholinergic
Chem. class.: Tertiary amine
Legal class.: POM

Action: Acts on acetylcholine receptors in CNS, which decrease involuntary movements

Uses: Parkinson symptoms, including those induced by anti-dopaminergic drugs

Dosage and routes:
• *Adult:* By mouth 2.5 mg three times a day after meals, titrated to patient response, not to exceed 60 mg/day IV (in acute dystonia) IM 5–10 mg once repeated after 20 mins if necessary, maximum 20 mg daily

Available forms include: Tablets 5 mg, injection 5 mg/ml, syrup 2.5, 5 mg/5 ml

Side effects/adverse reactions:
CNS: Confusion, anxiety, restlessness, irritability, delusions, hallucinations, incoherence, dizziness
EENT: Blurred vision, photo-

phobia, dilated pupils, difficulty swallowing
CV: Palpitations, tachycardia, postural hypotension
GI: Dryness of mouth, constipation, nausea, vomiting, abdominal distress, paralytic ileus
GU: Hesitancy, retention
INTEG: Flushing, dry skin
Contraindications: Tardive dyskinesia
Precautions: Pregnancy, elderly, lactation, prostatic hypertrophy, glaucoma, GI/GU obstruction, hepatic and renal impairment, cardiovascular disease. NB: Abuse potential
Pharmacokinetics:
By mouth: Onset 30−45 mins, duration 4−6 hr, plasma half-life 12 hr
Interactions/incompatibilities:
• Decreased action of: haloperidol, phenothiazines, buccal formulations (dry mouth), cisapride, ketoconazole
• Increased anticholinergic effect: antihistamines, MAOIs, phenothiazines, tricyclic antidepressants, other anticholinergic drugs
Treatment of overdose: Gastric lavage if recently ingested, supportive treatment including diazepam for convulsions
NURSING CONSIDERATIONS
Administer:
• With or after meals for GI problems, including a dry mouth; may be given with any fluid before for dry mouth; may be given with fluids other than water
Perform/provide:
• Mouthwashes, frequent drinks, to relieve dry mouth
Evaluate:
• Therapeutic response
• Parkinsonism: shuffling gait, muscle rigidity, involuntary movements
• Urinary hesitancy, retention
• Constipation; increase fluids, bulk, exercise if this occurs
• For tolerance over long-term therapy; dose may need to be increased or changed
• Mental status: affect, mood, CNS depression, worsening of mental symptoms during early therapy
Teach patient/family:
• Not to discontinue this drug abruptly; to taper off over 1 week
• To avoid non-prescribed medication: cough, cold preparations with alcohol, antihistamines unless directed by clinician

---

progesterone

Cyclogest, Gestone
Func. class.: Progestogen
Chem. class.: Steroid hormone
Legal class.: POM

Action: Prepares uterus to receive fertilised ovum, stimulates growth of mammary tissue, anti-neoplastic action against endometrial cancer
Uses: Amenorrhoea, premenstrual syndrome, abnormal uterine bleeding
Dosage and routes:
Amenorrhoea/uterine bleeding
• *Adult:* IM 5−10 mg daily for 5−10 days until 2 days before anticipated onset of menstruation
PMS
• *Adult:* Rectal suppository/vaginal suppository 200−400 mg twice a day from day of symptom appearance to start of bleed
Available forms include: Injection IM 25, 50 mg/ml; rectal/vaginal suppository 200, 400 mg
Side effects/adverse reactions:
CNS: Dizziness, headache, migraines, depression, fatigue, insomnia
CV: Oedema
GI: Nausea, vomiting, anorexia, cramps, cholestatic jaundice; with

rectal administration diarrhoea, flatulence
EENT: Diplopia, loss of vision, retinal lesions
GU: Amenorrhoea, cervical erosion, breakthrough bleeding, dysmenorrhoea, vaginal candidiasis, breast changes
INTEG: Rash, urticaria, acne, hirsutism, alopecia, oily skin, seborrhoea, pain at injection site
META: Weight gain, catabolism
Contraindications: Breast cancer, hypersensitivity, reproductive cancer, undiagnosed vaginal bleeding, high risk of arterial disease; rectal use in colitis; vaginal use in vaginal infection, immediately postpartum or with recurrent cystitis
Precautions: Pregnancy, lactation, hypertension, congestive cardiac failure, diabetes mellitus, bone disease, depression, migraine headache, convulsive disorders, hepatic disease, renal disease
Pharmacokinetics:
IM: Duration 24 hr
Excreted in urine, faeces, metabolised in liver
Interactions/incompatibilities:
• Vaginal preparation interferes with barrier contraceptives
• Raises plasma cyclosporin levels
Treatment of overdose: Unlikely to be of significance, treatment symptomatic
NURSING CONSIDERATIONS
Assess:
• Baseline observations especially BP and weight
• Urinalysis to detect undiagnosed diabetes
Evaluate:
• Therapeutic response: decrease abnormal uterine bleeding, absence of amenorrhoea
• BP and weight during therapy
• Mood changes
• For side effects
Teach patient/family:
• All aspects of drug usage, including Cushingoid symptoms
• About potential side effects including breast lumps, vaginal bleeding, oedema, jaundice, dark urine, clay-coloured stools, dyspnoea, headache, blurred vision, abdominal pain, numbness or stiffness in legs, chest pain; male to report impotence or gynaecomastia
• Oral preparation to be taken with food/milk
• To report suspected pregnancy promptly

---

promazine HCl

Sparine
Func. class.: Antipsychotic, neuroleptic
Chem. class.: Phenothiazine
Legal class.: POM

Action: Depresses cerebral cortex, hypothalamus, limbic system, which control activity, aggression; blocks neurotransmission produced by dopamine at synapse; exhibits a strong α-adrenergic, cholinergic blocking action; as anti-emetic, inhibits medullary chemoreceptor trigger zone; mechanism for antipsychotic effects is unclear
Uses: Short-term management of psychomotor agitation; agitation, restlessness in elderly
Dosage and routes:
Psychomotor agitation
• *Adult:* 100−200 mg 4 times daily
Agitation and restlessness
• *Elderly:* 25−50 mg up to 4 times daily
Available forms include: Syrup 50 mg (as embonate)/5 ml; injection IV, IM 50 mg/ml
Side effects/adverse reactions:
RESP: Respiratory depression
CNS: Extrapyramidal symptoms: pseudoparkinsonism, akathisia,

dystonia; tardive dyskinesia, drowsiness, headache, seizures, confusion, excitement, agitation, nightmares, insomnia

HAEM: Anaemia, leucopenia, leucocytosis, agranulocytosis

INTEG: Rash, photosensitivity, dermatitis, pallor, vascular spasm if injected IV undiluted

EENT: Blurred vision, nasal congestion, lens changes

GI: Dry mouth, nausea, vomiting, anorexia, constipation, jaundice

GU: Urinary retention, impotence

ENDO: Amenorrhoea, gynaecomastia

CV: Orthostatic hypotension, cardiac arrest, ECG changes, tachycardia

SYST: Neuroleptic malignant syndrome, hypothermia

Contraindications: Hypersensitivity, coma, child, brain damage, lactation, pregnancy

Precautions: Seizure disorders, blood dyscrasias, bone marrow depression, hepatic disease, cardiac disease, respiratory disease, renal failure, epilepsy, narrow angle glaucoma, hypothyroidism, myasthenia gravis, phaeochromocytoma, prostatic hypertrophy, parkinsonism

Pharmacokinetics:

By mouth: Onset erratic, peak 2−4 hr

IM: Onset 15 min, peak 1 hr, duration 4−6 hr

Metabolised by liver, excreted in urine, enters breast milk

Interactions/incompatibilities:

• Oversedation: other CNS depressants, alcohol, barbiturates

• Decreased absorption: aluminium hydroxide or magnesium hydroxide antacids

• Decreased effects of: lithium, levodopa, bromocriptine, lysuride, pergolide, anticonvulsants

• Increased effects of: antihypertensives

• Increased anticholinergic effects: anticholinergics, tricylic antidepressants

• Increased risk of arrhythmias with anti-arrhythmics

• Increased hypotension with anaesthetics

• Decreased absorption of tetracyclines with sparine suspension

Clinical assessment:

• Reduce dose to minimum and use for minimum time

• Stop treatment if jaundice develops

• Carry out immediate haematological investigation if signs of unexplained fever/infection

Treatment of overdose: Lavage if orally ingested, no specific antidote, supportive treatment of convulsions, hypotension, hypothermia

NURSING CONSIDERATIONS

Assess:

• Fluid balance

• Establish baseline BP, pulse and respiratory rate

Administer:

• With flavours to mask taste (citrus, chocolate)

• IM injection into large muscle mass

Perform/provide:

• Decreased noise input by dimming lights, avoiding loud noises

• Supervised ambulation until stabilised on medication; do not involve in strenuous exercise program because fainting is possible; patient should not stand still for long periods of time

• Increased fluids to prevent constipation

• Sips of water, mouthwashes for dry mouth

Evaluate:

• Therapeutic response: decrease in emotional excitement, hallucinations, delusions, paranoia, reorganization of patterns of thought, speech

• Swallowing of oral medication; check for hoarding or giving of medication to other patients
• Effect, orientation, level of consciousness, reflexes, gait, co-ordination, sleep pattern disturbances
• BP (standing and lying); pulse, respirations, 4 hrly during initial treatment; report drops of 30 mmHg
• Dizziness, faintness, palpitations, tachycardia on rising
• Uncoordinated movements including akathisia (inability to sit still, no pattern to movements), tardive dyskinesia (bizarre movements of jaw, mouth, tongue, extremities), pseudoparkinsonism (rigidity, tremors, pill rolling, shuffling gait)
• Constipation, urinary retention daily, if these occur increase bulk and water in diet

Teach patient/family:
• That postural hypotension occurs frequently, and to rise from sitting or lying position gradually
• To remain lying down after IM injection for at least 30 min
• To sit down in bathroom; avoid standing for long periods
• To avoid hot baths, hot showers, or stand up washes since hypotension may occur
• To avoid abrupt withdrawal of this drug or tremors may result; drugs should be withdrawn slowly
• To avoid non-prescribed preparations (cough, hayfever, cold) unless approved by clinician since serious drug interactions may occur; avoid use with alcohol or CNS depressants, increased drowsiness may occur
• To use a sunscreen during sun exposure to prevent burns
• Regarding compliance with drug regimen
• About possibility of unco-ordinated movements and need to

inform clinician immediately if these occur. Necessity for meticulous oral hygiene since oral candidiasis may occur
• To report sore throat, malaise, fever, bleeding, mouth sores; if these occur, full blood count should be taken and drug discontinued

---

promethazine HCl
promethazine theoclate

Avomine, Phenergan, Sominex
Func. class.: Antihistamine, H₁-receptor antagonist
Chem. class.: Phenothiazine derivative
Legal class.: Tablets P, Injection POM

Action: Acts on blood vessels, GI, respiratory system by competing with histamine for H₁-receptor site; decreases allergic response by blocking histamine
Uses: Motion sickness, rhinitis, allergy symptoms, sedation, nausea, pre-operative and post-operative sedation
Dosage and routes:
Nausea
• *Adult and child over 10 yr:* By mouth/IM 25 mg up to 4 times a day
• *Child:* By mouth every 6−8 hr, 2−5 yr 5 mg; 5−10 yr 10 mg or 6.25−12.5 mg IM
Motion sickness
• *Adult and child over 10 yr:* By mouth 25 mg once or twice a day, first dose at least 1 hr before travelling
• *Child 5−10 yr:* By mouth 12.5−25 mg twice a day
Allergy/rhinitis
• *Adult and child over 10 yr:* By mouth 10−25 mg 3−4 times a day; slow IV, diluted, in emergency 25−50 mg

• *Child:* By mouth once or twice a day, 2−5 yr 5−15 mg; 5−10 yr 10−25 mg

Sedation

• *Adult and child over 10 yr:* By mouth/IM 25−50 mg at bedtime

• *Child:* By mouth at bedtime, 2−5 yr 15−20 mg; 5−10 yr 20−25 mg

Sedation (pre-operative/postoperative)

• *Adult:* By mouth/IM 25−50 mg

• *Child 1−5 yr:* By mouth 15−20 mg; 5−10 yr, by mouth 20−25 mg, IM 6.25−12.5 mg

Available forms include: Tablets 10, 25 mg; syrup 5 mg/5 ml; injection 25 mg/ml

Side effects/adverse reactions:

CNS: Dizziness, drowsiness, poor coordination, fatigue, confusion, neuritis, restlessness, headache, nightmares, hyperactivity in children, tremor, tics, dyskinesias

CV: Hypotension, palpitations, arrythmias

RESP: Increased thick secretions

HAEM: Thrombocytopenia, agranulocytosis, haemolytic anaemia

GI: Dry mouth, nausea, vomiting, anorexia, constipation, diarrhoea, jaundice

INTEG: Rash, urticaria, photosensitivity, pain at injection site

GU: Retention, dysuria, frequency

EENT: Blurred vision, dilated pupils, tinnitus, nasal stuffiness

SYST: Allergic reactions including anaphylaxis

Contraindications: Hypersensitivity to H_1-receptor antagonist, lower respiratory tract disease, coma, CNS depression, neonates, porphyria, patients receiving MAOIs within 14 days

Precautions: Renal disease, cardiac disease, bronchial asthma, seizure disorder, hyperthyroidism, bronchitis, prostatic hypertrophy, bladder neck obstruction, pregnancy, lactation, narrow angle glaucoma

Pharmacokinetics:

By mouth: Onset 20 min, duration 4−6 hr, metabolised in liver, excreted by kidneys, GI tract (inactive metabolites)

Interactions/incompatibilities:

• Increased CNS depression: barbiturates, narcotics, hypnotics, tricyclic antidepressants, alcohol

• Increased anticholinergic effects with: anticholinergics, tricyclic antidepressants

Lab. test interferences:

False negative: Skin allergy tests

False positive/negative: Urine pregnancy test

Treatment of overdose: Administer ipecacuanha syrup or lavage, no specific antidote, provide symptomatic treatment, ensure adequate respiratory, circulatory status, diazepam for convulsions

NURSING CONSIDERATIONS

Assess:

• Fluid balance

• Urinalysis before treatment

Administer:

• IV; in an emergency by slow intravenous injection 25 mg over 2 min, after dilution of its volume. Maximum parenteral dose 100 mg

• Deep IM in large muscle; rotate site

• With meals if GI symptoms occur, absorption may slightly decrease

• When used for motion sickness, 30 min before travel

Perform/provide:

• Sips of water, mouthwashes for dryness

• Ensure oral medication is swallowed by elderly

Evaluate:

• When used as a sedative for elderly. Variations in dosage may be necessary if desired effect is to be obtained

• Therapeutic response: absence

of running or congested nose or rashes, nausea and absence of motion sickness
• Respiratory status: rate, rhythm, increase in bronchial secretions, wheezing, chest tightness
• Cardiac status: palpitations, increased pulse, hypotension
• Be alert for retention, frequency or dysuria. Discontinue drugs if these occur

Teach patient/family:
• Avoid prolonged sunlight as photosensitive skin reaction may occur
• Ambulant patients when first using drug should not drive or operate machinery as drowsiness and disorientation may occur
• To notify clinician if confusion, over-sedation, hypotension occur

---

propafenone hydrochloride

Arythmol
Func. class.: Anti-arrhythmic
Legal class.: POM

Action: Class 1C anti-arrhythmic with basic local anaesthetic activity and membrane-stabilising effects. Some beta-blocking activity has been reported
Uses: Prophylaxis and treatment of ventricular arrhythmias
Dosage and routes:
• *Adult:* By mouth initially 150 mg, three times a day, increasing at intervals of not less than 3 days to 300 mg twice daily, maximum 300 mg three times a day
• *Children:* Not recommended
Available forms include: Tablets 150 mg, 300 mg
Side effects/adverse reactions:
GI: Nausea, vomiting, constipation, diarrhoea, dry mouth, cholestasis, bitter taste
CNS: Dizziness, fatigue, head-

ache, blurred vision, seizures
HAEM: Blood dyscrasias
CV: Bradycardia, sinoatrial, atrio-ventricular or intraventricular blocks. Proarrhythmic effects. Postural hypotension
INTEG: Allergic skin reactions, lupus syndrome
Contraindications: Uncontrolled congestive heart failure, cardiogenic shock (except arrhythmia-induced), severe bradycardia, uncontrolled electrolyte disturbances, severe obstructive pulmonary disease, marked hypotension. Sinus node dysfunction, atrial conduction defects, second degree or greater atrio-ventricular block, bundle branch block or distal block unless patients are paced adequately. Pregnancy, myasthenia gravis, lactation, obstructive airways disease
Precautions: The weak negative inotropic effect of propafenone may assume importance in patients with cardiac failure. A reduction in dose is recommended in patients weighing less than 70 kg, and may also be necessary if liver or renal function is impaired. Elderly patients may respond to a lower dose
Pharmacokinetics: Peak levels after 2 to 3 hr
Interactions/incompatibilities:
• Propafenone potentiated by: other local anaesthetic type agent, cimetidine, quinidine. Reduced propafenone blood levels with: rifampicin
• Propafenone increases blood levels of: digoxin, warfarin, propranolol, metoprolol
Clinical assessment:
• Monitor concurrent therapy with oral anticoagulants closely; dose adjustment probably needed
• Halve dose of concurrent digoxin therapy and monitor levels
NURSING CONSIDERATIONS:

Assess:
- Baseline vital signs, ECG

Administer:
- Tablets should be swallowed whole with a drink after food

Perform/provide:
- Therapy should be initiated under hospital conditions with ECG monitoring and cardiovascular surveillance

Evaluate:
- Therapeutic effect
- BP continuously for fluctuations. Report changes to clinician
- For all side effects

Teach patient/family:
- That they should take special care if driving, operating machinery or performing any other hazardous task
- About potential side effects
- To report any change to clinician
- Rise slowly to sitting or standing position to minimise hypotension
- Not to stop medication without medical advice

---

propantheline bromide

Pro-Banthine

Func. class.: Gastrointestinal anticholinergic

Chem. class.: Synthetic quaternary ammonium compound

Legal class.: POM

Action: Inhibits muscarinic actions of acetylcholine at postganglionic parasympathetic neuroeffector sites

Uses: Treatment of peptic ulcer disease, irritable bowel syndrome, gastrointestinal conditions characterised by smooth muscle spasm, hyperhidrosis, enuresis

Dosage and routes:
- *Adult:* By mouth 15–30 mg up to four times a day before meals

Available forms include: Tablets 15 mg

Side effects/adverse reactions:

CNS: Confusion, stimulation in elderly, headache, insomnia, dizziness, drowsiness, anxiety, weakness, hallucinations, depression

GI: Dry mouth, constipation, paralytic ileus, heartburn, nausea, vomiting, dysphagia

GU: Hesitancy, retention, impotence

CV: Palpitations, tachycardia

EENT: Blurred vision, photophobia, mydriasis, cycloplegia, increased ocular tension

INTEG: Urticaria, rash, pruritus, anhidrosis, fever, flushing

SYST: Anaphylaxis, angioedema

Contraindications: Hypersensitivity to anticholinergics, narrow-angle glaucoma, GI obstruction, myasthenia gravis, paralytic ileus, GI atony, toxic megacolon, severe ulcerative colitis, obstruction of urinary tract, hiatus hernia with reflux oesophagitis

Precautions: Hyperthyroidism, coronary artery disease, arrhythmias, congestive heart failure, ulcerative colitis, hypertension, hepatic disease, renal disease, elderly, prostatic hypertrophy, pregnancy, breast-feeding

Pharmacokinetics:

By mouth: Onset 30–45 min, duration 4–6 hr, plasma half-life 2–3 hr; metabolised by liver, GI system, excreted in urine, bile

Interactions/incompatibilities:
- Increased anticholinergic effect: amantadine, tricyclic anti-depressants, MAOIs, other anticholinergics, phenothiazines
- Decreased plasma levels of: phenothiazines
- Reduced GI effects of: domperidone, metoclopramide, cisapride
- Reduced effect of any concurrent buccal tablets (dry mouth)

Treatment of overdose: Emesis/gastric lavage and activated charcoal, no specific antidote, treat-

ment supportive, diazepam for CNS stimulation, consider physotigmine 500 mcg−2 mg IV in severe cases

NURSING CONSIDERATIONS
Assess:
• Baseline vital signs, cardiac status: checking for arrhythmias, increased rate, palpitations
Administer:
• ½−1 hr before meals for better absorption
• Decreased dose to elderly patients; their metabolism may be slowed
Perform/provide:
• Frequent sips of water, mouthwashes for dryness of oral cavity
• Increased fluids, bulk, exercise to patient's lifestyle to decrease constipation
• Frequent mouth washes
Evaluate:
• Therapeutic response: absence of epigastric pain, bleeding, nausea, vomiting
• GI complaints: pain, bleeding (frank or occult), nausea, vomiting, anorexia
Teach patient/family:
• Avoid driving or other hazardous activities until stabilised on medication
• Avoid alcohol or other CNS depressants; will enhance sedating properties of this drug

---

propranolol HCl

Angilol, Apsolol, Berkolol, Sloprolol, Inderal, Propanix, Bedranol SR, Betadur CR
Func. class.: Antihypertensive, antianginal
Chem. class.: β-Adrenergic blocker
Legal class.: POM

Action: Decreases preload, afterload, which is responsible for decreasing left ventricular end diastolic pressure, systemic vascular resistance

Uses: Hypertension, arrhythmias, migraine prophylaxis, thyrotoxic crisis, anxiety, anxiety-induced tachycardia, chronic stable angina pectoris, prophylaxis of angina pain, essential tremor

Dosage and routes:
Hypertension
• *Adult:* By mouth 80 mg twice a day increasing at weekly intervals if required, maintenance usually 160−320 mg daily

Angina
• By mouth 40 mg two or three times a day, increased at weekly intervals until response seen, usual range 120−240 mg/day

Arrhythmias/Thyrotoxicosis
• IV 1 mg over 1 min, repeat at 2 min intervals. (Maximum 10 mg conscious patient, 5 mg under anaesthesia.) By mouth 10−40 mg, three or four times a day

Anxiety
• By mouth 40 mg daily in short-term situational anxiety, 40 mg 2 or 3 times daily in generalised anxiety

Phaeochromocytoma
• By mouth 60 mg daily for 3 days before surgery; 30 mg daily in inoperable cases, use with α-blocker

Migraine prophylaxis essential tremor
• By mouth 40 mg two or three times a day increased at weekly intervals according to patient response, usual range 80−160 mg day

Note: Oral doses described above can be given as once or twice daily doses using modified release preparations

Child:
• *Arrhythmias:*, phaeochromocytoma, thyrotoxicosis
• By mouth (as a guide) 0.25−

0.5 mg/kg 3 or 4 times a day; IV 25−50 mcg/kg
• Injected slowly 3−4 times daily under ECG control

Migraine
• By mouth, under 12 yr, 20 mg 2 or 3 times daily; over 12 yr, adult dose

Available forms include: Capsules modified release 80, 160 mg; tablets 10, 40, 80, 160 mg; injection 1 mg/ml

Side effects/adverse reactions:
RESP: Dyspnoea, bronchospasm
CV: Bradycardia, hypotension, congestive heart failure
HAEM: Agranulocytosis, thrombocytopenia
GI: Nausea, vomiting, diarrhoea, constipation, cramps, dry mouth
INTEG: Rash, pruritus, fever
CNS: Depression, hallucinations, dizziness, fatigue, lethargy, paraesthesias, nightmares
EENT: Dry eyes
MISC: Cold extremities
MS: Muscle fatigue

Contraindications: Hypersensitivity, cardiogenic shock, 2nd or 3rd degree heart block, bronchospastic disease, metabolic acidosis, prolonged fasting

Precautions: Diabetes mellitus, pregnancy, renal disease, lactation, congestive heart failure, hyperthyroidism, chronic obstructive airways disease, elderly

Pharmacokinetics:
By mouth: Onset 30 min, peak 1−1½ hr, duration 6 hr
IV: Onset 2 min, peak 15 min, duration 3−6 hr
Half-life 3−5 hr, metabolised by liver, crosses blood−brain barrier, excreted in breast milk

Interactions/incompatibilities:
• Risk of severe hypotension, asystole if verapamil is injected during propranolol therapy−avoid; risk less when given by mouth, but only if myocardium well preserved
• Severe hypertension with nor-adrenaline, adrenaline and if switched abruptly from clonidine
• Bradycardia, AV block with diltiazem, digoxin, amiodarone
• Severe hypotension, heart failure with nifedipine
• Enhanced effect of: hypoglycaemic agents (and masked hypoglycaemic symptoms), antihypertensives, chlorpromazine
• Increased toxicity with: lignocaine
• Hypotensive effects enhanced by: alcohol, anaesthetics, diuretics anxiolytics, hypnotics, fluvoxamine cimetidine
• Hypotensive effects reduced by: corticosteroids, oestrogens, rifampicin, thyroxine
• Reduced effects of: neostigmine, pyridostigmine
• Increased peripheral vasoconstriction with: ergotamine

Clinical assessment:
• Consider stopping treatment if skin rashes, dry eyes appear

Lab. test interferences:
• Determination of catecholamines by fluorescence, serum bilirubin by diazo method

Treatment of overdose: Gastric lavage; atropine 1−2 mg IV to counter bradycardia; glucagon 10 mg IV as cardiac stimulant repeated if needed; β-agonist if glucagon fails

NURSING CONSIDERATIONS
Assess:
• Baseline BP, pulse, respirations
• Weight
• Fluid balance
Administer:
• With full glass of water on empty stomach (oral tablet)
Evaluate:
• Pain: duration, time started, activity being performed, character

- Tolerance if taken over long period of time
- Therapeutic response; degree of palpitations, breathlessness and anxiety levels
- BP, heart and respiratory rates
- Observe for postural hypotension

Teach patient/family:
- That dose must be taken with a glass of water
- That drug may be taken before stressful activity: exercise, sexual activity
- That sublingual area may sting when drug comes in contact with mucous membranes
- To seek medical advice if dizziness, breathlessness or any other side effects are experienced
- To avoid hazardous activities if dizziness occurs
- Stress patient compliance with complete medical regimen
- To change position changes slowly to prevent fainting
- Decrease dosage over 2 weeks to prevent cardiac damage

---

propylthiouracil

Func. class.: Thyroid hormone antagonist
Chem. class.: Thioamide
Legal class.: POM

Action: Blocks synthesis of T_3, T_4 (triiodothyronine, thyroxine), inhibits organification of iodine
Uses: Hyperthyroidism
Dosage and routes:
- *Adult:* By mouth 300−450 mg daily in divided doses
Available forms include: Tablets 50 mg
Side effects/adverse reactions:
ENDO: Enlarged thyroid
INTEG: Rash, urticaria, pruritus, alopecia, hyperpigmentation,
GU: Irregular menses, nephritis

CNS: Drowsiness, headache, vertigo, fever
HAEM: Agranulocytosis, leucopenia, thrombocytopenia, hypothrombinaemia, lymphadenopathy
GI: Nausea, diarrhoea, vomiting, jaundice, hepatitis
MS: Myalgia, arthralgia
MISC: Lupus-like syndrome, fetal goitre
Contraindications:
Hypersensitivity
Precautions: Bone marrow depression, hepatic disease, pregnancy, renal disease, lactation, large goitre
Pharmacokinetics:
By mouth: Rapidly absorbed, half-life 1−2 hr, excreted in urine, bile, breast milk, cross placenta
Clinicial assessment:
- Triiodothyronine, thyroxine, which is decreased; serum thyroid stimulating hormone, which is increased; free thyroxine index, which is increased if dosage is too low; discontinue drug 3−4 weeks before radioactive iodine uptake
- Blood for blood dyscrasias: leucopenia, thrombocytopenia, agranulocytosis
- Lowest dose that relieves symptoms
Treatment of overdose: No symptoms likely from single large dose, supportive
NURSING CONSIDERATIONS
Assess:
- Pulse, BP, temperature and night pulse
- Input and output of fluids
- Height, growth rate if given to children
- Weight daily prior to initial treatment at weekly intervals
Administer:
- Orally
- At same time daily in divided doses to maintain drug level
- Lowest dose that relieves symptoms

• With meals to decrease GI upset
Perform/provide:
• Fluids to 3−4 litres/day, unless contraindicated
• Removal of medication 4 weeks before radioactive iodine uptake test
Evaluate:
• Therapeutic effect: weight gain, decreased pulse, thyroxine and BP
• Overdose: peripheral oedema, heat intolerance, sweating, palpitations, arrhythmias, severe tachycardia, increased temperature, delirium, CNS irritability
• Hypersensitivity: rash, enlarged cervical lymph nodes, drug may need to be discontinued
• Hypoprothrombinaemia: bleeding, petechiae, ecchymosis
• Bone marrow depression: sore throat, fever, fatigue
Teach patient/family:
• To abstain from breast feeding after delivery
• Report redness, swelling, sore throat, mouth lesions, which indicate blood dyscrasias
• To keep graph of weight, pulse, mood
• That seafood, other iodine products may be restricted
• Not to discontinue this medication abruptly; thyroid crisis may occur; stress patient response
• That response may take several months if thyroid is large
• Symptoms/signs of overdose: periorbital oedema, cold intolerance, mental depression
• Symptoms of inadequate dose: tachycardia, diarrhoea, fever, irritability, weight loss
• That surgery may be necessary
• To only take other medication if directed by clinician
• That children show immediate behaviour personality changes

protamine sulphate

Prosulf
Func. class.: Heparin antagonist
Chem. class.: Low molecular weight protein
Legal class.: POM

Action: Produces stable complex when combined with heparin
Uses: Heparin overdose

Dosage and routes:
• *Adult:* IV 1 mg of protamine neutralises 100 U heparin (mucus) or 80 U heparin (lung), administer slowly 1−3 min; do not exceed 50 mg/10 min
• Reduce dose if given more than 15 mins after heparin as heparin is rapidly excreted
Available forms include: Injection IV 10 mg/ml

Side effects/adverse reactions:
CV: Hypotension, bradycardia
INTEG: Rash, dermatitis, urticaria, alopecia, flushing
HAEM: Bleeding (in overdose)
RESP: Dyspnoea
Contraindications: Hypersensitivity
Precautions: Pregnancy, breast feeding

Pharmacokinetics:
IV: Onset 5 min, duration 2 hr

Clinical assessment:
• Coagulation tests (activated partial thromboplastin time, ACT) 15 min after dose, then in several hours

NURSING CONSIDERATIONS
Assess:
• Vital signs
• Degree of bleeding

Perform/provide:
• Ensure dilution in saline or 5% dextrose

Evaluate:
• Vital signs, BP every 30 min per first 3 hr

- Therapeutic response, diminution of bleeding
- Skin rash, urticaria, derma

protirelin

TRH, TRH-ROCHE
Func. class.: Thyrotrophin-releasing hormone
Chem. class.: Tripeptide
Legal class.: POM

Action: Stimulates secretion of thyroid stimulating hormone
Uses: Assessment of thyroid function and thyroid stimulating hormone reserve in hypopituitarism
Dosage and routes:
- *Adult:* IV injection 200 mcg
- *Child:* IV 1 mcg/kg
Available forms include: Injection 100 mcg/ml; 2-ml ampoule
Side effects/adverse reactions:
CNS: Dizziness
CV: Syncope, bronchospasm, tachycardia, hypertension
GI: Nausea, strange taste
GU: Desire to micturate
INTEG: Flushing
Precautions: Severe hypopituitarism, cardiac insufficiency, bronchial asthma, obstructive airways disease, pregnancy
Pharmacokinetics: IV: metabolised in plasma, possibly tissues, half-life 5–6 min
Interactions/incompatibilities: Not to be diluted
Clinical assessment:
- Take blood at 20, 60 min postinjection to detect peak/delayed TSH response
Treatment of overdose: Doses of up to 1 mg have not resulted in symptoms of overdose
NURSING CONSIDERATIONS
Assess:

- Pulse and BP; night pulse if possible
- Weight for children
Administer:
- After blood sample for control thyroid-stimulating hormone
- Intravenously, directly in vein as a single bolus injection
- Take a blood sample 20 min after injection for peak thyroid-stimulating hormone level
- 60 min after injection blood sample taken to detect a delayed thyroid-stimulating hormone level
Evaluate:
- Interpretation of results, by the response to protriptyline HCl from the basal values
- Effect of any other medication
- Side effects: usually mild and transient; nausea, desire to micturate, flushing, hypertension
Teach patient/family:
- Advise on result of test

protriptyline HCl

Concordin
Func. class.: Antidepressant, tricyclic
Chem. class.: Dibenzocyclohepatene — secondary amine
Legal class.: POM

Action: Blocks reuptake of noradrenaline, serotonin into nerve endings, increasing action of noradrenaline, serotonin in nerve cells
Uses: Depression
Dosage and routes:
- *Adult:* By mouth 15–40 mg daily in divided doses, may increase to 60 mg daily
- *Elderly:* By mouth, initially 5 mg 3 times a day, exceed 20 mg daily with caution
Available forms include: Tablets 5, 10 mg

Side effects/adverse reactions:

ENDO: Gynaecomastia, breast enlargement, galactorrhoea, changes in libido, changes in blood sugar

HAEM: Agranulocytosis, thrombocytopenia, eosinophilia, leucopenia

CNS: Dizziness, drowsiness, confusion, headache, anxiety, tremors, stimulation, weakness, insomnia, nightmares, extrapyramidal symptoms (elderly), increased psychiatric symptoms, paraesthesia, hallucinations, peripheral neuropathy, ataxia

GI: Diarrhoea, dry mouth, nausea, vomiting, paralytic ileus, decreased appetite, cramps, epigastric distress, jaundice, hepatitis, stomatitis, constipation, peculiar taste, black tongue

GU: Retention, impotence

INTEG: Rash, urticaria, sweating, pruritus, photosensitivity, flushing alopecia

CV: Orthostatic hypotension, ECG changes, tachycardia, hypertension, palpitations, myocardial infarction, stroke, heart block

EENT: Blurred vision, tinnitus, mydriasis

SYST: Hyperpyrexia, oedema, fever, weight gain/loss

Contraindications: Hypersensitivity to tricyclic antidepressants, recovery phase of myocardial infarction, heart block, severe liver disease, concurrent use of MAOIs, children under 16 yr, cardiac, arrhythmias, mania, marked agitation, breast feeding

Precautions: Prostatic hypertrophy, suicidal patients, increased intra-ocular pressure, narrow-angle glaucoma, urinary retention, hepatic disease, hyperthyroidism, electroshock therapy, elective surgery, pregnancy, epilepsy, elderly, CV disorders

Pharmacokinetics:

By mouth: Peak plasma levels 8–12 hr, therapeutic effect 2–3 weeks; metabolised by liver, excreted by kidneys, half-life 54–198 hr

Interactions/incompatibilities:
- Decreased effects of: guanethidine, clonidine, debrisoquine, bethanidine, anticonvulsants, buccal medications (dry mouth)
- Increased effects of: alcohol, barbiturates, benzodiazepines, CNS depressants
- Hyperpyretic crisis, convulsions, hypertensive episode: MAOIs
- Inhalational anaesthetics increase risk of hypotension and arrhythmias
- Hypertension and/or arrhythmias with: sympathomimetic agents e.g. noradrenaline, adrenaline, ephedrine, phenylpropanolamine, isoprenaline
- Increased anticholinergic effects: anticholinergics, antihistamines, phenothiazines

Clinical assessment:
- ECG for flattening of T wave, bundle branch block, atrioventricular block, dysrhythmias in cardiac patients

Treatment of overdose: ECG monitoring, induce emesis, lavage, activated charcoal, administer anticonvulsant, dialysis ineffective

NURSING CONSIDERATIONS

Administer:
- Increased fluids, bulk in diet if constipation, urinary retention occur
- With food or milk for GI symptoms
- Dosage before bedtime if oversedation occurs during day; may take entire dose at bedtime; elderly may not tolerate once daily dosing
- Frequent mouthwashes, sips of water for dry mouth

Perform/provide:
- Assistance with movement

during beginning therapy if drowsiness/dizziness occurs

Evaluate:
• Weight weekly, appetite may increase with drug
• Uncontrolled movements primarily in elderly: rigidity, dystonia, akathisia
• Mental status: mood, sensorium, affect, suicidal tendencies, increase in psychiatric symptoms: depression, panic
• Urinary retention, constipation
• Withdrawal symptoms: headache, nausea, vomiting, muscle pain, weakness; do not usually occur unless drug was discontinued abruptly

Teach patient/family:
• That therapeutic effects may take 2−3 weeks
• Use caution in driving or other activities requiring alertness because of drowsiness, dizziness, blurred vision
• To avoid alcohol ingestion, other CNS depressants unless prescribed
• Not to discontinue medication quickly after long-term use, may cause nausea, headache, malaise
• To wear sunscreen or large hat since photosensitivity may occur

---

proxymetacaine HCl (ophthalmic)

Ophthaine
Func. class.: Anaesthetic, ocular (short acting)
Chem. class.: Ester
Legal class.: POM

Action: Decreases ion permeability by stabilising neuronal membrane
Uses: Cataract extraction, tonometry, gonioscopy, removal of foreign bodies, suture removal, glaucoma surgery
Dosage and routes:

Glaucoma surgery and cataract extraction
• *Adult and child:* Instil 1 drop every 5−10 min for 5−7 doses
Tonometry/gonioscopy/suture removal
• *Adult and child:* Instil 1−2 drops 3 min before procedure
Available forms include: Solution 0.5%
Side effects/adverse reactions:
EENT: Blurred vision, stinging, burning, lacrimation, photophobia, conjunctival redness, iritis, stromal oedema, pupil dilation, corneal erosion (in chronic use), allergic keratitis
INTEG: Contact dermatitis
Contraindications: Hypersensitivity
Precautions: Abnormal levels of plasma esterases, allergies, hyperthyroidism, hypertension, cardiac disease
Pharmacokinetics:
Instil: Onset 13−30 seconds, duration 15−20 min
NURSING CONSIDERATIONS
Perform/provide:
• Protective covering for eye
• Storage in refrigerator
Teach patient/family:
• To report change in vision, with blurring or loss of sight, trouble breathing, sweating, flushing
• Not to touch or rub eye, which may further damage eye

---

pseudoephedrine HCl/ pseudoephedrine sulphate

Sudafed SA, Galpseud, NHS many combination products
Func. class.: Sympathomimetic
Chem. class.: Substituted phenylethylamine
Legal class.: P

Action: Stimulates vascular

adrenergic receptors causing vaso-constriction resulting in decongestant action particularly in nasal sinuses. May also stimulate heart and cause hypertension

Uses: Decongestant, nasal congestion

Dosage and routes:
• *Adult:* By mouth 60 mg 8 hrly, modified release capsules 120 mg 12 hrly
• *Child 6−12 yr:* By mouth 30 mg 8 hrly
• *Child 2−6 yr:* By mouth 15 mg 8 hrly

Available forms include: Capsules modified release 120 mg; syrup 30 mg/5 ml; tablets 60 mg

Side effects/adverse reactions:
CNS: Tremors, anxiety, insomnia, headache, dizziness, confusion, hallucinations, sleep disturbances
EENT: Dry nose, irritation of nose and throat
CV: Palpitations, tachycardia, hypertension
GI: Anorexia, nausea, vomiting
RESP: Depression
INTEG: Rashes
GU: Retention

Contraindications: Hypersensitivity to sympathomimetics, concurrent use of MAOIs, severe hypertension, coronary artery disease

Precautions: Pregnancy, cardiac disorders, hyperthyroidism, diabetes mellitus, prostatic hypertrophy, elevated intraocular pressure, breast feeding, hypertension

Pharmacokinetics:
By mouth: Onset 15−30 min, duration 4−6 hr, 8−12 hr (modified release), plasma half-life 5−8 hr metabolised in liver, excreted in breast milk

Interactions/incompatibilities:
• Do not use with MAOIs, β-blockers or tricyclic antidepressants, hypertensive crisis may occur

• Decreased effects of: hypotensive agents especially guanethidine, debrisoquine, bethanidine

Treatment of overdose: Gastric lavage and supportive measures, anticonvulsants and bladder catheterisation if necessary. Acid diuresis, dialysis speed elimination

NURSING CONSIDERATIONS
Assess:
• Respirations, pulse, BP
• Vital signs
Perform/provide:
• Refrigerated storage of reconstituted solution if refrigerated for no longer than 24 hr
• Do not use discoloured solutions
Evaluate:
• Paraesthesias and coldness of extremities, peripheral blood flow may decrease
• Insomnia, anxiety, dizziness, any urinary retention
• Therapeutic response: decreased nasal and sinus congestion
Teach patient/family:
• Reason for drug administration
• To only take other medication if directed by clinician

---

pyrantel embonate

Combantrin
Func. class.: Anthelmintic
Chem. class.: Pyrimidine derivative
Legal class.: POM

Action: Causes paralysis in worm by neuroblockade, worms are expelled by normal peristalsis

Uses: Threadworm, hookworm, roundworms

Dosage and routes:
• *Adult and child over 6 months:* By mouth 10 mg/kg as a single dose, minimum 125 mg, maximum 1 g; repeat on 3 consecutive days for *Necator*

Available forms include: Tablets 125 mg

Side effects/adverse reactions:
INTEG: Rash
CNS: Dizziness, headache, drowsiness, insomnia, weakness
GI: Nausea, vomiting, anorexia, diarrhoea, distension, elevations of liver enzymes
Contraindications: Hypersensitivity
Precautions: Hepatic disease, pregnancy
Pharmacokinetics:
By mouth: Poorly absorbed, metabolised in liver. More than 50% excreted in faeces, urine (unchanged/metabolites)
Interactions/incompatibilities:
• Antagonised by piperazine
Treatment of overdose: Gastric lavage supportive treatment

NURSING CONSIDERATIONS
Assess:
• Stools during entire treatment; specimens must be sent to lab while still warm; gloves must be worn whilst handling stools
Administer:
• Orally after meals to avoid GI symptoms
Perform/provide:
• Storage in tight, light-resistant containers in cool environment
Evaluate:
• For therapeutic response: expulsion of worms, 3 negative stool cultures after completion of treatment
• For allergic reaction: rash
• For diarrhoea during expulsion of worms
• Anorexia can result so observe diet and fluid intake
Teach patient/family:
• Proper hygiene after bowel movements including handwashing technique; wash hands before meals, tell patient to avoid putting fingers in mouth
• To take a bath or shower in the morning on rising, not to shake bed linen, to change bed linen daily, wash in hot water
• To clean toilet daily with disinfectant
• Importance of compliance with dosage schedule, duration of treatment
• To drink fruit juice to help expel worms
• To wear shoes, wash all fruits, vegetables well before eating
• Wear gloves when handling stools
• Avoid hazardous activity if drowsiness occurs

---

pyrazinamide

Zinamide
Func. class.: Antitubercular
Chem. class.: Pyrazinoic acid amide
Legal class.: POM

Action: Bactericidal interference with lipid, nucleic acid biosynthesis
Uses: Tuberculosis, as an adjunctive to other drugs
Dosage and routes:
• *Adult:* By mouth 20−35 mg/kg/day in 3−4 divided doses, not to exceed 3 g/day
Available forms include: Tablets 500 mg
Side effects/adverse reactions:
INTEG: Photosensitivity, urticaria
CNS: Anorexia, malaise
GI: Hepatotoxicity, abnormal liver function tests, aggravation of peptic ulcer, nausea, vomiting
GU: Urinary difficulty, increased uric acid
HAEM: Sideroblastic anaemia
SYST: Fever
MS: Arthralgia, gout
Contraindications: Hypersensitivity, hepatic damage, lactation hyperuricaemia, gouty arthritis, porphyria
Precautions: Pregnancy, child,

renal insufficiency, diabetes mellitus

Pharmacokinetics:

By mouth: Peak 2 hr, half-life 9−10 hr; metabolised in liver, excreted in urine (metabolites/unchanged drug)

Interactions/incompatibilities:

• Antagonises effects of probenicid, sulphinpyrazone as uricosurics

Clinical assessment:

• Liver function tests prior to therapy and every 2−4 weeks during therapy

• Renal status before, monthly, during therapy, including blood urate

Lab. test interferences:

• Certain urine dip-tests for ketones

Treatment of overdose: Gastric lavage, supportive treatment; high-carbohydrate, low-fat diet, probenecid for hyperuricaemia

NURSING CONSIDERATIONS

Assess:

• Temperature, baseline BP, pulse

• Culture and sensitivity prior to therapy

Administer:

• With meals to decrease GI symptoms

Evaluate:

• Hepatic status: decreased appetite, jaundice, dark urine, fatigue

Teach patient/family:

• The importance of compliance with regimen

• Inform about side effects. Patients must tell clinician immediately if these occur

• That scheduled appointments must be kept or relapse may occur

• Avoid alcohol while taking this drug

---

pyridostigmine bromide

Mestinon

Func. class.: Cholinergic

Chem. class.: Tertiary amine carbamate

Legal class.: POM

Action: Inhibits destruction of acetylcholine, which increases concentration at sites where acetylcholine is released; this facilitates transmission of impulses across myoneural junction

Uses: Myasthenia gravis, paralytic ileus, post-operative urinary retention

Dosage and routes:

Myasthenia gravis

• *Adult:* By mouth 30−120 mg two to four times a day, usually daily dose 300−1200 mg

• *Child over 6 yr:* Initially 60 mg, usual dose 30−360 mg daily

• *Child under 6 yr:* Initially 30 mg, usual dose range 30−360 mg daily

Other indications:

• *Adult:* By mouth 60−240 mg, frequency determined by patient needs

• *Child:* By mouth 15−60 mg, frequency determined by patient needs

Available forms include: Tablets 60 mg

Side effects/adverse reactions:

INTEG: Rash, urticaria, sweating

CNS: Confusion, weakness, convulsions, paralysis

GI: Nausea, diarrhoea, vomiting, cramps, involuntary defaecation

CV: Bradycardia, hypotension

GU: Frequency, incontinence

RESP: Bronchospasm, excessive secretions

EENT: Miosis, blurred vision, lacrimation, salivation

Note: Most effects described are dose-related and indicative of overdose

Contraindications: Obstruction of intestine, urinary tract

Precautions: Seizure disorders, bronchial asthma, coronary occlusion, hyperthyroidism, arrhythmias, peptic ulcer, pregnancy, lactation, parkinsonism, hypotension, vagotonia, bradycardia

Pharmacokinetics:

By mouth: Onset, 1−2 hr, duration 2½−4 hr, poorly absorbed, plasma half-life 3−4 hr

Metabolised in liver, excreted in urine largely unchanged

Interactions/incompatibilities:

• Decreased action of: gallamine, pancuronium, tubocurarine, atropine

• Increased action of: suxamethonium chloride

• Decreased action of aminoglycosides, anaesthetics, procainamide, quinidine, clindamycin, lincomycin, propranolol, lithium

NURSING CONSIDERATIONS

Assess:

• Vital signs, respiration 4 hrly

• Fluid balance, check for urinary retention or incontinence

Administer:

• Smaller doses required after thymectomy or when additional therapy (steroids, immunosuppressants) are given

• Larger doses after exercise or fatigue

• Dose titration needed to give best therapeutic response with minimum toxicity

• With food or milk to decrease GI symptoms

• On empty stomach for better absorption

Evaluate:

• Therapeutic response: increased muscle strength, hand grasp, improved gait, absence of laboured breathing (if severe)

• Bradycardia, hypotension, bronchospasm, headache, dizziness, convulsions, respiratory depression; drug should be discontinued if toxicity occurs

Teach patient/family:

• That drug is not a cure, it only relieves symptoms

• Emphasise importance of taking drug at time prescribed

• All aspects of drug: action, side effects, dose, symptoms of both over and under usage, when to notify clinician

• To wear ID specifying myasthenia gravis, drugs taken

---

pyridoxine HCl (vitamin B$_6$)

Benadon, Complement Continus

Func. class.: Vitamin B$_6$, water soluble

Chem. class.: Methylpyridine derivative

Legal class.: Tablets: P. Injectable: POM

Action: Necessary for fat, protein, carbohydrate metabolism; enhances glycogen release from liver and muscle tissue; needed as co-enzyme for metabolic transformations of a variety of amino acids

Uses: Vitamin B$_6$ deficiency associated with inborn errors of metabolism, seizures, isoniazid therapy, or oral contraceptives, premenstrual syndrome

Dosage and routes:

Deficiency states

• *Adult:* By mouth 25−50 mg up to three times a day

Isoniazid neuropathy

• *Prophylaxis:* By mouth 10 mg

• *Therapeutic:* By mouth 50 mg three times a day

Idiopathic sideroblastic anaemia

• *Adult:* By mouth 100−400 mg daily in divided doses

Premenstrual syndrome
• *Adult:* By mouth 50−100 mg daily
Available forms include: Tablets 10, 20, 50 mg; tablets modified release 100 mg; injection IM/IV 50 mg (with Vitamins B and C)
Side effects/adverse reactions:
SYST: Serious allergic reactions possible with Vitamins B and C injection
Contraindications:
Hypersensitivity
Pharmacokinetics:
By mouth/injection: Half-life 2−3 weeks, metabolised in liver, excreted in urine
Interactions/incompatibilities:
• Decreased effects of: levodopa
NURSING CONSIDERATIONS
Assess:
• Baseline vital signs
Evaluate:
• Therapeutic response: absence of nausea, vomiting, anorexia, skin lesions, glossitis, stomatitis, oedema, convulsions, restlessness
• Nutritional status:
• Pyridoxine levels during treatment
• Vital signs 4-hrly
• For hypersensitivity
Teach patient/family:
• Good dietary habits; foods such as brown bread, cereals, green vegetables, pulses, meat
• To avoid vitamin supplements unless directed by clinician

---

pyrimethamine

Daraprim, Fansidar (with sulfa-doxine), Maloprim (with dapsone)
Func. class.: Antimalarial
Chem. class.: Folic acid antagonist
Legal class.: (Daraprim) P; combinations POM

Action: Inhibits folic acid metabolism in parasite, prevents transmission by stopping growth of fertilised gametes
Uses: Malaria, prophylaxis in conjunction with other agents
Dosage and routes:
Prophylaxis of malaria
Daraprim/Maloprim
• *Adults:* 1 tablet weekly
• *Child over 10 yr:* 1 tablet weekly
• *Child 5−10 yr:* ½ tablet weekly
Fansidar (not recommended by UK experts for prophylaxis)
• *Adults:* 1 tablet weekly
• *Child 9−14 yr:* ¾ tablet weekly
• *Child 4−8 yr:* ½ tablet weekly
• *Child under 4 yr:* ¼ tablet weekly
Acute attacks of malaria
Fansidar
• *Adult:* By mouth 2−3 tablets as a single dose alone or with quinine
• *Child 10−14 yr:* 2 tablets
• *Child 7−9 yr:* 1½ tablets
• *Child 4−6 yr:* 1 tablet
• *Child under 4 yr:* ½ tablet
Available forms include: Tablets 25 mg; 25 mg with 500 mg sulfadoxine; 12.5 mg with 100 mg dapsone
Side effects/adverse reactions:
Pyrimethamine alone:
INTEG: Rash
HAEM: Megaloblastic anaemia
Additionally, with dapsone:
HAEM: Agranulocytosis, met-haemoglobinaemia
Additionally, with sulfadoxine:
INTEG: Alopecia, Stevens−Johnson syndrome, Lyell's syndrome
GI: Nausea, vomiting, stomatitis, feeling of fullness, hepatitis
HAEM: Leucopenia, thrombocytopenia, agranulocytosis
RESP: Pulmonary infiltration
CNS: Fatigue, headache, polyneuritis
SYST: Fever
Contraindications: Hypersensitivity, allergy to sulphonamides (Fansidar, Maloprim), megaloblastic anaemia caused by folate

deficiency. Fansidar only (sulfa-doxine): prophylactic use in patients with severe renal/liver damage or blood dyscrasias, lactation. Dapsone only: G6PD deficiency

Precautions: Pregnancy

Pharmacokinetics:

By mouth: Peak 2 hr, half-life 111 hr; metabolised in liver, highly protein bound, excreted in urine (metabolites)

Interactions/incompatibilities:

• Increased antifolate effect when given with: cotrimoxazole, tri-methoprim, phenytoin, metho-trexate

• Theoretical risk of increased blood levels of oral anticoagu-lants, sulphonylurea, hypogly-caemics, phenytoin with Fansidar (sulfadoxine)

Treatment of overdose: Gastric lavage, anticonvulsant and respir-atory support if needed

NURSING CONSIDERATIONS

Administer:

• Before or after meals at same time each day to maintain drug level and to decrease GI symptoms

• Stop treatment immediately if signs of muco-cutaneous toxicity (seen with Fansidar)

• Give folinic acid supplements during pregnancy

Teach patient/family:

• To report visual problems, fever, fatigue, bruising, bleeding; may indicate blood dyscrasias

• To take frequent rest periods when fatigued

• To take avoidance measures against mosquito bites e.g. repel-lants, nets

---

quinalbarbitone sodium

Seconal Sodium, combination product

Func. class.: Sedative/hypnotic (short-acting)

Chem. class.: Barbiturate

Legal class.: CD (Sch 2) POM

Action: Depresses activity in brain cells primarily in reticular acti-vating system in brainstem; selectively depresses neurones in posterior hypothalamus, limbic structures

Uses: Severe, intractable insomnia

Dosage and routes:

• *Adult:* By mouth 50−100 mg at bedtime

Available forms include: Capsules 50, 100 mg

Side effects/adverse reactions:

CNS: Lethargy, drowsiness, hangover, dizziness, confusion, agitation, anxiety, psychiatric disturbances, nightmares, halluci-nations, headache, dependence, CNS depression, ataxia

GI: Nausea, vomiting, constipation

INTEG: Rash, urticaria, angi-oedema, exfoliative dermatitis

CV: Hypotension, bradycardia

RESP: Respiratory depression

HAEM: Megaloblastic anaemia (long-term treatment)

Contraindications: Hypersensi-tivity to barbiturates, history of drug/alcohol abuse, acute/chronic pain, debilitated patients, preg-nancy, lactation, dyspnoea or res-piratory obstruction, severe liver impairment, porphyria, children/young adults, elderly, use for more than 14 days

Precautions: Mental depression, hepatic or renal dysfunction, shock, respiratory depression

Pharmacokinetics: Well absorbed by mouth. Metabolised by liver, excreted by kidneys (metabolites); half-life 15−40 hr

Interactions/incompatibilities:
• Increased CNS depression: alcohol, MAOIs, sedative, narcotics
• Decreased effect of these drugs: oral anticoagulants, calcium channel blockers, corticosteroids, disopyramide, griseofulvin, quinidine, oral contraceptives, phenytoin, tricyclic antidepressants, tetracyclines

Treatment of overdose: Supportive care; in severe poisoning consider haemodialysis or haemoperfusion

NURSING CONSIDERATIONS

Administer:
• ½−1 hr before bedtime for sleeplessness
• On empty stomach for best absorption

Perform/provide:
• Assistance with mobility after receiving dose; drug causes drowsiness

Evaluate:
• Therapeutic response: ability to sleep at night, decreased amount of early morning awakening if taking drug for insomnia
• Unresolved pain, as drug may cause severe stimulation if pain is present
• Mental status: mood, memory (long, short)
• Physical dependency: more frequent requests for medication, shakes, anxiety

Teach patient/family:
• That hypersensitivity is common, particularly in elderly: headache, hangover, drowsiness, dizziness, excitement, occasionally confusion
• Best taken 30 min before retiring to bed
• That drug is indicated only for short-term treatment of insomnia and is probably ineffective after 2 weeks
• That physical dependency may

result when used for extended periods of time (45−90 days depending on dose)
• To avoid driving or other activities requiring alertness
• To avoid alcohol ingestion or CNS depressants; serious CNS depression may result
• Not to discontinue medication quickly after long-term use; drug should be tapered over 1−2 weeks
• That withdrawal insomnia may occur after short-term use
• That effects may take 2 nights for benefits to be noticed
• Alternate measures to improve sleep (reading, warm bath, warm milk, TV, self-hypnosis, deep breathing)

quinapril

Accupro

Func. class.: Antihypertensive
Chem. class.: Angiotensin converting enzyme inhibitor, non-sulphydryl
Legal class.: POM

Action: Selectively suppresses renin-angiotensin-aldosterone system; the active metabolite quinaprilat inhibits angiotensin converting enzyme, prevents conversion of angiotensin I to angiotensin II

Uses: Adjunct to diuretics or cardiac glycosides in congestive heart failure; hypertension where standard therapy is ineffective or inappropriate

Dosage and routes:
Congestive heart failure
• *Adult:* By mouth initially in hospital 2.5 mg/day, adjusted according to response; usual maintenance, 10−20 mg/day in two divided doses with concomitant

therapy; up to 40 mg/day may be given
• *Children:* Not recommended

Hypertension
• *Adult:* Initially 5 mg/day, adjusted according to response; maintenance usually 20−40 mg/day, in single or divided doses; up to 80 mg/day has been given. Initial dose with concurrent diuretics or in renal impairment, 2.5 mg/day
• *Children:* Not recommended
• *Elderly:* Initially 2.5 mg/day

Available forms include: Tablets 5 mg, 10 mg, 20 mg

Side effects/adverse reactions:
CNS: Headache, dizziness, insomnia, paraesthesia, nervousness, fatigue
RESP: Cough, upper respiratory tract infection, rhinitis
MS: Myalgia, weakness, back pain
GI: Nausea, vomiting, dyspepsia, abdominal pain
CV: Chest pain, hypotension
INTEG: Angioedema (discontinue immediately), rash
EENT: Sinusitis, pharyngitis, taste disturbances
GU: Renal impairment

Contraindications: Pregnancy, porphyria, aortic stenosis, outflow obstruction, or renovascular disease

Precautions: Severe heart failure, renal insufficiency, peripheral vascular disease, atherosclerosis, dehydration, low sodium diet

Interactions/incompatibilities:
• May decrease effect of: tetracyclines
• Possibly increased toxicity: lithium, potassium salts, potassium sparing diuretics, non-steroidal anti-inflammatory agents
• Increased effect of: alcohol, anaesthetics, other antihypotensives, β-blockers, diuretics, phenothiazines
• Decreased effect of: non-steroidal anti-inflammatory agents, corticosteroids, oestrogens, oral contraceptives

Clinical assessment:
• Monitor: renal function before or during therapy in renal insufficiency
• White cell count in collagen vascular disorders or with leucopenic drugs. Use relevant points as for captopril

NURSING CONSIDERATIONS

Assess:
• Baseline vital signs
• Apical/radial pulse before administration; notify physician of any significant changes
• Urinalysis for protein daily, in first morning specimen, if protein is increased, 24 hr urinary protein should be collected

Administer:
• First dose under medical supervision in hospital
• IV infusion of 0.9% NaCl (as ordered) to expand fluid volume if severe hypotension occurs

Perform/provide:
• Supine or Trendelenburg position for severe hypotension, especially in early treatment

Evaluate:
• Therapeutic response
• BP, pulse every 4 hr; note rate, rhythm, quality during initial therapy
• Symptoms of congestive cardiac failure: oedema, dyspnoea
• Renal symptoms: polyuria, oliguria, frequency

Teach patient/family:
• Administer 1 hr before meals
• Not to discontinue drug abruptly
• Not to use non-prescribed (cough, cold, or allergy) products unless directed by clinician
• Stress patient compliance with dosage schedule, even if feeling better
• To rise slowly to sitting or

standing position to minimise orthostatic hypotension

• Notify clinician of: persistant dry cough, sore throat, swelling of hands or feet, irregular heartbeat, chest pain, signs of angioedema

• May cause dizziness, fainting; light-headedness may occur during first few days of therapy

---

quinidine bisulphate/ quinidine sulphate

Kiditard, Kinidin

Func. class.: Antiarrhythmic (Class IA)
Chem. class.: Quinine dextro isomer
Legal class.: POM

Action: Stabilises cardiac membrane and prolongs action potential duration

Uses: Atrial fibrillation, supraventricular and ventricular tachyarrhythmias

Dosage and routes:

• *Adult:* By mouth 200 mg (sulphate) or 250 mg (bisulphate) as a test dose, then 200−400 mg (sulphate) 3 or 4 times daily or 500−1250 mg (bisulphate) as controlled release capsules or tablets twice daily

Available forms include: Capsules modified release 250 mg (bisulphate); Tablets modified release 250 mg (bisulphate); Tablets 200 mg (sulphate)

Side effects/adverse reactions:

CNS: Headache, dizziness, confusion, vertigo (signs of cinchonism)

EENT: Tinnitus, blurred vision, hearing loss (signs of cinchonism)

GI: Nausea, vomiting, abdominal pain, diarrhoea, granulomatous hepatitis

CV: Heart block, extrasystole, ventricular arrhythmias, widened QRS complex, cardiac arrest, hypotension

HAEM: Thrombocytopenia, haemolytic anaemia, aplastic anaemia

RESP: Asthma (hypersensitivity)

INTEG: Rash, urticaria, pruritus, purpura (signs of hypersensitivity); photosensitivity, lupus, flushing

SYST: Fever

Contraindications: Hypersensitivity, acute infection, severe heart block

Precautions: Pregnancy, lactation, hypotension, liver disease, uncompensated cardiac failure, partial heart block, myocardial damage, conductive tissue disease, myasthenia gravis

Pharmacokinetics:

By mouth: Onset 2−3 hr, peak 1−3 hr, duration 6−8 hr; half-life 6−7 hr, metabolised in liver, excreted unchanged by kidneys

Interactions/incompatibilities:

• May increase effects of: neuromuscular blockers, digoxin, anticoagulants, β-blockers

• May increase effects of quinidine: cimetidine, verapamil, diuretics, antacids

• May decrease effects of: neostigmine, pyridostigmine

• May decrease effects of quinidine: rifampicin, antiepileptics, barbiturates

Clinical assessment

• ECG continuously at high doses

• Blood levels at higher doses

Treatment of overdose: Symptomatic supportive care; monitor CV, respiratory, and renal function and blood electrolytes

NURSING CONSIDERATIONS

Assess:

• BP, temp, pulse, respiration, ECG prior to therapy

Evaluate:

• Cardiac and respiratory rate, temperature, BP

- Observe for potential tachypnoea, tachycardia, pyrexia and changes in BP
- CNS effects: may cause dizziness, confusion, psychosis paraesthesias, convulsions
- Inform clinician if any of the above occur. Therapy may be discontinued

---

quinine bisulphate/ quinine dihydrochloride/ quinine hydrochloride/ quinine sulphate

Func. class.: Antimalarial
Chem. class.: Cinchona tree alkaloid
Legal class.: POM

Action: Inhibits parasite replications, transcription of DNA to RNA by forming complexes with DNA of parasite

Uses: *Plasmodium falciparum* malaria, nocturnal leg cramps

Dosage and routes:

Malaria

- *Adults:* By mouth 600 mg (dihydrochloride, hydrochloride, or sulphate) 8 hrly for 7 days (with pyrimethamine/sulfadoxine or tetracycline); IV infusion, loading dose of 20 mg/kg (of salts as above) over 4 hrs then 10 mg/kg (up to maximum 700 mg) over 4 hr; every 8−12 hr, until course can be completed by mouth. Reduce every 8−12 hr, until course can be completed by mouth. Maintenance to 5−7 mg/kg if given more than 72 hr
- *Child:* By mouth 10 mg/kg of salts as above 8 hrly for 7 days (with pyrimethamine/sulfadoxine or tetracycline); IV infusion as for adult

Leg cramps

- *Adult:* By mouth 200 mg (sulphate) or 300 mg (bisulphate) at night

Available forms include: Tablets 300 mg (bisulphate, dihydrochloride, hydrochloride, sulphate) 125 mg (sulphate), 200 mg (sulphate); IV infusion (dihydrochloride) 300 mg/ml

Side effects/adverse reactions:

RESP: Asthma (hypersensitivity)

INTEG: Pruritus, rashes, purpura, angioedema (signs of hypersensitivity)

HAEM: Thrombocytopenia, agranulocytosis, hypothrombinaemia, haemolysis

CNS: Headache, confusion, vertigo, dizziness (signs of cinchonism)

EENT: Visual disturbances including temporary blindness, tinnitus, deafness (signs of cinchonism)

GI: Nausea, vomiting, diarrhoea, abdominal pain, hepatitis

CV: Heartblock, ventricular, arrhythmias, hypotension, circulatory failure

ENDO: Hypoglycaemia

GU: Renal failure

SYST: Fever

Contraindications: Hypersensitivity, haemolysis, optic neuritis, tinnitus, haemoglobinuria

Precautions: Pregnancy (avoid except in life threatening disease), atrial fibrillation, heart block or other cardiac disease, severe hepatic disease, myasthenia gravis, G6PD deficiency

Pharmacokinetics:

By mouth: Peak 1−3 hr, metabolised in liver, excreted in urine, half-life 4−5 hr

Interactions/incompatibilities:

- May increase effects of quinine: cimetidine
- May increase effects of: digoxin, neuromuscular blockers, anticoagulants

Treatment of overdose: Symptomatic supportive care; monitor CV, respiratory, and renal function

NURSING CONSIDERATIONS
Assess:
• BP, pulse
Administer:
• Before/after meals at same time each day to maintain drug level
• At night if taking for leg cramps (nocturnal)
Perform/provide:
• Urinalysis for haemoglobin
Evaluate:
• Therapeutic effect: relief of symptoms
• If administered IV, watch for hypotension, tachycardia
• Signs of rhinitis, nausea, rashes, abdominal pain, visual disturbances
Teach patient/family:
• To avoid non-prescribed preparations: cold preparations, tonic water
• To inform prescribing clinician if already on anticoagulant therapy or digoxin
• To take regular exercise if experience night cramps

---

rabies vaccine

Merieux Inactivated Rabies Vaccine
Func. class.: Inactivated human diploid cell vaccine
Chem. class.: Inactivated Wistar Pm/Wl 38 1503−3M virus strain
Legal class.: POM

Action: Promotes development of rabies specific antibodies
Uses: Active immunisation as prophylactic measure to personnel at risk of contracting rabies e.g. staff at animal quarantine stations, animal handlers, veterinary surgeons, field workers at risk of being bitten by wild animals, staff in attendance upon a patient suspected of or known to be suffering from rabies; post-exposure treatment of previously unvaccinated patients

Dosage and routes:
Prophylaxis
• Deep subcutaneous, IM injection initially 1 ml, then further 1 ml after 1 month, then further 1 ml after 6−12 months; reinforcing doses 1 ml every 2−3 yr depending on risk of infection
Staff in attendance on patients with rabies
• Intradermally, 4 doses of 0.1 ml injected at different sites on the same day
• For further advice contact Duty Medical Officer, Central Public Health Laboratory, Colindale Avenue, Colindale, London NW9 5HT, Tel 081−200 4400
Post-exposure treatment (no, or inadequate prophylaxis)
• Deep subcutaneous, IM injection 1 ml on day of exposure then 1 ml after 3, 7, 14, 30 and 90 days; rabies immunoglobulin should be given concurrently on day 0
Available forms include: Injection, 2.5 International Units single dose vial
Side effects/adverse reactions:
INTEG: Pain, erythema and induration of injection site, pruritus, nausea
SYST: Fever, malaise or myalgia. Anaphylaxis
Interactions/incompatibilities:
• Reduced effect of vaccine: steroids, immunosuppressants
Clinical assessment:
• Do not wait for confirmation of rabies before administering first vaccination
• Cease injections if animal is found to be not rabid
• Use with care in allergy to neomycin (traces are present in vaccine)
• Prescribe protection against

tetanus and infection for those with serious bites
• All contacts of a rabid subject should be vaccinated

NURSING CONSIDERATIONS
Administer:
• Use immediately after reconstitution
• Discard any vaccine unused within an hour of reconstitution
• Administer deep subcutaneous or IM into deltoid region — avoid the gluteal region
• Ensure adrenaline is readily available in case of anaphylactic reaction
• Ensure bite wounds are thoroughly cleansed with soapy water

Evaluate:
• For anaphylaxis
• For signs of local skin reactions and mild fever or malaise

Teach patient/family:
• That local and systemic side effects are common within 48 hr but are usually mild
• That all contacts will need vaccination if subject is rabid
• If vaccination is given prophylactically, further immunisation will be required if patient is exposed to rabies virus

---

ranitidine

Zantac
Func. class.: Antihistamine — H_2 receptor antagonist
Legal class.: POM

Action: Inhibits histamine at H_2 receptor site in parietal cells, which inhibits gastric acid secretion
Uses: Duodenal ulcer, Zollinger-Ellison syndrome, benign gastric ulcer, reflux oesophagitis, prophylaxis for stress ulcer, Mendelson's syndrome

Dosage and routes:
• *Adult:* By mouth 150 mg twice a day or 300 mg at bedtime for 4–8 weeks; maybe increased to 300 mg twice a day. Maintenance if required 150 mg at bedtime. IV bolus 50 mg diluted to 20 ml over 5 min every 6–8 hr. IV intermittent infusion 50 mg/100 ml over 2 hr every 6–8 hr, IM injection 50 mg 6–8 hrly. Continuous IV infusion in severely ill patients 0.125–0.25 mg/kg/hr

Zollinger-Ellison syndrome
• *Adult:* By mouth 150 mg 3 times a day increasing if required to maximum 6 g daily

Mendelson's syndrome
• *Adult:* By mouth pre-operative: 150 mg 2 hr before induction and, preferably night before; IM or slow IV 50 mg, 45–60 min before anaesthesia
• *Obstetric*: By mouth 150 mg on commencement of labour then 150 mg 6 hrly; administer antacid prior to anaesthesia

Available forms include: Tablets 150, 300 mg; injection 25 mg/ml IM, IV; syrup 75 mg in 5 ml; dispersible tablets 150 mg

Side effects/adverse reactions:
CNS: Headache, dizziness, confusion, hallucination
GI: Hepatotoxicity
CV: Bradycardia, atrioventricular block, asystole
HAEM: Leucopenia, thrombocytopenia, agranulocytosis
INTEG: Urticaria, rash, swelling/discomfort in breast (men)
SYST: Anaphylaxis, fever

Contraindications: Hypersensitivity
Precautions: Pregnancy, lactation, use in children is limited therefore caution is necessary, renal disease, may mask symptoms of undiagnosed gastric carcinoma

Pharmacokinetics:
By mouth: Peak 2–3 hr, metabolised by liver, excreted in urine

largely unchanged, breast milk, half-life 2−3 hr

Interactions/incompatibilities:
• Decreased absorbtion of: itraconazole, ketoconazole

Treatment of overdose: No problem expected in overdose, supportive treatment only

NURSING CONSIDERATIONS

Assess:
• Establish baseline pulse then monitor pulse rate frequently
• Fluid balance

Teach patient/family:
• That gynaecomastia may occur but is reversible
• Avoid driving or other hazardous activities until patient is stabilised on this medication
• About appropriate diet
• To avoid black pepper, caffeine, alcohol, harsh spices, extremes in temperature of food
• To avoid non-prescribed preparations: aspirin, cough, cold preparations

---

rauwolfia alkaloids

Hypercal

Func. class.: Antihypertensive
Chem. class.: Antiadrenergic agent
Legal class.: POM

Action: Inhibits noradrenaline release, depleting noradrenaline stores in adrenergic nerve endings

Uses: Hypertension

Dosage and routes:
• *Adult:* By mouth initial 4 mg at night or in 2 divided doses

Available forms include: Tablets 2 mg

Side effects/adverse reactions:
CV: Bradycardia, chest pain, arrhythmias
HAEM: Prolonged bleeding time, thrombocytopenia, purpura
CNS: Drowsiness, fatigue, lethargy, dizziness, depression, anxiety, headache, increased dreaming, nightmares, convulsions, Parkinsonism, extrapyramidal symptoms (high doses)
GI: Nausea, vomiting, cramps, peptic ulcer, dry mouth, increased appetite, anorexia, diarrhoea, haematemisis
INTEG: Rash, alopecia, flushings, warm feeling, pruritus, ecchymosis
EENT: Lacrimation, miosis, blurred vision, ptosis, dry mouth, epistaxis, glaucoma, nasal congestion
GU: Impotence, dysuria, nocturia
SYST: Sodium/water retention, oedema
ENDO: Breast engorgement, galactorrhoea, gynaecomastia
RESP: Bronchospasm, dyspnoea, cough, rales

Contraindications: Hypersensitivity; depression/suicidal patients, peptic ulcer, ulcerative colitis, phaeochromocytoma, bronchial asthma, thyrotoxicosis, Parkinson's Disease, epilepsy

Precautions: Pregnancy, lactation, heart failure, arteriosclerosis

Pharmacokinetics:
By mouth: Peak 3−6 hr, duration 2−6 weeks, half-life 50−100 hr, metabolised by liver, excreted mostly unchanged in urine, faeces, blood−brain barrier, excreted in breast milk. Times refer to reserpine, the most active constituent of the product

Interactions/incompatibilities:
• Increased extrapyramidal side-effects: Antipsychotics, metoclopramide
• Decreased effects of: Levodopa, amantadine
• Increased bradycardia: β-blockers
• Decreased hypotension: Non-steroidal anti-inflammatory drugs, corticosteroids, sex steroids,

sympathomimetics, tricyclic anti-depressants
• Increased hypotension: diuretics, alcohol, anaesthetics, other antihypertensives, anxiolytics, hypnotics, levodopa, nitrates
• Excitation, hypertension: MAOIs
• Increased CNS depression: barbiturates, alcohol, narcotics

Lab. test interferences:
Interferences: 17-ketosteroids in urine, urinary catecholamines measured fluorimetrically

Treatment of overdose: Lavage, IV atropine for bradycardia, supportive therapy

NURSING CONSIDERATIONS
Assess:
• Baseline BP, pulse, weight and fluid balance
Administer:
• Orally at night or in 2 divided doses
• With food or milk if GI symptoms occur
Perform/provide:
• Frequent drinks to prevent a dry month
Evaluate:
• Therapeutic response: decreased BP check for hypotension and bradycardia
• Pulse, BP regularly until therapeutic response obtained
• Weigh weekly during treatment
• Oedema in feet and legs
• Effect of any other medication
• Symptoms of congestive cardiac failure, bronchospasm
• Report excessive bruising haematemisis, bleeding from mucous membranes or pin-prick bruising immediately
Teach patient/family:
• To avoid driving, hazardous activities if drowsiness occurs
• Not to discontinue drug abruptly
• To report bradycardia, dizziness, confusion, depression, fever,

breathing difficulties, excessive bruising
• That impotence, enlarged breasts may occur but is reversible
• To rise slowly to sitting or standing position to minimise hypotension
• That therapeutic effect may take 2−6 weeks
• To take other medication only if directed by clinician
• To avoid alcohol
• To give up smoking and encourage a healthy diet

---

reproterol HCl

Bronchodil
Func. class.: Adrenergic β-2 bronchodilator
Chem. class.: Theophylline
Legal class.: POM

Action: Selective β_{-2} stimulation of receptors in respiratory smooth muscle producing bronchodilation
Uses: Reversible airways obstruction, bronchial asthma, chronic bronchitis and emphysema
Dosage and routes:
• *Adult:* Inhalation (aerosol) 0.5−1 mg (1−2 puffs), repeated after 3−6 hr if necessary; maintenance therapy 1 mg (2 puffs) 3 times daily
• *Child 6−12 yr:* Inhalation (aerosol) 0.5 mg (1 puff) every 3−6 hr; maintenance therapy 0.5 mg (1 puff) three times a day
Available forms include: Aerosol inhalation, 500 mcg metered dose inhaler
Side effects/adverse reactions:
CNS: Fine tremor, headache, nervous tension
CVS: Tachycardia
Precautions: Hyperthyroidism, pregnancy, myocardial infarction, phaeochromocytoma

Interactions/incompatibilities:
• May inhibit action of this drug: other β-blockers

Clinical assessment:
• Monitor blood potassium levels before, during long-term therapy

Treatment of overdose:
Symptomatic relief only necessary

NURSING CONSIDERATIONS

Assess:
• Baseline pulse rate; tachycardia may occur

Perform/provide:
• Store aerosol canister away from heat, do not puncture even when empty
• Replace nebuliser solutions daily

Evaluate:
• Patient technique with aerosol inhaler — poor technique may be mistaken for poor drug action
• For side effects of digital tremor, restlessness — children may need reassurance when these occur
• Therapeutic response — easier breathing
• Need for further measures if usual degree of relief not obtained

Teach patient/family:
• Correct technique — this should be re-assessed occasionally
• Not to exceed prescribed dose
• Children should always be supervised by responsible adult when using aerosol/nebuliser
• Check with clinician before taking unprescribed preparations
• Report to clinician at once if usual degree of relief is not obtained or if asthma is severe

---

rifampicin

Rifadin, Rimactane,
Func. class.: Anti-tubercular
Chem. class.: Rifamycin derivative
Legal class.: POM

Action: Inhibits DNA-dependent RNA polymerase, bactericidal

Uses: Pulmonary tuberculosis, leprosy, brucellosis, Legionnaires' Disease. Prophylaxis of meningococcal meningitis, *H. influenzae*

Dosage and routes:
Tuberculosis
• *Adult:* By mouth: 450−600 mg/day as single dose 1 hr before food; IV infusion: 600 mg over 2−3 hr
• *Child:* By mouth 10−20 mg/kg/day as single dose 1 hr before meals not to exceed 600 mg/day

Leprosy
• *Adult:* By mouth 600 mg once per month

Brucellosis, Legionnaires' disease, serious staphylococcal infection
• *Adult:* By mouth 600−1200 mg in 2−4 divided doses

Prophylaxis of meningococcal meningitis
• *Adult:* By mouth 600 mg twice daily for 2 days
• *Child (1−12 yr):* By mouth 10 mg/kg twice daily for 2 days
• *Child (3 months−1 yr):* By mouth 5 mg/kg twice daily for 2 days

Prophylaxis of H. influenzae
• *Adult and children in exposed household:* By mouth 20 mg/kg (maximum 600 mg) once daily for 5 days

Available forms include: Capsules 150, 300 mg; Syrup, 100 mg/5 ml; IV infusion, 300, 600 mg

Side effects/adverse reactions:
CV: Hypotension, shock
CNS: Headache, drowsiness, lethargy, confusion, peripheral neuropathy, psychosis
GU: Acute renal failure
EENT: Blurred vision, optic neuritis, photophobia, conjunctivitis
HAEM: Haemolytic anaemia, thrombocytopenia, leucopenia, purpura, eosinophilia
GI: Anorexia, nausea, vomiting,

diarrhoea, abdominal discomfort, pseudomembranous colitis, liver damage
INTEG: Rash, flushing
MISC: Flu-like syndrome, red colouration of body fluids
RESP: Wheezing, dyspnoea
MS: Myopathy
Contraindications: Hypersensitivity, jaundice
Precautions: Pregnancy, hepatic impairment, alcoholism, breast feeding, soft contact lenses (permanent red staining), for treatment should always be given in combination to prevent resistance occurring, porphyria
Pharmacokinetics:
By mouth: Peak 2−3 hr, duration greater than 24 hr, half-life 2−5 hr (dose dependent) metabolised in liver (active/inactive metabolites), excreted mostly in bile, also in urine as free drug excreted in breast milk
Interactions/incompatibilities:
• Decreased effect of: barbiturates, clofibrate, corticosteroids, dapsone, anticoagulants, oral antidiabetics, hormones, digoxin, PAS, oral contraceptives, digitalis, vitamin D, phenytoin, quinidine, mexiletine, methadone, theophylline, chloramphenicol, ketoconazole, cyclosporin A, azathioprine, β-blockers, verapamil, cimetidine
Clinical assessment:
• Liver function tests before treatment and at regular intervals
• Regular blood counts during prolonged therapy
• Do not restart therapy stopped because of serious toxicity
• Reduce dose to 8 mg/kg in heppatic impairment
• If restarting therapy after a break, start at dose of 75 mg/day and increase towards therapeutic dose by 75 mg/day. Side effects more likely upon restarting

Lab. test interferences:
Interference: Folate level, vitamin B_{12}, bromsulphthalein, radiographic gall bladder studies
Treatment of overdose: Gastric lavage, activated charcoal, consider forced diuresis, haemodialysis, general supportive measures
NURSING CONSIDERATIONS
Assess:
• Signs of anaemia including regular blood count Hb
• Pulse, BP, respirations and temperature
• Input and output of fluids, check for decrease in output, urinalysis
• Weight
Administer:
• Orally before meals or 2 hr after
• IV by infusion only over 2−3 hr
• Antiemetics if vomiting occurs
• With food if severe GI upset, but absorption of rifampicin decreased
Evaluate:
• Therapeutic effect: containment and decreased infection. Prophylaxis use for contacts preventing diseases
• Hepatic status, decreased appetite, jaundice, dark urine, fatigue
• Hypotension, shock, confusion, psychosis
• Anaemia, purpura, thrombocytopenia
• Nausea, vomiting, rash, flushing, flu-like symptoms
• Effects of other drugs increased or decreased
• Culture and sensitivity to detect resistance
Teach patient/family:
• To report purpura and any signs of bleeding immediately
• To report signs of jaundice — yellowing skin, eyes, dark urine and faeces
• Women using oral contraception require another method of contraception

• That tests and treatment may take many months, but correct dosage will be scheduled and must be taken as directed
• That permanent red staining of soft contact lenses can occur during therapy
• That urine, faeces, saliva, sputum, sweat, tears may be coloured red-orange

---

rimiterol hydrobromide

Pulmadil, Pulmadil Auto
Func. class.: Bronchodilator
Chem. class.: Sympathomimetic, adrenergic β2 stimulant
Legal class.: POM

Action: Selective β_2 stimulation of receptors in respiratory smooth muscle producing bronchodilation
Uses: Reversible airways obstruction, especially when short action required
Dosage and routes:
• *Adult and child:* Inhalation (aerosol) 200−600 mcg (1−3 puffs) up to 8 times daily; do not repeat in less than 30 mins
Available forms include: Aerosol inhalation, 200 mcg metred dose inhaler
Side effects/adverse reactions:
CNS: Headache
INTEG: Rash
META: Hypokalaemia
RESP: Paradoxical bronchospasm
Precautions: Pregnancy
Pharmacokinetics: Readily absorbed, subject to first pass metabolism and metabolism by catechol-*O*-methyltransferase. Very short half-life of less than 5 min
Interactions/incompatibilities:
• May inhibit effect β-blockers
Clinical assessment:
• Regular serum potassium monitoring

Treatment of overdose: Symptomatic relief only necessary
NURSING CONSIDERATIONS
Assess:
• Baseline pulse; Tachycardia may occur
Administer:
• Shake before use to disperse particles
Perform/provide:
• Do not puncture or burn container
Evaluate:
• Patient's technique to ensure correct
• Therapeutic response—improvement in respiratory status
Teach patient/family:
• Correct technique for administration—this should be checked periodically
• Administration of drug to children must always be supervised by a responsible adult
• Wait for 1 min between inhalations to allow assessment of response
• Not to administer more than eight treatments in any 24 hr
• Not to take any non-prescribed medication without consulting clinician
• Seek medical advice if the usual degree of symptomatic relief is not obtained

---

ritodrine HCl

Yutopar
Func. class.: Uterine relaxant
Chem. class.: β_2-adrenergic agent
Legal class.: POM

Action: Reduces frequency, intensity of uterine contractions by stimulation of the β_2 receptors in uterine smooth muscle
Uses: Preterm labour, fetal asphyxia in labour where it is desired to obtain uterine relaxation

Dosage and routes:
• *Adult:* IV infusion 50 mcg/min, increased gradually by 50 mcg/min every 10 min until desired response or control maternal heart rate reaches 140 beats per minute, usually 150−350 mcg/min continue 12−48 hr after contractions have ceased. By mouth 10 mg given ½ hr before termination of IV, then 10 mg every 2 hr for 24 hr, then 10−20 mg every 4−6 hr, not to exceed 120 mg/day. IM 10 mg every 3−8 hrs continued 12−48 hr after contractions have ceased
Available forms include: Tablets 10 mg; IV/IM injection 10 mg/ml
Side effects/adverse reactions:
META: Hyperglycaemia in diabetics
CNS: Headache, anxiety, nervousness, tremor
GI: Nausea, vomiting, anorexia, malaise
CV: Tachycardia palpitation, hypotension
INTEG: Flushing, sweating
Contraindications: Hypersensitivity, antepartum haemorrhage which requires immediate delivery, eclampsia and severe pre-eclampsia, intra-uterine fetal death, chorioamnionitis, maternal cardiac disease, cord compression
Precautions: Heart disease, first 16 weeks of pregnancy, diabetes, hypertension, mild to moderate pre-eclampsia, hyperthyroidism
Pharmacokinetics:
Metabolised in liver, excreted in urine
Interactions/incompatibilities:
• Increased risk of hypokalaemia: potassium depleting diuretics, corticosteroids, theophylline
• Pulmonary oedema: corticosteroids
• Increased effects of: general anaesthetics
Clinical assessment:

• Maternal heart rate during infusion, maintain below 140 beats per minute
• Monitor blood glucose during IV infusion in diabetics
NURSING CONSIDERATIONS
Assess:
• Maternal, pulse rate
• For premature labour
• Intensity, length of uterine contractions
• Blood glucose in diabetics
Administer:
• By infusion pump, and monitor carefully
Perform/provide:
• Explanation of procedure
• Call bell
• Continuous CTG
Evaluate:
• Therapeutic response: decreased intensity, length of contraction, absence of preterm labour, decreased BP
• Maternal pulse rate
• Foetal heart rate
• Dilatation of cervix
Teach patient/family:
• To remain in bed during infusion
• Relevance of treatment
• Possible side effects

salcatonin

Calsynar, Miacalcic
Func. class.: Thyroparathyroid agent (calcium regulator)
Chem. class.: Synthetic polypeptide hormone
Legal class.: POM

Action: Decreases: bone resorption, blood calcium levels; increases deposits of calcium in bones
Uses: Hypercalcaemia, postmenopausal osteoporosis, Paget's Disease, bone cancer
Dosage and routes:

Hypercalcaemia
• IM/Subcutaneous up to 8 units/kg 6−8 hrly adjusted as required; IV Infusion 5−10 units/kg over at least 6 hr in 500 ml physiological saline

Paget's disease
• IM/Subcutaneous initially 50−100 units 3 times weekly increased to daily if needed for 3−6 months

Bone pain (neoplastic disease)
• IM/Subcutaneous 200 units 6-hrly or 400 units 12-hrly for 24−48 hr

Post-menopausal osteoporosis
• IM/Subcutaneous 100 units/day plus calcium and vitamin D

Available forms include: Injectable Subcutaneous/IM 50, 100, 200 units/ml; injectable IV 50, 100 units/ml

Side effects/adverse reactions:
INTEG: Rash, flushing, irritation at injection site
CNS: Dizziness
GU: Diuresis, calcitonin antibody formation
GI: Nausea, diarrhoea, vomiting, unpleasant taste
MS: Tingling of hands
SYST: Anaphylactic and other allergic reactions

Contraindications: Hypersensitivity, lactation

Precautions: Renal disease, pregnancy, children

Pharmacokinetics:
IM/Subcutaneous: Onset 15 min, peak 1 hr, elimination half-life 70−90 min, metabolised by kidneys, excreted as inactive metabolites
IV: Plasma half-life less than 15 min

Interactions/incompatibilities:
• Theoretically may enhance toxicity of cardiac glycosides by producing rapid change serum electrolytes
• Dilution for IV use results in potency loss of approximately 20%

Clinical assessment:
• Reductions in serum alkaline phosphatase, urinary hydroxyproline denote response in Paget's Disease; lowered serum calcium in hypercalcaemia. Check for response, continued response

Treatment of overdose: Not likely to be significant, treatment supportive.

NURSING CONSIDERATIONS
Assess:
• Nutritional status; diet for sources of vitamin D (milk, some seafood), calcium (dairy products, dark green vegetables), phosphates
• Systemic allergic reaction to drug: skin test before first dose

Perform/provide:
• Urinalysis
• Storage in refrigerator
• Restriction of sodium, potassium if required

Evaluate:
• Local reaction at injection site
• GI symptoms, polyuria, flushing, tingling, headache

Teach patient/family:
• Avoid non-prescribed medicines
• All aspects of drug: action, side effects, dose, when to notify clinician

---

salicylic acid

Func. class.: Keratolytic
Legal class.: GSL

Action: Corrects abnormal keratinization and causes peeling of skin

Uses: Dandruff, seborrhoeic dermatitis, psoriasis, multiple superficial epitheliomatoses, hyperkeratosis, tinea, removal of warts

Dosage and routes:
• *Adult and child:* Apply as needed, cover at night

Available forms include: Ointment 2%, Collodion 12%; Plaster 20%, 40%; Lotion 2%. Also many combination products

Side effects/adverse reactions:

INTEG: Irritation, drying

CNS: Salicylism: hearing loss, tinnitus, dizziness

Contraindications:

Hypersensitivity

Treatment of overdose: Overdose not likely in normal use

NURSING CONSIDERATIONS

Administer:

• Only to intact skin, do not use on inflamed, denuded skin

• After wetting skin, wash thoroughly each morning after treatment

• Using an occlusive dressing to increase absorption

Evaluate:

• Therapeutic response: decrease in dandruff, size of lesions

• Salicylism: tinnitus, hearing loss, dizziness

• Allergic reactions: irritation, redness

Teach patient/family:

• To avoid contact with eyes, mucous membranes

• To apply lotion if drying occurs

---

selegiline

Eldepryl

Func. class.: Antiparkinson agent

Chem. class.: Monoamine-oxidase-*B* inhibitor

Legal class.: POM

Action: Prevents breakdown of dopamine in the brain, inhibits re-uptake of dopamine at the pre-synaptic dopamine receptor, thus prolonging the effect of endo-genous dopamine and levodopa

Uses: Adjunctive treatment in Parkinson's disease

Dosage and routes:

• *By mouth:* 10 mg in morning or 5 mg at breakfast time and 5 mg at midday alone or as an adjunct to levodopa therapy

Available forms include: Tablets 5 mg

Side effects/adverse reactions:

CNS: Confusion, agitation, psychosis

CV: Hypotension

GI: Nausea, vomiting

Contraindications: Pregnancy

Precautions: Side effects of levodopa may be increased; concurrent levodopa dose may need to be reduced by 25−50%

Pharmacokinetics:

By mouth: Rapidly and completely absorbed, plasma half-life 39 hr, metabolised in liver, excreted in urine

Interactions/incompatibilities:

• Risk of hypertensive crises with: non-selective MAOIs

• Note: Selegiline does not require dietary restrictions of the type needed with non-specific MAOIs

Clinical assessment:

• Reduce concurrent levodopa dose if side-effects are increased with selegiline

Treatment of overdose: Low toxicity, observe 24−48 hr, symptomatic treatment

NURSING CONSIDERATIONS

Assess:

• Baseline BP − hypotension may occur

Evaluate:

• Check to ensure patient has swallowed tablet

• Confusion: patient may need reassurance and careful explanations if confused

• Therapeutic response: reduction in parkinsonian symptoms

selenium sulphide

Selsun, Lenium
Func. class.: Antibiotic, topical
Legal class.: P

Action: Unknown
Uses: Dandruff, seborrhoea in scalp
Dosage and routes:
• *Adult and child:* Topical wash hair with 1–2 tsp, leave on 2–3 min; rinse, repeat, use twice a week for 2 weeks then once a week or as needed
Available forms include: Shampoo 2.5%
Side effects/adverse reactions:
INTEG: Oiliness of hair/scalp, alopecia, discolouration of hair
Contraindications: Hypersensitivity, inflamed skin
Precautions: Child under 5 yr, pregnancy
Interactions/incompatibilities:
• Do not use within 2 days of dyeing, tinting, waving the hair
Treatment of overdose:
Unknown in normal use. If swallowed induce vomiting/gastric lavage, supportive treatment
NURSING CONSIDERATIONS
Perform/provide:
• Thorough hair rinsing after use
Evaluate:
• Toxicity: tremors, perspiration, pain in abdomen, weakness, anorexia
• Area of body involved, including time involved, what helps or aggravates condition
Teach patient/family:
• To avoid contact with eyes, genital area
• To discontinue use if rash or irritation occurs
• That drug may damage jewellery, remove before application
• That drug is not to be taken internally

• Should not be used within 48 hr of applying hair colouring or perm solution

senna

NHS Senokot
Func. class.: Laxative
Chem. class.: Anthraquinone glycoside
Legal class.: P/GSL (small packs)

Action: Stimulates peristalsis by action on Auerbach's plexus
Uses: Constipation, bowel preparation for surgery or examination, avoidance of straining after cerebral and cardiovascular disease
Dosage and routes:
• *Adult:* By mouth 2–4 tablets, 1–2 5 ml spoonfuls granules, 10–20 ml syrup at bedtime
• *Child (over 6 yr):* Half adult doses taken in the morning
• *Child (2–6 yr):* ½–1 5 ml spoonful syrup
Available forms include: Tablets 7.5 mg; granules 15 mg/5 ml; syrup 7.5 mg/5 ml, (as sennoside B)
Side effects/adverse reactions:
GI: Nausea, vomiting, anorexia, cramps, diarrhoea, loss of bowel tone
META: Hypokalaemia
Contraindications: Hypersensitivity, bowel obstruction, abdominal pain (undiagnosed), acute surgical abdomen
Pharmacokinetics:
By mouth: Onset 6–24 hr; metabolised by liver, excreted in faeces
Interactions/incompatibilities:
None known
Clinical assessment:
• Physical examination if 3 days of increasing dose fail to produce bowel motion

• Blood electrolytes if drug is used often by patient

Treatment of overdose: Supportive, plenty of fluid for diarrhoea

NURSING CONSIDERATIONS

Assess:

• Fluid balance

Administer:

• In morning or evening (oral dose)

Evaluate:

• Therapeutic response: return to normal bowel habit

• Cause of constipation; identify whether fluids, fibre, or exercise is missing from lifestyle

• Cramping, rectal bleeding, nausea, vomiting; seek medical advice if these occur

Teach patient/family:

• That normal bowel movements do not always occur daily

• That shortage of fluids, fibre, and lack of exercise contribute to constipation

• Not to use laxatives for long-term therapy; bowel tone will be lost

• Do not use in presence of abdominal pain, nausea, vomiting

• Notify clinician if constipation unrelieved or if symptoms of electrolyte imbalance occur: muscle cramps, pain, weakness, dizziness

---

silver nitrate

Func. class.: Keratolytic
Legal class.: P

Action: Possesses antiinfective, astringent, caustic properties

Uses: Cauterisation of lesions, warts, over-granulation of wounds

Dosage and routes:

• *Adult and child:* Apply as directed by clinician

Available forms include: Sticks

Side effects/adverse reactions:

INTEG: Skin discolouration

Contraindications: Hypersensitivity

NURSING CONSIDERATIONS

Administer:

• To apply to lesion only after protecting surrounding tissue with petroleum jelly

• After moistening stick with water

Evaluate:

• Therapeutic response: absence of lesions

Teach patient/family:

• To handle very carefully with dry hands or wearing surgical gloves

• To avoid contact with healthy tissue

• To avoid contact with clothing

• Not to moisten with saliva

• Keep away from children

---

silver sulphadiazine (topical)

Flamazine
Func. class.: Antibiotic, topical
Chem. class.: Sulphonamide
Legal class.: POM

Action: Interferes with bacterial cell wall synthesis

Uses: Burns (2nd, 3rd degree), infected leg ulcers, pressure sores

Dosage and routes:

• *Adult and child:* Topical apply to affected area once to twice daily; leg ulcers apply at least 3 times a week

Available forms include: Cream 1%

Side effects/adverse reactions:

INTEG: Rash, urticaria, stinging, burning, itching

HAEM: Leucopenia

Contraindications: Hypersensitivity, premature infants and newborn

Precautions: Impaired renal function, pregnancy, impaired hepatic function, lactation

Pharmacokinetics: Up to 10% absorbed from large wounds, metabolism slow

Interactions/incompatibilities:
• Increased blood levels of: oral hypoglycaemics, phenytoin

NURSING CONSIDERATIONS

Administer:
• Using aseptic technique
• After cleansing debris before each application
• Analgesic before application if needed
• Enough medication to cover burns, leg ulcers completely, keep covered with medication at all times

Evaluate:
• Allergic reaction: burning, stinging, swelling, redness
• Therapeutic response: development of granulation tissue

Teach patient/family:
• That drug may be continued until graft can be done
• To move digits inside the plastic
• That grey coloured exudate is normal

---

simvastatin ▼

Zocor
Func. class.: Hypolipidaemic agent
Legal class.: POM

Action: Competitive inhibitor of HMG CoA reductase

Uses: Primary hypercholesterolaemia unresponsive to other therapy, with a cholesterol level in excess of 7.8 mmol/l

Dosage and routes:
• *Adult:* By mouth initially 10 mg at night, adjusted at intervals of not less than 4 weeks; usual range 10−40 mg once daily at night
Available forms include: Tablets 10 mg, 20 mg

Side effects/adverse reactions:
CNS: Headache, fatigue
GI: Constipation, flatulence;

nausea, dyspepsia, abdominal cramps, diarrhoea, raised liver enzymes
INTEG: Rash
MS: Myopathy

Contraindications: Active liver disease; pregnancy, women must be adequately protected by non-hormonal contraceptive methods; lactation

Precautions: Avoid conception for 1 month after treatment, history of liver disease/alcohol abuse

Pharmacokinetics: Simvastatin is activated by extensive first-pass metabolism to form active metabolites. Mainly excreted in the bile

Interactions/incompatibilities:
• Increased risk of myositis when given with: nicotinic acid, fibric acid derivatives, cyclosporin, other immunosuppressants
• Increased effects of: oral anticoagulants

Clinical assessment:
• Liver function tests before treatment then periodically
• Monitor serum creatine phosphokinase regularly in patients on drugs increasing risk of myositis

Treatment of overdose:
Supportive measures, monitor liver function

NURSING CONSIDERATIONS

Assess:
• For signs of vitamin A, D, K deficiency

Administer:
• Drug with meals if GI symptoms occur

Evaluate:
• Therapeutic response
• Bowel pattern daily; increase bulk, water in diet if constipation develops

Teach patient/family:
• To take tablet at night or with meals to reduce incidence of GI complications
• To have good fibre/fluid intake if prone to constipation

- To report any rash to clinician
- To remain on low fat diet to help the tablet work effectively

---

sodium aurothiomalate

Myocrisin
Func. class.: Rheumatic disease suppressant
Chem. class.: Gold complex
Legal class.: POM

Action: Anti-inflammatory action unknown; may decrease phagocytosis, lysosomal activity, prostaglandin synthesis
Uses: Active progressive, rheumatoid arthritis, juvenile chronic arthritis
Dosage and routes:
- *Adult:* Deep IM injection, 10 mg test dose in the first week followed by weekly doses of 50 mg until signs of remission. Benefit is not expected until 300 to 500 mg has been given. The dose is continued at 2-week intervals until full remission. The interval between injections is then gradually increased to 4 weeks, after 18 months to 2 yrs to 6 weeks and then continued for 5 yr. If there is no remission after 1 g has been given and no signs of gold toxicity are present, 6 injections of 100 mg at weekly intervals may be given. If after this time no signs of remission occur alternative treatments should be considered
- *Child:* Progressive juvenile chronic arthritis, deep IM injection 1 mg/kg weekly to a maximum dose of 50 mg weekly. A test dose corresponding to one-tenth to one-fifth of calculated dose should be given for 2−3 weeks. The dosing interval should be gradually increased to 4 weeks according to response and continued for 1−5 yr

Available forms include: IM injection 10, 20, 50 mg in 0.5 ml
Side effects/adverse reactions:
EENT: Gold deposits in the eye
HAEM: Thrombocytopenia, agranulocytosis, aplastic anaemia, leucopenia, eosinophilia
INTEG: Rash, pruritus, dermatitis, exfoliative dermatitis, angioneurotic oedema
GI: Stomatitis, nausea, vomiting, alopecia, diarrhoea, metallic taste, jaundice, hepatitis
GU: Proteinuria, haematuria, nephrosis
RESP: Pulmonary fibrosis
CNS: Weakness, flushing
CV: Palpitations
INTEG: Local irritation at injection site
Contraindications: Hypersensitivity to gold, systemic lupus erythematosus, exfoliative dermatitis, pregnancy, severe renal disease, severe liver disease, blood disorders, porphyria
Precautions: Decreased tolerance in elderly, necrotising enterocolitis, pulmonary fibrosis, diabetes mellitus
Interactions/incompatibilities:
- Increased risk blood dyscrasias: when given in combination with other therapy, capable of inducing blood disorders; oxyphenbutazone, phenylbutazone
Clinical assessment:
- Before each injection, full blood count and test urine for albumin
- Annual chest X-ray should be carried out
NURSING CONSIDERATIONS
Assess:
- Urinalysis for protein before each injection
Administer:
- By deep IM injection followed by gentle massage of the area
Evaluate:
- Improvement in disease symptoms after 6−8 weeks

- Proteinuria
- Slow rashes or mouth ulcers

Teach patient/family:
- If appropriate to test own urine and record it
- Report any skin rashes or mouth ulcers
- Full effectiveness after approximately 2 months
- Importance of regular injections
- Gold card to be carried
- May experience change in taste
- May get itchy skin
- May get heavy periods
- May get easy bruising or bleeding gums or nose
- Must report symptoms to clinician

---

sodium bicarbonate

Func. class.: Alkalinizer
Chem. class.: $NaHCO_3$
Legal class.: GSL, Injection POM

Action: Orally neutralises gastric acid, which forms water, NaCl, CO_2; increases plasma bicarbonate, which buffers hydrogen ion concentration; reverses acidosis

Uses: Acidosis (metabolic), cardiac arrest, alkalinisation (systemic/urinary), antacid

Dosage and routes:
Acidosis
- *Adult and child:* Slow IV injection, a strong solution (up to 8.4%) or by continuous IV infusion sodium bicarbonate (1.26%) may be infused with isotonic sodium chloride determined by blood gas values. Seek clinician's advice

Cardiac arrest
- *Adult and child:* IV bolus injection 50 ml of 8.4% or according to blood gas results. Seek clinician's advice
- *Infant:* Seek clinician's advice

Urinary alkalinisation
- *Adult:* 3 g in water every 2 hr until urinary pH exceeds 7, maintenance of alkaline urine 5−10 g daily

Antacid
- *Adult:* By mouth tablets: 2−6 tablets sucked when required; powder: 1−5 g in water when required

Available forms include: Tablets 300 mg; powder, ear drops
Injection: 8.4%, 4.2%
Infusion: 1.26%, 4.2%, 8.4%

Side effects/adverse reactions:
CNS: Irritability, headache, confusion, stimulation, tremors, twitching, tetany, weakness, convulsions, hypertonicity
CV: Irregular pulse, cardiac arrest
GI: Flatulence, belching, distension
META: Alkalosis
RESP: Shallow, slow respirations, cyanosis, apnoea
INTEG: Tissue necrosis at injection site

Contraindications: Hypertension, peptic ulcer, eclampsia, hypernatraemia, hypoventilation

Precautions: Congestive cardiac failure, hepatic and renal impairment

Pharmacokinetics:
By mouth: Onset 2 min, duration 10 min
IV: Onset 15 min, duration 1−2 hr, excreted in urine

Interactions/incompatibilities:
- Increases effects: salicylates, quinidine
- Reduces effects: 4-quindones; lithium, tetracyclines, penicillamine
- Do not mix solution with other drugs

Clinical assessment:
- Respiratory rate, rhythm, depth, notify clinician of abnormalities
- Electrolytes, blood pH, PO_2, bicarbonate, during treatment

• Alkalosis: irritability, confusion, twitching, hypertonicity, slow respirations, cyanosis, irregular pulse
• Milk-alkali syndrome: confusion, headache, nausea, vomiting, anorexia, urinary stones, hypercalcaemia

NURSING CONSIDERATIONS
Assess:
• Vital signs
• Blood gas analysis
• Acidotic balance
Evaluate:
• For side effects
• Vital signs, respiratory function
• Blood gas analysis
• Urinary output
Teach patient/family:
• To suck antacid tablets and drink with 200 ml water
• Not to take antacid with milk, or milk-alkali syndrome may result
• Not to use antacid for more than 2 weeks

---

sodium cellulose phosphate

Calcisorb
Func. class.: Antihypercalcaemic
Chem. class.: Phosphorylated cellulose
Legal class.: P

Action: Decreases hypercalcium by binding with calcium in lumen of stomach and intestine and facilitates excretion
Uses: Reduces calcium absorption from diet in treatment of hypercalciuria and recurrent formation of renal stones, and in osteopetrosis. Also used for idiopathic hypercalcaemia of infancy, hypercalcaemic sarcoidosis and treatment of vitamin D intoxication
Dosage and routes:
• *Adult:* By mouth 15 g/day divided as three 5 g doses with each meal

• *Child:* 10 g daily in divided doses with meals
Available forms include: Powder 5 g packets
Side effects/adverse reactions:
GU: Hypomagnesuria
GI: Nausea, anorexia, diarrhoea, dyspepsia
Contraindications: Renal failure, congestive cardiac failure, pregnancy, lactation
Precautions: Children
Clinical assessment:
• Any associated increase in serum phosphate may be harmful
Interactions/incompatibilities:
• May decrease action of this drug: magnesium preparations
• Calcium and magnesium levels (serum, urinary) throughout treatment
NURSING CONSIDERATIONS
Administer:
• Powder may be dispersed in water, juice; taken with meals; sprinkled on food
Perform/provide:
• Increase fluids to 3 litres/day; urinary output should be over 2 litres/day
Evaluate:
• Therapeutic response: absence of renal stone formation
Teach patient/family:
• To decrease calcium in diet; dairy products; decrease sodium, citrus fruits in diet; increased excretion of drug will occur; decrease oxalate (chocolate, tea, spinach) rhubarb, beetroot

---

sodium cromoglycate

Opticrom
Func. class.: Anti-allergic drug
Chem. class.: Mast cell stabilizer
Legal class.: POM

Action: Inhibits degranulation of mast cells after contact with antigens, which decreases release of histamine and slow-releasing-substance of anaphylaxis (SRS-A) from mast cell

Uses: Allergic and vernal conjunctivitis

Dosage and routes:
• *Adult:* Instil 1−2 drops in both eyes 4 times a day; ointment apply 2 or 3 times daily

Available forms include: Aqueous solution 2%, 4% ointment

Side effects/adverse reactions:
EENT: Stinging, transient blurring of vision with eye ointment

Contraindications: Hypersensitivity to benzalkonium chloride

Interactions/incompatibilities: Soft contact lenses should not be worn during treatment with the eye drops. The eye ointment should not be used if contact lenses are worn

NURSING CONSIDERATIONS

Teach patient/family:
• Method of instillation, and not to touch dropper or take nozzle to eye
• Blurring of vision may occur following instillation of ointment
• To report stinging, burning, itching, lacrimation, puffiness
• Not to wear soft contact lens, use may be reinstituted 4−6 hr after therapy is discontinued

---

sodium cromoglycate

Intal, Rynacrom
Func. class.: Antiasthmatic, antiallergic agent
Chem. class.: Mast cell stabiliser
Legal class.: POM (Intal) P (Rynacrom)

Action: Inhibits histamine, slow-reacting substance of anaphylaxis release from mast cells in respiratory tract; this decreases allergic response

Uses: Prophylaxis of asthma and allergic rhinitis

Dosage and routes:
Allergic rhinitis
• *Insufflation:* 10 mg each nostril up to 4 times a day
• *Drops:* Instil 2 drops each nostril 6 times a day
• *Spray:* 1 squeeze each nostril 4−6 times a day

Prophylaxis of asthma
• Regular use is necessary
• *Aerosol inhalation:* 10 mg (2 puffs) 4 times daily increased up to 6−8 times daily. Additional dose may also be taken before exercise; maintenance 5 mg (1 puff) 4 times daily
• *Powder inhalation:* 20 mg 4 times a day, increased to 6−8 times daily in severe cases
• *Nebuliser solution:* 20 mg inhaled 4 times a day up to 6 times daily

Available forms include: Insufflation cartridges, 2.0% w/v nasal drops and spray, capsules for inhalation 20 mg, inhaler (5 mg per dose), nebuliser solution 20 mg/2 ml

Side effects/adverse reactions:
EENT: Throat irritation, cough, nasal congestion, transient bronchospasm

Contraindications: Hypersensitivity to this drug or lactose, status asthmaticus

Precautions: Pregnancy, lactation

Pharmacokinetics:
Inhalation: Peak 15 min, duration 4−6 hr, excreted unchanged in faeces, half-life 80 min

NURSING CONSIDERATIONS

Administer:
• By inhalation/nebuliser only; not to be given by mouth
• Gargle, sips of water to decrease irritation in throat
• If nebuliser solution is mixed with other drugs, any unused solution should be discarded im-

mediately and the nebuliser chamber thoroughly cleaned

Evaluate:
• Therapeutic response
• Respiratory status: respiratory rate, rhythm, characteristics, cough, wheezing, dyspnoea

Teach patient/family:
• To clear mucus before using
• Proper inhalation technique for each device
• That therapeutic effect may take up to 4 weeks
• Not to swallow capsule
• Not to use for asthma attack
• To continue regular usage

---

sodium fluoride

Fluor-A-Day, En-De-Kay, Fluorigard, Zymafluor, Oral-B Fluoride
Func. class.: Trace elements
Chem. class.: Fluoride ion
Legal class.: P

Action: Necessary for hard tooth enamel, and for resistance to periodontal disease; reduces acid production by dental bacteria

Uses: Prevention of dental caries

Dosage and routes:
• Dosage should be adjusted for fluoride content of the drinking water, diet and age
Child:
• Water content less than 300 mcg/l, up to 6 months, none; 6 months–2 years, 0.55 mcg daily (250 mcg fluoride ions)
• 2–4 yr, 1.1 mg daily (500 mcg fluoride ions)
• Over 4 yr, 2.2 mg daily (1 mg fluoride ions)
• Water content between 300 and 700 mcg/l up to 2 yr, none;
• 2–4 yr, 0.55 mg daily (250 mcg fluoride ions)
• Over 4 yr, 1.1 mg daily (500 mcg fluoride ions)
• Water content over 700 mcg/l

• No supplementation recommended

Available forms include: Tablets; 0.55 (250 mcg fluoride ions) 1.1 mg (500 mcg fluoride ions) 2.2 mg (1 mg fluoride ions) Drops; 0.5 mg/0.15 ml (250 mcg fluoride ions) 0.275 mg/drop (125 mcg fluoride ions) 0.15% (250 mcg fluoride ions in 8 drops) Rinse; 2%, 0.05%, 0.2%

Side effects/adverse reactions:
Acute overdosage: Black tarry stools, bloody vomit, diarrhoea, hypocalcaemia, other metabolic and electrolyte disturbances, tremors, hyperreflexia, paraesthesia, tetany, cardiac arrhythmias, shock, respiratory arrest, cardiac failure
Chronic overdosage: Gastric complaints, joint pain, stiffness, discolouration of teeth (white, yellowish-brown, black)

Contraindications: Hypersensitivity, areas where drinking water is fluoridated

Pharmacokinetics:
By mouth: Excreted in urine and faeces, breast milk

Interactions/incompatibilities:
• Avoid use with dairy products

Treatment of overdose: Gastric lavage, maintenance of high urine output and other symptomatic and supportive measures

NURSING CONSIDERATIONS

Assess:
• Use in children

Administer:
• Drops after meals with fluids or undiluted

Evaluate:
• Therapeutic response: absence of dental caries
• Nutritional status: increase fluoride content of water, decrease carbohydrate snacks, increase fish, tea, mineral water

Teach patient/family:
• Tablets should be sucked or dis-

solved in the mouth, do not swallow whole
• To monitor children using gel or rinse; not to be swallowed
• Not to drink, eat, or rinse mouth for at least ½ hr
• To apply after brushing and flossing at bedtime
• Store out of children's reach

---

sodium fusidate

Fucidin
Func. class.: Antibiotic, narrow-spectrum
Chem. class.: Fusidic acid salt
Legal class.: POM

Action: Inhibits bacterial protein synthesis and may be bacteriostatic or bactericidal
Uses: Staphylococcal infections, especially osteomyelitis, resistant to penicillins
Dosage and routes:
• By mouth: *Adult:* 500 mg 8-hrly; double dose for severe infections or use appropriate combined therapy; suspension: 15 ml 3 times a day
Child: 0−1   yr,   1   ml suspension/kg daily in 3 divided doses: 1−5 yr, 5 ml 3 times daily; 5−12 yr, 10 ml 3 times a day
• By slow IV infusion:
Adults greater than 50 kg: 580 mg diethanolamine fusidate 3 times daily, infusion over 6 hr
Children and adult less than 50 kg: 6−7 mg of diethanolamine fusidate per kg 3 times a day, infusion over 6 hr
GEL: Careful curettage of abscess followed by filling with gel and cover with dressing
Available forms include: Tablets 250 mg (sodium fusidate); suspension 250 mg/5 ml (as fusidic acid); infusion powder for reconsti-

tution 500 mg with buffer (as diethanolamine fusidate); gel: for injection into cavities, 2%
Side effects/adverse reactions:
GI: Nausea, vomiting
HAEM: Hypocalcaemia (high doses of I/V)
INTEG: Rashes, jaundice (reversible)
Contraindications: Hypersensitivity. Avoid IM or subcutaneous injections
Precautions: Hepatic impairment, pregnancy, lactation. Preterm infants, jaundice, acidotic infants
Pharmacokinetics: Mainly excreted in the bile. Suspension is fusidic acid and has only 70% bioavailability compared to the tablets which are the salt, sodium fusidate. Doses stated for suspension take this into account, and to avoid underdosing must be adhered to (e.g. 750 mg/15 ml fusidic acid is equivalent to 500 mg sodium fusidate)
Interactions/incompatibilities:
• Infusion should not be mixed with amino-acid solutions or blood
Clinical assessment:
• Perform liver function tests periodically when high oral doses used over a long period and in patients with liver dysfunction
• Urea and electrolytes, liver function tests
• For severe or deep seated infections additional concurrent anti-staphylococcal antibiotic therapy may be necessary
Treatment of overdose: Symptomatic and supportive therapy
NURSING CONSIDERATIONS
Assess:
• Baseline fluid balance
Administer:
• By infusion into a large vein
• Over prescribed period
• Shake suspension before use
• Reconstitute powder for IV use

with care and according to enclosed instructions
• Discard any unused IV solution once reconstituted
Evaluate:
• For local reaction at intravenous site
• For jaundice — if this persists (stop drug in consultation with medical staff)
• For other side effects
• For resistance (narrow spectrum antibiotic)
• Regular liver function tests
• Fluid balance
• Venospasm, thromboplebilis and haemolysis (excessive doses)

---

sodium nitrite

Sodium Nitrite Injection (Special orders)
Func. class.: Cyanide antidote
Legal class.: POM

Action: Sodium nitrite converts haemaglobin to methaemaglobin; which competes with cytochrome oxidase for cyanide with the formation of cyanomethaemaglobin; thiosulphate aids the conversion or inactivation of cyanide to thiocyanate
Uses: In conjunction with sodium thiosulphate for emergency treatment of cyanide poisoning
Dosage and routes:
• IV injection 10 ml over 3 min, followed by 25 ml sodium thiosulphate injection 50% by IV injection 10 min
Available forms include: Injection 3% (30 mg/ml) in water for injections
Side effects/adverse reactions:
CV: Vasodilation
CNS: Headache
INTEG: Flushing

Clinical assessment:
• This drug is toxic if cyanides are not present
• Cyanide toxicity: blood screen
• Use only in conjunction with sodium thiosulphate
NURSING CONSIDERATIONS
Assess:
• Pulse, BP, respiration, check for apnoea
• ECG, blood gases, blood count
• Flushed face, red lips, cherry red mucous membranes
Administer:
• By IV injection, slowly over at least 3 min
• With resuscitation equipment available for assisted ventilation
Evaluate:
• For signs of vasodilation including flushing and headache
• Therapeutic response: normal blood gases, decreased carboxy-haemoglobin levels

---

sodium nitroprusside

Nipride
Func. class.: Antihypertensive
Chem. class.: Peripheral vasodilator
Legal class.: POM (available to hospitals only)

Action: Directly relaxes arteriolar, venous smooth muscle; resulting in reduction in cardiac preload, after-load
Uses: Hypertensive crisis, controlled hypotension in surgery, acute or chronic heart failure
Dosage and routes:
• Dissolve 50 mg in 2 ml of Dextrose 5%, then dilute in 250–1000 ml of Dextrose 5%, sodium chloride 0.9%, compound sodium lactate IV infusion
Hypertensive crisis
• In patients not already receiving

antihypertensives. Adults, IV infusion only; 0.3–1 mcg/kg/min initially, then adjusted; usual range 0.5–6 mcg/kg/min (20–400 mcg/min)
• Maximum 8 mcg/kg/min
Lower doses will be required for those already being treated with antihypertensives

Controlled hypotension in surgery
• *Adults:* IV infusion; maximum dose should not exceed 1.5 mcg/kg/min

Cardiac failure
• *Adults:* By IV infusion, initially 10–15 mcg/min, increased every 5–10 min in 10–15 mcg/min increments as necessary. Usual range 10 to 200 mcg/min; maximum 280 mcg/min (4 mcg/kg/min)
Available forms include: Injection IV 50 mg

Side effects/adverse reactions:
GI: Nausea, vomiting, abdominal pain, retro-sternal discomfort
CNS: Dizziness, headache, agitation, twitching, restlessness, apprehension
EENT: Tinnitus, blurred vision
CVS: Palpitations
INTEG: Pain, irritation at injection site, sweating
METAB: Acidosis
Contraindications: Hypertension compensatory, Vitamin B_{12} deficiency, liver disease, Leber's optic atrophy
Precautions: Pregnancy, lactation, children, fluid, electrolyte imbalances, hepatic disease, severe renal impairment, impaired cerebral circulation, hypothyroidism, elderly

Pharmacokinetics:
IV: Onset 1–2 min, duration 1–10 min after IV dose, half-life 4 days in patients with normal renal function; metabolised in liver, excreted in urine

Interactions/incompatibilities:
• Severe hypotension: anaesthetic agents, nitrates, other antihypertensives
• Do not mix with any drug in syringe or solution
Clinical assessment:
• Electrolytes: potassium, sodium, chloride, CO_2, bicarbonate, lactate
• Assess renal and hepatic function
• BP by direct means if possible, check ECG continuously
• Thiocyanate levels daily if on long-term treatment
• Monitor plasma-cyanide concentration
• Administer depending on BP reading every 15 min
Treatment of overdose: Cyanide intoxication; immediately
1. Stop infusion
2. Administer cyanide antidote either IV administration of sodium thiosulphate or dicobalt edetate
3. Institute auxiliary treatment to support respiration

NURSING CONSIDERATIONS
Assess:
• Baseline vital signs, weight, renal function, electrolyte and bicarbonate levels
Administer:
• By infusion pump only
Perform/provide:
• Protect from direct sunlight with foil or brown paper, discard if gross colour changes in fluid
• Solution should not be used after a period of 24 hr from the time of preparation
Evaluate:
• Therapeutic response: decreased BP, absence of bleeding
• Nausea, vomiting, diarrhoea, abdominal pain
• Oedema in feet, legs daily
• Pain at infusion site
• Skin turgor, dryness of mucous membranes for hydration status
Teach patient/family:
• To report dizziness, headache, nausea or other side effects

sodium valproate

Epilim
Func. class.: Anticonvulsant
Chem. class.: Carboxylic acid
derivative
Legal class.: POM

Action: Increases levels of gamma-aminobutyric acid (GABA) in brain

Uses: All forms of epilepsy

Dosage and routes:
• *Adults:* By mouth initially 600 mg daily in divided doses preferably after food, increasing by 200 mg/day at 3 day dose intervals to a maximum of 2.5 g daily in divided doses according to the patient's needs; usual maintenance 1−2 g daily (20−30 mcg/kg daily)
• *Child over 20 kg:* initially 400 mg daily in divided doses increased gradually to 20−30 mg/kg daily in divided doses according to patient's needs. Maximum 35 mg/kg daily
• *Child under 20 kg:* initially 20 mg/kg daily in divided doses, increased gradually to 40 mg/kg daily providing plasma concentrations monitored

Available forms include: Enteric Coated (EC) tablets 200, 500 mg, crushable tablets 100 mg, syrup 200 mg/5 ml, liquid (sugar free) 200 mg/5 ml; Injection 400 mg/vial

Side effects/adverse reactions:
HAEM: Thrombocytopenia, leucopenia, increased prothrombin time, inhibition of platelet aggregation, red cell hypoplasia
CNS: Sedation, incoordination, hallucinations, behavioural changes, tremors, lethargy, confusion
GI: Nausea, vomiting, gastric irritation, anorexia, cramps, hepatic failure, pancreatitis. Increased appetite and weight gain
INTEG: Rash, alopecia, bruising
GU: Amenorrhoea
METAB: Hyperammonaemia
CVS: Oedema

Contraindications: Active liver disease, porphyria

Precautions: Renal disease, pregnancy, lactation, children and patients with a history of liver disease, major surgery, diabetics, avoid sudden withdrawal

Pharmacokinetics:
By mouth: Onset 15−30 min, peak 1−4 hr, duration 4−6 hr
By mouth: Onset slow, duration 4−6 hr
Metabolised by liver, excreted by kidneys, faeces, excreted in breast milk, half-life 8−20 hr

Interactions/incompatibilities:
• Increased effects: MAOIs and other antidepressants
• Increased toxicity: salicylates, warfarin
• Dosage adjustment may be required in combination with other anticonvulsants

Clinical assessment:
• Full blood count and coagulation studies prior to undergoing surgery
• Liver function tests for first six months on therapy for patients most at risk or with prior history of liver disease
• Blood levels: therapeutic level 40−100 mg/litre (depending on time or sampling and presence of co-medication)

Lab. tests interferences: False positives in urine testing for possible diabetics

Treatment of overdose: Induced vomiting, gastric lavage assisted ventilation and other supportive measures may be necessary in massive overdose

NURSING CONSIDERATIONS
Administer:
• Tablets whole
• Liquid alone; do not dilute with carbonated beverage
Evaluate:

• For signs of nausea, transient alopecia, false ketonuria, weight gain, purpuric rash/bruising
• Mental status: mood, alertness, affect, memory (long, short)
• Respiratory dysfunction: respiratory depression, character, rate, rhythm; hold drug if respirations are under 12/min or if pupils are dilated

Teach patient/family:
• That physical dependency may result when used for extended periods
• To avoid driving, other activities that require alertness
• Not to discontinue medication quickly after long-term use; convulsions may result
• To inform prescribing clinician if already taking anti-convulsants, especially phenobarbitone

---

sotalol HCl

Beta-Cardone, Sotacor, Sotazide, Tolerzide
Func. class.: Antihypertensive
Chem. class.: β-adrenergic blocker
Legal class.: POM

Action: Decreases preload, afterload, which is responsible for decreasing left ventricular end diastolic pressure, systemic vascular resistance. Cardiac work and oxygen consumption are diminished
Uses: Hypertension, angina, arrhythmias, prophylaxis after infarction, thyrotoxicosis
Dosage and routes: Generally advisable to start with a low dose, heart rate should not be reduced to less than 55 beats per minute
Hypertension/angina
• By mouth: Initially 160 mg/day in 1 or 2 doses; maintenance 160 mg/day increased to maximum of 600 mg/day if necessary

Arrhythmias
• By mouth 120−240 mg/day in single or divided doses
• Slow IV injection 20−60 mg over 2−3 mins with ECG monitoring, repeated if necessary with 10 min intervals between injections; maximum dose 100 mg over 3 min or longer
Prophylaxis after infarction
• By mouth 320 mg/day starting 5−14 days after infarction
Thyrotoxicosis
• By mouth 120−240 mg/day in single or divided doses
Available forms include: Tablets 40, 80, 160, 200 mg; injection 10 mg/ml, 4 ml ampoule
Side effects/adverse reactions:
CV: Heart failure, bradycardia, peripheral vasoconstriction, atypical ventricular arrhythmias (torsade de pointes)
RESP: Bronchospasm
GI: Gastric disturbances, diarrhoea
INTEG: Rash
EENT: Dry eyes
Contraindications: Heart failure, 2nd or 3rd degree heart block, asthma, cardiogenic shock, hypokalaemia, severe or persistent diarrhoea. Bronchospasm. Diabetic ketoacidosis or metabolic acidosis. Lactation
Precautions: Pregnancy (may cause fetal bradycardia), lactation, hepatic or renal impairment, avoid abrupt withdrawal in angina. In combined therapy clonidine should not be discontinued until several days after withdrawal of sotalol. Diabetes (may mask hypoglycaemic attack), anaesthesia, hypokalaemia, hypomagnesaemia
Pharmacokinetics: Completely absorbed from GI tract, peak plasma concentrations at 2−3 hr. Excreted unchanged in urine, not plasma protein bound. Plasma half-life 17 hr; low lipid solubility.

Interactions/incompatibilities:
• Increased effect: Adrenaline, amiodarone, amphetamines, anti-arrhythmics, diltiazem, ergotamine, nifedipine, prenylamine, sympathomimetic amines, verapamil, diuretics
Clinical assessment:
• Creatinine clearance if kidney damage is diagnosed
• If given with thiazide or loop diuretic avoid hypokalaemia (note combination products)
• Stop therapy if severe or persistent diarrhoea; risk of hypokalaemia/hypomagnesaemia
Lab. test interferences:
Decrease: Blood glucose
NURSING CONSIDERATIONS
Assess:
• Baseline BP, pulse, respirations
• Fluid balance (for IV administration)
Administer:
• With 8 oz glass of water on empty stomach
Perform/provide:
• Peak flow if patient is chesty, wheezy or short of breath
Evaluate:
• For headache, lightheadedness, decreased BP; may indicate need for decreased dosage
• Pain: duration, time started, activity being performed
• Weight gain; report if less than 2.5 kg
• Tolerance, if taken over a long period of time
Teach patient/family:
• That drug should be taken before stressful activity or exercise
• That if taken sublingually, mucous membranes may sting
• To avoid potentially hazardous activities if dizziness occurs
• Stress patient compliance with complete medical regime and to take medication as prescribed
• To make positional changes slowly to prevent fainting

• Decrease dosage over 2 weeks to prevent cardiac damage

---

spectinomycin hydrochloride

Trobicin
Func. class.: Antibiotic
Chem. class.: Aminoglycoside
Legal class.: POM

Action: Inhibits bacterial synthesis by binding to 30S subunit on ribosomes
Uses: Gonorrhoea
Dosage and routes:
• *Adult:* IM 2–4 g as single dose
• *Children over 2 yr:* 40 mg/kg, if no alternative treatment
Available forms include: Injection IM 2 g
Side effects/adverse reactions:
CNS: Dizziness, chills, fever, headache
HAEM: Anaemia
GI: Nausea, vomiting, increased blood urea nitrogen
GU: Decreased urine output
INTEG: Pain at injection site, urticaria, rash, pruritus, fever
SYST: Anaphylaxis
Contraindications: Hypersensitivity, syphilis
Precautions: Pregnancy
Pharmacokinetics:
IM: Peak 1–2 hr, duration up to 8 hr, half-life 1–3 hr, excreted in urine (active form)
Interactions/incompatibilities:
• Increases effect of lithium
Clinical assessment:
• Gonorrhoea culture after treatment
• Liver function tests; enzymes, aspartate aminotransferase, alanine aminotransferase, serum alkaline phosphatase following multiple doses
• Blood studies: haematocrit, Hb,

blood creatinine if multiple diag-
noses given
• Serologic test for syphilis 3
months after treatment
NURSING CONSIDERATIONS
Assess:
• Input and output of fluids, report
decreased output
• Allergies before treatment, re-
action of each medication
• Weight
• Gonorrhoea culture for sensi-
tivity taken before initial dose
Administer:
• No more than 2 grams per in-
jection site
• After shaking vial vigorously.
Add 3.2 ml water for injection to
vial. Final volume is 5 ml
• IM upper outer quadrant of
gluteal muscle
• With 20-gauge needle; no more
than 5 ml per site
Perform/provide:
• Storage at room temperature;
reconstituted solutions should be
discarded after 24 hr
Evaluate:
• Therapeutic response, decreased
dysuria, discharge
• Negative culture and sensitivity
• Side effects; dizziness, chills,
fever, nausea, urticaria and mild
discomfort at injection site
Teach patient/family:
• To avoid sexual contact with
other people until negative culture
is confirmed
• To treat sexual contacts simul-
taneously
• To practise safe sex
• That follow-up appointments are
necessary to ensure syphilis has
not been contacted and masked

spironolactone

Aldactone, Spirolone, Spiroctan,
Lasilactone, Aldactide
Func. class.: Potassium-sparing
diuretic
Chem. class.: Aldosterone antag-
onist
Legal class.: POM

Action: Competes with aldosterone
at receptor sites in renal tubule,
resulting in excretion of sodium
chloride, water, retention of potassium, phosphate
Uses: Congestive cardiac failure,
hepatic cirrhosis with ascites and
oedema. Nephrotic syndrome, malignant ascites, primary aldosteronism (diagnosis and treatment)
Dosage and routes:
Congestive heart failure
• *Adults:* By mouth 100 mg daily
increasing gradually if necessary
up to 400 mg daily. Maintain 75–
200 mg daily
Hepatic cirrhosis
• When with ascites and oedema,
urinary sodium/potassium ratio is
greater than 1, 100 mg daily; when
ratio is less than 1 then 200–
400 mg daily
Malignant ascites
• Initially 100–200 mg daily in
severe cases up to 400 mg daily
Nephrotic syndrome
• 100–200 mg daily
Primary aldosteronism
• Long test: 400 mg daily for 3–4
weeks
• Short test: 400 mg daily for
4 days
• Pre-surgery: 100–400 mg daily
prior to surgery
Available forms include: Tablets 25,
50, 100 mg; capsules 100 mg
Side effects/adverse reactions:
CNS: Headache, confusion,
drowsiness, lethargy, ataxia

GI: Diarrhoea, cramps, hepatic cirrhosis
INTEG: Rash, pruritus, urticaria, fever
ENDO: Impotence, gynaecomastia, menstrual irregularities, breast soreness, mild androgenic effects e.g. hirsutism, deepening voice
ELECT: Hyperchloraemic metabolic acidosis, hyperkalaemia, increased blood urea
Contraindications: Hypersensitivity, anuria, severe renal disease, rapidly deteriorating renal function, hyperkalaemia, acute renal insufficiency, Addison's disease, porphyria
Precautions: Dehydration, hepatic disease, pregnancy, lactation, hyponatraemia, elderly

Pharmacokinetics:
By mouth: Onset 24−48 hr, peak 48−72 hr; metabolised in liver, excreted in urine

Interactions/incompatibilities:
• Diuretic effect antagonised by aspirin and indomethacin
• Increased action of: antihypertensives, digoxin
• Increased hyperkalaemia: potassium sparing diuretics, potassium products or angiotensin converting enzyme inhibitors

Lab. test interferences:
Interfere: certain serum digoxin assays

Treatment of overdose: Monitor electrolytes, administer IV fluids and electrolytes as necessary

NURSING CONSIDERATIONS
Assess:
• Baseline weight, fluid balance
Administer:
• In morning to avoid interference with sleep
• With food, if nausea occurs; absorption may be decreased slightly
Perform/provide:

• Fluid balance daily to determine fluid loss
Evaluate:
• Therapeutic effect
• Improvement in oedema of feet, legs, sacral area daily if medication is being used in congestive cardiac failure
• Improvement in CVP readings
• Signs of metabolic acidosis: drowsiness, restlessness
• Rashes, temperature elevation daily
• Confusion, especially in elderly, take safety precautions if needed
• Hydration: skin turgor, thirst, dry mucous membranes
Teach patient/family:
• That drowsiness, ataxia, mental confusion may occur; observe caution in driving (elderly patients should probably not drive at all)
• To notify clinician of cramps, diarrhoea, lethargy, thirst, headache, skin rash, menstrual abnormalities, deepening voice, breast enlargement

---

stanozolol

Stromba
Func. class.: Androgenic anabolic steroid
Chem. class.: Halogenated testosterone derivative
Legal class.: POM

Action: Anabolic agent with fibrinolytic properties. Alter the functional level of plasma C1 esterase inhibitor; enzyme which is depressed in hereditary angiooedema. Protein building properties.
Uses: Prevention of hereditary angioedema, vascular manifestations of Behcet's disease
Dosage and routes:
Hereditary angiooedema
• *Adult:* By mouth 2.5−10 mg

daily to control attacks, reduced for maintenance (2.5 mg 3 times weekly may be sufficient)
• *Child 1−6 yr:* Initially 2−5 mg daily. 6−12 yr, initially 2.5−5 mg daily

Behcet's disease
• *Adult:* By mouth 10 mg daily
Available forms include: Tablets 5 mg

Side effects/adverse reactions:
INTEG: Rash, acneiform lesions, oily hair and skin, flushing, sweating, acne vulgaris, alopecia, hirsutism
CNS: Dizziness, headache, fatigue, tremors, paraesthesias, flushing, sweating, anxiety, lability, insomnia
MS: Cramps, spasms
CV: Increased BP
GU: Haematuria, amenorrhoea, vaginitis, decreased libido, decreased breast size, clitoral hypertrophy, testicular atrophy. In children prolonged use may lead to premature closure of the epiphyses
GI: Nausea, vomiting, constipation, weight gain, cholestatic jaundice, dyspepsia, peliosis hepatis, hepatic tumours
EENT: Voice change
Contraindications: Severe renal disease, severe cardiac disease, hepatic disease, hypersensitivity, pregnancy, lactation, prostate cancer, porphyria, premenopausal women except in lifethreatening situations
Precautions: Insulin dependent diabetes mellitus, cardiovascular disease
Pharmacokinetics: Metabolised in liver, excreted in faeces and urine. Highly protein bound
Interactions/incompatibilities:
• Increased effects of: oral anticoagulants and oral hypoglycaemic age
Clinical assessment:

• Electrolytes: potassium, sodium, chloride, calcium; cholesterol
• Liver function tests: enzymes, aspartate aminotransferase, alanine aminotransferase, bilirubin
• Thyroid function tests: Measure T_3 and T_4
Lab. test interferences:
Increase: Serum cholesterol, blood glucose, urine glucose
Decrease: Serum calcium, serum potassium, thyroxine, triiodothyranine, thyroid ^{131}I uptake test
Treatment of overdose: Observe and monitor liver function tests

NURSING CONSIDERATIONS
Assess:
• Weigh before initial treatment
• Input and output of fluids
Administer:
• Initial dose then reduce according to patient response. Lowest effective maintenance dose
• To children in short course with intervals between if possible
Perform/provide:
• Diet based on specific need of patient
• NB. This is a drug of abuse, particularly for athletes
Evaluate:
• Regular urinalysis
• Children in prolonged use for growth rate and premature closure of the epiphysis
• Weight gain greater than 2.5 kg a week
• Signs of masculinisation in female: increased libido, deepening of voice, breast tissue, enlarged clitoris, menstrual irregularities; male: gynaecomastia, impotence, testicular atrophy
• Therapeutic response, occurs in 4−6 weeks in osteoporosis, increased mobility. Control of angiooedema
• Effect of any other drug therapy e.g. anticoagulants increased
• Any adverse effects: report so increase, decrease or even discon-

tinuing of the drug may occur especially if voice changes

Teach patient/family:
• Drug needs to be combined with complete health plan: diet, rest, exercise
• To notify clinician if therapeutic response decreases
• Not to discontinue this medication abruptly
• To notify clinician if any voice changes occur
• To understand body changes may occur including breast in men
• To test urine
• To weigh weekly and report changes greater than 2.5 kg a week
• About potential abuse

---

stilboestrol

Apstil
Func. class.: Oestrogen
Chem. class.: Non-steroidal synthetic oestrogen
Legal class.: POM

Action: Suppresses androgenic hormonal activity in the management of androgen-dependent carcinomas. Carcinogenic potential
Uses: Carcinoma of prostate, metastatic post-menopausal carcinoma of breast

Dosage and routes:
Prostatic cancer
• *Adult:* By mouth 1−3 mg daily
Breast cancer
• *Adult:* By mouth 10−20 mg daily
Available forms include: Tablets 1, 5 mg

Side effects/adverse reactions:
CNS: Dizziness, headache, migraines, depression, elation
CV: Hypotension, venous thrombosis, oedema, thromboembolism, stroke, pulmonary embolism, myocardial infarction
GI: Nausea, vomiting, diarrhoea, anorexia, pancreatitis, cramps, constipation, increased appetite, increased weight, cholestatic jaundice
EENT: Contact lens intolerance, increased myopia, astigmatism
GU: Amenorrhoea, cervical erosion, breakthrough bleeding, dysmenorrhoea, vaginal candidiasis, breast changes, gynaecomastia, testicular atrophy, impotence, increased risk of endometrial carcinoma
INTEG: Rash, urticaria, acne, hirsutism, alopecia, oily skin, seborrhoea, purpura, melasma
META: Folic acid deficiency, hypercalcaemia, hyperglycaemia
Contraindications: Premenopausal breast cancer, thromboembolic disorders, oestrogen-dependent neoplasms, genital bleeding (abnormal, undiagnosed), pregnancy, children, porphyria, hepatic disease, herpes gestationis, severe hypertension, thromboembolic disease, fibroids (uterine), hyperlipoproteinaemia
Precautions: Hypertension, asthma, blood dyscrasias, gallbladder disease, congestive cardiac failure, diabetes mellitus, migraine, epilepsy, depression, cardiac failure, contact lenses, cholestatic jaundice, renal dysfunction
Interactions/incompatibilities:
• Decreased action of: anticoagulants, oral hypoglycaemics, insulin
Clinical assessment:
• Liver function studies, including aspartate aminotransferase, alanine aminotransferase, bilirubin, alkaline phosphatase
• Monitor BP regularly, look for signs of thrombosis
Lab. test interferences:
Increase: Protein bound iodine retention test, T_4, thyroxine-binding globulin (TBG), prothrombin, factors VII, VIII, IX, X, triglycerides
Decrease: Glucose tolerance test
Treatment of overdose: Gastric

lavage. Monitor plasma electrolytes, symptomatic support. Oestrogen-withdrawal bleeding may occur in female child

NURSING CONSIDERATIONS

Assess:

• Input and output of fluids, check for oedema and fluid retention

• Weigh before initial treatment and at weekly intervals

• Regular urinalysis

Administer:

• Titrated dose, use lowest effective dose

• Suitable analgesics and diuretics

• Orally with food or milk to decrease GI symptoms

Perform/provide:

• Store below 25°C in dry, light proof container

• Diet suitable to enhance each patients good health and aid any medical problems

Evaluate:

• Therapeutic response: decrease in tumour size in prostatic and breast cancer

• Oedema, hypertension, cardiac symptoms, jaundice, venous thrombosis

• Mental status: affect, mood, behavioural changes, aggression

• Signs of feminizing in men; impotence, testicular atrophy, enlarged breasts

• Females; withdrawal bleeding

• Effect of any other drug therapy e.g. decreased action of anticoagulants

Teach patient/family:

• To weigh weekly, report gain over 2 kg or weight losses more than 2 kg

• To report breast lumps, vaginal bleeding, oedema, jaundice, dark urine, clay coloured stools, dyspnoea, headache, blurred vision, abdominal pain, numbness or stiffness in legs, chest pain

• To avoid sunlight or wear sunscreen; photosensitivity can occur

• To understand body changes may occur

• To test urine for glucose

• Drug needs to be combined with complete health plan: diet, rest, exercise

---

streptokinase

Kabikinase, Streptase
Func. class.: Thrombolytic enzyme
Chem. class.: β-Haemolytic streptococcus filtrate (purified)
Legal class.: POM

Action: Activates conversion of plasminogen to plasmin (fibrinolysin): plasmin is able to dissolve clots (fibrin), fibrinogen, plasma proteins; induces dissolution of intravascular thrombi and emboli

Uses: Deep vein thrombosis, pulmonary embolism, arterial thromboembolism, arteriovenous cannula occlusion, lysis of coronary artery thrombi after myocardial infarction

Dosage and routes:

• *Adult:* IV infusion 250,000 units over 30 mins, then 100,000 units/hr or $24-72$ hr depending on condition (seek specialist advice)

• Myocardial infarction, 1,500,000 units over 60 min followed by aspirin 150 mg by mouth for at least 4 weeks (seek specialist advice)

• Local application in blocked haemodialysis shunts, $10,000-25,000$ units deposited in clotted section, seal on venous side. Repeat after $30-45$ min if necessary

• *Child:* Reduce standard dose according to circulating volume (seek specialist advice)

Available forms include: Injection IV 100,000, 250,000, 600,000, 750,000, 1.5 million unit vials

Side effects/adverse reactions:

HAEM: Decreased haematocrit, bleeding

INTEG: Rash, urticaria, phlebitis at IV infusion site, itching, flushing, headache

CNS: Headache, fever, intracerebral haemorrhage

GI: Nausea, vomiting

RESP: Altered respirations, shortness of breath, bronchospasm

MS: Low back pain

CV: Hypertension, arrhythmias, hypotension

EENT: Periorbital oedema

Contraindications: Surgery or invasive procedure during proceeding 10 days, GI bleeding in previous 6 months. Thrombocytopenia, hepatic or renal disease, CVA, hypotension. Parturition (last 10 days). Ulcerative colitis, visceral carcinoma, menstrual bleeding, first 18 weeks of pregnancy (specialist advice). Subacute bacterial endocarditis, GU diseases associated with bleeding. Pulmonary disease with cavitation, acute pancreatitis, severe diabetes mellitus, severe hypertension (200 systolic or 100 diastolic)

Precautions: Arterial emboli from left side of heart, subsequent regimens may require test dose, elderly, pregnancy, mitral valve defects, atrial fibrillation, repeated therapy 5 days–12 months previously, recent streptococcal infections

Pharmacokinetics:

IV: Excreted in bile, urine, half-life under 20 min

Interactions/incompatibilities:

• Bleeding potential: Aspirin, indomethacin, phenylbutazone, anticoagulants, thyroid hormones, volatile oils, quinidine, allopurinol, sulphonamide, tetracyclines, valproic acid, dextrans

Clinical assessment:

• Blood studies (haematocrit, platelets, partial thromboplastin time, prothrombin time, thrombin time, activated partial thromboplastin time) before starting therapy; prothrombin time or activated partial thromboplastin time must be less than twice control before starting therapy. Measure thrombin time or prothrombin time every 3–4 hr during treatment

• Not effective if: deep vein thrombosis more than 14 days olds, occlusion of central retinal arteries more than 6–8 hr old, and thrombosis of central retinal vein more than 10 days old

• Anticoagulation with heparin or aspirin may be recommended after stop taking

• Streptokinase should not be given to same patient 5 days to 12 months since last dose

• Risk of allergic reaction, measure streptokinase serum antibody level

• Urokinase may be an alternative

Lab. test interferences:

Increase: Prothrombin time, activated partial thromboplastin time, thrombin time

Treatment of overdose: Haemorrhage controlled at site of injection as required. Serious life threatening haemorrhage controlled with aprotinin or IV tranexamic acid therapy (10 mg/kg slow IV injection)

NURSING CONSIDERATIONS

Assess:

• Vital baseline signs

Administer:

• By infusion over 1 hr in 100 mls Normal Saline, whilst observing for reperfusion arrhythmias [fairly common] for myocardial infarction

• By prescribed infusion intra-arterially, in specialist area, for arterial thrombosis

Perform/provide:

• Continuous electrocardiogram monitoring before, during and after infusion — particularly if post-myocardial infarction

• Resuscitation equipment as

cardiac arrest/arrhythmias may occur
• Continuous observation of all puncture sites, IV sites for bleeding and general signs of bruising
• Daily urinanalysis
• Bed-rest during and after (under medical supervision) treatment
• Prescribed pain relief

Evaluate:
• BP, pulse; respirations, neurological signs, 4 hrly temperature
• 12 lead ECG and signs for cardiac history if post-myocardial infarction
• Therapeutic response. Avoidance of invasive procedures
• Pressure to bleeding sites — report immediately
• Allergy: fever, rash, loin pain, hypotension; stop infusion, seek medical advice, may need anaphylaxis treatment before recommencement

Teach patient/family:
• Issue advice card: teach about further effects and health education issues relating to diagnosis

---

streptomycin sulphate

Func. class.: Antibiotic
Chem. class.: Aminoglycoside
Legal class.: POM

Action: Interferes with protein synthesis in bacterial cell by binding to ribosomal subunit, causing inaccurate peptide sequence to form in protein chain, causing bacterial death

Uses: Sensitive strains of *M. tuberculosis*; non-tuberculous infections such as septicaemia, bacterial endocarditis, chronic respiratory infections and pneumonia caused by sensitive strains of *K. pneumoniae*, and urinary tract infections due to *E. coli*

Dosage and routes:
Tuberculosis
• *Adult:* IM 1 g daily for 2−3 months, then 1 g 2−3 times a week given with other antitubercular drugs. Under 50 kg, over 40 yr age 500−750 mg IM daily, then 750 mg 3 times a week
• *Child:* IM 30 mg/kg daily up to 1 g given with other antitubercular drugs, then 30 mg/kg 3 times a week

Tuberculous meningitis
• IM 30−40 mg/kg (maximum 1 g) daily; intrathecal 50 mg daily (adult) or 1 mg/kg daily (children)

Non-tuberculous infections
• *Adult:* IM 1 g daily for 3−7 days
• *Child:* IM 22−40 mg/kg daily (may use divided doses)

Available forms include: Injection vial 1 g

Side effects/adverse reactions:
GU: Oliguria, haematuria, renal damage, renal failure, nephrotoxicity
CNS: Confusion, depression, numbness, tremors, convulsions, neurotoxicity
EENT: Ototoxicity, deafness, visual disturbances, paraesthesia of mouth
GI: Nausea, vomiting, anorexia, increased alanine aminotransferase, aspartate aminotransferase, bilirubin, hepatomegaly, hepatic necrosis, splenomegaly
CV: Hypotension, myocarditis
INTEG: Rash, burning, urticaria, photosensitivity, dermatitis

Contraindications: Severe renal disease, hypersensitivity, suppurative otitis media, labyrinthine disturbances, pregnancy, myasthenia gravis

Precautions: Neonates, renal disease, lactation, hearing deficits, elderly

Pharmacokinetics:
IM: Onset rapid, peak 1−2 hr; plasma half-life 1−3 hr, not

metabolised, excreted unchanged in urine

Interactions/incompatibilities:
• Increased ototoxicity, neurotoxicity, nephrotoxicity: other aminoglycosides, amphotericin B, polymyxin, vancomycin, ethacrynic acid, frusemide, mannitol, methoxyflurane, cisplatin, cephalosporins
• Decreased effects of: parenteral penicillins
• Increased effects: non-depolarising muscle relaxants

Clinical assessment:
• Serum peak, drawn at 60 min after IM injection, trough level drawn just before next dose
• For elderly, 24 hr serum level should not exceed 1 mcg/ml
• For renal impairment, initial dose 250−500 mg IM injection. No further dose given until serum level less than 20 mcg/ml. If 24 hr serum level greater than 3 mcg/ml reduce dose

Treatment of overdose: Haemodialysis, monitor serum levels of drug

NURSING CONSIDERATIONS
Assess:
• Fluid balance
• Weight before treatment; calculation of dosage is usually done based on ideal body weight, but may be calculated on actual body weight
• Hearing levels

Administer:
• After specimens have been taken for culture and sensitivity
• By deep IM injection in large muscle mass, rotate injection sites
• Drug in evenly spaced doses to maintain blood level
• Concentration of drug in injection must not exceed 5 mg/ml
• Intrathecally through spinal tap. After withdrawal of equal volume of cerebrospinal fluid, inject very slowly (at least 10 min) and observe vital signs. Watch for blood pressure and pulse changes
• Using gloves to avoid skin sensitisation to the powder when reconstituting

Perform/provide:
• Adequate fluids of 2−3 litres daily unless contraindicated to prevent irritation of tubules
• Supervise mobility, observe balance
• Dehydration: high specific gravity, decrease in skin turgor, dry mucous membranes, dark urine
• Overgrowth of infection: increased temperature, malaise, redness, pain, swelling, perineal itching, diarrhoea, stomatitis, change in cough, sputum
• Vestibular dysfunction: nausea, vomiting, dizziness, headache; drug should be discontinued if severe

Evaluate:
• Therapeutic effect, absence of fever, draining wounds, clear sputum, painless micturition, negative culture and sensitivity after treatment
• Close attention to input and output of fluids
• Urinalysis daily for proteinuria, cells, casts; report sudden change in urine output
• Urine pH if drug is used for urinary tract infection; urine should be kept alkaline
• Renal impairment by securing urine for creatinine clearance testing, blood urea, serum creatinine; in renal impairment (creatinine clearance less than 80 ml/min) lower dosage should be given
• Deafness by audiometric testing, ringing, roaring in ears, vertigo. Assess hearing before, during, after treatment

Teach patient/family:
• To report headache, dizziness, symptoms of overgrowth of infection, renal impairment

• To report loss of hearing, ringing, roaring in ears, fullness in head
• To drink plenty of fluids for urinary infection. Water, milk, tea etc

---

sucralfate

Antepsin
Func. class.: Gastric protectant
Chem. class.: Aluminium hydroxide/sulphated sucrose
Legal class.: POM

Action: Forms a complex that adheres to ulcer site, inhibits pepsin, gastric juice, absorbs bile salts
Uses: Duodenal ulcer, gastric ulcer, chronic gastritis
Dosage and routes:
• *Adult:* By mouth 1 g 4 times a day 1 hr before meals at bedtime or 2 g twice daily taken on rising and at bedtime (maximum 8 g daily) for 4−6 weeks
Prophylaxis of GI haemorrhage from stress ulceration:
• By mouth 1 g 6 times a day (maximum 8 g daily)
Available forms include: Tablets 1 g; suspension 1 g/5 ml
Side effects/adverse reactions:
CNS: Drowsiness, dizziness, sleeplessness, vertigo
GI: Dry mouth, constipation, nausea, vomiting, diarrhoea, indigestion
INTEG: Urticaria, rash, pruritus
Contraindications: Hypersensitivity, severe renal impairment
Precautions: Pregnancy, renal dysfunction, lactation, children
Pharmacokinetics:
By mouth: Minimal amounts absorbed from GI tract
Interactions/incompatibilities:
• Decreased effect: antacids

• Decreased action of: tetracyclines, cimetidine, phenytoin, digoxin
Clinical assessment:
• Severe renal impairment, measure serum aluminium
• Monitor blood urea, creatinine
NURSING CONSIDERATIONS
Assess:
• Pain levels
• Fluid balance
Administer:
• Antacid should not be taken half an hour before or after a dose
• Allow 2 hr separation between sucralfate and other drugs
• Tablets may be dispensed in 10−15 ml of water
Evaluate:
• Therapeutic response: absence of pain, nausea and vomiting
• Ability to tolerate normal diet
Teach patient/family:
• To reassess diet and avoid some foods and alcohol
• To take 1 hr before meals
• To complete full course
• To take other medications only if directed by clinician

---

sulconazole nitrate

Exelderm
Func. class.: Topical antifungal
Chem. class.: Imidazole antimycotic
Legal class.: POM

Action: Alters the permeability of cell membranes of sensitive fungi
Uses: Fungal skin infections, tinea pedis, corporis, and cruris, pityriasis versicolor and candidiasis
Dosage and routes: Topical, apply 1−2 times daily continuing for 2−3 weeks after lesions have healed
Available forms include: Cream, 1%
Side effects/adverse reactions:

INTEG: Occasional skin irritation or sensitivity

Contraindications: Hypersensitivity

Precautions: Pregnancy

NURSING CONSIDERATIONS

Administer:

• After skin scrapings taken to confirm diagnosis

• Cleanse skin before application

• Massage gently into affected and surrounding skin areas

• Avoid contact with eyes

Evaluate:

• Sensitivity to drug — rashes, itching, discontinue drug

Teach patient/family:

• Correct method of application

• To avoid contact with eyes

• To inform clinician and stop using drug if sensitivity occurs

• To continue treatment for 2–3 weeks after improvement to prevent relapse

---

sulfametopyrazine

Kelfizine W

Func. class.: Antibiotic

Chem. class.: Sulphonamide

Legal class.: POM

Action: Long acting sulphonamide. Interferes with the synthesis of nucleic acids in sensitive organisms

Uses: Urinary tract infections, chronic bronchitis (including prophylaxis)

Dosage and routes:

• *Adult:* By mouth: 2 g as a single dose once per week

Available forms include: Tablets 2 g

Side effects/adverse reactions:

GI: Nausea, vomiting

HAEM: Eosinophilia, agranulocytosis, granulocytopenia, leucopenia, megaloblastic anaemia

INTEG: Erythema multiforme, rashes, epidermal necrolysis, purpura

Contraindications: Renal or hepatic failure, jaundice, blood disorders, children, pregnancy, hypersensitivity

Precautions: Hepatic or renal impairment, photosensitivity, elderly, lactation

Pharmacokinetics: Readily absorbed from GI tract; 60% bound to plasma protein. High degree of renal tubular resorption and low hepatic metabolism gives half-life of 65 hr

Interactions/incompatibilities:

• Potentiation: pyrimethamine, coumarin derivatives, sulphonylureas, trimethoprim

• Antagonism: PABA

Clinical assessment:

• Avoid prescribing to those sensitive to other sulphonamides

• Regular blood picture for disorders

Treatment of overdose:

• Increase fluid intake for seven days to increase excretion of drug

• Give potassium citrate mixture or sodium bicarbonate to render urine alkaline and increase excretion of drug

NURSING CONSIDERATIONS

Assess:

• Fluid balance

Perform/provide:

• Regular mouthcare/mouthwashes if vomiting occurs

• Regular urinalysis if long-term therapy

Administer:

• After sample taken for culture and sensitivity

• Stir tablet into a half tumblerfull of water or orange squash

• At least 2 litres daily fluid intake to avoid crystallisation in kidneys

• Anti-emetic for severe nausea and vomiting

Perform:

• Full blood count, urea and electrolytes, renal function

Evaluate:

- Urine — colour, fluid balance if drug given for urinary tract infection
- Signs of allergic reactions — rashes, erythema multiforme, dyspnoea
- Therapeutic response — absence of pain, fever, negative culture and sensitivity
- Blood dyscrasias — skin rash, fever, sore throat, bruising, bleeding, fatigue, joint pain

Teach patient/family:
- To dilute tablet in half tumblerful of fluid
- To take tablets only once per week
- To complete course of tablets even when symptoms improve or cease
- To avoid direct sunlight to skin — burning may occur
- To check with clinician before taking non-prescribed medication
- To notify clinician at once of rash, fever, sore throat, bruising, bleeding, joint pain

---

sulindac

Clinoril
Func. class.: Non-steroidal anti-inflammatory drug
Chem. class.: Indeneacetic acid derivative
Legal class.: POM

Action: Inhibits prostaglandin synthesis by inhibiting an enzyme needed for biosynthesis; possesses analgesic, anti-inflammatory, anti-pyretic properties
Uses: Osteoarthritis, rheumatoid arthritis, ankylosing spondylitis, bursitis, tendinitis, tenosynovitis, acute gout
Dosage and routes:
- *Adult:* By mouth 200 mg twice a day, dose reduction may be possible in some patients; acute

gout should respond within 7 days; limit treatment in peri-articular disorders to 7−10 days
Available forms include: Tablets 100, 200 mg
Side effects/adverse reactions:
GI: Nausea, anorexia, vomiting, dyspepsia, convulsions, diarrhoea, jaundice, cholestatic hepatitis, constipation, flatulence, cramps, dry mouth, peptic ulcer, gastro-intestinal bleeding/perforation
CNS: Dizziness, drowsiness, fatigue, tremors, confusion, psychosis, insomnia, anxiety, depression, headache, vertigo, paraesthesia
CV: Peripheral oedema, palpitations, dysrhythmias, hypertension, congestive heart failure
INTEG: Purpura, rash, pruritus, sweating, alopecia, photosensitivity, toxic epidermal necrolysis
GU: Nephrotoxicity: dysuria, haematuria, oliguria, azotaemia, crystalluria, vaginal bleeding
HAEM: Blood dyscrasias
RESP: Bronchospasm, dyspnoea
EENT: Tinnitus, hearing loss, blurred vision, metallic taste, epistaxis
MISC: Allergic reactions including anaphylaxis
Contraindications: Hypersensitivity, severe renal disease, severe hepatic disease, active GI bleeding peptic ulcer, children, pregnancy, lactation
Precautions: Elderly, cardiac disorders, hypersensitivity to other non-steroidal anti-inflammatory drugs, renal impairment, liver dysfunction, history of GI bleeding/peptic ulcer/kidney stones
Pharmacokinetics:
By mouth: Peak 2 hr, half-life 7−8 hr; activated by metabolism in liver (active sulphide metabolite half-life 16−17 hr, excreted in urine (metabolites), excreted in breast milk

Interactions/incompatibilities:
• May increase action of: oral anticoagulants, oral hypoglycaemics, lithium
• Decreased effect of sulindac, risk of peripheral neuropathy: dimethyl sulphoxide
• Increased risk of nephrotoxicity: cyclosporin, methotrexate, diuretics
• Decreased effect of sulindac: aspirin, diflunisal

Clinical assessment:
• Renal, liver function tests, before treatment, periodically thereafter if abnormality suspected
• Stop treatment permanently if patient develops unexplained fever, rash, liver changes, constitutional symptoms

Treatment of overdose: Empty stomach, activated charcoal, symptomatic treatment, no specific antidote

NURSING CONSIDERATIONS
Administer:
• With food to decrease GI symptoms
• With plenty of fluid if patient has history of renal stones

Evaluate:
• Therapeutic response: decreased pain, stiffness, swelling in joints, ability to move more easily
• For eye, ear problems: blurred vision, tinnitus (may indicate toxicity)
• Report any persistant indigestion and black tarry stools

Teach patient/family:
• To report blurred vision or ringing, roaring in ears (may indicate toxicity)
• To avoid driving or other hazardous activities if dizziness or drowsiness occurs
• To take with food or milk
• To report change in urine pattern, weight increase, oedema, pain increase in joints, fever, blood in urine (indicates nephrotoxicity)

• That therapeutic effects may take up to 1 month
• Report any persistant indigestion or black tarry stools

---

sulphacetamide sodium (ophthalmic)

Albucid, Minims, Sulphacetamide Sodium
Func. class.: Antibiotic
Chem. class.: Sulphonamide
Legal class.: POM

Action: Inhibits bacterial growth by preventing PABA conversion to folic acid
Uses: Conjunctivitis, superficial eye infections
Dosage and routes:
• *Adult and child:* Instil 2–4 drops 2–6 hrly
Available forms include: Sterile ophthalmic solution 10%
Side effects/adverse reactions:
EENT: Burning, stinging, swelling
Contraindications: Hypersensitivity to sulphonamides
NURSING CONSIDERATIONS
Administer:
• After washing hands, cleanse crusts or discharge from eye before application
Perform/provide:
• Storage at room temperature
Evaluate:
• Therapeutic response: absence of redness, inflammation, tearing
• Allergy: itching, lacrimation, redness, swelling
Teach patient/family:
• To use drug exactly as prescribed
• Not to rub eye
• Not to use eye makeup, towels, washcloths, eye medication of others; reinfection may occur
• That drug container tip should not be touched to eye
• To report itching, increased red-

ness, burning, stinging; drug should be discontinued
• That blurred vision may occur when ointment is applied

---

sulphadiazine

Func. class.: Antibiotic
Chem. class.: Sulphonamide
Legal class.: POM

Action: Interferes with bacterial biosynthesis of proteins by competitive antagonism of para-aminobenzoic acid (PABA). Bacteriostatic antibiotic

Uses: Meningococcal meningitis and other gram-negative and -positive infections sensitive to sulphonamides

Dosage and routes:
• *Adult:* IM/IV 2 g initially, then 1 g 6-hrly for 2 days, then by mouth 1 g 6-hrly for 5 days
• *Child over 2 months:* IM/IV 50 mg/kg once then 25 mg/kg 6-hrly for 2 days then by mouth 25 mg/kg 6-hrly for 5 days

Available forms include: Tablets 500 mg, IM/IV injection 250 mg/ml (as sodium salt)

Side effects/adverse reactions:
SYST: Anaphylaxis, cyanosis
GI: Nausea, vomiting, abdominal pain, hepatitis, glossitis, diarrhoea, jaundice, anorexia
CNS: Headache, confusion, insomnia, hallucinations, depression, vertigo, fatigue, anxiety, drug fever, chills
HAEM: Leucopenia, thrombocytopenia, agranulocytosis, haemolytic anaemia, eosinophilia
INTEG: Rash, urticaria, Stevens-Johnson syndrome, erythema, photosensitivity, pain and inflammation at injection site
GU: Renal failure, toxic nephrosis, crystalluria, haematuria

CV: Vasculitis

Contraindications: Hypersensitivity to sulphonamides, pregnancy at term, premature/newborn babies under 6 weeks, severe renal or hepatic disease, porphyria

Precautions: Pregnancy, lactation, impaired hepatic or renal function, severe allergy, elderly

Pharmacokinetics:
By mouth: Rapidly absorbed, peak 3–6 hr; 30%–50% bound to plasma proteins, half-life 8–16 hr, excreted in urine, breast milk

Interactions/incompatibilities:
• Increased hypoglycemic response: sulphonylurea agents
• Increased anticoagulant effects: oral anticoagulants
• Decreased renal excretion of: methotrexate
• Increased renal toxicity of: cyclosporin
• Reduced effect of sulphadiazine: PABA, procaine and related local anaesthetics

Clinical assessment:
• Kidney function studies; blood urea, creatinine, urinalysis before and during treatment
• Monitor cotreatment with oral anticoagulants, sulphonylureas
• Discontinue if crystalluria followed by haematuria/oliguria occurs; increase fluid input, alkalinise urine with sodium bicarbonate

Treatment of overdose: Forced alkaline diuresis, symptomatic treatment

NURSING CONSIDERATIONS

Administer:
• After samples have been sent for culture and sensitivity (repeat after full course complete)
• With full glass of water to maintain adequate hydration; increase fluids to 2 litres daily to decrease crystallisation in kidneys
• Do not administer subcutaneously or intrathecally

Perform/provide:
• Resuscitation equipment; severe allergic reactions may occur

Evaluate:
• Therapeutic response: absence of pain, fever, culture and sensitivity negative
• Blood dyscrasias: skin rash, fever, sore throat, bruising, bleeding, fatigue, joint pain
• Allergic reaction: rash, dermatitis, urticaria, pruritus, dyspnoea, bronchospasm

Teach patient/family:
• To take each oral dose with full glass of water to prevent crystalluria
• To complete full course of treatment to prevent superimposed infection
• To avoid sunlight or use sunscreen to prevent burns
• To avoid non-prescribed medicines (aspirin, vitamin C) unless directed by the clinician
• To use alternative contraceptive measures; decreased effectiveness of oral contraceptives may result
• To notify clinician if skin rash, sore throat, fever, mouth scores, unusual bruising, bleeding occur

---

sulphadimidine sodium

Sulphadimidine
Func. class.: Antibiotic
Chem. class.: Sulphonamide
Legal class.: POM

Action: Short acting, interferes with the synthesis of nucleic acids in sensitive microorganisms

Uses: Urinary tract infections, prophylaxis of meningococcal meningitis

Dosage and routes:
Urinary tract infections
• *Adult and child over 8 yr:* By mouth, initially 2 g then 0.5–1 g every 6–8 hr

Meningococcal prophylaxis (sensitive strains only)
• *Adult:* By mouth 1 g every 12 hr for 2 days
• *Child:* 3–12 months: By mouth 250 mg every 12 hr for 2 days over 1 yr: By mouth 500 mg every 12 hr for 2 days
Over 1 yr: By mouth 500 mg every 12 hr for 2 days

Available forms include: Tablets 500 mg

Side effects/adverse reactions:
SYST: Anaphylaxis, cyanosis
GI: Nausea, vomiting, abdominal pain, hepatitis, glossitis, diarrhoea, jaundice, anorexia
HAEM: Eosinophilia, agranulocytosis, leucopenia, thrombocytopenia, haemolytic anaemia
INTEG: Rashes, epidermal necrolysis, photosensitivity
CNS: Headache, confusion, insomnia, hallucinations depression, vertigo, fatigue, anxiety, drug fevers, chills
GU: Renal failure, toxic nephrosis, crystalluria, haematuria
CV: Vasculitis

Contraindications: Severe renal or hepatic disease, pregnancy at term, premature or newborn infants under 6 weeks, hypersensitivity to sulphonamides, porphyria

Precautions: Renal or hepatic impairment, elderly, lactation, pregnancy

Pharmacokinetics: Readily absorbed from GI tract, 50% bound to plasma protein. It penetrates into CSF, 40% of plasma concentration is as acetyl derivative. 50% of the dose will be excreted in the urine in 2 days

Interactions/incompatibilities:
• Potentiation of: oral anticoagulants, sulphonylureas
• Decreased renal excretion of: Methotrexate

• Increased renal toxicity of: cyclosporin
• Reduced effect of sulphadimidine: PABA, procaine and related local anaesthetics
Clinical assessment:
• Kidney function studies, before and during treatment if impairment expected
• Blood counts at intervals during long-term treatment
• Discontinue if crystalluria develops; increase fluid input, alkanise urine with sodium bicarbonate
• Monitor cotreatment with oral anticoagulants, sulphonylureas
Treatment of overdose: Alkalinisation of the urine, with high fluid intake to produce at least 1.5 litres urine daily
NURSING CONSIDERATIONS
Assess:
• Fluid balance, urinalysis
Administer:
• After sample taken for culture and sensitivity (repeat after full course completed)
• At least 2 litres fluid/day to avoid crystallisation in kidneys
• Anti-emetic for severe nausea and vomiting
Evaluate:
• Fluid balance if drug given for urinary tract infection
• Urinalysis for crystals and blood
• Signs of allergic reactions — rashes, erythema multiforme, dyspnoea
• Therapeutic response — absence of pain, fever, negative culture and sensitivity
• Blood dyscrasias — skin rash, fever, sore throat, bruising, bleeding, fatigue, joint pain
Teach patient/family:
• Complete course of tablets even when symptoms improve or cease
• Drink plenty of fluids
• Avoid direct sunlight to skin — burning may occur
• Check with clinician before taking non-prescribed preparations
• Notify clinician at once of rash, fever, sore throat, bruising, bleeding, joint pain

---

sulphamethoxazole

Chemotrim, Comox, Laratrim, Comixco, Fectrim, Septrin, Bactrim (all in conjunction with trimethoprim as co-trimoxazole)
Func. class.: Antibiotic
Chem. class.: Sulphonamide
Legal class.: POM

Action: Interferes with bacterial biosynthesis of proteins by competitive antagonism of PABA. Synergistic with trimethoprim; only available as co-trimoxazole (1 part trimethoprim, 5 parts sulphamethoxazole)
Uses: Urinary tract infections, systemic infections, otitis media, gonorrhoea, *Pneumocystis carinii*
Dosage and routes:
(As co-trimoxazole)
• *Adult and child over 12 yr:* By mouth, IM/IV infusion 960 mg twice a day increasing to 1.44 g in severe infections, reducing to 480 mg twice a day if treated for more than 14 days
• *Child over 6 weeks:* By mouth/IV infusion 120 mg twice a day
• *Child 6 months to 6 yr:* By mouth/IV infusion 240 mg twice a day
• *Child over 6 yr:* By mouth/IV infusion 480 mg twice a day
Gonorrhoea
• *Adult:* 1.92 g twice a day for 2 days or 2.4 g once plus 2.4 g after 8 hr and stop
Pneumocystis carinii
• By mouth, IM/IV infusion 20 mg/kg daily in divided doses for 14 days
Available forms include: (As

co-trimoxazole) Tablets 120, 480, 960 mg; dispersible tablets 120, 480 mg; suspension 240, 480 mg/5 ml; IM injection 320 mg/ml; IV infusion 96 mg/ml (for dilution)

Side effects/adverse reactions (see also trimethoprim):

SYST: Anaphylaxis, cyanosis

GI: Nausea, vomiting, abdominal pain, stomatitis, hepatitis, glossitis, diarrhoea, enterocolitis jaundice, anorexia

CNS: Headache, confusion, insomnia, hallucinations, depression, vertigo, fatigue, anxiety, drug fever, chills

HAEM: Leucopenia, thrombocytopenia, agranulocytosis, haemolytic anaemia, eosinophilia

INTEG: Rash, urticaria, Stevens–Johnson syndrome, erythema, photosensitivity, pain/inflammation at injection site

GU: Renal failure, toxic nephrosis, crystalluria, haematuria

CV: Vasculitis

Contraindications: Hypersensitivity to sulphonamides, pregnancy at term, infants under 6 weeks, renal or hepatic failure

Precautions: Pregnancy, lactation, renal/hepatic impairment, elderly

Pharmacokinetics:

By mouth: Rapidly absorbed, peak 2–4 hr, 50%–70% bound to plasma proteins, half-life 7–12 hr, excreted in urine (unchanged 70%), breast milk

Interactions/incompatibilities:

• Increased hypoglycaemic response: sulphonylurea agents

• Increased anticoagulant effects: oral anticoagulants

• Decreased renal excretion of: methotrexate

• Increased renal toxicity of: cyclosporin

• Reduced effect of sulphamethoxazole: PABA, procaine and related local anaesthetics

• Decreased hepatic clearance of: phenytoin (given as co-trimoxazole)

Clinical assessment:

• Renal function tests before treatment if impairment expected, especially if high dose treatment planned

• Blood counts during long-term therapy. Give folinic acid for signs of folate deficiency (with co-trimoxazole)

• Urinalysis during high-dose therapy

• Monitor sulphamethoxazole blood levels during *Pneumocystis* treatment (therapeutic range 120–150 mcg/ml)

• Monitor cotreatment with oral anticoagulants, sulphonylureas, phenytoin

• Discontinue if crystalluria occurs; increase fluid input, alkalinise urine

Treatment of overdose: Gastric lavage, forced diuresis. If taken as co-trimoxazole, folinic acid to overcome folate antagonism

NURSING CONSIDERATIONS

Assess:

• Fluid balance, urinalysis

Administer:

• With full glass of water to maintain adequate fluid intake; increase fluids to 2 litres/day to decrease crystallisation in kidneys

• After sample taken for culture and sensitivity; repeat culture and sensitivity after full course completed

Evaluate:

• Therapeutic response: absence of pain, culture and sensitivity negative

• Fluid balance—note colour, character, pH of urine if drug administered for urinary tract infections. Output should be 800 ml less than intake; if urine is highly acidic, alkalisation may be needed

• Blood dyscrasias: skin rash,

fever, sore throat, bruising, bleeding, fatigue, joint pain
• Allergic reaction: rash, dermatitis, urticaria, pruritus, dyspnoea, bronchospasm

Teach patient/family:
• Take each oral dose with full glass of water to prevent crystalluria
• Complete full course of treatment to prevent superimposed infection
• Avoid sunlight or use sunscreen to prevent burns
• Avoid unprescribed medication (aspirin, vitamin C) unless directed by clinician
• Use alternative contraceptive measures; decreased effectiveness of oral contraceptives may result
• To notify clinician if skin rash, sore throat, fever, mouth sores, unusual bruising, bleeding occur

---

sulphasalazine

Salazopyrin
Func. class.: Anti-inflammatory
Chem. class.: Aminosalicylate/sulphonamide complex
Legal class.: POM

Action: Metabolised by gut bacteria to release 5-aminosalicylate which has local anti-inflammatory action
Uses: Ulcerative colitis and Crohn's disease, active rheumatoid arthritis
Dosage and routes:
Ulcerative colitis, Crohn's disease
• *Adult:* By mouth, acute attack 1−2 g 4 times a day; maintenance 2 g daily in divided doses 6 hrly; suppositories 2 per rectum morning and at bedtime alone or with oral therapy; enema 1 daily at bedtime
• *Child over 2 years:* By mouth, acute attack. 40−60 mg/kg daily in

divided doses; maintenance 30 mg/kg daily in 4 doses
Rheumatoid arthritis
• *Adult:* By mouth, 0.5 g daily increased by 0.5 g at weekly intervals to a maximum of 3 g daily in 2 divided doses
Available forms include: Tablets 500 mg; oral suspension 250 mg/5 ml; enteric coated tablets 500 mg; suppository 500 mg; retention enema 3 g/100 ml single dose
Side effects/adverse reactions:
SYST: Anaphylaxis, lupus-like syndrome
GI: Nausea, vomiting, abdominal pain, stomatitis, hepatitis, glossitis, pancreatitis, diarrhoea, exacerbation of colitis, anorexia
CNS: Headache, confusion, insomnia, hallucinations, depression, vertigo, fatigue, anxiety, convulsions, drug fever, chills, neurotoxicity
HAEM: Leucopenia, neutropenia, thrombocytopenia, agranulocytosis, haemolytic anaemia, Heinz body anaemia, methaemoglobinaemia, hypoprothrombinaemia, folate deficiency anaemia
INTEG: Rash, urticaria, Stevens-Johnson syndrome, erythema, photosensitivity
GU: Renal failure, haematuria, nephrotic syndrome, crystalluria, azoospermia, orange urine
CV: Allergic myocarditis, allergic vasculitis
RESP: Pneumonitis
EENT: Staining of soft contact lenses, tinnitus
Contraindications: Hypersensitivity to sulphonamides or salicylates, children under 2 years, porphyria
Precautions: Impaired renal/hepatic function, severe allergy, G6PD deficiency, pregnancy
Pharmacokinetics:
By mouth: Partially absorbed, largely metabolised to 5-amino-

salicylic acid and sulphapyridine by gut bacteria. Sulphapyridine mostly absorbed, excreted in urine; 5-aminosalicylic acid mostly excreted in faeces

Interactions/incompatibilities:
• Decreased absorption of: digoxin, folic acid
• Increased hypoglycaemic response: sulphonylurea agents
• Increased anticoagulant effects: oral anticoagulants
• Decreased renal excretion of: methotrexate
• Increased renal toxicity: cyclosporin

Clinical assessment:
• Liver function tests, full blood count monthly for first 3 months of treatment
• Renal function tests if impairment anticipated
• Monitor cotreatment with oral anticoagulants, sulphonylureas, digoxin

Treatment of overdose: Gastric lavage, supportive treatment, no specific antidote

NURSING CONSIDERATIONS
Assess:
• Fluid balance if acute attack ulceration colitis or Crohn's disease

Administer:
• Give with food or milk
• With full glass of water to maintain adequate fluid intake; increase fluids to 2 litres daily to decrease crystallisation in kidneys
• Total daily dose in evenly spaced doses to help minimise GI intolerance

Perform/provide:
• Resuscitation equipment; severe allergic reactions may occur

Evaluate:
• Therapeutic response
• Blood dyscrasias: skin rash, fever, sore throat, bruising, bleeding, fatigue, joint pain
• Allergic reaction: rash, dermatitis, urticaria, pruritus, dyspnoea, bronchospasm

Teach patient/family:
• To take with food or milk
• Take each oral dose with full glass of water to prevent crystalluria
• That drug may discolour urine orange−yellow
• That extended wear soft contact lenses may be permanently stained. Daily wear soft contacts and gas permeable lenses should respond to standard cleaning
• To complete full course of treatment to prevent superimposed infection
• To avoid sunlight or use sunscreen to prevent burns
• To notify clinician if skin rash, sore throat, fever, mouth sores, unusual bruising, bleeding occur
• May cause temporary infertility in men reversible on discontinuance of drug
• Full effectiveness of drug reached in several weeks

sulphinpyrazone

Anturan
Func. class.: Uricosuric
Chem. class.: Pyrazolone
Legal class.: POM

Action: Inhibits tubular reabsorption of urates, with increased excretion of uric acid
Uses: Gout, hyperuricaemia
Dosage and routes:
Gout
• *Adult:* By mouth 100−200 mg then increased to 600 mg daily over 2−3 weeks, not to exceed 800 mg/day. Reduce dose once serum uric acid levels normal
Available forms include: Tablets 100, 200 mg
Side effects/adverse reactions:
GU: Renal calculi, renal colic,

impaired renal function

GI: Gastric irritation, nausea, vomiting, hepatic necrosis, GI bleeding, jaundice

INTEG: Rash, pruritus, fever, photosensitivity

HAEM: Blood dyscrasias

RESP: Apnoea, irregular respirations

SYST: Sodium/water retention, precipitation of acute gout

Contraindications: Hypersensitivity to pyrazolone derivatives, or non-steroidal anti-inflammatories, severe hepatic disease, blood dyscrasias, severe renal disease, active peptic ulcer

Precautions: Pregnancy, lactation, healed peptic ulcer, latent heart failure, impaired renal function

Pharmacokinetics:

By mouth: Peak 1−2 hr, half-life 3 hr, metabolized by liver, excreted in urine. 98% protein bound

Interactions/incompatibilities:

• Increased effect of: oral anti-coagulants, sulphonylureas, phenytoin

• Decreased blood levels of: theophylline

• Effect reduced by: aspirin, pyrazinamide

Clinical assessment:

• Serum uric acid levels

• Full blood counts, renal function tests at regular intervals

Lab. test interferences:

Phenolsulphonphthalein, aminohippuric acid tests of renal function

Treatment of overdose: Empty stomach, gastric lavage, supportive treatment, no specific antidote

NURSING CONSIDERATIONS

Assess:

• Fluid balance; increase fluid intake to at least 2 litres in 24 hours

• Urinalysis

Administer:

• With glass of water

• With food for GI symptoms

Perform/provide:

• Ensure urine is alkaline

Evaluate:

• Therapeutic response: absence of pain, stiffness in joints

• Signs of renal impairment

Teach patient/family:

• To avoid high purine foods

• To avoid non-prescribed medicines, especially aspirin

• To report side-effects

---

suxamethonium chloride

Anectine, Scoline

Func. class.: Depolarising neuromuscular blocker

Legal class.: POM

Action: Inhibits transmission of nerve impulses by binding with cholinergic receptor sites, antagonising action of acetylcholine. Short acting depolarisation

Uses: Facilitation of endotracheal intubation, skeletal muscle relaxation during mechanical ventilation, surgery, or general anaesthesia

Dosage and routes:

• *Adult:* IV 20−100 mg repeated every 5−10 min as needed or followed by 2.5−4 mg/min by continuous infusion according to patients need, not to exceed 500 mg/hr

• *Child:* IV 1−2 mg/kg initially then as for adult adjusted to body weight

Available forms include: Injection IV 50 mg/ml

Side effects/adverse reactions:

SYST: Anaphylaxis

CV: Bradycardia, tachycardia, increased, decreased BP, sinus arrest, arrhythmias

RESP: Prolonged apnoea, bronchospasm, cyanosis, respiratory depression

EENT: Increased secretions, increased intraocular pressure
GI: Increased secretions, increased bowel movement
MS: Weakness, muscle pain, fasciculations, prolonged relaxation
HAEM: Myoglobulinaemia
INTEG: Rash, flushing, pruritus, urticaria
ELECT: Transient hyperkalaemia
Contraindications: Hypersensitivity, family history of/current malignant hyperthermia, severe liver disease, decreased plasma pseudo-cholinesterase, myasthenia gravis, major muscle wasting, muscular dystrophy, ophthalmic procedures when the anterior chamber of the eye is open, hyperkalaemia, patients with severe burns, recovering from major trauma, myotonia
Precautions: Pregnancy, cardiac disease, fractures — fasciculations may increase damage, dehydration, severe anaemia, malnutrition, neuromuscular disease, elderly, mothers within 6 weeks of giving birth, severe infection, phaeochromocytoma
Pharmacokinetics:
IV: Onset 1 min, peak 2–3 min, duration 6–10 min
IM: Onset 2–3 min
Hydrolysed in plasma, excreted in urine
Interactions/incompatibilities:
• Increased neuromuscular blockade: aminoglycosides, clindamycin, lincomycin, quinidine, local anaesthetics, polymyxin antibiotics, lithium, narcotic analgesics, oxytocin, procainamide, phenothiazines, phenelzine, alkylating agents, amphotericin, anticholinesterases (including organo-phosphorus pesticides and demecarium/ecothiopate eye drops), ketamine, quinine, verapamil
• Increased risk of cardiac arrhythmias given with: digoxin, other cardiac glycosides
• Reduced neuromuscular blockade: diazepam, propranolol
Clinical assessment:
• For electrolyte imbalances (potassium, magnesium); may lead to increased action of this drug
Treatment of overdose: Maintain airway, ventilate mechanically; consider anticholinesterase for secondary non-depolarising block
NURSING CONSIDERATIONS
Assess:
• History of malignant hyperthermia, myasthenia gravis or scolinic apnoea
• Vital signs (BP, pulse, respirations, airway)
Administer:
• Using nerve stimulator by anaesthetist to determine neuromuscular blockade
• By slow IV over 1–2 min (only by specially qualified person, usually an anaesthetist)
Perform/provide:
• Storage in light-resistant container at 4°C or less and do not resterilise
• Reassurance if communication is difficult during recovery from neuromuscular blockade
Evaluate:
• Vital signs, degree of respiratory function
• Check for urinary retention
• Therapeutic response: paralysis of jaw, eyelid, head, neck, rest of body
• Recovery: decreased paralysis of face, diaphragm, leg, arm, rest of body
• Allergic reactions: rash, fever, respiratory distress, pruritus; drug should be discontinued
Teach patient/family:
• That some muscular pain may occur during recovery

talampicillin HCI

Talpen
Func. class.: Broad spectrum β-lactam antibiotic
Chem. class.: Ampicillin ester
Legal class.: POM

Action: Interferes with biosynthesis of bacterial cell wall
Uses: Bacterial infections due to sensitive organisms, including urinary tract infections, otitis media, chronic bronchitis, invasive salmonellosis, gonorrhoea, ear, nose, throat skin and soft tissue infections
Dosage and routes:
• *Adult:* By mouth, 250−500 mg every 8 hr
• *Child 2−10 yr:* 125−250 mg every 8 hr
• *Child less than 2 yr:* 3−7 mg/kg every 8 hr
Gonorrhoea
• *Adult:* By mouth 1.5−2 g as a single dose
Available forms include: Tablets, 250 mg; Syrup, 125 mg(as napsylate)/5 ml when reconstituted with water
Side effects/adverse reactions:
GI: Diarrhoea, nausea, colitis
INTEG: Rashes, urticaria (signs of possible hypersensitivity)
MS: Joint pains
SYST: Fever, anaphylactic shock
Contraindications: Penicillin hypersensitivity, severe hepatic or renal failure
Precautions: History of allergy, pregnancy, glandular fever, HIV, or lymphatic leukaemias (increased risk of skin reactions); treatment should be discontinued if rash develops
Pharmacokinetics: Well absorbed through GI tract, rapidly hydrolysed to give high blood levels of ampicillin. Peak plasma concentrations are obtained 40−60 mins after oral dose. Not affected by presence of food in stomach. 50% of dose excreted as ampicillin in urine, within 6 hr
Interactions/incompatibilities
• Possibly decreased effect of: oral contraceptives
• Possibly decreased effect of talampicillin: tetracyclines
• Increased antibacterial effect: aminoglycosides
NURSING CONSIDERATIONS
Assess:
• For known sensitivity to penicillin group
Administer:
• After culture and sensitivity tests
• With or before food
• With probenecid for gonorrhoea
Perform/provide:
• Storage in damp-proof container
Evaluate:
• Therapeutic result
• For all known side effects; rashes, urticaria, GI disturbance
Teach patient/family:
• That full course must be taken as prescribed
• To report any side-effects
• Technique for administering syrup to children

tamoxifen

Nolvadex, Tamofen, Noltam, Emblon, Oestrifen
Func. class.: Anti-neoplastic
Chem. class.: Hormone, anti-oestrogen
Legal class.: POM

Action: Inhibits cell division by binding to cytoplasmic oestrogen receptors
Uses: Breast cancer, anovulatory infertility
Dosage and routes:
Breast cancer

- *Adult:* By mouth 20−40 mg daily
Infertility
- *Adult:* By mouth 20 mg daily on days 2−5 of cycle, increasing if necessary to 40 mg and then 80 mg daily in subsequent cycles

Available forms include: Tablets 10, 20, 40 mg (as citrate)

Side effects/adverse reactions:
HAEM: Transient thrombocytopenia, deep vein thrombosis
GI: Gastrointestinal disturbances
GU: Vaginal bleeding, pruritus vulvae, cystic ovarian swelling (premenopausal women)
INTEG: Rash, dry skin
CNS: Headache, dizziness, depression, confusion
EENT: Ocular lesions, retinopathy, corneal opacity, blurred vision
ENDO: Hot flushes, amenorrhoea (in premenopausal women)
SYST: Fluid retention, tumour flare

Contraindications: Hypersensitivity, pregnancy, porphyria

Pharmacokinetics:
By mouth: Peak 4−7 hr, half-life 7−14 hr (1 week terminal), extensively metabolised, excreted in faeces, urine

Interactions/incompatibilities:
- Increased effect of: coumarin anticoagulants

NURSING CONSIDERATIONS
Evaluate:
- Bleeding: haematuria, bruising, petechiae, mucosa or orifices daily if in acute condition
- Side effects especially if adding to patient's distress
- Symptoms indicating severe allergic reactions: rash, pruritus, urticaria, purpuric skin lesions, itching, flushing

Teach patient/family:
- To report any complaints, side effects to nurse or clinician
- That vaginal bleeding, pruritus, hot flashes, ocular lesions can oc-

cur, are reversible after discontinuing treatment

---

teicoplanin

Targocid
Func. class.: Antibiotic
Chem. class.: Glycopeptide
Legal class.: POM

Action: Bactericidal antibiotic which acts by binding to peptidoglycan units in the bacterial cell wall; with activity against both aerobic and anaerobic Gram-positive bacteria

Uses: Potentially serious Gram-positive infections including endocarditis, dialysis-associated peritonitis and serious infection due to multiply-resistant staphylococci

Dosage and routes:
Moderate infections
- *Adult:* IV injection (as a bolus or a 30-min infusion) 400 mg initially, maintenance IV or IM 200 mg/day
- *Children (under 14 yr):* 6 mg/kg every 12 hr for the first 3 doses followed by 3 mg/kg daily
Severe infections
- *Adult:* IV injection every 12 hr for 3 doses initially, 400 mg, maintenance IV or IM 400 mg/day
- *Children under 14 yr:* IV injection 6 mg/kg every 12 hr for 3 doses initially, maintenance IV or IM 6 mg/kg/day

Available forms include: Injection 200 mg, 400 mg

Side effects/adverse reactions:
CNS: Dizziness, headache
EENT: Hearing loss, tinnitus, vestibular disturbances
INTEG: Erythema and local pain, thrombophlebitis, rash, pruritus
HAEM: Eosinophilia, leucopenia, neutropenia, thrombocytopenia, thrombocytosis

GU: Transient elevations of serum creatinine

GI: Nausea, vomiting, diarrhoea, raised liver enzyme values

RESP: Bronchospasm

SYST: Fever, anaphylaxis

Contraindications:
Hypersensitivity

Precautions: Hypersensitivity to vancomycin, pregnancy, lactation, renal insufficiency (renal and auditory function should be monitored if therapy prolonged; dosage reduction required)

Pharmacokinetics: IV serum concentration exceeding typical MICs persist for 24 hr. 90 to 95% bound to serum albumin. Excreted unchanged by the kidney

Clinical assessment:
• Determination of teicoplanin serum concentrations may optimise therapy

NURSING CONSIDERATIONS

Assess:
• Fluid balance
• Bowel pattern

Administer:
• After specimens have been sent for culture and sensitivity
• Prepare injection by slowly adding diluent to the drug vial, and rolling the vial gently until the powder is completely dissolved, taking care to avoid the formation of foam
• If the solution becomes foamy allow to stand for about 15 mins before use
• Reconstituted vials should be used immediately
• If this is not possible, keep at 4°C and discard within 24 hr
• Duration of therapy depends on infection; in endocarditis and osteomyelitis, treatment of 3 weeks or longer is recommended

Evaluate:
• For side effects
• Therapeutic response

• Observe injection site for signs of inflammation

Teach patient/family:
• To report side effects, tinnitus, etc.

---

temazepam

Func. class.: Sedative/hypnotic
Chem. class.: Benzodiazepine
Legal class.: CD (Sch 4) POM

Action: Produces CNS depression at limbic, thalamic, hypothalamic levels of the CNS; may be mediated by neurotransmitter gamma-aminobutyric acid (GABA); results are sedation, hypnosis, skeletal muscle relaxation, anticonvulsant activity, anxiolytic action

Uses: Insomnia (short term), premedication

Dosage and routes:
Insomnia
• *Adult:* By mouth 10−30 mg at bedtime increasing to 40−60 mg if needed; elderly patients may respond to 5−15 mg
Premedication
• *Adult:* By mouth 20−40 mg, 30−60 mins before surgical procedure

Available forms include: Capsules 10, 15, 20, 30 mg; Tablets 10, 20 mg; Elixir 10 mg/5 ml

Side effects/adverse reactions:
CNS: Drowsiness, dizziness, confusion, depression, restless sleep, vivid dreams or nightmares, headache, dependence

GI: Gastro-intestinal disturbances

CV: Hypotension, palpitations

INTEG: Rash

EENT: Dry mouth

Contraindications: Hypersensitivity to benzodiazepines, children, acute pulmonary insufficiency; psychotic states

Precautions: Hepatic disease, renal

disease, suicidal individuals, history of drug abuse, personality disorder, elderly, seizure disorders, pregnancy, lactation, arteriosclerosis; do not use for more than 2−4 weeks

Pharmacokinetics:

By mouth: Onset 30−45 min, duration 6−8 hr, half-life 8 hr; metabolised by liver, excreted by kidneys, excreted in breast milk

Interactions/incompatibilities:

• Increased sedative effects of alcohol, anaesthetics, antihistamines, antidepressants: cimetidine, disulfiram, narcotic analgesics

• Possibly reduced effect of: levodopa

NURSING CONSIDERATIONS

Administer:

• ½−1 hr before bedtime for sleeplessness

• On empty stomach for fast effect, but may be taken with food if GI symptoms occur

Evaluate:

• Therapeutic response: ability to sleep at night, decreased amount of early morning awakening if taking drug for insomnia

• Mental status: mood, alertness, affect, memory (long, short)

Teach patient/family:

• To avoid driving or other activities requiring alertness until drug is stabilized

• To avoid alcohol ingestion or CNS depressants; serious CNS depression may result

• That effects may take 2 nights for benefits to be noticed

• Alternative measures to improve sleep: reading, exercise several hours before bedtime, warm bath, warm milk, TV, self-hypnosis, deep breathing

• Hangover is common in elderly, but less common than with barbiturates

temocillin ▼

Temopen
Func. class.: Antibiotic
Chem. class.: Synthetic penicillin
Legal class.: POM

Action: Interferes with biosynthesis of bacterial cell wall. It is active against many β-lactamase producing Gram-negative aerobes

Uses: Septicaemia, urinary tract infection, lower respiratory tract infections involving susceptible Gram-negative bacilli. Not active against Gram-positive bacteria

Dosage and routes:

• *Adult:* IM, IV injection, intermittent IV infusion, 1 to 2 g every 12 hr. In acute uncomplicated urinary tract infections 1 g daily, as single or divided doses

Available forms include: Injection 500 mg, 1 g (as sodium salt)

Side effects/adverse reactions:

INTEG: Pain at site of IM injection, rashes

GI: Diarrhoea

MS: Joint pains (hypersensitivity)

SYST: Anaphylactic shock, fever (hypersensitivity)

Contraindications: Hypersensitivity to penicillin

Precautions: Pregnancy, breast feeding, renal insufficiency, history of allergy

Pharmacokinetics: Half-life 4 to 5 hr. 70% to 80% excreted in urine unchanged

Interactions/incompatibilities:

• Possibly decreased effect of: oral contraceptives

• Possibly decreased effect of temocillin: tetracyclines

• Increased antibacterial effect: aminoglycosides

NURSING CONSIDERATIONS

Assess:

• For known allergies to penicillin group

- Fluid balance
- Bowel pattern

Administer:
- After culture and sensitivity tests
- IV: By slow injection over 3−4 min or infusion over 30−40 min (drug is compatible with water, sodium chloride 0.9% or dextrose 5%)
- IM: By deep IM injection (may be mixed with lignocaine hydrochloride 0.5 to 1.0% if pain is experienced at site of injection)

Evaluate:
- Therapeutic response
- For allergic response, rashes, diarrhoea

tenoxicam

Mobiflex
Func. class.: Non-steroidal anti-inflammatory
Chem. class.: Oxicam
Legal class.: POM

Action: Inhibits prostaglandin synthesis; has marked anti-inflammatory and analgesic activity and some antipyretic activity
Uses: Osteoarthrosis, rheumatoid arthritis
Dosage and routes:
- *Adult:* By mouth, 20 mg daily
Available forms include: Tablets 20 mg
Side effects/adverse reactions:
GI: Nausea, dyspepsia, abdominal pain, constipation, diarrhoea, flatulence, stomatitis, peptic ulcer, GI haemorrhage
HAEM: Blood dyscrasias
CNS: Headache, dizziness, depression, confusion, paraesthesia, vertigo, somnolence
INTEG: Rashes, erythema, pruritus, alopecia, photosensitivity
EENT: Swelling and irritation of eyes, blurred vision, tinnitus
CV: Palpitations
RESP: Dyspnoea
SYST: Weight changes, oedema
Contraindications: History of, or active peptic ulcer, GI bleeding, gastritis; hypersensitivity to non-steroidal anti-inflammatory agents; pregnancy
Precautions: Renal or hepatic insufficiency, congestive heart failure, elderly
Pharmacokinetics:
By mouth: Rapidly and completely absorbed, extensively bound to plasma protein, elimination half life about 72 hr, extensively metabolised, excreted in urine and bile
Interactions/incompatibilities:

- Possibly increased toxicity: cyclosporin, diuretics, lithium, salicylates
- Possibly increased effects of: anticoagulants, anti-diabetic agents (sulphonylureas)

NURSING CONSIDERATIONS

Administer:
- With food to decrease GI symptoms; best taken on empty stomach to facilitate absorption

Evaluate:
- Therapeutic response: decreased pain, stiffness, swelling in joints, ability to move more easily
- For eye, ear problems: blurred vision, tinnitus (may indicate toxicity)

Teach patient/family:
- To report blurred vision, ringing, roaring in ears (may indicate toxicity)
- To avoid driving or other hazardous activities if dizziness or drowsiness occurs
- To report change in urine pattern, weight increase, oedema, pain increase in joints, fever, blood in urine (indicates nephrotoxicity)
- That therapeutic effects may take up to 1 month

---

terbutaline sulphate

Bricanyl, Monovent

Func. class.: β_2-adrenergic stimulant
Chem. class.: Catecholamine
Legal class.: POM

Action: Causes bronchodilation by acting on β-receptors in bronchus and lung; has relatively little effect on cardiac receptors

Uses: Bronchospasm, premature labour

Dosage and routes:

Bronchospasm
- *Adult:* By mouth 5 mg two or three times a day; subcutaneous/IM/slow IV injection 250−500 mg up to four times a day; IV infusion, solution of 3−5 mcg/ml at 1.5−5 mcg/min; inhalation powder 500 mcg as required (max. 4 inhalations/24 hr); nebulizer solution 5−10 mg up to four times a day; aerosol inhalation 250−500 mcg every 6 hr if necessary, maximum 8 inhalations/24 hr
- *Child: 3−7 yr:* By mouth 0.75−1.5 mg three times a day
- *7−15 yr:* By mouth 2.5 mg two or three times a day; subcutaneous slow IV/IM: 2−15 yr 10 mcg/kg (maximum 300 mcg)

Inhalation, nebuliser solution:
- *up to 3 yr:* 2 mg two to four times a day
- *3−6 yr:* 3 mg two to four times a day
- *6−8 yr:* 4 mg two to four times a day
- *over 8 yr:* 5 mg two to four times a day

Premature Labour
- *Adult:* IV infusion: 10 mcg/min for 1 hr, increased by 5 mcg every 10 min to maximum 25 mcg/min, reduced once then subcutaneous contractions stop; injection 250 mcg four times daily for 3 days and by mouth 5 mg three times daily until 37th week of pregnancy

Available forms include: Tablets 5 mg; tablets modified release 7.5 mg; aerosol 0.25 mg/actuation; syrup 0.3 mg/ml; injection 0.5 mg/ml; nebuliser solution 2.5, 10 mg/ml; Aerosol inhaler 0.25 mg/inhalation; powder inhaler 0.5 mg/inhalation

Side effects/adverse reactions:
CNS: Tremors, anxiety, headache
CV: Palpitations, tachycardia, arrhythmias
GI: Nausea
META: Hypokalaemia, hyperglycaemia

MS: Cramp

Contraindications: Hypersensitivity to sympathomimetics

Precautions: Pregnancy, cardiac disorders, hyperthyroidism, diabetes mellitus, hypertension, elderly patients

Pharmacokinetics:

By mouth: Onset ½ hr, duration 4−8 hr

Subcutaneous: Onset 6−15 min, duration 1½−4 hr

Inhalation: Onset 5−30 min, duration 3−6 hr

Interactions/incompatibilities:

• Increased effects of both drugs: other sympathomimetics

• Decreased action: β-blockers

• Increased risk of hypokalaemia: corticosteroids, diuretics, xanthines

Treatment of overdose: Supportive symptomatic care; a cardioselective β-blocker may be helpful in arrhythmias, at the risk of inducing bronchoconstriction

NURSING CONSIDERATIONS

Evaluate:

• Therapeutic response: absence of dyspnoea, wheezing

• Tolerance over long-term therapy, dose may need to be increased or changed

Teach patient/family:

• Not to use non-prescribed medications; extra stimulation may occur

• Use of inhaler, review package insert with patient

• To avoid getting solution in eyes

• On all aspects of drug; avoid smoking, smoke-filled rooms, persons with respiratory infections

---

terfenadine

Triludan

Func. class.: Antihistamine

Chem. class.: Butyrophenone derivative

Legal class.: P

Action: Acts peripherally on blood vessels, GI, respiratory system by competing with histamine for H_1-receptor site; decreases allergic response by blocking histamine

Uses: Allergic symptoms such as hayfever, rhinitis, and skin reactions

Dosage and routes:

• *Adult and child over 12 yr:* By mouth 60 mg twice a day or 120 mg in the morning

• *Child 6−12 yr:* By mouth 30 mg twice a day

• *Child 3−6 yr:* By mouth 15 mg twice a day

Available forms include: Tablets 60, 120 mg; suspension 30 mg/5 ml

Side effects/adverse reactions:

CNS: Dizziness, headache, depression, convulsions, confusion, insomnia, nightmares, paraesthesia, tremor

CV: Palpitations, arrhythmias

RESP: Bronchospasm

GI: Abdominal pain, dyspepsia, jaundice, liver dysfunction

INTEG: Rash, alopecia photosensitivity, sweating, angioedema

GU: Menstrual disturbances

EENT: Visual disturbances

MS: Muscle pain

SYST: Anaphylaxis

Contraindications: Hypersensitivity, porphyria

Precautions: Pregnancy, lactation, hepatic impairment

Pharmacokinetics:

By mouth: Peak 1−2 hr, 97% bound to plasma proteins, half-life is biphasic 3½ hr, 16−23 hr

Interactions/incompatibilities:

• Increased effect (reduced metabolism of terfenadine): ketoconazole, macrolide antibiotics

NURSING CONSIDERATIONS
Administer:
• 30 min before travel if used for motion sickness
Evaluate:
• Therapeutic response: absence of running or congested nose or rashes
Teach patient/family:
• All aspects of drug use; to notify clinician if confusion, sedation occurs
• To avoid driving or other hazardous activity if drowsiness occurs

---

testosterone

Func. class.: Androgenic anabolic steroid
Chem. class.: Steroid
Legal class.: POM

Action: Increases weight by building body tissue, increases potassium, phosphorus, chloride, nitrogen levels, increases bone development; controls development and maintenance of male sexual characteristics
Uses: Hypogonadism (male) menopausal disorders
Dosage and routes:
Hypogonadism
• *Adult:* By implantation 600 mg every 6 months
Menopausal disorders
• *Adult:* By implantation 50−100 mg every 4−8 months
Available forms include: Implant 100, 200 mg
Side effects/adverse reactions:
INTEG: Rash, acneiform lesions, oily hair, alopecia, hirsutism
MS: Closure of epiphyses in prepubertal males, increased bone growth

GU: Amenorrhoea, decreased female libido, decreased breast size, clitoral hypertrophy, prostatism in elderly men, testicular atrophy, suppression of spermatogenesis, priapism, precocious sexual development in prepubertal males
GI: Jaundice, hepatitis
META: Hypercalcaemia, sodium and fluid retention
Contraindications: Nephrosis, hypersensitivity, pregnancy, lactation, hypercalcaemia, breast cancer (men), prostatic carcinoma
Precautions: Ischaemic heart disease, cardiac, renal or hepatic impairment, epilepsy, migraine, skeletal metastases, hypertension, prepubertal males
Interactions/incompatibilities:
• Increased effects of: oral anticoagulants

NURSING CONSIDERATIONS
Assess:
• Baseline weight and BP
• Drug can be one of abuse, particularly by athletes
Perform/provide:
• Diet with increased calories and protein; decrease sodium if oedema occurs
Evaluate:
• Growth rate in children since growth rate may be uneven (linear/bone growth) when used for extended period
• Therapeutic response
• Cardiac symptoms, jaundice
• Observe for fluid retention
• Mental status: affect, mood, behavioural changes, aggression
• Signs of masculinisation in female: increased libido, deepening of voice, breast tissue, enlarged clitoris, menstrual irregularities; male: gynaecomastia, impotence, testicular atrophy
Teach patient/family:
• Drug needs to be combined with complete health plan: diet, rest, exercise

- To notify clinician if therapeutic response decreases
- Do not discontinue this medication abruptly
- Teach patient all aspects of drug usage, including changes in sex characteristics
- Women to report menstrual irregularities
- Drug can be abused

testosterone decanoate/ testosterone enanthate/ testosterone isocaproate/ testosterone phenylpropionate/ testosterone propionate/ testosterone undecanoate

Primoteston Depot, Restandol, Sustanon, Virormone
Func. class.: Androgenic anabolic steroid
Chem. class.: Steroid
Legal class.: POM

Action: Increases weight by building body tissue, increases potassium, phosphorus, chloride, nitrogen levels, increases bone development; controls development and maintenance of male sexual characteristics
Uses: Androgen deficiency, such as in hypogonadism (male), delayed puberty or cryptorchidism; breast cancer (female)
Dosage and routes:
Delayed puberty, cryptorchidism
- *Adult:* IM 50 mg (propionate) weekly
Breast cancer
- *Adult:* IM 100 mg (propionate) 2−3 times weekly; or 250 mg (enanthate) every 2 weeks
Hypogonadism
- *Adult:* IM 50 mg (propionate) 2−3 times weekly; or 250 mg (enanthate) every 2−3 weeks, reduced to every 3−6 weeks for maintenance; or 100 mg (isocaproate/phenylpropionate/propionate 2:2:1) every 2 weeks; or 250 mg (decanoate/isocaproate/phenylpropionate/propionate 10:6:6:3) every 3 weeks; By mouth 120−160 mg (undecanoate) daily for 2−3 weeks, then adjust in range 40−120 mg daily according to response
Available forms include: Capsules 40 mg (undecanoate); Injection 250 mg (enanthate)/ml, 50 mg (propionate)/ml, 100 mg (isocaproate 40 mg, phenylpropionate 40 mg, propionate 20 mg)/ml, 250 mg (decanoate 100 mg, isocaproate 60 mg, phenylpropionate 60 mg, propionate 30 mg)/ml
Side effects/adverse reactions:
INTEG: Rash, acneiform lesions, oily hair, skin, alopecia, hirsutism
MS: Closure of epiphyses in prepubertal males, increased bone growth
GU: Amenorrhoea, decreased female libido, decreased breast size, clitoral hypertrophy, prostatism in elderly man, testicular atrophy, suppression of spermatogenesis, priapism, precocious sexual development in prepubertal males
GI: Jaundice, hepatitis
META: Hypercalcaemia, sodium and fluid retention
Contraindications: Hypercalcaemia, nephrosis, breast cancer (men), prostatic carcinoma, hypersensitivity, pregnancy, lactation
Precautions: Ischaemic heart disease, cardiac, renal or hepatic impairment, hypertension, epilepsy, migraine, prepubertal males
Pharmacokinetics:
By mouth: Metabolised in liver, excreted in urine, breast milk

Interactions/incompatibilities:
• Increased effects of: oral anticoagulants

NURSING CONSIDERATIONS
Assess:
• Baseline weight and BP
• Growth rate in children since growth rate may be uneven (linear/bone growth) used for extended periods of time

Administer:
• Titrated dose; use lowest effective dose
• IM deep into large muscle mass

Perform/provide:
• Diet with increased calories, protein; decrease sodium if oedema occurs as medically directed
• Give iron in anaemia

Evaluate:
• Therapeutic response: occurs in 4−6 weeks in osteoporosis
• Weight daily, notify clinician if weekly weight gain is over 2 kg
• BP 4 hrly
• Fluid balance; be alert for decreasing urinary output, increasing oedema
• Oedema, hypertension, cardiac symptoms, jaundice
• Mental status: affect, mood, behavioural changes, aggression
• Signs of masculinisation in female: increased libido, deepening of voice, breast tissue, enlarged clitoris, menstrual irregularities; male: gynaecomastia, impotence, testicular atrophy
• Hypercalcaemia: lethargy, polyuria, polydipsia, nausea, vomiting, constipation; drug may need to be decreased
• Hypoglycaemia in diabetics, since oral anticoagulant action is decreased

Teach patient/family:
• Drug needs to be combined with complete health plan: Diet, rest, exercise
• To notify clinician if therapeutic response decreases
• Not to discontinue this medication abruptly
• Aspects of drug usage, including changes in sex characteristics
• Women to report menstrual irregularities
• That 1−3 month course is necessary for response in breast cancer
• That drug can be abused

tetanus vaccine; tetanus vaccine, adsorbed

Tet/Vac/FT, Tet/Vac/Ads, Clostet, Tetavax
Func. class.: Vaccine
Legal class.: POM

Action: Produces specific antibodies to tetanus
Uses: Prevention of tetanus (adsorbed vaccine preferred)
Dosage and routes:
• *Adult and child:* IM or deep subcutaneous injection 0.5 ml repeated twice at intervals of 4 weeks. Reinforcing doses may be given every 10 yr
Side effects/adverse reactions:
INTEG: Local pain, redness and swelling at injection site
MS: Myalgia
SYST: Pyrexia, anaphylaxis
CNS: Headache, lethargy
Contraindications: Hypersensitivity, active infection, immunosuppression, patients who have received a booster in the preceding year
NURSING CONSIDERATIONS
Assess:
• Tetanus toxoid status
• History of reactions to vaccinations
Administer:
• Preferably by IM injection into deep muscle mass
Perform/provide:

• Record dose and lot number on notes
• Ensure patient has record card with dose, batch no and dates of next due injection or booster

Teach patient/family:
• Of importance of completing of primary course; second injection 6 weeks after first dose; booster
• That some local reaction may occur particularly if injection is given subcutaneously (swollen, red injection site)

---

tetrabenazine

Nitoman
Func. class.: Suppressor of choreiform movements
Chem. class.: Quinolizinone
Legal class.: POM

Action: Thought to deplete nerve endings of dopamine
Uses: Disorders of movement caused by Huntingdon's chorea, senile chorea, and related neurological conditions
Dosage and routes:
• *Adult:* By mouth; initially 12.5–25 mg 3 times daily, gradually increased by 12.5–25 mg/day every 3–4 days; maximum daily dose 200 mg
Available forms include: Tablets 25 mg
Side effects/adverse reactions:
CNS: Drowsiness, extrapyramidal symptoms, depression
CVS: Hypotension
GI: Disturbances
Contraindications: Lactation
Precautions: Pregnancy
Interactions/incompatibilities:
• CNS excitation, hypertension: MAOIs (within 14 days)
• Diminished effects of: reserpine, levodopa
Clinical assessment:

• Consider withdrawal of drug if patient becomes depressed
Treatment of overdose:
• Empty stomach; symptomatic treatment
NURSING CONSIDERATIONS
Assess:
• Baseline BP
Evaluate:
• Therapeutic response — improvement in movement disorders
• Onset of depression — drug may need to be withdrawn
• Side-effects, including hypotension
Teach patient/family:
• Rise slowly as fainting may occur
• Avoid potentially dangerous tasks requiring alertness (e.g. driving) as drowsiness may occur
• Check with clinician before taking non-prescribed preparations

---

tetracosactrin

Synacthen, Synacthen Depot
Func. class.: Corticotrophin analogue
Chem. class.: Synthetic polypeptide
Legal class.: POM

Action: Stimulates adrenal cortex to produce, secrete glucocorticoids, mineralocorticoids and, to a lesser extend, androgens
Uses: Testing adrenocortical function, short-term replacement of corticosteroids in Crohn's disease, rheumatoid arthritis
Dosage and routes:
Investigation of adrenocortical function
• *Adult:* IM/IV 250 mcg solution (short test) or 1 mg depot (long test)
• *Child:* IM/IV 250 mcg/1.73 m^2

body surface area solution (short test)

Depot injection for therapeutic purposes
• *Adult:* IM 1−2 mg daily reduced to 1 mg every 2−3 days then 1 mg weekly
• *Child:* IM 1 month−2 yr, initially 250 mcg daily reduced to 250 mcg every 2−8 days;
• *2−5 yr:* IM initially 250−500 mcg daily reduced to 250−500 mcg every 2−8 days
• *5−12 yr:* IM initially 0.25−1 mg daily reduced to 0.25−1 mg every 2−8 days

Available forms include: Injection 250 mcg/ml; depot injection 1 mg/ml (both as acetate)

Side effects/adverse reactions:
INTEG: Rash, urticaria, pruritus, flushing
CV: Sodium, water retention
SYST: Significant risk of anaphylaxis

Contraindications: Hypersensitivity, history of allergic disorders e.g. asthma. Depot also contraindicated in: acute psychosis, infectious disease, Cushing's syndrome, peptic ulcer, refractory heart failure, adrenogenital syndrome, as therapy for adrenocortical insufficiency

Pharmacokinetics:
IV/IM: Onset 5 min, peak 1 hr, duration 2−4 hr
Depot preparations: Peak effect 8 hr, duration greater than 24 hr

Clinical assessment:
• When using diagnostically, take blood samples for cortisol levels 30 min after injection and also at hourly intervals up to 5 hr if depot preparation used

Treatment of overdose:
Symptomatic

NURSING CONSIDERATIONS
Assess:
• Weight
Administer:

• IV or IM with equipment/drugs in case of anaphylaxis
Perform/provide:
• Storage in a refrigerator at 2−8°C
• All equipment to deal with anaphylaxis
Evaluate:
• For all side effects including water retention
Teach patient/family:
• Of necessity to carry "Steroid ID" card at all times

---

tetracycline HCl

Achromycin, Panmycin, Sustamycin, Tetrabid-Organon, Tetrachel
Func. class.: Antibiotic, broad-spectrum
Chem. class.: Tetracycline
Legal class.: POM

Action: Inhibits protein synthesis in microorganisms
Uses: Early syphilis, chlamydial infections (trachoma, lymphogranuloma venereum, psittacosis, salpingitis, urethritis), *Mycoplasma* (respiratory and genital infections), exacerbations of chronic bronchitis, acne, refractory periodontal disease, brucellosis, rickettsia and other infections due to tetracycline-sensitive organisms. Malignant or cirrhotic pleural effusions
Dosage and routes:
• *Adult:* By mouth 250−500 mg every 6 hr or 250 mg modified release capsules 2 as one dose, then 1 every 12 hr; IM, 100 mg every 8−12 hr or 4−6 hr in severe infections; IV infusion 500 mg 12 hrly maximum 2 g daily
Non-gonococcal urethritis
• *Adult:* By mouth 500 mg every 6 hr for 10−21 days four times a day

Acne
• *Adult:* By mouth 250 mg three times a day for 3–4 weeks then 250 mg twice a day for 4 months or modified release capsules 250 mg once daily

Early syphilis
• *Adult:* By mouth 500 mg every 6 hr for 14 days

Pleural effusions
• *Adult:* Via chest drain 500 mg IV preparation in 30–50 ml saline

Available forms include: Capsules 250 mg, modified release 250 mg; tablets 250 mg; powder for injection IM 100 mg; IV 250, 500 mg

Side effects/adverse reactions:

CNS: Headache, benign intracranial hypertension

HAEM: Eosinophilia, neutropenia, thrombocytopenia, haemolytic anaemia

EENT: Glossitis, decreased calcification and staining of deciduous teeth, oral candidiasis, visual disturbances

GI: Nausea, vomiting, diarrhoea, anorexia, enterocolitis, hepatotoxicity, flatulence, abdominal cramps, epigastric burning, pseudomembranous colitis, oesophageal ulceration

GU: Nephrotoxicity

INTEG: Rash, urticaria, photosensitivity, erythema, pruritus, pain and irritation of injection site

Contraindications: Hypersensitivity to tetracyclines, children under 12 yr severe renal insufficiency, pregnancy, lactation, systemic lupus erythematosus

Precautions: Renal disease, hepatic disease

Pharmacokinetics:

By mouth: Peak 2–4 hr, only partially absorbed, half-life 6–10 hr; excreted in urine and faeces, excreted in breast milk, 20%–60% protein bound

Interactions/incompatibilities:
• Decreased absorption of tetracycline: antacids, dairy products, iron, quinapril, calcium salts, sucralfate, bismuth, zinc
• Increased effect of: oral anticoagulants
• Decreased effect: penicillins
• Nephrotoxicity enhanced by: methoxyflurane
• Reduced effect of: oral contraceptives

Clinical assessment:
• Monitor renal/hepatic function if pre-existing problems

Lab. test interferences:
False increase: Urinary catecholamines

Treatment of overdose: Gastric lavage, administer milk or antacid, supportive treatment

NURSING CONSIDERATIONS

Assess:
• Bowel pattern
• Fluid balance

Administer:
• After specimens have been obtained and sent for culture and sensitivity
• 1 hr before or 2 hr after ferrous or milk products; 3 hr after antacid

Evaluate:
• Therapeutic response: decreased temperature, absence of lesions, negative culture and sensitivity
• Allergic reactions: rash, itching, pruritus, angioneurotic oedema
• Nausea, vomiting, diarrhoea; administer anti-emetic, antacids as ordered
• Overgrowth of infection: increased temperature, malaise, redness, pain, swelling, drainage, perineal itching, diarrhoea, changes in cough or sputum

Teach patient/family:
• Avoid sun exposure since burns may occur; sunscreen does not seem to decrease photosensitivity
• That all prescribed medication must be taken to prevent superimposed infection

• To avoid taking milk products at same time as tetracycline

---

tetracycline HCl (otic, ophthalmic)

Achromycin, Eye and Ear Ointment
Func. class.: Antibiotic
Chem. class.: Tetracycline
Legal class.: POM

Action: Inhibits bacterial cell-wall synthesis
Uses: Infection of eye, external otitis, trachoma
Dosage and routes:
• *Adult and child:* Ointment: apply every 2 hr
Trachoma
• *Adult and child:* Apply to eye 3 times daily for 6 weeks
Available forms include: Ointment 1%
Side effects/adverse reactions:
EENT: Poor corneal wound healing, overgrowth of non-susceptible organisms
Contraindications: Hypersensitivity
Precautions: Antibiotic hypersensitivity
Clinical assessment:
• Serious infections may require systemic treatment, especially trachoma
NURSING CONSIDERATIONS
Administer:
• After samples have been sent for culture and sensitivity
• After washing hands, cleanse crusts or discharge from eye before application
Evaluate:
• Therapeutic response: absence of redness, inflammation, tearing
• Allergy: itching, lacrimation, redness, swelling
Teach patient/family:
• To use drug exactly as prescribed
• Do not use eye make-up, towels, washclots, or eye medication of others, or reinfection may occur
• That drug container tip should not be touched to eye
• To report itching, increased redness, burning, stinging, swelling; drug should be discontinued
• That drug may cause blurred vision when ointment is applied
• Discard unused ointment 28 days after opening

---

tetracycline HCl (topical)

Topicycline, Achromycin
Func. class.: Antibiotic, topical
Chem. class.: Tetracycline
Legal class.: POM

Action: Interferes with microorganism phosphorylation, protein synthesis
Uses: Acne. Superficial pyogenic infections, prevention of wound infection caused by susceptible organisms
Dosage and routes:
Superficial infections
• *Adult and child:* Topical, apply ointment to affected area 1—3 times a day
Acne
• *Adult:* Apply solution twice a day
Available forms include: Ointment 3%; solution 0.22%
Side effects/adverse reactions:
INTEG: Rash, urticaria, stinging, burning, overgrowth of resistant organisms
Contraindications: Hypersensitivity
Precautions: Pregnancy, lactation
Clinical assessment:
• Systemic therapy may be required in serious infections
NURSING CONSIDERATIONS
Administer:
• After cleansing with soap, water before each application, dry well

- Enough medication to cover lesions completely
- Avoid eyes, nose and mouth

Perform/provide:
- Storage in a cool place (8−15°C)

Evaluate:
- Allergic reaction: burning, stinging, swelling, redness
- Therapeutic response: decrease in size, number of lesions

Teach patient/family:
- Wash hands thoroughly before, after each application
- Apply with glove to prevent further infection
- Avoid use of non-prescribed creams, ointments, lotions unless directed by clinician

---

theophylline, theophylline sodium glycinate

Biophylline, Labophylline, Lasma, Nuelin, Nuelin SA, Pro-vent, Slo-Phyllin, Theo-Dur, Uniphyllin-continus, combination products

Func. class.: Bronchodilator
Chem. class.: Xanthine
Legal class.: Oral formulations P; injectable POM

Action: Relaxes smooth muscle of respiratory system by blocking phosphodiesterase, which increases cyclic AMP

Uses: Asthma, bronchospasm associated with chronic bronchitis, reversible airway obstruction

Dosage and routes:
Note: The dosage of theophylline varies considerably with the formulation of the product. Due to the potential toxicity of theophylline it is essential to maintain plasma concentrations at 10−20 mg/litre, this may require adjustment of doses outside of ranges specified below.

Dosage and route for each product are shown below:

Biophylline
Available forms: Syrup 125 mg theophylline hydrate (as sodium glycinate) per 5 ml; modified-release tablets 350, 500 mg
Dosage:
- *Adult:* By mouth, syrup 125−250 mg 3 or 4 times a day; modified-release tablets, patient over 70 kg 500 mg every 12 hr, under 70 kg, 350 mg every 12 hr
- *Child 7−12 yr:* By mouth, syrup 62.5−125 mg 3 or 4 times a day
- *Child 2−6 yr:* By mouth 62.5 mg three or four times a day

Labophylline
Available forms: Injection 20 mg/ml
Dosage:
The initial doses that follow should be reduced by 50% in patients who have received oral xanthines in the previous 24 hr. Maintenance doses should be reduced in the elderly, heart failure
- *Adult:* Initial dose slow IV injection 200 mg over 15 min or IV infusion 4 mg/kg over 20−30 min Maintenance: 0.5 mg/kg/hr for 12 hr then 0.4 mg/kg/hr
- *Child:* Initial dose slow IV injection 4 mg/kg (over 15 min) Maintenance: over 6 yr 0.75 mg/kg/hr for 12 hr then 0.5 mg/kg/hr; 6 months−6 yr 1−0.8 mg/kg/hr for 12 hr then 0.6 mg/kg/hr

Lasma
Available forms: Modified-release tablets 300 mg
Dosage:
- *Adult:* 300 mg every 12 hr or 600 mg at night in nocturnal asthma increased to 900 mg per day after 1 week in patients over 70 kg. Adjust dose in 150 mg increments

Nuelin
Available forms: Tablets 125 mg, liquid 60 mg theophylline hydrate (as sodium glycinate) per 5 ml

Dosage:
• *Adult:* By mouth, tablets 125 mg 3 or 4 times a day after meals increasing to 250 mg if required; liquid 120–240 mg 3 or 4 times a day
• *Child 7–12 yr:* By mouth, tablets 62.5–125 mg 3 or 4 times a day after meals; liquid, 90–120 mg 3 or 4 times a day
• *Child 2–6 yr:* By mouth, liquid 60–90 mg 3 or 4 times a day
Nuelin SA
Available forms: modified-release tablets 175, 250 mg (SA 250)
Dosage:
• *Adults:* By mouth 175–350 mg or 250–500 mg (SA 250) every 12 hr
• *Child over 6 yr:* By mouth 175 mg or 125–250 mg (SA 250) every 12 hr
Pro-Vent
Available forms: Capsules modified-release 300 mg
Dosage:
• *Adult:* By mouth 300 mg every 12 hr with a further 300 mg once daily if required
Slo-Phyllin
Available forms: Capsules modified-release 60, 125, 250 mg
Dosage:
• *Adult:* By mouth 250–500 mg every 12 hr
• *Child 6–12 yr:* By mouth 125–250 mg every 12 hr
• *Child 2–6 yr:* By mouth 60–120 mg every 12 hr
Theo-Dur
Available forms: Modified-release tablets 200, 300 mg
Dosage:
• *Adult:* By mouth 200–300 mg every 12 hr
• *Child over 35 kg:* 200 mg every 12 hr
• *Child under 35 kg:* 100 mg every 12 hr
Uniphyllin-continus

Available forms: Tablets modified-release 200, 300, 400 mg
Dosage:
• *Adult:* By mouth, under 70 kg, 200 mg every 12 hr increasing to 300 mg 12 hrly after 1 week; over 70 kg, 300 mg every 12 hr increasing to 400 mg 12 hrly after 1 week
• *Child:* By mouth 9 mg/kg twice a day increasing if needed to maximum 16 mg/kg twice a day

Side effects/adverse reactions:
CNS: Anxiety, restlessness, insomnia, dizziness, convulsions, headache, light-headedness, delirium
CV: Palpitations, sinus tachycardia, other dysrhythmias
GI: Nausea, vomiting, anorexia, diarrhoea, dyspepsia, GI bleeding
RESP: Increased rate
Contraindications: Hypersensitivity to xanthines, concurrent use of other xanthines, porphyria
Precautions: Elderly, congestive cardiac failure, cor pulmonale, hepatic disease, active peptic ulcer disease, hyperthyroidism, hypertension, cardiac arrhythmias, alcoholism, epilepsy, lactation
Pharmacokinetics: By mouth, free drug rapidly and completely absorbed; kinetics dependent upon formulation, metabolised in liver, excreted in urine, breast milk

Interactions/incompatibilities:
• Increased theophylline plasma levels: allopurinol, disulfiram, frusemide, thiabendazole, oral contraceptives cimetidine, propranolol, erythromycin, viloxazine, mexiletine, ciprofloxacin, enoxacin, norfloxacin, diltiazem, verapamil
• Increased clearance of theophylline: barbiturates, carbamazepine, lithium, phenytoin, rifampicin, aminoglutethimide, sulphinpyrazone, smoking, alcohol, primidone, interferon

• Increased risk of arrhythmias with: halothane
• Increased risk of hypokalaemia with: β-agonists
• Reduced plasma levels of: lithium
• Antagonism of: adenosine

Clinical assessment:
• Theophylline blood levels (therapeutic level is 10−20 mg/litre); toxicity may occur with small increase above 20 mg/litre

NURSING CONSIDERATIONS

Assess:
• Baseline vital signs

Administer:
• By mouth; with or after meals to decrease GI symptoms; absorption may be affected
• Swallow modified release tablets whole at prescribed regular intervals

Evaluate:
• Heart rate; tachycardia can occur
• Monitor fluid balance; diuresis occurs, dehydration may result in elderly or children
• Respiratory rate, rhythm, depth
• Allergic reactions: rash, urticaria; if these occur, consult medical staff; drug may be discontinued

Teach patient/family:
• Avoid non-prescribed medications that contain theophylline or its derivatives
• To avoid hazardous activities; dizziness may occur
• Aspects of drug therapy: dosage, routes, side effects, when to notify the clinician
• If GI upset occurs, to take drug with water; seek advice if nausea/vomiting persists
• To swallow tablets whole

thiabendazole

Mintezol
Func. class.: Anthelmintic
Chem. class.: Benzimadazole derivative
Legal class.: POM

Action: Inhibits vital enzyme in worm

Uses: Strongyloidiasis, trichinosis, cutaneous and visceral larva migrans, dracontiasis; secondary treatment for threadworm when mixed with above infestations; adjunct in hookworm, whipworm, roundworm

Dosage and routes:
• *Adult and child:* By mouth 25 mg/kg (maximum 1.5 g) twice a day for variable number of days according to disease:
Strongyloides
• 2 days
Cutaneous larva migrans
• 2 days, repeated if necessary
Visceral larva migrans
• 7 days
Trichinosis
• 2−4 days
Dracontiasis
• 1 day (double dose in multiple infection)

Side effects/adverse reactions:
SYST: Anaphylaxis, collapse, angioneurotic oedema
GU: Haematuria, nephrotoxicity, crystalluria, enuresis, abnormal smell of urine
INTEG: Rash, pruritus, fever, flushing, perinal rash, dry mucous membranes, Stevens−Johnson syndrome
CNS: Dizziness, headache, drowsiness, weariness, irritability, convulsions, behavioural changes
EENT: Tinnitus, blurred vision, xanthopsia
GI: Nausea, vomiting, anorexia,

diarrhoea, jaundice, liver damage, epigastric distress
CV: Hypotension
HAEM: Transient leucopenia
Contraindications: Hypersensitivity, pregnancy, lactation
Precautions: Severe malnutrition, hepatic disease, renal disease, anaemia, severe dehydration
Pharmacokinetics
By mouth: Well absorbed, peak 1−2 hr, metabolised completely by liver, excreted in faeces, urine
Interactions/incompatibilities:
• Increased plasma levels of: theophylline, other xanthines
Treatment of overdose: Induce emesis or gastric lavage, supportive treatment, no specific antidote
NURSING CONSIDERATIONS
Assess:
• Stools periodically during entire treatment; gloves must be worn when handling stools
Administer:
• By mouth with meals to avoid GI symptoms chewed before swallowing
Teach patient/family:
• Proper hygiene after bowel movement including handwashing technique; tell patient to avoid putting fingers in mouth
• To observe diet and fluid intake
• That infected person should sleep alone and change bed linen daily
• Not to shake bed clothing
• To take a bath or shower with hot water each morning
• To clean toilet daily with disinfectant
• To wear gloves when handling stools
• Need for compliance with dosage schedule, duration of treatment
• To drink fruit juice to remove mucus that intestinal tapeworms burrow in; aids in expulsion of worms

• To avoid hazardous activities if drowsiness occurs
• To wash all fruit and vegetables
• To wear shoes

thiamine HCl (vitamin B₁)

NHS Benerva, many combination products, (Parentrovite injection)
Func. class.: Vitamin B₁
Chem. class.: Water-soluble vitamin
Legal class.: Tablets P; Injection POM

Action: Used for pyruvate metabolism
Uses: Thiamine deficiency: beri-beri, Wernicke-Korsakoff syndrome; prophylactic in impaired absorption or where requirements are increased
Dosage and routes:
Prophylaxis
• *Adult:* By mouth 3−10 mg daily
Mild chronic deficiency
• By mouth 10−25 mg daily
Severe deficiency
• By mouth 200−300 mg daily
Seek specialist advice for dosage by injection
Available forms include: Tablets 25, 50, 100, 300 mg; injection IM, IV 250 mg (as part of vitamins B and C injection). Many combination products
Side effects/adverse reactions:
CNS: Weakness, restlessness
INTEG: Angioneurotic oedema, cyanosis, sweating, warmth (all primarily after injection)
SYST: Anaphylaxis (primarily after injection)
Contraindications: Hypersensitivity
Pharmacokinetics: Unused amounts excreted in urine (unchanged)
NURSING CONSIDERATIONS

Assess:
• Thiamine level
• Prophylactic or therapeutic treatment

Administer:
• Tablets orally with a drink or food
• Dilution with normal saline for IV infusion. Flush tubing before and after
• Intramuscular and intravenous preparation are combined vitamin preparations, and may not be interchangeable

NB: Do not give IM as an IV injection. IM rotate deep muscle sites. IV inject slowly into vein

Perform/provide:
• Storage of injections in light-resistant container and refrigerate
• Local treatment for any painful muscle sites after injection

Evaluate:
• Therapeutic response: absence of nausea, vomiting, anorexia, insomnia, tachycardia, paraesthesia, depression, muscle weakness
• After IM and IV treatment observe patient for anaphylaxis; cyanosis, sweating

Teach patient/family:
• To eat varied diet rich in vitamin B, includes yeast, pulses, whole wheat, vegetables
• To seek help for alcoholism
• Not to discontinue treatment without medical advice

---

thiethylperazine maleate, thiethylperazine malate

Torecan
Func. class.: Anti-emetic
Chem. class.: Phenothiazine, piperazine derivative
Legal class.: POM

Action: Acts centrally by blocking chemoreceptor trigger zone, which in turn acts on vomiting centre

Uses: Severe nausea, vomiting, vertigo, labyrinthine disorders

Dosage and routes:
• *Adult:* By mouth/IM 10 mg two to three times a day; rectally 10 mg morning and at bedtime
Available forms include: Tablets 10 mg; suppositories 10 mg; injection (as malate) 10 mg/ml

Side effects/adverse reactions:
CNS: Euphoria, depression, drowsiness, somnolence, tardive dyskinesia, restlessness, tremor, convulsions, extrapyramidal symptoms
GI: Constipation, cramps, liver damage
CV: Circulatory failure, postural hypotension
RESP: Respiratory depression
SYST: Neuroleptic malignant syndrome
EENT: Nasal congestion

Contraindications: Hypersensitivity to phenothiazines, severely depressed or coma states, children under 15 yr

Precautions: Pregnancy, elderly, lactation, young adults

Pharmacokinetics:
By mouth: Onset 45−60 min
Rectal: Onset 45−60 min, metabolised by liver, excreted by kidneys, excreted in breast milk

Interactions/incompatibilities:
• Decreased effect of thiethylperazine: antacids
• Increased anticholinergic action: anticholinergics, tricyclic antidepressants
• Potentiates effect of sedatives and alcohol
• Enhanced hypotensive effect with: anaesthetics, antihypertensives
• Antagonism of: dopaminergic antiparkinsonians, anticonvulsants (lowered seizure threshold)
• Increased risk of extrapyramidal effects and possibly neurotoxicity with: lithium

• Do not mix with other drug in syringe or solution

Clinical assessment:
• Withdraw treatment if tardive dyskinesia, neuroleptic malignant syndrome develops

Treatment of overdose: Gastric lavage, supportive · treatment, diazepam for convulsions, anticholinergic for severe extrapyramidal symptoms

NURSING CONSIDERATIONS
Assess:
• Severity of vomiting
• Vital signs, BP; check patients with cardiac disease more often

Administer:
• IM injection in large muscle mass

Evaluate:
• Therapeutic response: absence of nausea, vomiting
• Respiratory status before, during, after administration of emetic; check rate, rhythm, character; respiratory depression can occur rapidly with elderly or debilitated patients

Teach patient/family:
• Avoid hazardous activities, activities requiring alertness; dizziness may occur

---

thioguanine

Lanvis
Func. class.: Cytotoxic agent
Chem. class.: Purine analogue
Legal class.: POM

Action: Interferes with synthesis, utilization of purine nucleotides; effect is related to substitution of defective ribonucleotides into DNA

Uses: Acute myeloblastic, acute lymphoblastic and chronic granulocytic leukaemias

Dosage and routes:
• *Adult and child:* By mouth 2–2.5 mg/kg/day initially usually in combination with other cytotoxic agents

Available forms include: Tablets 40 mg

Side effects/adverse reactions:
HAEM: Thrombocytopenia, leucopenia, anaemia
GI: Nausea, vomiting, anorexia, diarrhoea, stomatitis, hepatotoxicity, gastritis
GU: Renal failure, hyperuricaemia, oliguria, haematuria, crystalluria
INTEG: Rash, dermatitis, dry skin
SYST: Fever

Contraindications: Prior drug resistance, lactation

Precautions: Liver disease, bone marrow suppression, concurrent infections, pregnancy, potential carcinogen, teratogen

Pharmacokinetics: Oral form absorbed only 30%, metabolised in liver, excreted in urine as metabolites

Interactions/incompatibilities:
• Increased toxicity: radiation, other anti-neoplastics

Clinical assessment:
• Full blood count, differential, platelet count at least weekly; withhold drug if excessive myelosuppression occurs
• Renal function tests, during therapy
• Liver function tests before, during therapy

Treatment of overdose: Gastric lavage, monitor blood picture. Supportive treatment including transfusion, filgrastim

NURSING CONSIDERATIONS
Assess:
• Baseline vital signs, fluid balance

Administer:
• In accordance with local cytotoxic policy
• Other medications by oral route if possible; avoid IM, subcutaneous, IV routes to prevent infections

• Antacid before oral agent; give drug after evening meal before bedtime
• Anti-emetic 30−60 min before giving drug to prevent vomiting
• Allopurinol or sodium bicarbonate to maintain uric acid levels, alkalinisation of urine
• Antibiotics for prophylaxis of infection

Perform/provide:
• Strict medical asepsis, protective isolation if WBC levels are low
• Increase fluid intake to 2−3 litres/day to prevent urate deposits, calculi formation, unless contraindicated
• Strict oral hygiene with prescribed mouth washes
• Nutritious diet with iron, vitamin supplements as ordered

Evaluate:
• Fluid balance. Report fall in urine output to less than 30 ml/hr
• Temperature 4 hrly. Increase may indicate beginning of infection
• Bleeding: haematuria, bruising, petechiae, mucosa or orifices 8 hrly
• Hepatotoxicity: yellowing of skin, sclera, dark urine, clay-coloured stools, pruritus, abdominal pain, fever, diarrhoea
• Buccal cavity 8 hrly for dryness, sores, ulceration, white patches, oral pain, bleeding, dysphagia
• Symptoms indicating severe allergic reaction: rash, urticaria, itching, flushing

Teach patient/family:
• Why protective isolation precautions are needed
• To report any complaints, side effects to nurse or clinician: black tarry stools, chills, fever, sore throat, bleeding, bruising, cough, shortness of breath, dark, bloody urine
• To avoid foods with citric acid, hot or rough texture if stomatitis is present
• To report stomatitis: any bleeding, white spots, ulcerations in mouth; tell patient to examine mouth daily, report symptoms
• Contraceptive measures are recommended during therapy
• To drink 10−12 glasses of fluid/day
• To avoid vigorous brushing of teeth

thiopentone sodium

Intraval Sodium, Add-A-Med Thiopentone, Min-I-Mix Thiopentone
Func. class.: Anaesthetic, general
Chem. class.: Barbiturate
Legal class.: POM

Action: Acts by depressing CNS to produce anaesthesia

Uses: Short general anaesthesia, induction anaesthesia before other anaesthetics

Dosage and routes:
• *Adult:* IV 100−150 mg (4−6 ml of 2.5% solution) over 10−15 secs repeated if necessary after 30 sec; *or* up to 4 mg/kg
• *Child:* Induction IV 4−8 mg/kg
Available forms include: Powder for injection IV 2.5 g/100 ml diluent (2.5%), 5.0 g/200 ml diluent (2.5%), 0.5 g/20 ml diluent (2.5%), 1 g/20 ml diluent (5%)

Side effects/adverse reactions:
RESP: Respiratory depression, bronchospasm
CNS: Retrograde amnesia, prolonged somnolence
CV: Tachycardia, hypotension, myocardial depression, arrhythmias
EENT: Sneezing, coughing, laryngeal spasm
INTEG: Chills, *shivering*, necrosis and pain at injection site, rash,
MS: Arthralgia
SYST: Fever, allergic reactions

Contraindications: Hypersensitivity, porphyria

Precautions: Drug addiction, elderly, adrenocortical insufficiency, cachexia and severe toxaemia, diabetes, raised plasma potassium or urea, severe cardiovascular disease, renal disease, hypotension, liver disease, myxoedema, dehydration, thyrotoxicosis, myasthenia gravis, asthma, increased intracranial pressure, muscular dystrophies, pregnancy, hypovolaemia, severe anaemia, status asthmaticus, severe haemorrhage, burns

Pharmacokinetics:
IV: Onset 30−40 sec; half-life 4−12 hr metabolised in liver

Interactions/incompatibilities:
• Increased action of thiopentone: CNS depressants, sulphonamides
• Do not mix with any other drug in solution or syringe
• Increased risk of arrhythmias with: tricyclic antidepressants, verapamil
• Increased hypotension with: antihypertensives, antipsychotics, β-blockers, verapamil

Treatment of overdose: Supportive
NURSING CONSIDERATIONS
Assess:
• Starvation status
• Vital signs and conciousness level before and 3−5 min after administration

Administer:
• Only with resuscitative equipment nearby
• IV slowly
• Discard unused solution within 24 hr
• Do not mix with any other drug in solution or syringe

Perform/provide:
• Sterile water to reconstitute powder

Evaluate:
• Therapeutic response to induction
• Arrhythmias or myocardial depression

• Signs of hypotension or bronchospasm in asthmatics
Teach patient/family:
• That patient will feel drowsy, disoriented before 'falling asleep'

---

thioridazine HCl

Melleril
Func. class.: Antipsychotic, neuroleptic
Chem. class.: Phenothiazine, piperidine
Legal class.: POM

Action: Depresses cerebral cortex, hypothalamus, limbic system, which control activity, aggression; blocks neurotransmission produced by dopamine at synapse; exhibits strong α-adrenergic, anticholinergic blocking action; mechanism for antipsychotic effects is unclear. Less sedating; produces less extrapyramidal effects than other phenothiazines
Uses: Psychotic disorders, schizophrenia, severe behavioral problems in children, (alcohol withdrawal), agitation in elderly, short-term adjunct in anxiety
Dosage and routes:
Psychosis
• *Adult:* By mouth 150−600 mg daily in divided doses, maximum dose 800 mg a day in hospitalised patients (maximum 4 weeks) dose is gradually increased to desired response, then reduced to minimum maintenance
Severe mental/behavioural problems, non-psychotic emotional disturbances
• *Adult:* By mouth 75−200 mg daily
• *Child 1−5 yr:* By mouth 1 mg/kg daily
• *5−12 yr:* By mouth 75−150 mg daily (severe cases up to 300 mg daily)

Anxiety, agitation in elderly
• *Adult:* By mouth 30–100 mg daily

Available forms include: Tablets 10, 25, 50, 100 mg; suspension 25, 100 mg (thioridazine base)/5 ml; syrup 25 mg/5 ml

Side effects/adverse reactions:
CNS: Extrapyramidal symptoms (rare): pseudoparkinsonism, akathisia, dystonia, tardive dyskinesia; seizures, headache, sedation, mental dulling, dizziness, confusion, agitation, excitement
HAEM: Leucopenia, agranulocytosis
INTEG: Rash, photosensitivity, dermatitis
EENT: Blurred vision, glaucoma, nasal congestion decreased visual acuity, pigmentary retinopathy
GI: Dry mouth, nausea, vomiting, anorexia, constipation, diarrhoea, jaundice, weight gain, hepatitis
GU: Urinary retention, impotence, retrograde ejaculation
ENDO: Amenorrhoea, gynaecomastia, galactorrhoea
CV: Orthostatic hypotension, hypertension, cardiac arrest, ECG changes, tachycardia, arrhythmias, oedema

Contraindications: Hypersensitivity, history of blood dyscrasias, coma, porphyria, CNS depression, children under 1 yr, lactation

Precautions: Pregnancy, hepatic disease, cardiac disease, severe respiratory disease, renal failure, parkinsonism, narrow angle, glaucoma, prostatic hypertrophy, myasthenia gravis, epilepsy, phaeochromocytoma

Pharmacokinetics:
By mouth: Onset erratic, peak 2–4 hr; metabolised by liver, excreted in urine, enters breast milk, half-life 6–40 hr

Interactions/incompatibilities:
• Enhanced sedation with: alcohol, barbiturates other CNS depressants
• Decreased absorption of thioridazine: aluminium hydroxide or magnesium hydroxide antacids
• Decreased effects of: levodopa, antiepileptics (lowered seizure threshold), dopamine agonists
• Increased risk of extrapyramidal effects and neurotoxicity with: lithium
• Increased anticholinergic effects: anticholinergics, tricyclic antidepressants
• Increased hypotensive effect: anaesthetics, antihypertensives
• Increased risk of cardiac arrhythmias with: antiarrhythmias

Clinical assessment:
• Full blood counts monthly for first 3–4 months and if any unexplained infection, fever develops
• Liver function tests before, during treatment if abnormality suspected
• Stop treatment if tardive dyskinesias develop

Lab. test interferences:
False positive: Pregnancy tests
False negative: Urinary 5-hydroxy-indolocetic acid

Treatment of overdose: Lavage if orally injested, provide an airway, supportive treatment including plasma expanders for acute hypotension

NURSING CONSIDERATIONS
Assess:
• Establish baseline BP, pulse and respiratory rate
• Urinalysis is recommended before and during prolonged therapy
Administer:
• Antimuscarinic agent, if ordered; to be used if extrapyramidal symptoms occur
Perform/provide:
• Decreased noise input by dimming lights, avoiding loud noises
• Supervised ambulation until

stabilised on medication; do not involve in strenuous exercise program because fainting is possible; patient should not stand still for long periods of time
• Increased fluids to prevent constipation
• Frequent sips of water for dry mouth
Evaluate:
• Swallowing of oral medication; check for hoarding or giving of medication to other patients
• Therapeutic response: decrease in emotional excitement, hallucinations, delusions, paranoia, reorganisation of patterns of thought, speech
• Affect, orientation, level of consciousness, reflexes, gait, coordination, sleep pattern disturbances
• BP (standing and lying) pulse and respirations 4 hrly during initial treatment; report drops of 30 mmHg
• Dizziness, faintness, palpitations, tachycardia on rising
• Extrapyramidal symptoms including akathisia (inability to sit still, no pattern to movements), tardive dyskinesia (bizarre movements of jaw, mouth, tongue, extremities), pseudoparkinsonism (rigidity, tremors, pill rolling, shuffling gait)
• Constipation, urinary retention daily; if these occur, increase bulk, water in diet
Teach patient/family:
• Postural hypotension occurs frequently; to rise from sitting or lying position gradually
• To avoid hot baths, hot showers, since hypotension may occur
• To avoid abrupt withdrawal of this drug or rapid relapse may result; drugs should be withdrawn slowly
• To avoid non-prescribed preparations (cough, hayfever, cold)

unless approved by clinician since serious drug interactions may occur; avoid use with alcohol or CNS depressants, increased drowsiness may occur
• To use a sunscreen during sun exposure to prevent burns
• Compliance with drug regimen
• Necessity for meticulous oral hygiene since oral candidiasis may occur
• To report sore throat, malaise, fever, bleeding, mouth sores; if these occur, full blood count should be drawn and drug discontinued

thiotepa

Func. class.: Anti-neoplastic
Chem. class.: Alkylating agent
Legal class.: POM

Action: Alkylates DNA, RNA; inhibits enzymes that allow synthesis of amino acids in proteins; also responsible for cross-linking DNA strands
Uses: Breast, bladder, cancer, neoplastic effusions
Dosage and routes:
Breast cancer
• *Adult:* IM 15−30 mg 3 times a week for 2 weeks or 15 mg daily for 4 days
Neoplastic effusions
• *Adult:* Intracavity 10−65 mg in 20−60 ml sterile water repeated at weekly or 2 weekly intervals
Bladder cancer
• *Adult:* Instil up to 60 mg/60 ml water instilled in bladder once weekly for 4 weeks
Available forms include: Injection 15 mg, powder for injection
Side effects/adverse reactions:
CNS: Dizziness, headache
HAEM: Thrombocytopenia, leucopenia, pancytopenia
GI: Nausea, vomiting, anorexia

GU: Cystitis and rarely haemorrhagic cystitis
INTEG: Rash, pruritus, alopecia
Contraindications: Hypersensitivity, WBC under 3000 and/or platelets under 100,000
Precautions: Radiation therapy, bone marrow suppression, pregnancy, lactation, children
Pharmacokinetics:
Onset slow, metabolised in liver, excreted in urine
Clinical assessment:
• Full blood count, differential, platelet count weekly; withhold drug if WBC is under 3000 or platelet count is under 100,000
Treatment of overdose: Gastric lavage, general supportive measures, blood transfusions if indicated
NURSING CONSIDERATIONS
Assess:
• Baseline temp, pulse, respiration, fluid balance
• Nutritional status
• Reconstitution and administration by trained personnel. NB. Should not to be handled by pregnant staff
Administer:
• Following local cytotoxic policy
• Other medications by oral route; if possible, avoid IM, subcutaneous, IV routes to prevent infections
• Anti-emetic 30−60 min before giving drug to prevent vomiting
• Antibiotics for prophylaxis of infection
Perform/provide:
• Storage in light-resistant container, refrigerate
• Strict medical asepsis, protective isolation if WBC levels are low
• Special skin care
• Nutritious diet as tolerated
• Increased fluid intake to 2−3 litres/day to prevent urate deposits, calculi formation
• Scrupulous care of catheter

• Good mouth care
• Warm compresses at injection site for inflammation
Evaluate:
• Fluid balance and adequate fluid intake
• All side effects including GI disturbance
• Skin and mucosal condition
Teach patient/family:
• Of protective isolation precautions
• To report any complaints or side effects to nurse or clinician

---

thyroxine sodium

Eltroxin
Func. class.: Thyroid hormone
Legal class.: POM

Action: Increases metabolic rates, increases cardiac output, O_2 consumption, body temperature, blood volume, growth, development at cellular level
Uses: Hypothyroidism
Dosage and routes:
• *Adult:* By mouth 0.025−0.1 mg daily, increased by 0.025−0.1 mg every 1−4 weeks until desired response; maintenance dose 0.1−0.2 mg daily
• *Elderly:* Not advised to exceed maximum by mouth 0.05 mg daily initially
• *Child:* By mouth 0.01−0.05 mg daily, may increase 0.025−0.05 mg every 1−4 weeks until desired response
Available forms include: Tablets 0.025, 0.05, 0.1 mg
Side effects/adverse reactions:
INTEG: Sweating, flushing
CNS: Insomnia, headache, restlessness
CV: Tachycardia, palpitations, arrhythmas, angina
GI: Nausea, diarrhoea
MS: Muscular weakness, cramps in skeletal muscle

Contraindications: Hypersensitivity, thyrotoxicosis

Precautions: Elderly (reduced dose may be required), angina, pectoris, hypertension, ischaemia, myocardial insufficiency, diabetes mellitus/insipidus, cardiac disease, adrenal insufficiency

Pharmacokinetics:
Peak 12−48 hr, half-life 6−7 days; distributed throughout body tissues. 100 mcg thyroxine is equivalent in activity to 20−30 mcg liothyronine or 60 mg thyroid BP

Interactions/incompatibilities:
• Decreased absorption of this drug: cholestyramine
• Increased effects of: anticoagulants, sympathomimetics, tricyclic antidepressants, phenytoin
• Toxicity: digitalis preparations, catecholamines

Clinical assessment:
• Serum thyroxine and serum thyrotrophin levels in younger patients

Treatment of overdose: Gastric lavage or emesis if patient seen within several hours of taking dose. Treatment thereafter symptomatic. Thyroxine can recommence at lower dosage after a few days

NURSING CONSIDERATIONS

Assess:
• BP, pulse before each dose
• Weight
• Pretherapy ECG

Administer:
• Orally before breakfast as a single dose to decrease sleeplessness, and adjusted at 1−4 week intervals until normal metabolism maintained
• At same time daily to maintain drug level
• Lowest dose that relieves symptoms

Perform/provide:
• Store in childproof, light-resistant container
• Removal of medication 4 weeks before radio active iodine uptake test

Evaluate:
• Therapeutic response; increase in mental and physical ability, increased weight loss, diuresis, appetite and absence of depression, constipation, peripheral oedema, cold intolerance, pale, cool, dry skin, brittle nails, alopecia, night blindness, paraesthesia, syncope, stupor, coarse hair, menorrhagia, coma, carot-enaemia, skin, rosy cheeks
• Input and output of fluids to determine fluid loss
• Weigh before and during initial treatment
• Too rapid an increase in metabolism caused by excessive dosage/overdose; restlessness insomnia, sweating, flushing, headache cardiac arrhythmias, palpitation, tachycardia, diarrhoea, excessive weight loss, cramps in skeletal muscle and muscular weekness−stop treatment

Teach patient/family:
• Report nervousness, excitability, irritability, anxiety, may indicate too large a dose/overdose
• That children show immediate behaviour personality changes
• To read drug labels and avoid non-prescribed drugs containing iodine
• To avoid iodine food, salt iodinised, soy beans, tofu, turnips, some seafood, some bread

---

tiaprofenic acid

Surgam, Surgam SA
Func. class.: Non-steroidal anti-inflammatory drug
Chem. class.: Propionic acid derivative
Legal class.: POM

Action: Has both analgesic and anti-inflammatory effects

Uses: Pain and inflammation in rheumatic disease and other musculoskeletal disorders and soft tissue injury

Dosage and routes:
• By mouth 600 mg daily in 2−3 divided doses; modified release 600 mg at night

Available forms include: Tablets 200, 300 mg; capsules modified release 300 mg

Side effects/adverse reactions:
GI: Discomfort constipation, flatulence, bleeding, nausea, diarrhoea, dyspepsia, vomiting, anorexia, stomatitis
CV: Angioneurotic oedema
CNS: Headache, drowsiness
RESP: Asthma
INTEG: Rashes, photosensitivity, pruritus, alopecia
META: Fluid retention

Contraindications: Active peptic ulceration, children, hypersensitivity

Precautions: Elderly patients, history of peptic ulceration, allergic disorders, asthma, renal, cardiac, hepatic impairment (reduce dosage to 200 mg twice daily), pregnancy

Pharmacokinetics:
Readily absorbed from GI tract. Short half-life of 2 hr, highly bound to plasma protein. Excreted predominantly in the urine with smaller amounts in the bile

Interactions/incompatibilities:
Anticoagulants, antihypertensives, cardiac glycosides, diuretics, hypoglycaemic agents, phenytoin, lithium

Clinical assessment:
• Renal and liver function tests, blood studies before treatment, periodically thereafter: blood urea, creatinine, aspartate aminotransferase, alanine aminotransferase, Hb

NURSING CONSIDERATIONS
Administer:
• With food or milk to decrease GI symptoms

Evaluate:
• Therapeutic response: decreased pain, stiffness, swelling in joints, ability to move more easily

Teach patient/family:
• To report change in urine pattern, weight increase, oedema, pain increase in joints, fever, blood in urine (indicates nephrotoxicity)
• Report any unresolved indigestion or black tarry stools

---

ticarcillin disodium

Ticar
Func. class.: Antibiotic, antipseudomonal
Chem. class.: Broad-spectrum penicillin
Legal class.: POM

Action: Interferes with cell wall replication of susceptible organisms; osmotically unstable cell wall swells, bursts from osmotic pressure

Uses: Respiratory, soft tissue, urinary tract infections, bacterial septicaemia, general system infections, peritonitis, intra-abdominal sepsis, endocarditis effective for Gram-positive cocci (*S. aureus, S. faecalis, S. pneumoniae*), Gram-negative cocci (*N. gonorrhoeae*), Gram-positive bacilli (*C. perfringens, C. tetani*), Gram-negative bacilli (*Bacteroides* spp, *F. nucleatum, E. coli, P. mirabilis, Salmonella* spp, *M. morganii, P. rettgeri, Enterobacter* spp, *P. aeruginosa, Serratia* spp, *Peptococcus* spp, *Peptostreptococcus* spp, *Eubacterium* spp)

Dosage and routes:
• *Adult:* IV/IM 15−20 g daily in divided doses every 4−8 hr, infuse over ½−2 hr. For the treatment of uncomplicated urinary tract infec-

tions 3−4 g daily in divided doses every 4−8 hr
• *Child:* IV/IM 200−300 mg/kg daily in divided doses every 4−8 hr. For treatment of uncomplicated urinary tract infections 50−100 mg/kg daily in divided doses every 4−8 hr
Available forms include: Injection IM, IV 1, 5 g; IV infusion 5 g
Side effects/adverse reactions:
HAEM: Increased bleeding time, eosinophilia
GI: Nausea, vomiting, diarrhoea
META: Hypokalaemia
INTEG: Skin rashes
Contraindications: Hypersensitivity to penicillins
Precautions: Pregnancy, renal dysfunction (reduce dosage)
Pharmacokinetics:
IM: Peak 1 hr, duration 4−6 hr
IV: Peak 30−45 min, duration 4 hr, Half-life 70 min, small amount metabolised in liver, excreted in urine, breast milk
Interactions/incompatibilities:
• Increased antimicrobial effect of this drug: aminoglycosides, may be due to synergy
• Increased penicillin concentrations: probenecid
Clinical assessment:
• Blood studies: WBC, RBC, bleeding time
• Renal studies: urinalysis, protein, blood
• Culture and sensitivity before drug therapy
• Do not mix in some syringe with aminoglycosides
Treatment of overdose: Drug removed by haemodialysis, symptomatic support as required, increased risk of bleeding
NURSING CONSIDERATIONS
Assess:
• Baseline pattern
• Fluid balance
• Allergies before initiation of treatment, reaction of each medication; highlight allergies on patient's chart
Administer:
• By slow IV or infusion, lower doses
Perform/provide:
• Storage at 2 to 8°C; reconstituted solution for 24 hr at room temperature or 3 days refrigerated
Evaluate:
• Therapeutic response: absence of fever, purulent drainage, redness, inflammation
• Bowel pattern during treatment
• Fluid balance; report haematuria, oliguria since penicillin in high doses is nephrotoxic
• Skin eruptions after administration of penicillin to 1 week after discontinuing drug
Teach patient/family:
• To report sore throat, fever, fatigue: could indicate superimposed infection
• To wear or carry ID if allergic to penicillins

ticarcillin disodium/ clavulanate potassium

Timentin
Func. class.: Antibiotic, antipseudomonal
Chem. class.: Broad-spectrum penicillin
Legal class.: POM

Action: Interferes with cell wall replication of susceptible organisms; osmotically unstable cell wall swells, bursts from osmotic pressure
Uses: Respiratory, soft tissue, and urinary tract infections, bacterial septicaemia, general systemic infections, peritonitis, intra-abdominal sepsis, endocarditis, effective for gram-positive cocci (*S. aureus, S. faecalis, S. pneumoniae*), gram-negative cocci

(*N. gonorrhoeae*), gram-positive bacilli (*C. perfringens, C. tetani*), gram-negative bacilli (*Bacteroides, F. nucleatum, E. coli, P. mirabilis, Salmonella, M. morganii, P. rettgeri, Enterobacter, P. aeruginosa, Serratia, Peptococcus, Peptostreptococcus, Eubacterium*)

Dosage and routes:
• *Adult:* IV infusion 1 vial containing ticarcillin 3 g, clavulanate potassium 0.2 g every 4−8 hr, infuse over 30 min
• *Child:* 80 mg/kg every 6−8 hr; in infants 80 mg/kg every 12 hr during perinatal period
Available forms include: Injection IM, IV, 1.6 g and 3.2 g

Side effects/adverse reactions:
HAEM: Increased bleeding time, eosinophilia
GI: Nausea, vomiting, diarrhoea, hepatitis, cholestatic jaundice
INTEG: Skin rash
META: Hypokalaemia
Contraindications: Hypersensitivity to penicillins
Precautions: Neonates, severe hepatic dysfunction, renal impairment (reduce dosage)

Pharmacokinetics:
IV: Peak 30−45 min, duration 4 hr, half-life 64−68 min. Both components are well distributed in body fluids and tissue

Interactions/incompatibilities:
• Increased antimicrobial effect of this drug: aminoglycosides IV (mixed) due to synergy
• Increased penicillin concentrations: probenecid

Clinical assessment:
• Liver function tests
• Blood studies: WBC, RBC, hct, bleeding time
• Renal tests: urinalysis, protein, blood
• Culture and sensitivity before drug therapy
Treatment of overdose: Increased rate of bleeding, may be removed from circulation by dialysis

NURSING CONSIDERATIONS
Assess:
• Allergies before initiation of treatment, reaction of each medication; highlight allergies on chart, Kardex
• Fluid balance
• Bowel pattern
• Previous hypersensitivity to penicillins
Administer:
• After sample has been sent for culture and sensitivity
Perform/provide:
• Storage at room temperature, reconstituted solution for up to 24 hr at room temperature in water for injections or 3 days refrigerated
Evaluate:
• Therapeutic response: absence of fever, purulent drainage, redness, inflammation
• Bowel pattern before, during treatment
• Fluid balance; report haematuria, oliguria since penicillin in high doses is nephrotoxic
• Any patient with compromised renal system, since drug is excreted slowly in poor renal system function; toxicity may occur rapidly
• Skin eruptions after administration of penicillin to 1 week after discontinuing drug
• Respiratory status: rate, character, wheezing, and tightness in chest
Teach patient/family:
• To report sore throat, fever, fatigue; could indicate superimposed infection
• To wear or carry ID if allergic to penicillins

timolol maleate (ophthalmic)

Timoptol
Func. class.: Antihypertensive, ocular
Chem. class.: Non-selective β-adrenergic blocker
Legal class.: POM

Action: Reduces production of aqueous humour

Uses: Elevated intra-ocular pressure, chronic open-angle glaucoma, secondary glaucoma, aphakic glaucoma, ocular hypertension

Dosage and routes:
• *Adult:* Instil 1 drop of 0.25% solution in affected eye twice a day, then 1 drop for maintenance; may increase to 1 drop of 0.5% solution twice a day if needed

Available forms include: Solution 0.25%, 0.5%

Side effects/adverse reactions:
CV: Bradycardia, arrhythmia, hypotension, syncope, heart block, CVA, cerebral ischaemia, congestive heart failure, palpitation, cardiac arrest
RESP: Bronchospasm, respiratory failure, dyspnoea
CNS: Weakness, fatigue, depression, anxiety, headache, confusion
EENT: Eye irritation, conjunctivitis, keratitis, visual disturbances
INTEG: Rash, urticaria

Contraindications: Hypersensitivity, asthma, 2nd/3rd degree heart block, severe obstructive pulmonary disease, sinus bradycardia, cardiac failure, cardiogenic shock, children

Precautions: Pregnancy, soft contact lenses

Pharmacokinetics:
INSTIL: Onset 15−30 min, peak 1−2 hr, duration 24 hr

NURSING CONSIDERATIONS

Teach patient/family:
• To report change in vision, with blurring or loss of sight, trouble breathing, sweating, flushing
• Method of instillation, and not to touch dropper to eye
• That long-term therapy may be required
• That blurred vision will decrease with continued use of drug
• Discard remaining eye drops 28 days after opening

timolol maleate

Blocadren, Betim, Prestim, Moducren
Func. class.: Antihypertensive
Chem. class.: Non-selective β-blocker
Legal class.: POM

Action: Competitively blocks stimulation of β-adrenergic receptor within vascular smooth muscle; produces chronotropic, inotropic activity (decreases rate of SA node discharge, increases recovery time), slows conduction of AV node, decreases heart rate, which decreases O_2 consumption in myocardium; also, decreases renin−aldosterone−angiotensin system, at high doses inhibits β2 receptors in bronchial system

Uses: Mild to moderate hypertension, prophylaxis after infarction, prophylaxis of angina pectoris, migraine

Dosage and routes:
Hypertension
• *Adult:* By mouth 5 mg twice a day, or 10 mg daily, may increase by 10 mg every 2−3 days, not to exceed 60 mg/day
Angina
• *Adult:* By mouth initially 5 mg two to three times a day maintenance 15−45 mg daily
Myocardial infarction
• *Adult:* 5 mg twice a day initially

then 10 mg twice a day 7−28 days after infarction (acute phase)

Migraine prophylaxis
- *Adult:* By mouth 10−20 mg daily

Available forms include: Tablets 10 mg

Side effects/adverse reactions:

CV: Hypotension, bradycardia, heart failure, heart block, coldness of limb extremities

CNS: Insomnia, dizziness, hallucinations, fatigue, insomnia, depression, paraesthesiae, disorientation, vertigo, nightmares

GI: Nausea, vomiting, abdominal pain, retroperitoneal fibrosis

INTEG: Rash, pruritus

RESP: Bronchospasm, dyspnoea

MS: Arthralgia

Contraindications: Hypersensitivity to β-blockers, cardiogenic shock, heart block (2nd, 3rd degree), sinus bradycardia, cardiac failure. Bronchospasm, severe pulmonary disease, asthma, patients on MAOIs, sicksinus syndrome, peripleural vascular disease, Raynaud's disease, congestive heart failure

Precautions: Pregnancy, lactation, diabetes mellitus, renal disease, cardiac failure/insufficiency, children

Pharmacokinetics:

By mouth: Peak 2−4 hr; half-life 3−4 hr, excreted 30%−45% unchanged, 60%−65% is metabolised by liver, excreted in breast milk

Interactions/incompatibilities:
- Increased hypotension, bradycardia: reserpine, hydralazine, methyldopa, prazosin, anticholinergics, alcohol, anaesthetics, anti-arrhythmics
- Decreased antihypertensive effects: indomethacin, NSAIDs
- Increased hypoglycaemic effects: insulin, anti-diabetics
- Decreased bronchodilation: theophyllines

Clinical assessment:
- Baselines in renal, liver function tests before therapy begins
- Reduced dosage in renal dysfunction

Treatment of overdose: Lavage, activated charcoal, IV atropine for bradycardia, IV β_2 stimulants for bronchospasm, administer vasopressor (noradrenaline), glucagon can reverse the effects of excessive beta blockade

NURSING CONSIDERATIONS

Assess:
- Baseline vital signs, weight and fluid balance
- Apex/radial pulse before administration; notify clinician of any significant changes

Administer:
- Orally, before meals, before bedtime

Perform/provide:
- Storage in dry area in a cool place, do not freeze

Evaluate:
- Therapeutic response: decreased BP after 1−2 weeks
- Oedema in feet, legs daily
- Fluid balance, weight daily if at risk of heart failure
- BP, pulse 4 hrly; note rate, rhythm, quality

Teach patient/family:
- Not to discontinue drug abruptly
- Not to use non-prescribed products containing α-adrenergic stimulants (nasal decongestants, cold preparations) unless directed by clinician/pharmacist
- To report bradycardia, dizziness, confusion, depression, fever, sore throat, shortness of breath to clinician
- To avoid alcohol, smoking, high sodium intake
- To avoid hazardous activities if dizziness is present
- To report symptoms of congestive heart failure: difficult breathing, especially on exertion or when

lying down, night cough, swelling of extremities
• Take medication at bedtime to decrease effect of postural hypotension if it occurs

tinidazole

Fasigyn
Func. class.: Antibiotic
Chem. class.: Imidazole
Legal class.: POM

Action: Penetration of the drug into the cell of the micro-organism and subsequent damage of DNA strands or inhibition of their synthesis
Uses: Anaerobic bacterial and protozoal infections
Dosage and routes:
Anaerobic infections
• *Adult and child over 12 yr:* By mouth initially 2 g as single dose, then 1 g daily, as single or 2 equal doses, for 5−6 days
Non-specific vaginitis, trichomoniasis, giardiasis, acute ulcerative gingivitis
• *Adult:* By mouth 2 g as single dose possible to repeat dose on day 2
• *Child:* By mouth 50−75 mg/kg as single dose may repeat dose
Intestinal amoebiasis
• *Adult:* By mouth 2 g/day for 2−3 days
• *Child:* By mouth 50−60 mg/kg/day for 3 days
Amoebic involvement of liver
• *Adult:* By mouth 1.5−2 g daily for 3−5 days
• *Child:* By mouth 50−60 mg/kg/day for 5 days
Prophylaxis of infection in abdominal surgery
• *Adult and children over 12 yr:* By mouth 2 g as single dose approx 12 hr before surgery

Available forms include: Tablets 500 mg
Side effects/adverse reactions:
CNS: Headache, drowsiness
HAEM: Leucopenia
GI: Nausea, vomiting, furry tongue, anorexia, metallic taste, diarrhoea
INTEG: Rashes, pruritus, urticaria, angioneurotic oedema
GU: Dark urine
Contraindications: Blood dyscrasias; organic neurological disorders, hypersensitivity; pregnancy, lactation
Precautions: Hepatic impairment
Pharmacokinetics: Completely absorbed through GI tract, peak plasma levels after 2 hr. Half-life is 12−14 hr. Plasma protein binding is approximately 12%
Interactions/incompatibilities:
• Reduced effect of: phenobarbitone
• Potentiation: nicoualone, phenytoin, warfarin, lithium
• Increased plasma concentrations: cimetidine
• Psychotic reactions: alcohol, disulfiram
Clinical assessment:
• Full blood count
Treatment of overdose:
• Gastric lavage if soon after ingestion
• Symptomatic and supportive treatment
NURSING CONSIDERATIONS
Administer:
• Tablets with or after food to minimise GI disturbances
Perform/provide:
• Mouthwashes to relieve furry tongue
Evaluate:
• Dizziness, lack of coordination, pruritus, joint pains. Discontinue drug
• Allergic reactions—fever, rigour, rash, itching. Discontinue drug

Teach patient/family:
- Take tablets with or after food
- Urine may turn dark red−brown
- Avoid alcohol−it may cause vomiting and abdominal cramps
- Proper hygiene and handwashing following bowel movements
- Report any side effects to clinician
- Check with clinician before taking non-prescribed preparations

---

tobramycin (ophthalmic)

Tobralex
Func. class.: Antibiotic
Chem. class.: Aminoglycoside
Legal class.: POM

Action: Inhibits bacterial cell wall in organism by preventing amino acid and nucleotide incorporation into cell wall

Uses: Infection of eye

Dosage and routes:
- *Adult and child:* Instil 1−2 drops every 1−4 hr depending on infection

Available forms include: Solution 0.3%

Side effects/adverse reactions:
EENT: Lid itching, conjunctival erythema

Contraindications: Hypersensitivity, use of soft contact lenses

Precautions: Antibiotic hypersensitivity, prolonged use may result in antibiotic overgrowth of non-susceptible organisms including fungi

NURSING CONSIDERATIONS

Administer:
- After samples have been sent for culture and sensitivity
- After washing hands, cleanse crusts or discharge from eye before application
- Apply pressure on lacrimal sac for 1 min

Perform/provide:
- Storage of eye drops at 8−25°C, discard 28 days after opening, sterile until opened

Evaluate:
- Therapeutic response: absence of redness, inflammation, tearing
- Allergy: itching, lacrimation, redness, swelling

Teach patient/family:
- To use drug exactly as prescribed
- Not to use eye make-up, towels, washcloths, and eye medication of others, or reinfection may occur
- That drug container tip should not be touched to eye
- To report itching, increased redness, burning, stinging; drug should be discontinued
- That drug may cause blurred vision when ointment is applied
- Discard 28 days after opening

---

tobramycin sulphate

Nebcin
Func. class.: Antibiotic
Chem. class.: Aminoglycoside
Legal class.: POM

Action: Interferes with protein synthesis in bacterial cell by binding to ribosomal subunit, causing inaccurate peptide sequence to form in protein chain, causing bacterial death

Uses: Severe systemic infections of CNS, respiratory, GI, urinary tract, bone, skin, soft tissues caused by susceptible organisms

Dosage and routes:
- *Adult:* IM/IV 3 mg/kg/day in divided doses every 8 hr; may give up to 5 mg/kg/day in divided doses every 6−8 hr
- *Child:* IM/IV 6−7.5 mg/kg/day in 3−4 equally divided doses
- *Neonates under 1 week:* IM up to 4 mg/kg/day in divided doses every 12 hr; IV up to 4 mg/kg/day in divided doses every 12 hr diluted

in 50−100 ml 0.9% sodium chlorid or Dextrose 5%, given over 20−60 min

Available forms include: Injection IM, IV 10, 40 mg/ml. Volume of diluent for adults 50−100 ml; for children, should be proportionately less

Side effects/adverse reactions:

GU: Oliguria, haematuria, renal damage, proteinuria, renal failure, nephrotoxicity

CNS: Confusion, vertigo, numbness, headache, fever

EENT: Ototoxicity, deafness, visual disturbances, tinnitis

HAEM: Agranulocytosis, thrombocytopenia, leucopenia, eosinophilia, anaemia

GI: Nausea, vomiting, diarrhoea, increased aspartate aminotransferase, alanine aminotransferase, bilirubin

INTEG: Rash, burning, urticaria

Contraindications: Intrathecal administration, hypersensitivity

Precautions: Neonates, renal disease (reduce dose) pregnancy, myasthenia gravis, lactation, hearing deficits parkinsonism, extensive burns

Pharmacokinetics:

IM: Onset rapid, peak 1−2 hr

IV: Onset immediate, peak 1−2 hr. Plasma half-life 1−3 hr, not metabolised, excreted unchanged in urine

Interactions/incompatibilities:

• Increased ototoxicity, neurotoxicity, nephrotoxicity: other aminoglycosides, amphotericin B, polymyxin, vancomycin, ethacrynic acid, frusemide, mannitol, cisplatin, cephalosporins

• Do not mix in solution or syringe: carbenicillin, ticarcillin, amphotericin B, cephalothin, erythromycin, heparin

• Increased effects: non-depolarising muscle relaxants

Clinical assessment:

• Serum peak, drawn at 30−60 min after IV infusion or 60 min after IM injection, trough level drawn just before next dose; blood level should not exceed 12 mg/l for prolonged periods; trough levels above 2 mg/l may indicate tissue accumulation

Treatment of overdose: Haemodialysis, monitor serum levels of drug

NURSING CONSIDERATIONS

Assess:

• Fluid balance

• Bowel pattern

• Weight before treatment; calculation of dosage is usually done based on ideal body weight, but may be calculated on actual body weight

Administer:

• After sample has been sent for culture and sensitivity

• IM injection in large muscle mass, rotate injection sites

• Drug in evenly spaced doses to maintain blood level

• Bicarbonate to alkalinise urine if ordered in treating urinary tract infection, as drug is most active in an alkaline environment

• Culture and sensitivity before starting treatment to identify infecting organism

Perform/provide:

• Adequate fluids of 2−3 litres/day unless contraindicated to prevent irritation of tubules

• Vital signs during infusion, watch for hypotension, change in pulse

• Flush IV line with or Dextrose 5% after infusion

• Supervised ambulation, other safety measures

Evaluate:

• IV site for thrombophlebitis including pain, redness, swelling ½-hrly, change site if needed; apply warm compresses to discontinued site

- Fluid balance, urinalysis daily for proteinuria, cells, casts; report sudden change in urine output
- Urine pH if drug is used for urinary tract infection; urine should be kept alkaline
- Therapeutic effect: absence of fever, draining wounds, negative culture and sensitivity after treatment
- Renal impairment (by securing urine for creatinine clearance testing)
- Deafness by audiometric testing, ringing, roaring in ears, vertigo; assess hearing before, during, after treatment
- Dehydration: decrease in skin turgor, dry mucous membranes, dark urine
- Overgrowth of infection: increased temperature, malaise, redness, pain, swelling, perineal itching, diarrhoea, stomatitis, change in cough, sputum
- Vestibular dysfunction: nausea, vomiting, dizziness, headache, drug should be discontinued if severe
- Injection and infusion sites for redness, swelling, abscesses; use warm compresses at site

Teach patient/family:
- To report headache, dizziness, symptoms of overgrowth of infection, renal impairment
- To report loss of hearing, ringing, roaring in ears, feeling of fullness in head

tocainide HCl

Tonocard
Func. class.: Anti-arrhythmic
Chem. class.: Lignocaine analogue
Legal class.: POM

Action: Increases electrical stimulation threshold of ventricale, His—Purkinje system, which stabilizes cardiac membrane

Uses: Ventricular tachycardia, arrhythmias, symptomatic and life threatening

Dosage and routes:

Acute treatment
- *Adult:* IV (slow or infusion) 500−750 mg, over 15−30 min with ECG monitoring followed by 800 mg by mouth

Maintenance
- *Adult:* By mouth 400 mg three times a day

Chronic ventricular arrhythmias
- *Adult:* 1200 mg daily in 3 divided doses increasing to 1800−2400 mg daily if required

Available forms include: Tablets 400, 600 mg IV injection 50 mg/ml

Side effects/adverse reactions:

CNS: Headache, dizziness, involuntary movement, confusion, psychosis, restlessness, irritability, paraesthesias, tremor, convulsions

EENT: Tinnitus, blurred vision, hearing loss

GI: Nausea, vomiting, anorexia, diarrhoea

CV: Hypotension, bradycardia, angina, heart block, cardiovascular collapse (at high plasma concentrations), arrest, congestive heart failure

RESP: Dyspnoea, respiratory depression

HAEM: Agranulocytosis, aplastic anaemia, thrombocytopenia

INTEG: Rash, urticaria, oedema, swelling

Contraindications: Hypersensitivity to amides, 2nd or 3rd degree AV block (in the absence of a pacemaker)

Precautions: Pregnancy, lactation, children, renal disease, liver disease, respiratory depression, myasthenia gravis, uncompensated congestive heart failure, concurrent anti-arrhythmic agents, congestive heart failure

Pharmacokinetics:

By mouth: Peak 1 hr; half-life 10−17 hr, metabolised by liver, excreted in urine

Interactions/incompatibilities:

• May increase effects when used with: propranolol, quinidine

Clinical assessment:

• Chest X-ray, pulmonary function test during treatments

• Blood count weekly during first 12 wks of treatment

• Drug blood levels (therapeutic level 4−10 mcg/ml)

• Lung fields, bilateral rales may occur in congestive heart failure patient

Lab. test interferences:

Increase: Creatinine phosphokinase

Treatment of overdose: O_2, artificial ventilation, ECG, inotropic support

NURSING CONSIDERATIONS

Assess:

• Baseline BP and fluid balance

Administer:

• IV infusion under direction of anaesthetist with resuscitation facilities available

Evaluate:

• Toxicity: fine tremors, dizziness

• Fatigue, sore throat, fever, bruising, increased temperature

• Cardiac rate, respiration: rate, rhythm, character, ½ hrly

• Fluid balance ratio; check for decreasing output

tolazamide

Tolanase
Func. class.: Hypoglycaemic, oral
Chem. class.: Sulphonylurea (1st generation)
Legal class.: POM

Action: Causes functioning β-cells in pancreas to synthesise and release insulin, leading to drop in blood glucose levels; stimulation of insulin results in increased insulin binding; this drug not effective if patient lacks functioning β-cells

Uses: Maturity onset diabetes, mild to moderate severity

Dosage and routes:

• *Adult:* By mouth 100−250 mg/day; dose should be titrated to patient response maximum 1 g daily in divided doses if necessary

Available forms include: Tablets 100, 250 mg

Side effects/adverse reactions:

CNS: Headache, weakness, fatigue, lethargy, dizziness, vertigo

GI: Nausea, vomiting, diarrhoea, constipation, flatus, hepatotoxicity, jaundice, anorexia

HAEM: Leucopenia, thrombocytopenia, agranulocytosis, aplastic anaemia, pancytopenia, haemolytic anaemia

INTEG: Rash (rare) allergic reactions, pruritus, urticaria, eczema, photo-sensitivity), erythema

ENDO: Hypoglycaemia

Contraindications: Hypersensitivity to sulphonylureas, juvenile or brittle diabetes, renal disease, hepatic disease, pregnancy, surgery, trauma, ketosis, acidosis, coma daily in divided doses

Precautions: Elderly, cardiac disease, thyroid disease, severe hypoglycaemic reactions

Pharmacokinetics:

By mouth: Completely absorbed by GI route; onset 1 hr, peak 4−

8 hr, duration 20 hr; half-life 7 hr, metabolised in liver, excreted in urine (metabolites), breast milk, highly protein bound

Interactions/incompatibilities:

• May increase effects when taken with insulin, MAOIs, cimetidine, phenylbutazone and other NSAIDs, sulphonamides, chloramphenicol, probenecid, coumarin anticoagulants, β-blockers

• Decreased action of this drug: calcium channel blockers, corticosteroids, oral contraceptives, thiaide diuretics, thyroid preparations, oestrogens, phenothiazines, phenytoin, rifampicin, isoniazid

Treatment of overdose: Conscious patient, administer glucose or 3–4 lumps of table sugar with water. Repeat if necessary. Comatosed patient, administer IV glucose infusion or glucagon 1 mg by SC or IM injection to produce consciousness

NURSING CONSIDERATIONS

Administer:

• Drug 30 min before meals

Evaluate:

• Therapeutic response: decrease in polyuria, polydipsia, polyphagia, alertness, absence of dizziness, stable gait

• Hypoglycaemic/hyperglycaemic reaction that can occur soon after meals

Teach patient/family:

• To check for symptoms of cholestatic jaundice (dark urine, pruritus, yellow sclera); if these occur notify clinician

• To use a capillary blood glucose test while on this drug

• To avoid alcohol; disulfiram type reaction with alcohol

• To test urine glucose levels approximately 2 hr after each meal

• The symptoms of hypo/hyperglycaemia, what to do about each

• That this drug must be continued on a daily basis; explain consequence of discontinuing drug abruptly

• To take drug in morning to prevent hypoglycaemic reactions at night

• To avoid non-prescribed medications

• That diabetes is a life-long illness, drug will not cure disease

• That all food included in diet plan must be eaten in order to prevent hypoglycaemia

• To carry medic alert ID as a diabetic

---

tolbutamide

Rastinon

Func. class.: Hypoglycaemic, oral
Chem. class.: Sulphonylurea
Legal class.: POM

Action: Causes functioning β-cells in pancreas to synthesise and release insulin, leading to drop in blood glucose levels; stimulation of insulin results in increased insulin binding; this drug is not effective if patient lacks functioning β-cells

Uses: Maturity onset diabetes mild to moderate; NIDDM patients who have failed to be controlled by dietary means

Dosage and routes:

• *Adult:* By mouth 0.5–1.5 g (maximum 2 g) daily in divided doses, titrated to patient response

Available forms include: Tablets 500 mg

Side effects/adverse reactions:

CNS: Headache, weakness, paraesthesia

GI: Nausea, fullness, heartburn, hepatotoxicity, cholestatic jaundice

HAEM: Leucopenia, thrombocytopenia, agranulocytosis, aplastic anaemia, increased aspartate aminotransferase, alanine amino-

transferase, alkaline phosphatase
INTEG: Rash, allergic reactions, pruritus, urticaria, eczema, photosensitivity, erythema
ENDO: Hypoglycaemia
MS: Joint pains

Contraindications: Hypersensitivity to sulphonylureas, juvenile or brittle or insulin dependent, diabetes, renal disease, hepatic disease, impairment of adrenocortical function

Precautions: Pregnancy, elderly, cardiac disease, thyroid function, previous history of ketoacidosis, surgery, trauma, pregnancy, severe hypoglycaemic reactions

Pharmacokinetics:
By mouth: Completely absorbed by GI route; onset 30−60 min, peak 3−5 hr, duration 24 hr; half-life 7 hr, metabolised in liver, excreted in urine (metabolites), breast milk, 90%−95% is plasma protein bound

Interactions/incompatibilities:
• Increased effects of this drug: insulin, MAOIs, dicoumarol, salicylates, β-blockers, sulphonamides. NSAIDs, chloramphenicol
• Decreased action of this drug: calcium channel blockers, corticosteroids, oral contraceptives, thiazide diuretics, thyroid preparations, oestrogens, adrenaline, lithium, rifampicin, cyclophosphamide

Treatment of overdose: Conscious patient, administer glucose or 3−4 lumps of table sugar with water. Repeat if necessary. If comatosed patient, administer IV glucose infusion or glucagon 1 mg by subcutaneous or IM injection to produce consciousness

NURSING CONSIDERATIONS
Administer:
• Drug 30 min before meals
Perform/provide:
• Storage in tight container in cool environment, protected from light

Evaluate:
• Therapeutic response: decrease in polyuria, polydipsia, polyphagia, alertness, absence of dizziness, stable gait
• Hypoglycaemic/hyperglycaemic reaction that can occur soon after meals

Teach patient/family:
• To check for symptoms of cholestatic jaundice (dark urine, pruritus, yellow sclera); if these occur a clinician should be notified
• To use a capillary blood glucose test while on this drug
• To test urine glucose levels approximately 2 hr after each meal
• The symptoms of hypo/hyperglycaemia; what to do about each
• That this drug must be continued on a daily basis; explain consequence of discontinuing drug abruptly
• To take drug in morning to prevent hypoglycaemic reactions at night
• To avoid non-prescribed medications
• That diabetes is a life-long illness, drug will not cure disease
• That all food included in diet plan must be eaten in order to prevent hypoglycaemia (usually low fat, low carbohydrate diet)
• To carry a radioactive iodine uptake ID for emergency purposes
• Discuss with clinician if any of the following symptoms occur: dizziness, confusion, weakness, sweating, nausea, vomiting, skin rash

tolmetin sodium

Tolectin
Func. class.: Non-steroidal anti-inflammatory agent
Chem. class.: Pyrrole acetic acid derivative
Legal class.: POM

Action: Inhibits prostaglandin synthesis by decreasing an enzyme needed for biosynthesis; possesses analgesic, anti-inflammatory, antipyretic properties

Uses: Osteoarthritis, rheumatoid arthritis, ankylosing spondylitis, fibrositis, bursitis, juvenile arthritis

Dosage and routes:
• *Adult:* By mouth 400 mg three or four times a day, maximum 30 mg/kg daily, not to exceed 1.8 g/ day in 2−4 divided doses

Juvenile arthritis
• *Child:* By mouth 20−25 mg/kg daily in 3−4 divided doses; maximum 30 mg/kg daily up to 1.8 g/day

Available forms include: Capsules 200 mg, 400 mg

Side effects/adverse reactions:
GI: Nausea, anorexia, vomiting, diarrhoea, jaundice, cholestatic hepatitis, constipation, flatulence, cramps, dry mouth, peptic ulcer
CNS: Dizziness, drowsiness, fatigue, tremors, confusion, insomnia, anxiety, depression
INTEG: Purpura, rash, pruritus, sweating
GU: Nephrotoxicity
HAEM: Blood dyscrasias
EENT: Tinnitus, hearing loss, blurred vision

Contraindications: Hypersensitivity to this drug or other anti-inflammatory drugs, asthma, active peptic ulcer, or history of upper gastrointestinal tract disease, gastrointestinal bleeding. Avoid in patients currently receiving warfarin or oral anticoagulant drugs

Precautions: Pregnancy, lactation, bleeding disorders, GI disorders, cardiac disorders, elderly, renal/hepatic disease

Interactions/incompatibilities:
• May increase action of coumarin, phenytoin, sulphonamides when used with this drug

Clinical assessment:
• Renal, liver tests, blood count: serum urea, creatinine, aspartate aminotransferase, alanine aminotransferase, Hb before treatment, periodically thereafter
• Audiometric, ophthalmic examination before, during, after treatment

NURSING CONSIDERATIONS

Administer:
• With food or milk to decrease GI symptoms

Evaluate:
• Therapeutic response: decreased pain, stiffness, swelling in joints, ability to move more easily
• For eye, ear problems: blurred vision, tinnitus (may indicate toxicity)

Teach patient/family:
• To report blurred vision or ringing, roaring in ears (may indicate toxicity)
• To avoid driving or other hazardous activities if dizziness or drowsiness occurs
• To report change in urine pattern, weight increase, oedema, pain increase in joints, fever, blood in urine (indicates nephrotoxicity)
• That therapeutic effects may take up to 1 month to develop
• Avoid over the counter preparations; these may contain Aspirin

tranexamic acid

Cyklokapron
Func. class.: Haemostatic, anti-fibrinolytic
Legal class.: POM

Action: Competitively inhibits the activation of plasminogen to plasmin

Uses: Prophylaxis and treatment of haemorrhage following prosta-tectomy, conisation of the cervix, surgery in haemophiliacs, menor-rhagia, traumatic hyphaema, management of dental extractions in haemophiliacs, hereditary angioneurotic, oedema, epistaxis, complications of thrombolysis, disseminated intravascular coagulation with predominant inacti-vation of the fibrinolytic system

Dosage and routes:
Seek specialist advice for treat-ment areas
• *Adult:* By mouth, 1−1.5 g 2−4 times daily depending on condition
• Slow IV injection, 1 g 3 times daily. Adjust dose in renal impairment

Available forms include: Tablets 500 mg, injection 100 mg/ml, syrup 500 mg/5 ml

Side effects/adverse reactions:
GI: Nausea, vomiting, abdominal cramps, diarrhoea
CV: Hypotension with too rapid injection

Contraindications: Hypersensi-tivity, history of thromboembolic disease

Precautions: Renal disease, preg-nancy, lactation, upper urinary tract infection, haematuria

Clinical assessment:
• Fluid balance. If urinary output decreases the clinician must be in-formed and the drug discontinued
• Blood tests: clotting factors, platelets, signs and symptoms of thrombophlebitis
• Blood pressure and tachycardia
• Creatinine phosphokinase, urin-alysis
• Liver function tests

NURSING CONSIDERATIONS
Assess:
• Baseline vital signs
Administer:
• Initial intravenous dose should be given over 30 mins to avoid hypotension. A plastic syringe should be used
• Drug may be given after dilution with normal saline, Dextrose 5%, Dextran 40, Dextran 70
Evaluate:
• Allergy, fever, rash, itching, jaundice
• Myopathy, weakness, fever, myoglobinaemia or oliguria, which indicate that drug should be discontinued
• Bleeding from mucous mem-branes, epistaxis, ecchymosis, petechiae, haematuria, haema-temesis
• Blood pressure and tachycardia
Teach patient/family:
• Any signs of bleeding must be reported e.g. from gums, sub-cutaneously, in urine, stools or vomit
• To rise slowly when standing or sitting to avoid postural hypotension

tranylcypromine sulphate

Parnate
Func. class.: Antidepressant, (MAOI)
Chem. class.: Non-hydrazine MAOI
Legal class.: POM

Action: Increases concentrations of endogenous adrenaline, nor-adrenaline, serotonin, dopamine in storage sites in CNS by inhibition of monoamine oxidase; increased concentration reduces depression

Uses: Depressive illness, when uncontrolled by other means

Dosage and routes:
• *Adult:* By mouth 10 mg twice a day, may increase the second daily dose to 20 mg after 1 week. Usual maintenance dose: 10 mg daily

Available forms include: Tablets 10 mg

Side effects/adverse reactions:
HAEM: Dyscrasias
CNS: Dizziness, drowsiness, confusion, headache, anxiety, tremors, stimulation, weakness, hyperreflexia, mania, insomnia, restlessness, increased appetite, peripheral neuritis, dependence, fatigue
GI: Constipation, dry mouth, nausea, vomiting, diarrhoea, liver dysfunction
GU: Change in libido, frequency, difficulty in micturition
INTEG: Rash, flushing, increased perspiration
CV: Orthostatic hypotension, hypertension, dysrhythmias, hypertensive crisis (see Interactions below), palpitation
EENT: Blurred vision
SYST: Weight gain, oedema

Contraindications: Hypersensitivity to MAOIs, suspected cerebrovascular disease, blood dyscrasias, severe hepatic disease, phaeochromocytoma, porphyria, hyperthyroidism concurrent or within 1 week of other MAOIs or antidepressant drugs

Precautions: Convulsive disorders, hyperactivity, diabetes mellitus, pregnancy, lactation, elderly, surgery, alcohol/drug abuse, cardiovascular disease, concurrent electroconvulsive therapy

Pharmacokinetics:
Metabolised by liver, excreted by kidneys, elimination half-life 2–3 hr, excreted in breast milk. May take 3 weeks to start working, 5 weeks for maximal effect

Interactions/incompatibilities:
• CNS excitation or depression given with: pethidine and possibly other opiates, nefopam
• Serious CNS toxicity and/or hypertensive crisis given with, shortly before or after: other antidepressants including other MAOIs, rauwolfia alkaloids, oxypertine, sumatriptan, buspirone, tetrabenazine
• Hypertensive crisis with: levodopa, amphetamines, dexfenfluramine, diethylpropion, dopamine, dopexamine, ephedrine, fenfluramine, isometheptene, mazindol, pemoline, phentermine, phenylephrine, phenylpropanolamine, pseudoephedrine, other sympathomimetics, high tyramine foods (see below)
• Effect of oral hypoglycaemics, insulin reduced

Clinical assessment:
• Phentolamine for severe hypertension
• Check hepatic function if impairment suspected before, during treatment

Treatment of overdose: Lavage, activated charcoal, symptomatic and supportive treatment including phentolamine for severe hypertension

NURSING CONSIDERATIONS

Assess:
• Baseline vital signs
• BP (lying, standing), pulse

Administer:
• Increased fluids, bulk in diet if constipation, urinary retention occur
• With food or milk for GI symptoms
• Crushed if patient is unable to swallow medication whole

• Dosage at bedtime if oversedation occurs during day
• Mouthwashes, frequent sips of water for dry mouth

Perform/provide:
• Storage in tight container in cool environment
• Assistance with ambulation during beginning therapy since drowsiness/dizziness occurs
• Safety measures including cot sides
• Checking to see oral medication swallowed

Evaluate:
• Toxicity: increased headache, palpitation, discontinue drug immediately; prodromal signs of hypertensive crisis
• Mental status: mood, sensory, affect, memory (long, short), increase in psychiatric symptoms
• Urinary retention, constipation, oedema. Weight weekly
• Withdrawal symptoms: headache, nausea, vomiting, muscle pain, weakness

Teach patient/family:
• That therapeutic effects may take 1–4 weeks
• To avoid driving or other activities requiring alertness
• To avoid alcohol ingestion, CNS depressants or non-prescribed medications; particularly for colds, coughs, hay fever
• Not to discontinue medication quickly after long-term use
• To avoid high tyramine foods: mature cheese, sour cream, beer, wine, Marmite, Bovril, heavy red wines, broad beans, non-alcoholic beer, pickled products, liver, raisins, bananas, figs, avocados, meat tenderizers, chocolate, yogurt
• Report headache, palpitation, neck stiffness

trazodone HCl

Molipaxin
Func. class.: Antidepressant
Chem. class.: Triazolopyridine derivative
Legal class.: POM

Action: Unclear, may potentiate noradrenaline and antagonise serotonin in the brain
Uses: Depression, depression accompanied by anxiety
Dosage and routes:
• *Adult:* By mouth 150 mg/day in divided doses after meals, may be increased to 300 mg/day, or maximum 600 mg/day for hospitalised patients
Available forms include: Capsules 50, 100, tablets 150 mg, tablets modified release 150 mg, liquid 50 mg/5 ml
Side effects/adverse reactions:
CNS: Dizziness, drowsiness, confusion, headache, tremor, stimulation, weakness, insomnia
GI: Diarrhoea, dry mouth, nausea, vomiting
GU: Priapism
INTEG: Rash
CV: Orthostatic hypotension, tachycardia, bradycardia
EENT: Blurred vision
SYST: Weight loss, oedema
Contraindications: Hypersensitivity
Precautions: Cardiovascular disease, hepatic disease, pregnancy, epilepsy, renal disease, lactation
Pharmacokinetics:
Metabolised by liver, excreted by kidneys, faeces; half-life 5–13 hr
Interactions/incompatibilities:
• Decreased effects of: guanethidine, clonidine
• Increased effects of: alcohol, barbiturates, benzodiazepines, and other CNS depressants
• Hyperpyretic crisis, convulsions,

hypertensive episode given with or within 14 days of: MAOIs

Clinical assessment:
• Check hepatic and renal function if significant impairment considered likely

Treatment of overdose: Induce emesis, lavage, activated charcoal, symptomatic and supportive treatment

NURSING CONSIDERATIONS

Assess:
• BP (lying, standing), pulse
• Baseline weight

Administer:
• Increased fluids, fibre in diet if constipation, urinary retention occur
• After food
• In divided doses or entire daily dose may be given at night
• Mouthwashes, frequent sips of water for dry mouth

Perform/provide:
• Storage in tight, light-resistant container at room temperature
• Assistance with ambulation during beginning therapy since drowsiness/dizziness occurs
• Safety measures including side-rails, primarily in elderly
• Checking to see oral medication swallowed

Evaluate:
• Weight weekly, appetite may increase with drug
• Uncoordinated movements primarily in elderly: rigidity, dystonia, akathisia
• Mental status: mood, sensory, affect, suicidal tendencies, increase in psychiatric symptoms: depression, panic
• Cardiovascular side-effects, particularly with high doses
• Urinary retention, constipation
• Withdrawal symptoms: headache, nausea, vomiting, muscle pain, weakness; do not usually occur unless drug was discontinued abruptly

Teach patient/family:
• That therapeutic effects may take 2−3 weeks
• Use caution in driving or other activities requiring alertness because of drowsiness, dizziness, blurred vision
• To avoid alcohol ingestion, other CNS depressants; drug enhances the effect of alcohol
• Not to discontinue medication quickly after long-term use, may cause nausea, headache, malaise

---

treosulfan

Treosulfan
Func. class.: Anti-neoplastic alkylating
Chem. class.: Busulphan derivative
Legal class.: POM

Action: Alkylates DNA, RNA; inhibits enzymes that allow synthesis of proteins; is also responsible for cross linking DNA strands

Uses: Ovarian carcinoma

Dosage and routes:
• By mouth 1 g daily in 4 divided doses to provide total dose of 21−28 g over initial 8 weeks
• Injection: 5−15 g IV every 1−3 weeks depending on blood count and concurrent chemotherapy. Doses below 5 g may be given as bolus, above 5 g give as infusion

Available forms include: Capsules 250 mg; injection, powder for reconstitution 5 g

Side effects/adverse reactions:
HAEM: Thrombocytopenia, leucopenia, pancytopenia, acute myeloid leukaemia
GI: Nausea, vomiting, diarrhoea, abdominal pain, weight loss
INTEG: Alopecia, dermatitis, skin pigmentation, local pain and necrosis following extravasation of IV infusion

---

Contraindications: Hypersensitivity, pregnancy, lactation
Precautions: Radiotherapy, bone marrow depression, renal impairment, liver failure
Pharmacokinetics:
Activated *in vivo* by non-enzymic conversion to epoxide compounds
Clinical assessment:
• Prescribe anti-emetic to combat nausea and vomiting
• Monitor blood picture every 1–2 weeks
• Withdraw drug if white blood cell count is below 3×10^9/litre or platelet count below 100×10^9/litre
Treatment of overdose: Symptomatic and supportive treatment, including blood transfusion and filgrastim if appropriate

NURSING CONSIDERATIONS
Administer:
• Capsule must be swallowed whole and not allowed to disintegrate in mouth
• Other medication by mouth if possible; avoid IM, SC routes to prevent infection
• In accordance with local cytotoxic policy
• Avoid contact with eyes and skin
• Use solution immediately discarding any unused material safely
• Anti-emetic as prescribed for nausea and vomiting
Perform/provide:
• Avoid extravasation into tissues as local pain and tissue damage will occur
• Analgesics as appropriate
Evaluate:
• IV site for signs of extravasation. Discontinue at once if this happens and use a different vein for remaining solution
Teach patient/family:
• To expect nausea and vomiting—take anti-emetics as prescribed

• Swallow capsules whole—do not allow to disintegrate in mouth
• About all side effects of drug and to report these immediately
• Reversible alopecia may occur

---

tretinoin

Retin-A, Retin-A Forte
Func. class.: Keratolytic
Chem. class.: Retinoid
Legal class.: POM

Action: Decreases cohesiveness of follicular epithelial cells, decreases microcomedone formation
Uses: Acne vulgaris in which comedones, papules and pustules predominate
Dosage and routes:
• *Adult and child:* Topical, cleanse area, apply to cover area lightly once or twice daily
Available forms include: Gel 0.01, 0.025%; lotion 0.025%; cream 0.025%, 0.05%
Side effects/adverse reactions:
INTEG: Rash, stinging, warmth, erythema, peeling, contact dermatitis, hypo/hyperpigmentation, photosensitivity
Contraindications: Hypersensitivity, family history of cutaneous epithelioma, pregnancy, sunburn
Precautions: Eczema, avoid application to broken skin
Pharmacokinetics:
Topical: Poor absorption, excreted in urine
Interactions/incompatibilities:
• Increased skin peeling when used with: medications containing agents such as sulphur, benzoyl peroxide, resorcinol, salicylic acid
• Do not apply at the same time as other skin medications
• Use with caution medicated or abrasive soaps or cleansers that have drying effect, products with

high concentrations of alcohol astringent

Treatment of overdose: Gastric emptying if significant oral ingestion occurs

NURSING CONSIDERATIONS

Administer:

• Avoid oversaturation or contact with eyes, accumulation in angles of the nose

Perform/provide:

• Wash hands after application

Evaluate:

• Therapeutic response: decrease in size and number of lesions

• Area of body involved, including time involved, what helps or aggravates condition

Teach patient/family:

• To avoid application on normal skin or getting cream in eyes, nose, or other mucous membranes

• To avoid sunlight or sunlamps

• Treatment may cause warmth, stinging; dryness, peeling will occur

• Cosmetics may be used over drug, not to use shaving lotions

• That rash may occur during first 1−3 weeks of therapy

• That drug does not cure condition, only relieves symptoms

---

triamcinolone/ triamcinolone acetonide/ triamcinolone hexacetonide

Adcortyl, Kenalog, Lederspan, Ledercort

Func. class.: Corticosteroid
Chem. class.: Synthetic fluorinated glucocorticoid
Legal class.: POM

Action: Decreases inflammation by suppression of migration of polymorphonuclear leucocytes, fibroblasts, reversal to increase capillary permeability and lysosomal stabilization. Immediate action

Uses: Severe inflammation, pain and stiffness associated with rheumatoid arthritis or osteoarthrosis, neoplasms, asthma (steroid dependent), bursitis, tendinitis, lichen planus, lichen simplex, collagen disorders, severe dermatitis and Stevens−Johnson syndrome, nephrotic syndrome, tenosynovitis, epicondylitis, hypertrophic scars, granuloma annulare, keloids, alopecia areata, seasonal or perennial allergic rhinitis, endocrine disorders, autoimmune haematological disorders, neoplastic disorders

Dosage and routes:

Bronchial asthma, rheumatoid arthritis, dermatoses

• *Adults and children over 34 kg:* By mouth 8−16 mg/day

• *Children less than 34 kg:* By mouth 4−12 mg/day

• *Adults and children over 6 yr:* By deep IM injection 40 mg (acetonide)

Rheumatic fever with severe carditis, nephrotic syndrome

• *Adult:* By mouth initially 16−20 mg/day

Collagen diseases e.g. systemic lupus erythematosus

• *Adult:* By mouth, initially 20−30 mg/day

All doses should be adjusted according to individual requirements

Local joint inflammation or pain

• *Adult:* Intra-articular injection, small joint 2.5−10 mg (acetonide), large joint 5−40 mg (acetonide). A maximum of 80 mg over several sites can be given

• *Adult:* Intra-articular injection, small joint 2−6 mg (hexacetonide). Large joint 10−30 mg. Adjust dose and frequency according to individual requirements

Lichen simplex or planus, granuloma annulare, keloids, alopecia areata, hypertrophic scars
• *Adult:* Intradermal injections 2−3 mg (acetonide) depending on the size of the lesion. Maximum of 5 mg per site or total of 30 mg at several sites. Repeat if necessary at intervals of 1−2 weeks
• *Adult:* For intralesional or sublesional use 0.5 mg or less per square inch of affected skin (as hexacetonide)
Available forms include: Tablets 2, 4 mg; injection 10, 40 mg/ml acetonide; injection 5, 20 mg/ml hexacetonide

Side effects/adverse reactions:
INTEG: Acne, poor wound healing, bruising, striae, telangiectasia, ecchymosis, petechiae, weight gain, hirsutism, Cushingoid features
CNS: Depression, headache, mood changes intracranial hypertension, insomnia, aggravation of schizophrenia, dizziness
META: Sodium and water retention, hypokalaemic alkalosis, growth suppression in children, menstrual irregularity and amenorrhoea, impaired carbohydrate tolerance
CV: Hypertension, thrombophlebitis, thromboembolism, tachycardia
HAEM: Thrombocytopenia, leucocytosis
MS: Fractures, osteoporosis, sterile abscess, hyper- or hypopigmentation and subcutaneous and cutaneous atrophy at site of intradermal injection, weakness, proximal myopathy, avascular osteonecrosis, tendon rupture, local fat atrophy
GI: Diarrhoea, nausea, abdominal distension, peptic ulceration with perforation and haemorrhage, dyspepsia, GI haemorrhage, increased appetite, pancreatitis, oesophageal candidiasis, oesophageal ulceration
EENT: Opportunistic infections, increased intraocular pressure, glaucoma, papilloedema, cataracts, blurred vision, corneal or scleral thinning, exacerbation of ophthalmic viral disease

Contraindications: Psychosis, hypersensitivity, exacerbation of viral disease, child less than 6 years, active tuberculosis, herpes simplex
Precautions: Pregnancy, diabetes mellitus, intestinal anastomoses, tuberculosis, viral, bacterial or fungal infection, hypertension, epilepsy, glaucoma, osteoporosis, ulcerative colitis, congestive heart disease, myasthenia gravis, acute glomerular nephritis, steroid myopathy, thrombophlebitis, peptic ulcer, epilepsy. Psychosis, elderly, chronic nephritis, metastatic carcinoma

Interactions/incompatibilities:
• Decreased effects of this drug: cholestyramine, colestipol, barbiturates, ripampicin, carbamazepine, phenytoin, theophylline
• Decreased effects of: anticoagulants, antidiabetics, antihypertensives, loop and thiazide diuretics, acetazolamide, vaccines
• Increased side effects: alcohol, salicylates, indomethacin

Clinical assessment:
• Serum potassium, blood sugar, urine glucose while on long-term therapy; hypokalaemia and hyperglycaemia
• Plasma cortisol levels during long-term therapy (normal level: 136−690 nmol/litre when drawn at 08.00)

NURSING CONSIDERATIONS
Assess:
• Baseline weight, BP, pulse rate
• BP, pulse 4 hrly; notify clinician if chest pain occurs
• Fluid balance ratio, be alert for

decreasing urinary output and increasing oedema

Administer:

• After shaking suspension (parenteral)

• Titrated dose, use lowest effective dose

• IM injection deeply in large muscle mass; rotate sites, avoid deltoid, use appropriate gauge needle

• In one dose in morning to prevent adrenal suppression. Avoid subcutaneous administration; damage may be done to tissue

• With food or milk to decrease GI symptoms

Perform/provide:

• Assistance with ambulation in patient with bone tissue disease to prevent fractures

Evaluate:

• Weight daily, notify clinician if weekly gain is over 2−3 kg

• Therapeutic response: ease of respirations, decreased inflammation

• Infection: increased temperature, WBC, even after withdrawal of medication. Drug masks infection symptoms

• Potassium depletion: paraesthesias, fatigue, nausea, vomiting, depression, polyuria, dysrhythmias, weakness

• Oedema, hypotension, cardiac symptoms

• Mental status: affect, mood, behavioural changes, aggression

Teach patient/family:

• That ID card as steroid user should be carried

• To notify clinician if therapeutic response decreases; dosage adjustment may be needed

• Not to discontinue this medication abruptly or adrenal crisis can result

• To avoid non-prescribed products: salicylates, alcohol in cough products, cold preparations unless directed by clinician

• Teach patient all aspects of drug use, including Cushingoid symptoms

• Symptoms of adrenal insufficiency: nausea, anorexia, fatigue, dizziness, dyspnoea, weakness, joint pain

---

triamcinolone acetonide (topical)

Adcortyl, Ledercort (with neomycin), Adcortyl with Graneodin

Func. class.: Corticosteroid, topical

Chem. class.: Synthetic fluorinated glucocorticoid

Legal class.: POM

Action: Possesses anti-pruritic, anti-inflammatory actions

Uses: Psoriasis of the scalp, palms or soles only, eczema, contact dermatitis, pruritus, neurodermatitis

Dosage and routes:

• *Adult and child:* Apply sparingly to affected area two to four times a day

Available forms include: Ointment 0.1%; cream 0.1%. With neomycin 0.1%

Side effects/adverse reactions:

INTEG: Burning, dryness, itching, increased sweating, lupus erythematosus like lesions, ecchymoses, irritation, hirsutism, atrophy, striae, secondary infection, impaired wound healing, facial erythema and telangiectasia, purpura, acneiform eruptions, petechiae, thinning of the skin

Contraindications: Hypersensitivity to corticosteroids, fungal, viral or bacterial skin infections, tuberculosis, acne vulgaris, facial rosacea, perioral dermatitis or napkin eruptions

Precautions: Pregnancy, lactation, viral infections, bacterial infections, children (maximum of 5 days treatment)

NURSING CONSIDERATIONS

Administer:
• Only to affected areas; do not get in eyes
• Medication, then cover with occlusive dressing (only if prescribed), seal to normal skin, change 12 hrly; use occlusive dressing with extreme caution (group II potency)
• Only to dermatoses; do not use on weeping, denuded, or infected area

Perform/provide:
• Cleansing before application of drug
• Treatment for a few days after area has cleared

Evaluate:
• Therapeutic response: absence of severe itching, patches on skin, flaking
• Temperature; if fever develops, drug should be discontinued

Teach patient/family:
• To avoid sunlight on affected area; burns may occur
• That rebound exacerbation may occur

---

triamcinolone acetonide (oral)

Adcortyl in Orabase
Func. class.: Corticosteroid
Chem. class.: Synthetic fluorinated glucocorticoid
Legal class.: POM

Action: Anti-inflammatory, antipruritic
Uses: Aphthous ulcers, ulcerative or denture stomatitis, desquamative gingivitis, erosive lichen planus, lesions of traumatic origin

Dosage and routes:
• *Adult and child:* Apply to the affected area two to four times a day. Do not rub in

Available forms include: Paste 0.1%
Side effects/adverse reactions:
INTEG: Irritation, sensitization
Contraindications: Hypersensitivity, to presence of fungal, viral, or bacterial infections of mouth or throat (unless treated), tuberculosis
Precautions: Child (maximum of 5 days), sepsis, pregnancy, prolonged usage

NURSING CONSIDERATIONS

Administer:
• After cleansing oral cavity
• Do not rub in

Evaluate:
• Allergy: rash, irritation, reddening, swelling
• Therapeutic response: absence of pain in affected area
• Infection: if affected area is infected, do not apply

Teach patient/family:
• To report rash, irritation, redness, swelling
• How to apply paste

---

triamterene

Dytac
Func. class.: Potassium-sparing diuretic
Chem. class.: Diuretics
Legal class.: POM

Action: Acts on distal tubule to inhibit reabsorption of sodium, chloride
Uses: Oedema; in cardiac failure, cirrhosis of the liver, or nephrotic syndrome and that associated with corticosteroid treatment, may be used with other diuretics

Dosage and routes:

• *Adult:* By mouth 150—250 mg daily in divided doses after meals, reduce to alternate days after 1 week. Lower initial doses when given with other diuretics

Available forms include: Capsules 50 mg

Side effects/adverse reactions:

GI: Nausea, diarrhoea, vomiting, dry mouth, jaundice and elevated serum levels of liver enzymes

ELECT: Hyperkalaemia, hyponatraemia, metabolic acidosis

CNS: Weakness, headache

INTEG: Photosensitivity, rash

HAEM: Thrombocytopenia, megaloblastic anaemia

Contraindications: Hypersensitivity, anuria, severe renal disease, severe hepatic disease, hyperkalaemia, Addison's disease. Do not routinely administer with angiotensin converting enzyme (ACE) inhibitors

Precautions: Dehydration, pregnancy, hepatic disease, lactation, renal disease, cirrhosis, gout, other hypotensive agents as an additive effect may result

Pharmacokinetics:

By mouth: Onset 2 hr, peak 6—8 hr, duration 12—16 hr; half-life 3 hr; metabolised in liver, excreted in urine

Interactions/incompatibilities:

• Enhanced action of: antihypertensives

• Increased hyperkalaemia: other potassium sparing diuretics, potassium products, ACE inhibitors, NSAIDs, cyclosporin

Clinical assessment:

• Serum electrolytes: potassium, sodium, chloride; include serum urea, blood sugar, full blood count, serum creatinine, blood pH, arterial blood gases

Lab. test interferences:

Interfere: Bioassay of folic acid

Treatment of overdose: Lavage if taken orally, monitor electrolytes, administer IV fluids, dialysis

NURSING CONSIDERATIONS

Assess:

• Baseline weight

• Postural hypotension

Administer:

• With food

Perform/provide:

• Fluid balance daily to determine fluid loss; effect of drug may be diminished if taken daily

Evaluate:

• Improvement in oedema of feet, legs, sacral area daily if medication is being used in congestive heart failure

• Improvement in CVP and BP recordings

• Signs of metabolic acidosis: drowsiness, restlessness

• Rashes, temperature elevation daily

• Confusion, especially in elderly, take safety precautions if needed

• Hydration: skin turgor, thirst, dry mucous membranes

Teach patient/family:

• To take medication after meals

• To avoid prolonged exposure to sunlight since photosensitivity may occur

• Urine may appear blue in certain lights

• To notify clinician if weakness, headache, nausea, vomiting, dry mouth, fever, sore throat, mouth sores, unusual bleeding or bruising occurs

• Rise slowly from lying to sitting position

---

trientine dihydrochloride

Func. class.: Heavy metal antagonist

Chem. class.: Chelating agent (thiol compound)

Legal class.: POM

Action: Binds with ions of lead,

mercury, copper, iron, zinc to form a water-soluble complex excreted by kidneys

Uses: Wilson's disease (in patients intolerant of penicillamine)

Dosage and routes:
• *Adult:* By mouth 1.2−2.4 daily in 2−4 divided doses before food

Available forms include: Capsules 300 mg

Side effects/adverse reactions:
HAEM: Anaemia, iron deficiency
INTEG: Urticaria, fever
SYST: Hypersensitivity
GI: Nausea

Contraindications: Hypersensitivity
Precautions: Pregnancy

Pharmacokinetics:
By mouth: Peak 1 hr, metabolised in liver, excreted in urine

Interactions/incompatibilities:
• Decreased action: mineral supplements

Clinical assessment:
• Monitor hepatic renal studies: aspartate aminotransferase, alanine aminotransferase, alkaline phosphatase, blood urea, creatinine−CSM requests special records kept by pharmacist
NB. Special records must be kept by the pharmacist for this drug

NURSING CONSIDERATIONS

Assess:
• Fluid balance and urinalysis
• Baseline full blood count
• Dietary habits

Administer:
• On an empty stomach, ½−1 hr before meals
• Vitamin B$_6$ daily; depleted when this drug is used

Evaluate:
• Therapeutic response: improvement in neurologic, psychiatric symptoms
• Signs of anaemia
• Blood dyscrasias
• Side-effects, nausea
• Urinalysis regularly

Teach patient/family:

• That therapeutic effect may take 1−3 months
• To avoid diet containing copper; this includes offal, shellfish, nuts, dried legumes, chocolate, wholegrain cereal
• That penicillamine-induced systemic lupus erythematosus may not resolve

---

trifluoperazine HCl

Stelazine
Func. class.: Antipsychotic, neuroleptic
Chem. class.: Piperazine, Phenothiazine
Legal class.: POM

Action: Depresses cerebral cortex, hypothalamus, limbic system, which control activity, aggression; blocks neurotransmission produced by dopamine at synapse; exhibits strong α-adrenergic, anticholinergic blocking action; mechanism for antipsychotic effects is unclear

Uses: Psychotic disorders, non-psychotic anxiety, schizophrenia, symptomatic treatment of nausea and vomiting, severe psychomotor agitation

Dosage and routes:
Psychotic disorders
• *Adult:* By mouth 5 mg twice a day (high dosage) or 10 mg daily in modified-release form, increase to 15 mg daily after 1 week, then increasing at 5 mg intervals every 3 days. IM 1−3 mg in divided doses up to maximum 6 mg daily
• *Child:* By mouth initial dose not to exceed 5 mg in divided doses; IM *not recommended for children*, but 1 mg per 20 kg may be given daily in divided doses
Non-psychotic anxiety
• *Adult:* By mouth 1−2 mg twice a

day (low dosage), not to exceed 6 mg/day

• *Child 3–5 yr:* By mouth up to 1 mg daily in divided doses; 6–12 yr: By mouth maximum 4 mg daily in divided doses

Available forms include: Tablets 1, 2, 5 mg; Spansule 2, 10, 15 mg; syrup concentrate 10 mg/ml for dilution prior to use, injection IM 1 mg/ml, Syrup 1 mg/5 ml

Side effects/adverse reactions:

RESP: Laryngospasm, dyspnoea, respiratory depression

CNS: Extrapyramidal symptoms: pseudoparkinsonism, akathisia, dystonia, tardive dyskinesia, seizures, headache, drowsiness, insomnia, restlesness, hyperpyrexia

HAEM: Leucopenia, pancytopenia; thrombocytopenia agranulocytosis

INTEG: Rash, photosensitivity, pigmentation

EENT: Blurred vision, glaucoma

GI: Dry mouth, nausea, vomiting, anorexia, constipation, diarrhoea, jaundice, weight gain

GU: Urinary retention, urinary frequency, enuresis, impotence, amenorrhoea, gynaecomastia

CV: Orthostatic hypotension, hypertension, cardiac arrest, ECG changes, tachycardia

MS: Muscular weakness

Contraindications: Hypersensitivity, coma, blood dyscrasias, severe hepatic disease

Precautions: Breast cancer, epilepsy, Parkinson's disease, narrow angle glaucoma, pregnancy, lactation, children, elderly, cardiovascular disease, angina, prostatic hypertrophy, myasthenia gravis

Pharmacokinetics:

By mouth: Onset rapid, peak 2–3 hr, duration 12 hr, modified-release form. 60% released over 6–8 hr

IM: Onset immediate, peak 1 hr, duration 12 hr

Metabolised by liver, excreted in urine, enters breast milk

Interactions/incompatibilities:

• Oversedation: other CNS depressants, alcohol, barbiturate anaesthetics

• Decreased absorption: aluminium hydroxide or magnesium hydroxide antacids

• Decreased effects of: levodopa, anti-epileptics

• Increased effects of both drugs: antihypertensives, alcohol

• Increased anticholinergic effects: anticholinergics

Clinical assessment:

• Bilirubin, full blood count, liver function tests monthly

• Urinalysis is recommended before and during prolonged therapy

Treatment of overdose: Lavage if orally ingested, provide an airway; *do not induce vomiting*

NURSING CONSIDERATIONS

Assess:

•Swallowing of oral medication; check for hoarding or giving of medication to other patients

• Fluid balance

• Baseline vital signs including BP standing and lying

Perform/provide:

• Decreased noise input by dimming lights, avoiding loud noises

• Supervised ambulation until stabilised on medication; do not involve in strenuous exercise programme

• Increased fluids to prevent constipation

• Sips of water, mouthwashes for dry mouth

Evaluate:

• Therapeutic response: decrease in emotional excitement, hallucinations, delusions, paranoia, reorganization of patterns of thought, speech

• Affect, orientation, level of con-

sciousness, reflexes, gait, co-ordination, sleep pattern disturbances
• BP standing and lying; also pulse, respirations 4 hrly during initial treatment; report drops of 30 mmHg
• Dizziness, faintness, palpitations, tachycardia on rising
• Extrapyramidal symptoms including akathisia (inability to sit still, no pattern to movements), tardive dyskinesia (bizarre movements of jaw, mouth, tongue, extremities), pseudoparkinsonism (rigidity, tremors, pill rolling, shuffling gait)
• Skin turgor daily
• Constipation, urinary retention daily

Teach patient/family:
• That orthostatic hypotension occurs frequently, and to rise from sitting or lying position gradually
• To remain lying down after IM injection for at least 30 min
• To avoid abrupt withdrawal of this drug or extrapyramidal symptoms may result; drugs should be withdrawn slowly
• To avoid non-prescribed preparations (cough, hayfever, cold) unless approved by clinician since serious drug interactions may occur; avoid use with alcohol or CNS depressants, increased drowsiness may occur
• To use a sunscreen during sun exposure to prevent burns
• Regarding compliance with drug regimen
• To report sore throat, malaise, fever, bleeding, mouth sores; if these occur, full blood count should be drawn and drug discontinued
• In hot weather, heat stroke may occur; take extra precautions to stay cool
• To take additional fibre in diet and fluids if constipated
• Not to stand still for long periods of time

---

trifluperidol

Triperidol
Func. class.: Antipsychotic
Chem. class.: Butyrophenone
Legal class.: POM

Action: Depresses cerebral cortex, hypothalamus, limbic system, which controls aggression; blocks neurotransmission produced by dopamine at synapse; exhibits strong α-adrenergic, anticholinergic blocking action

Uses: Schizophrenia and related psychoses, particularly mania

Dosage and routes:
• *Adult:* By mouth initially 500 mcg/day, adjusted by 500 mcg every 3–4 days according to response; maximum dose 6–8 mg/day
• *Child 5–12 yr:* By mouth initially 250 mcg/day adjusted according to response; maximum dose 2 mg/day

Available forms include: Tablets 500 mcg, 1 mg

Side effects/adverse reactions:
CNS: Extrapyramidal symptoms, tardive dyskinesia, sedation, drowsiness, apathy, nightmares, insomnia, depression, agitation, headache
CV: Hypotension
GU: Difficulty with micturition, menstrual disturbances, impotence
META: Galactorrhoea, gynaecomastia, changes in weight
INTEG: Photosensitization, contact sensitization, rashes, jaundice
GI: Nausea, loss of appetite, dyspepsia

Contraindications: Pregnancy, lactation, comatose states

Precautions: Parkinsonism, epilepsy, renal or hepatic impairment, elderly patients, closed angle glaucoma

Interactions/incompatibilities:
• Oversedation: alcohol, other CNS depressants, barbiturates, anaesthetics
• Decreased absorption: antacids
• Decreased effects of: levodopa, anti-epileptics
• Increased effects of: anti-hypertensives

Clinical assessment:
• Bilirubin, full blood count, liver function tests monthly

Treatment of overdose: Supportive measures and anti-parkinsonian drugs as necessary

NURSING CONSIDERATIONS

Assess:
• Swallowing of oral medication, check for hoarding or giving medication to other patients
• Fluid balance
• Urinalysis, before and during therapy

Perform/provide:
• Decreased noise input by dimming lights, avoiding loud noises
• Supervised ambulation until stabilised on medication: do not involve in strenuous exercise programme because fainting is possible: patient should not stand still for long periods of time
• Increased fluids to prevent constipation
• Sips of water or mouthwashes for dry mouth

Evaluate:
• For extrapyramidal symptoms
• Orientation, level of consciousness, reflexes, coordination, sleep pattern; report any disturbances to clinician
• BP standing/lying; pulse and respirations 4-hrly during initial treatment; report drop in BP of 30 mmHg
• For constipation, urinary retention; if these occur, increase fibre and water in diet
• Therapeutic response: decrease in emotional excitement

Teach patient/family:
• That hypotension occurs; to rise from sitting or lying position gradually
• To avoid abrupt withdrawal of the drug — should be withdrawn slowly
• To avoid non-prescribed medication unless approved by clinician
• Avoid use with alcohol
• Keep to drug regime
• To report sore throat, malaise, fever, mouth sores

trimeprazine tartrate

Vallergan
Func. class.: Antihistamine
Chem. class.: Sedative antihistamines
Legal class.: POM

Action: Acts on blood vessels, GI, respiratory system by competing with histamine for H_1-receptor site; decreases allergic response by blocking histamine. Central sedative effect

Uses: Pruritus, premedication for anaesthesia

Dosage and routes:
Urticaria/Pruritus
• *Adult:* By mouth 10 mg two or three times a day up to 100 mg (in intractable cases). Reduce dosage in elderly 10 mg once or twice a day
• *Children:* By mouth 2.5−5 mg three or four times a day

Premedication
• *Child:* Maximum dosage of Vallergan or Vallergan Forte syrup is 2 mg/kg

Available forms include: Tablets 10 mg; syrup 7.5 mg/5 ml, Forte syrup 30 mg 15 ml

Side effects/adverse reactions:
CNS: Drowsiness, insomnia, agitation, akathesia, Parkinsonism, tardive dyskinesia, dystonia
CV: Hypotension, tachycardia A-V block, atrial arrhythmia, ventricular fibrillation
RESP: Respiratory depression
HAEM: Agranulocytosis, leucopenia
GI: Dry mouth, jaundice
INTEG: Rash, urticaria, photosensitivity
ENDO: Hyperprolactinaemia, neuroleptic malignant syndrome
EENT: Nasal stuffiness, dry nose, throat, mouth
Contraindications: Hepatic or renal dysfunction, epilepsy, Parkinsonism, hypothyroidism, phaeochromocytoma, myasthenia gravis, prostatic hypertrophy, narrow angle glaucoma, hypersensitivity to H_1-receptor antagonist
Precautions: Children under 2 yr, pregnancy, elderly
Interactions/incompatibilities:
• Increased CNS depression: barbiturates, hypnotics, tricyclic antidepressants, alcohol
• Decreased effect of: amphetamine, levodopa, clonidine, guanethidine, adrenaline, hypoglycaemic drugs
• Increased effect of this drug: MAOIs, anticholinergic drugs
• Increased effect of: antihypotensive drugs
• Decreased absorption of this drug: antacids, lithium
Clinical assessment:
• WBC during long-term therapy
Treatment of overdose: Administer lavage, activated charcoal, maintain airway

NURSING CONSIDERATIONS
Assess:
• Fluid balance
Administer:
• Preoperatively; 1−2 hrs before anaesthesia
• With meals if GI symptoms occur; absorption may be slightly decreased
Perform/provide:
• Sips of water, frequent rinsing of mouth for dryness (except when used for premedication)
Evaluate:
• Therapeutic response: decreased itching associated with pruritus
Teach patient/family:
• All aspects of drug use; to notify clinician if side effects occur
• To avoid driving or other hazardous activity if drowsiness occurs
• To avoid concurrent use of alcohol or other CNS depressants

---

trimethoprim

Ipral, Monotrim, Syraprim, Trimogal, Trimopan
Func. class.: Antibiotic, urinary
Chem. class.: Folate antagonist
Legal class.: POM

Action: Prevents bacterial synthesis by blocking enzyme reduction of dihydrofolic acid
Uses: Urinary tract infection, acute and chronic bronchitis, bronchopneumonia and lobar pneumonia
Dosage and routes:
• *Adult:* Acute infection by mouth 200 mg every 12 hr, IV infusion 200 mg every 12 hr. Urinary tract 300 mg daily or 200 mg twice a day. Chronic infections, and prophylaxis: 100 mg at bedtime
• *Child:* By mouth 2−5 months, 25 mg twice a day; 6 months−5 yr 50 mg twice a day; 6 yr−12 yr 100 mg twice a day IV or IV infusion: 6−9 mg/kg daily in 2−3 divided doses
Available forms include: Tablets 100, 200, 300 mg; suspension 50 mg/5 ml; injection 20 mg (lactate)/ml

Side effects/adverse reactions:
INTEG: Pruritus, rash
HAEM: Depression of haemopoiesis
GI: Nausea, vomiting
Contraindications: Hypersensitivity, renal disease, pregnancy, neonates, megaloblastic anaemia, lactation, blood dyscrasias
Precautions: Folate deficiency, mild or moderate renal disease
Pharmacokinetics:
By mouth: Peak 1–4 hr, half-life 8–11 hr, metabolised in liver, excreted in urine (unchanged 60%), breast milk
Interactions/incompatibilities:
• Increased concentration of procainamide
• Increased effect of anti-coagulants
• Elimination of digoxin and phenytoin may be enhanced
Clinical assessment:
• Nocturia; may indicate drug resistance
• Creatinine, urine cultures
Treatment of overdose: Gastric lavage and symptomatic treatment as necessary
NURSING CONSIDERATIONS
Administer:
• With full glass of water
• Culture and sensitivity before drug therapy; drug may be taken as soon as culture is taken
Perform/provide:
• Adequate intake of fluids (2 litres) to decrease bacteria in bladder
Evaluate:
• Therapeutic response: absence of pain in bladder area, negative culture and sensitivity
• Skin eruptions
• Allergies before treatment, reaction of each medication; note allergies on chart, Kardex in bright red letters; notify all people giving drugs
Teach patient/family:

• Aspects of drug therapy: need to complete entire course of medication to ensure organism death (10–14 days); culture may be taken after completed course of medication
• To notify if nausea, vomiting

---

trimipramine maleate

Surmontil
Func. class.: Antidepressant, tricyclic
Chem. class.: Tertiary amine
Legal class.: POM

Action: Selectively inhibits serotonin uptake by brain; potentiates behavioural changes
Uses: Depression, particularly where sedation is required
Dosage and routes:
• *Adult:* By mouth 50–75 mg daily 2 hr prior to bedtime or 25 mg midday and 50 mg evening. Increased as necessary to maximum of 300 mg daily in divided doses
• *Elderly:* By mouth 10–25 mg three times a day, not recommended for use in children
Available forms include: Tablets 10, 25 mg; capsules 50 mg
Side effects/adverse reactions:
HAEM: Agranulocytosis, depression of bone marrow
CNS: Dizziness, drowsiness, tremors, peripheral neuropathy, increase in psychiatric symptoms convulsions
GI: Dry mouth, nausea, vomiting, jaundice, constipation
GU: Retention, interference with sexual function
INTEG: Rash, urticaria, sweating
CV: Orthostatic hypotension, tachycardia, palpitations
EENT: Blurred vision
Contraindications: Hypersensitivity to tricyclic antidepressants, recovery phase of myocardial in-

farction, concurrent use or within 2 weeks of monoamine oxidase inhibitor treatment. Lactation, mania, severe liver disease, any degree of heart block or other cardiac arrhythmia

Precautions: Suicidal patients, severe depression, increased intra-ocular pressure, narrow-angle glaucoma, urinary retention, cardiac disease, hepatic disease, hyperthyroidism, elderly prostatic hypertrophy, epilepsy, pregnancy, concurrent use of anaesthetics (arrhythmias and hypotension)

Pharmacokinetics: Metabolised by liver, excreted by kidneys, steady state 2−6 days; half-life 7−30 hr

Interactions/incompatibilities:
• Decreased effects of: guanethidine, debrisoquine, bethanidine, clonidine, antiepileptics
• Increased effects of: sympathomimetics (adrenaline, noradrenaline, ephedrine, isoprenaline, phenylephrine, phenylpropanolamine), alcohol, barbiturates, benzodiazepines, CNS depressants, antihistamines
• Hyperpyretic crisis, convulsions, hypertensive episode: MAOIs

Clinical assessment:
• Blood studies: Full blood count, leucocytes, differential, cardiac enzymes if patient is receiving long-term therapy
• Hepatic studies: aspartate aminotransferase, alanine aminotransferase, bilirubin, creatinine
• ECG for flattening of T wave bundle branch block, AV block arrhythmias in cardiac patients

Treatment of overdose: ECG monitoring, induce emesis, lavage, activated charcoal, administer anticonvulsant, treat acidosis with 20 ml/kg sodium lactate

NURSING CONSIDERATIONS

Assess:
• BP lying, standing
• Baseline weight

Administer:
• Increased fluids, fibre in diet if constipation, urinary retention occur
• Frequent sips of water; mouthwashes for dry mouth

Perform/provide:
• Assistance with ambulation during beginning therapy since drowsiness/dizziness occurs
• Safety measures, including side-rails primarily in elderly
• Checking to see oral medication swallowed

Evaluate:
• BP (lying, standing), pulse 4 hrly; if systolic BP drops 20 mmHg hold drug, notify clinician; take vital signs 4 hrly in patients with cardiovascular disease
• Weight weekly; appetite may increase with drug
• Mental status: mood, sensory affect, suicidal tendencies, increase in psychiatric symptoms: depression, panic
• Urinary retention, constipation
• Cardiovascular side effects, particularly with high doses
• Withdrawal symptoms: headache, nausea, vomiting, muscle pain, weakness; do not usually occur unless drug was discontinued abruptly
• Alcohol consumption; if alcohol is consumed, hold dose until morning (drug enhances effect of alcohol)

Teach patient/family:
• That therapeutic effects may take 2−3 weeks
• Use caution in driving or other activities requiring alertness because of drowsiness, dizziness, blurred vision
• To avoid alcohol ingestion, other CNS depressants and non-prescribed medications
• Not to discontinue medication

quickly after long-term use, may cause nausea, headache, malaise

---

triprolidine HCl

Pro Actidil
Func. class.: Antihistamine
Chem. class.: Alkylamine, H_1-receptor antagonist
Legal class.: P

Action: Acts on blood vessels, GI, respiratory system, by competing with histamine for H_1-receptor site; decreases allergic response by blocking histamine
Uses: Allergy e.g.: hay fever and urticaria
Dosage and routes:
• *Adult:* By mouth 10 mg early evening or 5−6 hr before retiring increased to 20 mg daily if symptoms severe
• *Child:* Not recommended
Available forms include: modified release tablets 10 mg
Side effects/adverse reactions:
CNS: Drowsiness
INTEG: Rash, urticaria, photosensitivity
Contraindications: Hypersensitivity to H_1-receptor antagonist, severe hepatic or renal dysfunction
Precautions: Increased intraocular pressure, prostatic hypertrophy, pregnancy, lactation
Pharmacokinetics:
By mouth: Onset 20−60 min, duration 8−12 hr, detoxified in liver, excreted by kidneys (metabolites/free drug), half-life 20−24 hr
Interactions/incompatibilities:
• Increased CNS depressants: barbiturates, narcotics, hypnotics, tricyclic antidepressants, alcohol
• Decreased effect of: betahistine
Treatment of overdose: Gastric lavage, diazepam, vasopressors
NURSING CONSIDERATIONS

Administer:
• With meals if GI symptoms occur; absorption may slightly decrease
Perform/provide:
• Sips of water, frequent rinsing of mouth for dryness
• Storage in tight container at room temperature
Evaluate:
• Therapeutic response: decreased itching associated with urticaria
Teach patient/family:
• All aspects of drug use; to notify clinician if side effects occur
• To avoid driving or other hazardous activity if drowsiness occurs
• To avoid concurrent use of alcohol or other CNS depressants while taking this drug

---

tropicamide (ophthalmic)

Mydriacyl, Minims
Func. class.: Mydriatic, cycloplegic, anticholinergic
Chem. class.: Belladonna alkaloid
Legal class.: POM

Action: Paralysis of ciliary muscle, dilation of pupil
Uses: Fundus examination, cycloplegic refraction
Dosage and routes:
• *Adult and child:* Instil 1−2 drops of 1% solution, repeat in 5 min (refraction) or 1−2 drops of 0.5% solution 15−20 min before exam (fundus examination)
Available forms include: Solution 0.5%, 1%
Side effects/adverse reactions:
EENT: Raised intraocular pressure, stinging of eyes, photophobia, local hyperaemia, oedema
INTEG: Rash in children, dry skin, flushing
GI: Abdominal distension in in-

fants, dry mouth, constipation, vomiting
CV: Bradycardia, tachycardia, palpitations, arrhythmias
GU: Urinary urgency, retention
CNS: Behavioural disturbances in children, giddiness, staggering
Contraindications: Hypersensitivity, narrow angle glaucoma
Precautions: Infants, soft contact lenses, pregnancy, elderly, ocular hyperaemia
Pharmacokinetics:
INSTIL: Peak 15−20 min, (mydriasis), 20 min (cycloplegia), duration 2−6 hr (cycloplegia), 7 hr (mydriasis)
Interactions/incompatibilities:
Soft contact lenses (preparations with preservative)
NURSING CONSIDERATIONS
Evaluate:
• Eye pain, discontinue use
Teach patient/family:
• To report change in vision, with blurring or loss of sight, trouble breathing, sweating, flushing
• Method of instillation, including pressure on lacrimal sac for 1 min, and not to touch dropper to eye
• That blurred vision will decrease with repeated use of drug
• Not to engage in hazardous activities until able to see
• Wait 5 min to use other drops
• Contact lense wearers should seek advice from clinician before starting drops

---

tubocurarine chloride

Jexin, Tubarine
Func. class.: Non-depolarising muscle relaxant
Chem. class.: Curare alkaloid
Legal class.: POM

Action: Inhibits transmission of nerve impulses by binding to cholinergic receptor sites,

antagonising action of acetylcholine
Uses: Facilitation of endotracheal intubation, skeletal muscle relaxation during mechanical ventilation, surgery, or general anaesthesia, tetanus
Dosage and routes:
• *Adult:* IV bolus injection based upon initial dose of 10−30 mg (maximum 40 mg), supplementary doses of 5 mg as needed
• *Child:* IV bolus injection initial dose of 0.3−0.5 mg/kg, then 60−100 mcg/kg as required
Available forms include: Injection IV 10 mg/ml
Side effects/adverse reactions:
CV: Bradycardia, tachycardia, decreased BP
RESP: Prolonged apnoea, bronchospasm, collapse, respiratory
INTEG: Rash, flushing, pruritus, urticaria, pain at injection site
Contraindications: Hypersensitivity, respiratory insufficiency, renal or hepatic impairment, asthma
Precautions: Pregnancy, lactation, respiratory disease, myasthenia gravis, gross obesity, myopathy, after poliomyelitis, repeat dose within 24 hr, family history of malignant hyperthermia
Pharmacokinetics:
IV: Onset 3−5 min, duration ½−hr; half-life 1−3 hr, degraded in liver, mainly excreted in urine unchanged
Interactions/incompatibilities:
• Increased hypotension: halothane
• Increased neuromuscular blockade: aminoglycosides, clindamycin, lincomycin, quinidine, volatile anaesthetics, polymyxin antibiotics, lithium, narcotic analgesics, thiazides, azlocillin, mezlocillin, nifedipine, verapamil, parenteral magnesium salts, β-blockers, tetracyclines
• Concurrent administration with

depolarising relaxant may cause relaxation which is not reversible by neostigmine
• Neuromuscular blockade reduced by: azathioprine, mercaptopurine, lymphocytic antiglobulin
• Neuromuscular blockade reversed by: anticholinesterases

Clinical assessment:
• For electrolyte imbalances (potassium, magnesium); may lead to increased action of this drug

Treatment of overdose: Edrophonium or neostigmine, atropine, monitor, mechanical ventilation, monitor CV, electrolyte, respiratory status

NURSING CONSIDERATIONS

Assess:
• Vital signs (BP, pulse, respirations, airway)
• Anaesthetic history—NOT to be given to asthmatics, patients with renal or liver impairment
• Electrolyte levels

Perform/provide:
• Storage in light-resistant area

Evaluate:
• Therapeutic response: level and degree of paralysis
• Vital signs, particularly respiratory rate
• Allergic reactions: rash, fever, respiratory distress, pruritus; drug should be discontinued

---

typhoid vaccine (injectable)

Typhoid Vaccine BP (whole, killed bacteria)
Typhim Vi (purified polysaccharide)
Func. class.: Monovalent vaccine
Legal class.: POM

Action: Promotes development of antibodies specific to *Salmonella typhi*
Uses: Active immunization against typhoid fever

Dosage and routes:
Typhoid Vaccine BP
Primary immunization
• *Adult:* Deep subcutaneous/IM injection, initially 0.5 ml; 2nd dose after 4–6 weeks 0.5 ml (or 0.1 ml intradermal)
• *Child 1–10 yr:* Deep subcutaneous/IM: unit 0.25 ml: 2nd dose 0.25 ml (or 0.1 ml intradermal)
Reinforcement of immunity
• Further doses every 3 yr approx on continued exposure
Typhim Vi
Primary immunization
• *Adult:* Deep subcutaneous/IM injection 0.5 ml single dose

Available forms include:
Typhoid Vaccine BP: Injection suspension, 1.5 ml vial containing more than 1,000 million organisms per ml *S. typhi*
Typhim Vi: Prefilled, single-dose syringe 25 mcg of *S. typhi*: Vi polysaccharide in 0.5 ml

Side effects/adverse reactions:
INTEG: Swelling, pain, tenderness at injection site
SYST: Malaise, fever, nausea, pyrexia
CNS: Headache. With Typhoid Vaccine BP: polyneuritis, myelitis
Contraindications: History of anaphylaxis, hypersensitivity, acute infection, children less than 1 yr, pregnancy
Precautions: Debilitated patients especially with previous history of typhoid vaccination

NURSING CONSIDERATIONS

Administer:
• Shake vial well before withdrawing dose
• Discard unused vaccine
• Record title, dose and batch no. of vaccine and date of administration
• Avoid administration during acute illness

Perform/provide:

• Ensure facilities available for management of anaphylaxis
Teach patient/family:
• That side effects, including nausea, malaise and headache may be acute and require cessation of normal activities. These usually subside within 36 hr
• Report any neurological signs to clinician at once

typhoid vaccine (oral)

Vivotif
Func. class.: Oral vaccine
Chem. class.: Live attenuated organisms of *Salmonella typhi*
Legal class.: POM

Action: Promotes development of antibodies to *S. typhi*
Dosage and routes:
Primary immunization
• *Adult and child over 6 yr:* By mouth, 1 capsule, 1 hr before meals with a cold drink on alternate days for 3 doses
Reinforcement of immunity
• *Adult and child over 6 yr:* After a course of capsules protection exists for at least three years, though in typhoid endemic areas an annual booster is recommended. Booster courses consist of 3 doses, identical to primary immunization
Available forms include: Packs of 3 enteric coated capsules each containing at least 2,000 million viable organisms of attenuated *S. typhi* Ty 21a
Side effects/adverse reactions:
GI: Nausea, vomiting, diarrhoea, abdominal cramps
INTEG: Urticarial exanthema
Contraindications: Hypersensitivity, congenital or acquired immune deficiency including treatment with immunosuppressive

drugs, acute febrile or gastro-intestinal illness
Precautions: Pregnancy
Pharmacokinetics: Not applicable
Interactions/incompatibilities:
Vaccine inactivated by: Mefloquine (do not give within 12 hr), sulphonamides, antibiotics
Risk of systemic infection: Immunosuppressive drugs
Treatment of overdose: Not applicable

NURSING CONSIDERATIONS
Administer:
• Avoid administration during acute illness
Perform/provide:
• Record title, dose and batch no. of vaccine and date of administration
Teach patient/family:
• That side effects, including nausea, malaise and headache may be acute and require cessation of normal activities. These usually subside within 36 hr
• Report any neurological signs to clinician immediately

urea hydrogen peroxide

Exterol
Func. class.: Cerulytic
Chem. class.: Urea compound
Legal class.: P

Action: Foaming action facilitates removal of impacted cerumen
Uses: Removal of impacted cerumen in ear, urea soften cerumen
Dosage and routes:
• *Adult and child:* Instil 5–10 drops once or twice daily for 3–4 days
Available forms include: Solution 5%
Side effects/adverse reactions:

EENT: Itching, irritation in ear, redness

Contraindications: Hypersensitivity, ear surgery, perforated eardrum

NURSING CONSIDERATIONS

Administer:

• By allowing drops to enter ear canal, do not touch dropper to ear

• Then irrigate ear if appropriate and necessary to remove wax

Evaluate:

• Therapeutic response: loosened cerumen, ability to hear better

Teach patient/family:

• Method of instillation, using aseptic technique

• Patients may experience effervescent feeling in ear after using drops

---

urofollitrophin

Metrodin

Func. class.: Gonadotrophin: human follicle stimulating hormone
Chem. class.: Peptide hormone
Legal class.: POM

Action: Stimulates ovarian follicular growth

Uses: Induction of ovulation in infertile women with hypopituitarism or who have not responded to clomiphene and induction of multiple follicular growth in women undergoing assisted conception

Dosage and routes:

Hypothalamic-pituitary dysfunction

• IM initially 75−150 IU/day or 225−375 IU on alternate days increasing by 75 IU daily or 75−150 IU on alternate days until response optimal, then 10,000 IU human chorionic gonadotrophin 1−2 days after last dose. Re-assess if unsuccessful after 6 ovulatory cycles

Assisted conception

• IM 150−225 IU, adjusted according to response, from day 5 of cycle until follicular development achieved in combination with clomiphene and human chorionic gonadotrophin. Other regimens are used

Available forms include: Powder for injection 75 IU/ampoule

Side effects/adverse reactions:

GI: Abdominal pain

INTEG: Rash, local reactions at injection site

GU: Multiple ovulation, ovarian hyperstimulation leading to ovarian rupture and peritoneal haemorrhage, multiple pregnancy

Contraindications: Hypersensitivity

Precautions: Ovarian cysts, adrenal or thyroid disease, hyperprolactinaemia, pituitary tumour

Pharmacokinetics: Metabolised in liver, excreted in faeces, stored in fat

Clinical assessment:

• Titrate dose to response assessed by measuring plasma/urinary oestrogen, or pelvic ultrasound scans

Treatment of overdose: Monitor degree of ovarian enlargement, give symptomatic relief, hospitalise if ovaries enlarged beyond 12 cm in diameter

NURSING CONSIDERATIONS

Assess:

• At the same time every day

Administer:

• By deep IM injection

Teach patient/family:

• Multiple births have been reported following treatment with this drug

• To inform clinician if low abdominal pain is experienced, as this may indicate the presence of an ovarian cyst, or rupture of a cyst

• Teach patient how to take and chart early morning temperature

to determine if ovulation has occurred
• If pregnancy is suspected the clinician should be informed at once

urokinase

Ukidan
Func. class.: Thrombolytic enzyme
Chem. class.: Protein
Legal class.: POM

Action: Promotes thrombolysis by acting directly on endogenous fibrinolytic system to change plasminogen to plasmin

Uses: Vitreous haemorrhage, clotted AV shunts and IV cannulae, pulmonary embolism, deep vein thrombosis, peripheral vascular occlusion

Dosage and routes:
Pulmonary embolism
• *Adult:* IV infusion, initially 4400 IU/kg in 15 ml over 10 min, then 4400 IU/kg/hr for 12 hr
Deep vein thrombosis
• *Adult:* IV infusion, initially 4400 IU/kg in 15 ml over 10 min, then 4400 IU/kg/hr for 12–24 hr
Peripheral vascular occlusion
• Seek specialist advice
AV shunts
• *Adult:* Instil 5000–37,500 IV in 2–3 ml 0.9% sodium chloride clamp off × 2–4 hr
Intraocular
• Intraocular injection: 5000–37,500 IV in 2 ml 0.9% sodium chloride
Available forms include: Powder for injection 5000, 25,000, 100,000 IU vials

Side effects/adverse reactions:
HAEM: Bleeding
INTEG: Local pain when injected into AV shunt
GI: Nausea, vomiting
GU: Haematuria
SYST: Elevated temperature following liberation of lysis products

Contraindications: Vitreous haemorrhage complicated by severe retinal disturbances e.g. (retinal detachment), active bleeding, severe hypertension, recent surgery, pregnancy, severe hepatic or renal disease

Precautions: Known GI lesions prone to bleeding, multiple cardiac puncture as a consequence of cardio-pulmonary resuscitation, history of cerebro-vascular disease

Pharmacokinetics:
IV: Half-life 10–20 min, small amounts excreted in urine

Interactions/incompatibilities:
• Increased risk of bleeding given with: Aspirin and other non-steroidal anti-inflammatories, anticoagulants
• Incompatible with: dextrose solutions when mixed
• Action prolonged by: dextrans

Clinical assessment:
• As soon as thrombi identified; not useful for thrombi over 1 week old

Treatment of overdose: Aprotinin, tranexamic acid or aminocaproic acid to antagonise. Clotting factors, red cells, whole blood for severe haemorrhage

NURSING CONSIDERATIONS
Assess:
• Baseline vital signs, BP, pulse, respiration, neurological signs, temperature, ECG

Administer:
• After reconstituting with 2 ml of 0.9% sodium chloride or water for injection; do not shake

Perform/provide:
• Bed rest during entire course of treatment
• Careful handling of patient to avoid bruising
• Avoidance of invasive pro-

cedures: injections, rectal temperature
• Treatment of fever with paracetamol or aspirin
• Pressure for 30 sec to minor bleeding sites; inform clinician if haemostasis not attained, apply pressure dressing

Evaluate:
• Vital signs, ECG and neurological observations
• Allergy: fever, rash, itching, chills, mild reaction may be treated with antihistamines
• Bleeding during first hr of treatment (most likely from site of injection but also haematuria, haematemesis, bleeding from mucous membranes, epistaxis, ecchymosis)
• Side effects: nausea, vomiting

Teach patient/family:
• About effects of drug
• To report any change indicating bleeding

---

ursodeoxycholic acid

Destolit, Ursofalk
Func. class.: Bile acid
Chem. class.: 7β-epimer of chenodeoxycholic acid
Legal class.: POM

Action: Dissolves cholesterol gallstones through desaturation of bile by cholesterol
Uses: Dissolution of radiolucent cholesterol gallstones
Dosage and routes:
• By mouth 8–12 mg/kg daily (up to 15 mg/kg daily in obese patients) in divided doses or as single dose at bedtime, for up to 2 yr; treatment should be continued for 3–4 months after stones dissolve
Available forms include: Tablets 150 mg; capsules 250 mg
Side effects/adverse reactions:
GI: Diarrhoea

INTEG: Pruritus
Contraindications: Radio-opaque stones, active gastric or duodenal ulcer, non-functioning gallbladder, chronic liver disease, inflammatory diseases of small intestine or colon, pregnancy
Pharmacokinetics: Absorbed through GI-tract and undergoes enterohepatic recycling, excreted in faeces largely unchanged, some bacterial breakdown
Interactions/incompatibilities:
• Reduced effect of ursodeoxycholic acid: oestrogenic hormones, oral contraceptives, cholestyramine, colestipol
Treatment of overdose: Low toxicity, symptomatic relief only

NURSING CONSIDERATIONS
Assess:
• GI symptoms before commencing treatment
Administer:
• During meals for better absorption
• Whole—not to be crushed or chewed
Evaluate:
• GI symptoms, nausea, vomiting, abdominal pain, cramps, diarrhoea
Teach patient/family:
• Diarrhoea may occur initially; if persistent to consult clinician
• To take good, balanced diet, low in cholesterol
• That medication may need to be continued for up to 2 years

---

vancomycin HCl

Vancocin
Func. class.: Antibiotic
Chem. class.: Tricyclic glucopeptide
Legal class.: POM

Action: Inhibits cell wall bacterial synthesis

Uses: Resistant staphylococcal infections, pseudomembranous colitis, staphylococcal enterocolitis, endocarditis, prophylaxis for dental procedures

Dosage and routes:

Serious staphylococcal infections

Doses should be adjusted according to plasma drug concentration

• *Adult:* IV infusion 500 mg every 6 hr or 1 g every 12 hr

• *Child:* IV infusion 40 mg/kg/day divided every 6 hr

• *Neonates:* IV 10 mg/kg every 12 hr

Pseudomembranous/staphylococcal enterocolitis

• *Adult:* By mouth 500 mg twice a day or 125 mg every 6 hr for 7−10 days (Maximum 2 g total daily dose)

• *Child:* By mouth 40 mg/kg/day in divided doses every 6−8 hr

Available forms include: Capsules 125, 250 mg; powder for injection IV 500 mg; injection may be given orally

Side effects/adverse reactions:

Serious side effects are unusual following oral dosing

CV: Cardiac arrest and vascular collapse after rapid infusion, vasculitis

EENT: Ototoxicity, permanent deafness, tinnitus

HAEM: Eosinophilia, neutropenia, thrombocytopenia

GI: Nausea

RESP: Wheezing, dyspnoea after rapid infusion

SYST: Anaphylaxis

GU: Nephrotoxicity: increased blood urea nitrogen, creatinine, albumin

INTEG: Chills, fever, rash, necrosis and thrombophlebitis at injection site, after rapid infusion; urticaria, pruritus

Contraindications:

Hypersensitivity

Precautions: Renal disease (adjust dose), pregnancy, lactation, elderly, neonates, decreased hearing

Pharmacokinetics:

Little oral absorption. After IV administration: peak 2 hr, half-life 3−13 hr, excreted in urine (active form). Therapeutic plasma levels: peak 18−26 mg/litre, trough 5−10 mg/litre

Interactions/incompatibilities:

• Ototoxicity or nephrotoxicity: aminoglycosides, cephalosporins notably cephalothin, colistin, polymyxin, bacitracin, cisplatin, amphotericin, loop diuretics

• Do not mix in solution or syringe with other drugs; check product information

• Exaggerated infusion reactions when given concomitantly with: anaesthetic agents

Clinical assessment:

• Blood levels at regular intervals

• Monitor renal function at regular intervals, adjust dose in renal impairment

• Signs of ototoxicity

• Blood studies: WBC

• Culture and sensitivity before drug therapy; drug may be taken as soon as culture is taken. Use less toxic agents where possible

Treatment of overdose: Supportive care with maintenance of glomerular filtration

NURSING CONSIDERATIONS

Assess:

• Fluid balance

• Bowel pattern

• Allergies before treatment, reaction of each medication; note allergies in nursing care plan in bright red letters; notify all people giving drugs

Administer:

• After samples have been sent for culture and sensitivity

• After reconstitution with 10 ml sterile water for injection 500 mg/100 ml; further dilution is needed for IV

- Infusion over 60 min; avoid extravasion

Perform/provide:
- Storage at 0−6°C — for up to 24 hr after reconstitution
- Adrenaline, resuscitation equipment on unit; anaphylaxis may occur
- Adequate intake of fluids (2 litres) to prevent nephrotoxicity
- Fluid balance ratio; report haematuria, oliguria since nephrotoxicity may occur
- BP during administration; sudden drop may indicate "red man" syndrome

Evaluate:
- Therapeutic response: absence of fever, sore throat
- Hearing loss, ringing, roaring in ears; drug should be discontinued
- Skin eruptions
- Respiratory status: rate, character, wheezing, tightness in chest

Teach patient/family:
- Aspects of drug therapy: need to complete entire course of medication to ensure organism death (7−10 days); culture may be taken after completed course of medication
- To report sore throat, fever, fatigue; could indicate superimposed infection
- That drug must be taken in equal intervals around clock to maintain blood levels

---

vasopressin (antidiuretic hormone)/(argipressin)

Pitressin
Func. class.: Pituitary hormone
Chem. class.: Lysine vasopressin
Legal class.: POM

Action: Promotes reabsorption of water by action on renal tubular epithelium, contracts smooth muscle

Uses: Pituitary diabetes insipidus, bleeding oesophageal varices

Dosage and routes:
Diabetes insipidus
- *Adult:* IM/subcutaneous 5−20 units every 4 hr as needed

Oesophageal varices
- IV 20 units in 100 ml dextrose 5% infused over 15 min

Available forms include: Injection IV, IM, subcutaneous 20 units/ml

Side effects/adverse reactions:
CNS: Drowsiness, headache, lethargy, tremor, vertigo
GU: Vulval pain, uterine cramp
GI: Nausea, cramps, belching, vomiting, urge to defecate
CV: Increased BP, anginal attack
INTEG: Sweating, pallor, urticaria
SYST: Anaphylaxis, water intoxication

Contraindications: Hypersensitivity, vascular disease (with extreme caution), chronic nephritis

Precautions: Epilepsy, migraine, asthma, congestive cardiac failure

Pharmacokinetics: Not absorbed orally, plasma half life 5−15 min

Interactions/incompatibilities:
- Increased antidiuretic effect: chlorpropamide, carbamazepine, clofibrate, tricyclic antidepressants
- Decreased antidiuretic effect: alcohol, lithium

Treatment of overdose: Monitor fluid balance carefully, hypertonic solutions for water intoxication, nitrates for angina pain

NURSING CONSIDERATIONS

Assess:
- Fluid balance
- Weight
- Pulse, BP, when giving drug IV or IM

Perform/provide:
- Store injection between 2−8°C

Evaluate:
- Therapeutic response: absence

of severe thirst, decreased urine output, osmolality
• Fluid balance ratio, weight daily, check for oedema in extremities, if water retention is severe, diuretic may be prescribed
• Water intoxication: lethargy, behavioural changes, disorientation, neuromuscular excitability
Teach patient/family:
• All aspects of drug: action, side effects, dose, when to notify clinician

vecuronium bromide

Norcuron
Func. class.: Non-depolarising neuromuscular relaxant
Chem. class.: Piperidinium derivative
Legal class.: POM

Action: Inhibits transmission of nerve impulses by binding with cholinergic receptor sites, antagonising action of acetylcholine
Uses: Facilitation of endotracheal intubation, skeletal muscle relaxation during mechanical ventilation, surgery, or general anaesthesia
Dosage and routes:
• *Adult and child:* IV bolus 0.08–0.10 mg/kg; incremental doses, 0.03–0.05 mg/kg, IV infusion 0.05–0.08 mg/kg/hr
Available forms include: Powder for IV use 10 mg vial and diluent (5 ml)
Side effects/adverse reactions:
RESP: Bronchospasm
EENT: Increased secretions
INTEG: Irritation at injection site
SYST: Anaphylaxis
Contraindications: Hypersensitivity
Precautions: Pregnancy, lactation, electrolyte imbalances, dehydration, neuromuscular disease, myasthenia gravis, obesity, after poliomyelitis
Pharmacokinetics:
IV: Onset 1–2 min, duration 20–30 mins; half-life 30–70 min, not metabolised, excreted in faeces
Interactions/incompatibilities:
• Increased neuromuscular blockade: aminoglycosides, clindamycin, lincomycin, quinidine, volatile anaesthetics, polymyxin antibiotics, lithium, narcotic analgesics, thiazides, azlocillin, mezlocillin, nifedipine, verapamil, parenteral magnesium salts, β-blockers, tetracyclines
• Neuromuscular blockade reduced by: chronic corticosteroids, azathioprine, mercaptopurine
• Neuromuscular blockade reversed by: anticholinesterases
• Concurrent administration with depolarising relaxant may cause relaxation which is not reversible by neostigmine
Clinical assessment:
• For electrolyte imbalances (potassium, magnesium); may lead to increased action of this drug
Treatment of overdose: Neostigmine, atropine, monitor vital signs; may require mechanical ventilation
NURSING CONSIDERATIONS
Assess:
• Baseline vital signs
Administer:
• Slowly over 1–2 minutes (by qualified anaesthetic personnel only)
• With resuscitation equipment nearby
Perform/provide:
• Storage in light-resistant area
• Nerve stimulator
Evaluate:
• Therapeutic response; degree of paralysis (jaw, neck, respiratory function)
• Heart rate for signs of distress

• Vital signs (BP, pulse, respirations, airway) until fully recovered; rate, depth, pattern of respirations, strength of hand grip
• Fluid balance; check for urinary retention, frequency, hesitancy

Administer:
• Using nerve stimulator by anaesthetist to determine neuromuscular blockade
• Anticholinesterase to reverse neuromuscular blockade
• By slow IV over 1−2 min (only by specially qualified person, usually an anaesthetist)
• Only slightly discoloured solution

Perform/provide:
• Reassurance if communication is difficult during recovery from neuromuscular blockade

Evaluate:
• Therapeutic response: paralysis of jaw, eyelid, head, neck, rest of body
• Recovery: decreased paralysis of face, diaphragm, leg, arm, rest of body
• Allergic reactions: rash, fever, respiratory distress, pruritus; drug should be discontinued

---

verapamil HCl

Berkatens, Cordilox, Securon, Securon SR, Univer
Func. class.: Calcium-channel blocker, class IV anti-arrhythmic
Legal class.: POM

Action: Inhibits calcium ion influx across cell membrane during cardiac depolarisation; produces relaxation of coronary vascular smooth muscle, dilates coronary arteries
Uses: Chronic stable angina pectoris, vasospastic angina, supraventricular arrhythmias, hypertension

Dosage and routes:
Hypertension
• *Adult:* By mouth 240−480 mg daily in 2−3 divided doses or modified release initially 120 mg daily increasing to 240−480 mg daily in one or two doses
• *Child:* By mouth up to 10 mg/kg/day in divided doses
Angina
• *Adult:* By mouth 80−120 mg three times a day or modified release 240−480 mg daily in one or two doses
Supraventricular arrhythmias (non-acute)
• *Adult:* By mouth 40−120 mg three times a day according to severity
• *Child under 2 yr:* By mouth 20 mg two to three times a day
• *Over 2 yr:* By mouth 40−120 mg two to three times a day according to age
(Acute)−IV injection
• *Adult:* Tachyarrhythmias: IV bolus 5−10 mg Paroxysmal tachyarrhythmias: IV bolus 5−10 mg followed by 5 mg after 5−10 min if required
• *Child:* Newborn: IV bolus 0.75−1 mg
Under 1 yr: IV bolus 0.75−2 mg
1−5 yr: IV bolus 2−3 mg
6−15 yr: IV bolus 2.5−5 mg
Available forms include: Tablets 40, 80, 120, 160 mg; IV injection 2.5 mg/ml; tablets modified release 240 mg; capsules modified release 120, 180, 240 mg

Side effects/adverse reactions:
CV: Arrhythmias, oedema, worsening bradycardia, hypotension, heart block, asystole. Adverse CV effects much more likely after IV administration
GI: Nausea, vomiting, constipation, impaired liver function
INTEG: Rash, pruritus, flushing, photosensitivity
CNS: Headache, fatigue, dizziness

EENT: Gingival hyperplasia
ENDO: Gynaecomastia
Contraindications: Sick sinus syndrome, 2nd or 3rd degree heart block, hypotension, bradycardia (under 50 beats per minute), uncompensated heart failure, combination with β-blockers in patients with poor ventricular function (cardiogenic shock), porphyria
Precautions: Congestive heart failure, IV route in patients taking β-blockers, 1st degree heart block, atrial flutter or fibrillation complicating Wolff Parkinson White syndrome, myocardial infarction, pregnancy
Pharmacokinetics:
IV: Onset 3 min, plasma half-life 2−8 hr
By mouth: Onset 1−2 hr, half-life (biphasic) 4−12 hr (terminal)
Metabolised by liver, excreted in urine (96% as metabolites), 90% protein bound
Interactions/incompatibilities:
• Increased hypotensive effects with: general anaesthetics, other antihypertensives, quinidine, antipsychotics
• Increased risk of bradycardia, heart block, myocardial depression with: amiodarone
• Increased effects of: carbamazepine, imipramine, non-depolarising muscle relaxants
• Severe hypotension, heart block, bradycardia, asystole with: β-blockers, especially if either agent given IV
• Increased blood levels of: digoxin, cyclosporin, theophylline
• Increased heart block and bradycardia with: cardiac glycosides
• Increased neurotoxicity with: lithium
• Cardiac status, ECG
• Blood levels of co-administered digoxin, theophylline
Treatment of overdose: Defibril-lation, cardiac massage for asystole, atropine for AV block, vasopressor for hypotension

NURSING CONSIDERATIONS
Assess:
• Vital signs
• Baseline BP and respiratory rate
Perform/provide:
• Continuous ECG monitoring if given IV
Evaluate:
• Therapeutic response: decreased anginal pain
• BP, pulse, respiration
Teach patient/family:
• How to take pulse before taking drug; record or graph should be kept
• To avoid hazardous activities until dizziness is no longer a problem
• To limit caffeine consumption
• To avoid non-prescribed medicines unless approved by clinician
• Patient compliance with all areas of medical regimen: diet, exercise, stress reduction, drug therapy
• To report any side effects, headache, dizziness or fatigue

vigabatrin ▼

Sabril
Func. class.: Anticonvulsant
Chem. class.: GABA analogue
Legal class.: POM

Action: Selective irreversible inhibitor of GABA-transaminase, raises brain GABA levels
Uses: Treatment of epilepsy not satisfactorily controlled by other anti-epileptic drugs
Dosage and routes:
• *Adult:* Initially 2 g daily in single or 2 divided doses. The dose may be increased or decreased in 500 mg or 1 g increments as necess-

ary. Increasing the dose above 4 g per day does not usually result in improved efficacy
• *Child 3–9 yr:* Starting dose 1 g. Older children 2 g
• *Child under 3 yr:* Not recommended
Available forms include: Tablets 500 mg
Side effects/adverse reactions:
GI: Minor disturbances, changes in liver enzymes
CNS: Drowsiness, fatigue, dizziness, nervousness, irritability, depression, headache, confusion, aggression, psychosis, memory disturbance, paradoxical increase in seizure frequency. Excitation and agitation have been seen in children
HAEM: Slight decrease in haemoglobin
EENT: Diplopia
MISC: Weight gain
Contraindications: Pregnancy, breastfeeding
Precautions: Impaired renal function, elderly, history of psychosis, behavioural problems. Abrupt withdrawal may lead to rebound seizures. If treatment is to be discontinued it is recommended that the dose is reduced gradually over 2–4 weeks
Pharmacokinetics:
By mouth: Peak levels within 2 hr. Elimination half-life 5–8 hr via kidneys, not metabolised
Interactions/incompatibilities:
• Reduced blood levels of: phenytoin
NURSING CONSIDERATIONS
Assess:
• Baseline weight
• Renal function
Evaluate:
• Weight gain
• GI disturbance
• Neurological function
Teach patient/family:
• That drug is to be taken in conjunction with other anti-epileptic drugs
• About side-effects
• Not to discontinue drug suddenly; rebound seizures can occur
• Not to undertaken hazardous activity associated with machinery

---

vinblastine sulphate

Velbe
Func. class.: Antineoplastic
Chem. class.: Vinca rosea alkaloid
Legal class.: POM

Action: Inhibits mitotic activity, arrests cell cycle at metaphase; inhibits RNA synthesis
Uses: Breast, testicular cancer, leukaemias neuroblastoma, Hodgkin's and non-Hodgkin's lymphomas, mycosis fungoides, histiocytosis-X, renal cell carcinoma, methotrexate—resistant choriocarcinoma and other sensitive tumours
Dosage and routes:
• *Adult and child:* IV 6 mg/m^2 usually no more frequently than every 7 days, for testicular tumours may increase dose to 0.2 mg/kg on each of two consecutive days every 3 weeks. Should normally be given as part of a recognised cancer treatment protocol
Available forms include: Injection IV 1 mg/ml, powder for IV injection 10 mg and 10 ml diluent
Side effects/adverse reactions:
HAEM: Thrombocytopenia, leucopenia, anaemia
GI: Nausea, vomiting, anorexia, stomatitis, constipation, abdominal pain, haemorrhagic enterocolitis, rectal bleeding, diarrhoea, pharyngitis, adynamic ileus
INTEG: Rash, alopecia, pain and necrosis following extravasation

CV: Orthostatic hypotension, hypertension
CNS: Paraesthesias, peripheral neuropathy, depression, headache, convulsions, malaise, dizziness, weakness
ENDO: Inappropriate antidiuretic hormone secretion
MS: Myalgia, jaw pain, bone pain
Contraindications: Hypersensitivity, pregnancy, lactation, bacterial infection, granulocytopenic patients. Intrathecal administration
Precautions: Hepatic disease
Pharmacokinetics: Terminal half-life in plasma 19 hr, metabolised in liver, excreted in urine, faeces, does not cross blood−brain barrier, 99% protein bound
Interactions/incompatibilities:
• Do not use with irradiation of liver
• Risk of bronchospasm, pulmonary infiltration and fibrosis with: mitomycin C
Clinical assessment:
• Liver function tests before, during therapy as needed or monthly
• Stop treatment if neurotoxicity develops
• Full blood count prior to each treatment, withhold if neutropenic
Treatment of overdose: Supportive treatment including anticonvulsants, transfusion products, filgrastim, cathartics
NURSING CONSIDERATIONS
Assess:
• Fluid balance, report fall in urine output of 30 ml/hr
• Monitor temperature 4 hrly may indicate beginning infection
Administer:
• Other medications by oral route if possible; avoid IM, subcutaneous, IV routes to prevent infections if thrombocytopenic
• Anti-emetic 30−60 min before giving drug to prevent vomiting

• Antibiotics for prophylaxis of infection
• IV infusion using appropriate gauge needle; administer by slow IV infusion. Use Luer lock fittings
• Topical or systemic analgesics for pain
• Local or systemic drugs for infection
• Transfusion for anaemia
• Antispasmodic
Perform/provide:
• Trained personnel should reconstitute the drug in a designated area, adequate protective measures required. Avoid contact with eyes
• Not to be handled by pregnant personnel
• Strict medical asepsis, protective isolation if WBC levels are low
• Increase fluid intake to 2−3 litres/day to prevent urate deposits, calculi formation
• Strict oral hygiene with prescribed mouthwashes
• Brushing of teeth 2−3 times day with soft brush or cotton-tipped applicators for stomatitis; use unwaxed dental floss
• Warm compresses at injection site for inflammation
• Nutritious diet with iron, vitamin supplements
• Elevate head of bed to facilitate breathing
Evaluate:
• Bleeding: haematuria, guaiac, bruising or petechiae, mucosa of orifices 8 hrly
• Dyspnoea, rales, unproductive cough, chest pain, tachypnoea, fatigue, increased pulse, pallor, lethargy
• Effects of alopecia on body image; discuss feelings about changes in body image
• Oedema in feet, joint pain, stomach pain, shaking
• Inflammation of mucosa, breaks in skin

- Yellowing of skin and sclera, dark urine, clay-coloured stools, itchy skin, abdominal pain, fever, diarrhoea
- Buccal cavity 8 hrly for dryness, sores or ulceration, white patches, oral pain, bleeding, dysphagia
- Local irritation, pain, burning, discolouration at injection and infusion site
- Symptoms indicating severe allergic reaction: rash, pruritus, urticaria, purpuric skin lesions, itching, flushing
- Frequency of stools and characteristics: cramping, acidosis; signs of dehydration: rapid respirations, poor skin turgor, decreased urine output, dry skin, restlessness, weakness

Teach patient/family:
- Of protective isolation precautions
- To report any complaints or side effects to the nurse or clinician
- That impotence or amenorrhoea can occur, are reversible after discontinuing treatment
- To report any changes in breathing or coughing
- That hair may be lost during treatment, a wig or hairpiece may be available on the NHS; tell patient that new hair may be different in colour, texture
- To avoid foods with citric acid, hot or rough texture
- To report any bleeding, white spots or ulcerations in mouth to clinician; tell patient to examine mouth daily

---

vincristine sulphate

Oncovin
Func. class.: Antineoplastic
Chem. class.: Vinca alkaloid
Legal class.: POM

Action: Inhibits mitotic activity, arrests cell cycle at metaphase; inhibits RNA synthesis

Uses: Breast, lung cancer, lymphomas, neuroblastoma, Hodgkin's and non-Hodgkin's lymphomas, acute lymphoblastic and other leukaemias, rhabdomyosarcoma, Wilms' tumour, osteogenic and other sarcomas, and other sensitive tumours

Dosage and routes:
- IV 1.4–1.5 mg/m^2/wk not to exceed 2 mg/week
Available forms include: Injection IV 1 mg/ml, 1, 2, 5 mg vials; 1 mg, 2 mg, pre-filled syringes; powder for IV use 1, 2, 5 mg vials

Side effects/adverse reactions:
HAEM: Granulocytopenia, rarely anaemia and thrombocytopenia
GI: Nausea, vomiting, anorexia, stomatitis, constipation, paralytic ileus, abdominal pain, diarrhoea
INTEG: Alopecia, rash, pain and necrosis following extravasation
SYST: Weight loss, fever, anaphylaxis
EENT: Optic atrophy
CV: Orthostatic hypotension, hypertension
CNS: Decreased reflexes, numbness, weakness, motor difficulties, CNS depression, cranial nerve palsies paralysis, neuritic pain, paraesthesia, difficulty walking, slapping gait, ataxia, foot drop, convulsions
MS: Muscle wasting, pain in limbs, bone, pharynx, jaw, myalgia
ENDO: Inappropriate secretion of antidiuretic hormone
GU: Polyuria, dysuria, retention, risk of uric acid nephropathy secondary to tumour lysis

Contraindications: Hypersensitivity, pregnancy. Intrathecal administration, patients with demyelinating form of Charcot–Marie–Tooth syndrome

Precautions: Hepatic disease,

neuromuscular disease, infection, granulocytopenia

Pharmacokinetics: Terminal half-life 85 hr metabolised in liver, excreted in faeces, urine; does not cross blood−brain barrier, extensively protein bound

Interactions/incompatibilities:
• Do not use with irradiation of liver
• Risk of bronchospasm, pulmonary infiltration and fibrosis with: mitomycin
• Excretion slowed by: asparaginase (possibility of increased toxicity)

Clinical assessment:
• Liver function tests before, during therapy as needed or monthly
• Stop treatment if neurotoxicity develops
• Full blood count before each treatment, consider treatment carefully if neutropenic

Treatment of overdose: Supportive treatment including anticonvulsants, transfusion products, cathartics. Folinic acid may be protective in first 24 hr

NURSING CONSIDERATIONS

Assess:
• Baseline vital signs and fluid balance

Administer:
• In accordance with local cytotoxic policy
• Other medications by oral route if possible; avoid IM, subcutaneous, IV routes to prevent infections if thrombocytopenic
• Anti-emetic 30−60 min before giving drug to prevent vomiting
• Antibiotics for prophylaxis of infection
• IV infusion using appropriate gauge needle; administer by slow IV infusion; use Luer lack fittings (vesicant drug)
• Topical or systemic analgesics for pain

• Local or systemic drugs for infection
• Transfusion for anaemia
• Antispasmodic

Perform/provide:
• Trained personnel, should reconstitute the drug in a designated area, adequate protective measures required. Avoid contact with the eyes
• Not to be handled by pregnant personnel
• Strict medical asepsis, protective isolation if WBC levels are low
• Special skin care
• Strict oral hygiene with prescribed mouth washes
• Brushing of teeth 2−3 times day with soft brush or cotton-tipped applicators for stomatitis; use unwaxed dental floss
• Warm compresses at injection and infusion site for inflammation
• Nutritious diet with iron, vitamin supplements

Evaluate:
• Fluid balance, report fall in urine output of 30 ml/hr
• Monitor temperature 4 hrly may indicate beginning infection
• Bleeding: haematuria, bruising or petechiae, mucosa of orifices 8 hrly
• Dyspnoea, rales, unproductive cough, chest pain, tachypnoea, fatigue, increased pulse, pallor, lethargy
• Effects of alopecia on body image, allow patient to discuss feelings about changes in body image
• Oedema in feet, joint pain, stomach pain, shaking
• Inflammation of mucosa, breaks in skin
• Yellowing of skin and sclera, dark urine, clay-coloured stools, itchy skin, abdominal pain, fever, diarrhoea
• Buccal cavity 8 hrly for dryness, sores or ulceration, white patches,

oral pain, bleeding, dysphagia
• Local irritation, pain, burning, discolouration at injection site
• Symptoms indicating severe allergic reaction: rash, pruritus, urticaria, purpuric skin lesions, itching, flushing
• Frequency of stools, characteristics: cramping, acidosis; signs of dehydration: rapid respirations, poor skin turgor, decreased urine output, dry skin, restlessness, weakness

Teach patient/family:
• About protective isolation precautions when indicated
• To report any complaints or side effects to nurse or clinician
• To report any bleeding, white spots or ulcerations in mouth to clinician; tell patient to examine mouth daily
• Good oral hygiene techniques; avoid vigorous brushing of teeth

---

vindesine sulphate

Eldisine
Func. class.: Antineoplastic
Chem. class.: Vinca alkaloid
Legal class.: POM

Action: Inhibits mitotic activity, arrests cell cycle at metaphase; inhibits RNA synthesis

Uses: Breast cancer, acute lymphoblastic, blastic crises of chronic myeloid leukaemia, malignant melanoma, and other sensitive tumours

Dosage and routes:
• *Adult:* IV 3 mg/m^2 every 7 days. Provided there is no granulocytopenia dosage may be increased in 0.5 mg/m^2 steps at weekly intervals to maximum 4 mg/m^2
• *Child:* IV 4 mg/m^2 every 7 days
Available forms include: Powder for IV injection 5 mg and 5 ml diluent

Side effects/adverse reactions:

HAEM: Thrombocytopenia, leucopenia, anaemia, thrombocytosis
INTEG: Alopecia, pain and necrosis following extravasation
GI: Nausea, vomiting, anorexia, constipation, stomatitis, paralytic ileus, abdominal pain, dysphagia, dyspepsia, diarrhoea
MS: Jaw pain, myalgia, bone and joint pain
CNS: Neuritis, paraesthesia, mental depression, loss of deep tendon reflexes, foot drop, headache, convulsions

Contraindications: Granulocytopenia, bacterial infection, demyelinating form of Charcot–Marie–Tooth syndrome, hypersensitivity, pregnancy, intrathecal administration

Precautions: Renal disease, hepatic disease, neuromuscular disease

Pharmacokinetics: Terminal half-life greater than 20 hr, metabolised in liver, excreted in urine and bile, does not cross blood–brain barrier

Interactions/incompatibilities:
• Do not use with irradiation of liver
• Risk of bronchospasm, pulmonary infiltration and fibrosis with: mitomycin C

Clinical assessment:
• Liver function tests before, during therapy as needed or monthly
• Full blood count prior to each treatment, withhold if neutropenic
• Stop treatment if neurotoxicity develops

NURSING CONSIDERATIONS
Assess:
• Baseline fluid balance
Administer:
• In accordance with local cytotoxic policy
• Other medications by oral route if possible; avoid IM, subcutaneous, IV routes to prevent infections

• Anti-emetic 30−60 min before giving drug to prevent vomiting
• Antibiotics for prophylaxis of infection
• By slow IV infusion using appropriate gauge needle
• Topical or systemic analgesics as appropriate

Perform/provide:
• Should not be handled by pregnant staff
• Store at 2−8°C
• Reconstituted solutions stable for 30 days if refrigerated
• Strict medical asepsis, protective isolation if WBC levels are low
• All good supportive care including that of mouth and skin
• Warm compresses at injection and infusion site for inflammation
• Nutritious diet as tolerated

Evaluate:
• GI disturbances and abdominal bloating
• Signs of neuropathy
• Food preferences; list likes, dislikes
• Effects of alopecia on body image, discuss feelings about changes in body image
• All changes in condition

Teach patient/family:
• Of protective isolation precautions
• To report any complaints or side effects to nurse or clinician
• That hair may be lost during treatment, a wig or hairpiece may be available on the NHS; tell patient that new hair may be different in colour, texture
• That if neurological side effects occur they are usually reversible

vitamin A (retinol)

Many combination products
Func. class.: Vitamin, fat soluble
Chem. class.: Retinol
Legal class.: POM

Action: Needed for epitheleal development, visual dark adaptation, skin and mucosal tissue repair

Uses: Vitamin A deficiency and prophylaxis

Dosage and routes:
Deficiency
• *Adults:* IM 100,000 units once monthly or in acute deficiency once weekly
• *Child:* IM 50,000 units monthly

Available forms include: Injection 100,000 units (as palmitate) in 2 ml, oral combination products

Side effects/adverse reactions:
Except for anaphylaxis to injection, described effects are symptoms of overdose
GI: Nausea, vomiting, anorexia, abdominal pain, jaundice, liver enlargement
CNS: Headache, increased intracranial pressure, lethargy, malaise
EENT: Gingivitis, papillaoedema, exophthalmos, inflammation of tongue and lips, tinnitus, visual disturbances
INTEG: Drying of skin and hair, pruritus, alopecia, erythema
MS: Arthraglia, retarded growth, bone pain and swelling
META: Hypercalcaemia
HAEM: Raised ESR
SYST: Anaphylaxis (after injection), weight loss

Contraindications: Hypersensitivity to vitamin A or injection vehicle, pregnancy

Precautions: Liver disease

Pharmacokinetics:
By mouth/injection: Stored in

liver, fat; excreted (metabolites) in urine, faeces

Interactions/incompatibilities:
• Decreased absorption of this drug: liquid paraffin, cholestyramine, neomycin

Treatment of overdose: Discontinue drug

NURSING CONSIDERATIONS

Assess:
• Vitamin A deficiency: decreased growth, night blindness, dry, brittle nails, hair loss, urinary stones, increased infection

Administer:
• With food (orally) for better absorption

Evaluate:
• Therapeutic response: increased growth rate, weight; absence of dry skin and mucuous membranes, night blindness

Teach patient/family:
• Not to use mineral oil while taking this drug
• To notify clinician of nausea, vomiting, lip cracking, loss of hair, headache
• Not to take more than the prescribed amount
• To take a Vitamin A-rich diet

---

vitamin D (cholecalciferol, vitamin D₃ or ergocalciferol, vitamin D₂)

Func. class.: Vitamin, fat soluble
Legal class.: Tablets P, Injection POM

Action: Needed for regulation of calcium, phosphate levels, normal bone development, parathyroid activity, neuromuscular functioning

Uses: Vitamin D deficiency, rickets, renal osteodystrophy, hypoparathyroidism

Dosage and routes:
Simple deficiency
• *Adult and children:* By mouth 400 units daily
Malabsorption/liver disease
• By mouth/IM up to 40,000 units daily
Hypoparathyroidism
• *Adult and child:* By mouth/IM up to 100,000 units daily

Available forms include: Tablets 400 (with 2.4 mmol calcium) 10,000 50,000 units; injection 300,000 units/ml

Side effects/adverse reactions:
Described effects are symptoms of overdose

GI: Nausea, vomiting, anorexia, cramps, diarrhoea, constipation, metallic taste, dry mouth
CNS: Fatigue, weakness, drowsiness, convulsion, headache, vertigo
GU: Polyuria, nocturia, haematuria, albuminuria, renal failure
CV: Hypertension, dysrhythmias
MS: Decreased bone growth, bone pain, early muscle pain
INTEG: Pruritus, photophobia, sweating
MISC: Ectopic calcification
META: Raised serum and urine calcium and phosphate, thirst, weight loss

Contraindications: Hypersensitivity, hypercalcaemia

Precautions: Lactation, cardiovascular disease, renal calculi, renal dysfunction

Pharmacokinetics:
By mouth/injection: Well absorbed orally, stored in muscle, fat, liver, metabolised in liver and kidneys, excreted in bile (metabolites) and urine

Interactions/incompatibilities:
• Decreased effects of this drug: cholestyramine, colestipol, phenobarbitone, phenytoin, rifampicin

Clinical assessment:
• Blood calcium at regular in-

tervals (initially weekly) and if nausea or vomiting present, also in patients receiving high dose therapy

Treatment of overdose: Empty stomach following recent bulk ingestion, monitor serum calcium, supportive treatments including IV fluids, calcitonin

NURSING CONSIDERATIONS

Assess:
• Nutritional status

Administer:
• IM injection in deep muscle mass, administer slowly

Evaluate:
• Therapeutic response: absence of rickets/osteomalacia, decrease in bone pain

Teach patient/family:
• Necessary foods to be included in diet: egg yolk, dairy products
• To avoid vitamin supplements unless directed by clinician
• To keep clinician's appointments to assess risk of toxicity/therapeutic benefit
• To report weakness, lethargy, headache, anorexia, loss of weight, nausea, vomiting, abdominal cramps, diarrhoea, constipation, excessive thirst, polyuria, muscle and bone pain

---

vitamin E (alpha tocapheryl acetate)

Ephynal, Vita-E, many combination products
Func. class.: Vitamin, fat soluble
Chem. class.: Tocopherols
Legal class.: GSL

Action: Anti-oxidant, co-factor for metabolic reactions

Uses: Vitamin E deficiency, in malabsorption syndrome. Need for supplementation in adults doubtful

Dosage and routes:
Cystic fibrosis
• *Adult:* By mouth 100−200 mg daily
• *Child (over 1 yr):* By mouth 100 mg daily
• *Child (under 1 yr):* By mouth 50 mg daily
Abetaliproteinaemia
• *Adult and child*: By mouth 50−100 mg/kg daily

Available forms include: Capsules 75, 200, 400 units. Chewable tablets 75 units; tablets (succinate) 50, 200 units; suspension 500 mg/5 ml

Side effects/adverse reactions:
CNS: Headache, fatigue
GI: Nausea, cramps, diarrhoea

Contraindications: Hypersensitivity

Pharmacokinetics:
By mouth: Metabolised in liver, excreted in bile

Interactions/incompatibilities:
• Increased action of: oral anticoagulants

Treatment of overdose: Supportive only, not likely to be significant

NURSING CONSIDERATIONS

Assess:
• Nutritional status

Evaluate:
• Clotting disturbances in patients previously stabilised on oral anticoagulants
• Therapeutic response: improvement in skin lesions, decreased oedema

Teach patient/family:
• Necessary foods to be included in diet: wheat germ, dark green leafy vegetables, nuts, eggs, liver, vegetable oils, dairy products, cereals
• To avoid vitamin supplements unless directed by clinician

warfarin sodium

Marevan
Func. class.: Anticoagulant
Chem. class.: Coumarin derivative
Legal class.: POM

Action: Interferes with blood clotting by indirect means; depresses hepatic synthesis of vitamin K-dependent coagulation factors (II, VII, IX, X)

Uses: Prophylaxis is of embolisation in rheumatic heart disease and atrial fibrillation. Prophylaxis after insertion of prosthetic heart valve. Prophylaxis and treatment of venous thrombosis and pulmonary embolism. Transient ischaemic attacks

Dosage and routes:
• *Adult:* By mouth 10−15 mg daily, then titrated to prothrombin time daily

Available forms include: Tablets 1 (Brown), 3 (Blue), 5 mg (Pink)

Side effects/adverse reactions:
GI: Diarrhoea, nausea, vomiting, pancreatitis
INTEG: Rash, alopecia
CNS: Fever
HAEM: Haemorrhage
EENT: Epistaxis

Contraindications: Hypersensitivity, potential haemorrhagic conditions, peptic ulcer disease, hepatic disease (severe), renal disease (severe), severe hypertension, subacute bacterial endocarditis, pregnancy

Precautions: Alcoholism, elderly, decreased dietary intake of Vitamin K, hepatic/renal dysfunction, concurrent administration of salicylates and other highly plasma protein-bound drugs

Pharmacokinetics:
By mouth: Onset 24 hr, peak 36−48 hr, duration 3−5 days, half-life ½−3 days; metabolised in liver, excreted in urine/faeces (active/inactive metabolites)

Interactions/incompatibilities:
• Increased action: allopurinol, chloramphenicol, clofibrate, amiodarone, diflunisal, heparin, steroids, cimetidine, disulfiram, thyroxine, glucagon, metronidazole, quinidine, sulindac, sulphinpyrazone, sulphonamides, tricyclic antidepressants, inhalation anaesthetics, salicylates, ethacrynic acid, indomethacin, mefenamic acid, oxyphenbutazone, phenylbutazone
• Decreased action: barbiturates, griseofulvin, haloperidol, carbamazepine, rifampicin, cholestyramine
• Increased or decreased action: chloral hydrate, glutethimide, sulphinpyrazone, triclofos sodium, alcohol

Clinical assessment:
• Blood counts (haematocrit, platelets, occult blood in stools) every 3 months
• International Normalised Ratio; use local laboratory guidelines to establish required ratio

Treatment of overdose: Administer Vitamin K and/or fresh frozen plasma

NURSING CONSIDERATIONS

Assess:
• Blood count, especially prothrombin time

Administer:
• At same time each day to maintain steady blood levels
• Alone; NOT to be given with food
• Avoid all IM injections that may cause bleeding

Evaluate:
• Therapeutic response: decrease of deep vein thrombosis
• Signs of bleeding; gums, black tarry stools, haematuria, epistaxis
• Fever, skin rash, urticaria

Teach patient/family:

• To avoid non-prescribed preparations that may cause serious drug interactions unless approved by clinician/pharmacist
• To carry an ID identifying drug taken
• Stress patient compliance
• On all aspects of: dosage, route, action, side effects, when to notify clinician
• To report any signs of bleeding: gums, under skin, urine, stools or epigastric pain
• To avoid hazardous activities (football, hockey, skiing) or dangerous work (driving)

---

xamoterol

Corwin
Func. class.: Inotropic sympathomimetic
Chem. class.: β₁-adrenoceptor partial agonist
Legal class.: POM

Action: Acts on β₁-receptors; in mild heart failure it improves ventricular function with no increase in myocardial oxygen demand
Uses: Restricted by CSM to chronic mild heart failure in patients not breathless at rest but limited by symptoms on exertion
Dosage and routes: Treatment to be initiated in hospital after full assessment
• *Adult:* By mouth 200 mg for 1 week, then 200 mg twice daily
Available forms include: Tablets 200 mg (as fumarate)
Side effects/adverse reactions:
CNS: Headache, dizziness
CV: Chest pain, palpitations
GI: Disturbances
INTEG: Rashes
MS: Muscle cramp
Contraindications: Moderate to severe heart failure, lactation,

children (seek specialist advice)
Precautions: Cardiac outflow obstruction, arrhythmias, maintain concurrent digoxin in atrial fibrillation, chronic obstructive airways disease, bronchospasm, development of asthma, cardiac symptoms at rest, renal impairment, pregnancy, deterioration of heart failure (withdraw)
Interactions/incompatibilities:
• Beta-blockers—antagonism of effect of xamoterol and reduced beta-blockade
• Beta-agonists—competition for receptors
Clinical assessment:
• Fully assess severity of heart failure before starting treatment
• Monitor cardiac function
Treatment of overdose: Symptomatic conservative management
NURSING CONSIDERATIONS
Assess:
• Baseline vital signs
• Fluid balance
Administer:
• With meals to prevent GI symptoms
Evaluate:
• BP regularly
• Therapeutic response
• Exercise range—ease of breathing and respiration rate
• Coldness of extremities—peripheral blood flow may decrease
Teach patient/family:
• On all aspects of drug—avoid smoking and smoke-filled rooms
• Report any chest pain or palpitations, bronchospasm
• Not to drive as dizziness may occur

xipamide

Diurexan
Func. class.: Diuretic
Chem. class.: Thiazide related
Legal class.: POM

Action: Diuresis. Probably reduces peripheral vascular resistance. Reduces reabsorption of electrolytes from renal tubules increasing excretion of sodium and chloride ions and thereby water

Uses: Oedema, including congestive heart failure, hypertension

Dosage and routes: Adults by mouth

Oedema

• Initially 40 mg in morning increased to 80 mg if necessary; maintenance 20 mg in morning

Hypertension

• 20 mg in morning (may be increased to 40 mg if necessary but if other anti-hypertensive therapy being given initial dose should not exceed 20 mg daily)

Available forms include: Tablets, scored 20 mg

Side effects/adverse reactions:

GU: Slight gastrointestinal disturbances

CNS: Mild dizziness

Contraindications: Hypercalcaemia, severe renal and hepatic impairment, Addison's disease, children, severe electrolyte deficiency, porphyria

Precautions: Pregnancy, diabetes, gout, renal or hepatic impairment, may cause hypokalaemia, prostatic hypertrophy, lactation

Pharmacokinetics: Absorption is rapid, peak plasma concentrations within 1−2 hr, 99% bound to plasma protein, plasma half-life 5−8 hr, excreted in urine, diuretic effect lasts up to 12 hr, antihypertensive effect lasts up to 24 hr or more

Interactions/incompatibilities:

• Increased toxicity of NSAIDs, calcium salts, cardiac glycosides, lithium

• If hypokalaemia increased toxicity and side effects of: amiodarone disopyramide, flecainide, quinidine, pimozide, sotalol, cardiac glycosides

• If hypokalaemia decreased effect of: lignocaine, mexiletine, tocainide

• Antagonise diuresis: NSAIDs, carbenoxolone, corticosteroids, oestrogens and combined oral contraceptives

• Reduced absorption caused by: cholestyramine, colestipol

• Decreased effect of: antidiabetics

• Enhanced hypotension: tricyclic antihypertensives (NB: α-blockers and ACE inhibitors)

• Increased risk of hypokalaemia: indapamide, corticosteroids, carbenoxolone, other diuretics

Clinical assessment:

• Lower or increase dose to achieve adequate control

• Monitor plasma electrolytes especially potassium

Treatment of overdose: Maintain BP, restore blood volume, Correct electrolyte imbalance

NURSING CONSIDERATIONS

Assess:

• Baseline BP

Administer:

• In morning to avoid nocturia

• Ensure patient has ready access to toilet facilities

• With food if nausea occurs

Perform/provide:

• Weigh daily

Evaluate:

• Therapeutic effect: reduced oedema, lower blood pressure, reduction in weight

• For side effects — GI disturbance and mild dizziness

• Urine output for signs of acute urinary retention

• For signs of oedema
Teach patient/family:
• To take in morning to avoid nocturia
• To ensure toilet facilities readily available
• Not to perform tasks requiring alertness until sure they are not affected by dizziness
• To check with GP before taking other medications

---

xylometazoline HCl (nasal)

Otrivine
Func. class.: Nasal decongestant
Chem. class.: Sympathomimetic agent
Legal class.: GSL

Action: Marked α-adrenergic activity. Vasoconstrictor with rapid and prolonged action—decreases congestion
Uses: Nasal congestion
Dosage and routes:
Intranasal
• *Adult and child over 12 yr:* Instil 2—3 drops or 1—2 sprays in each nostril 2—3 times daily (0.1%) when required
• *Child under 12 yr and over 3 months:* Instil 1—2 drops in each nostril once or twice a day (0.05%) when required
Available forms include: Nasal drops 0.1%, 0.05%, nasal spray 0.1%
Side effects/adverse reactions:
EENT: Irritation, sneezing, stinging, dryness, headache
CNS: In children—restlessness, sleep disturbance
After excessive use: tolerance and rebound congestion
Contraindications: Hypersensitivity to sympathomimetic amines, infants under 3 months, trans-

sphenoidal hypophysectomy or surgery exposing the dura mater
Precautions: Avoid excessive use—do not use for more than 7 consecutive days, cardiovascular disease
Pharmacokinetics:
INSTIL: Onset 5—10 min, duration 5—6 hr; systemic absorption may occur
Treatment of overdose: No specific treatment—supportive measures

NURSING CONSIDERATIONS
Administer:
• Not more than 4 hrly
• For less than 7 consecutive days
Perform/provide:
• Environmental humidification to decrease nasal congestion, dryness
Evaluate:
• Redness, swelling, pain in nasal passages
Teach patient/family:
• To avoid contamination of container
• Stinging may occur for a few applications; drying of mucosa may be decreased by environmental humidification
• To notify doctor if irregular pulse, insomnia, dizziness, or tremors occur
• Proper administration to avoid systemic absorption

---

yellow fever vaccine

Yellow Fever Vaccine, Live, Arilvax
Func. class.: Live attenuated vaccine 17D strain
Legal class.: POM

Action: Promotes development of antibodies specific to yellow fever virus
Uses: Active immunisation against yellow fever virus. Certificate of vaccination, in case of primary vaccination, is valid 10 yr from the 10th day after vaccination for re-

vaccination within 10 yr, certificate is valid at once

Dosage and routes:
• *Adults and children over 9 months:* subcutaneous injection, 0.5 ml
Available forms include: Freeze-dried live vaccine 1-, 5-, 10-dose vial with diluent contains neomycin and polymyxin sulphates

Side effects/adverse reactions:
INTEG: Redness, swelling
CNS: Risk of encephalitis in infants under 9 months, headache

Contraindications: Presence of acute infection, impaired immune response, pregnancy, sensitivity to eggs or chick protein, neomycin or polymyxin, malignant conditions or other tumours of reticulo-endothelial system. History of serious reaction to previous dose

Precautions: Infants under 9 months, within 6 weeks of administration of immune globulin. Allow minimum of 2 weeks after yellow fever vaccine before giving immune globulin. Interval of at least 3 wks between administration of other live vaccines. If not possible give simultaneously at different sites

Pharmacokinetics: Active immunity usually established within 10 days of primary vaccination and persists for many years

Interactions/incompatibilities:
• Not to be given while patient is being treated with corticosteroids, other immunosuppressive drugs
• Concurrent (within 3 wks) of other live vaccines

Clinical assessment:
• The decision to vaccinate during pregnancy or infants under 9 months must depend on the risk of exposure to the disease
• Do not prescribe for those sensitive to eggs or to neomycin or polymyxin
• Avoid vaccination within 6 weeks of immunoglobulin administration
• An interval of 3 weeks should lapse between administering any two live vaccines

NURSING CONSIDERATIONS
Assess:
• Active or suspected infection
• History of allergies, especially hypersensitivity to penicillin or eggs

Administer:
• Subcutaneously
• 5 ml for all ages
• With adrenaline 1:1000 and resuscitative equipment available
• Reconstitute with suitable sterile Arilvax solutions only
• After reconstitution keep cool and protect from light for up to one hr

Provide:
• Store at 2−3°C protected from light
• Dispose of remaining vaccine by incineration
• A record of injection, dose, lot number of vaccine, and date of administration

Evaluate:
• For anaphylaxis: dyspnoea, bronchospasm, tachycardia, profuse sweating, collapse
• History of allergies
• For local effects of soreness and redness at vaccination site

Teach patient/family:
• That there could be local effects of soreness and redness at vaccination site
• Immunity after primary injection commences after 10 days and lasts 10 yr reinforcing dose would then be required

zidovudine (formerly azidothymidine or AZT)

Retrovir
Func. class.: Antiviral
Chem. class.: Thymidine analogue
Legal class.: POM

Action: Inhibits replication of HIV virus by interfering with transcription of RNA and DNA

Uses: Management of advanced HIV disease such as AIDS or AIDS-related complex; early symptomatic or asymptomatic HIV infection with markers indicating risk of disease progression

Dosage and routes:

Asymptomatic

• *Adult:* Orally, 500 mg−1500 mg daily depending on the individual patient

Symptomatic

• *Adult:* Orally, 200 mg every 4 hr, decreasing to 100 mg every 4 hr in advanced disease, if not well tolerated. IV infusion 2.5 mg/kg every 4 hr for a maximum of 2 weeks

• *Children over 3 months:* Orally 180 mg/m^2 body surface area every 6 hr

• In haematological toxicity a brief interruption of therapy (2−4 weeks) or dose reduction may be necessary

• In hepatic impairment dosage reduction may be necessary, according to plasma levels

Available forms include: Capsules 100 mg, 250 mg, syrup 50 mg in 5 ml, injection (for dilution and infusion) 20 mg per ml (10 ml)

Side effects/adverse reactions:

HAEM: Neutropenia, leucopenia, anaemia

CNS: Fever, headache, malaise, asthenia, dizziness, insomnia, sweating, paraesthesia, somnol-ence, chills, anxiety, depression, loss of mental acuity

GI: Nausea, vomiting, diarrhoea, abdominal pain, anorexia, dyspepsia, flatulence

RESP: Dyspnoea, cough

EENT: Taste change

INTEG: Rash, pruritus, urticaria

MS: Myalgia

GU: Frequency

General: Chest pain, influenza-like syndrome, generalised pain

Contraindications: Hypersensitivity, neutrophils less than 0.75 × 10^9/litre or haemoglobin less than 7.5 g/decilitre; avoid in breast feeding

Precautions: Pregnancy, children, renal and hepatic impairment, elderly, haematological toxicity, adjust dose if anaemia or myelosuppression. Pre-existing bone marrow compromise (lower dose)

Pharmacokinetics: In healthy adults

By mouth: Rapidly absorbed from GI tract, peak ½−1½ hr, metabolised in liver (inactive metabolites) and intracellularly, plasma half-life − 1 hr, excreted by kidneys (some tubular secretion). Plasma protein binding is relatively low

Interactions/incompatibilities:

• Limited experience − care with all combined regimes

• Increased risk of toxicity: amphotericin, doxorubicin, dapsone, flucytosine, ganciclovir (profound myelosuppression), interferon, vincristine, vinblastine, pentamidine, probenecid, and all nephrotoxic and myelosuppressive drugs

• Increased risk of: paracetamol, neutropenia

• Altered blood levels of: phenytoin

• Altered metabolism of zidovudine: aspirin, codeine, morphine, indomethacin, ketoprofen,

naproxen, oxazepam, lorazepam, cimetidine, clofibrate, dapsone, isoprinosine, paracetamol
• Antagonise antiviral effect of zidovudine: nucleoside analogues
• Extreme lethargy: IV acyclovir
• Profound myelosuppression: ganciclovir

Clinical assessment:
• Full blood counts at least every 2 wks for first 3 months, thereafter at least monthly; if low, dose adjustments may be necessary or therapy may need to be discontinued and restarted after haematologic recovery; blood transfusions may be required
• Monitor plasma zidovudine (and its glucuronide) levels in renal and hepatic impairment
• Watch for signs of intolerance

Treatment of overdose: Observe closely for evidence of toxicity and give necessary supportive therapy. Haemodialysis enhances elimination of glucuronide metabolite but limited effect on zidovudine elimination

NURSING CONSIDERATIONS
Administer:
• By mouth, capsules should be swallowed whole
• Trimethoprim-sulfamethoxazole, pyrimethamine, or acyclovir as prescribed to prevent opportunistic infections; if these drugs are given, watch for neurotoxicity

Perform/provide:
• Storage in cool environment, protect from light

Evaluate:
• Blood dyscrasias (anaemia, granulocytopenia): bruising, fatigue, bleeding, poor healing

Teach patient/family:
• Drug is not cure for AIDS, but will control symptoms
• To call clinician if sore throat, swollen lymph nodes, malaise, fever occur since other infections may occur

• That even with drug administration, patient is still infective and may pass HIV on to others
• That follow-up visits must be continued since serious toxicity may occur, blood counts must be done every 2 weeks
• That drug must be taken every 4 hr around clock even during night
• That serious drug interactions may occur if non-prescribed products are ingested, check with clinician first
• That other drugs may be necessary to prevent other infections

---

zinc sulphate (ophthalmic)

Func. class.: Astringent
Chem. class.: Zinc salt
Legal class.: P

Action: Vasoconstriction occurs by action on conjunctiva
Uses: Excessive lacrimation
Dosage and routes:
• *Adult and child over 2 yr:* INSTIL 1−2 drops two or three times a day
Available forms include: Solution — eye-drops 0.25% 10 ml
Side effects/adverse reactions:
EENT: Eye irritation, burning
NURSING CONSIDERATION
Teach patient/family:
• To report change in vision, or irritation
• Method of instillation; tilt head backward, hold dropper over eye, drop medication inside lower lid, using pressure on inside corner of eye, hold 1 min, do not touch dropper to eye

zinc sulphate

Solvazinc, Zincomed, Z Span, many combination products
Func. class.: Trace element
Legal class.: P

Action: Needed for adequate healing, bone and joint development. Zinc is a constituent of many enzyme systems and an integral part of insulin

Uses: Demonstrated zinc deficiency

Dosage and routes:
• *Adult:* By mouth. Depends on individual formulation, 45−50 mg zinc 1−3 times daily

Available forms include: Effervescent tablets 200 mg (45 mg zinc); capsules 220 mg (50 mg zinc); modified-release capsules 61.8 mg (monohydrate) (22.5 mg zinc)

Side effects/adverse reactions:
GI: Abdominal pain, dyspepsia, GI irritation

Precautions: Renal failure

Pharmacokinetics: Partially absorbed from GI tract, excreted in faeces traces in urine

Interactions/incompatibilities:
• Reduced absorption of: ciprofloxacin tetracycline, oral iron, penicillamine
• Reduced absorption of zinc: tetracyclines, oral iron

Treatment of overdose: In gross overdose is corrosive; avoid gastric lavage or emesis; give demulcents (e.g. milk); chelating agents (e.g. dimercaprol, penicillamine, edetic acid) have been recommended. Absorption of zinc slowed by modified release. Give symptomatic and supportive therapy

NURSING CONSIDERATIONS
Administer:
• With meals to decrease gastric upset; avoid dairy products

Evaluate:
• Zinc levels during treatment
• Therapeutic response: absence of zinc deficiency

Teach patient/family:
• That element will need to be taken for 2 months to be effective
• To immediately report nausea, diarrhoea, rash, severe vomiting, restlessness

zinc undecenoate and undecenoic acid (topical)

Mycota
Func. class.: Antibiotic, topical; antifungal
Legal class.: GSL

Uses: Skin infections, particularly tinea pedis

Dosage and routes:
• *Adult and child:* Topical apply to affected areas once or twice a day

Available forms include: Cream (undecanoate 20% undecenoic acid 5%), dusting powder (undecanoate 20%, undecenoic acid 2%), spray application (undecenoic acid 2.5%, dichlorophen 0.25%)

Side effects/adverse reactions:
None common

Contraindications:
Hypersensitivity

Precautions: Pregnancy, lactation

NURSING CONSIDERATIONS
Administer:
• Enough medication to cover lesions completely
• After cleansing with soap, water before each application, dry well

Evaluate for:
• Allergic reaction: burning, stinging, swelling, redness
• Therapeutic response: decrease in size, number of lesions

Teach patient/family:

- To apply with glove to prevent further infection
- To avoid use of non-prescribed creams, ointments, lotions unless approved by clinician
- To use medical asepsis (hand washing) before, after each application
- Not to walk barefoot

zopiclone ▼

Zimovane
Func. class.: Hypnotic
Chem. class.: Cyclopyrrolone
Legal class.: POM

Action: Non-benzodiazepine hypnotic with high affinity for CNS binding sites of GABA macromolecular receptor complex
Uses: Short-term treatment of insomnia
Dosage and routes:
- *Adult:* By mouth 7.5 mg shortly before retiring, may be increased to 15 mg if patient does not respond. Reduce dose in hepatic impairment
- *Elderly:* Initial dose of 3.75 mg nightly
Available forms include: Tablets 7.5 mg (scored)
Side effects/adverse reactions:
GI: A mild bitter or metallic aftertaste, nausea, vomiting
CNS: Irritability, confusion, anterograde amnesia, depressed mood, drowsiness on working, hallucinations, dizziness, lightheadedness, dependence, behavioural disturbances, incoordination
Contraindications: Avoid in pregnancy and lactation, children
Precautions: Hepatic insufficiency, monitor withdrawal, elderly, history of drug abuse and psychiatric illness, avoid prolonged use (avoid abrupt withdrawal thereafter)

Pharmacokinetics: Short elimination half-life 3.5 to 6 hr
Interactions/incompatibilities:
- Enhanced sedative effect: CNS depressants, alcohol, anaesthetics, opioid analgesics, antidepressants, antihistamines, α-blockers, antipsychotics, baclofen, nabilone
- May decrease antidepressant activity of trimipramine
Clinical assessment:
- Monitor therapeutic effect and effect on alertness
- Monitor length of treatment—should be no longer than 4 weeks
Treatment of overdose: Supportive and in response to clinical signs and symptoms

NURSING CONSIDERATIONS
Administer:
- At bedtime
Perform/provide:
- Mouthwash, drink to dispel bitter, metallic taste
Evaluate:
- Therapeutic effect
- GI disturbance including nausea, vomiting
Teach patient/family:
- Not to drive or operate machinery the day after treatment until established that performance is unimpaired
- Long-term continuous treatment is not recommended. A course of treatment should last no longer than 4 weeks
- Not to discontinue abruptly; rebound insomnia may occur

zuclopenthixol acetate

Clopixol, Acuphase
Func. class.: Antipsychotic, neuroleptic
Chem. class.: Thioxanthene
Legal class.: POM

Action: Believed to be related to

dopamine receptor blocking effect

Uses: Short-term management of acute psychosis, mania or exacerbations of chronic psychosis

Dosage and routes:

• Treatment duration should not exceed 2 weeks

• *Adult:* By deep IM injection, 50–150 mg (elderly 50–100 mg), if necessary repeated after 2–3 days (1 additional dose may be needed 1–2 days after the first injection); maximum cumulative dose 400 mg per course and maximum 4 injections, if maintenance treatment necessary change to oral therapy 2–3 days after last injection or to a longer acting antipsychotic depot injection given concomitantly with last injection of zuclopenthixol acetate

Available forms include: Injection (oily) 50 mg per ml, 1 ml, 2 ml

Side effects/adverse reactions:

CNS: Extrapyramidal symptoms, sedation, confusional states, epileptic fits, drowsiness. Impaired temperature regulation

EENT: Dry mouth, nasal congestion, blurred vision

ENDO: Menstrual disturbances, gynaecomastia, galactorrhoea, amenorrhoea, hyperprolactinaemia, oligomenorrhoea

GI: Constipation

GU: Difficulty with micturition or retention

CV: Postural hypotension, tachycardia

INTEG: Pain, nodule formation at injection site

Contraindications: Children, Parkinsonism, coma, lactation, porphyria. Acute alcohol, barbiturate or opiate poisoning

Precautions: Treatment should not exceed 2 weeks. Hepatic impairment, advanced renal disease, elderly, pregnancy, convulsive disorders, cardiovascular disease

Pharmacokinetics: Acetate is slowly released from oil depot and rapidly hydrolysed to release zuclopenthixol. Onset of sedation shortly after injection. Antipsychotic action persists 2–3 days. Metabolised in liver. Excreted in urine and faeces

Interactions/incompatibilities:

• Enhanced sedative effect: alcohol, anxiolytics and hypnotics, barbiturates and other CNS depressants

• Enhanced hypotensive effect: anaesthetics, antihypertensives (NB: ACE inhibitors), calcium-channel blockers

• Enhanced antimuscarinic effects: tricyclics, antimuscarinics

• Antagonism: anti-epileptics (convulsive threshold lowered), bromocriptine, levodopa, lysuride, pergolide, adrenergics

• Increased risk of extrapyramidal effects: methyldopa, metirosine, rauwolfia alkaloids, metoclopramide, lithium, tetrabenazine, piperazine

• Possible neurotoxicity: lithium

• Increased risk of ventricular arrhythmias: anti-arrhythmics which prolong QT interval

• Possible enhanced effect of zuclopenthixol: cimetidine

• Blocked antihypertensive effect of guanethidine and similarly acting compounds

• Mutual inhibition of metabolism: tricyclics antidepressants

• Reduced absorption of zuclopenthixol: antacids

• Do not mix in syringe with other injection fluids

Clinical assessment:

• Prescribe anticholinergic drugs only if Parkinsonian symptoms are a problem, and reassess requirements at regular intervals

• Monitor liver function

Treatment of overdose: No specific antidote. Symptomatic and supportive treatment. Support respiratory and cardiovascular systems. Adrenaline should not be given

NURSING CONSIDERATIONS

Assess:
• Baseline vital signs and fluid balance

Administer:
• With care; contact sensitisation can occur
• Do not mix with other injection fluids in syringe
• Ensure, by aspiration before injecting, that drug not given intravascularly
• Not more than 2—3 ml only injection at any one site
• Do not stop drug abruptly — withdrawal must be slow

Evaluate:
• BP (lying and standing) — postural hypotension may occur
• Pulse — tachycardia and arrhythmias may present
• Temperature — hypothermia may occur
• Urine output and intake — urinary retention may occur
• Monitor therapeutic effect and side effects and adjust dose accordingly
• Monitor length of treatment — should not be more than 2 weeks
• Monitor accumulated dose given — should not exceed 400 mg and no more than 4 injections
• Check mouth to ensure patient swallowed tablets
• Patient may need help with walking and other tasks if blurred vision occurs
• For Parkinsonian symptoms — give anticholinergic drugs as prescribed
• Therapeutic response — improvement of schizophrenic state, reduction of aggression, agitation, hostility

NB: Stop drug and inform clinician at once if signs of neuroleptic malignant syndrome occur (hyperthermia, fluctuating consciousness, muscular rigidity, pallor, tachycardia, labile BP, sweating, urinary incontinence)

Teach patient/family:
• Rise slowly as fainting may occur
• Avoid alcohol
• Avoid driving and other activities requiring alertness until certain that drowsiness does not occur
• Check with clinician before taking non-prescribed preparation
• Side effects may include menstrual disturbances or impotence
• Not to stop taking drug suddenly
• Report any side effects to clinician
• That contact sensitisation can occur

zuclopenthixol decanoate

Clopixol, Clopixol Conc
Func. class.: Antipsychotic, neuroleptic
Chem. class.: Thioxanthene
Legal class.: POM

Action: Believed to be related to dopamine receptor blocking effect

Uses: Maintenance in schizophrenia and other psychoses, particularly with aggression and agitation, where compliance with oral medication is a problem

Dosage and routes:
• Deep IM into upper outer buttock or related thigh
• *Adult:* Test dose initially 100 mg then after 7—28 days 100—200 mg

or more, followed by 200–400 mg repeated at intervals of 2–4 weeks adjusted according to response; maximum 600 mg per week

Available forms include: Injection (oily) 200 mg per ml, 1 ml and 10 ml 500 mg per ml, 1 ml

Side effects/adverse reactions:

CNS: Tardive dyskinesia (carefully assess risk as may be irreversible). Extrapyramidal symptoms, sedation, confusional states, epileptic fits. Impaired temperature regulation

EENT: Dry mouth, nasal congestion, blurred vision

META: Alteration in weight, oedema

HAEM: Blood dyscrasias

ENDO: Menstrual disturbances, gynaecomastia, hyperprolactinaemia, oligomenorrhoea, galactorrhoea, amenorrhoea

INTEG: Erythema, swelling, pain, nodule formation at injection site

CV: Postural hypotension, tachycardia

GI: Constipation

GU: Difficulty with micturition or retention

Contraindications: Children, Parkinsonism, coma, lactation, apathetic or withdrawn states—confusional states, porphyria. Acute alcohol, barbiturate or opiate poisoning

Precautions: Pregnancy, cardiovascular or severe respiratory disease, hepatic or renal disease, elderly, arrhythmias, convulsive disorders, arteriosclerosis, phaeochromocytoma, hypothyroidism, myasthenia gravis, prostatic hypertrophy, personal or family history of narrow angle glaucoma, thyrotoxicosis, extrapyramidal disorders

Pharmacokinetics: Decanoic ester is slowly released from the oil depot and is rapidly hydrolysed to release zuclopenthixol which is relatively short-acting. Metabolised in liver. Excreted in urine and faeces

Interactions/incompatibilities:
• Enhanced sedative effect: alcohol, anxiolytics and hypnotics, barbiturates and other CNS depressants
• Enhanced hypotensive effect: anaesthetics, antihypertensives (NB: ACE inhibitors), calcium-channel blockers
• Enhanced antimuscarinic effects: tricyclics, antimuscarinics
• Antagonism: anti-epileptics (convulsive threshold lowered), bromocriptine, levodopa, lysuride, pergolide, adrenergics
• Increased risk of extrapyramidal effects: methyldopa, metirosine, rauwolfia alkaloids, metoclopramide, lithium, tetrabenazine, piperazine
• Possible neurotoxicity: lithium
• Increased risk of ventricular arrhythmias: anti-arrhythmics which prolong to QT interval
• Possible enhanced effect of zuclopenthixol: cimetidine
• Blocked antihypertensive effect of guanethidine and similarly acting compounds
• Mutual inhibition of metabolism: tricyclic antidepressants
• Reduced absorption of zuclopenthixol: antacids
• Do not mix in syringe with other injection fluids

Clinical assessment:
• Perform blood count
• Monitor liver function
• Prescribe anticholinergic drugs only if Parkinsonian symptoms are a problem, and reassess requirement at regular intervals

Treatment of overdose: Institute measures to support respiratory and cardiovascular systems. Adrenaline should not be given. There is no specific antidote

NURSING CONSIDERATIONS

Assess:
• Baseline vital signs and fluid balance
Administer:
• With care: contact sensitisation can occur
• Protect tablets from light and moisture and injection from light
• Ensure, by aspiration before injecting, that drug not given intravascularly
• Not more than 2−3 ml only injection at any one site
• Do not stop drug abruptly — withdrawal must be slow
Evaluate:
• BP (lying and standing) — postural hypotension may occur
• Pulse — tachycardia and arrhythmias may present
• Temperature — hypothermia may occur
• Urine output and intake — urinary retention may occur
• Therapeutic effect and side effects and adjust dose accordingly
• Monitor accumulated dose given (see dose)
• Monitor blood pressure (lying and standing)
• Check mouth to ensure patient swallowed tablets
• Patient may need help with walking and other tasks if blurred vision occurs
• For Parkinsonian symptoms — give anticholinergic drugs as prescribed
• Therapeutic response — improvement of schizophrenic state, reduction of aggression, agitation, hostility

NB: Stop drug and inform clinician at once if signs of neuroleptic malignant syndrome occur (hyperthermia, fluctuating consciousness, muscular rigidity, pallor, tachycardia, labile BP, sweating, urinary incontinence

Teach patient/family:
• Rise slowly as fainting may occur
• Avoid alcohol
• Avoid driving and other activities requiring alertness until certain that drowsiness does not occur
• Check with clinician before taking non-prescribed preparation
• Side effects may include menstrual disturbances or impotence
• Not to stop taking drug suddenly
• Report any side effects to clinician
• That contact sensitisation can occur

zuclopenthixol dihydrochloride

Clopixol
Func. class.: Antipsychotic, neuroleptic
Chem. class.: Thioxanthene
Legal class.: POM

Action: Believed to be related to dopamine receptor blocking effect
Uses: Schizophrenia and other psychoses, particularly when associated with agitated, aggressive or hostile behaviour
Dosage and routes:
• *Adult:* By mouth, initially 20−30 mg daily in divided doses increasing to maximum 150 mg daily if necessary; usual maintenance dose, 20−50 mg daily
Available forms include: Tablets, 2 mg, 10 mg, 25 mg (as dihydrochloride)
Side effects/adverse reactions:
GI: Constipation
GU: Difficulty with micturition or retention
META: Alteration in weight, oedema
HAEM: Blood dyscrasias
CNS: Tardive dyskinesia (carefully assess risk as may be irrever-

sible), extrapyramidal symptoms, sedation, confusional states, epileptic fits. Impaired temperature regulation

EENT: Dry mouth, nasal congestion, blurred vision

ENDO: Menstrual disturbances, gynaecomastia, hyperprolactinaemia, oligomenorrhoea, galactorrhoea, amenorrhoea

CV: Postural, hypotension, tachycardia

Contraindications: Children, Parkinsonism, coma, lactation, porphyria, apathetic or withdrawn states. Acute alcohol, barbiturate or opiate poisoning. Patients who cannot tolerate oral neuroleptic drugs

Precautions: Pregnancy, cardiovascular or severe respiratory disease, hepatic or renal disease, elderly, arrhythmias, convulsive disorders, arteriosclerosis, phaeochromocytoma, hypothyroidism, myasthenia gravis, prostatic hypertrophy, personal or family history of narrow angle glaucoma, thyrotoxicosis, extrapyramidal disorders

Pharmacokinetics: Metabolised in gut wall and in liver. Excreted in urine and faeces

Interactions/incompatibilities:
• Enhanced sedative effect: alcohol, anxiolytics and hypnotics, barbiturates and other CNS depressants
• Enhanced hypotensive effect: anaesthetics, antihypertensives (NB: ACE inhibitors), calcium-channel blockers
• Enhanced antimuscarinic effects: tricyclics, antimuscarinics
• Antagonism: anti-epileptics (convulsive threshold lowered), bromocriptine, levodopa, lysuride, pergolide, adrenergics
• Increased risk of extrapyramidal effects: methyldopa, metirosine, rauwolfia alkaloids, metoclopramide, lithium, tetrabenazine, piperazine
• Possible neurotoxicity: lithium
• Increased risk of ventricular arrhythmias: anti-arrhythmics which prolong a QT interval
• Blocked antihypertensive effect of guanethidine and similarly acting compounds
• Mutual inhibition of metabolism: tricyclic antidepressants
• Reduced absorption of zuclopenthixol: antacids
• Do not mix in syringe with other injection fluids

Clinical assessment:
• Perform blood count
• Monitor liver function
• Prescribe anticholinergic drugs only if Parkinsonian symptoms are a problem, and reassess requirement at regular intervals

Treatment of overdose: Measures to support the respiratory and cardiovascular systems should be instituted. Adrenaline should not be given. There is no specific antidote

NURSING CONSIDERATIONS
Assess:
• Baseline vital signs and weight before commencing medication

Administer:
• With care; contact sensitisation can occur
• Protect tablets from light and moisture
• Do not stop drug abruptly — withdrawal must be slow

Evaluate:
• BP (lying and standing) — postural hypotension may occur
• Pulse — tachycardia and arrhythmias may present
• Temperature — hypothermia may occur
• Urine output and intake — urinary retention may occur
• Therapeutic effect and side effects and adjust dose accordingly

- Monitor blood pressure (lying and standing)
- Check mouth to ensure patient has swallowed tablets
- Patient may need help with walking and other tasks if blurred vision occurs
- For Parkinsonian symptoms — give anticholinergic drugs as prescribed
- Therapeutic response — improvement of schizophrenic state, reduction of aggression, agitation, hostility
- For side effects

NB: Stop drug and inform clinician at once if signs of neuroleptic malignant syndrome occur (hyperthermia, fluctuating consciousness, muscular rigidity, pallor, tachycardia, labile BP, sweating, urinary incontinence

---

Teach patient/family:
- Rise slowly as fainting may occur
- Avoid alcohol
- Avoid driving and other activities requiring alertness until certain that drowsiness does not occur
- Check with clinician before taking non-prescribed preparation
- Side effects may include menstrual disturbances or impotence
- Not to stop taking drug suddenly
- Report any side effects to clinician
- That contact sensitisation can occur

Appendices

Appendix 1: Exemptions from the Controls on Retail Sale: Midwives

There are certain exemptions from the restrictions that apply to General Sale List Medicines, Pharmacy Medicines or Prescription Only Medicines. The classes of persons and the bodies exempted, the medicinal products to which the exemptions apply, and the conditions (if any) which attach to the sale, supply or administration by these exempted persons [include midwives and the activities associated with their professional practice] . . .

Retail pharmacists may sell by wholesale to the exempted persons provided the sale constitutes no more than an inconsiderable part of the business, otherwise a wholesale dealers' licence is required.

Midwives: Sale or Supply

The restrictions do not apply to the supply or sale (but not offer for sale) of certain medicinal products by a certified midwife in the course of her professional practice.

The medicinal products to which this exemption applies are: (i) all medicinal products on a General Sale List and all Pharmacy Medicines; (ii) Prescription Only Medicines containing any of the following substances but no other Prescription Only Medicine: chloral hydrate, dichloralphenazone, ergometrine maleate (only when contained in a medicinal product which is not for parenteral administration), pentazocine hydrochloride, and triclofos sodium.

Midwives: Administration

Certified midwives may also administer parenterally in the course of their professional practice Prescription Only Medicines containing any of the following substances: ergometrine maleate, levallorphan tartrate, lignocaine, lignocaine hydrochloride, naloxone hydrochloride, oxytocins (natural and synthetic), pentazocine lactate, pethidine, pethidine hydrochloride, phytomenadione and promazine hydrochloride (in the case of lignocaine, lignocaine hydrochloride and promazine hydrochloride only while attending on a woman in childbirth).

Medicines, Ethics and Practice. A Guide for Pharmacists (1992), No. 9, October: Royal Pharmaceutical Society of Great Britain. Reproduced with the permission of the Controller of HMSO.

Appendix 2: Guide to therapeutic drug monitoring

Drug	Ideal sampling time	Plasma half-life (hrs)	Time to steady state	Comments on half-life	Accepted therapeutic range
Digoxin	At least 6–8 hrs after an IV or oral dose, or predose	36–51	7–14 days	Prolonged in renal failure and/or CCF	0.8–2.2 mcg/l
Carbamazepine		5–27	Initiation of therapy 2–4 weeks, Chronic therapy: 4 days	Start with low doses as high levels seen on initiating therapy prior to auto-induction of liver enzymes. Altered by other antiepileptics. (Reduced in children.)	Multiple antiepileptics 4–8 mg/l\n\nSingle drug 8–14 mg/l
Phenobarbitone	Immediately before an oral dose	50–120	3 weeks	Altered by other antiepileptics. (Reduced in children.)	9–25 mg/l (paediatrics) 15–40 mg/l (adults) greater than 15 mg/l (febrile convulsions)
Valproic acid		6–17	3 days	Altered by other antiepileptics. (Reduced in children.)	50–100 mg/l
Phenytoin		20–50	2–4 weeks	Dose dependent kinetics. Altered by other antiepileptics. (Reduced in children.)	7–16 mg/l

Theophylline	Aminophylline/ Theophylline 1 Slow release pre-paration 8 hrs after a dose or pre-dose 2 During a continuous IV infusion, prefer-ably at 6 and 18 hrs	4–16	2 days	Prolonged in cardiac failure and/or cirrhosis. Reduced in smokers. (Reduced in children.)	10–20 mg/l (adults and paediatrics) 8–15 mg/l (neonates)
Lithium	12 hrs post dose	18–36	3–4 days	Prolonged by factors reducing GFR or renal function.	0.5–1.0 mmol/l minimum effective concentration mania prophylaxis potentially toxic concentration greater than 1.5 mmol/l

Note:

Ideal sampling time: This should be adhered to whenever possible. Drug levels taken at these times provide more meaningful information.

Time to steady state: This is the earliest time a drug level should be measured either following initiation of therapy or a change of dosage (unless therapeutic failure or toxicity is suspected).

Accepted therapeutic range: This is the range associated with optimal efficiency and minimal toxicity for the majority of patients. It is important to recognise that some patients will require levels outside of the quoted response.

Department of Clinical Pharmacy, Guy's Hospital

Appendix 3: District and regional drug information services

The following regional and district drug information services will provide information and advice on drugs, and drug therapy by request:

England

Birmingham		021-311 1974
	or	021-378 2211
		(extn 2296 /2297)
Bristol		0272 282867
Guildford		0483 504312
Ipswich		0473 704430
	or	0473 704431
Leeds		0532 430715
Leicester		0533 555779
Liverpool		051-236 4620 (extn 2126 /2127/2128)

London

Guy's Hospital		071-955 5000 (extn 3594/5892)
	or	071-378 0023
London Hospital		071-377 7487
	or	071-377 7488
Northwick Park		081-869 3973
Manchester		061-225 2063
	or	061-276 6270
Newcastle		091-232 1525

Oxford		0865 221808
	or	0865 221836
Southampton		0703 796908
	or	0703 796909

Northern Ireland

Belfast	0232 248095
Londonderry	0504 45171 (extn 3262)

Scotland

Aberdeen		0224 681818 (extn 52316)
Dundee		0382 60111 (extn 2351)
Edinburgh		031-229 2477 (extn 2094 /2416/2443)
	or	031-229 3901
Glasgow		041-552 4726
Inverness		0463 234151 (extn 288)
	or	0463 220157

Wales

Cardiff	0222 742979

For information on poisons and in some cases advice on laboratory analytical services, the following services are available:

Belfast		0232 240503
Birmingham		021-554 3801
Cardiff		0222 709901
Dublin		0001 379964
	or	0001 379966
Edinburgh		031-229 2477
		031-228 2441 (Viewdata)

Leeds		0532 430715
	or	0532 432799
London		071-635 9191
	or	071-955 5095
Newcastle		091-232 5131

Appendix 4: Immunisation against infectious diseases

The Department of Health, Welsh Office, Scottish Office and DHSS (Northern Ireland) publishes an informative and readable handbook, *Immunisation against Infectious Diseases*. The 1992 edition contains details of some important changes and additions of which the most noteworthy is probably the introduction of Haemophilus influenzae b vaccine [Editor].

Immunisation for foreign travel

Introduction

Health advice for travellers is becoming increasingly complex as more people travel to more remote parts of the world and new, and sometimes, unfamiliar vaccines have to be considered. This [appendix] summarises those vaccines to be considered for foreign travel. Full details are contained in the individual chapters.

Advice to an individual traveller will depend on not only the country or countries to be visited, but also the area, the season, the type of holiday, the length of stay and the age and previous health of the traveller. It must also take into account entry regulations for each country if travelling to more than one, and must allow for last minute excursions.

It is also important to remember that the commonest illnesses acquired abroad are preventable by measures other than vaccines:

(a) *Diarrhoea* occurs in up to 50% of travellers abroad. It and other diseases related to poor hygiene and sanitation such as hepatitis A and typhoid, are largely preventable by keeping to simple rules regarding personal hygiene and the food and drink consumed.

(b) *Malaria* – about 2000 cases of malaria are reported in the UK each year in travellers. Most are due to failure to take, or poor compliance with, malarial chemoprophylaxis.

Vaccines

See table for summary of vaccines, doses and intervals.

Recommendations

(a) *For all travellers*

This is an ideal opportunity to check that adults have completed tetanus and polio immunisations and that childhood immunisations are up to date.

(b) *For areas where there is still indigenous poliomyelitis, such as Africa, Asia and Eastern Europe*

Poliomyelitis vaccine

(c) *For areas of poor hygiene*

Typhoid

Hepatitis A

(d) *For some countries, as a condition of entry*

Yellow fever

Meningococcal meningitis

(e) *For visits to infected areas of a country*
Yellow fever
Meningococcal menigitis
(f) *For infected areas, in some circumstances*
Cholera – to satisfy unofficial border demands
Rabies – remote travel out of reach of medical attention
Japanese encephalitis – stays of more than one month in rural areas in the months during and after rainfall, usually June–September.
Tick-borne encephalitis – camping/walking in warm forested areas of North Europe in late spring-summer.
BCG – stays over one month; close contact with local population

Whenever possible, the recommended intervals between doses and between vaccines should be followed. Most travellers' needs can be accommodated in two visits four to six weeks apart:

First visit
Yellow fever
Typhoid – 1st dose
Tetanus – booster
Hepatitis A – 1st dose if vaccine indicated (see below)
Second visit
Typhoid – 2nd dose
Polio – booster
Meningitis
Hepatitis A immunoglobulin – (or 2nd dose of vaccine)

For short-term travel and single holiday trips, one dose of immunoglobulin gives adequate protection against hepatitis A. Hepatitis A vaccine is an alternative for those who need longer-term protection or who travel frequently to endemic areas.

Where there is less than three weeks before departure, yellow fever and polio should be given on the same day.

If the polio and tetanus doses are the first, rather than boosters, the courses should be started earlier. If time does not allow this, the 2nd and 3rd doses can be completed after travel.

If rabies and/or Japanese encephalitis vaccines are required, at least one additional visit will be required.

For most vaccines, if time is short, a single dose will afford some useful protection.

Bibliography
International Travel and Health, Vaccination Requirements and Health Advice, WHO Geneva, Published every year.
A guide on safe food for travellers, WHO, Geneva, Switzerland.

Useful telephone numbers
CDSC Travel Unit (for enquiries from the medical profession); Tel. 081-200 6868.
Malaria Reference Laboratory, pre-recorded message: 071-636 7921; (Egypt, Morocco, Turkey) 071-637 0248
For professional advice: 9.00–10.30am and 2.00–3.00pm 071-636 3924
Hospital for Tropical Diseases Travel Clinic (for enquiries from the medical profession): Tel. 071-637 9899.

Immunisation for foreign travel				
	Primary course	**Interval between doses**	**Reinforcing doses**	**Comments**
Diphtheria less than 10 years	3 doses usually as DTP	4 weeks	On exposure to a case	
greater than 10 years	Low dose vaccine 3 doses of 0.5ml SC or IM	4 weeks		
Tetanus less than 10 years	3 doses usually as DTP 0.5ml SC or IM	4 weeks	1 At school entry or 3 yrs after last dose 2 Before leaving school	
greater than 10 years	3 doses adsorbed vaccine of 0.5ml SC or IM	4 weeks	1 10 yrs after primary course 2 10 yrs later	
Poliomyelitis OPV	3 doses	4 weeks	1 At school entry 2 Before leaving school 3 Every 10 years if at continuing risk	Faecal excretion of vaccine virus up to 6/52; may be longer in immune suppressed
IPV	3 doses 0.5ml SC or IM	4 weeks	As above	
Hepatitis A (vaccine adults only)	2 doses 1.0ml IM	2–4 weeks	Single booster 6-12 months after primary course	
Immuno-globulin less than 10 yrs	2/12 protection: 125mg	3-5/12 protection 250mg IM		
greater than 10 yrs	2/12 protection: 250mg	3-5/12 protection 500mg IM		

Immunisation for foreign travel				
	Primary course	**Interval between doses**	**Reinforcing doses**	**Comments**
Typhoid Heat killed phenol preserved greater than 10 yrs	0.5ml SC or IM then 0.5ml SC or IM or 0.1 ml ID	4-6 weeks Valid greater than 10 days	0.5ml IM or SC or 0.1ml ID every 3 yrs	
1–10 yrs Vi antigen	0.25ml SC or IM then 0.25 ml SC or IM or 0.1ml ID		0.25ml IM or SC or 0.1ml ID every 3 yrs or as required for travel	
Cholera greater than 10 yrs	1 dose 0.5ml SC or IM		1.0ml	
1-10 yrs	0.3ml SC or IM		0.5ml	
1-5 yrs	0.1 MC or IM		0.3ml every 6 months or as required for travel	
Yellow fever greater than 9/12	1 dose 0.5ml SC		Every 10 yrs	Given at designated centres only
Meningo-coccal A + C greater than 2/12	1 dose 0.5ml SC or IM		Every 3 yrs	May be less effective if less than 2 yrs of age

Immunisation for foreign travel				
	Primary course	**Interval between doses**	**Reinforcing doses**	**Comments**
Rabies greater than 1 yr	3 doses 1.0ml SC or IM or 0.1m ID	0, 7 and 28 days	Every 2-3 yrs	
Japanese Encephalitis children less than 3 yrs half dose	3 doses 1.0ml SC	0, 7-14 and 28 days	greater than 3 yrs × 1	Unlicensed vaccine — named patient only
	2 doses 1.0ml SC	4 weeks	greater than 1 yr × 1	Gives immunity for 1 yr
Tick Borne Encephalitis	3 doses 0.5ml IM	0, 4-12 weeks then 9-12 months	Single dose × 1 up to 6 yrs greater than 10 course	Unlicensed vaccine – named patients only
	2 doses 0.5ml IM	4-12 weeks	Protection 1 year	
BCG	1 (greater than Heaf testing) 0.1ml ID		None	Valid after 2 months

Immunisation against Infectious Diseases (1992), **Department of Health Welsh Office, Scottish Office and Health Department DHSS (Northern Ireland): Reproduced with permission of the Controller of HMSO.**

Appendix 5: Weights, measures and units

Metric measures in SI units (International System of Units): abbreviation

picogram (pg)	1 picogram	= 0.000 000 000 001 gram
nanogram (ng)	1 nanogram	= 0.000 000 001 gram
microgram (mcg/µg)	1 microgram	= 0.000 001 gram
milligram (mg)	1 milligram	= 0.001 gram
gram (g)	1 gram	= 1.0 gram
kilogram (kg)	1 kilogram	= 1 000.0 grams

(1 mg = 1 000 000.0 grams)

Common symbols and conversions

1 gram	= 0.035 of an ounce
1 kilogram	= 2.2 pounds
1 ounce (oz)	= 28.35 grams
1 pound (lb)	= 453.6 grams
1 stone (st)	= 6.35 kilograms

Molecular units

mol	= mole – for molecular substances, this is the molecular weight in grams
millimole (mmol)	= 0.001 of a mole
micromole (µmol)	= 0.000 001 of a mole
nanomole (n mol)	= 0.000 000 001 of a mole

Length

millimetre (mm)	= 0.001 of a metre
centimetre (cm)	= 0.01 of a metre
metre (m)	= 1.0 metre

25.4 mm	= 1 inch
2.54 cm	= 1 inch
0.30 m	= 1 foot
0.91m	= 1 yard

Pressure

The unit of pressure is a pascal.

micropascal (µPa)	= 0.000 001 of a pascal
millipascal (mPa)	= 0.001 of a pascal
kilopascal (kPa)	= 1.0 pascal
megapascal (MPa)	= 1 000 000 pascal
gigapascal (GPa)	= 1 000 000 000 pascal

This unit should be used in place of measuring mm Hg (mercury) in measuring blood pressure.

1 mm Hg = 133.3; Pa 150 mm Hg = 20 kilopascal

Thermometric equivalents

Celsius	Fahrenheit
35.0°	= 95.0°
36.2°	= 97.2°
36.8°	= 98.2°
37.8°	= 100.0°
38.4°	= 101.0°
39.0°	= 102.2°
39.8°	= 103.6°
40.2°	= 104.4°
41.0°	= 105.8°

To convert °F to °C: subtract 32, and multiply by $5/9$,
     e.g. $101°F - 32 = 69 \times 5/9 = 38.3°C$.

To convert °C to °F: multiply by $9/5$ and then add 32,
     e.g. $37°C \times 9/5 = 66.6 + 32 = 98.6°F$.

Volume

millilitre (ml)	= 0.001 of a litre
litre (l)	= 1.0 litre
1 fluid ounce	= 28.4 ml
1 pint	= 568.0 ml

Latin abbreviations

a.c.	= ante cibum (before food)
b.d.	= bis die (twice daily)
o.d.	= omni die (daily)
o.m.	= omni mane (in the morning)
o.n.	= omni nocte (at night)
p.c.	= post cibum (after food)
p.r.n.	= pro re nata (when required)
q.d.s.	= quater die sumendus (four times daily)
q.i.d.	= quater in die (four times daily)
q.q.h.	= quarta quaque hora (every four hrs)
t.d.s.	= ter die sumendus (three times daily)

Appendix 6: Weight conversion table (stones and pounds to kilograms)

	0	1	2	3	4	5	6	7	8	9	10	11	12	13
												Pounds		
0		0.45	0.91	1.36	1.81	2.27	2.72	3.18	3.63	4.08	4.54	4.98	5.44	5.89
1	6.35	6.80	7.26	7.71	8.16	8.62	9.07	9.53	9.98	10.43	10.89	11.33	11.79	12.24
2	12.70	13.15	13.61	14.06	14.51	14.97	15.42	15.88	16.33	16.78	17.24	17.68	18.12	18.59
3	19.05	19.50	19.96	20.41	20.86	21.32	21.77	22.23	22.68	23.13	23.59	24.03	24.49	24.94
4	25.40	25.85	26.31	26.76	27.21	27.67	28.12	28.58	28.03	29.48	29.94	30.38	30.84	31.29
5	31.75	32.20	32.66	33.11	33.56	34.02	34.47	34.93	35.38	35.83	36.29	36.73	37.19	37.64
6	38.10	38.55	39.01	39.46	39.91	40.37	40.82	41.28	41.73	42.18	42.64	43.08	43.54	43.99
7	44.45	44.90	45.36	45.81	46.26	46.72	47.17	47.63	48.08	48.53	48.99	49.43	49.89	50.34
8	50.80	51.25	51.71	52.16	52.61	53.07	53.52	53.98	54.43	54.88	55.34	55.78	56.24	56.69
9	57.15	57.60	58.06	58.51	58.96	59.42	59.87	60.33	60.78	61.23	61.69	62.13	62.59	63.04
10	63.50	63.95	64.41	64.86	65.31	65.77	66.22	66.68	67.13	67.58	68.04	68.48	68.94	69.39
11	69.85	70.30	70.76	71.21	71.66	72.12	72.57	73.03	73.48	73.39	74.39	74.83	75.39	75.74
12	76.20	76.65	77.11	77.56	78.01	78.47	78.92	79.38	79.83	80.28	80.74	81.18	81.64	82.09
13	82.55	83.00	83.46	83.91	84.36	84.82	85.27	85.73	86.18	86.63	86.99	87.53	87.99	88.44
14	88.90	89.35	89.81	90.26	90.71	91.17	91.62	92.08	92.53	92.98	93.44	93.88	94.34	94.79
15	95.25	95.70	96.16	96.61	97.06	97.52	97.97	98.43	98.88	99.33	99.79	100.23	100.69	101.14
16	101.60	102.05	102.51	102.96	103.41	103.87	104.32	104.78	105.23	105.68	106.14	106.58	107.04	107.49
17	107.95	108.40	108.86	109.31	109.76	110.22	110.67	111.13	111.58	112.03	112.49	112.93	113.39	113.84
18	114.30	114.75	115.21	115.66	116.11	116.57	117.02	117.48	117.93	118.38	118.84	119.28	119.74	120.19

Professional Nurse: Drug Update, July 1992

Appendix 7: Height/weight– adults (desirable)

Men

Average weight in pounds and kilograms (in indoor clothing)

| Height (in shoes) | | 17–19 yr | | 20–24 yr | | 25–29 yr | | 30–39 yr | | 40–49 yr | | 50–59 yr | | 60–69 yr | |
cm	ft in	kg	lb	kg	lb	kg	lb	kg	lb	kg	lb	kg	lb	kg	lb
157.5	5 2	54	119	58.1	128	60.8	134	62.1	137	63.5	140	64.4	142	63	139
160	5 3	55.8	123	59.9	132	62.6	138	64	141	65.3	144	65.8	145	64.4	142
162.6	5 4	57.6	127	61.7	136	64	141	65.8	145	67.1	148	67.6	149	66.2	146
165.1	5 5	59.4	131	63	139	65.3	144	67.6	149	68.9	152	69.4	153	68.4	154
167.6	5 6	61.2	135	64.4	142	67.1	148	69.4	153	70.8	156	71.2	157	69.9	154
170.2	5 7	63	139	65.8	145	68.5	151	71.2	157	73	161	73.5	162	72.1	159
172.7	5 8	64.9	143	67.6	149	70.3	155	73	161	74.8	165	75.3	166	73.9	163
175.3	5 9	66.7	147	69.4	153	72.1	159	74.8	165	76.7	169	77.1	170	76.2	168
177.8	5 10	68.5	151	71.2	157	73.9	163	77.1	170	78.9	174	79.4	175	78.5	173
180.3	5 11	70.3	155	73	161	75.8	167	78.9	174	80.8	178	81.6	180	80.8	178
182.9	6 0	72.6	160	75.3	166	78	172	81.2	179	83	183	83.9	185	83	183
185.4	6 1	74.4	164	77.1	170	80.3	177	83	183	84.8	187	85.7	189	85.3	188
188	6 2	76.2	168	78.9	174	82.6	182	85.3	188	87.1	192	88	194	87.5	193
190.5	6 3	78	172	80.8	178	84.4	186	87.5	193	89.4	197	90.3	199	89.8	198
193	6 4	79.8	176	82.1	181	86.2	190	90.3	199	92.1	203	93	205	92.5	204

Average weight in pounds and kilograms (in indoor clothing)

Height (in shoes)		17–19 yr		20–24 yr		25–29 yr		30–39 yr		40–49 yr		50–59 yr		60–69 yr	
cm	ft in	kg	lb	kg	lb	kg	lb	kg	lb	kg	lb	kg	lb	kg	lb
147.3	4 10	44.9	99	46.3	102	48.5	107	52.2	115	55.3	122	56.7	125	57.6	127
149.9	4 11	46.3	102	47.6	105	49.9	110	53.1	117	56.2	124	57.6	127	58.5	129
152.4	5 0	47.6	105	49	108	51.3	113	54.4	120	57.6	127	59	130	59.4	131
154.9	5 1	49.4	109	50.8	112	52.6	116	55.8	123	59	130	60.3	133	60.8	134
157.5	5 2	51.3	113	52.2	115	54	119	57.2	126	60.3	133	61.7	136	62.1	137
160	5 3	52.6	116	53.5	118	55.3	122	58.5	129	61.7	136	63.5	140	64	141
162.6	5 4	54.4	120	54.9	121	56.7	125	59.9	132	63.5	140	65.3	144	65.8	145
165.1	5 5	56.2	124	56.7	125	58.5	129	61.2	135	64.9	143	67.1	148	67.6	149
167.6	5 6	57.6	127	58.5	129	60.3	133	63	139	66.7	147	68.9	152	69.4	153
170.2	5 7	59	130	59.9	132	61.7	136	64.4	142	68.5	151	70.8	156	71.2	157
172.7	5 8	60.8	134	61.7	136	63.5	140	66.2	146	70.3	155	72.6	160	73	161
175.3	5 9	62.6	138	63.5	140	65.3	144	68	150	72.1	159	74.4	164	74.8	165
177.8	5 10	64.4	142	65.3	144	67.1	148	69.9	154	74.4	164	76.7	169	—	—
180.3	5 11	66.7	147	67.6	149	69.4	153	72.1	159	76.7	169	78.9	174	—	—
182.9	6 0	68.9	152	69.9	154	71.7	158	74.4	164	78.9	174	81.6	180	—	—

Women

Professional Nurse: *Drug Update*, July 1992

Appendix 8: Height/weight – children (desirable)

Boys					Girls			
Height		Weight		Age	Height		Weight	
cm	in	kg	lb	yrs	cm	in	kg	lb
75.2	29.6	10.1	22.2	1	74.2	29.2	9.8	21.5
87.5	34.4	12.6	27.7	2	86.6	34.1	12.3	27.1
96.2	37.9	14.6	32.2	3	95.7	37.7	14.4	31.8
103.4	40.7	16.5	36.4	4	103.2	40.6	16.4	36.2
111.3	43.8	19.4	42.8	5	109.7	43.2	18.8	41.4
117.5	46.3	21.9	48.3	6	115.9	45.6	21.1	46.5
124.1	48.9	24.5	54.1	7	122.3	48.1	23.7	52.2
130.0	51.2	27.3	60.1	8	128.0	50.4	26.3	58.1
135.5	53.3	29.9	66.0	9	132.9	52.3	28.9	63.8
140.3	55.2	32.6	71.9	10	138.6	54.6	31.9	70.3
144.2	56.8	35.2	77.6	11	144.7	57.0	35.7	78.8
149.6	58.9	38.3	84.4	12	151.9	59.8	39.7	87.6
155.0	61.0	42.2	93.0	13	157.1	61.9	44.9	99.1
162.7	64.1	48.8	107.6	14	159.6	62.8	49.2	108.4
167.8	66.1	54.5	120.1	15	161.1	63.4	51.5	113.4
171.6	67.6	58.8	129.7	16	162.2	63.9	53.1	117.0

Professional Nurse: *Drug Update*, July 1992

Appendix 9: Blood normal values (adult)

Investigation	Value	Standard units	x factor	Value	SI units
Alkaline phosphatase	3–13	KA units/100ml	6.7	20–90	iu/l
Acetoacetate plus acetone	0.3–2.0	mg/100ml	10	3–20	mg/l
Albumin	4.0–5.0	g/100ml	10	40–50	g/l
Aldolase	0.7–4.5	mU/ml	16.67	12–75	$nmol.s^{-1}/l$
Amino-nitrogen (N)	3.0–5.5	mg/100ml	0.7138	2.1–3.9	mmol/l
Ammonia	80–110	µg/100ml	0.5872	47–65	µmol/l
Amylase	4–25	units/l	1.0	4–25	
Antinuclear antibodies	0	Absent/present	1.0	0	
Ascorbic acid	0.5–1.5	mg/100ml	56.77	28–85	µmol/l
Autoantibodies	negative	–/+	1.0	0	
Barbiturates	0	mg/100ml	43.06	0	µmol/l
Bilirubin (direct)	up to 0.4	mg/100ml	17.10	up to 7	µmol/l
Bilirubin (total)	more than 1.0	mg/100ml	17.10	more than 17	µmol/l
Bleeding time	3–8	minutes	0.06	0.18–0.48	ks
Blood volume	8.5–9.0	% body weight	9.4	80–85	ml/kg
Bromide	0	mEq/l	1.0	0	mmol/l
Calcitonin	0	pg/ml	1.0	0	ng/l
Calcium	8.5–10.5	mg/100ml	0.2495	2.1–2.6	mmol/l
CO_2 content	24–30	mEq/l	1.0	24–30	mmol/l
Carbon monoxide	0	% saturation	0.01	0	l
Carotenoids	0.8–4.0	µg/ml	1.863	1.5–7.4	µmol/l
Ceruloplasmin	27–37	mg/100ml	0.0667	1.8–2.5	µmol/l
Chloride	100–106	mEq/l	1.0	100–106	mmol/l

Investigation	Value	Standard units	x factor	Value	SI units
Cholesterol (total)	120–232	mg/100ml	0.02586	3.1–6.0	mol/l
Cholesterol LDL	more than 154.8	mg/100ml	0.02586	more than 4	mmol/l
Cholesterol HDL	30.96–73.53	mg/100ml	0.02586	0.8–1.9	mmol/l MALE
Cholesterol HDL	34.83–85.14	mg/100ml	0.02586	0.9–2.2	mmol/l FEMALE
Cholesterol esters	60–75	% total	0.01	0.60–0.75	1
Cholinesterase	0.5 or more/h	pH units	1.0	0.5 or more	
Clot reaction	50/100	% per 2 hr	1.0	50–100	
Clotting time	less than 15	minutes	0.06	less than 0.90	ks
Coagulation factors					
Fibrinogen (FI)	0.15–0.35	g/100ml	29.41	4.0–10.0	μmol/l
Prothrombin (FII)	70–130	%	0.01	0.70–1.30	1
Accelerator globulin (FV)	70–130	%	0.01	0.70–1.30	1
Proconvertin-Stuart (FVII)	70–130	%	0.01	0.70–1.30	1
Stuart factor (FX)	70–130	%	0.01	0.70–1.30	1
Antihaemophilic globulin (FVIII)	50–200	%	0.01	0.50–2.00	1
Thromboplastic factor (FIX)	70–130	%	0.01	0.70–1.30	1
Thromboplastic antecedent (FXI)	70–130	%	0.01	0.70–1.30	1
Hageman factor (FXII)	70–130	%	0.01	0.70–1.30	1
Complement	150–250	units/ml	1.0	150–250	
Congo-red test	more than 60	% retention	0.01	more than 0.60	1
Copper	100–200	g/100ml	0.1574	16–31	μmol/l
Cortisol	5–25	μg/100ml	0.02759	0.15–0.70	μmol/l
Creatine phosphokinase	5–35	mU/ml	0.01667	0.08–0.58	$\mu mol. S^{-1}$l

Investigation	Value	Standard units	x factor	Value	SI units
Creatinine	0.7–1.5	mg/100ml	88.40	62–132	µmol/l
Cryoglobulins	0		1.0	0	
Deoxycortisol	more than 10	µg/100ml	0.02903	more than 0.30	µmol/l
Diphenylhydantoin	0	µg/ml	3.964	0	µmol/l
Erythrocyte count	4.2–5.9	Million per mm³	10⁶	4.2–5.9	10¹²/l
Erythrocyte sedimentation rate	1–13	mm/hour	1.0	1–13	
Ethanol	0	%	217.1	0	mmol/l
Euglobulin lysis time	0	lysis/no lysis	1.0	0	
Fatty acids	190–420	mg/100ml	0.01	1.9–4.2	g/l
Foeto-protein	0	absent/present	1.0	0	
Fibrinogen split products (1)	more than 1:2	dilution -ve reaction	1.0	2	
Fibrinogen split products (2)	more than 1:8	dilution +ve reaction	1.0	8	
Foetal haemoglobin	less than 2	%	0.01	less than 0.02	1
Folic acid	6–15	ng/ml	2.266	14–34	nmol/l
Globulin	2.0–3.0	g/100ml	10	20–30	g/l
Glutethimide	0	mg/100ml	46.03	0	µmol/l
Gastrin	0–200	pg/ml	1.0	0–200	ng/l
Glucose	70–100	mg/100ml	0.05551	3.9–5.6	mmol/l
Glucose 6-phosphate dehydrogenase	5–15	units	1.0	5–15	
Glutathione reductase	9–13	units	1.0	9–13	
Growth hormone	less than 5	ng/ml	1.0	less than 5	µg/l
Haematocrit	42–50	%	0.01	0.42–0.50	1

Investigation	Value	Standard units	x factor	Value	SI units
Haemoglobin	13–16	g/100ml	0.6205	8.1–9.9	mmol/l
Haemoglobin, met- and sulphaemoglobin	0	absent/present	1.0	0	
Haptoglobin	100–300	mg/100ml	0.01	1.0–3.0	g/l
Immunoglobulins					
S-IgG	720–1500	mg/100ml	0.01	7.2–15.0	g/l
S-IgA	90–325	mg/100ml	0.01	0.9–3.3	g/l
S-IgM	45–150	mg/100ml	0.01	0.45–1.50	g/l
Insulin	6–26	μU/ml	1.0	6–26	10^{-2}iu/l
Iron	50–150	μg/100ml	0.1791	9.0–26.9	mol/l
Iron binding capacity	250–410	μg/100ml	0.1791	44.8–73.4	μmol/l
Lactic acid	0.6–1.8	mEq/l	1.0	0.6–1.8	mmol/l
Lactic dehydrogenase	60–120	mU/ml	0.01667	1.00–2.00	μmol.s^{-1}/l
Lead	up to 50	μg/100ml	0.04826	up to 2.4	μmol/l
Leukocyte count	4800–10800	per mm^3	10^6	4.8–10.8	10^9 /l
Lipase	up to 2	units/ml	1.0	up to 2	
Lithium	0	mEq/l	1.0	0	mmol/l
Lupus anticoagulant	0	absent/present	1.0	0	
Luteinising hormone	6–18	mU/ml	1.0	6–18	iu/l
Magnesium	1.5–2.5	mEq/l	0.5	0.8–1.3	mmol/l
Mean corpuscular volume (MCV)	80–94	u^3	1.0	80–94	fl
Mean corpuscular haemoglobin concentration (MCH)	27–32	pg	0.06205	1.7–2.0	fmol
Mean corpuscular haemoglobin concentration (MCHC)	33–38	%	0.6205	20–24	mmol/l

Investigation	Value	Standard units	x factor	Value	SI units
Methanol	0	mg/100ml	0.3121	0	mmol/l
Muramidase	4–12	µg/ml	1.0	4–12	mg/l
Nucleotidase	0.3–3.2	Bodansky	89.67	27–287	nmol.s^{-1}/l
Osmolality	280–295	mosm/kg	1.0	280–295	mmol/kg
Osmotic fragility (RBCs)	no haemolysis	increase/decrease	1.0	1	
Oxygen saturation	96/100	%	0.01	0.96–1.00	1
Parathyroid hormone	less than 15	µl equiv	1.0	less than 15	
Partial thromboplastin	22–37	seconds	1.0	22–37	
PCO_2	35–45	mmHg	0.1333	4.7–6.0	kPa
Peroxide haemolysis	less than 10	%	1.0	less than 10	
Phospholipids	9–16	mg/100ml	0.3229	2.9–5.2	mmol/l
pH	7.35–7.45		1.0	7.35–7.45	1
PO_2	75–100	mmHg	0.133	10.0–13.3	kPa
Phenylalanine	0–2	mg/100ml	60.54	0–120	µmol/l
Phosphatase (acid)	0.13–0.63	Sigma	278.4	36–175	nmol.s^{-1}/l
Phosphatase (alkaline)	2.0–4.5	Bodansky	0.08967	0.18–0.40	nmol.s^{-1}/l
Phosphogluconate dehydrogenase	2.5	units	1.0	2–5	
Phosphorus (inorganic)	3.0–4.5	mg/100ml	0.3229	1.0–1.5	mmol/l
Plasminogen	3–5	casein/u/ml	1.0	3–5	
Platelet count	200 000–350 000	mm^3	10^6	200–350	10^9/l
Platelet aggregation	Full response		1.0	1	
Platelet factor 3	33–57	seconds	1.0	33–57	s
Potassium	3.5–5.0	mEq/l	1.0	3.5–5.0	mmol/l

Investigation	Value	Standard units	x factor	Value	SI units
Primidone	0	µg/ml	4.582	0	mmol/l
Protein (total)	6.0–8.0	g/100ml	10	60–80	g/l
Prothrombin time	Countol ±2	seconds	1.0	control ±2	1
Protein electrophoresis albumin	50–60	% total	0.01	0.50–0.60	1
globulin ∝1	4.2–7.2	% total	0.01	0.04–0.07	1
∝ 2	6.8–12.	% total	0.01	0.07–0.12	1
β	9.3–15	% total	0.01	0.09–0.15	1
γ	13–23	% total	0.01	0.13–0.23	1
Pyruvate kinase	2–3	units	1.0	2–3	
Pyruvic acid	0–0.11	mEq/l	1000	0–110	µmol/l
Quinidine	1.1 0.8	µg/ml	3.082	0	µmol/l
Renin activity	0.5–1.5	ng/ml/hour	0.2777	0.3 0.2	ng.l⁻¹/s
Reticulocyte count	0	% red cells	0.01	0.005–0.015	1
Salicylate	0	mg/100ml	0.07240	0	mmol/l
Sodium	135–145	mEq/l	1.0	135–145	mmol/l
Sulfobromophthalein retention	less than 5%	%	0.01	less than 0.05	1
Sulphate	0.5–1.5	mg/100ml	104.1	52–156	µmol/l
Sulphonamide	0	mg/100ml	58.07	0	µmol/l
Testosterone	more than 0.30	µmol/l	34.67	more than 10	nmol/l
Thermolabile haemoglobin	negative	–/+	1.0	0	
Thrombin time	Control ±5	seconds	1.0	control±5	
Thymol turbidity	0–4	Maclagan	1.0	0–4	
Thyroid stimulating hormone (TSH)	1.6±1.2	µU/ml	1.0	1.6±1.2	10⁻³iu/l

Investigation	Value	Standard units	x factor	Value	SI units
Thyroxine binding globulin capacity (TBG)	15–25	µg/100ml	12.87	193–321	nmol/l
Thyroxine, total	4–11	µmol/l	12.87	51–141	nmol/l
Thyroxine, free	0.8–2.4	ng/100ml	0.01287	0.01–0.03	nmol/l
Total lipids	450–1000	mg/100ml	0.01	4.5–10.0.	g/l
Transaminase (SGOT)	10–40	KARMEN	0.008051	0.08–0.32	$\mu mol.s^{-1}/l$
Triglycerides	40–150	mg/100ml	0.01	0.4–1.5	g/l
Triglycerides (fasting)	8–200	mg/100ml	0.01	0.8–2.0	g/l
Tri-iodothyronine	150–250	ng/100ml	0.01538	2.3–3.9	nmol/l
Urea nitrogen	8–25	mg/100ml	0.3569	2.9–8.9	mmol/l
Uric acid	3.0–7.0	mg/100ml	0.05948	0.18–0.42	mmol/l
Vitamin-A	0.15–0.6	mg/ml	3.497	0.5–2.1	µmol/l
Vitamin B_{12}	200–800	pg/ml	0.738	147–590	pmol/l
Viscosity	1.4–1.8	relative to water	1.0	1.4–1.8	
Whole blood clot lysis time	0	lysis/no lysis	1.0	0	

Professional Nurse: Drug Update, July 1992

Appendix 10: Urine normal values (adult)

Investigation	Value	Standard units	x factor	Value	SI units
Acetoacetate plus acetone	0	mg/100ml	10	0	mg/l
Aldosterone	5–19	µg/day	2774	14–53	nmol/24h
Ascorbic acid loading test control	0.2–2.0	mg/h	1.577	0.3–3.2	nmol/s
after loading	24–49	mg/h	1.577	38–77	nmols/s
Amino nitrogen	64–199	mg/day	0.07138	4.6–14.2	mmol/24h
Amylase	24–76	units/ml	1.0	24–76	
Bence-Jones protein	0	absent/present	1.0	0	
Calcium	up to 150	mg/day	0.02495	up to 3.8	mmol/24h
Chorionic gonadotrophin	negative	–/+	1.0	0	
Cortisol	20–70	µg/day	2.759\	55–193	nmol/24h
Copper	0–100	µg/day	0.01574	0–1.6	umol/24h
Coproporphyrin	50–250	µg/day	1.527	76–382	nmol/24h
Creatine	less than 100	mg/day	0.007625	less than 0.75	mmol/24h
Creatinine	15–222	mg/kg/day	0.008840	0.13–0.22	mmol.kg^{-1}/24h
Creatinine clearance	150–180	l/day	0.01157	1.7–2.1	ml/s
Cystine/cysteine	negative	–/+	1.0	0	
Epinephrine	less than 10	µg/day	5.458	less than 55	nmol/24h
Follicle stimulating hormone	5–20	IU/day	1.0	5–20	int. unit/24h
Fructose	0	mg/100ml	0.05551	0	mmol/l
Glucose (quantitative)	0	g/100ml	55.51	0	mmol/l
Haemoglobin/myoglobin	negative	–/+	1.0	0	
Homogenitisic acid	negative	–/+	1.0	0	
Hydroxysteroids	3–8	mg/day	2.759	8–22	µmol/l

Investigation	Value	Standard units	x factor	Value	SI units
Norepinephrine	less than 100	μg/day	5.911	less than 590	nmol/24h
Pentose	0	mg/100ml	0.06661	0	mmol/l
Phenolsulphonphthalein (PSP)	25	%	0.01	0.25	1
Phenylpyruvic acid	neg	–/+	1.0	0	
Phosphorus (inorganic)	1	g/day	32.29	32	mmol/24h
Porphobilinogen	neg	–/+	1.0	0	
Protein (quantitative)	less than 150	mg/day	0.001	less than 0.15	g/24h
Titratable acidity	20–40	mEq/day	1.0	20–40	mmol/24h
Urobilinogen	up to 1.0	Ehrlich	1.0	up to 1.0	
Uroporphyrin	0	mg/day	1.2	0	nmol
Vanilmandelic acid	up to 9	mg/day	5.05	up to 45	μmol/24h

Professional Nurse: Drug Update, July 1992

Bibliography

ABPI Data Sheet Compendium (1991–1992): Datapharm Publications Ltd.

American Hospital Formulary Service. Drug Information 92 (1992): American Society of Hospital Pharmacists.

British National Formulary (BNF) (1992), No 24, September: British Medical Association and the Royal Pharmaceutical Society of Great Britain.

Dollery, Professor, Sir C.T. (ed.) *Therapeutic Drugs* (1991), Vols 1 and 2: Churchill Livingstone.

Goodman Gilman, A., Rall, T.W., Nies, A.S., Taylor, P. (eds) *The Pharmacological Basis of Therapeutics* (1990): Pergamon Press, Inc.

Immunisation against Infectious Diseases (1992), Department of Health Welsh Office, Scottish Office and Health Department DHSS (Northern Ireland).

Martindale, The Extra Pharmacopoeia (1989), 29th edn: Pharmaceutical Press.

Medicines, Ethics and Practice. A Guide for Pharmacists (1992), No. 9, October: Royal Pharmaceutical Society of Great Britain.

Stockley, I.H. *Drug Interactions* (1991), 2nd edn: Blackwell Scientific Publications.

Index of generic drugs and trade names

Index of generic drugs by functional classes

Anaesthesia

Anaesthetics, general
Etomidate, 250
Fentanyl citrate/droperidol combination, 259
Ketamine, 368
Methohexitone, 425
Midazolam, 451
Thiopentone, 676

Anaesthetics, local
Bupivacaine, 87
Cocaine, 154
Lignocaine, 378
    with prilocaine, 379
Prilocaine, 577
Procaine, 583
Proxymetacaine, 601

Muscle relaxants
Alcuronium, 16
Atracurium, 52
Gallamine, 293
Pancuronium, 516
Suxamethonium, 654
Tubocurarine, 713
Vecuronium, 721

Antidotes, antagonists, and chelating agents

Acetylcysteine, 6
Desferrioxamine, 184
Digoxin-specific antibody fragments (Fab), 205
Dimercaprol, 208
Flumazenil, 271
Folinic acid, 289
Mesna, 416
Naloxone, 468
Pralidoxime, 571
Protamine, 598
Sodium nitrite, 631
Trientine, 704

Blood and nutrition

Blood/plasma products
Albumin, human serum, 14
Dextran, 191
Hetastarch, 318

Fluids and electrolytes
Dextrose, 193
Potassium, 568
Sodium bicarbonate, 626

Haematinics
Ferrous fumarate, 260
Ferrous gluconate, 261
Ferrous sulphate, 263
Iron dextran, 357

Minerals
Calcium, 93
Sodium fluoride, 629
Zinc sulphate, 738

Nutrition
Amino acid solution, 28
Fat emulsions, 254

Vitamins
Ascorbic acid, 48
Calcitriol, 91
Folic acid, 288
Hydroxocobalamin, 328
Nicotinamide, 480
Nicotinic acid, 482
Phytomenadione, 545
Pyridoxine, 605
Thiamine, 673
Vitamin A, 729

Central nervous system disorders

Ear, nose and throat disorders

Endocrine system disorders

Infections

Methocarbamol, 423

Obstetrics, gynaecology and urinary tract disorders

Contraceptives
Oral contraceptives, combined, 501

Prostaglandins and oxytocics
Dinoprost, 209
Dinoprostone, 210
Ergometrine, 238
Gemeprost, 295
Oxytocin, 512

Uterine relaxants
Isoxsuprine, 364
Ritodrine, 618
Terbutaline, 661

Respiratory system disorders

Anti-asthma agents
Ketotifen, 371
Nedocromil, 471
Sodium cromoglycate, 628

Antihistamines
Acrivastine, 7
Cetirizine, 112
Chlorpheniramine, 126
Clemastine, 143
Cyclizine, 165
Cyproheptadine, 172
Hydroxyzine, 332
Promethazine, 591
Terfenadine, 662
Trimeprazine, 708
Triprolidine, 712

Bronchodilators
Aminophylline, 31
Choline theophyllinate, 137
Ipratropium, 356
Isoprenaline, 361
Orciprenaline, 503

Pirbuterol, 554
Reproterol, 615
Rimiterol, 618
Terbutaline, 661
Theophylline, 670

Mucolytics and expectorants
Acetylcysteine, 5
Guaiphenesin, 311

Respiratory stimulants
Doxapram, 223

Skin disorders

Anti-acne agents
Benzoyl peroxide, 70
Isotretinoin, 363
Tretinoin, 699

Antipsoriatic and anti-eczema agents
Dithranol, 219
Etretinate, 252

Antiseptics and disinfectants
Chlorhexidine, 120
Hexachlorophane, 319
Hydrogen peroxide, 328
Povidone-iodine, 571

Keratolytics
Podophyllum resin, 563
Salicylic acid, 621
Silver nitrate, 623

Parasiticides
Lindane, 381

Vaccines and immunological agents

Anti-D (Rho) Immunoglobulin, human, 48
BCG vaccine, 61
Botulism antitoxin, 82
Cholera vaccine, 134
Hepatitis B vaccine, 317
Immunoglobulin, human, 344

Notes

Notes

Notes

Notes

Notes

Notes

Notes